Library
Knowledge pa
R C spit

DULCAN'S
TEXTBOOK OF
Child and Adolescent Psychiatry

DULCAN'S
TEXTBOOK OF
Child and Adolescent Psychiatry

Edited by

Mina K. Dulcan, M.D.

Osterman Professor of Child Psychiatry and Head of Child and Adolescent
Psychiatry at Children's Memorial Hospital; Head of the Warren Wright
Adolescent Center at Northwestern Memorial Hospital; and
Professor of Psychiatry and Behavioral Sciences and Pediatrics
at Northwestern University's Feinberg School of Medicine,
Chicago, Illinois

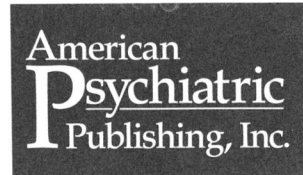

American Psychiatric Publishing, Inc.

Washington, DC
London, England

If you would like to buy between 25 and 99 copies of this or any other APPI title, you are eligible for a 20% discount; please contact APPI Customer Service at appi@psych.org or 800-368-5777. If you wish to buy 100 or more copies of the same title, please e-mail us at bulksales@psych.org for a price quote.

Manufactured in the United States of America on acid-free paper
13 12 11 10 09   5 4 3 2 1
First Edition

Typeset in Adobe Book Antiqua and Optima.

American Psychiatric Publishing, Inc.
1000 Wilson Boulevard
Arlington, VA 22209-3901
www.appi.org

Library of Congress Cataloging-in-Publication Data
Dulcan's textbook of child and adolescent psychiatry / edited by Mina K. Dulcan.—1st ed.
    p. ; cm.
  Includes bibliographical references and index.
  ISBN 978-1-58562-323-5 (alk. paper)
  1. Child psychiatry—Textbooks. 2. Adolescent psychiatry—Textbooks. I. Dulcan, Mina K. II. Title: Textbook of child and adolescent psychiatry.
  [DNLM: 1. Mental Disorders. 2. Adolescent. 3. Child. 4. Infant. WS 350 D881 2010]
  RJ499.D843 2010
  618.92'89—dc22
                                                                                                2009028001

British Library Cataloguing in Publication Data
A CIP record is available from the British Library.

Contents

PART I
A Developmental View of Assessment

PART II
Diagnosis and Approaches to Assessment

PART III
Developmental Disorders

PART VIII
Special Topics

PART XI
Psychosocial Treatments

PART XII
Consultation

Contributors

Ann J. Abramowitz, Ph.D.
Associate Professor of Psychiatry and Behavioral Sciences, and Senior Lecturer in Psychology, Department of Psychology, Emory University, Atlanta, Georgia

L. Eugene Arnold, M.D., M.Ed.
Professor Emeritus of Psychiatry, The Ohio State University, Columbus, Ohio

Miya R. Asato, M.D.
Assistant Professor of Pediatrics and Psychiatry, University of Pittsburgh School of Medicine, Children's Hospital of Pittsburgh, Division of Child Neurology, Pittsburgh, Pennsylvania

William R. Beardslee, M.D.
Director, Baer Prevention Initiatives; Chairman Emeritus, Department of Psychiatry, Children's Hospital Boston, Boston, Massachusetts

Deborah C. Beidel, Ph.D., A.B.P.P.
Professor of Psychology, Department of Psychology, University of Central Florida, Orlando, Florida

Tami Benton, M.D.
Assistant Professor of Psychiatry, Department of Psychiatry, University of Pennsylvania School of Medicine; Director of Education for Psychiatry, The Children's Hospital of Philadelphia, Philadelphia, Pennsylvania

Gail A. Bernstein, M.D.
Endowed Professor in Child and Adolescent Anxiety Disorders and Head, Program in Child and Adolescent Anxiety and Mood Disorders, Division of Child and Adolescent Psychiatry, University of Minnesota Medical School, Minneapolis, Minnesota

Joseph Biederman, M.D.
Professor of Psychiatry, Harvard Medical School; Chief, Clinical and Research Programs in Pediatric Psychopharmacology and Adult ADHD, Massachusetts General Hospital, Boston, Massachusetts

Boris Birmaher, M.D.
Professor of Psychiatry, Endowed Chair in Early Onset Bipolar Disease, University of Pittsburgh School of Medicine; Codirector, Child and Adolescent Bipolar Services, Western Psychiatric Institute and Clinic, Pittsburgh, Pennsylvania

David A. Brent, M.D.
Professor of Psychiatry, Pediatrics, and Epidemiology and Endowed Chair in Suicide Studies, University of Pittsburgh School of Medicine; Academic Chief, Child and Adolescent Psychiatry, Western Psychiatric Institute and Clinic, Pittsburgh, Pennsylvania

Larry K. Brown, M.D.
Director of Child and Adolescent Psychiatry Research, Department of Psychiatry, Rhode Island Hospital; Professor of Psychiatry and Human Behavior, Warren Alpert School of Medicine at Brown University, Providence, Rhode Island

Oscar G. Bukstein, M.D., M.P.H.
Associate Professor of Psychiatry, Western Psychiatric Institute and Clinic, Department of Psychiatry, University of Pittsburgh School of Medicine, Pittsburgh, Pennsylvania

Sharon Cain, M.D.
Associate Professor of Child and Adolescent Psychiatry; Director, Division of Child and Adolescent Psychiatry; Director, Child and Adolescent Psychiatry Residency Training Program, University of Kansas Medical Center, Kansas City, Kansas

Lee Carlisle, M.D.
Assistant Professor, Division of Child and Adolescent Psychiatry, Department of Psychiatry and Behavioral Sciences, University of Washington, Seattle, Washington

Gabrielle A. Carlson, M.D.
Professor of Psychiatry and Pediatrics and Director, Child and Adolescent Psychiatry, Stony Brook University School of Medicine, Stony Brook, New York

Marcia L. Caron, M.A.
Doctoral Student, Department of Psychology, Clinical Program, Emory University, Atlanta, Georgia

Teresa Marino Carper, M.S.
Doctoral Candidate in Clinical Psychology, Department of Psychology, University of Central Florida, Orlando, Florida

Anil Chacko, Ph.D.
Assistant Professor of Psychology, Queens College of City University of New York; Assistant Clinical Professor of Psychiatry, Mount Sinai School of Medicine, New York, New York

Colleen Cicchetti, Ph.D.
Director of Advocacy and Community-Linked Mental Health Services, Department of Child and Adolescent Psychiatry, Children's Memorial Hospital; Assistant Professor, Feinberg School of Medicine, Northwestern University, Chicago, Illinois

Judith A. Cohen, M.D.
Professor of Psychiatry, Drexel University College of Medicine; Medical Director, Center for Traumatic Stress in Children and Adolescents, Allegheny General Hospital, Pittsburgh, Pennsylvania

Brent Collett, Ph.D.
Assistant Professor, University of Washington School of Medicine; Attending Psychologist, Department of Child Psychiatry and Behavioral Medicine, Children's Hospital and Regional Medical Center, Seattle, Washington

Sucheta D. Connolly, M.D.
Associate Professor of Clinical Psychiatry and Director, Pediatric Stress and Anxiety Disorders Clinic, Department of Psychiatry, University of Illinois at Chicago, Chicago, Illinois

Daniel F. Connor, M.D.
Lockean Distinguished Professor of Psychiatry and Division Chief of Child and Adolescent Psychiatry, Department of Psychiatry, University of Connecticut School of Medicine, Farmington, Connecticut

Christoph U. Correll, M.D.
Medical Director, Recognition and Prevention (RAP) Program; Director, Adverse Events Unit, Advanced Center for Intervention and Services Research, The Zucker Hillside Hospital, North Shore–Long Island Jewish Health System, Glen Oaks, New York; Associate Professor of Psychiatry and Behavioral Sciences, Albert Einstein College of Medicine, Bronx, New York

Paul Croarkin, D.O.
Assistant Professor of Psychiatry, University of Texas Southwestern Medical Center, Department of Psychiatry, Dallas, Texas

Steven P. Cuffe, M.D.
Professor and Chair, University of Florida College of Medicine–Jacksonville, Jacksonville, Florida

Eric Daleiden, Ph.D.
President, Kismetrics LLC, Satellite Beach, Florida

Arman Danielyan, M.D.
Resident in Psychiatry, The University of Cincinnati Medical Center, Cincinnati, Ohio

Peter T. Daniolos, M.D.
Associate Professor and Residency Training Director, Department of Psychiatry and Behavioral Sciences, Children's National Medical Center; Assistant Professor of Psychiatry and Behavioral Sciences and Pediatrics, George Washington University School of Medicine, Washington, D.C.

Deborah Deas, M.D, M.P.H.
Professor of Psychiatry, Medical University of South Carolina, Charleston, South Carolina

Mary Lynn Dell, M.D., M.T.S., Th.M.
Associate Professor of Psychiatry and Bioethics, Case Western Reserve University School of Medicine, Cleveland, Ohio

Jon Dennis, M.D., M.P.H.
Pediatrics, CentraCare Clinic, Saint Cloud, Minnesota

Mina K. Dulcan, M.D.
Osterman Professor of Child Psychiatry and Head, Child and Adolescent Psychiatry, Children's Memorial Hospital; Head, Warren Wright Adolescent Center, Northwestern Memorial Hospital; Professor of Psychiatry and Behavioral Sciences and Pediatrics, Northwestern University, Feinberg School of Medicine, Chicago, Illinois

Kamryn T. Eddy, Ph.D.
Postdoctoral Fellow, Massachusetts General Hospital, Harvard University, Boston, Massachusetts

Graham J. Emslie, M.D.
Professor of Psychiatry, University of Texas Southwestern Medical Center, Department of Psychiatry, Dallas, Texas

Robert L. Findling, M.D.
Director, Child and Adolescent Psychiatry, University Hospitals Case Medical Center; Professor of Psychiatry and Pediatrics, Case Western Reserve University School of Medicine, Cleveland, Ohio

Mary A. Fristad, Ph.D., A.B.P.P.
Professor, Psychiatry and Psychology, The Ohio State University, Columbus, Ohio

Daniel A. Geller, M.B.B.S., F.R.A.C.P.
Director, Pediatric OCD Program, Massachusetts General Hospital; Associate Professor of Psychiatry, Harvard Medical School, Child and Adolescent Psychiatry, Boston, Massachusetts

Mary Margaret Gleason, M.D., F.A.A.P.
Assistant Professor, Warren Alpert Brown Medical School, Institute of Infant and Early Childhood Mental Health, Tulane University School of Medicine, New Orleans, Louisiana

Tina R. Goldstein, Ph.D.
Assistant Professor, Psychiatry, Western Psychiatric Institute and Clinic, University of Pittsburgh Medical Center, Pittsburgh, Pennsylvania

Karen R. Gouze, Ph.D.
Associate Professor of Psychiatry and Behavioral Sciences, Northwestern University, Feinberg School of Medicine; Director of Training in Psychology at Children's Memorial Hospital, Chicago, Illinois

Meredith L. Gunlicks-Stoessel, Ph.D.
Assistant Professor of Clinical Psychology in Psychiatry, Columbia University College of Physicians and Surgeons, New York State Psychiatric Institute, Division of Child and Adolescent Psychiatry, New York, New York

Jeffrey M. Halperin, Ph.D.
Distinguished Professor of Psychology, Queens College of City University of New York; Professorial Lecturer, Mount Sinai School of Medicine, New York, New York

John Hamilton, M.D., M.Sc.
Senior Physician, The Permanente Medical Group of California, Inc., Sacramento, California

David Herzog, M.D.
Professor of Psychiatry, Massachusetts General Hospital, Harvard University, Boston, Massachusetts

Anna Ivanenko, M.D., Ph.D.
Assistant Professor of Clinical Psychiatry and Behavioral Sciences, Northwestern University Feinberg School of Medicine, Division of Child and Adolescent Psychiatry, Children's Memorial Hospital, Chicago, Illinois; Pediatric Sleep Medicine Director, Central DuPage Hospital, Winfield, Illinois

Iliyan Ivanov, M.D.
Assistant Professor of Psychiatry, Mount Sinai School of Medicine, New York, New York

Rachel H. Jacobs, Ph.D.
Department of Psychiatry and Behavioral Sciences, Northwestern University Feinberg School of Medicine, Chicago, Illinois

Kyle P. Johnson, M.D.
Associate Professor, Departments of Psychiatry and Pediatrics, Oregon Health and Science University; Codirector, OHSU Sleep Disorders Program, Portland, Oregon

Paramjit T. Joshi, M.D.
Endowed Professor and Chair, Department of Psychiatry and Behavioral Sciences, Children's National Medical Center; Professor of Psychiatry and Behavioral Sciences and Pediatrics, George Washington University School of Medicine, Washington, D.C.

Nina M. Kaiser, Ph.D.
Postdoctoral Fellow, Department of Psychiatry, University of California, San Francisco, California

Myra M. Kamran, M.D.
Deputy Clinical Director, Child and Adolescent Services, Division of Mental Health, Illinois Department of Human Services, Chicago, Illinois

Amy Kim, M.D.
Attending Psychiatrist and Assistant Training Director, Department of Psychiatry, The Children's Hospital of Philadelphia, Philadelphia, Pennsylvania

Bryan H. King, M.D.
Professor and Vice Chair of Psychiatry and Behavioral Sciences and Director of Child and Adolescent Psychiatry, University of Washington and Seattle Children's Hospital, Seattle, Washington

Alexander Kolevzon, M.D.
Assistant Professor of Psychiatry and Pediatrics; Clinical Director, Seaver and New York Autism Center of Excellence; Associate Director of Residency Training, Division of Child and Adolescent Psychiatry, Mount Sinai School of Medicine, New York, New York

Robert A. Kowatch, M.D., Ph.D.
Professor of Psychiatry and Pediatrics, Cincinnati Children's Hospital Medical Center and The University of Cincinnati Medical Center, Cincinnati, Ohio

Louis Kraus, M.D.
Woman's Board Professor of Child Psychiatry and Chief, Section of Child and Adolescent Psychiatry, Rush University Medical Center, Chicago, Illinois

Jon S. Kuniyoshi, M.D., Ph.D.
Acting Assistant Professor, Division of Child and Adolescent Psychiatry, Department of Psychiatry and Behavioral Sciences, University of Washington, Seattle, Washington

Anlee D. Kuo, J.D., M.D.
Assistant Clinical Professor, The Children's Center at Langley Porter and the Psychiatry and the Law Program, University of California, San Francisco, California

John V. Lavigne, Ph.D., A.B.P.P.
Chief Psychologist, Department of Child and Adolescent Psychiatry, Children's Memorial Hospital, Children's Memorial Research Center, and Smith Child Research Center; Professor of Psychiatry and Pediatrics, Feinberg School of Medicine, Northwestern University, Chicago, Illinois

Alison Leary, Ph.D.
Psychologist, Evidence-Based Treatment Centers of Seattle, Seattle, Washington

Daniel Le Grange, Ph.D.
Professor of Psychiatry and Behavioral Neuroscience and Director, Eating Disorders Program, The University of Chicago, Chicago, Illinois

Kelly Walker Lowry, Ph.D.
Medical Psychologist, Children's Memorial Hospital, Chicago, Illinois

Joan Luby, M.D.
Infant/Preschool Psychiatrist and Professor of Child Psychiatry; Founder and Director, Early Emotional Development Program, Washington University School of Medicine, St. Louis, Missouri

Anthony P. Mannarino, Ph.D.
Professor of Psychiatry, Drexel University College of Medicine; Vice President, Department of Psychiatry, and Program Director, Center for Traumatic Stress in Children and Adolescents, Allegheny General Hospital, Pittsburgh, Pennsylvania

Jacqueline L. Martin, Ph.D.
Project Director, Baer Prevention Initiatives, Department of Psychiatry, Children's Hospital Boston, Boston, Massachusetts

D. Richard Martini, M.D.
Chief, Division of Behavioral Health, Department of Pediatrics; Director, Child and Adolescent Psychiatry, Primary Children's Medical Center; Professor of Pediatrics and Psychiatry, University of Utah School of Medicine, Salt Lake City, Utah

Taryn L. Mayes, M.S.
Faculty Associate, University of Texas Southwestern Medical Center, Department of Psychiatry, Dallas, Texas

Jon M. McClellan, M.D.
Professor, Division of Child and Adolescent Psychiatry, Department of Psychiatry and Behavioral Sciences, University of Washington, Seattle, Washington

James J. McGough, M.D.
Professor of Clinical Psychiatry and Biobehavioral Sciences, David Geffen School of Medicine and Semel Institute for Neuroscience and Human Behavior at UCLA, Los Angeles, California

Amy N. Mendenhall, Ph.D., M.S.W.
Assistant Professor, The School of Social Welfare, The University of Kansas, Lawrence, Kansas

Stephanie E. Meyer, Ph.D.
Former Director, Pediatric Mood Program, Division of Child and Adolescent Psychiatry, Department of Psychiatry and Behavioral Neurosciences, Cedars Sinai Medical Center, Los Angeles, California

Edwin J. Mikkelsen, M.D.
Associate Professor of Psychiatry, Harvard Medical School; Medical Director, The MENTOR Network, Boston, Massachusetts

Noah L. Miller, M.D.
Director of Inpatient Psychiatry, University Hospitals Rainbow Babies and Children's Hospital, Case Western Reserve University School of Medicine, Cleveland, Ohio

Laura Mufson, Ph.D.
Director of Clinical Child Psychology in Child Psychiatry and Associate Professor of Clinical Psychology in Psychiatry, Columbia University College of Physicians and Surgeons; Director, Department of Clinical Psychology, New York State Psychiatric Institute, New York, New York

Kathleen Myers, M.D., M.P.H.
Associate Professor, University of Washington School of Medicine; Director, Psychiatry Consultation and Liaison Service; Director, TeleMental Health Service, Department of Child Psychiatry and Behavioral Medicine, Children's Hospital and Regional Medical Center, Seattle, Washington

Paul Nagy, M.S., L.P.C., L.C.A.S., C.C.S.
Program Director, Duke Addictions Program; Clinical Associate, Duke University Department of Psychiatry and Behavioral Sciences, Duke University Medical Center, Durham, North Carolina

Stanley F. Nelson, M.D.
Professor, Department of Human Genetics, David Geffen School of Medicine and Semel Institute for Neuroscience and Human Behavior at UCLA, Los Angeles, California

Jeffrey H. Newcorn, M.D.
Associate Professor of Psychiatry and Pediatrics and Director, Child and Adolescent Psychiatry, Mount Sinai School of Medicine, New York, New York

Wanjiku Njoroge, M.D.
Attending Psychiatrist, Infant Psychiatry Program, The Children's Hospital of Philadelphia, Philadelphia, Pennsylvania

John D. O'Brien, M.D.
Clinical Professor of Psychiatry and Director, Residency Training in Child and Adolescent Psychiatry and Triple Board Program, Mount Sinai School of Medicine, New York, New York

April A. Peters, M.Div.
Research Coordinator, Bradley/Hasbro Children's Research Center, Providence, Rhode Island

Theodore A. Petti, M.D., M.P.H.
Professor of Psychiatry and Director, Division of Child and Adolescent Psychiatry, Robert Wood Johnson Medical School–University of Medicine and Dentistry, Piscataway, New Jersey

Linda J. Pfiffner, Ph.D.
Professor of Psychiatry, Department of Psychiatry, University of California, San Francisco, California

Karen Pierce, M.D.
Assistant Professor of Psychiatry, Northwestern University Medical School, Chicago, Illinois

Sigita Plioplys, M.D.
Attending Child Psychiatrist, Department of Child and Adolescent Psychiatry, Children's Memorial Hospital; Associate Professor of Psychiatry, Department of Psychiatry and Behavioral Sciences, Feinberg School of Medicine at Northwestern University, Chicago, Illinois

Steven R. Pliszka, M.D.
Professor and Vice Chair; Chief, Division of Child and Adolescent Psychiatry, Department of Psychiatry, The University of Texas Health Science Center at San Antonio, San Antonio, Texas

Yann Poncin, M.D.
Assistant Professor, Yale University School of Medicine, Yale Child Study Center, New Haven, Connecticut

Kayla Pope, M.D., J.D.
Child and Adolescent Psychiatry Research Fellow, Children's National Medical Center/National Institute of Mental Health, Washington, D.C.

Mark A. Reinecke, Ph.D.
Professor and Chief Psychologist, Department of Psychiatry and Behavioral Sciences, Northwestern University Feinberg School of Medicine, Chicago, Illinois

Jay A. Salpekar, M.D.
Associate Professor and Director of Outpatient Services, Department of Psychiatry and Behavioral Sciences, Children's National Medical Center; Associate Professor of Psychiatry and Behavioral Sciences and Pediatrics, George Washington University School of Medicine, Washington, D.C.

Lawrence Scahill, M.S.N., Ph.D.
Professor of Nursing and Child Psychiatry, Yale University Child Study Center and School of Nursing, New Haven, Connecticut

John B. Sikorski, M.D.
Clinical Professor, The Children's Center at Langley Porter and the Psychiatry and the Law Program, University of California, San Francisco, California

Thomas J. Spencer, M.D.
Associate Professor of Psychiatry, Harvard Medical School; Associate Chief, Clinical and Research Program, Pediatric Psychopharmacology, Massachusetts General Hospital, Boston, Massachusetts

Liza M. Suárez, Ph.D.
Assistant Professor of Clinical Psychology, Department of Psychiatry, University of Illinois at Chicago, Chicago, Illinois

L. Read Sulik, M.D.
Assistant Commissioner, Chemical and Mental Health Services Administration, Minnesota Department of Human Services, Saint Paul, Minnesota

Mini Tandon, D.O.
Child psychiatrist and Postdoctoral Research Fellow, Washington University School of Medicine, St. Louis, Missouri

Peter E. Tanguay, M.D.
Ackerly Endowed Chair in Child and Adolescent Psychiatry (Emeritus), Department of Psychiatry and Biobehavioral Sciences, Division of Child and Adolescent Psychiatry, University of Louisville School of Medicine, Louisville, Kentucky

Lenore Terr, M.D.
Clinical Professor of Psychiatry, University of California San Francisco School of Medicine, San Francisco, California

Christopher R. Thomas, M.D.
Robert L. Stubblefield Professor of Child Psychiatry, Department of Psychiatry and Behavioral Sciences, University of Texas Medical Branch at Galveston, Galveston, Texas

Karen Toth, Ph.D.
Assistant Professor of Psychiatry and Behavioral Sciences, University of Washington and Seattle Children's Hospital, Seattle, Washington

Kenneth E. Towbin, M.D.
Chief, Clinical Child and Adolescent Psychiatry, Mood and Anxiety Disorders Program, Emotion and Development Branch, NIMH-IRP, National Institutes of Health, U.S. Department of Health and Human Services; Clinical Professor, Department of Psychiatry and Behavioral Sciences, The George Washington University School of Medicine, Washington, D.C.

Andrea M. Victor, Ph.D.
Assistant Professor, Division of Child and Adolescent Psychiatry, University of Minnesota Medical School, Minneapolis, Minnesota

Froma Walsh, Ph.D.
Mose and Sylvia Firestone Professor Emerita and Co-director, Center for Family Health, School of Social Service Administration and Department of Psychiatry, Pritzker School of Medicine, The University of Chicago, Chicago, Illinois

Heather J. Walter, M.D., M.P.H.
Professor of Psychiatry and Pediatrics and Vice-Chair, Psychiatry (for Child and Adolescent Psychiatry), Boston University School of Medicine; Chief, Child and Adolescent Psychiatry, Boston Medical Center, Boston, Massachusetts

Richard Wendel, D.Min.
Assistant Professor of Clinical Psychiatry and Behavioral Sciences, Northwestern University, Feinberg School of Medicine; Adjunct Faculty of the Family Institute at Northwestern University; Allied Health Professional at Children's Memorial Hospital, Chicago, Illinois

Alexander Westphal, M.D.
Research Fellow in Child Psychiatry, Yale University School of Medicine, Yale Child Study Center, New Haven, Connecticut

Laura B. Whiteley, M.D.
Psychiatry Resident, Warren Alpert School of Medicine at Brown University, Butler Hospital, Providence, Rhode Island

Timothy E. Wilens, M.D.
Staff, Clinical and Research Programs in Pediatric Psychopharmacology, and Associate Professor of Psychiatry, Harvard Medical School; Director of Substance Abuse Services, Clinical and Research Program, Pediatric Psychopharmacology, Massachusetts General Hospital, Boston, Massachusetts

Joseph Woolston, M.D.
Albert J. Solnit Professor, Child Psychiatry and Pediatrics, Yale University School of Medicine, Yale Child Study Center, New Haven, Connecticut

Charles H. Zeanah, M.D.
Sellars-Polchow Professor of Psychiatry, Institute of Infant and Early Childhood Mental Health, Tulane University School of Medicine, New Orleans, Louisiana

Kenneth J. Zucker, Ph.D.
Psychologist-in-Chief, Centre for Addiction and Mental Health; Head, Gender Identity Service, Child, Youth, and Family Program; Professor, Departments of Psychology and Psychiatry, University of Toronto, Toronto, Ontario, Canada

Disclosure of Interests

The following contributors to this book have indicated a financial interest in or other affiliation with a commercial supporter, a manufacturer of a commercial product, a provider of a commercial service, a nongovernmental organization, and/or a government agency, as listed below:

L. Eugene Arnold, M.D., M.Ed. *Research funding:* Novartis, Noven, Lilly, Oelgen, Shire, Sigmatau, and Targacept; *Consultant:* Novartis, Noven, Organon, and Shire; *Speaker's bureau:* McNeil, Novartis, and Shire.

Miya R. Asato, M.D. *Grants:* NINDS K23 NS052234; *Research consultant:* GlaxoSmithKline (epilepsy and patient adherence).

Joseph Biederman, M.D. *Research support:* Abbott, Alza, AstraZeneca, Bristol-Myers Squibb, Celltech, Cephalon, Eli Lilly and Co., Esai, Forest, Glaxo, Gliatech, Janssen Pharmaceuticals, McNeil, Merck, NARSAD, New River, NIDA, NICHD, NIMH, Novartis, Noven, Neurosearch, Organon, Otsuka, Pfizer, Pharmacia, The Prechter Foundation, The Stanley Foundation, Shire, and Wyeth; *Consultant/Advisory board:* Abbott, AstraZeneca, Celltech, Cephalon, Eli Lilly and Co., Esai, Forest, Glaxo, Gliatech, Janssen, McNeil, NARSAD, NIDA, New River, Novartis, Noven, Neurosearch, Pfizer, Pharmacia, The Prechter Foundation, Shire, The Stanley Foundation, and Wyeth; *Speaker's bureau:* Abbott, AstraZeneca, Celltech, Cephalon, Eli Lilly and Co., Esai, Forest, Glaxo, Gliatech, Janssen, McNeil, NARSAD, NIDA, New River, Novartis, Noven, Neurosearch, Pfizer, Pharmacia, The Prechter Foundation, Shire, The Stanley Foundation, UCB Pharma, and Wyeth.

Boris Birmaher, M.D. *Research support:* National Institute of Mental Health; *Consultant:* Solvay Pharmaceuticals, Abcomm; *Speaker's bureau:* Solvay; Received royalties for a book *New Hope for Children and Teens with Bipolar Disorder,* published by Random House, Inc.; *Employed by:* The University of Pittsburgh and University of Pittsburgh Medical Center/Western Psychiatric Institute and Clinic.

Oscar G. Bukstein, M.D., M.P.H. *Research support:* Eli Lilly and Shire Pharmaceuticals; *Consultant:* McNeil Pediatrics, and Shire Pharmaceuticals; *Speaker's bureau:* Novartis, McNeil Pediatrics, and Shire Pharmaceuticals.

Gabrielle A. Carlson, M.D. *Research support:* Bristol-Myers Squibb, Eli Lilly, GlaxoSmithKline, Janssen, Otsuka, and Sanofi-Aventis; *Consultant:* Bristol-Myers Squibb, Eli Lilly, Janssen, Otsuka, Sanofi-Aventis, and Validus; *Speaker's bureau:* McNeil and Shire.

Judith A. Cohen, M.D. *Grant funding:* NIMH and SAMHSA. Receives royalty from Guilford Press.

Daniel F. Connor, M.D. *Grant support:* Janssen Pharmaceuticals; *Advisory Board:* Shire Pharmaceuticals.

Christoph U. Correll, M.D. *Research support:* The Zucker Hillside Hospital NIMH Advanced Center for Intervention and Services Research for the Study of Schizophrenia MH 074543–01; *Consultant/Advisor/ Lecturer:* AstraZeneca, Bristol-Myers Squibb, Cephalon, Eli Lilly, Intra-Cellular Therapeutics, Janssen Pharmaceutica, Otsuka, Pfizer, Schering-Plough, Solvay, Supernus, and Vanda; *Speaker's bureau:* AstraZeneca, Bristol-Myers Squibb, Otsuka, and Pfizer.

Steven P. Cuffe, M.D. *Speaker's bureau:* Synermed Communications.

Eric Daleiden, Ph.D. *Employed by:* Works as a paid consultant related to evidence-based behavioral health services and behavioral health system development. He is president of Kismetrics, LLC. Recent clients include the State of Hawaii Department of Health, PracticeWise, LLC, and Real Time Engines, LLC.

Mina K. Dulcan, M.D. *Advisory board:* APPI, Eli Lilly, and Strattera Global; *Consultant:* Comprehensive Neuroscience.

Graham J. Emslie, M.D. *Grant support:* Eli Lilly, Forest Laboratories, and Organon; *Consultant:* Eli Lilly, Forest Laboratories, GlaxoSmithKline, Pfizer, and Wyeth-Ayerst; *Speaker's bureau:* McNeil Consumer and Specialty Pharmaceuticals.

Robert L. Findling, M.D. *Research support, Consultant, Speaker's bureau:* Abbott, Addrenex, AstraZeneca, Biovail, Bristol-Myers Squibb, Celltech-Medeva, Forest, GlaxoSmithKline, Johnson and Johnson, KemPharm, Lilly, Lundbeck, New River, Neuropharm, Novartis, Organon, Otsuka, Pfizer, Sanofi-Aventis, Sepracore, Shire, Solvay, Supernus Pharmaceuticals, Validus, and Wyeth.

Mary A. Fristad, Ph.D., A.B.P.P. Receives royalties from a book (*Raising a Moody Child,* published by Guilford Press, Inc.); instrument (*Childrens Interview for Psychiatric Syndrome* from American Psychiatric Press, Inc.); DVD (*Beyond the Book: Bipolar Children and Their Families,* from CustomFlix, Inc.).

Daniel A. Geller, M.B.B.S., F.R.A.C.P. *Research support:* Bristol-Myers Squibb, Eli Lilly, Forest, McIngvale Family Foundation, NIH, NIMH, NINDS, Novartis, Obsessive Compulsive Foundation, Pfizer, and Shire, Tourette Syndrome Association, and Wallace Foundation; *Advisory board:* Bristol-Myers Squibb, Eli Lilly, Forest, Novartis, Pfizer, and Shire; *Speaker's bureau:* Bristol-Myers Squibb, Eli Lilly, Forest, Novartis, Pfizer, and Shire.

David Herzog, M.D. Receives royalties from a book (*Unlocking the Mysteries of Eating Disorders* (2007), with Dr. Debra Franko and Patricia Cable, published by McGraw-Hill) cited in her chapter.

Kyle P. Johnson, M.D. *Speaker's bureau:* GlaxoSmithKline, Sepracor, and Sanofi-Aventis.

Paramjit T. Joshi, M.D. *Research support:* NIMH (Treatment of Early Age Mania)

Robert A. Kowatch, M.D., Ph.D.   *Research support:* Bristol-Myers Squibb, NICHD, NIMH, and Stanley Research Foundation; *Consultant/Advisory board:* Abbott, Child Adolescent Bipolar Foundation, GSK, Medscape, Physicians Postgraduate Press, and Sanofi-Aventis; *Speaker's bureau:* AstraZeneca; *Editor:* Current Psychiatry.

Joan Luby, M.D.   *Research support:* NIMH and NARSAD; *Royalty:* Guilford Press.

James J. McGough, M.D.   *Grant/Research support:* Eli Lilly, McNeil Pharmaceuticals, Novartis Pharmaceuticals, and Shire Pharmaceuticals; *Consultant:* Eli Lilly, McNeil Pharmaceuticals, Novartis Pharmaceuticals and Shire Pharmaceuticals; *Speaker's bureau:* Eli Lilly, McNeil Pharmaceuticals, Novartis Pharmaceuticals and Shire Pharmaceuticals.

Kathleen Myers, M.D., M.P.H.   *Research support:* GlaxoSmithKline; Royalties received from a book (*Child and Adolescent Psychiatry: The Essentials*, with Keith Cheng, M.D., published by Lippincott, Williams, and Wilkins).

Jeffrey H. Newcorn, M.D.   *Research support:* Abbott, BioBehavioral Diagnostics, Eli Lilly and Company, McNeil/Janssen, Novartis, Psychogenics, Sanofi-Aventis, and Shire; *Consultant/Advisory board:* Abbott, BioBehavioral Diagnostics, Cephalon, Cortex, Eli Lilly and Company, Lupin, McNeil/Janssen, Novartis, Pfizer, Psychogenics, Sanofi-Aventis, and Shire; *Speaker's bureau:* Eli Lilly and Company, McNeil/Janssen, Novartis, and Shire.

Wanjiku Njoroge, M.D.   *Grant support:* Building Better Behavior and Pew Foundation.

Steven R. Pliszka, M.D.   *Research support:* Eli Lilly and Company and McNeil Pharmaceuticals; *Consultant:* Cephalon and Shire Pharmaceuticals; *Speaker's bureau/Honorarium:* McNeil Pharmaceuticals and Shire Pharmaceuticals.

Lawrence Scahill, M.S.N., Ph.D.   *Consultant:* Janssen, Bristol-Myers, and Supernus.

Thomas J. Spencer, M.D.   *Research support:* Cephalon, Eli Lilly and Company, GlaxoSmithKline, Janssen, McNeil Pharmaceutical, Novartis and Shire Laboratories; *Advisory board:* Cephalon, Eli Lilly and Company, GlaxoSmithKline, Janssen, McNeil Pharmaceutical, Novartis, Pfizer, and Shire Laboratories; *Speaker's bureau:* Eli Lilly and Company, GlaxoSmithKline, Janssen, McNeil Pharmaceutical, Novartis, and Shire Laboratories,

Timothy E. Wilens, M.D.   *Grant support:* Abbott, McNeil, Eli Lilly, NIH (NIDA), Merck, and Shire; *Consultant:* Abbott, McNeil, Eli Lilly, NIH, Novartis, Merck, and Shire; *Speaker's bureau:* Eli Lilly, McNeil, Novartis, and Shire.

The following contributors to this book have indicated no competing interests to disclose during the year preceding manuscript submission:

Ann J. Abramowitz, Ph.D.; William R. Beardslee, M.D.; Deborah C. Beidel, Ph.D., A.B.P.P.; Tami Benton, M.D.; Gail A. Bernstein, M.D.; David A. Brent, M.D.; Larry K. Brown, M.D.; Sharon Cain, M.D.; Lee Carlisle, M.D.; Marcia L. Caron, M.A.; Teresa Marino Carper, M.S.; Brent Collett, Ph.D.; Sucheta D. Connolly, M.D.; Arman Danielyan, M.D.; Mary Lynn Dell, M.D., M.T.S., Th.M.; Kamryn T. Eddy, Ph.D.; Mary Margaret Gleason, M.D., F.A.A.P.; Tina R. Goldstein, Ph.D.; Karen R. Gouze, Ph.D.; Meredith L. Gunlicks-Stoessel, Ph.D.; John Hamilton, M.D., M.Sc.; Anna Ivanenko, M.D., Ph.D.; Rachel H. Jacobs, Ph.D.; Nina M. Kaiser, Ph.D.; Myra M. Kamran, M.D.; Amy Kim, M.D.; Louis Kraus, M.D.; Jon S. Kuniyoshi, M.D., Ph.D.; Anlee D. Kuo, J.D., M.D.; John V. Lavigne, Ph.D., A.B.P.P.; Alison Leary, Ph.D.; Daniel Le Grange, Ph.D.; Kelly Walker Lowry, Ph.D.; Anthony P. Mannarino, Ph.D.; Jacqueline L. Martin, Ph.D.; D. Richard Martini, M.D.; Amy N. Mendenhall, Ph.D., M.S.W.; Stephanie E. Meyer, Ph.D.; Edwin J. Mikkelsen, M.D.; Noah L. Miller, M.D.; Paul Nagy, M.S., L.P.C., L.C.A.S., C.C.S.; Stanley F. Nelson, M.D.; John D. O'Brien, M.D.; Theodore A. Petti, M.D., M.P.H.; Linda J. Pfiffner, Ph.D.; Karen Pierce, M.D.; Yann Poncin, M.D.; Mark A. Reinecke, Ph.D.; Jay A. Salpekar, M.D.; Lawrence Scahill, M.S.N., Ph.D.; John B. Sikorski, M.D.; Mini Tandon, D.O.; Lenore Terr, M.D.; Christopher R. Thomas, M.D.; Karen Toth, Ph.D.; Kenneth E. Towbin, M.D.; Andrea M. Victor, Ph.D.; Froma Walsh, Ph.D.; Heather J. Walter, M.D., M.P.H.; Richard Wendel, D.Min.; Laura B. Whiteley, M.D.; Joseph Woolston, M.D.; Charles H. Zeanah, M.D.; Kenneth J. Zucker, Ph.D.

Preface

For even the most successful series of textbook editions, there comes a time for an ending and a new beginning. This book is just such a new beginning. Jerry Wiener's *Textbook of Child and Adolescent Psychiatry* was first published in 1991 as a joint project between the American Academy of Child and Adolescent Psychiatry and American Psychiatric Press. After more than 15 years and two subsequent editions, a fresh look at the field of child mental health was needed. I have preserved his vision of a clinically focused textbook that would encompass the state of the art and the science and that would be useful to trainees and practitioners in a variety of specialties while completely overhauling the organization of chapters, the selection of chapter authors, and the internal structure of each chapter. In that process, I have been able to apply what I have learned in 30 years as a training director and child and adolescent psychiatry division head and 10 years as Editor-in-Chief of the *Journal of the American Academy of Child and Adolescent Psychiatry*. Throughout the preparation of this book, I was constantly reminded of the teaching and example of Peter B. Henderson, M.D., and Richard L. Cohen, M.D. In addition, for nearly 35 years, countless teachers and colleagues from child and adolescent psychiatry, psychology, and social work; my residents and fellows (many of whom are now experts and academic leaders); and the children and parents who are our patients have been unfailingly generous with their experiences and insights. This text aims to communicate the clinical art and wisdom of child psychiatry, tied firmly to the science of our clinical disciplines. Each chapter highlights what we know about evidence-based practices in assessment and treatment. Sections titled "Research Directions" point toward what we need to know.

This text aims to be both scholarly and practical. It covers the most important topics in a format that is complete but efficient for the mental health professional in training or the clinician seeking an update. It is designed to be used as a core text for child and adolescent psychiatry fellowship training and will serve also as a reference for practicing child and adolescent psychiatrists, pediatricians, family physicians, general psychiatrists, child neurologists, psychologists, advanced practice nurses, and psychiatric social workers. As textbooks get bulkier and heavier and trainees and clinicians become increasingly mobile, access to the full-text electronic version of this book via Psychiatry Online (at Web site www.PsychiatryOnline.com) is a great bonus. Published by APPI as a companion volume, the *Study Guide to Child and Adolescent Psychiatry: A Companion to Dulcan's Textbook of Child and Adolescent Psychiatry* contains questions and answers based on this text.

In designing this "new and improved" text, I benefited greatly from the suggestions made by users and reviewers of *The American Psychiatric Publishing Textbook of Child and Adolescent Psychiatry*, 3rd edition, that Jerry Wiener and I edited. Especially valuable was Marty Drell's vision of the ideal text for child psychiatry fellows.

Some features of the table of contents remain from this book's predecessor. Chapters are organized by sections that include assessment, categories of diagnoses, and types of treatment, as well as special topics and special clinical circumstances. The 4 chapters in Part I, "A Developmental View of Assessment," address the clinical aspects of evaluating youth ranging in age from infancy to late adolescence. Part II, "Diagnosis and Approaches to Assessment," covers in 7 chapters the variety of methods and perspectives that may be considered in the clinical evaluation. The following five parts include 17 chapters on DSM-IV-TR disorders and 1 chapter on childhood obesity. These chapters have a consistent structure that includes definition and clinical description, diagnosis, epidemiology, comorbidity, etiology and risk factors, prevention, course and prognosis, evaluation, the variety of treatments, and research directions. Part VIII, "Special Topics," includes 9 chapters on evidence-based practice, child abuse and neglect, HIV, bereavement, cultural issues, suicide, gender and sexual orientation issues, aggression and violence, and the fundamentals of genetics as relevant to child mental health. The 6 chapters in Part IX, "Special Clinical Circumstances," cover psychiatric emergencies, family transitions, physically ill youth, children at risk due to ill parents, legal and ethical issues, and telepsychiatry. The parts on treatment have been greatly expanded, with 7 chapters on psychopharmacology, 1 chapter on brain-based innovative treatments, and 10 chapters on the range of psychosocial treatments that focus on individuals, families, systemic models of care, and therapeutic milieus. Finally, Part XII includes 3 chapters on consultation and collaboration with schools, primary care practitioners, and the juvenile justice system. Each chapter in the book ends with Summary Points—5 to 10 key learning points or take-home messages.

Of the 65 chapters in this book, only 9 chapters have the same lead author as in the book's predecessor. One more would have been Henrietta Leonard, who agreed to write the chapter on obsessive-compulsive disorder despite her illness. Sadly, she died all too soon. Dan Geller generously agreed to author that chapter. Three authors from the previous book appear here with new or additional chapters. All of the remaining lead authors are new—most from the current generation of senior faculty, ably assisted by their up-and-coming more junior colleagues. In selecting authors, I have celebrated the expertise of a variety of child mental health disciplines. The chapter authors exceeded my high expectations and responded patiently to my detailed copyediting and content suggestions. The most difficult part both for the authors and for me was to distill their great knowledge and expertise into the limited number of pages possible in a single volume.

Additional resources—books and Web sites—are provided for the reader following the Acknowledgments.

Onward and upward!

Acknowledgments

Both the Warren Wright endowment of Northwestern Memorial Hospital and the Osterman Chair of Child Psychiatry at Children's Memorial Hospital provided essential support for my work on this book over the entire 3 years from conception to delivery. My husband, Richard Wendel, not only contributed a chapter from his expertise in family therapy but also cheerfully interrupted his own academic work whenever a screech from my adjacent study signaled a need for his assistance when I was frustrated with the computer or a contributor. Tina Coltri-Marshall, APPI Publications Coordinator, supported every step of the process with precision and grace, from instructions to authors to assuring receipt of the final version of each and every chapter. Organizing this book and tracking all of the processes were major challenges that could not have been accomplished without her. Senior Editor Ann Eng ably managed the process at APPI that starts with submission of final chapter manuscripts. From idea to final book in hand, Bob Hales and John McDuffie both encouraged and supported me—all toward the goal we share of the best possible book.

Additional Resources

Selected Books for Professionals

Dulcan MK: Helping Parents, Youth, and Teachers Understand Medications for Behavioral and Emotional Problems: A Resource Book of Medication Information Handouts, 3rd Edition. Washington, DC, American Psychiatric Publishing, 2007

Findling, RL (ed): Clinical Manual of Child and Adolescent Psychopharmacology. Washington, DC, American Psychiatric Publishing, 2008

Hales RE, Yudofsky SC, Gabbard GO (eds): The American Psychiatric Publishing Textbook of Psychiatry, 5th Edition. Washington, DC, American Psychiatric Publishing, 2008

Petti TA, Salguero C (eds): Community Child and Adolescent Psychiatry: A Manual of Clinical Practice and Consultation. Washington, DC, American Psychiatric Publishing, 2006

Shaw RJ, DeMaso DR: Clinical Manual of Pediatric Psychosomatic Medicine: Mental Health Consultation With Physically Ill Children and Adolescents. Washington, DC, American Psychiatric Publishing, 2006

Web Sites for Professionals, Patients, and Families

American Academy of Child and Adolescent Psychiatry (AACAP)
Includes "Facts for Families," brief information sheets on a wide variety of topics in child and family development and mental health
www.aacap.org

American Academy of Pediatrics
www.aap.org

American Psychiatric Association
www.healthyminds.org

Autism Society of America
www.autism-society.org

Center for Mental Health Services (CMHS)
Information on child and adolescent mental health and on family mental health resources
www.mentalhealth.org

Child and Adolescent Bipolar Foundation
www.bpkids.org

Children and Adults With Attention-Deficit/Hyperactivity Disorder (CHADD)
www.chadd.org

National Alliance on Mental Illness (NAMI)
www.nami.org

National Institute of Mental Health
www.nimh.nih.gov

National Resource Center on AD/HD
A cooperative venture of CHADD and the Centers for Disease Control and Prevention
www.help4adhd.org/library.cfm

Online Asperger Syndrome Information and Support (OASIS)
www.aspergersyndrome.org

Parents Med Guide/Physicians Med Guide

Guides offering practical advice to parents of children and adolescents struggling with depression and information to general practitioners and pediatricians on pediatric depression treatment alternatives and the latest science

www.ParentsMedGuide.org

The Annenberg Foundation Trust at Sunnylands Adolescent Mental Health Initiative

Mental health site for teens; contains downloadable concise guides on psychiatric disorders in youth for teens, parents, and counselors (see the Mind Zone located on the site's drop-down menu)

www.CopeCareDeal.org

Tourette Syndrome Association

www.tsa-usa.org

PART I

A DEVELOPMENTAL VIEW OF ASSESSMENT

Chapter 1

Assessing Infants and Toddlers

Mary Margaret Gleason, M.D., F.A.A.P.
Charles H. Zeanah, M.D.

Assessing infants and toddlers is increasingly a requirement within clinical child mental health settings and often involves collaborating with a variety of other infant mental health professionals in assessments and in developing treatment plans. Infant psychiatry is a strength-based, prevention-focused subspecialty of child and adolescent psychiatry that has brought attention to the mental health needs of children from birth through the preschool years. Infant psychiatry focuses on early identification of risk contexts and mental health disorders in infants, young children, and their families and requires a different assessment approach than that used with older children and adolescents.

The field of infant mental health, which includes both mental health and allied health professionals involved with young children, explicitly considers the emotional functioning of infants and their families in their specific biological, developmental, relationship, and community contexts. Fundamentally, the focus is explicitly on the young child embedded in a complex set of contexts, ranging from the child's neurobiological endowment to the larger social and cultural contexts in which the child develops. This approach to families is founded upon an empirical base that demonstrates the importance of prenatal factors, developmental level, quality of relationships, and cumulative exposure to risk (and protective) factors in young children's current and future functioning (Sameroff and Fiese 2000). Infancy and toddlerhood are characterized by extraordinarily rapid development, which can be seen dramatically through brain imaging techniques that document peak cerebral metabolism, and rate of brain growth, as well as easily observable physical and emotional developmental milestones (Shonkoff and Phillips 2000; Vitiello 1998).

In early childhood, assessment focuses primarily on the child-caregiver relationship rather than on the young child as an individual. Characteristics of the child *and* parent(s) have their primary salience as important contributors to the child-caregiver relationships. In this chapter, we begin by proving a rationale for the relationship focus and then describe components and methods of the evaluation.

Relational Approach to Assessing Infants and Toddlers: Rationale and Implications

When working with young children and their families, the primary focus of assessment shifts from the child to the young child's important caregiving relationships. A primary reason for this is that the individual characteristics of the infant or toddler have limited predictive value for the child's future development. The child's important caregiving relationships, on the other hand, are far more predictive of subsequent outcomes (Shonkoff and Phillips 2000; Zeanah and Zeanah, in press; Zeanah et al. 2005). Infants who develop a secure attachment relationship with a primary caregiver during the first year of life are more likely to have positive relationships with peers, to be liked by their teachers, to perform better in school, and to be more resilient in the face of stress or adversity as preschoolers and later. Infants who develop an insecure attachment relationship, in contrast, are at risk for a more troublesome trajectory (Sroufe 2005). Because of the importance of the infant-caregiver relationship, any factors that affect this relationship strongly influence the emotional functioning of the young child. Thus, clinical assessment and treatment focus on changing young children's caregiving relationships as the most effective way to sustain meaningful changes in the child's adaptation.

A second reason for a relational focus is that through the caregiving relationships, infants begin to understand the social world, learn how to interact with others, and begin to develop a sense of competence and self-worth. If the relationship is disturbed, the relationship may need to change in order to help the child in these important domains. Even when risks to the young child's development derive from other sources, intervening through the relationship may be the most effective means of buffering the child against the risks.

Third, environmental risks exert their effect on the young child primarily through the caregiving relationship. Poverty, for example, is a well-known risk factor in young children (Knitzer and Perry, in press), but it means little to an infant to be poor except as poverty is experienced through the infant's primary caregiving relationships.

Fourth, intrinsic risk factors, such as many biological abnormalities, are moderated by the infant's caregiving relationships. For example, infants who experience the complications of prematurity have better outcomes when their caregiving environments are more supportive and have more problematic outcomes when their caregiving environments are less supportive (Sameroff and Fiese 2000). Difficult temperament in infants and toddlers, another biological risk factor, can be moderated through responsive, nurturing, and consistent caregiving experiences (van den Boom 1994).

Young children construct relationships with their caregivers based on experiences they have had with them. There is no evidence that children during the first 18 months to 2 years of life can even imagine what they have not experienced directly. Based on experience, young children may develop different kinds of relationships with different caregivers, as has been demonstrated in attachment research in which young children are found simultaneously to have different types of attachments to different caregivers.

Because the young child may have qualitatively different kinds of relationships with different caregiving adults, the child will be assessed in all of his or her important caregiving relationships. During the assessment process, the clinician always considers the possibility that a described or observed pattern of behaviors or symptoms is relationship specific. The more consistently a child's oppositional behavior, for example, is observed in different important relationships, the more confident the clinician can be that the problem is pervasive and not relationship specific. In contrast, in our experience, much symptomatic behavior observed in young children is relationship specific, requiring different kinds of intervention.

A relational approach requires focus on specific components of the relationship, such as the caregiver's perceptions of the child and the caregiver's interactive behavior with the child. Specific approaches to these components of the assessment are described below.

The final implication of this model is that clinically significant problems may derive primarily from within the child, primarily from within the parent, or from the unique pattern of interactions between the two. In most cases, all of these sources contribute to some degree. In any case, the intervention implemented will most likely use the parent-child relationship as a primary vehicle for change.

Diagnostic Issues Regarding Disorders of Early Childhood

In the psychiatric medical model, diagnosis is a primary determinant of treatment planning. In practical terms, it also drives third-party reimbursement for services. In infancy and early childhood, the issues of diagnosis deserve additional consideration. Much has been written about the limitations of DSM-IV (American Psychiatric Association 1994) in early childhood diagnoses—lack of developmentally sensitive criteria, failure to include young children in field trials, assuming young children have phenomenologically similar disorders as do adolescents and adults—leading to the development of alternative nosologies. The Research Diagnostic Criteria: Preschool Age (RDC:PA; American Academy of Child and Adolescent Psychiatry Task Force on Research Diagnostic Criteria 2003) was developed to increase consistency of application of diagnoses in research settings. This nosology applies evidence-based modifications to the DSM-IV criteria. The Diagnostic Criteria: Zero to Three (Revised) (DC:0–3R), which has incorporated some of the criteria from the RDC:PA, provides descriptions of clinical presentations commonly seen in infants and young children. Its multiaxial system emphasizes centrality of the parent-child relationship (Zero to Three Diagnostic Classification Task Force 2005).

Validity studies of psychiatric diagnoses in children younger than 3 years have grown substantially in the past decade, but they are still fewer in number than validity studies of disorders in even preschool children. While the evidence base for the RDC:PA and DC:0–3R is limited in children under 3 years, clinical application of a standard nosology can facilitate communication among providers and with third-party payers. Systematic use of these diagnoses in clinical settings can also facilitate clinical research that can inform further refinement of the criteria.

The use of the multiaxial system in infant psychiatry is as important as the consistent use of Axis I diagnosis. When applying the DSM-IV system, developmental status (Axis II), medical or biological conditions (Axis III), environmental factors (Axis IV), and child's level of functioning or impairment (Axis V) contribute to the understanding of the child and family. The DC:0–3R system includes a relationship classification axis (Axis II) and a social-emotional functioning axis (Axis V). Regardless of the classification system applied, caregiver-child relationship qualities, biological factors, environmental and family stressors and strengths, and child functioning all must be considered in the clinical formulation and treatment planning.

Assessment Settings

Assessments of infants and toddlers can occur in a number of different settings. In all clinical settings, collaboration and cross-specialty education for providers are important components of infant mental health services. Often, these assessments occur within an office-based mental health setting, with the child psychiatrist as sole practitioner or as leader of a clinical team. However, other clinical settings, such as early intervention programs, outpatient primary care practices, inpatient pediatric units, juvenile court settings, child care centers, or homeless shelters, also can provide infant mental health services. In these settings, the infant mental health assessment may be focused in the context of a larger comprehensive team evaluation or may respond to a specific clinical consultation question. The setting and specific question usually guide the approach to assessing infants and toddlers.

Wherever the assessment takes place, attention to the clinical environment can facilitate the therapist-parent relationship, even before the clinician sees the family. Waiting rooms and offices with child-size furniture and child activities (e.g., culturally appropriate reading material and baby books as well as parenting-focused magazines) may help the family feel welcome even before the assessment begins. Additionally, an office that supports breastfeeding (by having a breastfeeding room) is likely to feel most comfortable for young families.

Goals of Infant Mental Health Assessments

An important clinician role is to create a warm and welcoming environment for families and, early in the assessment, to develop a shared understanding of the goals and process of the assessment. Stigma can affect all clinical practice in child psychiatry, but its impact may be especially strong in early childhood. A first step in addressing these concerns may be to acknowledge some of the spoken or unspoken concerns a parent may have about the referral. Parents may be concerned that they are "bad parents" or that the referral indicates concerns that the infant is irremediably disordered. Among low-income or low-resource parents, for example, it is not unusual to be concerned that an early childhood mental health referral may result in losing custody of the child. Addressing these fears explicitly can be a useful step toward developing a collaborative relationship with the parents.

The clinician-parent relationship is central to the assessment and treatment process because the parent is the primary source of information about the child. A trusting relationship is necessary for the parent to share openly his or her observations and perceptions of the child. In addition, aspects of the clinician-parent relationship may serve as models for ongoing development of the parent-child relationship, especially for parents who have not experienced nurturing, consistent, warm relationships in the past.

Through the assessment, the clinician aims to understand the factors affecting a child's emotional and relationship development, in order to intervene early, reduce current distress and impairment, and positively influence the child's developmental trajectory. Assessments of infants and toddlers should provide sufficient information to develop a biopsychosocial formulation, with attention to multiple diagnostic axes and a specific focus on the parent-child relationship. Thus, an assessment of the relationship is used to understand the strengths and risks conveyed through the relationship and to identify the modalities that will be best suited for treating the dyad.

Comprehensive Assessment

Assessment of infants and toddlers ought to include multiple appointments, using multiple informants, and multiple modes of assessment, including formal and informal observational and history collection procedures (Table 1–1). Including the infant or toddler in all appointments can allow for extensive, informal ob-

servations of parent-child interactions and reduces the parent's need for child care during the appointments.

As in all psychiatric interviews, open-ended questions provide useful information. Questions about the child's personality and strengths can be a nonthreatening way to begin the interview, emphasize a strength-based perspective, and provide the clinician with a sense of the parent's ability to describe both the positive attributes and the concerning behaviors of the child. In taking the history of present illness, clinicians try to understand the chief complaint in detail, with attention to the child's behavior, the context and potential environmental influences of the behavior, and the parent's reaction (internal and external) to the behavior. Parental responses to a child's behaviors have the potential to help the child regulate behaviors or may exacerbate the pattern. The parent's attribution of meaning to a behavior is crucial. For example, although a 24-month-old's tantrums may seem developmentally appropriate to the clinician, they become an important clinical focus if the parent perceives the child as an aggressor or believes that these behaviors mean the child will follow the path of a psychiatrically disturbed relative.

A review of psychological and regulatory systems is critical in placing the chief complaint in context. It is helpful to understand the child's self-regulatory skills, including emotional regulation as well as biological processes such as sleep and feeding. These regulatory processes may be the most prominent patterns in young infants. In older toddlers, overall mood and patterns of mood changes, fears, activity level, impulsivity, aggression, and social interactions also contribute to the understanding of the child's emotional functioning. In the interview, it is useful to explore factors in the parent-child relationship, including 1) the child's developing attachment behaviors, such as seeking comfort in times of distress or new situations, as well as experiences of mutual enjoyment, and 2) the parent's expectations and hopes for the child. See the section "Formal Assessment Procedures" later in this chapter for more information.

Throughout the interview, the clinician attends to the parent's tone, his or her ability to consider events from the child's perspective or to recognize the child's needs, and the parent's sense of the child as having strengths as well as the problem that brought the family to the evaluation. When two parents are present, observing the way that the parents share the time in the interview, negotiate disagreements, and the similarities and differences in the way the parents perceive the child yields important information about family functioning.

TABLE 1–1. Key elements of the infant-toddler assessment

History (from all available sources)	Child observations	Parent-child interactions	Structured assessment tools
History of presenting problem	Dysmorphic features	Tone of interactions	Parent perception Interview
Review of systems	Size for age	Pacing of interactions	Structured parent-child interaction
Medical history	Regulatory capacity Behavior with parent vs. examiner	Mutual engagement and reciprocity Conflict	Behavior/emotion checklists
Developmental history	Activity level	Parent responsivity to child	Structured psychiatric interviews
Family history	Patterns of play	Separation and reunion (≥7 months old)	Questionnaires/interviews regarding competence
Social history	Vocalization	Child use of parent for help	

Medical History

A child's medical history can provide important information about biological influences on development and behavior, as well as events that could affect the infant's and family's emotional development. It is useful to begin the history in the preconception period. Pregnancy planning, including unwanted pregnancies and/or fertility problems, may influence a parent's expectations about a child. When a mother did not plan or want to be pregnant, it can be useful to understand what influenced her decision (or nondecision) to continue the pregnancy, and whether she changed her mind during the pregnancy. These topics can be included in other parts of the history but often can be easily incorporated into the medical history.

Illnesses during pregnancy, infections, substance use, violence exposure, and maternal psychopathology all may influence fetal growth and can influence later development (Koren et al. 1998; O'Connor et al. 2002; Yehuda et al. 2005). A history of prematurity, particularly if it included a stay in the neonatal intensive care unit, may have implications for the child's development and may be an early trauma impacting the parent-child relationship (Muller-Nix and Ansermet, in press). In addition to major medical events or hospitalizations, it is useful to explore any history of colic, failure to thrive, elevated serum lead levels, pica, head trauma, or other central nervous system events, which may be related to the infant's or toddler's pre-

sentation (Canfield et al. 2003; Coolbear and Benoit 1999).

Additionally, every child seen for an infant psychiatry assessment warrants an assessment of developmental milestones to understand the child in the context of his or her developmental pattern along with the chronological age. Standardized measures, such as the Ages and Stages Questionnaire, may be useful adjuncts to this clinical evaluation (Squires et al. 1999). Clinicians may use a low threshold for requesting a formal assessment of a child's development, as developmental status may greatly influence the clinical presentation.

Family History

The family psychiatric history can be of particular importance in the infant psychiatry assessment. It can be helpful to draw a multiple-generation genogram to clarify the relationships among family members, provide an opportunity to learn more about the parents' early caregiving environments, and identify potential genetic loading. When parents or other adults in the household have histories of psychiatric disorders, a sensitive exploration of their current symptoms and how the symptoms influence the child or the parent's caregiving style is warranted. Furthermore, when family histories are positive for certain disorders, parents may fear that the child's behavior problems are reflective of those disorders.

Social History

As noted, the context of early childhood development is the primary caregiving relationship. This relationship exists within a larger social context, with factors that can support or impair a child's social and emotional development. Thus, the social history in infant psychiatry ought to include attention to household members, extended family, cultural or spiritual influences, and community factors, including support systems or dangerous or frightening exposures. Family violence, including partner violence and child abuse, is a particularly important influence, which may not be shared spontaneously. Because perspectives on parenting and parent-child relationships may differ across cultures, even within ethnic groups, it can be useful to explore the family's expectations about the parent-child relationship and the types of interactions that are culturally acceptable or optimal. When these perspectives are not shared within the clinician-parent relationship, they may impede therapeutic progress because parents and therapists are moving toward different goals based on different implicit expectations.

Finally, the impact of community factors, parents' perceptions of safety within the home and community, and the degree to which the parents can meet the basic needs of their family can be strong influences on the clinical presentation and appropriate interventions. Some clinical infant mental health programs include provisions to meet the family's basic needs, with the recognition that a family may not be able to participate in needed therapy if the parents' primary concern relates to having enough food to feed their children or threats of eviction.

An example of such a program is Louisiana's Early Childhood Supports and Services program (www.ecssla.org), a state-funded program of the Office of Mental Health, that provides mental health evaluations for families with children 0–5 years old and also coordinates and enhances access to community services and short-term emergency financial assistance to families via case management services. This model facilitates family well-being by meeting immediate needs and enhances the therapeutic alliance by allowing clinicians to participate in meeting the family's prioritized needs.

Observations

In any infant psychiatry assessment, observations of parent-child interactions and clinician interactions with the child are important components of the evaluation. Observing the infant and parent-child interactions while taking the history allows the clinician to examine unscripted interactions. Additionally, it can be useful for clinicians to observe a specific activity in all assessments, such as a feeding in a young infant or a free-play period with toddlers. Observations of infants include noting the infant or young child's appearance, including the presence of stigmata of genetic syndromes or those associated with prenatal teratogenic exposures. Behavioral observations of infants and toddlers include level of activity; vocalizations or verbalizations; reciprocity; regulatory capacity (level of arousal, ability to reorganize after limit setting or frustration); and in toddlers, patterns of play and aggressive behaviors. Observable patterns of emotional development are described in Table 1–2.

Domains of parent-child interactions that can be observed informally include the child's use of the parent for assistance, joy sharing, comfort seeking, and play, as well as the parent's anticipation of the infant's needs, responsiveness to the child's cues, ability to structure the interactions to match the child's developmental needs, level of engagement in the interaction, and overall enjoyment of the child. While observing dyadic play, the evaluator can note the level of mutual engagement, shared attention, reciprocity, and, with verbal children, shared representational play themes (American Academy of Child and Adolescent Psychiatry 1997). The tone of the interaction and the dyad's comfort together, as well as the nature of affective interactions, also reflect the quality of the relationship.

With children whose developmental age is at least 7–9 months, it can be informative to negotiate a separation and reunion during the evaluation to provide an indicator of how the dyad reconnects following a brief separation. Parents can demonstrate sensitivity by preparing a child for the separation. However, the information most reflective of the quality of the attachment is the dyad's ability to resolve separation distress together during the reunion (Boris et al. 1997; Zeanah et al. 2000).

Formal Assessment Procedures

Parent-Child Relationship Assessments

A number of structured procedures can augment informal clinical history and observations. This section

TABLE 1–2. Clinically salient behaviors related to assessment

Domains	Birth–2 months	2–7 months	7–18 months	18–36 months
Social	Quiet, alert state evident for minutes at a time	Social smiling Sustained eye-to-eye contact	Stranger wariness Separation protest from attachment figures Social referencing	Awareness of relationship to group More emphasis on personal possessions
Emotional	Crying peaks at 6 weeks cross-culturally and then wanes	Joy, fear, surprise apparent	Affect attunement Greater differentiation of affective states	Moral emotions: shame, guilt, pride
Communicative	Crying indicates distress	Responsive cooing	Intentional communication; some protowords and some words	Expressive language blossoms
Gross motor	Tone improves	Rolls over (3–4 months); sits independently 6–8 months)	Walks (12–15 months)	Running (1½–2 years); jumping (2½–3 years)
Fine motor		Grasps with one hand (6 months)	Pincer grasp (7–9 months); transfers objects from one hand to other (12 months)	Hand dominance develops; able to stack two blocks at 18 months and eight blocks at 30 months; scribbles spontaneously; copies circle (36 months)
Growth	Regains birth weight by 2 weeks	Doubles birth weight by 4–6 months	Triples birth weight at 1 year	Quadruples birth weight at 2 years

will present one example of a structured interview and of an observational procedure that can be used in clinical settings.

The working model of the child interview is approximately a 1-hour interview focused on a parent's understanding of his or her child and of the relationship they share (available through www.infantinstitute.com/training.htm). During this interview, the parent is asked about the child's personality and the relationship he or she has with the child. The content of the parent's responses can be useful information about the parent's experience of the infant or toddler. Additionally, and often more saliently, a clinician can learn about the parent's internal representation of the child by attending to the characteristics of the narrative itself, including affective tone, level of emotional involvement, coherence of the responses, and the balance of parent's positive and negative descriptions about the child (Zeanah and Benoit 1995). The interview can be videotaped for further review. When the interview is formally coded for research purposes, parental representation differentiates between clinically referred and non–clinically referred infants (Benoit et al. 1997). Additionally, parents who present balanced representations of their child in the interview are likely to have children who have a secure attachment relationship with the parent, based upon the Strange Situation Procedure (Zeanah et al. 1994).

In the Crowell Procedure (Crowell and Feldman 1988), the parent and child (of at least 6 months developmental age) are observed in a series of activities including free play, cleanup, a bubbles sequence, and four puzzle tasks, as well as a separation and reunion (access at www.infantinstitute.org). The procedure provides a standardized method of assessing a number of domains of the parent-child relationship including reciprocal emotions, protection and safety, comforting and comfort seeking, teaching and learning, play, discipline and response to limits, and parental structure and child's self-regulation. The assessment can provide more depth of understanding of the dyad's interactions, capacity for joy, and ability to negotiate stressful situations. The process of separation and reunion provides valuable information about how the child uses the parent for comfort during a mild relationship stressor.

For younger infants (3–6 months), the still-face paradigm can also provide valuable information about dyadic emotional regulation. The procedure includes three phases including a naturalistic interaction, a 3-minute period when the parent maintains a nonreactive ("still") facial expression, and a 3-minute reengagement period when the parent interacts as usual. Responses to the still-face procedure correlate with maternal internal representation of the infant (Rosenblum et al. 2002) and predict future attachment classification. Clinically, the still-face paradigm may provide an opportunity to observe mutual regulatory capacities of an infant and parent.

Measures of Infant or Toddler Functioning

Diagnostic Interviews

Structured interviews may provide a systematic approach to assessing parent report of toddler symptoms and yield information to guide application of diagnoses. These interviews also provide critical information about the level of impairment associated with a child's symptoms and the degree to which a family has accommodated the child's symptoms. As with any single tool, the information provided by systematic interviews can add to the clinical impression and be incorporated into the diagnostic formulation, but they do not, independently, provide sufficient information to make a diagnosis. All parent-report measures provide information about the parent's experience and observations of the child and therefore are considered within the context of a larger assessment.

The Preschool Age Psychiatric Assessment (PAPA) is the only diagnostic interview for which reliability data have been published (Egger et al. 2006). The instrument is an interviewer-based psychiatric diagnostic interview focused on children 2–5 years old. The interview includes assessment of the symptoms included

in DSM-IV, RDC:PA, DC:0–3R, ICD-10, as well as behavioral patterns applicable to young children but not included in these nosologies. Importantly, the interview explores the impairment associated with the child's symptoms in a number of functional domains. The PAPA was developed as a research tool, and in its entirety may not be appropriate for clinical settings, although efforts to create an electronic version may facilitate its use in clinical settings.

The Diagnostic Infant Preschool Structured Interview (Scheeringa M: "Diagnostic Infant Preschool Structured Interview," unpublished manual, 2005) is a respondent-based interview of parents of children 18–60 months. Like the PAPA, the interview includes symptoms from the RDC:PA and DSM-IV. It also explores the degree to which parents have accommodated to their children's behavioral patterns. For example, a parent may not consider the child's sleeping patterns a problem, but only because the father now sleeps on a mattress next to the crib with his arm on the infant at all times.

Caregiver-Report Checklists

Parent- or child care provider–report measures can be useful ways of assessing the level of reported symptoms (Table 1–3). Validated, normed measures allow comparison of the child's symptom level to larger populations. Additionally, when completed by more than one reporter, they can be used to develop a multidimensional picture about the child in more than one context or relationship. Clinicians can also use these measures to track the symptoms or strengths across time. Although they are useful adjuncts to the clinical assessment, adult-report checklists share a number of limitations. Most notably, they reflect the specific subjective experiences and perceptions of the reporter. The best studied influence on parent-report measures is maternal depression. Maternal depression is associated with higher levels of reported symptoms than concurrent reports by child care providers, but is also associated with higher levels of clinician-observed symptoms in play, especially when mothers have comorbid psychopathology (e.g., Carter et al. 2001; Chilcoat and Breslau 1997; Dawson et al. 2003; Ingersoll and Eist 1998). Researchers and clinicians postulate that maternal depression may influence child behaviors within the relationship and child development in multiple domains, as well as parental sensitivity to challenging child behaviors. It is likely that a myriad of other factors also influence reporting patterns. Thus, these checklists are best considered within the context of the complete assessment.

TABLE 1–3.   Selected measures of early childhood symptoms

Measure	Ages, months	Domains	Format	Number of items	Validity	Reliability	Special characteristics
Ages and Stages Questionnaires: Social-Emotional (Squires et al. 2001)[a]	6–60	Self-regulation, compliance, communication, adaptive functioning, autonomy, affect, and interaction with people	3-point Likert scale Different forms for each age group (months): 6, 18, 24, 30, 36, 48, 60	22–36	Sensitivity in predicting a positive score on the CBCL and Vineland Social-Emotional Early Childhood scales, or a known diagnosis: 71%–85%; lower in younger age groups Specificity: 90%–98%.	Test-retest reliability after 1–3 weeks is excellent (r=0.91)	Screening measure; includes strength-based items; validity using broadly defined.
Child Behavior Checklist 1½–5 (Achenbach and Rescorla 2000)[b]	18–60	Internalizing, externalizing, and total problems	3-point Likert scale	99	Clinically referred children have higher scores than non-clinically referred children (effect size=0.3); 77% referred sample vs. 26%	1-week test-retest reliability: mean=0.85 (parent report), 0.81 (teacher report)	Computer scoring system; validated teacher rating form
Infant-Toddler Social and Emotional Assessment (Briggs-Gowan 1998)[c]	12–36	Internalizing, externalizing, dysregulation, and competence	3-point Likert scale	166	Correlation with CBCL total problem scores: r=0.47 (internalizing problems); r=−0.67 (externalizing problems) Correlation with observer ratings: r=0.20–0.31	Mean 1-month test-retest reliability: r=0.82–0.90 for domains;	Includes strengths; BITSEA screener (a companion measure) available

Note. BITSEA=Brief Infant-Toddler Social and Emotional Assessment; CBCL=Child Behavior Checklist.
[a]Purchasing information: www.brookespublishing.com/store/books/squires-asqse/index.htm
[b]Purchasing information: www.aseba.com
[c]Purchasing information: http://pearsonassess.com

Perhaps the best known adult-report measure about children's behavior is the Child Behavior Checklist (CBCL), for ages 1½–5 (Achenbach and Rescorla 2000). The CBCL has been used to track treatment outcomes as well as for assessment (e.g., Lieberman et al. 2005). It can be scored by hand or using a computer program, which also generates a profile with comparison norms.

The Infant-Toddler Social and Emotional Assessment (ITSEA; Briggs-Gowan 1998) and its companion, the Brief Infant-Toddler Social and Emotional Assessment (BITSEA; Briggs-Gowan and Carter 2002), assess problems and strengths in children 12–36 months, using a 3-point Likert scale. The ITSEA has strong evidence supporting its concurrent validity with well-accepted observational and parent-report measures (Carter et al. 1999). The BITSEA was developed as a brief screening tool. A BITSEA screen is considered positive if both the problem score and the competency score are outside of the cutoff score.

Parent-report checklists of younger children's social-emotional development are limited in number and perhaps in clinical utility. Reports of infant mental health patterns, even more than toddler mental health, can be considered only in the context of the parent-child relationship. To date, adult-report measures of the relationship have limited clinical utility. The Ages and Stages Questionnaire: Social-Emotional (ASQ:SE) screening system includes a 6-month screen, which focuses primarily on infant cues and regulation patterns related to calming the infant, feeding, sleeping, and stooling (Squires et al. 2002). The ASQ:SE tools show moderate concordance with the Vineland Social-Emotional Early Childhood Scale but have not yet been tested in their prediction of clinically assessed infant mental health problems.

Parent Symptoms

Some clinical problems within the infant-parent relationship may stem from parent distress or psychopathology. Structured tools, such as the Edinburgh Postnatal Depression Scale, can be administered in the

peripartum period (Cox et al. 1987). The Beck Depression Inventory–II (Beck et al. 1996) and the Parenting Stress Index—Short Form (Haskett et al. 2006) may be helpful in assessing the need for further parental assessment. Although maternal depression may be the best-studied form of parental psychopathology in the context of infant and early childhood well-being (e.g., Dawson et al. 2003; Seifer et al. 2001), comorbid conditions are the strongest predictor of adverse early childhood outcome (Carter et al. 2001). Other psychopathology, including substance abuse, psychotic illnesses, and anxiety, can affect the caregiving environment and young children's psychiatric presentation (Hipwell et al. 2000).

Research Directions

The field of infant and toddler mental health is growing and has an increasing evidence base. However, as a new field, there are areas for further research. First, while the DC:0–3R nosology presents a diagnostic approach to classifying psychopathology in very young children and their relationships, the field needs further research focused on the validity of these diagnostic criteria in children under 36 months, and especially under 24 months. In the future, clinically applicable diagnostic assessment strategies may improve consistency across assessments. Structured observations have been developed for assessment of specific disorders in preschoolers (e.g., Disruptive Behavior Diagnostic Observation Schedule [Wakschlag et al. 2008]). In the future, infant and toddler observation strategies may be structured in order to provide more consistent information to guide diagnostic and relationship assessment in very young children. Finally, while research assessments of the quality of parent-child relationship are fairly well validated, clinician-friendly assessment strategies are just beginning to be developed. Dissemination of such approaches will add important information to clinical assessments.

Summary Points

- The quality of the primary caregiving relationship is the strongest determinant of early childhood development.

- Use of systematic developmentally sensitive approaches to diagnosis in infancy and early childhood can assist with communication across providers and with consistency across patients, and may provide important data to allow the field to progress.

- Although assessment can take place in a variety of settings, every effort should be made to help a family feel comfortable by creating a welcoming physical environment and to help parents feel comfortable seeking mental health treatment.

- Assessment follows the rule of multiples: it takes place over multiple appointments, with multiple informants, using multiple forms of information gathering.

- Assessment in infancy and early childhood includes not just the usual components of a psychiatric assessment but also attention to parent-child interactions and the parent's perception of the child.

- Structured assessments can provide useful information to supplement a thorough clinical history and observation.

References

Achenbach T, Rescorla L: Manual for the ASEBA Preschool Form. Burlington, University of Vermont, 2000

American Academy of Child and Adolescent Psychiatry: Practice parameters for the psychiatric assessment of infants and toddlers (0–36 months). J Am Acad Child Adolesc Psychiatry 36(suppl):21S–36S, 1997

American Academy of Child and Adolescent Psychiatry Task Force on Research Diagnostic Criteria: Infancy Preschool: Research diagnostic criteria for infants and preschool children: the process and empirical support. J Am Acad Child Adolesc Psychiatry 42:1504–1512, 2003

American Psychiatric Association: Diagnostic and Statistical Manual of Mental Disorders, 4th Edition. Washington, DC, American Psychiatric Association, 1994

Beck A, Steer RA, Brown G: Beck Depression Inventory II. San Antonio, TX, Harcourt Assessment, 1996

Benoit D, Parker KCH, Zeanah CH: Mothers' representations of their infants assessed prenatally: stability and association with infants' attachment classifications. J Child Psychol Psychiatry 38:307–313, 1997

Boris NW, Fueyo M, Zeanah CH: The clinical assessment of attachment in children under five. J Am Acad Child Adolesc Psychiatry 36:291–293, 1997

Briggs-Gowan M: Preliminary acceptability and psychometrics of the Infant-Toddler Social and Emotional Assessment (ITSEA): a new adult-report questionnaire. Infant Ment Health J 19:422–445, 1998

Briggs-Gowan M, Carter AS: Brief Infant Toddler Social Emotional Assessment (BITSEA) Manual, Version 2.0. New Haven, CT, Yale University, 2002

Canfield RL, Henderson CR Jr, Cory-Slechta DA, et al: Intellectual impairment in children with blood lead concentrations below 10 micrograms per deciliter. N Engl J Med 348:1517–1526, 2003

Carter AS, Little C, Briggs-Gowan MJ, et al: The Infant-Toddler Social and Emotional Assessment (ITSEA): comparing parent ratings to laboratory observations of task mastery, emotion regulation, coping behaviors, and attachment status. Infant Ment Health J 20:375–392, 1999

Carter AS, Garrity-Rokous FE, Chazan-Cohen R, et al: Maternal depression and comorbidity: predicting early parenting, attachment security, and toddler social-emotional problems and competencies. J Am Acad Child Adolesc Psychiatry 40:18–26, 2001

Chilcoat HD, Breslau N: Does psychiatric history bias mothers' reports? An application of a new analytic approach. J Am Acad Child Adolesc Psychiatry 36:971–979, 1997

Coolbear J, Benoit D: Failure to thrive: risk for clinical disturbance of attachment? Infant Ment Health J 20:87–104, 1999

Cox JL, Holden JM, Sagovsky R: Detection of postnatal depression: development of the 10-item Edinburgh Postnatal Depression Scale. Br J Psychiatry 150:782–786, 1987

Crowell JA, Feldman SS: Mothers' internal models of relationships and children's behavioral and developmental status: a study of mother-child interaction. Child Dev 59:1273–1285, 1988

Dawson G, Ashman SB, Panagiotides H, et al: Preschool outcomes of children of depressed mothers: role of maternal behavior, contextual risk, and children's brain activity. Child Dev 74:1158–1175, 2003

Egger HL, Erkanli A, Keeler GM, et al: Test-retest reliability of the Preschool Age Psychiatric Assessment (PAPA). J Am Acad Child Adolesc Psychiatry 45:538–549, 2006

Haskett ME, Ahern LS, Ward CS, et al: Factor structure and validity of the Parenting Stress Index-Short Form. J Clin Child Psychol 35:302–312, 2006

Hipwell AE, Goossens FA, Melhuish EC, et al: Severe maternal psychopathology and infant-mother attachment. Dev Psychopathol 12:157–175, 2000

Ingersoll BD, Eist HI: Are depressed mothers biased reporters? J Am Acad Child Adolesc Psychiatry 37:681–682, 1998

Knitzer J, Perry D: Poverty and infant and toddler development: facing the complex challenges, in Handbook of Infant Mental Health, 3rd Edition. Edited by Zeanah CH. New York, Guilford, in press

Koren G, Pastuszak A, Ito S: Drugs in Pregnancy. N Engl J Med 338:1128–1137, 1998

Lieberman AFP, Van Horn PJ, Ippen CGP: Toward evidence-based treatment: child-parent psychotherapy with preschoolers exposed to marital violence. J Am Acad Child Adolesc Psychiatry 44:1241–1248, 2005

Muller-Nix C, Ansermet F: Prematurity: risk and protective factors, in Handbook of Infant Mental Health, 3rd Edition. Edited by Zeanah CH. New York, Guilford, in press

O'Connor TG, Heron J, Golding J: Maternal antenatal anxiety and children's behavioural/emotional problems at 4 years: report from the Avon Longitudinal Study of Parents and Children. Br J Psychiatry 180:502–508, 2002

Rosenblum KL, McDonough S, Muzik M, et al: Maternal representations of the infant: associations with infant response to the Still Face. Child Dev 73:999–1015, 2002

Sameroff AJ, Fiese BH: Models of development and developmental risk, in Handbook of Infant Mental Health, 2nd Edition. Edited by Zeanah CH. New York, Guilford, 2000, pp 3–19

Seifer R, Dickstein S, Sameroff A, et al: Infant mental health and variability of parental depressive symptoms. J Am Acad Child Adolesc Psychiatry 40:1375–1382, 2001

Shonkoff JP, Phillips DA: From Neurons to Neighborhoods: The Science of Early Childhood Development Committee on Integrating the Science of Early Childhood Development. Washington, DC, National Academy Press, 2000

Squires J, Potter L, Bricker D: The ASQ User's Guide, 2nd Edition. Baltimore, MD, Brooks Publishing, 1999

Squires J, Bricker D, Heo K, et al: Identification of social-emotional problems in young children using a parent-completed screening measure. Early Child Res Q 16:405–419, 2001

Squires J, Bricker D, Twombly E: Ages and Stages Questionnaires: Social-Emotional: A Parent-Completed, Child-Monitoring System for Social-Emotional Behaviors. 6 Month ASQ:SE Questionnaire (For Infants Ages 3 Through 8 Months). Baltimore, MD, Paul H. Brookes Publishing, 2002. Available at: http://eip.uoregon.edu/pdf/6month_asqse.pdf. Accessed August 10, 2007.

Sroufe L: Attachment and development: a prospective, longitudinal study from birth to adulthood. Attach Hum Dev 7:349–367, 2005

van den Boom DC: The influence of temperament and mothering on attachment and exploration: an experimental manipulation of sensitive responsiveness among lower-class mothers with irritable infants. Child Dev 65:1457–1477, 1994

Vitiello B: Pediatric psychopharmacology and the interaction between drugs and the developing brain. Can J Psychiatry 43:582–584, 1998

Wakschlag LS, Briggs-Gowan MJ, Hill C, et al: Observational assessment of preschool disruptive behavior, part II: validity of the Disruptive Behavior Diagnostic Observation Schedule (DB-DOS). J Am Acad Child Adolesc Psychiatry 47:632–641, 2008

Yehuda R, Engel SM, Brand SR, et al: Transgenerational effects of posttraumatic stress disorder in babies of mothers exposed to the World Trade Center attacks during pregnancy. J Clin Endocrinol Metab 90:4115–4118, 2005

Zeanah CH, Benoit D: Clinical applications of a parent perception interview in infant mental health. Child Adolesc Psychiatr Clin N Am 4:539, 1995

Zeanah CH, Zeanah PD: Infant mental health: the case for early experience, in Handbook of Infant Mental Health, 3rd Edition. Edited by Zeanah CH. New York, Guilford, in press

Zeanah CH, Benoit D, Hirschberg L, et al: Mothers' representations of their infants are concordant with infant attachment classifications. Developmental Issues in Psychiatry and Psychology 1:9–18, 1994

Zeanah CH, Larrieu JA, Valliere J, et al: Infant-parent relationship assessment, in Handbook of Infant Mental Health, 2nd Edition. Edited by Zeanah CH. New York, Guilford, 2000, pp 222–235

Zeanah PD, Stafford B, Nagle GN, et al: Addressing Social-Emotional Development and Infant Mental Health in the State Early Childhood Comprehensive Systems Initiative. Los Angeles, University of California, Los Angeles, 2005

Zero to Three Diagnostic Classification Task Force: Diagnostic Classification of Mental Health and Development Disorders of Infancy and Early Childhood: DC:0–3R. Washington, DC, Zero to Three Press, 2005

Chapter 2

Assessing the Preschool-Age Child

Joan Luby, M.D.
Mini Tandon, D.O.

It is necessary to use specialized techniques to conduct a developmentally valid mental health assessment of the preschool-age child (ages 2–6 years). The standard approaches used for older children and adolescents, while they may seem applicable, will not be sufficient to obtain an age-appropriate and clinically meaningful assessment. Significant developmental differences between a preschool- and school-age child require a tailored approach to obtaining a history and eliciting a mental status exam. The first, and perhaps most fundamental, principle is that the preschool child does not function as a psychologically autonomous individual and remains inextricably tied to the primary caregiver for adaptive and emotional functioning. This idea was succinctly expressed by Winnicott (1965), whose famous phrase, "There is no such thing as a baby," emphasized the importance of the dyad very early in life.

This adage remains applicable during the preschool period, despite the important developmental transitions in the primary relationship. Therefore, because the caregiver-child dyad more accurately represents the psychological status and functioning of the preschooler, the dyad is the most meaningful unit of observation or assessment. This means that, whenever possible, the mental status exam of a preschool child should be conducted with the child and caregiver together rather than with the child individually. While an individual play interview of the preschooler alone may be necessary in some circumstances (e.g., with preschoolers without the benefit of primary caregivers), observation of the child with the caregiver present is generally the most appropriate method.

The second developmentally driven principle is that the mental status exam of the preschooler must be conducted in the context of play. While this may seem an obvious component of any child assessment, it is essential to a valid preschool mental status exam. The facilitation and interpretation of play during the mental status exam will be discussed in more detail later in this chapter. Both the availability of age-appropriate toys to facilitate representational play, if the child is capable, and the examiner's willingness and ability to engage the child in play are essential. Concretely, this means the examiner should not wear a white coat or carry a chart or examination tools. The examiner should be able to adopt a playful posture, which often involves sitting on the floor, following the child's play, and assuming a more imaginative and whimsical demeanor. Clinicians unwilling or unable to engage in elaborate play will not be well suited to work with preschoolers.

Another key principle of preschool assessment is that due to significant state- and relationship-related variation in the mental status of the young child, it is necessary to observe a preschooler on more than one occasion and with more than one caregiver. For this reason, assessments are best done over a series of several sessions on different days and, whenever possible, with different caregivers. In general, this requires an extended evaluation conducted over several days or weeks. While this is more cumbersome to schedule, as well as burdensome for the family, changes in the child's behavior, evident within relationships and over time, are often invaluable in deriving an accurate diagnosis.

Socioeconomic and social pressures facing the clinician make such a comprehensive multisession assessment challenging. Insurance carriers or families are resistant to paying for the number of sessions required to conduct an appropriate assessment. It is inconvenient for families to schedule and attend multiple sessions and successfully involve multiple caregivers in the assessment process. However, it is critical that the clinician take a firm stance about the need for this kind of evaluation in order to obtain a valid diagnosis. More harm than good can come from conducting an assessment that is abbreviated and insufficient. The potential for greater efficacy for early intervention may prove that these techniques are cost-effective from a societal point of view.

Format of a Preschool Assessment

Based on the principles described above, a standard format for a preschool mental health assessment has been established in the Washington University School of Medicine Infant/Preschool Mental Health (WUSM IPMH) clinic. This format has been used successfully for nearly two decades; however, many variations on this format have been used in other clinics and may prove more feasible and equally useful. The WUSM IPMH clinic format (Table 2–1) is an example of one approach that incorporates all of the principles outlined. The preschool assessment is conducted in four 50-minute sessions over 4 consecutive weeks. In the first session, all primary caregivers (both parents, or grandparent and parent, if available) are asked to come in without the child to obtain a comprehensive history. This information is more expediently obtained when the child is not present, and, unlike with the assessment of the adolescent, there is little risk of damaging the rapport with the preschool child when caregivers are interviewed before the child.

The mental health history of the preschool child includes all of the components of a standard mental health history, such as chief complaint and history of present illness, as well as family and medical histories. In addition, detailed social and developmental histories are required. The developmental history includes milestone achievement in the following domains: motor, language, cognitive, sensory, social, and emotional. Details about eating and sleeping patterns are pertinent to the child's adaptation. Information about bedtime routines and rituals—for example, whether the child sleeps alone or with parents, whether the child can self-soothe during awakenings or requires comfort from caregivers—is important. Eating habits, such as limitations in the child's food repertoire, ability to sit down for family mealtimes, and food refusal, may be a chief complaint or related to other behavioral and emotional problems. Information about family eating habits and parental expectations for eating is relevant to this domain.

Details of pregnancy and perinatal history—both medical and psychological—are essential and often relevant to the chief complaint and current mental state. Premature birth or extended hospital stays may influence development, as well as the early relationship between parent and child. Exposure to drugs or alcohol in utero is of obvious relevance. Details of the maternal mental status during the perinatal period may be relevant to the presenting problems as maternal mental illness or psychosocial stressors could impair parent-child relationship development. As has been elaborated so eloquently by Selma Fraiberg (1980) and others, the primary caregivers' internal working models of the child as well as their expecta-

TABLE 2–1. Washington University School of Medicine Infant Preschool Mental Health clinic assessment paradigm

Session 1	Complete emotional, psychological, family, and developmental history of child obtained from caregivers
Session 2	Free-play observation with secondary caregiver
Session 3	Semistructured observation with primary caregiver: shared snack, mildly challenging cognitive task, dyadic play, and then separation and reunion
Session 4	Review of observations/findings, biopsychosocial formulation, differential diagnosis, and treatment plan

tions of the child are often key contributors to the child's symptoms and the family's reaction and coping. Open-ended questions about the parents' own experiences of being parented, as well as their expectations of the child and attributions about the etiology of the child's presenting problems, should be explored. The psychiatric history of the preschooler should also include questions about parental discipline and parenting practices.

Detailed information about the child's play is absolutely essential for the evaluation of a preschooler, including questions about the child's favorite toys, typical spontaneous play themes, and preferred play activities. It is often useful for a parent to describe the child in typical play. The capacity for symbolic or representational versus sensory-motor or mechanical play is important. When symbolic play is present, the complexity may illustrate the child's cognitive capacities. Perhaps more importantly, the thematic content of symbolic play may elucidate the preschooler's internal preoccupations. Information about the child's ability to enjoy play and his or her affective range during play is also important. The preschooler's interest in and capacity for parallel or interactive play with same-age peers, siblings, and others are also key components of the mental health assessment.

When focusing on the presence or absence of specific symptoms of disorders in DSM-IV (American Psychiatric Association 1994) and its text revision, DSM-IV-TR (American Psychiatric Association 2000), it is critical to ask caregivers detailed questions about age-appropriate manifestations of symptom states. The clinician must "translate" DSM-IV symptom criteria to address the life experiences and developmental abilities of the preschool-age child. Several structured psychiatric interviews are now available that have been designed for the research assessment of preschool children. In particular, the Preschool Age Psychiatric Assessment (PAPA; Egger et al. 1999, 2006) is a comprehensive interview with established reliability that includes symptoms from DSM-IV as well as commonly occurring symptoms that arise in young children and are not included in the DSM system. While a clinical version is not yet available, a review of this measure may be useful to the preschool clinician for ideas about how to assess age-appropriate symptom states.

Obtaining collateral information from multiple contexts—for example, from preschool, daycare, home, and another family member's home—is a key feature of the assessment of the young child. The need for approaches that combine reports from multiple informants across contexts has been empirically supported (Kraemer et al. 2003). Environment-specific behaviors may be important in understanding the nature of the presenting complaints. For example, the preschool child who is adjusting to a new preschool may act withdrawn or distressed according to the teacher but appear happy and engaged at home. Some DSM-IV diagnoses, such as attention-deficit/hyperactivity disorder (ADHD), require impairment in at least two settings for diagnosis. For example, if a child becomes hyperactive only at a grandparent's house when multiple peers are present, the problem may not represent clinical psychopathology.

Preparing the Preschooler for the Play Evaluation

Once a comprehensive history has been obtained, play-assessment sessions are the next step. At the completion of the session in which the history was obtained, it is very important to instruct the parents on how to prepare the child for the play session. If the child comes to the session with a basic knowledge of the purpose of the encounter, it is likely to be far more fruitful and productive. To inform the child about the assessment and the reasons for it in a nonjudgmental way, using clear, simple, and understandable language is the most important first step in the assessment as well as the therapeutic process. The clinician should encourage the parents to be as honest as possible with the child about the nature of the concern. This may be the first time that caregivers engage in a direct and candid exchange with the child about the problem. It is, of course, also important to make sure the child understands that the assessment will involve play and not any frightening or painful medical examinations or procedures. To avoid unnecessary anticipatory anxiety, and in keeping with limitations in the young child's sense of time, informing the child about the evaluation on the day prior may be most sensible. Further, it is also useful for parents, as well as the examiner, to disclose to the child that they have already met with the clinician to tell them about the child, the family, and the nature of the problem.

Dyadic Free-Play Assessment and Mental Status Examination, Part I

The child's experience of the first encounter in the clinical setting is important to set the stage for the evaluation, as well as his or her general feelings and attitudes about mental health treatment. For this reason, it is important to conduct a free-play session prior to any structured tasks that may involve minor stressors (detailed below). At the onset of the session, it is important for the clinician to communicate two basic principles. The first is to explain to the child the purpose of the session and to disclose what the therapist knows from meeting with the parent about the nature of the child's problems. The second is that the child may play with the toys however he or she would like. Since this session is conducted in a dyadic format with both the parent and clinician present in the playroom, it is imperative that the parent also be given instructions to play with the child "as they normally would at home." It is often necessary to redirect parents' natural attempts to engage in conversational exchanges with the therapist. This will derail the dyadic interaction, which is the central purpose of this session. Advise parents that there will be another time to ask questions and relay further details of history. In general, since the free-play session is thought to be less demanding than the semistructured play session, it should be con-

ducted when feasible with a secondary caregiver. The semistructured observation that follows is both more stressful and comprehensive and therefore more appropriate for the child and primary caregiver.

The role of the examiner in this dyadic free-play observation is to serve as a "participant-observer" in the play. That is, the examiner should be prepared to respond to any bids from the child to engage in play. The examiner, though, should follow and never lead the child's play. This requires a delicate balance of acting in a spontaneous and playful fashion while also seeking direction and narration from the child to inform his or her role in play. The primary purpose of the dyadic free-play session is to observe the child in play with the caregiver. The examiner should be cautious not to overshadow the parent in play yet be participatory at the same time. The examiner should respond fully if preferentially engaged by the child. It is necessary for the examiner to sit on the floor or at a table with the parent and child and to be fully attentive to the child and refrain from taking notes or charting.

It may be useful to enact a brief separation between parent and child midway through the free-play session. This allows observation of how the parent separates from the child, how the child responds to this separation, and how the parent and child reunite. Further, during the brief period that the parent is out of the room, the examiner has the opportunity to engage the child in individual play. In the event that the preschooler is highly resistant to the separation and/or expresses an intense emotional response, the attempt to separate the dyad can be abandoned (as important aspects of the dyadic relationship will have already been illuminated). The examiner should not give the parent detailed instructions about how to warn the child he or she is leaving but rather should leave it to the parent to do "what you think is best."

Semistructured Dyadic Play Assessment and Mental Status Examination, Part II

In keeping with the need to observe the preschooler on more than one occasion and with more than one caregiver, a second session is recommended with the primary caregiver. A semistructured format, in which the dyad is observed performing specific tasks, provides another useful method of observation for the preschool assessment. Observing the dyad sharing a snack, performing a mildly stressful structured cognitive task under time pressure, during a brief separation and reunion, and during free play are all useful exercises in the clinical setting.

Several standardized semistructured interviews, originally developed for research, are now available and may be useful in the clinical setting. In one such interview, the Parent-Child Early Relational Assessment (PCERA; Clark 1985), the clinician observes, through a one-way mirror, the dyad performing several tasks. The primary caregiver and child share a snack, and then perform a structured task in which block designs are made from sample cards. Next, they engage in free play, and, lastly, a brief separation and reunion is enacted. This interview provides an interesting and varied format in which the quality of parent-child relationship, parenting, and child's behaviors toward the caregiver are observed. The Crowell Procedure (Crowell and Fleischmann 1993) is a similar interview that adds blowing bubbles to specifically elicit affect in the child. Other similar useful dyadic observational assessments include "The Teaching Task" (Egeland et al. 1995), in which tasks of escalating difficulty are performed by the dyad while parent-child interactions are observed and videotaped for later review. Another useful clinical component of the semistructured interview is the review of a videotape of the interaction. The review of the interaction at a later point often leads the clinician to detect important interactions that might be missed during the live observation. The videotape is also a useful teaching tool, with appropriate written consent from the child's legal guardian.

Clinical Threshold: Differentiation From Developmental Norms

One of the challenges of the mental health assessment of preschoolers is making the distinction between developmentally normative behavioral extremes and clinically significant psychopathology. A comprehensive understanding of the rapid changes in social and emotional development that characterize the preschool period is required. For example, the preschooler's normal growing sense of autonomy commonly referred to as the "terrible twos" may mimic clinical oppositional behavior. Defiance or temper tantrums may bring care-

givers to seek clinical attention although these behavioral patterns may be developmentally appropriate. Belden et al. (2008) have shown that the frequency, intensity (e.g., hits others, breaks items), duration (e.g., tantrums last >20 minutes), and functional impairment across contexts (e.g., home, school, day care) are key factors in distinguishing normative from pathological temper tantrums.

Knowledge of developmental milestones, including gross and fine motor development, receptive and expressive language development, as well as social and emotional development, is essential for the assessment of the preschooler. The preschooler's developmental functioning in all of these domains can be ascertained through play observation. For example, simple symbolic or pretend play, where play objects are used in a representational fashion, should be evident at 18 months of age. Thematic symbolic play, such as enacting a tea party, becomes more elaborate as the child progresses through the preschool years (for review, see Siegler et al. 2003). Delays in play skills may signal cognitive and/or social reciprocal deficits characteristic of developmental delays or autistic spectrum disorders. Furthermore, developmental studies have demonstrated that preschoolers are more cognitively and emotionally competent than previously assumed. For example, it is not uncommon for 4-year-olds to personify or attribute human qualities to other organisms (Siegler et al. 2003), as in "my goldfish says he is hungry." Also characteristic of the preschool period and often reviewed in textbooks of development is Piaget's concept of egocentrism evident in the preschooler's inability to understand another's viewpoint (for review, see Shaffer 2002). In the assessment of the preschooler, the clinician must consider the range of individual variations that may be based on environment, context, or temperament. Several texts that elaborate on developmental norms and their variations specific to this age group may be helpful for review (Shaffer 2002; Siegler et al. 2003). Table 2–2 lists frequently used terms in the preschool period.

When significant cognitive delay is detected, organic and metabolic disorders must be ruled out. A neurological exam and an organic work-up, as well as referral to a geneticist and other specialists during both assessment and treatment, may be indicated (see Chapter 9, "Pediatric Evaluation and Laboratory Testing"; Chapter 10, "Neurological Examination, Electroencephalography, and Neuroimaging"; Chapter 11, "Psychological and Neuropsychological Testing"; and Chapter 38, "Genetics: Fundamentals Relevant to Child and Adolescent Psychiatry").

TABLE 2–2.   Frequently used terminology in the preschool period

Term	Description	Example
Symbolic play	Child uses play objects in a representational fashion	Uses banana as a telephone
Parallel play	Play alongside a peer that is not directly reciprocal or interactive	Child stacks blocks while peer is coloring in close proximity and child is aware of activity of peer
Reciprocal play	Interactive play that involves reciprocity	Child uses toy stethoscope to examine mom and then asks mom to listen to his heart
Attachment	The development of a stable internal representation of the availability of caregiver	Children display variations of secure to insecure attachment based on their own temperament and caregiver characteristics
Animism	Attributes living qualities to objects	Treats rock as a pet rock, which needs water
Egocentrism (Piaget)	Difficulty seeing another's visuospatial perspective	Child describes what he himself sees when asked what peer across the table sees
Dual representation (DeLoache)	Ability to think of an object simultaneously in two ways	Use of a map may be difficult as the preschooler cannot conceptualize that a piece of paper represents a location

Source.   Adapted from Shaffer 2002.

Accessing the Preschool Child as Informant in the Assessment

The clinician must use different strategies to access the internal emotional state of the preschooler than the direct interview methods used with older children and adults. Such direct approaches may even be counterproductive, causing the child to become more inhibited. A normally developing preschooler is unlikely to possess the verbal sophistication or insight to answer direct questions about emotional issues. Furthermore, a preschooler may fear reprisal or believe that negative feelings are not acceptable. Shorter attention span and greater suggestibility also limit the usefulness of direct questions. Several age-appropriate specialized assessment techniques, designed primarily for research, have been developed to avert these issues. Some of these techniques may also be fruitful when used in a clinical assessment.

Both direct and indirect methods for the assessment of the child's internal emotional state have been developed. The Berkeley Puppet Interview (BPI; Ablow and Measelle 1993) is a reliable and validated interview for young children that has been widely used in developmental research (Measelle et al. 1998). The BPI uses two puppets that make discrepant emotional statements, one of which the child selects as more representative of his or her own feelings. The BPI has symptom scales as well as scales that address family, social, and emotional functioning. While accessing a young child's self-report, the child is able to displace his or her emotion to the puppet, making the interview less confrontational. Preschoolers' reported depressive and anxiety symptoms on the BPI correlated with both teacher and parent ratings (Luby et al. 2007). Of note, however, and similar to correlations found in older children, preschooler's self-report and caregiver report were more highly correlated for internalizing compared to externalizing symptoms.

A more indirect, but potentially richly informative, semiprojective method that has been used in developmental research is the narrative or story stem. One form of this approach that has been used in clinical populations is the MacArthur Story Stem Battery (Bretherton I, Oppenheim D, Buchsbaum H, et al: "MacArthur Story Stem Battery," unpublished manuscript, Madison, University of Wisconsin, 1990). This instrument contains emotionally evocative story stems that the child completes. In research, scores are generated based on the thematic content and flow of the child's story completion. However, story completions may also be a useful play-assessment method in the clinical setting. Oppenheim et al. (1997) examined children's representations of their caregivers interpreted through narrative completion and found significant correlations between low levels of psychological distress and children's perception of caregivers as "positive" and "disciplinary." Belden et al. (2007) have also shown that narratives distinguish clinically referred from healthy preschoolers in their perceptions and representations of their caregivers.

Mental Status Examination of the Preschool Child

As noted above, observation of the preschool child in play is essential to the mental status exam. In addition to the thematic content of play, a number of other mental status observations can be made. Observation of the preschooler should include general appearance and initial behavior upon greeting the examiner, including cooperativeness, eye contact, social engagement, and social referencing. The assessment of developmental functioning during play is also highly feasible. Speech and all of its components, including articulation, prosody, rate, volume, and the presence of unique presentations such as echolalia, should be noted. Fine and gross motor skills can also be observed as the child moves around the playroom and manipulates the toys.

Flow of play, including perseveration or repetition of phrases or play themes as well as disorganization in play, may inform the differential diagnosis. Observation of the complexity and thematic content of play is essential. The clinician may note the child's preferences, including isolative, repetitive, violent, or aggressive themes in play, as well as how play figures behave toward each other. The child's ability to sustain attention to play is also of interest. The clinician, who serves as a participant-observer, may unobtrusively wonder about the play to help facilitate an understanding of what the child is enacting, by stating questions such as "I wonder why that baby is crying?" However, it is important for the clinician to refrain from leading the play or asking questions that require an answer from the child.

Furthermore, the mental status exam of a preschooler includes observation of the child's interaction with the primary caregiver as well as with the clinician. The child's ability to engage the caregiver and the caregiver's response are both noteworthy. The addition of a structured or mildly stressful task, as outlined above, can help elicit how child and caregiver interact under a variety of specific conditions. Key features of the mental status exam, such as mood and affect, can be gleaned during the series of play observations. As outlined above, several methods to access the child's internal emotional state, in addition to observation of dyadic free play, may be useful in the clinical evaluation.

The Infant and Toddler Mental Status Exam (ITMSE; American Academy of Child and Adolescent Psychiatry 1997) is a useful guide for the clinician, reflecting modifications of the adult mental status exam pertinent to the infant and young child, including attention to the child's sensory and state regulation. While the ITMSE has not undergone empirical testing, it was designed by a highly experienced infant and preschool clinician and may be a useful clinical guide.

Cultural Context of the Preschool Assessment

The comprehensive evaluation of a preschool child involves not only relational and contextual assessment, as emphasized above, but also a consideration for the cultural context of the preschooler and his or her family. Several authors have emphasized the need for a culturally sensitive evaluation (e.g., Garcia Coll and Meyer 1993). Lewis (2000) emphasizes the importance of the clinician's own awareness of personal theories and beliefs about childhood as well as the role of the caregiver. Lewis elaborates that the need for thorough assessment of culture should not be undermined by the strong provocation of emotion that these discussions may foster. In fact, understanding the cultural context may help to inform caregiver responsivity and sensitivity. Along this line, Grossman et al. (1985) reported that the cultural importance of fostering autonomy enhanced maternal sensitivity. The definition of an optimally "sensitive mother" may vary cross-culturally as well as intraculturally (Belsky and Isabella 1988; Nicholls and Kirkland 1996; Scheper-Hughes 1990). This association between maternal sensitivity and culture remains a topic of academic debate (Schaffer and Collis 1986) but nonetheless merits clinician awareness.

Differential Diagnosis in Preschoolers: Review of DSM-IV Preschool Disorders

A wide variety of psychopathological symptoms and categorical DSM-IV Axis I psychiatric disorders may present in the preschool period. These include ADHD, oppositional defiant disorder (ODD), and more rarely, conduct disorder. Affective disorders may also arise in preschool children including major depressive disorder and anxiety disorders, such as separation anxiety disorder, obsessive-compulsive disorder, and generalized anxiety disorder. Specific phobias may also be common, although relatively less impairing and therefore not often clinically significant. Further, there is also some evidence that bipolar disorder may arise as early as age 3; however, this remains an area in which further research is needed to inform the validity of this diagnosis in preschoolers. Sleep disorders and feeding disorders are also relatively common primary or secondary presenting problems.

Over the last decade, there has been an emerging body of empirical data investigating the nosology and validity of several DSM-IV Axis I disorders among preschoolers. In 2003, a task force was convened to review data on the diagnostic criteria for preschool disorders, which reviewed the empirical database, breaking down validity data into the various levels (e.g., face, descriptive, construct, and predictive) (Task Force on Research Diagnostic Criteria 2003). More recently, nine white papers on preschool disorders to inform DSM-V were published (Narrow et al. 2007). To summarize the findings, the diagnosis of ODD has been the most well studied disorder in preschoolers with well-established validity. ADHD and conduct disorder have also been well validated without modification to current DSM-IV criteria. There is also a substantial body of support for the diagnosis of major depressive disorder, although most findings to date are from a single site (Luby et al. 2002, 2003a, 2003b). Posttraumatic stress disorder has also been well studied, and findings suggest that some modification to the current DSM-IV criteria (fewer numbing and avoidance symptoms) is necessary for developmentally appropriate application to preschoolers (Scheeringa et al. 2001, 2003). The nosology and validity of reactive attachment disorder remain less clear, and further study is needed (Zeanah and Boris 2000). However, standard

criteria for DSM-IV reactive attachment disorder can often be applied in the clinical setting, particularly for preschoolers with histories of inadequate caregiving and/or multiple placements early in life. Sleep disorders (see Chapter 29, "Sleep Disorders") and feeding disorders (Chatoor and Ammaniti 2007) have also been investigated in young children but are not well integrated into the current DSM system.

The presence of functional impairment is key to crossing the clinical threshold, as defined by DSM-IV. However, impairment is more difficult to detect in a preschool-age child who does not function autonomously and may not be in structured preschool settings. The assessment of impairment must consider not only the individual functioning of the child but also how his or her symptoms are affecting the functioning of the family system (e.g., the mother cannot maintain a job because her preschool child has been expelled from several day care centers for aggression). Excessive fears that delay acquisition of developmental capacities (e.g., preschool child will not separate from mom and hence cannot start school or learn to sleep alone) should be considered in the assessment of impairment (Carter et al. 2004).

Overall, studies suggest that preschool diagnoses persist into school age and therefore warrant early intervention (Keenan and Wakschlag 2002; Lahey et al. 2004; Lavigne et al. 1998a, 1998b; Speltz et al. 1999). The finding of longitudinal stability is also pertinent to nosology and supports the validity of these early-onset disorders. Lavigne et al. (1998a) have demonstrated 4-year longitudinal stability of both disruptive and internalizing disorders in 2- to 5-year-old children. This study also suggested that the stability of a disruptive disorder increased with increasing age in early childhood. For example, about 50% of 2- to 3-year-olds continued to have disruptive disorders at follow-up compared with 65% of children who were first diagnosed between 4 and 5 years of age (Lavigne et al. 1998a). In fact, ADHD diagnosed in 4- to 6-year-old preschoolers persisted 3 years later into elementary school age (Lahey et al. 2004). Stability of preschool diagnoses was related to a number of factors including low family cohesion, socioeconomic status, and negative life events (Lavigne et al. 1998b).

Psychotic disorders are extremely rare at this early age. The assessment of psychosis in the preschooler is a challenge, given the limited capacity for expressive language, as well as the developmentally normative confusion between fantasy and reality. Preschool studies that review psychosis are essentially limited to case reports (Beresford et al. 2005). Nonetheless, it is essential for the preschool clinician to thoroughly investigate any behaviors suggestive of psychosis, which might include bizarre or disorganized play or descriptions of hallucinatory experiences. Assessment should rule out delirium, exposure to toxins or psychoactive substances, and febrile status. Hallucinations should be distinguished from normative phenomena such as imaginary companions, illusions, and elaborate fantasies common among preschoolers (Sosland and Edelsohn 2005). Accurate family history may help inform the differential diagnosis based on the finding that psychotic and affective disorders (in which psychotic symptoms may arise) are often familial.

Characteristics of Preschool Clinic Samples

Clinicians can anticipate a wide variety of referrals to a preschool mental health clinic, although externalizing disorders predominate (Hooks et al. 1988; Lee 1987; Luby and Morgan 1997). A university preschool clinic chart review of a sample of 116 patients revealed 66% with externalizing disorders or disruptive disorders, including ODD and ADHD; 24% with internalizing disorders, defined as depressive and anxiety disorders; and 11% as somatic disorders, including sleep and eating disorders, along with enuresis and encopresis as assessed by DSM-III-R (American Psychiatric Association 1987; Luby and Morgan 1997). Furthermore, 37% had developmental disorders, and autistic spectrum disorders (autism and pervasive developmental disorder) were found in 13% of the sample. Similarly, both Hooks et al. (1988) and Lee (1987) describe that boys presented more frequently than girls for evaluation and that externalizing symptoms, including aggression and oppositionality, were more common reasons for seeking care. Furthermore, both authors found that language delays were associated with higher rates of externalizing psychopathology. While the disruption of externalizing disorders prompts caregivers to seek care, the impact of internalizing symptoms on the child cannot be underemphasized and may be even more distressing.

Research Directions

Further empirical investigations of the nosology of DSM-IV Axis I disorders for the preschool-age group are needed. To facilitate this, measurement development and validity testing (to supplement reliability data) of age-appropriate measures of psychopathology and related areas of emotional development are also needed. Systematic methods to incorporate observational measures and child self-report into the diagnostic formulation process for preschoolers should be a specific area of focus.

Summary Points

- A comprehensive preschool assessment is ideally completed over several sessions on different days, with more than one caregiver.
- Use of both unstructured and semistructured observation is most informative.
- Observation of dyadic play is essential to the preschool evaluation.
- While disruptive behavior is the most common reason for seeking mental health assessment in the preschool period, it is also necessary to carefully assess for the presence of internalizing symptoms.
- Mental health disorders in preschoolers have been shown to be impairing and many have demonstrated longitudinal stability.

References

Ablow JC, Measelle JR: The Berkeley Puppet Interview. Berkeley, University of California, Berkeley, 1993

American Academy of Child and Adolescent Psychiatry: Practice parameters for the psychiatric assessment of infants and toddlers (0–36 months). J Am Acad Child Adolesc Psychiatry 36(suppl):21S–36S, 1997

American Psychiatric Association: Diagnostic and Statistical Manual of Mental Disorders, 3rd Edition, Revised. Washington, DC, American Psychiatric Association, 1987

American Psychiatric Association: Diagnostic and Statistical Manual of Mental Disorders, 4th Edition. Washington, DC, American Psychiatric Association, 1994

American Psychiatric Association: Diagnostic and Statistical Manual of Mental Disorders, 4th Edition, Text Revision. Washington, DC, American Psychiatric Association, 2000

Belden AC, Sullivan JP, Luby JL: Examining depressed and healthy preschoolers' representations of their caregivers through narratives: associations between preschoolers' internal representations and caregivers' behaviors one year later. Attach Hum Dev 9:1–16, 2007

Belden AC, Thompson NR, Luby JL: Temper tantrums in healthy versus depressed and disruptive preschoolers: defining tantrum behaviors associated with clinical problems. J Pediatr 152:117–122, 2008

Belsky J, Isabella R: Maternal infant and social-contextual determinants of attachment security, in Clinical Implications of Attachment. Edited by Belsky J, Nezworski T. Hillsdale, NJ, Erlbaum, 1988, pp 41–94

Beresford C, Hepburn S, Ross RG: Schizophrenia in preschool children: case reports with longitudinal follow up at 6 and 8 years. Clin Child Psychol Psychiatry 10:429–439, 2005

Carter AS, Briggs-Gowan MJ, Davis NO: Assessment of young children's social-emotional development and psychopathology: recent advances and recommendations for practice. J Child Psychol Psychiatry 45:109–134, 2004

Chatoor I, Ammaniti M: Classifying feeding disorders of infancy and early childhood, in Age and Gender Considerations in Psychiatric Diagnosis: A Research Agenda for DSM-V. Edited by Narrow WE, First MB, Sirovatka PJ. Washington, DC, American Psychiatric Association, 2007, pp 227–242

Clark R: The Parent-Child Early Relational Assessment, Manual and Instrument. Madison, University of Wisconsin Department of Psychiatry, 1985

Crowell J, Fleischmann MA: Use of structured research procedure in clinical assessments of infants, in Handbook of Infant Mental Health, 2nd Edition. Edited by Zeanah CH. New York, Guilford, 1993, pp 210–221

Egeland B, Weinfeld N, Hiester M, et al: Teaching Tasks Administration and Scoring Manual. Minneapolis, University of Minnesota Institute of Child Development, 1995

Egger HL, Ascher BH, Angold A: The Preschool Age Psychiatric Assessment: Version 1.1. Durham, NC, Center for Developmental Epidemiology, Department of Psychiatry and Behavioral Sciences, Duke University Medical Center, 1999

Egger HL, Erkanli A, Keeler GM, et al: Test-retest reliability of the Preschool Age Psychiatric Assessment (PAPA). J Am Acad Child Adolesc Psychiatry 45:538–549, 2006

Fraiberg S (ed): Clinical Studies in Infant Mental Health. New York, Basic Books, 1980

Garcia Coll CT, Meyer EC: The sociocultural context of infant development, in Handbook of Infant Mental Health. Edited by Zeanah CH. New York, Guilford, 1993, pp 56–69

Grossman K, Grossman KE, Spangler G, et al: Maternal sensitivity and newborns' orientation responses as related to quality of attachment in northern Germany, in Growing Points in Attachment Theory and Research. Monographs of the Society for Research in Child Development. Edited by Bretherton I, Waters E. Chicago, IL, University of Chicago Press, 1985, pp 233–256

Hooks MY, Mayes LC, Volkmar FR: Psychiatric disorders among preschool children. J Am Acad Child Adolesc Psychiatry 27:623–627, 1988

Keenan K, Wakschlag LS: Can a valid diagnosis of disruptive behavior disorder be made in preschool children? Am J Psychiatry 159:351–358, 2002

Kraemer HC, Measelle JR, Ablow JC, et al: A new approach to integrating data from multiple informants in psychiatric assessment and research: mixing and matching contexts and perspectives. Am J Psychiatry 160:1566–1577, 2003

Lahey BB, Pelham WE, Loney J, et al: Three-year predictive validity of DSM-IV attention deficit hyperactivity disorder in children diagnosed at 4–6 years of age. Am J Psychiatry 161:2014–2020, 2004

Lavigne JV, Arend R, Rosenbaum D, et al: Psychiatric disorders with onset in the preschool years, I: stability of diagnoses. J Am Acad Child Adolesc Psychiatry 37:1246–1254, 1998a

Lavigne JV, Arend R, Rosenbaum D, et al: Psychiatric disorders with onset in the preschool years, II: correlates and predictors of stable case status. J Am Acad Child Adolesc Psychiatry 37:1255–1261, 1998b

Lee BJ: Multidisciplinary evaluation of preschool children and its demography in a military psychiatric clinic. J Am Acad Child Adolesc Psychiatry 26:313–316, 1987

Lewis ML: The cultural context of infant mental health: the development niche of infant-caregiver relationships, in Handbook of Infant Mental Health, 2nd Edition. Edited by Zeanah CH. New York, Guilford, 2000, pp 91–107

Luby JL, Morgan K: Characteristics of an infant/preschool psychiatric clinic sample: implications for clinical assessment and nosology. Infant Ment Health J 18:209–220, 1997

Luby JL, Heffelfinger A, Mrakotsky C, et al: Preschool major depressive disorder: preliminary validation for developmentally modified DSM-IV criteria. J Am Acad Child Adolesc Psychiatry 41:928–937, 2002

Luby JL, Heffelfinger AK, Mrakotsky C, et al: The clinical picture of depression in preschool children. J Am Acad Child Adolesc Psychiatry 42:340–348, 2003a

Luby JL, Mrakotsky C, Heffelfinger AK, et al: Modification of DSM-IV criteria for depressed preschool children. Am J Psychiatry 160:1169–1172, 2003b

Luby JL, Belden A, Sullivan J, et al: Preschoolers' contribution to their diagnosis of depression and anxiety: uses and limitations of young child self-report of symptoms. Child Psychiatry Hum Dev 38:321–338, 2007

Measelle JR, Ablow JC, Cowan PA, et al: Assessing young children's views of their academic, social, and emotional lives: an evaluation of the self-perception scales of the Berkeley Puppet Interview. Child Dev 69:1556–1576, 1998

Narrow WE, First MB, Sirovatka PJ, et al: Age and Gender Considerations in Psychiatric Diagnosis: A Research Agenda for DSM-V. Washington, DC, American Psychiatric Association, 2007

Nicholls A, Kirkland J: Maternal sensitivity: a review of attachment literature definitions. Early Child Dev Care 120:55–65, 1996

Oppenheim D, Emde RN, Warren S: Children's narrative representations of mothers: their development and associations with child and mother adaptation. Child Dev 68:127–138, 1997

Schaffer HR, Collis GM: Parental responsiveness and child behavior, in Parental Behavior. Edited by Sluckin W, Herbert M. New York, Basil Blackwell, 1986, pp 283–315

Scheeringa MS, Peebles CD, Cook CA, et al: Toward establishing procedural, criterion, and discriminant validity for PTSD in early childhood. J Am Acad Child Adolesc Psychiatry 40:52–60, 2001

Scheeringa MS, Zeanah CH, Myers L, et al: New findings on alternative criteria for PTSD in preschool children. J Am Acad Child Adolesc Psychiatry 42:561–570, 2003

Scheper-Hughes N: Mother love and child death in northeast Brazil, in Cultural Psychology: Essays on Comparative Human Development. Edited by Stigler JW, Shweder RA, Herdt G. New York, Cambridge University Press, 1990, pp 542–568

Shaffer DR: Developmental Psychology, Childhood and Adolescence, 6th Edition. Belmont, CA, Wadsworth/Thompson Learning, 2002

Siegler R, DeLoache J, Eisenberg N: How Children Develop. New York, Worth Publishers, 2003

Sosland MD, Edelsohn GA: Hallucinations in children and adolescents. Curr Psychiatry Rep 7:180–188, 2005

Speltz ML, McClellan J, DeKlyen M, et al: Preschool boys with oppositional defiant disorder: clinical presentation and diagnostic change. J Am Acad Child Adolesc Psychiatry 38:838–845, 1999

Task Force on Research Diagnostic Criteria: Infancy and preschool: research diagnostic criteria for infants and preschool children: the process and empirical support. J Am Acad Child and Adolesc Psychiatry 42:1504–1512, 2003

Winnicott DW: The Maturational Process and the Facilitating Environment: Studies in the Theory of Emotional Development. New York, International Universities Press, 1965

Zeanah CH, Boris NW: Disturbances and disorders of attachment in early childhood, in Handbook of Infant Mental Health, 2nd Edition. Edited by Zeanah CH. New York, Guilford, 2000, pp 353–368

Chapter 3

Assessing the Elementary School–Age Child

Myra M. Kamran, M.D.
Colleen Cicchetti, Ph.D.

In the typical mental health setting, most presenting patients fall in the age range of "middle childhood," ages 6–12 years (Farmer et al. 2003). Clinicians evaluating these patients and their families should be familiar with expected childhood developmental progression and the more common developmental "deviations" or difficulties and psychopathology in middle childhood.

The key developmental milestones for this age group are focused upon the tasks of identity formation that are related to autonomy, peer identity, and social identity (Gemelli 1996). With cognitive development, children are more able to evaluate their own behaviors, modulate their emotional reactions, internalize social expectations, and anticipate reactions from others. The critical shift in energy toward autonomous social functioning provides much of the backdrop for clinical evaluation in this age group. Temperamental extremes (including shyness or a high activity level) that could be accommodated at home or in preschool can cause concern at the point of school entry. Additionally, students who fail to master social skills, emotional regulation, and behavioral skills struggle in a structured peer setting.

The purpose of the child psychiatric evaluation is to assess for the presence of psychopathology and to determine whether that psychopathology is causing dysfunction. This may affect the child alone (rarely), the family system, and/or the child's environment. Confirmation of child psychopathology and resultant distress and/or dysfunction at any of these levels are then followed by treatment planning. In this chapter we consider the evaluation process and the evaluation content.

The Evaluation Process

As noted in the opening to this chapter, the primary function of a psychiatric evaluation is determining whether the child exhibits the symptom pattern, severity, and impairment required to make a diagnosis. The evaluation content to be explored is discussed later in this chapter (in the section "The Evaluation Content").

It is essential to approach the psychiatric evaluation of such a child by including his or her parents and other adult caregivers. Eliciting history from adults familiar with the child in the school setting is usually appropriate and helpful. Assessing the child's functioning in the family as well as socially with peers and other adults is important and helps the evaluator to understand the child's development, as well as his or her psychiatric symptoms. During psychiatric assessment, the clinician also must consider the role of cultural and environmental issues related to a child's and family's functioning.

Key to the evaluation process is the establishment of a collaborative relationship between the clinician and the child and his or her family. This will increase the likelihood of gaining an accurate picture of the current difficulties and will also aid in establishing trust and in fostering an understanding of the evaluation process that will set the stage for accepting the case formulation and treatment recommendations. The establishment of a strong partnership with effective communication during the evaluation process will provide the foundation for all subsequent clinical work. Even if the ultimate decision is to refer a case to other professionals for further assessment or treatment, each new interaction with a mental health clinician affects the child and family's willingness to engage with professionals. It is critical that clinicians be aware of barriers to mental health services and work diligently to ensure that initial contact with children and their families helps to overcome any stigma and is conducted in a developmentally appropriate and culturally respectful manner.

Setting the Stage

The first step is to establish clear guidelines regarding the nature of the clinician's role, the procedures that will be followed, and the expectations of the family. Some of these expectations and procedures may be addressed by intake or administrative staff at the point of first contact. Nevertheless, it is important that the clinician discuss these issues during his or her first con-

tact with the family. This insures that the family understands the procedures and the clinician's rationale for these procedures and has an opportunity to discuss questions or concerns. In addition, these discussions begin to establish a working alliance and contract between the family and the clinician that respects the nature of the relationship and makes subsequent conversations regarding these matters more comfortable and appropriate.

The procedural information outlined in Table 3–1 helps to avoid surprises in the evaluation process. The clinician begins by informing and educating the parents about the process. While some families have experience with mental health services, many do not. The subtle differences between our standards of practice and those of general health practitioners, schools, and other social service agencies can be confusing and appear difficult to families. For example, when taking the child to a pediatrician, parents usually only provide some basic history and medical information. Laboratory tests and physical examinations provide the majority of the information necessary for diagnosis and treatment. Even medical treatments that include parental involvement and monitoring do not typically require the parents to share intimate details of their own personal life, nor to have their own behaviors and communication patterns discussed, evaluated, and potentially modified. Therefore, the mental health clinician must guide the parents toward establishing a more active collaborative and educational process, in which each party has particular goals, roles, and expertise and shares a mutual goal of fostering a child's healthy development.

Developmental Considerations for the Interview Process

Role of Parent and Child as Informants

In middle childhood, the specific roles of the parent and child in the process may vary with different clinical situations. It is therefore helpful to discuss the clinician's interview plan with the presenting family members and to ask for input from the parents. It is appropriate to ask them whether they would prefer to begin the substantive discussions in the presence of their child or separately. It is also helpful to ask the parents for input about what will make their child feel more comfortable: sitting in the room; remaining in the waiting room; or sitting nearby, outside of the office.

In the first session, it is critical to underscore to the parent that they are the experts on their child and that

TABLE 3–1. Key procedural information to cover in the first evaluation session

1.	Office/department procedures	*Cover* registration, payment, missed appointment policies, cancellations, appointment reminder calls, completion of research or clinical monitoring forms at subsequent appointments, and waiting room guidelines.
2.	Communication with clinician	*Cover* appropriate phone numbers, confidential voice mail, e-mail policies, clinician work schedule, and time frame for returning phone calls.
3.	Plan/process of the evaluation	*Plan* how interviews will be conducted (parent alone, child alone, combined sessions, involvement of other family members); the collection of information from other interested parties (school, primary care pediatrician, involved social service agencies, previous mental health providers); the anticipated time frame for completing the evaluation (number/frequency of sessions, time scheduled for appointments); and how feedback will be provided (discussion and/or written reports) to both family and referring parties.
4.	Confidentiality	*Review* the concepts and procedures related to confidentiality within the family, as well as with other interested and involved parties. Complete consents and explain nature of collecting information versus sharing diagnostic information and treatment recommendations.
5.	Safety plans	*Review* any safety concerns and agency or departmental procedures related to handling crisis situations and communication.
6.	Opportunity for questions about the process	*Allow* opportunities to offer other important information and for questions and concerns.

you welcome the opportunity to learn from them as much as possible. It can be helpful to frame your role as using your training and experience to understand their child's difficulties and then making recommendations to the family about how to foster healthy development and success with family, peers, school, and recreation.

Framing the Evaluation: Importance of Multiple Social Contexts

It is important to frame the evaluation process so that parents can understand the rationale for including multiple informants and gathering detailed family and social histories. Children in this age range would not typically seek mental health services on their own and are frequently referred for psychiatric assessment by outside agencies such as the school, social services, and courts. Pediatricians and other primary medical caregivers also refer children for psychiatric assessment and treatment. Unlike preschoolers and adolescents, who are typically referred by parents due to the stress that the child's behavior is causing at home, school-age children are frequently referred due to concerns raised by teachers. Parents may have little understanding of these difficulties. It is helpful to inquire directly about the reason that the family is seeking

help at this time and to determine who is most concerned about the child's behavior or emotions.

Understanding the motivation for seeking treatment and the perspective of all concerned parties is particularly important in the context of obtaining consents to gather information from other sources. For example, parents who feel that a teacher is blaming their child for more general peer-related problems in the school may be reluctant to give consent for communication with the school by the clinician. It is helpful to emphasize how information will be used. Most parents are willing to provide consent for release of information from the school if they are reassured that the initial contact will be purely to inform the school that parents are seeking an evaluation and to ask for behavioral and academic observations from the teacher and other professionals working with the child. Reassuring the parents that no feedback regarding diagnostic formulation or treatment recommendations will be shared with the school until after these findings are discussed with and agreed upon by parents is often sufficient. If parents continue to be reluctant to allow communication with the school, it may be best to inform the parent that this information will be critical in performing a comprehensive diagnostic assessment. In the meanwhile, continue with the initial child and parent interviews while gaining trust from the family through your professional conduct and use discretion before discussing consents further. This approach may also apply to social service agencies that have been involved with the family, including child welfare agencies. In these cases, an adversarial relationship may have developed that has impaired the parent's trust of professionals and/or sense of competence as a parent. Reestablishing trust and developing a collaborative relationship may be necessary before addressing consent issues.

Cultural Issues

Cultural issues influence the way in which families address a range of issues including privacy, family roles and boundaries, and trust of health care and mental health professionals. It is important for clinicians to acknowledge cultural differences and to defer to parents as the leaders in guiding understanding of their family values. As noted earlier, the information that is requested in a psychiatric evaluation includes information that many families consider private. They may be reluctant to share it between family members or with professionals. It is useful to acknowledge from the beginning that we will be asking for a lot of information about the child and family and to encourage the parents and child to inform us if they would like to discuss certain things separately. At times, modeling parent-child boundaries and exploring some topics with parents out of the presence of their child may be appropriate, particularly when discussing issues related to marital discord, domestic violence, divorce, or parental history of substance abuse, maltreatment, or psychiatric symptoms. When a parent openly discusses this type of information in front of the child, it provides information about family boundaries and communication patterns. It can be a useful intervention to introduce boundaries that may be protective for the child, for example: "These seem to be issues that are difficult for you to discuss without becoming upset. It may be helpful for us to talk about these while your child waits outside." Once the child leaves, the clinician can more appropriately support the parent and comment on how the child may be affected by hearing such discussions.

Family roles and boundaries are complex. It is useful to ask directly about who lives in the home as well as who are the other adults that are most involved in the child's care and daily life. This type of question may present opportunities to consider additional sources of information for the diagnostic process as well as elucidating important sources of conflict or support for the child and family. For example, an ex-

tended family member living in the home can be helpful for both child supervision and financial support. On the other hand, this can be stressful if parents feel evaluated and undermined as they balance multiple roles or if substance abuse or conflict is present. It can be very helpful to ask the child about his or her relationship with all of the adults and children living in the house.

Finally, it is useful to ask parents and children about their past experiences with professionals. You may ask them to share information about what works best for them to create a collaborative and trusting relationship. In discussing procedural issues, you may ask whether they have concerns about these expectations. It may be helpful to offer, "I have told you some of the things that I need from you to do my job. Maybe you can share with me your thoughts on what I can do to make you feel more comfortable with me or this process?" This may open up a discussion of the last therapist they saw and how he or she made them feel judged and evaluated. This type of question can create an understanding that you want them to play an active role in making this process a success, thereby avoiding premature termination due to miscommunication.

The Evaluation Content

The components of the evaluation of the school-age child and of the child mental status examination are summarized at the end of this chapter (see Appendix 3–1 and Appendix 3–2, respectively). A thorough evaluation process requires more than a single interview. The separate or combined interviews of the child, the parents and/or adult caregivers, obtaining collateral information, and providing a formulation and treatment plan at completion of the evaluation may require at least two to three visits (American Academy of Child and Adolescent Psychiatry 1995).

The following areas related to the *content* of the psychiatric evaluation of the school-age child warrant further commentary.

Mental Health Issues of the Elementary School–Age Child

Although a child in this age range may present with a multitude of psychiatric symptoms and diagnoses, the more common psychiatric illnesses are attention-deficit/hyperactivity disorder (ADHD), autism and the spectrum of pervasive developmental disorders, separation anxiety disorder, specific phobia, and oppositional defiant disorder (Lavigne et al. 1998; Rutter et al. 2003). There are some age-related concessions made by DSM-IV (American Psychiatric Association 1994) and its text revision, DSM-IV-TR (American Psychiatric Association 2000), allowing different presentations of certain psychiatric illnesses in children: an example of this is major depressive disorder (MDD) or dysthymia, where irritability can substitute for depressed mood. It is always important to evaluate for comorbid psychiatric conditions (Angold et al. 1999).

Reliability and Validity of Parent and Child Interviews

Studies have shown that obtaining factual information from a child is an important part of the clinical assessment (Herjanic and Reich 1982; see also Chapter 7, "Diagnostic Interviews"). It is now standard practice to obtain information from multiple informants regarding a child's functioning and symptoms and to realize that the information from these informants may not agree (see Chapter 7). Low correlation does not necessarily refute the validity of any of the reports; rather the reports are combined to best understand the child's symptoms and the impact of those symptoms on the child's functioning (Graham and Rutter 1968; Rutter and Graham 1968). For certain diagnoses, namely disruptive behavior disorders and the internalizing disorders, reports from the parent or the child (respectively) are more reliable. In assessing for ADHD, child symptom reports are not generally helpful (Loeber et al. 1991). In assessing for anxiety and depressive symptoms, the child's self-report is essential and may be more valid than that of the parent or teacher (Stanger and Lewis 1993).

Use of Rating Scales and Semistructured Interviews

The thorough assessment of the child and his or her family may be facilitated by the use of standardized tools such as symptom checklists, rating scales, and semistructured interviews (see Chapter 7, "Diagnostic Interviews," and Chapter 8, "Rating Scales"). Self- and parent-report instruments can be given to the child and/or adult caregivers to the evaluation and reviewed at the interview, or they may be given to the child and parent(s) during the evaluation process for

later review. These instruments can be broadly based and cover symptoms from multiple diagnostic categories, such as the Child Behavior Checklist (CBCL; Achenbach and Rescorla 2001), or they can be more specifically related to internalizing or externalizing symptoms. The Child Symptom Inventory–4 (CSI-4; Gadow and Sprafkin 1997) is a widely used questionnaire, formulated for children ages 5–12 years, that screens for 15 DSM-IV-based diagnoses. Structured interviews, though created for research purposes, have been increasingly adopted into usual clinical practice, reflecting the importance of assessing child psychopathology in a standardized way (see Chapter 7). Examples of these include the NIMH Diagnostic Interview Schedule for Children, Version IV (NIMH DISC-IV; Shaffer et al. 2000) and the Child and Adolescent Psychiatric Assessment (CAPA; Angold and Costello 2000). Clinicians also may create their own questionnaire forms to elicit factual information to expedite the interview process. Information gathered may include detailed previous psychiatric treatment history, past medical history, family constellation, and developmental milestones.

Obtaining Collateral Information

A school-age child is evaluated by considering his or her role and functioning in the family, in the school setting, and in peer interactions. Children in this age range function in multiple settings and interact with a range of adults and professionals including teachers, specialists, and recreational program leaders. Pediatricians and other primary medical caregivers also refer children for psychiatric assessment and treatment. Frequently children are receiving mental health services in other settings, especially in school settings (Briggs-Gowan et al. 2000). Consequentially, those referral sources are ones of valuable collateral information, and the thorough clinician will seek information from them. The process of obtaining proper legal releases allowing the clinician to contact and communicate with those sources must guide the effort to seek collateral information.

Obtaining Further Medical Evaluation

The clinician may seek additional medical evaluation for a child presenting with certain symptoms (see

Chapter 9, "Pediatric Evaluation and Laboratory Testing," and Chapter 10, "Neurological Examination, Electroencephalography, and Neuroimaging"). The process of obtaining additional medical evaluation, such as ordering lab tests or an electroencephalogram, should be considered carefully in a child of this age, since procedures can be distressing; however, this consideration alone should never preclude obtaining necessary medical evaluation. Further medical evaluation can be pursued directly by the clinician or through consultation with the patient's primary care provider or a specialist, such as a pediatric neurologist or geneticist (Zametkin et al. 1998). Recommendations should be discussed in detail with the child's parent(s), as well as with the child at an appropriate developmental level. Requesting recent medical evaluation results from a child's primary care provider is standard and can be helpful in understanding a child's health status and any recent changes.

Assessing Special Issues Common to the School-Age Child

School-age children may present with disorders or problems that do not parallel those of adult psychiatric disorders. Their presenting problems may represent failure of expected developmental progression and adaptation (Achenbach 1980). This section considers problems that commonly cause a child and/or his or her caregivers enough distress to seek clinical attention.

Behavioral Problems

The behavioral issues specific to school-age children reflect the developmental issues related to school entry and managing increased demands for social interactions and academic performance.

School Refusal/Social Anxiety

A common presenting problem in kindergarten and first grade is related to successfully negotiating the transition into the school environment. While a majority of children participate in some type of preschool experience, many of these experiences are brief, sporadic, and allow for parental presence and involvement. In addition, temperamental variables related to shyness and difficulty with separation are often ac-

commodated in a preschool setting. It is important when the transition to a formal school setting is a challenge to begin with an assessment of who is concerned about the child's behavior and to get a detailed history of involvement with nonfamilial structured settings. For some families, this transition presents a developmental challenge for both the child and the adult caregivers. Efforts to help the parent-child system to address separation anxiety and to begin a structured, gradual separation process should begin even during the evaluation process. This will address the problem promptly and test the family's ability to change. Collecting information about whether there is any adult history of social anxiety may also prove useful as there is growing evidence that a familial pattern is common and may be the result of both genetics and learned behaviors (Black and Uhde 1992; Kendler et al. 1992). It is also important to include a basic cognitive and language screen during the child interview. Language and cognitive delays can contribute to symptoms of anxiety, separation difficulty, and selective mutism that the child can present at this time. A referral for speech and language evaluation is often useful.

Academic Difficulties

Poor academic performance or lack of academic motivation may also manifest during this period. In most cases, a referral for psychiatric evaluation will occur only if these issues are present with comorbid concerns. The role of the clinician is to assess whether the academic concerns are primary or secondary. In many cases, externalizing behavior problems such as aggression, hyperactivity/impulsivity, and inattention can result from or mask underlying learning disabilities. The clinician advocates for assessment of general cognitive and academic abilities and educates both the family and school personnel about the importance of completing a comprehensive assessment (see Chapter 11, "Psychological and Neuropsychological Testing"). Many students who are labeled as a "behavior problem" have not received adequate evaluation. Therefore, advocacy related to obtaining a school-based evaluation or seeking a comprehensive psychoeducational assessment privately can be a critical component of the evaluation process and aid in establishing a collaborative relationship with the parent.

Peer Difficulties

Increasingly complex social demands are challenging for children experiencing behavioral and emotional difficulties. Frequent presenting complaints are related to either aggression and bullying toward peers and/or being the recipient of peer victimization and teasing, with subsequent social withdrawal or aggression. In these cases, the importance of collecting information from as many sources as possible is particularly critical. Children with aggressive behavior often exhibit a pattern of cognitive distortions, hostile bias, and inadequate repertoire of social problem-solving skills (Dodge 1986; Lochman 1992). These deficits make them extremely poor reporters regarding their peer difficulties. Further, parents receive most of their information about the peer difficulties either from their child's limited perspective or when contacted by school and recreational agencies after a specific incident. In response, the parents often adopt a defensive posture. By the time of evaluation, parents and school personnel often have become adversaries. The clinician must adopt a neutral stance related to these issues and continue to underscore the importance of working together to get the information necessary and to facilitate success for the child. Collecting information from school personnel in the form of rating scales and behavioral checklists is critical. Follow-up phone calls are also extremely helpful in assessing the schoolteacher's perspective on the child, the teacher's experience of working with the parents, and the teacher's flexibility and commitment to addressing the concerns. In optimal circumstances, attending a school meeting to help advocate for the child and family and to help both parents and school personnel to share concerns and develop a plan, by sharing your diagnostic formulation and school-based assessment or treatment recommendations, can be extremely helpful. This further establishes your relationship as a collaborator with and advocate for the child and family and models effective communication and teamwork.

Sexualized Behavior

A less common presenting problem in this age period is related to sexualized behavior between peers or siblings. In these situations, typically a parent or other adult has learned about these behaviors either by interrupting them or via a disclosure from an involved child. The request for evaluation is often surrounded by considerable anxiety and emotional response from the parent. In addition, if the behavior has occurred in a school or community setting, there may be other adults involved who are adding to the emotionality.

It is important that the clinician adopt a calm and professional response to these situations that provides a clear plan for how to proceed while also ensuring the safety and emotional well-being of all involved. De-

pending on the nature of the activity, the ages of the children involved, and the level of fear or intimidation surrounding these behaviors, the assessment and intervention may be very different. Any situation involving sexualized play requires an evaluation to explore the details of what occurred and the child's experience of the situation. It is important to also provide education to parents early in the process that this type of behavior is not uncommon and does not necessarily result in trauma, long-term effects on psychological functioning, or sexual identity issues (Goldman and Goldman 1988). Concerns about future sexuality can be particularly salient for parents when the sexualized behavior was between same-sex peers or siblings. It can be helpful to assure parents that sexual exploration between same-sex peers and siblings is common—and that in the absence of a power imbalance among those participating in the exploration, evidence of long-term influence of such activity on sexual preferences is rare.

Exploring the details with the child alone is critical. It is important to assess the child's experience of the interactions in order to determine the level of intimidation or fear involved and to process feelings related to both the behavior and the response that the disclosure (either accidental or voluntary) has evoked in others (Brown et al. 2006; Collins et al. 2004). (For more details, see American Academy of Child and Adolescent Psychiatry [1997b]; see also Chapter 22, "Posttraumatic Stress Disorder," and Chapter 31, "Child Abuse and Neglect").

Family and Community Issues Affecting Evaluations of the School-Age Child

Divorce

Many children presenting for evaluation will have experienced parental marital conflict, separation, and/or divorce. In separation or divorce cases, it is particularly critical that at the initial appointment the clinician discuss and establish plans and goals for completing the evaluation. Whether one or both parents accompany the child, it is critical to inquire about custody arrangements, including which parent has primary custody and health insurance responsibility and what are the guardianship visitation and custody-sharing arrangements. Requesting a copy of the custody agreement is advised. These discussions are critical for both establishing the fundamental collaborative relationship and clarifying the role of the clinician. It is important to address issues related to access to medical records, court involvement, and limitations related to roles. Custody evaluations are a highly specialized and contentious type of evaluation (see Chapter 43, "Legal and Ethical Issues"). Specialized training and procedures are standard practice for these evaluations (American Academy of Child and Adolescent Psychiatry 1997a). Clinicians need to be clear with parents about the limits upon our role if custody issues are involved and we are not providing a formal custody evaluation. Referrals to court mediators and custody evaluators are appropriate for these requests. However, even if the role of the clinician is not to conduct a custody evaluation, if custody disputes are ongoing, clinical records may be subpoenaed by the court. Although one parent may claim that the noncustodial parent has very little interest in or involvement with the child you are evaluating, it is good practice to attempt to include both parents in your information-gathering process. A direct request from a clinician regarding observations and concerns about the child may result in a very different response than was predicted by the other parent. In most cases, both parents do have some role with the child. Including both parents in the diagnostic process therefore underscores for the child and parents that both relationships are important and impact the child. In addition, it sets the stage for future therapeutic interventions that may necessitate coparenting despite the end of the marital relationship.

Trauma and Loss

The impact of trauma and loss for children presenting for evaluation also necessitates additional attention. In some cases, a specific traumatic event or loss will precipitate the request for evaluation. In these cases, it is critical to include assessment of the child and family functioning both before and after the event (see Chapter 33, "Bereavement and Traumatic Grief," for specific assessment and intervention strategies). In other cases, the child is brought for evaluation for behavioral or emotional issues and either a specific traumatic event or a chronically stressful environment is discovered. It is important that the clinician explore these issues in a context that avoids appearing judgmental to the family. It can be useful to introduce this line of questioning with comments like the following: "Many different types of situations can affect kids. Adults have ways of coping with stress or letting others know how they feel that kids may not have. Can you think of any situations or experiences that your child has experienced that may have been stressful or scary?" If this does not elicit a response, than it is useful to ask specifically about

losses including family members (immediate and extended), community members, or peers. It is also useful to explore episodes that may have occurred in their community that their child either witnessed or has experienced vicariously from other community members' responses. Adults often believe that unless a child was present for an event, it does not affect him or her. It can be useful to frame for the parent that children respond to both reports of particular events and the emotional response of the adults and peers around them.

Exposure to Violence and Sexual Images From the Media

The meaning of community for children is one that is changing partly due to the impact of electronic media. In many households, children are exposed to news channels, talk shows, and reality television that they may have little capacity to understand. Children watch television an average of 3 hours per day, some up to 16 hours in a row (Christakis and Zimmerman 2006). Adults often underestimate how much attention children are paying to shows that adults are watching in their presence. As such, they do not attempt to filter the programming or to discuss the details of the reports with their children. Children at this age are therefore exposed to both local and global news events with little understanding of where, when, or why things have happened. Stories of prison escapees or drive-by shootings in other states can evoke fear and trauma in children without parents recognizing the precipitant. For older children and adolescents, popular video games, music lyrics, and even prime-time television have graphic, violent, and sexual images that impact perception of normative behavior. It is therefore important to inquire about the amount of time and the types of shows, games, and Web sites that children and adolescents are exposed to both actively and passively. Providing education to parents that encourages more careful monitoring and supervision of media exposure may be a critical avenue for avoiding the risks associated with early initiation of sexual behavior and cybervictimization that are increasingly present (Hinduja and Patchin 2007).

Medical/Physical Issues in the School-Age Child

Enuresis

Enuresis is frequently encountered in child psychiatric evaluations. It is a complaint that warrants eliciting details including frequency of the episodes, duration, circumstances, and attempts to ameliorate. Referral for medical evaluation of enuresis may be warranted. (See Chapter 28, "Elimination Disorders.")

Medical Illness

Between 10% and 20% of children have some type of chronic medical illness, disability, or other type of health impairment. When helping a child and family to deal with either an acutely or chronically impairing medical illness, insure that you assess both the child's and the family's understanding of and emotions about the illness. (See Chapter 41, "Psychiatric Aspects of Chronic Physical Disorders.")

Sleep Problems

Sleep problems may include difficulties with bedtime, sleepwalking, sleeptalking, nightmares, night terrors, narcolepsy, and sleep apnea. Sleep problems may be part of a psychiatric illness, such as depression, anxiety, or bipolar disorder. Oppositional behavior may interfere with bedtime routines. Children with separation anxiety may have difficulty sleeping alone in their room. Some children have difficulty falling asleep simply because their bedtime is too early or late. Inquire about medication, such as stimulants, that might affect the child's sleep, as well as the child's caffeine intake. (See Chapter 29, "Sleep Disorders.")

Obesity

Over 30% of children in the United States are overweight (more than 20% above the ideal weight for height and age). Investigate the child's eating habits as well as the family's eating habits and the child's level of physical activity, and consider any medical and psychiatric issues possibly contributing to the obesity. (See Chapter 25, "Obesity.")

Research Directions

The process of psychiatrically evaluating and formulating diagnoses for a school-age child will likely be affected by the following trends. As stated earlier in this chapter, semistructured diagnostic interviews may be used more frequently in clinical settings as the understanding of the importance of standardized assessments of children increases (see Chapter 7, "Diagnostic Interviews"). Diagnostic understanding in our field is changing, and DSM-V may include laboratory findings among diagnostic criteria for some disorders (First and Zimmerman 2006). DSM-V will also address the phenomenon of extensive diagnostic co-occurrence, such as with anxiety and depressive disorders, including those in children and adolescents (Cole et al. 1997, 1998; Widiger and Clark 2000). In the future, settings in which children receive psychiatric evaluation and services will likely expand to allow more extensive provision of mental health care in school and pediatric primary care settings (American Academy of Child and Adolescent Psychiatry 2005; American Academy of Pediatrics 2004; Farmer et al. 2003; Rappaport 2001).

Summary Points

- An important goal of the evaluation process is to establish an alliance with the patient and family.

- Plan which topics will and will not be discussed in the child's presence.

- The key emotional developmental tasks for the school-age child are related to autonomy, peer identity, and social identity.

- The transition into the social/school domain has considerable impact upon the functioning of all school-age children. It is critical to consider the areas of school, community, peers, and culture in these evaluations and to use multiple informants from these settings to assess the child's functioning.

- Gathering clinical information from multiple informants and settings is also critical since there are some disorders in which research has shown that the symptom reports from either the child or parent are more reliable than that of the other party.

References

Achenbach TM: DSM-III in light of empirical research on the classification of child psychopathology. J Am Acad Child Psychiatry 19:395–412, 1980

Achenbach TM, Rescorla LA: Manual for the ASEBA School-Age Forms and Profiles. Burlington, VT, Research Center for Children, Youth, and Families, 2001. Available at: http://www.aseba.org. Accessed February 4, 2009.

American Academy of Child and Adolescent Psychiatry: Practice parameters for the psychiatric assessment of children and adolescents. J Am Acad Child Adolesc Psychiatry 31:1386–1402, 1995

American Academy of Child and Adolescent Psychiatry: Practice parameters for child custody evaluation. J Am Acad Child Adolesc Psychiatry 36(suppl):57S–68S, 1997a

American Academy of Child and Adolescent Psychiatry: Practice parameters for the forensic evaluation of children/adolescents who may have been sexually abused. J Am Acad Child Adolesc Psychiatry 36(suppl):37S–56S, 1997b

American Academy of Child and Adolescent Psychiatry: Practice parameter for psychiatric consultation to schools. J Am Acad Child Adolesc Psychiatry 44:1068–1084, 2005

American Academy of Pediatrics: Policy statement, school-based mental health services. Pediatrics 113:1839–1845, 2004

American Psychiatric Association: Diagnostic and Statistical Manual of Mental Disorders, 4th Edition. Washington, DC, American Psychiatric Association, 1994

American Psychiatric Association: Diagnostic and Statistical Manual of Mental Disorders, 4th Edition, Text Revision. Washington, DC, American Psychiatric Association, 2000

Angold A, Costello E: The Child and Adolescent Psychiatric Assessment (CAPA). J Am Acad Child Adolesc Psychiatry 39:39–48, 2000

Angold A, Costello EJ, Erkanli A: Comorbidity. J Child Psychol Psychiatry 40:57–87, 1999

Black B, Uhde TW: Elective mutism as a variant of social phobia. J Am Acad Child Adolesc Psychiatry 31:1090–1094, 1992

Briggs-Gowan MH, Horwitz SM, Schwab-Stone ME, et al: Mental health in pediatric settings: distribution of disorders and factors related to service use. J Am Acad Child Adolesc Psychiatry 39:841–849, 2000

Brown JD, Engle KL, Pardun CJ, et al: Sexy media matter: exposure to sexual content in music, movies, television and magazines predict black and white adolescents' sexual behavior. Pediatrics 117:1018–1027, 2006

Christakis DA, Zimmerman FJ: The Elephant in the Living Room: Making Television Work for Your Kids. New York, Rodale, 2006

Cole DA, Truglio R, Peeke L: Relation between symptoms of anxiety and depression in children: a multitrait-multi-method-multigroup assessment. J Consult Clin Psychol 65:110–119, 1997

Cole DA, Peeke L, Lachlan G, et al: A longitudinal look at the relation between depression and anxiety in children and adolescents. J Consult Clin Psychol 66:451–460, 1998

Collins RL, Elliot MN, Berry SH, et al: Watching sex on television predicts initiation of sexual behavior. Pediatrics 114:280–289, 2004

Dodge KA: A social information processing model of social competence in children, in Cognitive Perspectives on Children's Social and Behavioral Development. Minnesota Symposium on Child Psychology, Vol 18. Edited by Perlmutter M. Hillsdale, NJ, Lawrence Erlbaum, 1986, pp 77–125

Farmer EMZ, Burns BJ, Phillips SD, et al: Pathways into and through mental health services for children and adolescents. Psychiatr Serv 54:60–66, 2003

First MB, Zimmerman M: Including laboratory tests in DSM-V diagnostic criteria. Am J Psychiatry 163:2041–2042, 2006

Gadow KD, Sprafkin J: Child Symptom Inventory–4 Norms Manual. Stony Brook, NY, Checkmate Plus, 1997

Gemelli R: Normal Child and Adolescent Development. Washington, DC, American Psychiatric Press, 1996

Goldman R, Goldman J: Show Me Yours: Understanding Children's Sexuality. Middlesex, England, Penguin Books, 1988

Graham P, Rutter M: The reliability and validity of the psychiatric assessment of the child, II: interview with the parent. Br J Psychiatry 114:581–592, 1968

Herjanic B, Reich W: Development of a structural psychiatric interview for children: agreement between child and parent on individual symptoms. J Abnorm Child Psychol 10:307–324, 1982

Hinduja S, Patchin JW: Cyberbullying Research Summary: Emotional and Psychological Consequences, 2007. Available at: http://www.cyberbullying.us/cyberbullying_emotional_consequences.pdf. Accessed February 3, 2009.

Kendler KS, Neale MC, Kessler RC, et al: The genetic epidemiology of phobias in women: the interrelationship of agoraphobia, social phobia, situational phobia, and simple phobia. Arch Gen Psychiatry 49:273–281, 1992

Lavigne JV, Arend R, Rosenbaum D, et al: Psychiatric disorders with onset in the preschool years, II: correlates and predictors of stable case status. J Am Acad Child Adolesc Psychiatry 37:1255–1261, 1998

Lochman JE: Cognitive-behavioral intervention with aggressive boys: three year follow-up and preventive efforts. J Consult Clin Psychol 60:426–432, 1992

Loeber R, Green SM, Lahey BB, et al: Difference and similarities between children, mothers, and teachers as informants on disruptive child behavior. J Abnorm Child Psychol 19:75–95, 1991

McClellan JM, Hamilton JD: An evidence-based approach to an adolescent with emotional and behavioral dysregulation. J Am Acad Child Adolesc Psychiatry 45:489–493, 2006

Rappaport N: Psychiatric consultation to school-based health centers: lessons learned in an emerging field. J Am Acad Child Adolesc Psychiatry 40:1473–1475, 2001

Rutter M, Graham P: The reliability and validity of the psychiatric assessment of the child, I: interview with the child. Br J Psychol 114:563–579, 1968

Rutter M, Caspi A, Moffitt TE: Using sex differences in psychopathology to study causal mechanisms: unifying issues and research strategies. J Child Psychol Psychiatry 44:1092–1105, 2003

Schor E: Caring for Your School-Age Child: Ages 5 to 12: Complete and Authoritative Guide. New York, Bantam Books, 1999

Shaffer D, Fisher P, Lucus CP, et al: NIMH Diagnostic Interview Schedule for Children, Version IV (NIMH DISC-IV): description, differences from previous versions and reliability of some common diagnoses. J Am Acad Child Adolesc Psychiatry 39:28–38, 2000

Stanger C, Lewis M: Agreement among parents, teachers, and children on internalizing and externalizing behavior problems. J Clin Child Psychol 22:107–115, 1993

Widiger TA, Clark LA: Toward DSM-V and the classification of psychopathology. Psychol Bull 126:946–963, 2000

Zametkin AJ, Ernst M, Silver R: Laboratory and diagnostic testing in child and adolescent psychiatry: a review of the past 10 years. J Am Acad Child Adolesc Psychiatry 37:464–472, 1998

APPENDIX 3–1. Detailed outline for the psychiatric assessment of the school-age child

Informants and persons present	Some combination of the following individuals may be used as informants: • Child and parent(s) • Parent(s) and/or caregiver(s) without child • Child and other adult, such as a grandparent, designated by the guardian to accompany child to the evaluation visit • Child and other adult, such as social services case worker or guardian ad litem • Child alone (may occur more commonly in certain settings, such as an inpatient psychiatric unit) Additional information, including the mental status examination, will be obtained when the child is interviewed. If there are other adults present, ask who the person is, ascertain their relationship to the child and caregiver(s), and obtain a formal release of information from the legal guardian to allow that adult's participation in the evaluation.
Introduction	"Hi, Julie, I'm Dr. _____; you and your parent(s) are going to meet with me today to talk." "We are going into my office to talk together—I'll show you the way there." Remember, younger children in this age group usually experience well-child visits with their primary care doctors, at which times they may receive scheduled immunizations. Telling the child that you don't usually give "shots" in your office may help to ease their anxiety about what will happen during their initial visit with you.
Interview setting	Introduce parent(s) and child to your office if this is where you will evaluate the child. Have special areas for the child, such as smaller seats and table, toys, and an artwork area with supplies. In settings other than your office, such as in an emergency room or inpatient unit, attempt to make everyone comfortable.
Interview purpose	Evaluations of children in this age range may occur in different settings, each with a modified purpose: • Outpatient mental health setting • Emergency room or crisis setting • Pediatric setting, either inpatient or outpatient • School setting
Legal issues	If this has not already been addressed, ascertain who the child's legal guardian is. If the adult present at the initial appointment is not legally able to consent to an evaluation, the evaluation usually should not proceed until this issue is addressed and resolved.
Reason for referral	Understand from the parent(s)/caregiver(s) the "why now?" related to seeking psychiatric evaluation (e.g., what prompted arranging this initial evaluation?). Helpful questions: • "What brings you in today?" • "What can we do today to be helpful to you and your child?" • "Did someone recommend that you bring your child for an evaluation?" If the child is present: "What does your child understand is the reason you are here today?"

APPENDIX 3–1. Detailed outline for the psychiatric assessment of the school-age child *(continued)*

Identifying data	This information includes the following: • Child's name • Child's sex • Child's age in years and months • Child's race The clinician can also ascertain if the child has a nickname or abbreviated name that he or she prefers.
Vital signs	Depending on the setting of this initial interview, vital signs will not always be taken during the initial clinical contacts with the child and caregiver(s). If vital signs are taken, the following can be included: • Pulse and blood pressure • Temperature and respiratory rate (if indicated) • Height and weight Height and weight percentiles can be recorded on standardized growth charts for boys and girls in this age range. Body mass index can also be calculated for the patient using height and weight values.
Chief complaint and history of present illness	Allow the parent(s)/caregiver(s) to freely discuss the concern(s) for which they are seeking an evaluation. Gather the following information about the chief complaint or problem(s): • Onset • Frequency • Duration • Triggers • Ameliorators • Context • Impact on child's functioning • Impact on family system Guide the interview if necessary to ascertain the above details, including asking direct questions if necessary.
Psychiatric history	Includes all previous mental health contacts, whether through the child's school, primary care provider, or mental health providers: • "Has your child ever seen someone else for these concerns?" • "If so, what was the outcome of those contacts?" Obtaining the actual psychiatric evaluation and treatment history is important, as is understanding the parents' and the child's reactions to past psychiatric contacts and treatment. Detailed psychiatric history includes • Previous outpatient psychiatric evaluation and treatment • Past emergency-level evaluations and their outcome (e.g., hospitalization) • Past psychiatric hospitalizations • Previous and current psychotropic medication treatment and responses • Previous history of suicidal/homicidal statements, intent, and/or acts
Medical history	"Is your child healthy?" Pay special attention to past history related to potential neurological insult, such as seizure disorders, history of serious head injury, brain insults, and/or infections. Ascertain who is the child's primary care provider and the following related information: • Date of the child's last physical exam • Results of that exam

APPENDIX 3–1. Detailed outline for the psychiatric assessment of the school-age child *(continued)*

Medical history *(continued)*	This information is also important since collaboration with the primary care physician, with the parent(s)' consent, may be needed during psychiatric evaluation and/or treatment. Detailed medical history includes • Allergies to medications/environmental sources • Current medications • Potential neurological insults, including seizure disorders or symptoms, serious head injury, toxic brain insults • Review of systems, including cardiac, gastrointestinal, and pulmonary systems • Review of cardiac system should include history possible for congenital disease/structural abnormalities • Thyroid disease • Genetic disorders • Renal or hepatic disease • Sleep function • Appetite/weight changes/eating habits • Exercise/physical activity • Immunization history • Somatic complaints, including headaches and stomachaches • Any surgery, previous medical hospitalizations, procedures • Any previous serious injuries
Social history	Get to know the child's home environment, the child's role in the family, and the family's interactions with the child. Questions for the parent(s)/caregiver(s): • "Who lives in your home?" • "Who are the important grown-ups in your child's life?" Questions for the child: • "Who takes care of you at home?" All of the following information, if gathered, can help to understand the child's family situation: • Parent's (parents') age and occupation • Parent's (parents') level of education • Parent's (parents') own childhood and social circumstances and how these have influenced their parenting practices • Siblings/other children in the home, their ages, and functioning • Custody arrangements, if applicable • Parents' marital relationship, if applicable • Each parent's parenting style and compatibility with that of the other parent Inquire about individual and family stressors, past and present—for example: • Parental separation or divorce • Family loss/death • Illness in family • Financial stressors • Family conflict • Difficulties accessing mental health services • School dysfunction • School change(s) • Family moves How have these stressors impacted the child? the family?

APPENDIX 3–1. Detailed outline for the psychiatric assessment of the school-age child *(continued)*

Developmental history	"Have you ever had any concerns about your child's development?" Developmental history can be divided into these areas: • *Prenatal history* includes pregnancy complications, medication/substance exposure, infection • *Delivery history* includes complications, birth weight, method of delivery, Apgar scores • *Postnatal history* includes requirement of neonatal intensive care unit, approximate days in hospital, jaundice, early feeding difficulties • *Developmental milestones* can include age when spoke first words, crawled, walked, spoke in phrases and sentences; toilet training history • *Personality development* includes the child's temperament and how this temperament matches or does not match those of his or her parents (Schor 1999) • *Current developmental functioning* includes peer interactions and friendships, school functioning, family interactions, level of independence • *Physical development* includes assessing pubertal development since its onset is usually during the latter school-age years • *Developmental assessments*—Has the child received previous developmental assessment, such as through early intervention services, a developmental pediatrician, or specialist? • *Developmental interventions*—Has the child received a past speech and language evaluation or treatment, or occupational therapy evaluation and treatment?
Strengths, interests, and assets	This section can be one that especially helps the clinician to form an alliance with the child and the family. It helps the child and family to understand that the evaluation is not just problem-focused and that these areas are important too. Questions for the parent(s)/caregiver(s): • "What are your child's strengths?" • "What does your child do well?" Questions for the child: • "What do you like to play at home?" • "What do you do well at school?" • "What do you like best about yourself?"
Educational history	Includes the following detailed elements: • Current grade level • Name of school • Type of school (public, private, religiously based) • Grades • Past history of grade retention? • Any change in school functioning over the past year? Ascertain the child's functioning in the following broad areas: • Language arts • Mathematics • Writing Specialized educational services: • Is the child receiving these? • Has the child received any type of educational assessment through the school? • What were the results of this assessment? • Does the child have an individualized education plan? • What specialized services is the child receiving at school? • If the child is receiving services at school, how is the child responding to these interventions (i.e., is there improvement noted and reported?)? In general, understand the parent's and the child's impressions about how well the school is working with them to address the child's problems if they are school related.

APPENDIX 3–1. Detailed outline for the psychiatric assessment of the school-age child *(continued)*

Trauma history	Questions for the parent: • "Has your child been affected by any traumatic events in his or her life?" • "Do you have any concerns that your child may have been physically or sexually abused?" • "Has your child ever witnessed violence?" Questions for the child: • "Has anyone ever hurt you and you were afraid to tell your parent about it?" • "Has anything ever happened to you that really frightened you?" Be aware of your state's legal mandatory reporting requirements for any professional having concerns for possible child abuse and/or neglect. Be prepared to react appropriately to any such concerns for possible physical/sexual abuse and/or neglect. If the patient has a reported history of physical or sexual abuse, ascertain whether the child and family are interacting with the legal system to address the abuse. Has the family experienced any involvement with the department of social services? • "Has the department of social services ever taken custody of your child?" • "Has your child ever been in a foster placement?" Assess the level of media exposure the child has to violent and/or sexual content through television, computerized games, and the Internet.
Family psychiatric history	The following detailed information should be obtained as part of the family psychiatric history: • Presence of mental health diagnoses and treatment in parents, grandparents, and siblings, as well as other more distant relatives • Presence of substance use disorders and treatment in family members • History of psychiatric hospitalization and reasons for that hospitalization if known • History of legal involvement by family members, including family history of violent acts/threats and domestic violence • History of self-harmful threats and/or acts by family members If there is a positive mental health history found in close relatives, has this impacted the child and the family?
Family medical history	The following detailed information regarding family medical history should be obtained: • Family history of serious illnesses, including chronic illnesses, such as diabetes mellitus, and cancer • History of cardiac disease, including hypertension, infarctions, strokes, congenital heart disease • Inquire specifically about family history of sudden cardiac death and obtain details of this history if known, since this may be pertinent in the future if medications with potential adverse cardiac effects are considered • Neurological, developmental, and genetic disorders, such as seizures, fragile X syndrome, developmental delays, autism, mental retardation
Psychiatric review of symptoms	The major DSM-IV-TR (American Psychiatric Association 2000) diagnostic categories should be covered as appropriate. Some categories may be more appropriate to cover in greater detail than others.

APPENDIX 3–1. Detailed outline for the psychiatric assessment of the school-age child *(continued)*

Psychiatric review of symptoms *(continued)*	Many children may present with problems that do not "fall into" DSM-IV-TR categories. Examples of these problems may be the following, covered in more detail in this chapter: • School refusal • Poor social skills • Enuresis • Sleep problems Keep in mind that children may also present with symptoms that qualify under strict DSM-IV-TR criteria as a diagnosis, but the use of the diagnosis alone does not adequately define treatment needs or the level of resulting impairment (McClellan and Hamilton 2006).
Mental status examination	Refer to Appendix 3–2. The evaluating clinician is gathering data regarding the child's mental status throughout the clinical contact (American Academy of Child and Adolescent Psychiatry 1995). Many sections of the formal mental status examination are assessed through *observation*, such as the child's appearance, ability to separate from caregiver, affect, impulse control, and motor activity. Some sections are best assessed with *direct discourse* with the child, such as the child's mood report and thought content, as well as items covered in the next section of this appendix ("Risk assessment").
Risk assessment	The importance of assessing risk for a patient is highlighted by separating this topic into a separate section from the mental status examination. This assessment should address any possible issues of self-harm or harm to others, including presence of suicidal or homicidal thoughts or intent, violence exposure, and access to weapons including guns. Directly ask the child questions regarding possible suicidality: • "Have you ever thought of killing yourself?" • "Have you ever wished you were dead?" Understand the child's concept of death to aid in understanding his or her answers to such questions. Directly ask the parent(s)/caregiver(s) similar questions regarding the child's possible suicidality and homicidality as well.
Formulation	The formulation can be assimilated in the biopsychosocial model, addressing each area of this approach (American Academy of Child and Adolescent Psychiatry 1995): • Biological • Psychological • Social What are the patient's and family's assets and strengths that will aid in the treatment and recovery process?
Differential diagnosis	Often initial history and presentation do not allow the clinician to adequately confirm one or more DSM-IV-TR-based diagnoses. Further clinical contacts may need to occur, as well as collateral information gathered, before the clinician can adequately diagnose the condition(s).
Multiaxial diagnoses	Diagnoses, if present, should be given on Axis I through Axis V.

APPENDIX 3–1. Detailed outline for the psychiatric assessment of the school-age child *(continued)*

Treatment planning	The completed assessment should have identified target treatment areas through the biopsychosocial formulation.
	These treatment targets may be
	• The child's psychiatric symptoms
	• The child's and/or the family's dysfunction and distress related to those psychiatric symptoms
	• Developmental issues
	• Medical issues
	• Family systems issues
	• School issues
	• Community and cultural issues.
	Treatment targets may have to be prioritized based on acuity or on other more practical issues, such as the ability of the family to pursue psychiatric treatment or the paucity of psychiatric treatment resources in their local area.
Prognosis	This issue may be an especially important and sensitive area to the parents/caregivers seeking the initial psychiatric evaluation.
	Parents will often refer to this issue during the interview and may state: "We didn't seek help before now because we thought he or she would grow out of it."
	Questions helpful in understanding parents' hopes and fears for their child's future as impacted by a possible mental illness include
	• "What are your concerns about how this problem will affect your child in the next few years?"
	• "Have you observed this problem affecting your child's development?"
Further evaluation	Referrals may need to be made for the following additional evaluation(s) to aid in the evaluation process:
	• Psychological assessment, including psychological testing and neuropsychological testing; psychological testing is further described in detail in the section "Use of Rating Scales and Semistructured Interviews" in this chapter (see also Chapter 7, "Diagnostic Interviews," and Chapter 8, "Rating Scales")
	• Speech and language evaluation and services
	• Developmental assessment, including developmental testing

APPENDIX 3–2. Child mental status examination

Appearance	Is the child dressed neatly or disheveled? Is the child dressed appropriately for his or her age?
Eye contact	Does the child gaze at the interviewer curiously, or does the child avoid any eye contact with the interviewer?
Attitude and behavior	Is the child oppositional toward adult caregivers? Does the child separate from parents easily?
Speech and language	Does the child demonstrate normally developed speech for his or her age? Is the child's speech difficult to understand?
Mood and affect	How is the child feeling at the time of the visit? The interviewer may have to help the child answer this question with developmentally appropriate choices, such as "sad, mad, happy." Does the child's affect match his or her mood report?
Thought structure and content	Is the child's thinking organized and linear? Does the child's thinking demonstrate any abnormalities, such as delusions or paranoia?
Suicidality and homicidality	Does the child have any current or recent thoughts of wanting to hurt himself or herself? Does he or she have a plan and/or intent to do so? These are questions that a child in this age range can answer adequately. Assess for risk issues as covered in Appendix 3–1.
Attention and concentration	How is the child attending to and concentrating on activities in the interview setting? Does this child remain at his or her activity for several minutes, or is the child intrusive, moving about the office, and changing tasks frequently?
Orientation	Does the child know today's date? Is he or she developmentally advanced enough to be expected to know the date?
Cognitive functioning	How is the child's memory? Executive functions, such as attention and concentration, are described above (see "Attention and concentration").
Intellectual ability	Does intellect seem commensurate with parent reports of school performance?
Insight and judgment	Does the child's insight (or lack thereof) appear to be developmentally appropriate?

Chapter 4

Assessing Adolescents

Steven P. Cuffe, M.D.

The psychiatric assessment of adolescents is more similar to assessment of adults than is the assessment of younger children. Adolescents are able to give historical information, verbalize feelings, be introspective, and many are able to think abstractly. However, clinicians assessing adolescents should be aware that adolescents are not just younger adults. Adolescents live in a complex web of interdependent relationships within their family, peer group, school, agencies (e.g., social services, juvenile justice), and broader community and cultural groups. The assessment of adults typically relies almost solely on that adult's report of symptoms and problems. To do this with adolescents would be a grave mistake. Developmental considerations are of critical importance in the assessment of adolescents. The brain continues to develop into the early 20s, especially the areas involved in executive functions such as inhibition, impulse control, and critical decision making (see for example, Sowell et al. 2001). Developmental immaturity of the brain places adolescents at much higher risk for multiple prob-

lems, including violence and aggression, substance abuse, motor vehicle accidents, and risky sexual behavior.

Psychosocial developmental issues are also prominent in adolescents. Adolescents' development of a sense of self and identity is intimately connected with their striving for autonomy. Relationships with parents and family issues are pivotal in this process. The goal of parenting adolescents is to allow them to grow in independence and increase their decision-making authority within the context of a safe "container," with appropriate limits established by loving and supportive parents. Either absent/neglectful or overbearing and restrictive parenting styles can contribute to the development of problem behaviors in adolescents. Similarly, an adolescent's peer and community group can have a strong influence on the developing sense of identity (belonging) and subsequent behavior and choices. Emerging sexuality plays out in this context, as does experimentation with other "adult" behaviors such as substance use and driving habits.

Although there are some circumstances in which an assessment can be brief (hospital consults, emergency room evaluations, and so forth), this chapter will focus on how to conduct a thorough assessment of an adolescent. The clinician begins the assessment seeking to understand the adolescent's problems and symptoms within his or her genetic, developmental, family, peer, and community/cultural context. To accomplish this, a comprehensive assessment plan must be developed. Information from different sources must be obtained. Adolescents and parents have at best only modest agreement in their reporting of behaviors and symptoms (American Academy of Child and Adolescent Psychiatry 1995; Cantwell et al. 1997; Kramer et al. 2004). Parents tend to report more accurately on externalizing symptoms and behaviors, and adolescents tend to report more accurately on internalizing symptoms (Cantwell et al. 1997). Information from school and other agencies involved with the adolescent is also important.

Table 4–1 lists the elements involved in a comprehensive evaluation. The amount of time it takes to collect all the information (through record review, interviewing, phone calls, data collection by the use of standardized measures); establish relationships with parents and the adolescent (and other family members if needed); develop a case formulation and treatment plan; and present the plan to the parents and adolescent is highly variable and may range from 1 hour to many hours over multiple weeks. Clinicians from a variety of mental health and health care disciplines may perform these functions. It is optimal for a child and adolescent psychiatrist to be involved.

Deciding whom to interview may be complicated. Legal and family issues are important to discern. Are both parents available and do they maintain their parental rights? Are they both involved in important aspects of the child's life? Are divorce and custody issues involved? Are other adult caregivers taking primary roles in the care of the child? Establishing custody or guardianship is an important prerequisite to beginning an assessment. For children, usually the noncustodial parent has the right to participate in medical assessment and treatment but not to begin a treatment process unless it is emergent. Since laws vary between states, it is also critical to know the legal age for consent for medical treatment in your state. Many states have enacted laws allowing minors over the age of 14 or 16 to consent to most medical treatment (see Chapter 43, "Legal and Ethical Issues").

Involving as many informants as possible provides the broadest data set from which to base the diagnostic

TABLE 4–1. Elements of a comprehensive assessment

Parent interview

Adolescent interview

Interview with teachers as appropriate (could be by phone)

Family interview as appropriate

Interviews with other family members as needed (siblings, grandparents, other caretakers)

Medical records from primary care physician

Prior mental health treatment records

School records

Records from other involved agencies (e.g., social services, juvenile justice)

Standardized measures (rating scales, symptom checklists, diagnostic interviews) as needed to assess problem behaviors or symptoms

Psychological testing

assessment and proposed treatment plan. Mothers and fathers frequently have divergent views about the adolescent's problems and their underlying causes (Chess et al. 1966; Youngstrom et al. 2000). Whenever possible, both parents should be involved. They can be interviewed with the child, as a couple, or separately. Many times a combination of formats is best. Other primary caregivers can be included with the permission of the legal guardian. Similarly, prior records from the primary care physician, prior mental health treatment records, school records, and records from other involved agencies should be obtained as part of a comprehensive assessment. Data from rating scales, standardized diagnostic interviews, or psychological testing can also be helpful in establishing the correct diagnosis and an accurate problem list, leading to a plan of treatment.

Finally, understanding how the adolescent has been referred for treatment is an important piece of information to have prior to beginning the assessment. Did the parents self-refer? Was the school involved or the juvenile court? Do the parents or the adolescent believe there is a problem, or are they only following through on a forced assessment?

Beginning the Assessment

The first decision is whom to invite to the initial interview. Since autonomy issues and struggles for separation are frequently important issues, the way the initial interview is handled can have a significant effect, positive or negative, on the outcome of the assessment process. If the parent(s) is seen first, the adolescent may place the clinician in the role of "agent of the parent." Resistance and oppositional behavior from the adolescent are a frequent result. On the other hand, the clinician can choose to see the adolescent first. However, the adolescent may have little to say, so the result may be a quick session with little accomplished. The key is to engage both the adolescent and the parent in the assessment in a way that promotes a positive connection and thus a promising beginning to treatment.

In most cases, starting the initial assessment with parent(s) and adolescent together can be productive. How long to continue this interview is a decision based on the interaction of the parties. At a minimum, this allows the clinician to assess the relationship between the adolescent and the parent(s). An introduction to the problems causing the referral gives the clinician information on which to base the interview with the adolescent alone. The level of resistance and oppositional behavior can be seen. In order to minimize the perception of the clinician as solely a parental agent, this interview may be short and quickly transition to the adolescent alone. Maintaining this interview in the face of significant oppositional behavior can be counterproductive, as illustrated below.

Case Vignette

A clinician was administering a diagnostic interview to an adolescent referred for assessment to the outpatient clinic. The first part of the interview was to obtain consent from the parent and assent from the adolescent for participating in the assessment. The young girl, around age 15, was close-mouthed during the entire discussion. When it came time for her to sign the form, she refused. The clinician spent much time trying to convince this girl that it would be in her best interest to participate. Still, she dug her heels in even further. The mother and clinician both became frustrated and were at the point of terminating the interview. It was clear that the adolescent could not accept any possibility of giving her mother what she wanted. There was anger and defiance in her manner, and the initial interview was about to end in failure. A child and adolescent psychiatrist whose role was to observe decided to knock on the door. He spoke to the clinician and recommended she ask the mother to leave the room so she (the clinician) could speak to the adolescent alone. He further recommended she focus not on the task of assenting to the evaluation but on getting a rapport established with the teenager by getting the adolescent to talk about something, anything, about herself and her life. As soon as the mother left the room, the adolescent began to soften. Soon she was talking

about her life at home, school, and with friends. Within a few minutes, she readily signed the assent-to-treatment form, and the interview proceeded without further incident. Understanding when and how to involve the various parties in the assessment process can be critical to the success of the initial interview.

In the beginning of the assessment process, it is vital that both parent and adolescent understand the structure and process of the evaluation. Confidentiality issues must be explained to both the parent and adolescent. In order for adolescents to feel comfortable providing details about their life, symptoms, actions, and feelings, they need to know how much of what they disclose will be communicated to a parent. If adolescents assume that everything they say will be communicated directly to the parent, this places a huge roadblock on the flow of information. However, some will assume everything will be kept confidential, causing difficulties when significant issues need to be disclosed to parents. Conversely, parents often think it's their right to know every detail divulged by the adolescent in the interview. After all, they are bringing their underage child for assessment, and they are paying for it too! Coming to an understanding of just how confidentiality is handled will avoid some uncomfortable situations and allows for a much easier first interview with the adolescent.

What is the proper balance between confidentiality for the adolescent and sufficient communication with the parent? In order to facilitate communication by the adolescent, he or she should feel that the clinician is, at least in part, his or her advocate. Parents should be told the clinician will give them the overview of problems and diagnoses, without specific details of statements and behaviors reported by the adolescent, *unless the adolescent would be at risk of harm* if the parents were not informed. In cases of suicidal behaviors, dangerous sexual behaviors (multiple partners and/or unprotected sex), dangerous driving behaviors, and the like, the safety of the adolescent takes precedence over confidentiality. Where the line is drawn is up to the individual practitioner; however, it would be wise to give some examples of the limits of confidentiality for both the parent and the child. Parents can, at times, have unreasonable expectations.

Case Vignette

During my assessment of an adolescent boy, it became clear that substance abuse was a primary problem. His drug use involved marijuana and alcohol predominantly but also experimentation with cocaine on two occasions. The boy asked that this not be disclosed to his mother. I rather easily agreed to this since I felt fairly sure the youth was accurately reporting his use, and I also knew that I would be recommending random drug screens as part of the treatment—therefore, more extensive and dangerous use would be uncovered. When during the course of the treatment the youth disclosed his limited cocaine use to his mother, she became outraged that I hadn't told her about it and demanded he be hospitalized. I explained to her that his cocaine use was neither at a level I considered placed him at risk of harm, nor was it at a level warranting hospitalization. She responded with a question, "Can the ingestion of cocaine kill you?" Of course, the answer was "yes."

It is also important to note at the beginning of the assessment the limits of confidentiality posed by disclosures of abuse and neglect, and the legal "duty to report" such incidents to authorities (see Chapter 43, "Legal and Ethical Issues"). Laws vary somewhat by state, and all clinicians need to understand the laws under which they practice.

After dealing with confidentiality issues, the clinician should explain in general terms the structure anticipated in the first session: usually a joint interview to start, and then individual meetings with the adolescent and parent(s) to flesh out the presenting problems and history.

The Adolescent Interview

It is the rare adolescent who requests professional help. Most adolescents are brought for evaluation at least in part against their will. As a matter of fact, there is a significant decrease in the proportion of adolescents who receive an evaluation or treatment for psychiatric disorders as they age. As youth progress through adolescence, they are less likely to receive mental health evaluation or treatment (Cuffe et al. 2001). Many youth are forced into treatment by parents, social service agencies, schools, courts, and probation officers. How can an adolescent in such a position be successfully engaged?

An evidence-based approach that has been successfully used in adolescents, particularly teens with substance abuse, is called *motivational interviewing* or *motivational enhancement therapy* (see Chapter 60, "Motivational Interviewing"). Motivational interviewing uses Carl Rogers' client-centered approach, focusing on the person's current interests or concerns, and thus likely provides the adolescent with a more positive experience. This enhances the interviewer's role as advocate for the adolescent rather than agent of the parent.

However, as opposed to a true Rogerian therapy, motivational interviewing is directive. The approach specifically focuses on the resolution of ambivalence, guiding the person toward positive change. The interviewer elicits from the adolescent thoughts about change, reinforces them, and deals with resistance in ways intended to reduce it. The goal is to resolve ambivalence so that a person moves toward change.

In the first individual meeting with the adolescent, the key dialectic on which to focus is between rapport building and data collection. Both need to be accomplished. However, excessive focus on data collection can impede rapport building. In most cases, collecting data with the adolescent on the chief complaint and history of the present illness is off-putting and may result in both little development of rapport and poor collection of data. The primary focus at the start of the interview should be to begin to understand the adolescent from his or her interests and strengths. The adolescent generally feels comfortable discussing areas of strength, and this approach can break the ice for collecting data later in the interview.

After initial rapport building, the discussion of the adolescent's perception of why he or she has been brought for evaluation can proceed. It is important to try to elicit the adolescent's ideas as distinct from the parents' views. What does the adolescent see as the real problems? What is his or her view? How would he or she like to see change in himself or herself and the family? This approach can begin to show that the clinician is interested and that the adolescent's ideas are important. Elicit ideas about problems in the family, in the adolescent, and in the adolescent's peer relationships and school functioning. Begin with open-ended questions in order to obtain as broad and complete an idea as possible about the adolescent's views. Follow-up questions can be more focused and specific to elaborate and flesh out topics. The interview should feel more like a conversation than a question-and-answer session.

Frequently, an adolescent may deny any problems, or shrug and say "I don't know" when asked for ideas about problems. This is often a sign that the adolescent is not yet engaged. The interviewer may have to spend more time in the engagement process, perhaps using some motivational enhancement techniques, in order to move forward. The interview can be conceived as a cycle (Figure 4–1), consisting of the following:

1. Clinician engages the adolescent and seeks to understand his or her concerns, fears, and hopes.
2. Clinician conveys this understanding to the adolescent.

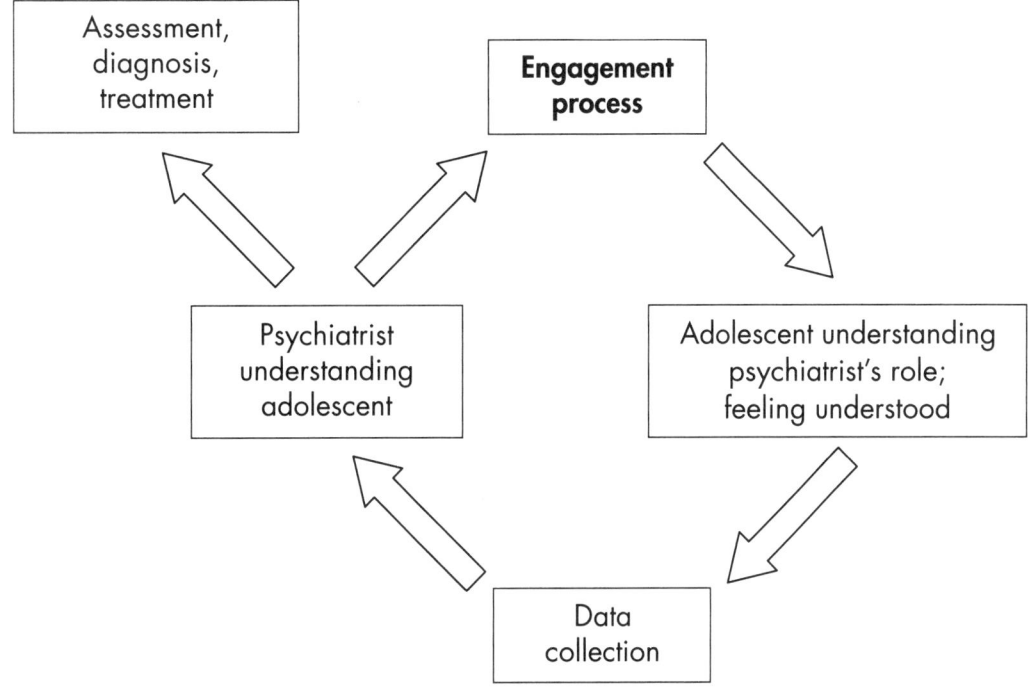

FIGURE 4–1. Adolescent interview.

Source. Adapted from Shea SC (ed): *Psychiatric Interviewing: The Art of Understanding.* Philadelphia, PA, W.B. Saunders, 1988, p. 8.

3. Adolescent begins to feel understood and to see clinician as an ally, leading to clinician's improved ability to collect accurate data.
4. Clinician uses data collection to increase understanding of patient's problems.
5. Clinician conveys this increased understanding to improve engagement with the adolescent.

Table 4–2 lists the elements of data collection that should be obtained during the course of one or more interviews with the adolescent. The history of present illness includes the timing, onset, severity, and variability of symptoms, including whether the adolescent has experienced a similar episode or episodes in the past. Comorbid psychiatric disorders should always be investigated. Comorbid diagnoses are extremely common in children and adolescents (Angold et al. 1999; Lewinsohn et al. 1995). One of the most common mistakes inexperienced interviewers make is to prematurely hone in on a diagnosis. This often excludes other diagnoses from consideration and results in an incomplete evaluation and inadequate treatment plan. All psychiatric diagnostic areas should be screened: affective disorders (unipolar, bipolar, dysthymia); anxiety disorders (generalized anxiety disorder, panic disorder, agoraphobia, social anxiety disorder, posttraumatic stress disorder, obsessive-compulsive disorder); psychotic disorders;

attention-deficit and disruptive behavior disorders; and so forth. This screen can be accomplished during the interview or by using structured diagnostic instruments or rating scales (discussed in the section "Standardized Measures" later in this chapter). If not explicitly determined during the history of present illness, an assessment of suicidal and homicidal ideation, plan, and intent should be obtained, in addition to other dangerous or risky behaviors.

The interview should end with a brief discussion with the adolescent of the clinician's initial impressions and a review with the adolescent of how the interview with parents will be conducted, what areas will be covered, and how confidentiality will be handled. If there are areas the psychiatrist feels must be reported to the parent from the first adolescent interview, these should be discussed.

Mental Status Examination

The mental status examination is an important element of any assessment. Many aspects of the mental status examination can be done during the course of the interview, reducing the need for formal testing. However, it is important to understand the basic ele-

TABLE 4–2. Elements of data collection during the adolescent interview

Chief complaint
History of present illness
Screening for psychiatric disorders
Substance use
Educational history
Family relationships
Peer relationships
Hobbies, interests, sports, music
Sexual history
Religious, spiritual, cultural history

TABLE 4–3. Elements of the mental status examination

Attitude and behavior
Hygiene and style of dress
Speech: fluency, rate, rhythm, prosody
Motor: gait, coordination, abnormal movements
Orientation (person, place, time, circumstance)
Affect (perceived by interviewer)
Mood (reported by adolescent)
Suicidal or homicidal ideation, plan, intent
Thought content (obsessions, delusions, looseness of associations)
Perceptions: auditory, visual, tactile, or olfactory hallucinations
Memory: immediate, recent, remote
Intellectual functioning: calculations, geography, presidents, etc.
Abstraction: proverbs, similarities
Judgment
Insight

ments of the mental status examination (listed in Table 4–3). Although the clinician can often get a sense of the level of cognitive functioning from the interview, the astute clinician looks in the history for areas of strength or weakness that may not be apparent in the interview.

The Parent Interview

The clinician should have multiple goals for the initial parent interview. First and foremost, this interview provides an opportunity for the clinician to establish a relationship with the parent(s) that sets the stage for the ongoing treatment of the adolescent, and possibly, for the success or failure of that treatment. Absent a positive, collaborative relationship with an adolescent's parent, treatment is arduous at best.

A second goal of the interview is to understand the presenting problems from the parent's point of view. This is best done without the presence of the adolescent. The adolescent has likely heard about his or her problems many times in the past. Hearing the recitation of problems in front of a stranger often creates a hostile, antagonistic, and resistive response from the adolescent. Conversely, many parents will not discuss their concerns about the adolescent frankly in the presence of their child. Therefore, an interview with the parent alone is crucial. However, information from the parent about the adolescent's current problems and functioning is frequently not complete and is sometimes not accurate. Some parents may deny a particular problem or be unable to accurately recall certain events (Chess et al. 1966). A secondary goal of the parent interview is thus to try to gain insight into the validity of the parent's report.

Data collection is a third primary aim of the parent interview. The present illness should be thoroughly explored from the parent's perspective. Similar to the adolescent interview, a screen for other psychiatric disorders should be completed with the parents. Following discussion of the present illness, clinicians should explore historical information about both the child and the family. Table 4–4 lists the data elements parents can provide. This provides depth for the clinician's understanding of the child's and family's problems. How did the problems develop? Creating a timeline of important events in the family's and child's life, including the development of psychiatric symptoms, can aid in the understanding of the patient and family. If, during the course of the parent interview, information is obtained that one or both parents have experienced psychiatric or emotional problems, the clinician should strongly consider individual interviews with each parent to further explore how these problems may have affected the adolescent. From child abuse and domestic violence to depression or psychotic disorders, parental emotional problems may have an immense impact on a developing child (Cuffe et al. 2005). Absence or unavailability of a parent may cause anxiety, particularly separation fears. Divorce, separations, and the deaths of important family members should all be explored. A thorough family history of mental disorders should be obtained. In complex families, a family genogram, a diagram of the family history and relationship patterns of three or more generations of family members (Hartman 1995; McGoldrick and Gerson 1985), is a helpful tool to organize this information. Conversely, it is also important for the clinician to try to understand how this child has affected the family. A child with serious emotional or behavioral problems can distort and impair the functioning of an otherwise healthy family. In some cases, the family's functioning improves once the impaired child is out of the home (Hechtman 1996).

At the conclusion of the initial interview with the parents, the clinician should provide to the parents an initial view of the strengths and weaknesses of their child and tell them how the evaluation will proceed. This presentation of initial findings is another time when the clinician can engage the parents in collaboration and further develop an alliance.

Family Assessment

The family assessment has already begun with the parent interview. In uncomplicated cases, there may be no need to interview each family member or see the entire family as a group. As a minimum requirement, the family assessment must include an observation of the child's interaction with caretakers (Josephson and AACAP Work Group on Quality Issues 2007). If there are clear indications that family interaction patterns, discipline style, or structure promote, precipitate, or perpetuate the adolescent's psychiatric or behavioral problems, a more thorough family evaluation should be undertaken. At this point, the assessment goals expand to include the meaning and function of the symptom in relation to the family (Josephson and AACAP Work Group on Quality Issues 2007).

For example, a family living in a small town once consulted me about their teenage daughter. The girl was acting out and oppositional. During my initial interview with her, she expressed anger at having to live in such a small town (they had recently moved from a large city). During the initial parent interview, it became clear that the daughter was acting out her mother's fury at her husband for having moved her to this town. The focus of the treatment, in order to be successful, had to include the treatment of the family to deal with this dynamic.

When a thorough evaluation of the family is indicated, the evaluation should adequately inform the clinician about the family's structure, communication,

TABLE 4–4. Elements of data collection from parents

Parental history
  How they met
  History of the relationship
  Problems in the relationship
  Decision to marry
  Having children: planned?
  Response to pregnancy: happy? anxious?
  Relationship after children
  Style of discipline
  Marital problems
Developmental history of the identified patient
  Problems during pregnancy
    Perinatal problems
    Birth and delivery
  Developmental milestones
    Feeding problems
    Motor development
    Language development
    Play
    Peer relationships
  Educational history: learning disabilities?
Sibling relationships
  Birth order
  Relationship with siblings
  Physical or emotional problems of siblings
Family history of mental illness
  Examination of each parent may be needed

belief systems, and regulatory processes (Josephson and AACAP Work Group on Quality Issues 2007; see also Chapter 56, "Family Therapy"). *Family structure* refers to the important relationships and boundaries within families and the transactional patterns that exist within these relationships (Minuchin 1974). Boundaries should exist between generational elements in the family, such as between parent and child. Elements of family structure include its ability to change and adapt to new circumstances (adaptability) and the degree of cohesion among the members of the family. Is there a correct balance between autonomy of family members and closeness or connectedness among family members? Is the family enmeshed or disorganized and chaotic? Do healthy family boundaries exist, or is there evidence of boundary violations? Has the family been able to adapt to changes such as childbirth, divorce, or the death of a family member? Are the family rules and discipline clear and consistent?

Family communication refers not only to the ability to communicate clearly and effectively both facts and emotional content but also to the ability to problem solve. Are family members able to identify problems, negotiate conflicts, and resolve issues in a way that enhances family functioning? Do family members feel part of the process, or is the decision making authoritarian? *Family beliefs* often influence the way in which families make decisions and function. Family beliefs are ideas about reality that are shared among family members and denote a kind of family memory system (Josephson and AACAP Work Group on Quality Issues 2007). Family beliefs often guide decision making. They may be healthy and promote positive action (family members protect each other in times of stress) or be unhealthy (men are alcoholic and abusive). These beliefs may show a generational pattern of continuity.

The final element of family functioning, *family regulatory processes,* refers to the ability of the family to meet the developmental needs of the children and promote healthy growth and development. Are family members able to nurture and support the children? At the conclusion of the family assessment, the clinician should be able to incorporate the family's strengths and problems into an overall formulation of the identified patient and be able to understand the reciprocal effects of the adolescent and the family on each other.

Standardized Measures

Psychological testing and standardized instruments that rate symptoms and behaviors can supplement data from the clinical interview and observations of the adolescent and family. Psychological testing, diagnostic interviews, and rating scales are discussed in detail in other chapters (see Chapter 7, "Diagnostic Interviews"; Chapter 8, "Rating Scales"; and Chapter 11, "Psychological and Neuropsychological Testing"). This chapter will briefly mention diagnostic interviews and symptom rating scales. Diagnostic interviews are generally modular and can be used to assess symptoms of a particular diagnostic category or to broadly screen across all diagnostic areas. It is important to note that they cannot replace the clinical interview but rather should be used to help focus the clinical interview on areas of concern. Compared to earlier periods, adolescence may be an optimal time for structured inter-

views. The adolescent is cognitively capable of completing the interviews either in a computer or interview format. Adolescents may also be more open and responsive in a diagnostic interview, particularly the less personal computer-administered format.

Diagnostic interviews allow a comprehensive assessment of psychiatric diagnoses and are of two primary types: interviewer-based and respondent-based interviews. The Schedule for Affective Disorders and Schizophrenia for School-Age Children (K-SADS; Ambrosini 2000; Chambers et al. 1985) and the Child and Adolescent Psychiatric Assessment (CAPA; Angold and Costello 2000) are examples of interviewer-based diagnostic interviews. These are semistructured interviews that allow the interviewer to make judgments during the interview. They require a clinician or highly trained interviewer and thus are more expensive to administer. Respondent-based interviews, such as the NIMH Diagnostic Interview Schedule for Children, Version IV (DISC-IV; Shaffer et al. 2000), are highly structured and use trained lay interviewers. The interviewer follows a predetermined script and is not allowed to deviate from the script or interpret the subject's response. The DISC-IV has also been formatted for computer administration and has a special program for adolescents to self-administer the interview (Voice DISC-IV; Lucas 2003; Shaffer et al. 2000).

Rating scales screen for problem symptoms or behaviors using parent, adolescent, or teacher reports. They should be used to help focus the clinician on problem areas to explore. These instruments generally compare responses for the individual being assessed to standardized population norms. Rating scales may be broad-band scales assessing problems across broad dimensions of behavior, such as the Child Behavior Checklist (CBCL; Achenbach and Rescorla 2001) and the Behavior Assessment System for Children (BASC; Kamphaus et al. 2007); or narrow-band scales focused on a dimension of behavior, such as depression or attention-deficit/hyperactivity. Rating scales place subjective reports from parents, teachers, or adolescents into a more objective form by comparing their responses to those of a normative population. This allows the clinician to better understand how deviant the adolescent's behavior is from other adolescents.

Presenting the Findings

At the conclusion of any assessment, whether it is a single interview or a highly complex assessment involving multiple interviews, the clinician analyzes the data obtained and uses his or her diagnostic skill and clinical acumen to develop an understanding of the problems and strengths of the adolescent and family. Using a biopsychosocial framework, the clinician should understand the predisposing, precipitating, and perpetuating factors at work in the case and develop a treatment plan to address those areas. Next, the clinician must convey the assessment and recommended plan to the adolescent and parents. The presentation of the findings is a critical aspect of the assessment process (Group for the Advancement of Psychiatry 1957) and should be done with care and empathy for those receiving the results. Coming for a psychiatric evaluation is difficult, and both the adolescent and parents may be anxious about the results, fearing that each will be identified as the cause of the problem. Parents feel guilty and fear their "failings as parents" will be exposed, while the adolescent is braced for more blows to his or her self-esteem. It is important, therefore, to be supportive and reassuring during this discussion (Cox 1994). In order to maintain and enhance the relationship with the adolescent, it is often best to meet with the adolescent first to let him or her hear the results. The adolescent can then respond without having to deal with the complicated relationships that may exist with parents. Following this, the clinician can meet with the parents, with or without the adolescent's presence.

The first part of the presentation should always focus on the strengths of both the adolescent and the parents. The psychiatrist might say, for example, "Mike is a bright and engaging boy…very creative and funny. He has a lot going for him." The important thing to keep in mind is that the positive attributes must reflect reality. Beginning this way helps to set everyone at ease. The clinician may also want to highlight problems *not* found, of which the parents or adolescent may have feared. Next, the clinician begins to discuss the problem areas uncovered during the assessment. It is important to convey not only what symptoms and diagnoses have been found but also a formulation of how the problems developed and are perpetuated. The clinician must not shy away from discussing parental or family factors. While it is important not to make the parents feel they are solely to blame for their child's problems, it is equally important that family and social issues are acknowledged and discussed frankly.

Finally, the clinician presents the plan for treatment. This should be done in a manner that encourages discussion and collaboration. In addition, the clinician should incorporate the strengths of the child and family into the discussion of the plan of treatment and prognosis. This allows the session to end on a positive and hopeful note. In this way, the discussion of the problems and difficulties are "sandwiched" between discussions of the positive attributes of the child and family, allowing the family to feel understood and supported at the end of the assessment, and, hopefully, setting the stage for a positive working relationship to begin the treatment.

Research Directions

Future research to improve diagnostic assessment of adolescents should focus on two major areas: interview techniques and improving the diagnostic classification of disorders in childhood and adolescence. The diagnosis a clinician makes is only as good as the diagnostic system available. How best to elicit the signs and symptoms of disorders is vital. Continuing research on promising interview techniques, such as motivational enhancement—and the dissemination of the research findings to practicing clinicians—will improve the diagnostic assessment and treatment of adolescents.

Summary Points

- Adolescents must be assessed from a developmental perspective and include family, school, peer, and community assessments.
- Reports from adolescents, mothers, fathers, teachers, and other caregivers show only modest agreement. Information should be collected from multiple sources.
- Confidentiality and consent to treatment should be explicitly discussed at the onset of the evaluation.
- Oppositional behavior is frequent among adolescents forced to participate by parents, school, or the legal system.

- Motivational interviewing is a promising tool to enhance the engagement of adolescents in the assessment and treatment process.

- Family assessment is crucial, and the adolescent should, at a minimum, be observed interacting with caregiver(s).

- Symptom or behavior rating scales make parent, teacher, and youth reports more objective by comparing responses to a normative population.

- Assessment of adolescents should result in a formulation of the biological, psychological, social, cultural, and spiritual factors predisposing, precipitating, and perpetuating the development of psychopathology in the adolescent and family.

- Presentation of the findings of the assessment should emphasize the strengths of the adolescent and family, in addition to the problems or weaknesses, and should be done in an empathic, supportive manner.

References

Achenbach TM, Rescorla LA: Manual for ASEBA School-Age Forms and Profiles. Burlington, University of Vermont, Research Center for Children, Youth, and Families, 2001

Ambrosini PJ: Historical development and present status of the Schedule for Affective Disorders and Schizophrenia for School-Age Children (K-SADS). J Am Acad Child Adolesc Psychiatry 39:49–58, 2000

American Academy of Child and Adolescent Psychiatry: Practice parameter for the psychiatric assessment of children and adolescents. J Am Acad Child Adolesc Psychiatry 34:1386–1402, 1995

Angold A, Costello E: The Child and Adolescent Psychiatric Assessment (CAPA). J Am Acad Child Adolesc Psychiatry 39:39–48, 2000

Angold A, Costello EJ, Erkanli A: Comorbidity. J Am Acad Child Adolesc Psychiatry 40:57–87, 1999

Cantwell DP, Lewinsohn PM, Rohde P, et al: Correspondence between adolescent report and parent report of psychiatric diagnostic data. J Am Acad Child Adolesc Psychiatry 36:610–619, 1997

Chambers WJ, Puig-Antich J, Hirsch M, et al: The assessment of affective disorders in children and adolescents by semistructured interview: test-retest reliability of the Schedule for Affective Disorders and Schizophrenia for School-Age Children. Arch Gen Psychiatry 42:696–792, 1985

Chess S, Thomas A, Birch HD: Distortions in developmental reporting made by parents of behaviorally disturbed children. J Am Acad Child Adolesc Psychiatry 5:226–234, 1966

Cox AD: Interviews with parents, in Child and Adolescent Psychiatry: Modern Approaches. Edited by Rutter M, Taylor E, Hersov L. Oxford, UK, Blackwell Scientific, 1994, pp 34–50

Cuffe SP, Waller JL, Addy CL, et al: A longitudinal study of adolescent mental health service use. J Behav Health Serv Res 28:1–11, 2001

Cuffe SP, McKeown RE, Addy CL, et al: Family and psychosocial risk factors in a longitudinal epidemiological study of adolescents. J Am Acad Child Adolesc Psychiatry 44:121–129, 2005

Group for the Advancement of Psychiatry: The Diagnostic Process in Child Psychiatry (Rep No 38). New York, Group for the Advancement of Psychiatry, 1957

Hartman A: Diagrammatic assessment of family relationships. Fam Soc 76:111–122, 1995

Hechtman L: Families of children with attention deficit hyperactivity disorder: a review. Can J Psychiatry 41:350–360, 1996

Josephson AM, AACAP Work Group on Quality Issues: Practice parameter for the assessment of the family. J Am Acad Child Adolesc Psychiatry 46:922–937, 2007

Kamphaus RW, VanDeventer MC, Brueggemann A, et al: Behavior Assessment System for Children, in The Clinical Assessment of Children and Adolescents: A Practitioner's Handbook. Edited by Smith SR, Handler L. Mahwah, NJ, Lawrence Erlbaum Associates, 2007, pp 311–326

Kramer TL, Phillips SD, Hargis MB, et al: Disagreement between parent and adolescent reports of functional impairment. J Child Psychol Psychiatry 45:248–259, 2004

Lewinsohn PM, Rohde R, Seeley JR: Adolescent psychopathology, III: the clinical consequences of comorbidity. J Am Acad Child Adolesc Psychiatry 34:510–519, 1995

Lucas CP: Use of structured diagnostic interviews in clinical child psychiatric practice, in Standardized Evaluation in Clinical Practice (Review of Psychiatry, Vol 22). Edited by First MB. Washington, DC, American Psychiatric Publishing, 2003, pp 75–101

McGoldrick M, Gerson R: Genograms in Family Assessment. New York, WW Norton, 1985

Minuchin S: Families and Family Therapy. Cambridge, MA, Harvard University Press, 1974

Shaffer D, Fisher P, Lucas CP, et al: NIMH Diagnostic Interview Schedule for Children, Version IV (NIMH DISC-IV): description, differences from previous versions, and reliability of some common diagnoses. J Am Acad Child Adolesc Psychiatry 39:28–38, 2000

Sowell ER, Thompson PM, Tessner KD, et al: Mapping continued brain growth and graymatter density reduction in dorsal frontal cortex: inverse relationships during postadolescent brain maturation. J Neurosci 21:8819–8829, 2001

Youngstrom E, Loeber R, Stouthamer-Loeber M: Patterns and correlates of agreement between parent, teacher, and male adolescent ratings of externalizing and internalizing problems. J Consult Clin Psychol 68:1038–1050, 2000

PART II

DIAGNOSIS AND APPROACHES TO ASSESSMENT

Chapter 5

Classification of Psychiatric Disorders

Mina K. Dulcan, M.D.

An ideal system of diagnostic classification implies etiology of disorders, predicts their course and prognosis, determines treatment, serves as a means of efficient communication for clinical and administrative purposes, and defines homogeneous groups of patients for treatment or research. To the extent possible, a system of classification should be based on observable and measurable characteristics and empirical research, and it should have been demonstrated to be reliable and valid in both clinical and epidemiological samples. For children and adolescents, a diagnostic system should have been tested with youth for reliability and validity and be constructed to be developmentally appropriate and allow for changes over the course of development in both the characteristics of the disorders and the symptoms shown by individual children and adolescents. The American Psychiatric Association *Diagnostic and Statistical Manual of Mental Disorders* (DSM) system

has undergone repeated changes in diagnostic categories and criteria as the use of each version for clinical care and research led to new knowledge that was incorporated into the next version. (See First et al. 2004 for more discussion of the principles and history of the successive versions of DSM.)

Categorical diagnoses may be defined by sets of rules and criteria (as in the current DSM) or a glossary of descriptions (as in the *International Classification of Diseases* [ICD]). A dimensional system would use ratings on a variety of dimensions or scales, often with normative comparisons and cutoff points.

Categorical diagnostic classification of childhood psychiatric disorders began with the publication by Leo Kanner (1935) of the first English-language textbook of child psychiatry, in which all disorders were placed in categories of "personality difficulties." In the third (and final) edition of his textbook, Kanner (1957) categorized personality problems as related to physical illness, psychosomatic problems, and behavior problems. The latter grouping was the largest, including categories such as eating behavior (e.g., anorexia nervosa, rumination), sleeping behavior (e.g., nightmares, sleepwalking, narcolepsy), speech and language habits, scholastic performance, sexual behavior, anger, jealousy, fear, anxiety attacks, hypochondriasis, obsession and compulsion, hysteria, delinquency (a large chapter), hospitalism, schizophrenia (including a chapter on Kanner's concept of early infantile autism), and suicide.

The developers of the first edition of DSM (American Psychiatric Association 1952) did not include child and adolescent psychiatrists. There were only four categories relating specifically to childhood or adolescence: 1) chronic brain syndrome associated with birth trauma; 2) schizophrenic reaction, childhood type; 3) special symptom reactions such as learning disturbance, enuresis, and somnambulism; and 4) the adjustment reactions (habit disturbance, conduct disturbance, neurotic traits) of infancy, childhood, and adolescence. An innovation in DSM-I compared to previous systems was the addition of a glossary that defined each of the diagnoses.

The Committee on Child Psychiatry of the Group for the Advancement of Psychiatry (GAP) developed a diagnostic system (Group for the Advancement of Psychiatry 1966) aimed at addressing DSM's shortcomings with regard to children and adolescents. The GAP classification provided a more detailed, broad, inclusive biopsychosocial and developmental framework within which to include etiologic and phenomenological considerations. Innovations were the introduction of categories of healthy response and developmental deviations in maturational rate or sequence, use of a symptom list, consideration of interaction with the environment, and modification of diagnoses as acute or chronic and mild, moderate, or severe.

DSM-II

DSM-II (American Psychiatric Association 1968) was intended to coincide with the *International Classification of Diseases,* 8th Revision (ICD-8; World Health Organization 1969), in the context of ongoing dialogue and constructive tension between the U.S. and international approaches to diagnostic classification in psychiatry. The developers of DSM-II tried to avoid terms that implied either the nature of a disorder or its causes and to be "explicit about causal assumptions when they are integral to a diagnostic concept" (p. viii). DSM-II reflected

the growing importance of biological theories and research findings in understanding mental disorders and decreased emphasis on psychoanalytic theory as either sufficiently or even predominantly explanatory. Descriptive phenomenology assumed a larger role than it had previously.

DSM-II made progress in the classification of child and adolescent disorders. Mental retardation was placed as the first category. Schizophrenia, childhood type, remained, as did an expanded section of "special symptoms" and transient situational disturbances. A new category, "behavior disorders of childhood and adolescence," recognized a range of psychopathologies in children and adolescents that was both broader and more specific than in DSM-I. It included:

- Hyperkinetic reaction of childhood (or adolescence)
- Withdrawing reaction of childhood (or adolescence)
- Overanxious reaction of childhood (or adolescence)
- Runaway reaction of childhood (or adolescence)
- Unsocialized aggressive reaction of childhood (or adolescence)
- Group delinquent reaction of childhood (or adolescence)
- Other reaction of childhood (or adolescence)

DSM-III

DSM-III (American Psychiatric Association 1980), highly controversial when it was introduced, represented and became the hallmark of the dramatic changes that had occurred in psychiatry during the previous 20 years. Except when etiology was clearly known, as in organic mental disorders, no assumptions about etiology were included. DSM-III was modeled on the Feighner criteria, developed at Washington University, and the subsequent related Research Diagnostic Criteria (RDC), developed as part of a National Institute of Mental Health (NIMH)–sponsored research project. Unfortunately, these were focused only on adults and were not well developed for children. DSM-III provided specific phenomenological diagnostic criteria for each disorder, in a first attempt to operationalize the diagnostic process. Some observers called this the "Chinese menu" approach, in contrast to the global clinical impressions of DSM-II. Each diagnosis had inclusion criteria, in which making a diagnosis required a specific number of criteria from a list of descriptive symptoms, as well as meeting duration and onset criteria. Exclusion criteria were also added. In the "splitter" approach (as contrasted with the ICD "lumper" preference), all diagnoses were given for which criteria were met (unless there was an explicit hierarchy excluding one specific diagnosis in the presence of another). DSM-III introduced a five-part multiaxial system that allowed for the coding of most psychiatric disorders on Axis I, personality and specific developmental disorders on Axis II, medical conditions on Axis III, and psychosocial stressors and the highest level of adaptive functioning in the past year on Axes IV and V, respectively. The intention of the multiple axes was to encourage comprehensive diagnosis, and therefore treatment, rather than focusing on only one disorder or omitting consideration of learning, personality, or medical disorders.

Although children and adolescents could be given a diagnosis in any section (if the same criteria used in adults were met), DSM-III introduced as its first Axis I category "Disorders Usually First Evident in Infancy, Childhood, or Adolescence," which included the following:

- Mental retardation
- Attention deficit disorder (ADD) (with or without hyperactivity)
- Conduct disorder (five subtypes)
- Anxiety disorders (separation anxiety, avoidant, and overanxious disorders)
- Other disorders of infancy, childhood, or adolescence (reactive attachment; schizoid, oppositional, and identity disorders; and elective mutism)
- Eating disorders
- Stereotyped movement disorders (tic disorders and Tourette's disorder)
- Other disorders with physical manifestations (stuttering, enuresis, encopresis, and sleepwalking and sleep terror disorders)
- Pervasive developmental disorders (including infantile autism)

"Specific developmental disorders" (e.g., developmental reading or arithmetic disorder) were to be coded on Axis II.

DSM-III-R

DSM-III-Revised (American Psychiatric Association 1987) was intended, as the title suggests, to be a modification of DSM-III rather than a radical departure. Inconsistencies were cleaned up. Research findings from studies using DSM-III and specially commissioned field trials were used to revise categories and criteria and to set cutoff points for the number of symptoms required to make each diagnosis. An additional goal was to provide input into the *International Classification of Diseases and Related Health Problems*, 10th Revision (ICD-10; World Health Organization 1992). Axis II was expanded to include mental retardation and pervasive developmental disorders (autistic disorder), as well as the DSM-III categories of specific developmental disorders (including academic, language, and motor skills disorders) and personality disorders. This seems to have been the most logical Axis II grouping of all the DSM versions. One could argue, of course, that enuresis, encopresis, and tic disorders should be on Axis III. However, when these patients present to mental health settings, it is appropriate to include the diagnoses on Axis I. Conceptually, research shows that psychiatric disorders and medical conditions have more similarities than differences, but focusing on the setting of care has some utility.

Some important changes occurred in the disorders usually first evident in infancy, childhood, or adolescence. In the ADDs, the new term *attention-deficit hyperactivity disorder* (ADHD), defined by a single list of symptom criteria, replaced the term attention-deficit disorder. ADD without hyperactivity was dropped (replaced by undifferentiated attention-deficit disorder). ADHD was grouped with oppositional defiant disorder (ODD) and conduct disorder (CD) as the "Disruptive Behavior Disorders" (DBDs). For several disorders, criteria changes resulted in apparent changes in prevalence when using DSM-III-R compared to DSM-III. Rates of ODD and CD were decreased, and ADHD was diagnosed at a higher rate than attention deficit disorder with hyperactivity (ADD-H).

DSM-IV

DSM-IV (American Psychiatric Association 1994) is a modification and refinement of its predecessor rather than a reconceptualization. The process of developing DSM-IV included committees that conducted literature reviews, reanalyzed existing data sets, and commissioned field trials to inform specific questions. There was even greater coordination with the ICD development process, and DSM-IV and ICD-10 agree more closely than their predecessors do.

In DSM-IV, disorders relevant to youth are listed in two ways: some in the section "Disorders Usually First Diagnosed in Infancy, Childhood, or Adolescence" and others in sections that are applicable to all age groups, in which almost the same diagnostic criteria as for adults are used. "The provision of a separate section for disorders that are usually first diagnosed in infancy, childhood, or adolescence is for convenience only and is not meant to suggest that there is any clear distinction between 'childhood' and 'adult' disorders....For most (but not all) DSM-IV disorders, a single criteria set is provided that applies to children, adolescents, and adults" (American Psychiatric Association 1994, p. 37).

Disorders usually first diagnosed in infancy, childhood, or adolescence include the following:

- Mental retardation
- Learning disorders (LDs)
- Motor skills disorder
- Communication disorders
- Pervasive developmental disorders (PDDs)
- Attention-deficit and disruptive behavior disorders (ADHD is no longer considered to be a DBD)
- Feeding and eating disorders of infancy or early childhood
- Tic disorders
- Elimination disorders
- Other disorders of infancy, childhood, or adolescence

A number of other changes in DSM-IV apply specifically to childhood. The overarching category of developmental disorders that was previously coded on Axis II was dropped. PDDs and LDs (formerly academic skills disorders), motor skills disorder, and communication disorders (formerly language and speech disorders) were moved to Axis I from Axis II. This move is not logically consistent with the way the axes were conceptualized, but that was the decision of the committee. Only personality disorders (rarely, if ever, used in children and adolescents) and mental retardation remain on Axis II.

PDDs in DSM-IV have additional subclassifications to improve differential diagnosis and provide greater specificity. PDDs now include:

- Autistic disorder
- Rett's disorder
- Childhood disintegrative disorder
- Asperger's disorder
- PDD not otherwise specified

The diagnostic criteria for LDs remain essentially the same as in DSM-III-R, but the terminology is simplified and the exclusion criteria have been modified

to allow for the presence of a neurological condition. LD now includes:

- Reading disorder (formerly developmental reading disorder)
- Mathematics disorder (formerly developmental arithmetic disorder)
- Disorders of written expression (formerly developmental expressive writing disorder)
- LD not otherwise specified

The communication disorders category now includes the previous two DSM-III-R categories of language and speech disorders and speech disorders not elsewhere classified and is subdivided into:

- Expressive language disorder (formerly developmental expressive language disorder)
- Mixed receptive-expressive language disorder (formerly developmental receptive language disorder)
- Phonological disorder (formerly developmental articulation disorder)
- Stuttering, including a much expanded criteria set and discussion (the term *cluttering* in DSM-III-R was eliminated from DSM-IV)
- Communication disorder not otherwise specified

The category "Attention-Deficit and Disruptive Behavior Disorders" replaced the DSM-III-R category of DBDs. This category now is subdivided into:

- Attention-deficit/hyperactivity disorder (ADHD)
  1. Combined type
  2. Predominantly inattentive type
  3. Predominantly hyperactive-impulsive type
- ADHD not otherwise specified
- Conduct disorder—DSM-III-R categories of group, solitary, and undifferentiated were dropped in favor of childhood-onset or adolescent-onset (after age 10 years) type; the criteria are reorganized into thematically related groups, and "stays out at night" and "intimidates others" have been added.
- Oppositional defiant disorder
- DBD not otherwise specified—new for DSM-IV

The category of anxiety disorders of childhood or adolescence was eliminated, with these disorders now falling under either other disorders of infancy, childhood, or adolescence or the general anxiety disorders category. Overanxious disorder (OAD) of childhood was eliminated, with generalized anxiety disorder

(GAD) (not exactly congruent) to be used instead. GAD requires "excessive" anxiety and worry rather than OAD's "unrealistic" worries.

The DSM-IV discussion of GAD's diagnostic features, age features, and criteria does include considerations specific or relevant to childhood onset. Identity disorder was also deleted.

Feeding and eating disorders of infancy or early childhood is a new category, reflecting the displacement of anorexia nervosa and bulimia nervosa to a separate eating disorders section (with criteria applicable to all ages). Feeding and eating disorders of infancy or early childhood, which focus on early-onset eating problems, include:

- Pica
- Rumination disorder
- Feeding disorder of infancy or early childhood

The category of gender identity disorders (GIDs) has been removed from disorders usually first diagnosed in infancy, childhood, or adolescence and reclassified under the section "Sexual and Gender Identity Disorders," with the categories "in children," "in adolescents or adults," and "not otherwise specified." The category of transsexualism was deleted and is subsumed under GID with specifiers.

The tic disorders category was left essentially unchanged in DSM-IV, except for a drop in the upper limit of age at onset from 21 to 18 years, and includes:

- Tourette's disorder
- Chronic motor or vocal tic disorder
- Transient tic disorder
- Tic disorder not otherwise specified

The elimination disorders category had relatively minor changes in duration specifiers and terminology and now includes:

- Encopresis (previously "functional encopresis")
  1. With constipation and overflow incontinence
  2. Without constipation and overflow incontinence
- Enuresis (previously "functional enuresis")
  1. Nocturnal only
  2. Diurnal only
  3. Nocturnal and diurnal

The category of other disorders of infancy, childhood, or adolescence was reorganized and now includes:

- Separation anxiety disorder
- Selective mutism (including new provisions to reduce false-positive diagnoses)
- Reactive attachment disorder of infancy or early childhood, with two new subtypes added for compatibility with ICD-10
  1. Inhibited type
  2. Disinhibited type (with indiscriminate and diffuse attachments)
- Stereotypic movement disorder (previously stereotypy/habit disorder)—the specifier "with self-injurious behavior" is added if the behavior results in self-damage requiring treatment
- Disorder of infancy, childhood, or adolescence not otherwise specified (It is not clear when this diagnosis would be used, if at all.)

In the DSM-IV section on anxiety disorders, social phobia subsumes the DSM-III-R category of avoidant disorder of childhood or adolescence. DSM-IV includes criteria and discussion for a childhood onset of social phobia.

Finally, there is a significant change in the use of Axis IV, which in DSM-III-R was termed "severity of psychosocial stressors" and included severity ratings, coding, and types of stressors to be considered. DSM-IV conceptualizes Axis IV as "psychosocial and environmental problems," grouped together as indicated in Table 5–1. Axis IV is to be used for recording external stressors, not for the impairment caused by symptoms of the disorder(s). The coding and severity rating scales for Axis IV are no longer used in DSM-IV. It is recognized that these psychosocial and environmental factors often play a role in the onset or exacerbation of a psychiatric disorder and inform the diagnosis, treatment, and prognosis of disorders. Identifying them is a key part of the biopsychosocial formulation. Often they are of particular urgency in the management of child and adolescent patients.

DSM-IV-TR

The text revision of DSM-IV, DSM-IV-TR (American Psychiatric Association 2000), was developed to reflect new research since the publication of DSM-IV. With very few exceptions, changes were made only in the text of the manual, not in the criteria themselves or in the grouping or names of diagnoses.

The goals were to correct errors and clarify ambiguities and to use empirical data to refine sections of

TABLE 5–1.   DSM-IV Axis IV psychosocial and environment problems

Problems with primary support group

Problems related to the social environment

Educational problems

Occupational problems

Housing problems

Economic problems

Problems with access to health care services

Problems related to interaction with the legal system/crime

Other psychosocial and environmental problems

the manual describing symptoms, associated features, etiology, comorbidity, course, and prognosis.

An exception to the rule of not changing criteria was made in the "Tic Disorders" section (including Tourette's disorder): The requirement for "clinically significant distress or impairment" (that had been added to the majority of disorders in DSM-IV) was removed.

In addition, the description of how to use the Global Assessment of Functioning (GAF) to rate Axis V was clarified. Generally, the lowest level of functioning in the past week is rated, with the score determined by the lowest area of functioning.

Other Diagnostic Criteria Sets

Two other diagnostic systems have been developed for populations of patients or professionals who have not been well served by either the DSM or ICD models. A collaboration between the American Academy of Pediatrics and the American Psychiatric Association (including representatives of the American Academy of Child and Adolescent Psychiatry) developed the *Diagnostic and Statistical Manual for Primary Care* (DSM-PC), Child and Adolescent Version (American Academy of Pediatrics 1996). This is designed to be used by pediatricians and family physicians to classify emotional and behavioral problems seen in office primary care practice. It includes a system for coding "Situation" that might be producing a child's symptoms and three clusters of "Child Manifestations": developmental variations, problems requiring intervention, and disorders (for those children who meet DSM-IV criteria for a disorder).

The DSM system has very limited utility for infants and toddlers. To address the need for diagnoses and criteria tailored for very young children, the Zero to Three/National Center for Clinical Infant Programs Diagnostic Classification Task Force (1994) developed a diagnostic classification system. This was recently revised (Zero to Three 2005) based on clinical experience using the 1994 system as well as empirical research. The goals of this system are to increase the recognition of mental health and developmental challenges in young children and to use diagnostic criteria effectively. It is aimed at a multidisciplinary group of professionals and emphasizes the contributions of relationships and developmental factors. It is intended to assist in developing treatment plans.

RDC for psychiatric disorders in infant and preschool children are being developed by a cadre of child psychiatrist and psychologist experts in psychopathology research in young children (Task Force on Research Diagnostic Criteria: Infancy Preschool 2003).

Future Directions: Toward DSM-V

Because each new version of DSM introduces discontinuities into clinical care, administrative systems, and research, and in order to commission and complete targeted research, a decision was made that DSM-V will be published no sooner than 2012. In 1999, a DSM-V Research Planning Conference was convened by the American Psychiatric Association and NIMH to work together on an agenda to expand the scientific basis for psychiatric diagnosis and classification. An additional goal is to unify the ICD-11 system for psychiatric disorders and DSM-V. In 2000, additional multidisciplinary conferences were held to set the research agenda. Planning work groups developed a series of white papers (Kupfer et al. 2002) setting out the issues to be considered for various age groups and diagnoses and to specify what new research is required to clarify and improve the validity and reliability of the diagnostic system. Each diagnosis has its own list of detailed questions (often controversial) to be answered (or at least addressed). Key topics identified as in need of research included:

- Improved understanding of specific versus shared risk factors, symptoms, and correlates among disorders currently considered to be discrete, but often found to be comorbid
- Age and gender considerations in how disorders are manifested and whether and how diagnostic criteria should differ with developmental stage
- How dimensional (scalar) approaches could improve DSM's categorical structure
- Incorporation of relational (interpersonal) processes and disorders to facilitate diagnosis and treatment

- Contributions from research in genetics, developmental neuroscience, brain imaging, postmortem brain studies, cognitive psychology, family studies, and animal models of behavior
- How culture should inform psychiatric diagnosis

Other issues that are of particular concern with respect to child and adolescent disorders include how to assess impairment, the effects of the multiple interactions between the child and the child's environment (an ecological model), and how best to integrate information from multiple reporters (youth, mother, father, teacher).

International meetings followed from 2004 to 2008. The task force to oversee the development of DSM-V was appointed in 2007, and the members of the 13 work groups for each diagnostic group were announced in 2008. Updates on the process are posted at http://www.dsmv.org.

Summary Points

- In DSM-IV, ADHD is no longer considered to be a disruptive behavior disorder.
- The ADHD subtypes combined, predominantly inattentive, and predominantly hyperactive-impulsive first appeared in DSM-IV.
- The only DSM-IV disorders coded on Axis II are mental retardation and personality disorders.
- The only criterion change made in the transition from DSM-IV to DSM-IV-TR was that the requirement of clinically significant distress or impairment was removed from all of the tic disorders.
- The Zero to Three/National Center for Clinical Infant Programs has developed a diagnostic classification system for psychiatric and developmental disorders in infants and toddlers.
- The creation of DSM-V will make use of a broad range of expertise, and the results will incorporate detailed reviews of existing studies as well as specifically commissioned research. Publication is anticipated in 2012.

References

American Academy of Pediatrics: The Classification of Child and Adolescent Mental Diagnoses in Primary Care: Diagnostic and Statistical Manual for Primary Care (DSM-PC), Child and Adolescent Version. Chicago, IL, American Academy of Pediatrics, 1996

American Psychiatric Association: Diagnostic and Statistical Manual: Mental Disorders. Washington, DC, American Psychiatric Association, 1952

American Psychiatric Association: Diagnostic and Statistical Manual of Mental Disorders, 2nd Edition. Washington, DC, American Psychiatric Association, 1968

American Psychiatric Association: Diagnostic and Statistical Manual of Mental Disorders, 3rd Edition. Washington, DC, American Psychiatric Association, 1980

American Psychiatric Association: Diagnostic and Statistical Manual of Mental Disorders, 3rd Edition, Revised. Washington, DC, American Psychiatric Association, 1987

American Psychiatric Association: Diagnostic and Statistical Manual of Mental Disorders, 4th Edition. Washington, DC, American Psychiatric Association, 1994

American Psychiatric Association: Diagnostic and Statistical Manual of Mental Disorders, 4th Edition, Text Revision. Washington, DC, American Psychiatric Association, 2000

First MB, Frances A, Pincus HA: DSM-IV-TR Guidebook. Washington, DC, American Psychiatric Publishing, 2004

Group for the Advancement of Psychiatry: Psychopathological Disorders in Childhood: Theoretical Considerations and a Proposed Classification, Vol 6. New York, Group for the Advancement of Psychiatry, 1966

Kanner L: Child Psychiatry. Baltimore, MD, Charles C Thomas, 1935

Kanner L: Child Psychiatry, 3rd Edition. Baltimore, MD, Charles C Thomas, 1957

Kupfer DJ, First MB, Regier DA: A Research Agenda for DSM-V. Washington, DC, American Psychiatric Publishing, 2002

Task Force on Research Diagnostic Criteria: Infancy Preschool: Research Diagnostic Criteria for Infants and Preschool Children: The process and empirical support. J Am Acad Child Adolesc Psychiatry 42:1504–1512, 2003

World Health Organization: International Classification of Diseases, 8th Revision. Geneva, Switzerland, World Health Organization, 1969

World Health Organization: International Statistical Classification of Diseases and Related Health Problems, 10th Revision. Geneva, Switzerland, World Health Organization, 1992

Zero to Three/National Center for Clinical Infant Programs Diagnostic Classification Task Force: Diagnostic Classification of Mental Health and Developmental Disorders of Infancy and Early Childhood. Arlington, VA, The Zero to Three/National Center for Clinical Infant Programs, 1994

Zero to Three: Diagnostic Classification of Mental Health and Developmental Disorders of Infancy and Early Childhood, Revised (DC:0–3R). Arlington, VA, The Zero to Three/National Center for Clinical Infant Programs, 2005

Chapter 6

The Process of Assessment and Diagnosis

John D. O'Brien, M.D.
Alexander Kolevzon, M.D.

The purpose of a psychiatric evaluation is to answer several fundamental questions: Does this child or adolescent have one or more psychiatric disorders? If the answer is yes, the next question confronting the clinician is, What is/are the disorder(s)? (Do the symptoms and their patterns fit a known recognizable clinical syndrome or diagnosis?) The next question is, How does this come to be? (What are the factors—biological, psychological, and social—that have influenced this child or adolescent and his family to be in their current state and present for evaluation?) The final fundamental question for the evaluation is, What is the recommended treatment (if any)?

These are very complex questions and require the collecting, sifting, and prioritizing of data from many sources. While there are several supplemental ways to gather information about a child and his family (e.g., agency reports, questionnaires, and rating scales), the clinical interview of both the parents and child is the primary source of information that will be used to come to a diagnosis, formulate a case, and provide a treatment plan. This chapter focuses on the process of assessment, diagnosis, and treatment planning. The direct interview of the child at various ages is covered in Chapter 1, "Assessing Infants and Toddlers"; Chapter 2, "Assessing the Preschool-Age Child"; Chapter 3, "Assessing the Elementary School–Age Child"; and Chapter 4, "Assessing Adolescents."

Some general comments must be kept in mind regarding the assessment process, which is too often focused on what is wrong with the child. It is essential to also look at the strengths and assets of the child, the family, and their environment. What are the factors that help to facilitate a child's normal developmental trajectory? Often a parent will come in with a litany of complaints about the child. It is important for the clinician to listen carefully but then to ask a question such as "What are the things your child does well?" or "What about your child makes you proud?"

No assessment is complete without including an evaluation of the impairment caused by the syndrome—often referred to as *severity*. This level of impairment or severity needs to be ascertained to answer the question of whether intervention is needed, what kind of intervention, and in what time frame. For example, for the symptom of aggression, is the aggression at home, at school, on the playground? Is the aggression toward the self, others, or both? How has this symptom affected the patient's relationships with family, peers, and so forth? The answers to these questions not only give the clinician a picture of the impact caused by the symptom but also point the way to various interventions. Severity often influences clinical decision making in assessing the urgency of intervention. Is the aggression affecting safety, of either self or others? If so, the clinician needs to act quickly to prevent harm.

The evaluation of any child requires the use by the clinician of a developmental framework. The clinician, through his or her knowledge of development, has in mind an idea of what the average expectable child will be like at any given age. The child will be compared to a developmental standard as the clinician seeks to discover if this child's behavior or degree of competence in any particular area differs significantly from that of the child's peers. The pediatrician uses height and weight charts to assess a child's physical growth. The psychiatric clinician does not have such specifics but applies the same process of evaluation of normality and deviation from it. The developmental perspective brings the clinician back to the aforementioned issue of impairment: How do the present impairments caused by the child's symptoms affect the developmental tasks of the child and the acquisition of new skills? Finally, does the current adaptation and set of problems reflect a disorder rooted in earlier developmental periods, and/or how will this current status affect later development? While these questions are paramount in the mind of the clinician, these are the same questions that parents will ask, particularly related to future functioning.

Comparison of Adult Assessment With Child Assessment

Sullivan's (1954) definition of an adult psychiatric interview is "a situation of primarily *vocal* communica-

tion in a *two-group*, more or less *voluntarily integrated*, on a progressively unfolding *expert-client* basis for the purpose of elucidating *characteristic patterns of living* of the subject person, the patient or client, which patterns he experiences as particularly troublesome or especially valuable, and in the revealing of which he expects to derive *benefit*" (p. 4).

The prime source of information in the evaluation of an adult is the person himself. There are some exceptions to this, particularly in the geriatric population where other informants, especially caregivers, are needed. Multiple sources, especially the parents, constitute the field for data collection with children. At the very least, Sullivan's "two group" becomes a three group or a four group (in intact families). Teachers, guidance counselors, and foster care workers all contribute essential data. The overwhelming majority of child assessments need information from the school regarding not only academic status but also social relatedness to peers and adults. It would be quite unusual for a psychiatrist to request information from the employer of an adult patient. A child psychiatrist sees contacting the school and other agencies as a necessary and vital part of a complete evaluation. Children are strongly affected by their environment, and the evaluation needs to take that into account.

The interchange between psychiatrist and adult patient is generally verbal, with some data gathered from nonverbal communication. While this is true for most adolescents, the younger the child, the more central is the role of play in the evaluation process. How a child plays and what he plays is a window to the child and his world. In assessing the infant or preschool child, there is less emphasis on verbal production, and the clinician needs to be well versed in the popular toys, video games, and so forth that form an important part of a child's life.

The issue of volitional participation is another area of difference. Children are brought to the evaluation; they rarely seek it out. Infants and children are brought because, in general, their behavior is bothersome to others, not necessarily to themselves. An old-fashioned example illustrates this point. If Johnny puts Mary's pigtail in the inkwell, who has the problem? If the individual does not see himself as having a problem, the person certainly will not seek help.

The concept of the psychiatrist as expert is not easily grasped by a child. Adults generally see the psychiatrist as someone from whom they can benefit, even though they may approach the process with trepidation. Generally, when children come to see a doctor, they have two associations—needles and white coats. As a result, this issue has to be dealt with in preparing the child for evaluation. Most children do not see the doctor as particularly helpful. In fact, children are wary of the experience and often see the psychiatrist as an annoyance, someone who takes them away from their baseball game, video game, etc. The usual positive expectations that provide motivation for the initial phases of adult evaluation are absent with children. Thus, the child and adolescent psychiatrist has to work much harder to establish rapport and a working relationship with the child, who often regards him or her with suspicion or even as an agent of the parents or the school. The primary purpose of the initial phase of an assessment is to put the child at ease, present to him in language he is able to understand the purpose of the assessment and why he is there, and establish a working relationship. It must be emphasized that the evaluation is a collaboration among the parents, the child, and the physician. All three parties work together to facilitate the psychiatric evaluation.

Data Collection

The assessment of children and adolescents must be multifaceted. The clinician assesses multiple domains and dimensions of functioning, regardless of the reason for referral. Information is gathered about various situations from diverse informants, using multiple methods.

In addition to focusing on the nature and type of the specific referral problem, the clinician should assess all areas of the child's functioning and various dimensions of the child's capabilities, including cognitive abilities and interpersonal relationships (home and peers). The clinician should also assess for other symptoms that may be comorbid with the presenting problem.

Information concerning child and adolescent functioning in four different areas (home, school, with peers, with himself or herself) needs to be gathered:

1. How does the child function at home? This information can be obtained from parents, the child himself, babysitters, siblings, grandparents, etc.
2. The school is the child's workplace, where he spends much time. Again the clinician looks to the child and parents. However, teachers, guidance counselors, and principals are the main sources of information in this area, with parental consent for contact. Not only does the clinician get data regarding academic progress from the school, but the school also can give valuable information regarding the child's peer relationships and relationships with those in authority.
3. The clinician gets data on peer relationships from parents, children themselves, and school reports. An opportunity to actually observe the child with peers provides uniquely valuable information. Peers have a great deal of knowledge about other children, but it is difficult to tap this source of information without breaking confidentiality. Knowledge about current and past relationships is crucial in assessing a child's social and interpersonal competence.
4. All too frequently neglected is how the child views himself. Collateral information can be gathered from parents and the school, but the major source of data is the child himself. Often this cannot be assessed directly. The clinician must use indirect means such as drawings, dreams, and fantasy questions.

What are the tools or instruments that the clinician uses to view these four domains? What do clinicians do in the clinical setting to complete an assessment? They use some or all of the following: an interview with the parents and/or significant others; observation and interview of the child; family interviews; behavioral ratings by parents, teachers, the child, and significant others; physical examination; neurological examination; psychological and neuropsychological testing; and various biological and laboratory measures.

The relative value of each of these components in evaluating a particular child varies with the child's age, developmental state, and presenting problems. Interviews with the parents, observation of and interviews with the child, and use of behavioral rating scales in different settings are essential for any psychiatric assessment done today. Each element can provide unique information. In certain cases, specialized psychological testing, laboratory measures, and physical and neurological exams may add useful information. The important point is that sufficient data be collected to assess all areas of current functioning of the child and, using a developmental history, to assess functioning from birth to the present.

Beginning the Process

The initial contact for the evaluation most likely begins with a telephone call from the parents, who may be acting on their own or in conjunction with or at the behest of an agency, such as the school. This initial contact is important because it sets a tone for the evaluation process to come. The person taking the call must remember that parents have many emotions related to this call, most commonly anxiety. The usual identifying data are taken about *both* the parents and child. In some instances, who has custody of the child and who can give permission for the evaluation to take place become an issue. This is particularly true for children in foster care and in divorce situations. A brief history of the reason for the referral is then taken. Obviously, the information gatherer needs to assess if the presenting problem constitutes an emergency, and if so, deal with that issue. (Emergencies are discussed in Chapter 39, "Psychiatric Emergencies.") The contact person explains to the parent in as succinct and clear a way as possible the process of the evaluation. Depending on a variety of factors, such as age and clinic policy, the parents may be seen first. For adolescents, the identified patient may be seen initially. In some instances the family as a whole will be seen. Whatever the process, it should be clearly explained. A general description of what will happen in each part of the evaluation is discussed, such as that the parents will be seen by the clinician to gather their ideas about the problem and a developmental history. Some estimate of the length of each session and who is expected to be there is given. If previous evaluations have been done or there is pertinent current collateral information, parents are asked to either send it in advance or bring it with them. When school problems are at issue, then report cards, special education evaluations, results of psychological testing, and so forth need to be included. It is helpful if previous data can be reviewed prior to the first meeting. Finally, payment, such as fees, insurance coverage, authorization, or other issues, needs to be discussed. Thoroughness and directness are necessary so that parents can be prepared for the process. It is important to ask if there are any questions and to inform the parents whom to contact with questions or additional information. Although this process may be lengthy, such completeness at the beginning saves time later and facilitates forming an alliance with parents that is crucial to the successful completion of the evaluation.

The Parent Interview

The purposes of the parental interview include gathering data about the current problem; what interven-

tions, if any, have been previously tried; and a detailed developmental history. The clinician aims to assess parental understanding of the problem and expectations of the assessment, as well as parenting strengths and weaknesses. For treatment planning, it is important to get a sense of how the parents might view treatment recommendations. For example, some parents may strenuously object to the use of medication. The parental interview also serves to gather information that may help the clinician in approaching the child, such as favorite activities, interests, and strengths. Finally, the parent interview gives the clinician an opportunity to determine what preparation, if any, the parents have given to the child for the evaluation and, if necessary, to recommend other approaches that may facilitate the child's participation. This process also gives clues to how the child is perceived in the family and the degree of thoughtfulness and caring the parents show their offspring.

It is extremely important to ascertain what the parents want from the evaluation and immediately deal with inappropriate expectations. The parents, child, referring agency, and so forth likely have different goals for the process.

Case Example

A mother of a 9-year-old boy sought evaluation because she felt the visitation schedule set out in the divorce settlement was a burden for her son and was affecting his schoolwork. I made it clear from the beginning that I would not get involved in revisiting the divorce agreement or testify in court. The mother herself was a lawyer. She agreed to my focus and said this is what she wanted. After much work evaluating the mother and her husband, the child's father, and the child alone and with each parent and discussions with the school, I proposed a plan that I felt would put the least onus on the child. The mother immediately rejected it. It became clear that her real purpose was to change the custody judgment and show her ex-husband to be a poor father (which was not the case). When the plan was not to her liking, she revealed her real reason for the evaluation and refused to pay for the last session. Even though what I would do was initially made clear, she had a very different expectation. Every effort should be made at the very outset to have a frank discussion of what the evaluation is for and what can or cannot be accomplished.

It is important to make it clear to the parents that this is not treatment but an evaluation and that the evaluation may or may not lead to intervention. The clinician needs to focus on getting the data, formulating the data, arriving at a diagnosis, and establishing a treatment plan (which may or may not involve the evaluating clinician). An alliance with the parents and child not only will form the basis for a good evaluation but will set the groundwork for whatever future work may be needed.

The confidentiality of the sessions between the child and the clinician needs to be discussed upfront with the parents and child. Parents are reminded that unless there is an overriding reason (such as a danger to self or others), the specifics of the interactions between the clinician and child are confidential. However, what is said between the parents and the therapist may be brought up with the child. It is not uncommon for parents to come to the clinician after the first session and ask how it went or if the child did or said this or that. The clinician might share in advance with the parents that they may be curious about the session but that details will not be reported back to them unless, for example, there is a safety concern.

Preparation of the Child for the Interview

The parents' preparation of the child for the interview can be crucial for its success or failure.

Case Example

In one instance, a parent sought consultation regarding her teenage son, who was presenting with a somatic symptom. It was a very complicated case, and the mother had not told her son she was seeking an evaluation. I discussed with her in great detail how to present to him the need and reason for evaluation. He had been seen by other medical subspecialists. She asked if she could tell him it was another medical evaluation (as opposed to a psychiatric one). I told her that would not work because the adolescent would feel deceived and tricked, which would negatively affect the process. I reinforced with her what I had said previously. The boy arrived promptly and we began speaking. I explained who I was and what I intended to do. He jumped up and said that he thought I was another type of specialist, that he certainly did not need to see a shrink, and ran from the room. His mother then confessed she had lied to him about my specialty and the purpose of the session. Despite strenuous efforts, he would not continue the evaluation.

Obviously, how the parents approach this issue will depend on the age of the child, the purpose of the evaluation, and the parent-child relationship. The idea that the child has nothing to fear from the evaluation and the doctor (e.g., no needles) needs to be conveyed by the parents and later the clinician. The best way to

do this is a forthright discussion of the symptom or issue at hand. The clinician works with children who have troubles at home, or at school, or with other children. He or she is an expert in children's troubles. He or she is a talking doctor and may also play and draw. This direct approach works well with most children. With younger children, the clinician is quite concrete about the problem and its consequences. With adolescents, it is helpful to discuss the effect the symptom has on their social and psychological lives.

Other Sources of Data

The clinician should obtain (with permission) information from others in the child's community. This information gives other viewpoints about the child. Bringing this information back to the interview with parents, child, or family may stimulate further disclosure and discussion essential to diagnosis and treatment. Asking parents what they think and how they feel about the various reports provides data on how they see the problem, their defensive maneuvers (denial, blaming, and so forth), their motivation for change, and how they may view treatment recommendations.

The most important of these "outside" reports is the school report. Teachers spend long periods of time with the child, and they observe the child's response to work demands and learning. They are able to compare the child with same-age peers. The school is also the natural setting for interactions with other children. At school, the child's behavior and symptoms can be different from anywhere else. The behavior in school must be compared with the behavior at home and in the office (on a one-to-one basis). Another important source of information is the pediatrician, who often contributes both a medical perspective and a longitudinal view of the child's and family's development. Particularly important is whether he or she had seen the need for and recommended psychiatric evaluation and how that recommendation was presented and received. Data can be gathered from other agencies, such as child welfare or protective services, foster care, and courts.

The clinician should remember to get information about hobbies, group activities, and athletics. These can help the clinician understand how the child organizes his life and follows rules, what his capacity to function as a team member is, what his competitive strategies are, and how he sees himself in relation to others. The child's willingness to accept delays, capacity to persevere, ability to organize a project, and creativity can be estimated from these activities.

Family Assessment

Some clinicians prefer to have a family interview as a part of the assessment process. This can be helpful in many ways, particularly if it is the initial contact beginning the evaluation. With the family together, the clinician can clarify why the child is being brought for evaluation and inform everyone about the evaluation process. On the other hand, such a meeting can be held at any time during the evaluation process or not at all. The Group for the Advancement of Psychiatry (1973) listed eight major reasons for a family interview: to establish "the nature of the family as a unit (stable, cohesive, divisive, close, distant), the family capacity for cooperation with treatment plans, the psychologic-mindedness of members of the family, the capacity for communication among family members, the degree of mental health or ill health of the family as a unit or in terms of the individual members, the role of the child's disorder in the psychic economy of the family (secondary gain, or family misuse of the child's disorder), the relationship of the family to the community (distant, isolated, involved) and the subcultural values dominant in the family."

In a family interview, the clinician is able to glimpse the ways the members of the family live with each other. Whether or not the family interactions contribute to the child's problems, they can be helpful or detrimental to a treatment proposal. Family members other than the identified patient may suffer from stressful interactions within the family or may be negatively affected by the child's symptoms. This is particularly true of siblings in a family with a developmentally disabled or chronically physically or emotionally ill child. Finally, in any family assessment interview, the clinician needs to establish that the group is embarking on an effort to find real solutions to real problems and not to assign blame.

Formulation

One of the most crucial phases of the evaluation process is the formulation, which is too often misunderstood or neglected. A common error is to simply repeat the history, instead of constructing a formulation of a case.

"The presence of symptoms is only a starting point, not sufficient by itself for us to understand the context, feelings or behavior behind them" (Jellinek and McDermott 2004, p. 914). Formulations are typically organized in one of two ways: using a biopsychosocial approach and/or a shortened form of a temporal axis (Ebert et al. 2000, pp. 520–521). In the biopsychosocial model, those variables that influence the child and family to present in their current state are grouped into three categories: biological, psychological, and social. Biological factors include, but are not limited to, genetic, pregnancy and birth factors, and medical illnesses. Some examples of psychological factors are the child's and family's level of development, self-esteem, and ego defenses. Social variables include family functioning, spiritual and cultural issues, and peers. Ebert et al. (2000) suggest another viewpoint—that of looking at factors along a time axis grouped as predisposing, precipitating, perpetuating, and prognostic. *Predisposing factors* are genetic heritability, intrauterine or perinatal insults, neglect, and so forth. *Precipitating factors* are defined as stressors (e.g., physical illness, loss, or divorce) that test the coping mechanisms and cause signs and symptoms to occur. *Perpetuating factors* (e.g., continuous trauma or parental style) are those that reinforce symptomatology. *Prognostic factors* are those that influence a child's symptom future, duration of illness, severity of illness, time of onset of illness, etc. Whatever the system the clinician uses, "a formulation is necessary to sift, prioritize, and integrate the data for treatment planning" (Jellinek and McDermott 2004, p. 913).

The formulation leads to a differential diagnosis wherein the clinician considers the most likely diagnoses and chooses one or more that are consistent with the data. The purpose of the entire process is to make treatment recommendations tailored for the child and the family.

Treatment Planning

The Group for the Advancement of Psychiatry (1973) puts forth this definition: "Differential treatment planning consists of selecting, in order of priority, curative, corrective, ameliorative or palliative approaches to the child patient, his family, and, when needed, his extended environment. Such planning takes the fullest advantage of the available assets of the child, his family and the community" (p. 546). Looney (1984) makes the case for treatment planning: "The skillful matching of a child's problems with appropriate interventions is as important as either an accurate assessment of the nature of those problems or a skillful application of any modality of treatment. A misalignment of a child's constellation of problems with an array of therapeutic interventions even if those interventions are artfully administered, may lead to an unsatisfactory outcome" (p. 529). Treatment planning is done by the clinician or clinical team after the formulation and differential diagnosis. The clinician has found a set of problems that besets the child, family, and/or community, as well as assets or strengths that can be used to help alleviate these problems. Both behavioral and psychodynamic paradigms are useful. In child work, a combination is usually done. These problems and interventions then need to be put in terms understandable to the family and child.

Ebert et al. (2000, pp. 523–524) put forth a highly structured approach to treatment planning, which is called Goal-Directed Treatment Planning. This approach emphasizes *pivotal foci,* which are "factors external or internal that activate, reinforce or perpetuate psychopathology." *Goals* are the aims a clinician wants to achieve. A goal is a focus preceded by a verb. For example, a focus might be depressed mood (the problem) preceded by a verb (e.g., alleviate depressed mood). There may be a variety of goals, which lead to different verbs, such as reduce the frequency or intensity of, stabilize, or facilitate. To these are added *objectives,* which are things "the patient will be able to do or exhibit at the end of that stage of treatment." For Ebert's group, the objective is stated in behavioral terms (e.g., the child will be able to not fight or hold his temper). Finally, "for each goal, the clinician selects a therapy or set of therapies, according to the following criteria: most empirical support, resource availability (i.e., clinical resource, time, finances), least risk, greatest economy (i.e., time, expense) and appropriateness to family values and intervention style." As treatment progresses, the goals are monitored and revised as necessary.

In summary, the process is to identify 1) the problems, 2) what changes in the problems the clinician wishes to see, 3) the order in which the clinician needs to deal with them, and 4) the interventions most appropriate not only to the problem but to this child and his family.

The order of interventions must be considered. Obviously, the acuity of a situation or safety issues will determine what is to be addressed first. However, in most cases the problems are semiacute or chronic. In some cases, a child may be so depressed that medication may be needed first before the child can use any other type of psychotherapy. Or in the reverse case, the clinician may need to start with psychotherapy to form an alliance with the patient so that he may become more disposed to take medication. In conjunction with the child and the family, the clinician may choose a problem of lesser severity to work on initially because it is more amenable to timely intervention. Thus the clinician has an experience of success to build on to approach more complex issues. Looney (1984) sees treatment planning as having two basic steps: "The first is to formulate the problems and to state them in a commonsense manner so that they can be understood by the child and those referring the child for treatment. In addition, problems should be formulated in such a way that points of intervention and a reasonable order of progression of treatment are clear. The second step is to choose treatment modalities which would be most powerful, most rapid, least restrictive and most cost effective" (p. 530). Supported by this process of thinking, the clinician approaches the next evaluation phase.

Interpretative or Feedback Interview

The purpose of the interpretive or feedback interview is to inform the parents and child what has been found and what the clinician, with their help, would recommend to address the issues for which they came. This often is more complicated than in adult psychiatry where the clinician generally has one patient. In the evaluation of a child, both parents and child need to hear and understand what the clinician says, and their participation in the process needs to be encouraged and enlisted. Also, the issues for which they came may be the tip of the iceberg and lead to discovery of other problems that were not initially apparent. For example, a child's fighting behavior in school may be a reaction to the loss of a beloved grandparent, with subsequent depression. This sequence needs to be identified and explained.

For the parents, it is useful to start with a summary of what has been done in the assessment process and proceed from there to the findings. It is very important to put the findings in language that is understood by the parents, and it is helpful to give concrete examples from the history as well as the interview to illustrate and support conclusions drawn. Parents may need help to understand that human behavior, especially children's behavior, is shaped by many interacting variables, not a single cause, and because of this complexity, multiple interventions may be needed.

For many, "the evaluation is a crisis for the family, for though they may be aware that something has been wrong for a long time, the diagnosis…confronts them with the reality" (O'Brien et al. 1992, p. 113). Often, the presentation of the results precipitates a state of anxiety akin to an acute stress reaction. There is shock, even numbness and loss of focus. The clinician needs to be as supportive as possible, explaining what the diagnosis means, how it affects present functioning, what factors contributed to the genesis of the problem, and what needs to be done. The clinician may have to repeat these points several times, because the emotional state of the parents affects their ability to process the information.

Often guilt and anger come to the fore. Parents may ask what they did wrong. At this time, the clinician returns to the statement that behavior is multidetermined. Parents may blame each other or the school. Under these circumstances, emphasis is put on the future, not the past. How can we alter relationships and attitudes to change the situation? Often it is necessary to allow parents to ventilate their feelings about the evaluation and their present situation (O'Brien et al. 1992): "It is not uncommon for the anxiety of making the unknown known to further solidify previous unhealthy patterns. Thus, an overprotective parent may become more intrusive and overinvolved in the child's life. This tendency should be discussed with the parents and examples in their behavior pointed out" (O'Brien et al. 1992, p. 115).

The interview needs to focus on collaboration among the various participants. What is *each participant*—parent(s), child, clinician, agencies, and so forth—going to do to address the issue? Obviously, major emphasis here will be on the family, child, and clinician. While the clinician addresses problems, the clinician should include the positive aspects of the child and family and how these can be used to deal with the problems and form a treatment plan.

The clinician shares with the family the process of treatment planning. What are the family's thoughts about the goals and objectives, and how realistic and applicable are they to the family situation? The more active the parents are in setting up the treatment, the more likely they are to participate in the treatment process and facilitate their child's participation.

A major objective of the feedback session is to help parents realistically appraise their situation and their child. This is especially true for children who have a developmental disability or a chronic illness. In these circumstances, parents need to reevaluate the child and their expectations of the child (O'Brien et al. 1992). For these parents, "the primary issue that has to be worked through is the loss and subsequent mourning of the idealized child" (O'Brien et al. 1992, p. 113).

The clinician should always ask the parents for their understanding of what has been said and how they feel about it. This gives the clinician a chance to see how much the parents heard and understood and to correct any distortions. Parents are urged to go home and discuss the recommendation together and, depending on the age of the child, with the child. Parents are encouraged to ask questions now and in the future. They are given the clinician's telephone number in case they have questions or concerns.

How the clinician talks with the child about the findings is related to the age of the child. With preschoolers, the emphasis is on helping do something or attain something, and considerable assistance is needed from the parents. With school-age children, the clinician deals with concrete issues, such as "help you learn better at school" or "help you get along better with other children." With this age group, the clinician may say, "You came here because of this issue, and this is how we intend to help you with the problem." With early school-age children, the clinician focuses on behavior and doing things. With later school-age children, the clinician can introduce concepts of emotions and inner emotional states (e.g., "We want to help you be happier and less sad"). With adolescents, the clinician addresses a mixture of behavior and feelings, particularly about the self (e.g., "We want you to feel less depressed and feel better about yourself"). Parents need to be told how the child is being approached so they can reinforce the process in the home.

The study by Yeh and Weisz (2001) raises an important point that needs to be considered in any assessment of a child and his or her family. According to their study, "more than 60% of the parent-child pairs failed to agree on even a single problem for which the child needed help" (p. 1022). Yeh and Weisz suggest that "it may be wise for clinicians to assess parent and child concerns independently and then bring parents and child together to formulate joint goals" (p. 1024). They caution that "whatever the response of therapists and clinics, our findings suggest that parent-child discrepancies in perceived problems can be so pronounced at the beginning of clinic care that it would be unwise to leave them unassessed and unaddressed" (pp. 1024–1025).

When communicating information to others, the clinician should be judicious. No information can be shared without parental (and sometimes adolescent) permission. It is wise for the clinician to summarize what he or she intends to say and even to show parents the reports that will be sent. A large percentage of referrals come at the behest of the school or indicate at least some difficulty at school. Information should be given that relates to school functioning only. Personal issues such as family history of mental illness or marital strife are not shared with school personnel. How to help the child academically, such as small class size, extra time to complete tasks, and sitting near the teacher, should be addressed. Some suggestions related to social interchanges and peer relationships may also be warranted. Information sent to the school is subject to distribution and discussion with numerous people and needs to be given with great care.

Feedback to pediatricians, again with parental knowledge and consent, should be prompt and specific to the question asked and not be a detailed description, especially about personal issues. What the clinician sees as the problem and what he or she intends to do and how he or she intends to do it should be the focus rather than how things came to be the way they are. Obviously, if the clinician is working closely with a pediatrician on a problem such as nonadherence in a diabetic child, parents and child need to know that there will be continuous and in-depth exchange of information with the pediatrician but that certain information will not be shared.

In working with any agency, parents need to know what the clinician feels are the goals for that agency, such as a more appropriate class or supervised visitation for relatives, and the best way to approach the agencies and work with them. The clinician and parents need to discuss how these goals will affect the child and the treatment plan. Thus, clinician and parents form an alliance to promote change for the child in his environment.

There is a very high rate of dropout in the treatment of children, adolescents, and their families. Establishing an accurate diagnosis through a complete evaluation and formulation and forming an alliance with parents and child through the process of evaluation are the surest ways of helping parents and child enter into treatment positively. A helpful experience in the evaluation process will motivate parents and child to follow through on the treatment that is recommended and bodes well for its success.

Summary Points

- The purpose of a psychiatric evaluation of a child (or adolescent) is to ascertain if the child has a psychiatric disorder and what the next step(s) should be. A child may present with a set of symptoms that may be reactions to environmental circumstances, either familial or school. Who is the patient? is an important question in the evaluation.

- Any evaluation must proceed from a developmental framework.

- A psychiatric evaluation of a child is different from that of an adult.

- Data must be collected from multiple sources, detailing the child's functioning at home, in school, with peers, and alone.

- The child and parental interviews, behavioral ratings, and a recent physical exam form the core of every evaluation. Psychological testing and the like may be needed in specialized cases. (See Chapter 9, "Pediatric Evaluation and Laboratory Testing"; Chapter 10, "Neurological Examination, Electroencephalography, and Neuroimaging"; and Chapter 11, "Psychological and Neuropsychological Testing.")

- The process begins with the first telephone call, and the importance of that tone-setting interchange cannot be overestimated.

- The parental interview has many purposes, chief among which is collecting data (regarding present, past, and expectations) and helping parents prepare the child for his interview. The parental interview gives the clinician the opportunity to form an alliance with the parents, which is crucial to forming an alliance with the child and for involvement in future treatment, if needed.

- The formulation categorizes the biological, social, and psychological factors critical to the genesis of, sustaining of, and future of the psychiatric syndrome.

- Treatment planning matches the problems of child and family with the appropriate interventions in a timely, cost-effective way.
- The feedback interview presents to parents and child what was found and invites their participation in the process. This interview sets the groundwork for building on the alliances formed throughout the evaluation so that treatment flows naturally and smoothly from the evaluation.

References

Ebert MH, Loosen PT, Nurcombe B: Current Diagnosis and Treatment in Psychiatry. New York, McGraw-Hill, 2000

Group for the Advancement of Psychiatry: From diagnosis to treatment: an approach to treatment planning for the emotionally disturbed child. Rep Group Adv Psychiatry 8:517–662, 1973

Jellinek MS, McDermott JF: Formulation: putting the diagnosis into a therapeutic context and treatment plan. J Am Acad Child Adolesc Psychiatry 43:913–916, 2004

Looney J: Treatment planning in child psychiatry. J Am Acad Child Psychiatry 23:529–536, 1984

O'Brien JD, Pilowsky D, Lewis O: Psychotherapies With Children and Adolescents: Adapting the Psychodynamic Process. Washington, DC, American Psychiatric Press, 1992

Sullivan HS: The Collected Works of Harry Stack Sullivan, Vol I: The Psychiatric Interview. Edited by Perry HS, Gawel ML. New York, WW Norton, 1954

Yeh M, Weisz JR: Why are we here at the clinic? Parent-child (dis)agreement on referral problems at outpatient treatment entry. J Consult Clin Psychol 69:1018–1025, 2001

Chapter 7

Diagnostic Interviews

Lee Carlisle, M.D.
Jon M. McClellan, M.D.

The clinical interview remains the primary diagnostic tool for psychiatry. Despite extensive international research efforts, no valid biological markers with clinical utility for classifying psychiatric syndromes have yet been identified. Thus, the diagnostic process remains embedded within consensus-based, criterion-derived categories, using traditional interview and mental status examinations that define traditional medicine.

The psychiatric interview has evolved over time. Historically, a nondirective approach was promoted, using observations of unfettered discourse and play (in children) to elicit information and characterize thought processes. However, comparisons of different approaches suggest that a more directive systematic approach, with sensitivity toward the respondent's issues and concerns, provides more factual information (Cox et al. 1981).

Since the advent of the *Diagnostic and Statistical Manual of Mental Disorders* (DSM) and *International Classification of Diseases* (ICD) diagnostic systems, the focus on interviewing has shifted to a more disease-oriented approach. This change was prompted in part by the lack of clinician reliability in diagnosing recognized illnesses (e.g., schizophrenia, autism) and in part by the lack of an etiologic model on which to base a diagnostic system (McClellan and Werry 2000). Psychiatric diagnoses are defined by using a medical model, wherein each illness is assumed to be a distinct psychopathological entity, with definable symptom criteria. This allows clinicians, researchers, and administrative bodies (e.g., third-party payers, medical records departments) to communicate broadly about diagnostic entities with some expectation that the disorders are the same, or at least similar, across settings.

The subjective and variable nature of the symptom reports used to generate psychiatric diagnoses remains a limitation. Information derived from patients, their families, and other observers (e.g., teachers) is subtle, complex, and often conflicting (Achenbach 1987). Clinicians' diagnoses are potentially fraught with numerous biases (Angold 1999), including

- Making diagnoses before all relevant information is collected
- Collecting information selectively when confirming and/or ruling out a diagnosis
- Neglecting to be systematic in collecting and organizing information
- Allowing the clinician's particular expertise to influence diagnosis assignment (e.g., a physician in a mood disorders clinic diagnosing most patients' disorders as depression, regardless of each patient's clinical presentation)
- Assuming correlations between symptoms and illnesses that in reality are spurious or nonexistent (e.g., equating all irritability with mania).

The creation of diagnostic criteria helped structure the diagnostic process. However, even when the same diagnostic criteria are used, disagreements may still arise due to differences in wording of the questions or variable interpretations of either the question or the response. Furthermore, the respondent may have different perspectives over time in regard to the severity or existence of a problem. This is particularly an issue for child psychiatry, where children's symptoms often are somewhat context dependent and may fluctuate over time.

To address these limitations, various diagnostic tools have been developed to enhance the reliability of the information gathered and the diagnosis assignment. The two types of diagnostic tools commonly used by clinicians and researchers are diagnostic interviews and questionnaires. Questionnaires are usually completed by patients, parents, or other significant individuals (e.g., teachers) and generally focus on broader domains of psychopathology but may focus more narrowly on specific illness states or symptoms. For a thorough discussion of questionnaires and checklists pertinent to child and adolescent psychopathology, see Chapter 8 ("Rating Scales").

Structured diagnostic interviews are designed to elicit information from children and/or their parents about various aspects of functioning and mental health, including specific inquiries about symptom criteria for psychiatric disorders. They are primarily used for psychiatric research, both in epidemiological surveys and in clinical studies. The instruments vary as to whether they are administered by clinicians or trained interviewers, although some researchers have research assistants administer measures originally designed for

use by clinicians. Structured interviews were first developed to examine mental health problems in adults; interviews for use with children and adolescents and their families were subsequently developed. Many of the available measures have evolved over several versions, dating back to DSM-III (American Psychiatric Association 1980).

Interview Characteristics and Relevant Concepts

There are several characteristics and concepts relevant to the development, choice, use, and interpretation of structured diagnostic interviews.

Validity

Validity reflects the degree to which a measure or classification system accurately characterizes the entity it is examining. Types of validity include

- *Face validity*, or how well a category as defined appears to describe a recognized illness
- *Predictive validity*, or how well the category predicts a pertinent aspect of care, such as treatment needs or prognosis
- *Construct validity*, or whether the category has meaning in terms of what it is designed to describe (see below).

Childhood psychiatric disorders generally have face validity but not necessarily construct or predictive validity (Spitzer 1980). Some categories are better than others, but only a few disorders have been adequately studied (e.g., attention-deficit/hyperactivity disorder). Diagnostic validity is difficult to assess in psychiatry. Given the lack of biological markers, diagnoses made using a structured interview are often compared with those made by experienced clinicians. This approach is problematic because clinicians are notoriously unreliable at diagnostic assessments and may not represent the gold standard (Robins 1985). Furthermore, because the same diagnostic criteria define both methods, the validity of a diagnostic tool is not independent from the diagnostic criteria it assesses.

Some authors assess the construct validity of their diagnostic instruments as a method of inferring validity. Comparison is often made with a series of other measures that assess predictive and/or concurrent features of the disorder, using a strategy referred to as a nomological network (Cronbach and Meehl 1955). For example, the results of a diagnostic interview are compared with several pertinent theoretically related attributes, such as patterns and stability of diagnoses, independent ratings of psychopathology, service utilization, and family psychiatric history. Thus, by a process akin to triangulation, researchers examine the validity of a measure by determining its proximity to that of other theoretically related measures or attributes. The inferred validity of each measure supports the validity of the entire construct.

This method avoids the problems associated with defining a diagnostic gold standard. However, the diagnostic construct is only as valid as the measures or attributes used to define it. Validity of diagnostic concepts and constructs is often examined by comparing the results of diagnostic interviews with related questionnaires (e.g., determining the association between a diagnosis of major depressive disorder on a structured interview and the score on a depression rating scale). Because the same symptoms are assessed by both measures, the instruments are not truly independent. This type of validity test is commonly used, but it represents a circular logic that risks reifying the diagnostic criteria rather than establishing the validity of the disorder or the measure.

Another challenge is distinguishing between syndrome specificity and severity. Many measures used to predict validity assess functional impact (e.g., academic or social impairment). Although a diagnosis may be a good indicator of impairment, this is not unexpected, because impairment is usually one of the diagnostic criteria. Furthermore, although functional impairment is an important health issue, it does not imply specificity. The actual validity of the disorder itself—or the diagnostic criteria that define it—remains illusory.

Reliability

Reliability reflects agreement, including how often different interviewers assign the same diagnosis (interrater reliability), how consistently respondents report the same symptoms or diagnoses over time (test-retest reliability), and how internally consistent the measure is (i.e., the degree to which different sections of the measure give similar information).

Differences in diagnostic reliability may be due to 1) differences in the information collected, 2) theoretical biases held by diagnosticians, and/or 3) variations

in symptoms that individuals with disorders will experience over time (Susser et al. 2006). Diagnostic tools must be reliable to be useful, but reliability does not ensure validity. The two concepts are often confused. A diagnostic category may be reliably defined but not valid. Conversely, a disorder may be valid, but the diagnostic criteria, or the instruments used to assess for its presence, may not be reliable.

For categorical variables, reliability is generally measured using either percent agreement or the kappa statistic for categorical variables (Susser et al. 2006). The kappa statistic is preferred because it controls for the fact that high rates of agreement may be misleading when a disorder is rare, because most of the agreement will be for noncases. For continuous variables, either the product-moment correlation coefficient (r) or the intraclass correlation coefficient (ICC) is used to measure rater agreement. Cronbach's coefficient alpha is used to assess the internal consistency of a scale, which reflects how well different items measure similar information (Susser et al. 2006).

The methods used by investigators to establish reliability on a diagnostic interview raise some interesting questions. For example, establishing reliability at one site often means establishing agreement with the senior investigator. Many studies simply have other examiners watch and score the same interviews. It is not difficult to reach agreement regardless of whether one agrees with the conclusions. There is no guarantee that the same results would be obtained at another program. This is especially true for diagnoses that are considered controversial (e.g., juvenile bipolarity). Although the interviews were designed to improve reliability, the rules used to interpret symptoms and assign a diagnosis remain in part dependent on the views of the person using the measure, with some instruments more prone to this influence than others (see below). Research is needed to establish the reliability of measures across different centers.

Defining Cases

The goal of the psychiatric interview is to identify whether an individual has an illness, and if so, which one(s). Theoretically, using the current categorical model, psychiatric disorders are either present or absent. However, in practice, how cases are defined will depend on the nature and application of diagnostic criteria. Therefore, in any sample, individuals will either have a disorder or not have a disorder (reflecting the true population prevalence rates) and will be classified as either cases or noncases (depending on the diagnostic criteria). Although it is hoped that these two concepts are related, being a case is not necessarily the same as truly having a disorder (Zarin and Earls 1993). This model assumes that the disorder actually does exist in nature, an assumption that may be challenged as the neuroscience underlying psychopathology sheds light on specific disorders.

In assessing a diagnostic instrument's utility at identifying cases, the following concepts are important:

- *Sensitivity:* The percentage of individuals in a sample who have the disorder who are accurately identified by the interview
- *Specificity:* The percentage of individuals in a sample who do not have the disorder who are accurately identified by the interview as not having the disorder
- *Predictive value positive:* The percentage of individuals in the defined sample positively identified by the interview who actually have the disorder
- *Predictive value negative:* The percentage of individuals in the defined sample identified by the interview as not having the disorder who, in fact, do not have the disorder

The predictive value, both positive and negative, is important because it represents the conditional probability of having or not having a disorder, on the basis of the assessment procedure results. These values are influenced by the overall prevalence of the condition being investigated, whereas sensitivity and specificity are theoretically independent of prevalence rates (although clinicians' awareness of prevalence rates, and therefore assumptions about the frequency with which a disorder is diagnosed, may influence sensitivity and specificity ratings) (Robins 1985). Therefore, the probability of correctly diagnosing a rare condition using a given diagnostic tool may be low, even if the tool has acceptable sensitivity and specificity ratings.

It is important to recognize that when a consensus-based diagnostic system is being used, there is an inherent trade-off between false positives and false negatives that is unavoidable. Changes in the number of criteria required, or the definition of severity or duration of illness, may greatly influence the prevalence of the disorder in the population (McClellan and Werry 2000). Diagnostic decision-making must prioritize whether it is better to recognize all cases and accept the risk of overdiagnosis or to establish more conservative criteria and risk false negatives.

Furthermore, it is also important to examine the impact of prevalence on reliability and diagnostic agreement. Prevalence rates greatly affect positive predictive values (i.e., the percentage of individuals classified as a case who truly have the condition). Figure 7–1 presents the impact of changing prevalence rates in a hypothetical population of 1,000 individuals, using a diagnostic instrument with sensitivity and specificity rates arbitrarily set to approximately 95% (which are far better than currently available for existing instruments). Using these parameters, only 16% of individuals identified as "cases" actually have the disorder if the true prevalence rate is 1%. The low accuracy rate is due to an inherent rate of false positives for rare disorders. Since the vast majority of individuals are not affected, a specificity rating of 95% still results in 5% of nonaffected individuals inaccurately characterized as having the disorder, a number that is larger than the total number of those truly affected. Note also that in these examples, the "low" prevalence rates (i.e., 1%–5%) reflect the rate of common psychiatric illnesses in the general population.

Types of Diagnostic Interviews

Each revision of DSM has been accompanied by a wave of new, adapted, and revised versions of structured and unstructured diagnostic interviews. The goals of revising include improving the wording of questions to more accurately capture the desired concepts and criteria, upgrading scoring algorithms, and expanding the versions available to target different populations and/or route of administration (e.g., computerized versions) (Robins and Cottler 2004). The ultimate goal is to enhance the overall reliability and uniformity of data collection, which affords greater accuracy for research and also hopefully improves patient care.

Interviews are usually described as either structured or semistructured, depending on how much freedom the interviewer has to ask questions and interpret the responses:

- **Structured diagnostic interview**—The interviewer must follow a set script of questions using specified wording and is required to record the subject's responses as given. These instruments typically were designed for epidemiological research and are administered by trained nonclinician interviewers.
- **Semistructured diagnostic interview**—The interviewer is allowed to use his or her own questions

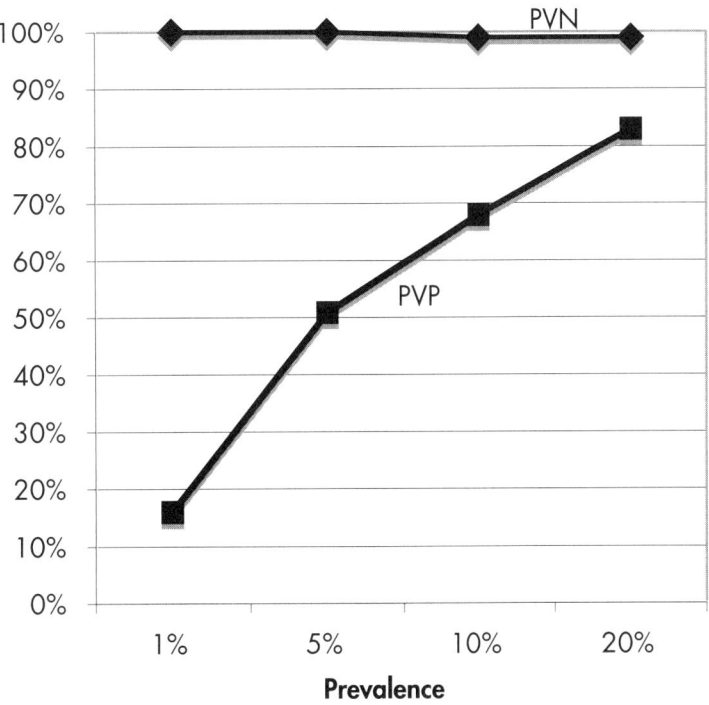

FIGURE 7–1. Impact of prevalence rates on predictive value positive and predictive value negative.

The predictive value positive (PVP) is the percentage of individuals identified as being a "case" who truly have the disorder. The predictive value negative (PVN) is the percentage of individuals identified as being a "noncase" who truly do not have the disorder. False positives are more likely with disorders that have low prevalence rates in the population. This simulation is based on a population of 1,000 individuals, using an assessment with 95% specificity and 95% sensitivity.

and incorporate other sources of information and interpret the responses. These instruments were developed for clinical research and community care and were designed for clinicians to administer. However, it is important to recognize that many clinical research projects use trained research assistants to administer these instruments, with the final diagnoses assigned after a review by the overseeing investigator.

Table 7–1 outlines characteristics of the structured diagnostic interviews most often used with children and adolescents. The choice of interview generally depends on the purpose (e.g., epidemiological vs. treatment study), type of interviewer (clinician vs. lay interviewer), training requirements, past familiarity or use of the instrument, and costs.

Discussion

Structured diagnostic interviews have helped advance the field by enhancing reliability and improving consistency of diagnostic practices. These assessment tools are important for research and also have potential utility for clinical settings. There are an increasing number of structured diagnostic interviews available to assess psychiatric illnesses in youth, many of which have been translated into different languages or can be administered via computers. The choice of instrument depends in part on the purpose (e.g., epidemiological vs. clinical intervention study), diagnoses to be addressed, training requirements, interviewer characteristics (lay interviewer vs. clinician), and time needed to administer.

It is important to recognize that no diagnostic instrument is perfect, nor does the use of structured interviews guarantee diagnostic uniformity and accuracy across clinicians or clinical settings. A meta-analytic review of child and adult studies found that agreement between structured interview diagnoses and clinician diagnoses is generally poor (Rettew et al. 2006). Agreement was best for eating disorders and substance abuse problems, and worse for disruptive behavior disorders, anxiety disorders, and mood disorders. This undoubtedly reflects the complicated nature of psychiatric conditions and limitations in both the assessment tools and clinical practices. Furthermore, the poor rates of agreement highlight the even

TABLE 7–1. Characteristics of structured diagnostic interviews frequently used with children and adolescents

Diagnostic instrument	Disorders covered	Type	Informant	Age range, years	Time, minutes	Inter-viewer	Special issues and comments
Schedule for Affective Disorders and Schizophrenia for School-Aged Children (K-SADS)	ANX, BEH, EAT, MOOD, SCH, SUB	SS	C, P	6–18	75–90	TC	Widely used in clinical research and treatment trials K-SADS available in Spanish (Ulloa et al. 2006), Hebrew (Shanee et al. 1997), Korean (Kim et al. 2004), and Farsi (Ghanizadeh 2006)
Schedule for Affective Disorders and Schizophrenia for School-Aged Children—Present and Lifetime (K-SADS-PL) www.wpic.pitt.edu/ksads	ANX, BEH, EAT, ELIM, MOOD, SCH, SUB, TIC	SS	C, P	6–18	75–90	TC	Widely used in clinical research and treatment trials
Washington University Schedule for Affective Disorders and Schizophrenia for School-Aged Children (WASH-U-KSADS)	ANX, BEH, EAT, MOOD, SCH, SUB; expanded definitions of mania	SS	C, P	6–18	75–90	TC	Widely used in clinical research and treatment trials
Schedule for Affective Disorders and Schizophrenia for School-Aged Children (Epidemiological; K-SADS-E)	ANX, BEH, EAT, MOOD, SCH, SUB	SS	C, P	6–18	75–90	TC	Widely used in clinical research and treatment trials
National Institute of Mental Health Diagnostic Interview Schedule for Children, Version IV (DISC-IV) Shaffer et al. 2000 disc@worldnet.att.net	ANX, BEH, EAT, ELIM, MOOD, SCH, SUB, TIC	S	C, P	6–18	70–120	TL	Computerized and Spanish versions available
Anxiety Disorders Interview Schedule for DSM-IV: Child and Parent Version (ADIS-CP) Silverman and Albano 1996 www.oup.com	ANX	SS	C, P	7–16	120	TC	Feelings Thermometer helps children quantify ratings of fear and interference with functioning
Diagnostic Interview for Children and Adolescents (DICA) Reich 2000 www.psychiatry.wustl.edu	ANX, BEH, EAT, ELIM, MOOD, PSYCH, SOM, SUB, TIC	SS, S	C, P	6–17	60–120	TL	Separate interviews for children (6–12 years old) and adolescents (13–17 years old)
Children's Interview for Psychiatric Syndromes (ChIPS) Weller 2000 www.wpspublish.com	ANX, BEH, EAT, ELIM, MOOD, SCH, SUB	S	C, P	6–18	40	TL	

TABLE 7–1. Characteristics of structured diagnostic interviews frequently used with children and adolescents *(continued)*

Diagnostic instrument	Disorders covered	Type	Informant	Age range, years	Time, minutes	Inter-viewer	Special issues and comments
Structured Clinical Interview for DSM-IV, Childhood Diagnoses (KID-SCID) http://cpmcnet.columbia.edu/dept/scid/info/kidscid.html	ANX, BEH, MOOD, SCH, SOM, SUB	SS	C, P	7–17	60–120	C	Adult version widely used in schizophrenia research
Child and Adolescent Psychiatric Assessment (CAPA) Angold and Costello 2000 http://devepi.mc.duke.edu	ANX, BEH, EAT, ELIM, MOOD, SCH, SOM, SUB, TIC	SS	C, P	9–17	60–150	BA, TL	Primarily used as screening tool
Preschool Age Psychiatric Assessment (PAPA) Egger et al. 2006		SS	P	3–6			Shows reliable test-test reliability with DSM-IV Spanish, Romanian, Norwegian, and electronic versions
Parent–Child Relationship Scale (PCRS) Wamboldt et al. 2001			C	9–18	Brief	TL	Assesses child's perspective of the parent-child relationship Adapted from CAPA
Interview Schedule for Children and Adolescents (ISCA) Sherrill and Kovacs 2000	ANX, BEH, EAT, ELIM, MOOD, PSYCH, SOM, SUB, TIC	SS	C, P	8–17	120 (P) 60 (C)	C	Organized around symptom reports
Dominic-R pictorial Valla et al. 2000	ANX, BEH, DEP		C	6–11	15–25	TL	Uses pictures to elicit symptom reports Versions for African American and French-speaking children available

Disorders covered: ANX=anxiety disorders (often includes posttraumatic stress disorder); BEH=disruptive behavior disorders; DEP=depressive disorders; EAT=eating disorders; ELIM=encopresis and enuresis; MOOD=mood disorders (depressive and bipolar); PSYCH=nondiagnostic screen for psychotic symptoms; SCH=schizophrenia and psychotic disorders; SOM=somatoform disorders; SUB=substance abuse/dependence; TIC=tic disorders.
Type of interview: S=structured, SS=semistructured.
Informant: C=child, P=parent.
Interviewer: BA=bachelor's level with training; C=clinician; TC=trained clinician; TL=trained lay interviewer.

greater challenge of developing accurate diagnostic processes in community systems of care.

There is a paucity of research comparing one structured diagnostic interview to another. Variations in wording or in how the instrument is scored may produce significant changes in prevalence estimates (Robins and Cottler 2004). Glossary-based interviews, such as the Child and Adolescent Psychiatric Assessment (CAPA; Angold and Costello 2000) and the Schedule for Affective Disorders and Schizophrenia for School-Aged Children (K-SADS), address this issue by developing clear definitions and training the interviewers to recognize the distinctions.

There are some specific developmental challenges noted when assessing youth. Children may misinterpret questions and respond positively to queries regarding symptoms that are rare and for which they have no inherent understanding, such as obsessive-compulsive, psychotic, or manic symptoms (Breslau 1987; Weller et al. 1996). In general, younger children lack the prerequisite attention span, abstract awareness (including timelines for duration criteria), and verbal skills necessary to understand many of the concepts involved in reporting psychiatric symptoms (Valla et al. 2000).

Poor agreement between different informants (e.g., parent-child, parent-teacher) represents another challenge (Achenbach 1987). Youth are thought to be better at describing their own internalizing states, whereas parents or teachers are better at describing acting-out behaviors in children, although research is needed to clarify when and if this is the case. Poor agreement does not necessarily imply error, since children's behavior depends to some extent on the setting and situation (Achenbach 1987).

Psychiatric decision making is dependent upon the integration of information from diverse sources and perspectives, including the patient and family interviews, the mental status examination, collateral informants (e.g., teachers), and other treatment providers. These are complex processes normally characterized as clinical judgment. However, there are no universally accepted algorithms dictating how to combine different types of information. For example, are both child and parent reports of symptoms necessary before making a diagnosis? If not, which informant's information takes precedence? How do the responses of other informants, such as teachers, influence the findings? Efforts are needed to quantify these decision-making processes in a manner that translates to different settings and situations.

The use of standardized assessment procedures is an important step toward evidence-based practices. By compelling clinicians to follow standard diagnostic and interviewing methods, structured interviews promote more consistent diagnostic practices and help justify therapeutic interventions and outcomes. Yet, the impact on clinical care and administrative issues needs to be more fully examined. For example, one study found that using the Anxiety Disorders Interview Schedule for DSM-IV: Child and Parent Version (ADIS-C/P) resulted in the identification of more anxiety disorders. The new process required more time and expense, and while patients and families responded well to the changes, the clinic's financial officers were concerned about the cost (Thienemann 2004). Another study of community mental health clinics found that practitioners were more likely to assign one diagnosis and less likely to assign zero diagnoses, while the National Institute of Mental Health Diagnostic Interview Schedule for Children, Version IV (DISC-IV) was more likely to assign zero or multiple diagnoses. This discrepancy was thought to be related to clinic policy (Jensen and Weisz 2002). Thus, as these instruments are incorporated into routine care, it will be important to assess clinical outcomes, impact on clinic functioning, and patient and family satisfaction.

Research Directions

The future development of structured psychiatric interviews will likely focus on strategies to better incorporate them into community care. This will require continued work to standardize instruments for clinical populations. Efforts are also needed to improve feasibility and access. For example, having the interviews available on CD-ROM or online will facilitate their use by psychiatrists and other community practitioners. Many interviews may need to be streamlined and translated into other languages in order to better serve the clinical populations in different settings.

Conclusion

There are now a variety of diagnostic instruments being used by different researchers, institutions, and clinicians. More studies are needed that systematically examine which instruments are best suited for specific research and clinical situations. Furthermore, it is also evident that the use of the same instrument does not ensure the same diagnostic conclusions. Standardization of diagnostic constructs, decision making, and treatment approaches is needed to reduce the large degree of variability evident in surveys of pediatric mental health care.

The days when structured diagnostic interviews were used only for research have passed. As evidence-based medicine continues making inroads into the field of psychiatry, there will be an ever increasing need for more evidence-based assessments. To this end, standardized diagnostic procedures, in some form or another, will likely soon be required by payers and policy makers to justify hospital admissions, length of stay, and reimbursements. And until something better comes along, the structured interview will continue to be the instrument/procedure to determine diagnoses in psychiatry. It behooves us all—whether our work is research-based or clinically based—to be well acquainted with the tools of our trade and to keep them sharp.

Summary Points

- Structured psychiatric interviews are designed to improve the reliability of obtaining diagnostic and clinical information from patients and families.

- Structured interviews are designed for epidemiological research and typically follow a set script, allowing them to be administered by trained nonclinical interviewers.

- Semistructured interviews are designed for clinical research and usually allow the interviewer some leeway in wording questions and interpreting responses. Information may also be incorporated from other sources (e.g., medical records). These instruments were developed for clinical research and are generally preferred by clinicians.

- The reliability of an instrument does not ensure validity. The validity of a structured interview is commonly assessed by comparing it with different but related sets of questionnaires and outcome measures. This is not truly an independent validation since the same symptom domains are being assessed by both methods.

- There is a high predictable rate of false positives when detecting disorders with low prevalence rates in large populations of individuals, even when using instruments that have excellent specificity ratings.

- When interviewing children, developmental challenges such as lack of prerequisite attention span, abstract awareness, and verbal skills may lead to children's misinterpretation of questions, especially for rare symptoms of which they may have no inherent understanding.

- A challenge in diagnostic assessment is the inherent variable agreement among children, parents, and teachers. Children appear better at reporting internalizing symptoms, whereas parents and other adults are often better at reporting externalizing symptoms.

- There are no universally accepted algorithms dictating how to combine different types of diagnostic information.

- Standardized assessment procedures are important in evidence-based practices.

- More research is needed that compares one structured diagnostic interview to another and to assess the utility of different instruments in community treatment settings.

References

Achenbach TE: Child/adolescent behavioral and emotional problems: implications of cross-informant correlations for situational specificity. Psychol Bull 101:213–232, 1987

American Psychiatric Association: Diagnostic and Statistical Manual of Mental Disorders, 3rd Edition. Washington, DC, American Psychiatric Association, 1980

Angold AF: Interviewer-based interviews, in Diagnostic Assessment in Child and Adolescent Psychopathology. Edited by Shaffer D, Lucas CP, Richters JE. New York, Guilford, 1999, pp 34–64

Angold A, Costello EJ: The Child and Adolescent Psychiatric Assessment (CAPA). J Am Acad Child Adolesc Psychiatry 39:39–48, 2000

Breslau N: Inquiring about the bizarre: false positives in Diagnostic Interview Schedule for Children (DISC), ascertainment of obsessions, compulsions and psychotic symptoms. J Am Acad Child Adolesc Psychiatry 26: 639–655, 1987

Cox A, Rutter M, Holbrook D: Psychiatric interviewing techniques V. Experimental study: eliciting factual information. Br J Psychiatry 139:29–37, 1981

Cronbach LJ, Meehl PE: Construct validity in psychological tests. Psychol Bull 52:281–302, 1955

Egger HL, Erkanli A, Keeler G, et al: Test-retest reliability of the Preschool Age Psychiatric Assessment (PAPA). J Am Acad Child Adolesc Psychiatry 45:538–549, 2006

Ghanizadeh A: Psychometric properties of the Farsi translation of the Kiddie Schedule for Affective Disorders and Schizophrenia—Present and Lifetime Version. BMC Psychiatry 6:10, 2006

Jensen AL, Weisz JR: Assessing match and mismatch between practitioner-generated and standardized interview-generated diagnoses for clinic-referred children and adolescents. J Consult Clin Psychol 70:158–168, 2002

Kim YS, Cheon KA, Kim BN, et al: The reliability and validity of Kiddie Schedule for Affective Disorders and Schizophrenia–Present and Lifetime Version–Korean version (K-SADS-PL-K). Yonsei Med J 45:81–99, 2004

McClellan JM, Werry JS: Introduction: research psychiatric diagnostic interviews for children and adolescents. J Am Acad Child Adolesc Psychiatry 39:19–27, 2000

Reich W: Diagnostic Interview for Children and Adolescents (DICA). J Am Acad Child Adolesc Psychiatry 39:59–66, 2000

Rettew DC, Doyle A, Achenbach TM, et al: Meta-analyses of agreement between clinical evaluations and standardized interviews. Poster presented at the annual meeting of the American Academy of Child and Adolescent Psychiatry, San Diego, CA, October 2006

Robins L: Epidemiology: reflections on testing the validity of psychiatric interviews. Arch Gen Psychiatry 42:918–924, 1985

Robins L, Cottler LB: Making a structured psychiatric diagnostic interview faithful to the nomenclature. Am J Epidemiol 160:808–813, 2004

Shaffer D, Fisher P, Lucas CP, et al: NIMH Diagnostic Interview Schedule for Children Version IV, (NIMH DISC-IV): description, differences from previous versions, and reliability of some common diagnoses. J Am Acad Child Adolesc Psychiatry 39:28–38, 2000

Shanee N, Apter A, Weizman A: Psychometric properties of the K-SADS-PL in an Israeli adolescent clinical population. Isr J Psychiatry Relat Sci 34:179–186, 1997

Sherrill JT, Kovacs M: Interview Schedule for Children and Adolescents (ISCA). Am Acad Child Adolesc Psychiatry 39:67–75, 2000

Silverman WK, Albano AM: The Anxiety Disorders Interview Schedule for DSM-IV: Child Interview Schedule. San Antonio, TX, Graywind Publications, 1996

Spitzer RL: The DSM-III classification of the psychiatric disorders of infancy, childhood and adolescence. J Am Acad Child Adolesc Psychiatry 19:356–370, 1980

Susser E, Schwartz S, Morabia A, et al: Psychiatric Epidemiology: Searching for Causes of Mental Disorders. New York, Oxford University Press, 2006

Thienemann M: Introducing a structured interview into a clinical setting. J Am Acad Child Adolesc Psychiatry 43:1057–1060, 2004

Ulloa RE, Ortiz S, Higuera F, et al: Interrater reliability of the Spanish version of Schedule for Affective Disorders and Schizophrenia for School-Age Children—Present and Lifetime Version (K-SADS-PL). Actas Esp Psiquiatr 34:36–40, 2006

Valla JP, Bergeron L, Smolla N: The Dominic-R: a pictorial interview for 6- to 11-year-old children. J Am Acad Child Adolesc Psychiatry 39:85–93, 2000

Wamboldt MZ, Wamboldt FS, Gavin L: A Parent–Child Relationship Scale derived from the Child and Adolescent Psychiatric Assessment (CAPA). J Am Acad Child Adolesc Psychiatry 40:945–953, 2001

Weller E: Children's Interview for Psychiatric Syndromes (ChIPS). J Am Acad Child Adolesc Psychiatry 39:76–84, 2000

Weller E, Weller RA, Svadjian H: Mood disorders, in Child and Adolescent Psychiatry: A Comprehensive Textbook, 2nd Edition. Edited by Lewis M. Baltimore, MD, Williams & Wilkins, 1996, pp 650–665

Zarin DA, Earls F: Diagnostic decision making in psychiatry. Am J Psychiatry 150:197–206, 1993

Chapter 8

Rating Scales

Alison Leary, Ph.D.
Brent Collett, Ph.D.
Kathleen Myers, M.D., M.P.H.

Functioning of Rating Scales

The term *rating scale* refers to any instrument that provides rapid assessment of a behavior or psychological dimension, yields a numerical score that is easily interpreted, and complements clinical care. This chapter presents rating scales that have high utility for disorders that are frequently treated in general psychiatric practice. The text discusses general issues regarding the use of the scales, including their strengths and weaknesses, and the tables provide information regarding the availability of psychometric data. Readers may also review the *Journal of Clinical Child and Adolescent Psychology* (Vol 34, Issue 3, 2005) for a special section devoted to evidence-based assessment practices.

Another excellent resource is *Assessment Scales in Child and Adolescent Psychiatry* (Verhulst and van der Ende 2006), which provides both descriptions of scales that are beyond the scope of this chapter and copies of several reproducible scales. From the large number of available scales, those presented here were selected on the basis of their frequency of use in clinical practice and the adequacy of their psychometric properties.

Advantages and Disadvantages

Rating scales provide systematic coverage and quantification of behaviors in order to compare youth with self and peers over time, setting, and context. In some cases, rating scales may allow youth to more easily reveal worrisome or covert symptoms. They also provide a cost-efficient means of documenting evidence-based treatment (Myers and Winters 2002a).

Problems arise if users of rating scales have unrealistic expectations of them or incorrectly assume that an elevated score equates to diagnosis. The data collected with rating scales should be considered in conjunction with other evaluation procedures and clinical judgment. When selecting a scale, it is important to evaluate its developmental suitability, particularly when working with special populations (e.g., individuals with developmental delays, very young children). Finally, many popular scales do not have sufficient data to determine how well the scales discriminate clinical groups, how reliable the scores are, and how suitable the scales may be for a youth or clinical population. For example, if a scale has been developed with a school-based sample, it may not function as well with a clinic-based sample.

Individual and situational factors can also affect a scale's performance. Youth who seek social acceptance may underreport (e.g., denial or lying), while those who feel overwhelmed may overreport symptoms (e.g., faking). Similarly, on observer-rated scales, adult respondents may convey their own distress with the youth by exaggerating the child's symptoms or minimizing the child's problems in an effort to protect him or her. Poor agreement is noted among adults who rate a youth in different settings (e.g., teachers and parents), and only moderate agreement is achieved among adults in the same environment (e.g., mothers and fathers). These disparities reflect both differences in reporters' perceptions and variations in youth behavior across settings. Not surprisingly, correlations between youth self-report and adults' reports are typically low. These differences highlight the need for information from multiple informants across settings and the importance of viewing scales as a means of communication when interpreting scores.

Psychometric Properties

Rating scales measure a construct, and all measurement is subject to error. Psychometric properties estimate this error to determine whether a scale is appropriate for an application.

Reliability refers to the consistency with which a scale's items measure the same construct, the same way, every time. Lack of reliability is termed *random error*. Although correlation coefficients exceeding 0.80 are typically considered adequate and support an instrument's reliability, this still leaves a considerable portion of the score that is attributable to random error.

There are several types of reliability to consider. *Internal reliability,* or internal consistency, represents the degree to which individual items are consistent with each other. Items that are not internally consistent detract from the scale. *Test-retest reliability,* or stability, assesses whether a scale is stable over time. If the construct measured has not changed, then repeated measurements should be similar. This might be difficult to determine for a state construct that is expected to wax and wane, such as suicidality, and easier to determine for a trait construct, such as hyperactivity. *Interrater reliability* represents the agreement, or concordance, between different informants. As noted above, even well-regarded scales may have relatively low interrater reliability.

Validity indicates whether the scale accurately assesses what it was designed to assess. Lack of validity is referred to as *systematic error. Content validity* assesses whether the scale's items represent the construct being measured. *Face validity* is a type of content validity that is determined by subjectively judging whether items measure the content area. *Criterion validity* is assessed in relation to other scales with established validity in measuring the same construct. There are two subtypes of criterion validity: *predictive validity* asks whether the scale correlates with an event that will occur in the future; *concurrent validity* refers to a scale's correlation with an event assessed at the same time the scale is administered. There are two types of concurrent validity: *discriminative validity* compares scores for groups that do and do not have a characteristic; *convergent validity* is the extent of correlation of related variables. In contrast, *divergent validity* measures the extent of divergence of two variables that are not expected to be correlated.

Even when a scale has solid technical properties, it is often appropriate to use more than one scale to tap various aspects of a problem. These selected scales should demonstrate at least fair convergent validity (>0.5), but not so high (>0.9) that they are redundant. Psychometric properties and other characteristics should be matched to the intended application. For example, screening requires an instrument with high sensitivity that is relatively brief to reduce respondent burden. Monitoring requires an instrument with good stability and a response format that is sensitive to response variation. Finally, cutoff scores vary according to youth developmental status, culture, and clinical status, but such information is often not available. Thus, caution is needed in using scales that were developed with groups that differ from the target subjects.

Broad-Band Rating Scales

Broad-band scales assess a variety of problems across broad dimensions of behavior and symptoms (Table 8–1). They have high utility for initial evaluation, as they can be completed by multiple informants in different settings, and results can be used to direct further evaluation. Broad coverage is important as youth referred for one concern generally have other problems needing attention. Despite these scales' utility, they have some limitations. To minimize respondent burden while still covering a broad range of problem areas, these scales contain few items per subscale. In other words, they lack depth. Further, because they are often lengthy and cover multiple problem areas, they are not as useful for some applications, such as screening and treatment monitoring. Thus, these scales are best used to identify problems needing further evaluation with interview, observation, or narrow-band scales.

Child Behavior Checklist

The Child Behavior Checklist (CBCL; Achenbach and Rescorla 2000, 2001) has been the gold standard for research and clinical work among broad-band behavior rating scales since its development in the 1960s. The CBCL includes multiple versions for different reporters and age groups, including the Teacher Report Form (TRF) for youth ages 6–18 years old, the CBCL for preschoolers (CBCL/1½–5), and the Caregiver-Teacher Report Form for preschoolers (C-TRF); there is also a Youth Self-Report (YSR) for youth over 11 years old. These scales were updated in 2001 with new normative data and several modifications to item content and subscale structure. In addition to the problem behavior domains familiar to users of earlier versions of the CBCL (e.g., anxious/depressed, somatic complaints, aggressive behavior), all of the newer scales can also be scored using factors that approximate the diagnostic criteria of DSM-IV (American Psychiatric Association 1994). In 2007, the CBCL/6–18, TRF, and YSR computer scoring profiles were updated to offer norms relevant to a number of different cultures (Achenbach and Rescorla 2007). Such information can be helpful when evaluating children who have recently immigrated and may help to avoid misinterpreting culture-based normative behavior.

The CBCL, TRF, and YSR include subscale scores for several specific problem areas, as well as composite scores for Internalizing, Externalizing, and Total Problems. There are also items to assess youth adaptive functioning in home, community, and school. The structure of the CBCL/1½-5 and C-TRF is comparable, with a few differences in subscales for this developmental stage and the inclusion of a language scale to screen for communication deficits.

A few issues with clinical interpretation of the CBCL scales warrant mention. Several problem behavior items in the CBCL system include blanks for respondents to provide specific examples. When interpreting scores, it is important to review these responses to ensure that the respondent has accurately understood the items. Also, labels for the CBCL subscales may be misleading. For example, the Aggressive Behavior subscale describes oppositional and defiant behaviors, with few items describing aggression. Scores on the Thought Problems subscale can be affected by various cognitive problems, and scores are not equivalent to a thought disorder. Such problems underscore the need to review a scale's items to ascertain what they really measure. Overall, the CBCL has high utility due to its rapid coverage of a wide range of problems in various settings, the inclusion of scales to assess adaptive functioning, recently published cross-cultural normative data, and its extensive use in the research literature. Computer scoring increases utility by easily integrating the various reporter forms.

Behavior Assessment System for Children, 2nd Edition

The Behavior Assessment System for Children, Second Edition (BASC-2; Reynolds and Kamphaus 2004) is an updated version of the BASC, a widely used broad-band measure of behavior problems. The BASC-2 includes a Parent Rating Scale (PRS) and Teacher Rating Scale (TRS). The Self-Report of Personality (SRP) scale is rarely used. In addition to individual clinical scales, the TRS and PRS provide composite scores for Internalizing, Externalizing, Adaptive Skills, and the Behavioral Symptom Index, an overall measure of problem behaviors. The similar items and structure of the PRS and TRS allow meaningful comparisons between different raters of youth behavior in school and at home.

A strength of the BASC-2 is its inclusion of subscales measuring specific components of adaptive functioning, such as social skills and functional communication, to allow a more comprehensive view of the child's strengths. The BASC-2 also includes a number of validity scales, including indices of "faking bad" and incon-

TABLE 8–1. Psychometric properties of broad-band rating scales

Scale (ages)	Type of scale, items, and factors	Availability of normative data and reliability data	Availability of validity data	Other
Child Behavior Checklist (CBCL)				
TRF (6–18 years) Achenbach and Rescorla 2001	Parent/teacher report 120 items 8 problem subscales 6 DSM-IV subscales 3 composite scales	Normative data available IC: Yes (parent and teacher) TR: Yes (parent and teacher) IR: Yes (parent-parent) Yes (teacher-teacher) Yes (parent-teacher)	CONV: Yes (parent and teacher with nonclinical samples) DIVG: NR DISC: Yes (parent and teacher for clinical vs. nonclinical samples)	Administration time: 15–20 min Computer scoring Extensive data available >60 translations
C-TRF (1½–5 years) Achenbach and Rescorla 2000	Parent, teacher, caregiver report 102 problem items 8 language items 310 vocabulary words 7 problem subscales 5 DSM-IV subscales 2 language subscales 3 composite scales	Normative data available IC: Yes (parent and teacher) TR: Yes (parent and teacher) IR: Yes (parent-parent) Yes (teacher-teacher) Yes (parent-teacher)	CONV: Yes (parent and teacher with various clinical and nonclinical samples) DIVG: NR DISC: Yes (parent and teacher for clinical vs. nonclinical samples; and for language delayed vs. nondelayed samples)	Administration time: 15–20 min Computer scoring Multiple translations
YSR (11–18 years) Achenbach and Rescorla 2000	Self-report 105 problem items 8 problem subscales 6 DSM-IV subscales 3 composite scales	Normative data available IC: Yes TR: Yes IR: Yes (youth-parent and youth-teacher, clinical and nonclinical samples)	CONV: NR DIVG: NR DISC: Yes (clinical vs. nonclinical samples)	Administration time: 15–20 min Computer scoring available Multiple translations
BASC-2 PRS/TRS (2½–5, 6–11, 12–18 years) Reynolds and Kamphaus 2004	Parent report/ teacher report PRS: 2½–5: 134 items 6–11: 160 items 12–18: 150 items TRS: 2½–5: 100 items 6–11, 12–18: 139 items 8–10 clinical subscales 3–6 adaptive subscales 4 composite scales	Normative data available IC: Yes (parent and teacher, clinical and nonclinical samples) TR: Yes (parent and teacher, clinical and nonclinical samples) IR: Yes (parent-teacher, clinical and nonclinical samples)	CONV: Yes (parent and teacher, clinical and nonclinical samples) DIVG: NR DISC: Yes (distinct profiles for children with clinical diagnoses)	Administration time: 20–30 min to complete and score Includes validity indices Computer administration and scoring available; telephone technical support available Spanish translation

TABLE 8–1. Psychometric properties of broad-band rating scales *(continued)*

Scale (ages)	Type of scale, items, and factors	Availability of normative data and reliability data	Availability of validity data	Other
CSI (3–5, 5–12, 12–18 years; 12–18 self-report) Gadow and Sprafkin 1997, 1998, 2002	Parent and teacher ECI-4: 3–5 years Parent and teacher CSI-4: 5–12 years Parent and teacher ASI-4: 12–18 years Adolescent self-report YI-4: 12–18 years 77–120 items depending on version	Normative data available IC: Yes (parent and teacher ECI-4; parent and teacher CSI-4; parent and teacher ASI-4; and YI-4) TR: Yes (variable time intervals and samples for parent and teacher ECI-4; parent and teacher CSI-4; and YI-4) IR: Yes (parent and teacher, teacher and child CSI-4; youth, parent, and teacher YI4)	CONV: Yes (parent and teacher ECI-4; parent and teacher CSI-4; parent and teacher ASI-4; YI-4) DIVG: NR DISC: Yes (parent ECI-4; parent and teacher CSI-4; YI-4) SENS: Yes (for several disorders in clinical samples for parent and teacher ECI-4; parent and teacher CDI-4; parent and teacher ASI-4; and YI-4)	Administration time: 15–20 min Scoring format varies from a 4-point to a 2-point scale depending on age group and informant ECI-4 also includes the Peer Conflict Scale and the Developmental Deficits Index Computer scoring available Spanish translation

Note. ASI-4=Adolescent Symptom Inventory-4; BASC-2=Behavior Assessment System for Children, Second Edition; C-TRF=Caregiver–Teacher Report Form for Ages 1½–5 years; CONV=convergent validity; CSI=Children's Symptom Inventories; CSI-4=Child Symptom Inventory-4; DISC=discriminative validity; DIVG=divergent validity; ECI-4=Early Childhood Inventory-4; IC=internal consistency reliability; IR=interrater reliability; NR=not reported; PRS=Parent Rating Scales; TR=test-retest reliability; TRF=Teacher Report Form; TRS=Teacher Rating Scales; YI-4=Youth's Inventory; YSR=Youth Self-Report.

sistency in responding. Such scales are rarely available in broad-band scales, and while they cannot unequivocally determine whether the informant answered truthfully, they identify unusual patterns of responding. Such information also helps to determine what the respondent is hoping to communicate to the clinician. Overall, the BASC-2 is a psychometrically sound broadband measure. It has found its greatest utility in nonclinical settings (e.g., schools).

Child Symptom Inventories

The Child Symptom Inventories (CSI; Gadow and Sprafkin 1997, 1998, 2002) are a series of scales based on DSM-IV diagnostic criteria for multiple disorders. The disorders covered vary by age group but include the most common disorders of childhood and adolescence as well as less common disorders such as schizophrenia, reactive attachment disorder, and somatization disorder. Parallel forms are available for different age groups (preschool, elementary school, high school) and informants (parents, teachers for all forms, and self-report for youth ages 12–18 years), which provide easy comparison of symptoms endorsed over time and among informants.

Two scoring procedures are available for these scales. The Symptom Severity procedure is simply the sum of items endorsed, which can then be compared to normative data. Some investigators have cautioned, however, that the moderate size and diversity of the scales' normative sample limit the utility of this dimensional scoring procedure (Kamphaus and Frick 2005). The Symptom Count procedure is more commonly used and allows the clinician to identify whether the child or adolescent is currently exhibiting the sufficient number of clinically relevant symptoms (i.e., rated as occurring "often" or "very often") necessary for DSM-IV diagnosis. While the scale directly corresponds to some DSM-IV diagnostic criteria, other criteria (e.g., age at onset, functional impairment) are not included.

Many clinicians and investigators prefer the use of these scales to other broad-band scales, especially when conducting diagnostic evaluations, as item responses can help to focus the diagnostic interview to the most likely categories while also highlighting potential comorbidities. Another strength is the inclusion of disorders that are severe in nature and rarely covered in other broad-band rating scales (such as schizophrenia and Asperger's disorder). As such, the CSI scales may be particularly helpful for use with children who present with more severe symptomatology. The psychometric properties of the CSI scales vary greatly by age group, informant, and disorder, but substantial data are available to guide users toward the most appropriate and effective use of these scales.

Rating Scales Assessing Externalizing Behaviors

Externalizing behaviors are publicly observable, and youth displaying these behaviors are referred because of problems they pose to parents and teachers. As a result, these disorders are especially well suited to assessment via rating scales (Table 8–2). Youth tend to underestimate their misbehaviors, and adults are generally considered the optimal informants on these narrow-band scales. Ratings are generally obtained from multiple adults to obtain varied perspectives and to assess the ecological aspects of youth behaviors. Many of these scales were developed with school-age children, and suitability is less clear for younger and older youth. Further, as research on externalizing behaviors has focused predominantly on boys, less is known about the suitability of these scales for girls. There are many scales developed to measure attention-deficit/hyperactivity disorder (ADHD), the most common and extensively studied externalizing disorder, and fewer scales assess oppositionality and conduct problems. Many of the ADHD scales are now based on DSM-IV criteria.

Conners' Rating Scale—Revised

The Conners' Rating Scale—Revised (CRS-R; Conners 2002) covers core ADHD subscales as well as comorbid problems, such as oppositional defiant disorder (ODD) and conduct disorder (CD). There are both regular and abbreviated versions for the parent, teacher, and youth self-report forms. The multiple indices of problem areas along with a normative base, strong psychometrics, and multiple uses make the CRS-R excellent for comprehensive assessment. Its strong sensitivity makes it a good choice for screening, although lower sensitivity for the teacher version may produce false negatives in school screening. Stability and availability of the abbreviated version facilitate efficient treatment monitoring (Kaplan et al. 2004). Relative disadvantages include the somewhat poorer functioning for the comorbidity indices and the poor discrimination of ADHD, ODD, and CD from one another.

TABLE 8–2. Psychometric properties of scales assessing externalizing behaviors

Scale (ages)	Type of scale, items, and factors	Availability of normative data and reliability data	Availability of validity data	Other
CRS-R (3–17 years) Conners 2002	Parent, teacher, and adolescent reports 80 items (parent) 59 items (teacher) 87 items (adolescent) 7 factors (parent) 6 factors (teacher) 6 factors (adolescent) Global index ADHD index DSM-IV symptom subscales	Normative data available IC: Yes (parent, teacher, adolescent for clinical and nonclinical samples) TR: Yes (parent, teacher, adolescent for clinical and nonclinical samples) IR: Yes (parent-teacher; parent-adolescent; teacher-adolescent; all for clinical and nonclinical samples)	CONV: NR DIVG: NR DISC: Yes (ADHD vs. nonclinical samples) SENS and SPEC: Yes (both for parent, teacher, adolescent versions)	Administration time: 20–30 min Quick-score forms; computer, fax, mail-in scoring French translation
VADPRS/VADTRS (school-age children) Wolraich 2003a, 2003b	Parent/teacher report 55/43 items 4 factors Includes Academic Performance and Behavioral Performance Scales	Limited normative data available IC: Yes (parent, clinical sample) Yes (teacher, nonclinical sample) TR: NR IR: Yes (parent-teacher, nonclinical sample)	CONC: Yes (parent, clinical sample) Yes (teacher, nonclinical sample) DIVG: NR DISC: NR SENS and SPEC: Limited data (within clinical sample)	Administration time: 20 min to complete and score German and Spanish translations
ADHD RS-IV (5–18 years) DuPaul et al. 1998	Home/school report 18 items 2 factors	Normative data available IC: Yes (home and school) 4-wk TR: Yes (home and school) IR: Yes (parent-teacher)	CONV: Yes (home and school) DISC: ADHD vs. nonclinical; ADHD vs. clinical control; ADHD-I vs. ADHD-C SENS: Yes (home and school) PPP: Yes (home and school) SPEC: Yes (home and school) NPP: Yes (home and school)	Administration time: 5–10 min Spanish translation
ECBI (2–16 years) Eyberg and Pincus 1999	Parent report 36 items 3 factors	Normative data available IC: Yes (nonclinical sample) TR: Yes (nonclinical sample) IR: Yes (mother-father)	CONV: Yes (clinical and nonclinical samples) DIVG: NR DISC: Yes (clinical and nonclinical samples) SENS and SPEC: Yes (clinical and nonclinical samples)	Administration time: 10–15 min to complete and score Rate for problems and intensity Multiple translations

TABLE 8–2. Psychometric properties of scales assessing externalizing behaviors *(continued)*

Scale (ages)	Type of scale, items, and factors	Availability of normative data and reliability data	Availability of validity data	Other
SESBI-R (2–16 years) Eyberg and Pincus 1999	Teacher report 38 items 1 factor	Normative data available IC: Yes (nonclinical samples) TR: Yes (nonclinical samples) IR: Yes (interteacher, nonclinical samples)	CONV: Yes (nonclinical samples) DIVG: NR DISC: Yes (nonclinical samples)	Administration time: 10–15 min to complete and score Rate for problems and intensity Multiple translations

Note.   ADHD=attention-deficit/hyperactivity disorder; ADHD-RS-IV=ADHD Rating Scale for DSM-IV; CONC=concurrent validity; CONV=convergent validity; CRS-R=Conners' Rating Scales—Revised; DISC=discriminative validity; DIVG=divergent validity; ECBI=Eyberg Child Behavior Inventory; IC=internal consistency reliability; IR=interrater reliability; NPP=negative predictive power; NR=not reported; PPP=positive predictive power; SENS=sensitivity; SESBI-R=Sutter-Eyberg Student Behavior Inventory—Revised; SPEC=specificity; TR=test-retest reliability; VADPRS=Vanderbilt ADHD Parent Rating Scale; VADTRS=Vanderbilt ADHD Teacher Rating Scale.

Recently, a third version of the CRS has been introduced (Conners 2008). The Conners 3 offers an updated normative sample, as well as screener items for anxiety and depression, validity scales, and measures of impairment. A measure of executive functioning is included, which is especially appealing due to the impulsivity of youth diagnosed with ADHD. Although there is little research yet available to evaluate the Conners 3, these upgrades are promising.

Vanderbilt ADHD Rating Scales

The Vanderbilt ADHD Teacher Rating Scale (VADTRS; Wolraich 2003b) and the Vanderbilt ADHD Parent Rating Scale (VADPRS; Wolraich 2003a) are DSM-IV-based scales that are free online (www.nichq.org). Similar to the Conners scales, both parent-report (Wolraich et al. 2003) and teacher-report (Wolraich et al. 1998) forms are available. Items cover the expected ADHD subscales of inattention and hyperactivity/impulsivity, as well as ODD and CD comorbidities. They also include a screening subscale for anxiety and depression. The VADTRS includes two subscales that assess school functioning: Academic Performance and Behavioral Performance. The VADPRS includes a comparable subscale to assess parents' perceptions of school and social functioning. These scales also have shorter versions to follow up ADHD symptoms, but they lack an ODD or CD scale.

The VADTRS performs well in a number of large, ethnically diverse samples. The VADPRS has not been as extensively studied, but in a high-risk, teacher-referred sample, the VADPRS demonstrated good reliability, internal consistency, and concurrent validity. The comorbidity scales evidenced adequate reliability, but lower convergent and discriminative validity may limit their utility. Overall, the VADTRS and VADPRS appear to be strong. They are particularly popular in primary care due to their no-cost availability, posting on a pediatric Web site (www.nichq.org), family-friendly wording, and an available Spanish version.

ADHD Rating Scale–IV

The ADHD Rating Scale-IV (ADHD-RS-IV; DuPaul et al. 1998) is a brief scale that is directly derived from DSM-IV criteria for ADHD with the expected ADHD subscales. It does not address comorbid disorders. It can be completed by parents (home form) and teachers (school form). Cutoff scores are provided for multiple percentiles to allow variable guidelines for interpretation. The ADHD-RS-IV is important in several regards. This is one of the most extensively studied ADHD scales with strong psychometric properties, including being one of few ADHD scales to have established test-retest reliability, considerable evidence of discriminative validity, sensitivity to medication effects, and cross-cultural validity (Dopfner et al. 2006; Swanson et al. 2006). There is a large, ethnically and geographically representative normative base consisting of parents' and teachers' ratings of 2,000 youth ages 5–18 years old. The scale's ethnic norms are important because scores may vary by ethnicity (DuPaul et al. 1998). Separate norms are available for males and females in four age groups: 5–7, 8–10, 11–13, and 14–18 years old. The ADHD-RS-IV also appears to perform well with preschool children.

Eyberg Child Behavior Inventory and Sutter-Eyberg Student Behavior Inventory—Revised

The Eyberg Child Behavior Inventory and Sutter-Eyberg Student Behavior Inventory—Revised (ECBI and SESBI-R; Eyberg and Pincus 1999) are well established scales for assessing externalizing behaviors corresponding to diagnoses of ADHD, ODD, and CD. The ECBI is completed by parents and the SESBI-R by teachers. These scales use the same format with item overlap. Respondents rate each item on two dimensions: an Intensity Scale assesses behavior frequency, and a Problem Scale assesses reporters' perception of whether the behavior is problematic. This format is clinically useful. Respondents may rate behaviors as problematic even though they occur at a normative rate, thus indicating a low threshold and/or developmentally inappropriate expectations. Conversely, a respondent may rate problem behaviors as frequent but not problematic, reflecting a high threshold.

The ECBI and SESBI-R have been extensively used to discriminate clinical samples of disruptive youth and to assess the efficacy of behavioral interventions (Burns and Patterson 2001; Hutchings et al. 2006). Although norms are available for youth up to age 16 years old, these scales do not assess CD in adolescents and are most suitable for younger children, with whom they have great utility. Disadvantages are minor.

Rating Scales Assessing Internalizing Symptoms

Internalizing symptoms may not be readily observable by others (Myers and Winters 2002b). They represent subjective distress and are best assessed by youth self-report. Many of these narrow-band scales have parallel parent-report and/or teacher-report forms that broaden the perspective of and provide context regarding youths' difficulties. Psychometric data for these observer-report scales often reveal adults' failure to appreciate youths' distress (i.e., youth generally endorse more symptoms than observers note, and interrater reliability is often low). Clinician-rated scales integrate youths' and adults' responses and may provide greater accuracy and reliability in treatment studies. Several factors intrinsic to internalizing symptoms affect the functioning of these scales. Youths' feelings of depression, anxiety, or suicidality wax and wane; therefore, it is best to use the same scales at different points in time. However, if the test-retest reliability of the scale is not established, then it is difficult to know whether observed change is due to a real clinical difference or random error in the scale. Additionally, each of these scales overlaps in detecting symptoms of other internalizing symptoms (e.g., depression rating scales detect anxiety and suicidality, and anxiety or suicidality rating scales detect depression). Thus, a scale with good discriminative and divergent validity is especially valuable. Psychometric properties of scales assessing internalizing symptoms are presented in Table 8–3.

Mood Symptoms

There are few depression rating scales specific to youth. The available scales appear to be better measures of distress than of depression. Also, discriminating clinically depressed youth can be difficult as depressive symptoms are common in both clinical and community samples.

Beck Depression Inventory–II

The Beck Depression Inventory–II (BDI-II; Beck 1996) is the most popular depression rating scale for adolescents. It assesses the same aspects of depression with adolescents that it assesses with adults: cognitive, behavioral, affective, and somatic. The BDI-II functions well, although less predictably, with clinical than with community samples. Most impressively, the BDI-II discriminates outpatient depressed teens from those with anxiety and CD. Decreasing scores as youth recover from depression also make the BDI-II useful for monitoring treatment. The BDI-II has been translated into several languages and used with various ethnic populations, but caution is warranted as cutoff scores vary with culture. However, the scale lacks an adult-report form to provide a contextual perspective. The BDI-II is likely most effective at assessing depression in adolescents. For younger children, use of the Children's Depression Inventory is more appropriate.

Children's Depression Inventory

The Children's Depression Inventory (CDI; Kovacs 1992) is a downward extension of the BDI to preadolescents, although it is also used with teens. It is the most studied and utilized scale of juvenile depression. Although there are five subscales (Dysphoric Mood, Acting Out, Loss of Personal and Social Interest, Self-Deprecation, Vegetative Symptoms), the role of the factors is unclear and total scores are usually used. The CDI functions well and has predictive validity. It has been translated into several languages and is used cross-culturally. However, sensitivity, specificity, and discriminative validity are suboptimal, and the CDI appears to measure youths' overall distress rather than actual depression.

Children's Depression Rating Scale— Revised

The Children's Depression Rating Scale—Revised (CDRS-R; Poznanski and Mokros 1999) is a clinician-rated scale patterned on the Hamilton Rating Scale for Depression but developed specifically for children and widely used with teens. It has three unique features: it integrates information from both the child and parent, it includes behaviors observed during the interview, and several items are not specific to depression. Thus, the CDRS-R construct of depression differs somewhat from that of DSM-IV. There is some evidence of discriminative validity. Its impressive interrater reliability supports the alleged superiority of clinician-rated scales over lay scales. The short form facilitates screening and repeated assessment. Use of the CDRS-R in combination with self-reports and global ratings offers comprehensive yet efficient assessment that is sensitive to treatment (Wagner et al. 2006).

TABLE 8–3. Psychometric properties of scales assessing internalizing symptoms

Scale (ages)	Type of scale, items, and factors	Availability of normative data and reliability data	Availability of validity data	Other
BDI-II (adolescents) Beck 1996	Self-report scale 21 items 3 factors	No normative data IC: Yes (clinical and nonclinical) TR: Yes (various clinical and nonclinical) IR: NR	CONV: Yes (clinical and nonclinical) DIVG: NR DISC: Yes (clinical and nonclinical) SENS and SPEC: Yes (clinical sample)	Administration time: <10 min to complete and score Brief version available No parent-report form Multiple translations
CDI (7–18 years) Kovacs 1992	Self-report scale 27 items 5 subscales	Normative data available IC: Yes (multiple clinical and nonclinical samples) TR: Yes (clinical and nonclinical samples) IR: Yes (various reporters, clinical and nonclinical samples)	CONV: Yes (multiple clinical and nonclinical samples) DIVG: NR DISC: Yes (multiple clinical and nonclinical samples) SENS and SPEC: Yes (multiple clinical and nonclinical samples)	Administration time: <20 min to complete and score Parent, teacher, brief versions available Multiple translations
CDRS (6–12 years) Poznanski and Mokros 1999	Clinician-administered scale 17 items 5 factors	No normative data available IC: Yes (nonclinical sample) TR: Yes (various clinical samples) IR: Yes (parent-child, various clinical samples)	CONV: Yes (various clinical samples) DIVG: NR DISC: Yes (clinical samples) SENS and SPEC: Yes (clinical samples)	Administration time: 45–70 min to complete and score Integrates youth and parent scores Brief version available Multiple translations
RADS (12–18 years) W.M. Reynolds 1987	Self-report 30 items 5 subscales	Normative data available IC: Yes (clinical and nonclinical samples) TR: Yes (clinical and nonclinical samples) IR: NR	CONV: Yes (clinical and nonclinical samples) DIVG: NR DISC: Yes (clinical and nonclinical samples) SENS and SPEC: Yes (clinical and nonclinical samples)	Administration time: 10–20 min to complete and score Multiple translations
RCDS (8–12 years) W.M. Reynolds 1989	Self-report 30 items 7 subscales	Normative data available IC: Yes (nonclinical samples) TR: Yes (nonclinical samples) IR: NR	CONV: Yes (nonclinical samples) DIVG: NR DISC: Yes (nonclinical samples) SENS and SPEC: Yes (nonclinical samples)	Administration time: 10–20 min to complete and score Multiple translations

TABLE 8–3. Psychometric properties of scales assessing internalizing symptoms *(continued)*

Scale (ages)	Type of scale, items, and factors	Availability of normative data and reliability data	Availability of validity data	Other
YMRS (adults, but being used with children and adolescents) Young et al. 1978	Clinician-administered scale 11 items 1 factor	Normative data available IC: Yes (clinical sample) TR: NR IR: NR	CONV: Yes (various clinical samples) DIVG: Yes (various clinical samples) DISC: Yes (various clinical samples) SENS and SPEC: Yes (various clinical samples)	Administration time: 15 min to complete and score, but considerable time to gather data Multiple translations
SIQ/SIQ-JR (14 years–adult/ 11–13 years) C.R. Reynolds 1987	Self-report scale 30/15 items 1–3 factors	Normative data available IC: Yes (clinical and nonclinical samples) TR: Yes (nonclinical sample) IR: NR	CONV: Yes (clinical and nonclinical samples) DIVG: NR DISC: Yes (clinical samples) PRED: Yes (clinical and nonclinical samples)	Administration time: 20–30 min to complete and score Chinese translation
BHS (adults and adolescents) Beck and Steer 1989	Self-report scale 20 items 3 subscales	No normative data available IC: Yes (clinical and nonclinical samples) TR: Yes (clinical and nonclinical samples) IR: NR	CONC: Yes (clinical and nonclinical samples) DIVG: NR DISC: Yes (clinical samples) PRED: Yes (clinical samples)	Administration time: <15 min to complete and score No parent report Multiple translations
HSC (children and adolescents) Kazdin et al. 1986	Self-report scale 17 items 2 factors	No normative data available IC: Yes (clinical and nonclinical samples) TR: Yes (clinical and nonclinical samples) IR: NR	CONC: Yes (clinical and nonclinical samples) DIVG: NR DISC: Yes (clinical samples) PRED: Limited data	Administration time: <15 min to complete and score Multiple translations
MASC (children and adolescents) March 1997	Self-report scale 39 items 4 factors	Normative data available IC: Yes (clinical and nonclinical samples) TR: Yes (clinical and nonclinical samples) IR: Yes (parent-child, clinical and nonclinical samples)	CONV: Yes (clinical and nonclinical samples) DIVG: Yes (clinical and nonclinical samples) DISC: Yes (clinical samples)	Administration time: <25 min to complete and score Parent and brief versions available Multiple translations

TABLE 8–3. Psychometric properties of scales assessing internalizing symptoms *(continued)*

Scale (ages)	Type of scale, items, and factors	Availability of normative data and reliability data	Availability of validity data	Other
SCARED (9–19 years) Birmaher et al. 1997	Self-report scale 41 items 5 factors	Normative data available IC: Yes (clinical and nonclinical samples) TR: Yes (clinical and nonclinical samples) IR: Yes (parent-child, clinical and nonclinical samples)	CONV: Yes (clinical and nonclinical samples) DIVG: Yes (nonclinical sample) DISC: Yes (clinical samples) SENS and SPEC: Yes (clinical samples)	Administration time: <15 min to complete and score Parent and brief versions available Multiple translations
SPAI-C (9–14 years) Beidel et al. 1988	Self-report scale 26 items 3 factors	Normative data available IC: Yes (clinical and nonclinical samples) TR: Yes (clinical and nonclinical samples) IR: NR	CONV: Yes (clinical and nonclinical) DIVG: Yes (clinical and nonclinical) DISC: NR SENS and SPEC: Yes (clinical and nonclinical)	Administration time: 30 min to complete and score Multiple translations
CPTS-RI Revision 2 (7–18 years) Rodriguez et al. 1998	Clinician-administered scale or self-report scale 48 items 3 factors	No normative data available IC: Yes (clinical sample of traumatized children) TR: Yes (clinical sample of traumatized teens) IR: Yes (parent-adolescent, clinical sample)	CONV: Yes (clinical samples) DIVG: NR DISC: NR SENS: Yes (clinical sample of traumatized children)	Administration time: 20–45 min to complete and score Parent-report version available Multiple translations

Note. BDI-II=Beck Depression Inventory, Second Edition; BHS=Beck Hopelessness Scale; CDI=Children's Depression Inventory; CDRS=Children's Depression Rating Scale; CONC=concurrent validity; CONV=convergent validity; CPTS-RI=Children's PTSD Reaction Index; DISC=discriminative validity; DIVG=divergent validity; HSC=Hopelessness Scale for Children; IC=internal consistency; IR=interrater reliability; MASC=Multidimensional Anxiety Scale for Children; NR=not reported; PRED=predictive validity; RADS=Reynolds Adolescent Depression Scale; RCDS=Reynolds Child Depression Scale; SCARED=Screen for Child Anxiety Related Emotional Disorders; SENS=sensitivity; SIQ=Suicidal Ideation Scale; SPAI-C=Social Phobia Anxiety Inventory for Children; SPEC=specificity; TR=test-retest; YMRS=Young Mania Rating Scale.

Reynolds Adolescent Depression Scale and Reynolds Child Depression Scale

The Reynolds Adolescent Depression Scale (RADS; (W.M. Reynolds 1987) and the Reynolds Child Depression Scale (RCDS; W.M. Reynolds 1989) are two related scales based on DSM-III (American Psychiatric Association 1980) criteria for depression. They have parent versions. These scales have shown very good reliability and convergent validity with multiple samples. They function well with diverse samples of ethnically heterogeneous community and clinical samples, although their main use has been in the schools. They offer the opportunity to assess children and adolescents with similar but developmentally suitable scales, making them useful for longitudinal applications. An advantage of these scales is their basis on a clear construct of depression. The disadvantage is that this construct has been replaced by DSM-IV criteria, although the two constructs are not very discordant. Therefore, if a scale with a clear construct of depression is needed, these scales have good utility.

Young Mania Rating Scale

The Young Mania Rating Scale (YMRS; Young et al. 1978; see also Yonkers and Samson 2008) is a very brief scale that assesses mania during the course of bipolar disorder. The YMRS is intended to be completed by the clinician after collecting data from the patient and relevant other individuals. The YMRS has been increasingly used with youth diagnosed with bipolar disorder, but the lack of consistent criteria for bipolar disorder with youth impedes interpretation of the studies. A parent-report version is available and shows good concordance with the clinician-administered YMRS (Youngstrom et al. 2004). The YMRS has shown some ability to discriminate bipolar disorder from ADHD, other disruptive behaviors, and depression (Gracious et al. 2002; Youngstrom et al. 2004). The YMRS has also shown some sensitivity to treatment with mood stabilizers. Overall, however, the YMRS has not been adequately examined to establish its utility for clinical applications with youth, despite its increasingly wide usage.

Suicidality and Hopelessness

Suicidality ranges from ideation to attempts to completed suicide, but it is unclear whether these manifestations comprise distinct, overlapping, or identical constructs (Winters et al. 2002). Suicidal ideation and attempts are relatively common, but rates of completed suicide are low. It is, therefore, difficult to attain strong predictive validity with suicide rating scales, and the goal is high sensitivity to identify youth for further assessment and intervention. There are few suicide rating scales specific to youth, and those developed for adults function variably with youth. By contrast, hopelessness strongly predicts suicidality, and scales measuring hopelessness are often used instead of, or in conjunction with, suicide rating scales.

Suicidal Ideation Questionnaire

The Suicidal Ideation Questionnaire (SIQ; C.R. Reynolds 1987) is available in two versions: the SIQ for high school and the SIQ-Jr for middle school students. The goal is suicide prevention in youth in the schools where these scales are mostly used, although they are appropriate to clinical settings. Both scales measure the intensity and frequency of suicidal ideation during the past month. Standardization was conducted with large normative samples, a major strength. Psychometric properties are quite good over various samples and across cultures. The large difference in scores between suicide attempters and other youth and the good sensitivity and specificity suggest discriminative validity. These scales have been used to elucidate the relationship of suicidality to hopelessness, depression, and loss. They have wide utility. How they function with self-harming, but nonsuicidal, youth is unknown.

Beck Hopelessness Scale

The Beck Hopelessness Scale (BHS; Beck 1988; available from the author at beckinst@gim.net) was developed for adults but has been widely used with adolescents as young as 12 years old. Hopelessness is correlated with depression but more powerfully predicts suicidal ideation and eventual suicide. Like suicidality, hopelessness measures a state, rather than trait, construct. The proposed subscales of the BHS—Feelings About the Future, Loss of Motivation, and Future Expectations—have not been consistently reported with adolescents (Aish and Wasserman 2001), and total scores are generally used. The BHS strongly discriminates suicidal from nonsuicidal adolescents and predicts serious suicide attempts independent of depression. The BHS has good utility for screening, group assignment, and longitudinal assessment. Its utility for monitoring treatment is less clear due to its response format and lack of stability data.

Hopelessness Scale for Children

The Hopelessness Scale for Children (HSC; Kazdin et al. 1986; available from the author at Alan.Kazdin@ yale.edu) is a downward modification of the BHS, developed with inpatient children. Although the HSC is widely used with teens, it functions better with children ages 6–13. Hopelessness in children relates to a negative attributional style fostered through aversive development and correlates with depression and suicidality, but not with anxiety. High scores on the HSC, along with high scores on measures of depression or distress, should alert clinicians to serious risk for self-harm. The HSC has discriminated suicidal from non-suicidal children, although this may be confounded by depression. Nonetheless, the HSC should function well in screening and phenomenological applications. The HSC has shown some sensitivity to treatment (Voelz et al. 2003). It has a long history of use with diverse psychiatric and medical samples, and an extensive literature supports its use with suicidal as well as nonsuicidal youth.

Anxiety Symptoms

Early anxiety rating scales were adapted from adult scales, had unclear suitability for youth, and focused on trait versus state anxiety (Myers and Winters 2002b). Newer scales have overcome these shortcomings and have focused on refining the construct of anxiety in youth.

Multidimensional Anxiety Scale for Children

The Multidimensional Anxiety Scale for Children (MASC; March 1997) was developed with diverse clinical and community samples. It assesses a spectrum of symptoms with four subscales, three of which can be further subdivided: Physical Symptoms (Tense/Restless and Somatic/Autonomic), Social Anxiety (Humiliation/Rejection and Public Performance Fears), Harm Avoidance (Perfectionism and Anxious Coping), and Separation Anxiety. Two factors match the DSM-IV diagnoses of social phobia and separation anxiety disorder, while the total score matches generalized anxiety disorder (GAD). The MASC validates the hypothesized division of anxiety into physical symptoms and approach-avoidance behaviors, and its construct of anxiety diverges from depression. Its other strengths include an Inconsistency Index that identifies invalid profiles, an Anxiety Disorders Index that discriminates anxious youth, and sensitivity to treatment. It offers strong psychometric properties and has been used effectively with several cultures throughout the world (Baldwin and Dadds 2007). The MASC has become the favored anxiety disorders rating scale for research and clinical work.

Screen for Child Anxiety Related Emotional Disorders

The Screen for Child Anxiety Related Emotional Disorders (SCARED; Birmaher et al. 1997; available from the author at birmaherb@msx.upmc.edu) was developed with youth presenting to a mood and anxiety disorders clinic. Its five factors conform to DSM-IV criteria for GAD, separation anxiety disorder, social phobia, somatic/panic disorder, and school phobia. This scale shows divergence from disruptive behaviors and, more impressively, from depression. It is sensitive to treatment effects (Cohen et al. 2006). The SCARED has been used cross-culturally (Wijsbroek et al. 2005) and functions well with both community and clinical samples. The SCARED could challenge the MASC due to its broader coverage, its basis on DSM-IV, and its no-cost availability.

Social Phobia and Anxiety Inventory for Children

The Social Phobia and Anxiety Inventory for Children (SPAI-C; Beidel et al. 1988) measures a specific anxiety construct: social anxiety. It has three subscales: Assertiveness, Traditional Social Encounters, and Public Performance. The SPAI-C has robust sensitivity, specificity, and construct validity (Inderbitzen-Nolan et al. 2004). It is impressive in its ability to discriminate among anxiety disorders. The SPAI-C correctly classifies 67% of youth with social phobia and 74% with other anxiety disorders. However, its sensitivity to treatment needs clarification as it has detected benefits of medication (Compton et al. 2001) but not psychotherapy (Masia et al. 2001). A parent-report version is available that shows good internal consistency (Higa et al. 2006). As for other scales assessing internalizing symptoms, the SPAI-P shows low correlation with the child version, indicating parents' unawareness of their children's suffering. Thus, the two scales should be used together. The special focus of this scale has found many uses with school and clinical samples.

Children's PTSD Reaction Index, Revision 2

The Children's PTSD Reaction Index, Revision 2 (CPTS-RI; Rodriguez et al. 1998), also referred to as the UCLA PTSD Index for DSM-IV, measures posttraumatic stress disorder (PTSD) symptoms in youth ages 7 years and older. It can be administered by the clinician or alternatively may be used as a self-report form. Child-, adolescent-, and parent-report versions are available. The scale includes items that are reflective of DSM-IV criteria as well as items related to feelings of guilt and fear of reoccurrence of the trauma. Sensitivity and specificity for a diagnosis of PTSD are moderate to good. Higher scores correlate with greater traumatization, and the CPTS-RI has shown sensitivity to psychotherapy (Feather and Ronan 2006). The utility of the scale has been demonstrated with a number of different ages, settings, cultures, and types of trauma, from abuse to medical procedures to war (Ellis et al. 2006). This flexible scale offers considerable utility in clinical and large-scale applications and has become the most widely used measure of PTSD symptoms in youth.

Rating Scales Assessing Autism Spectrum Disorders

Autism spectrum disorders (ASD), or pervasive developmental disorders, are characterized by deficits in social interaction, communication, and restricted interests or behaviors. There has been an increased emphasis on early diagnosis and treatment given the demonstrated efficacy of early interventions. While the diagnosis of ASD is best determined by a multidisciplinary, multimethod assessment, a number of scales are now available that can help in gathering relevant information about the child's behavior (Table 8–4). These screening scales aid in the identification of children who require more extensive diagnostic evaluation.

Social Communication Questionnaire

The Social Communication Questionnaire (SCQ; Rutter et al. 2003), previously known as the Autism Screening Questionnaire, is a parent-report measure used specifically to screen children for deficits in social skills or communication. It is based on the Autism Diagnostic Interview and items correspond to DSM-IV criteria for the diagnosis of autism. The SCQ is simple to complete and score. While the SCQ has demonstrated high specificity and sensitivity in identifying children with ASD, it may be less sensitive for children with high-functioning autism who are more verbal or who have highly developed cognitive abilities.

Modified Checklist for Autism in Toddlers

The Modified Checklist for Autism in Toddlers (M-CHAT; Robins et al. 2001) is a screening instrument for assessment of behaviors consistent with ASD in children between the ages of 18 months and 2 years. The M-CHAT was designed as a two-step process including 1) a parent questionnaire and 2) a clinical interview of the parent. The interview is structured to provide follow-up questions to clarify items that were "failed" (i.e., consistent with ASD) on the parent questionnaire. Use of the parent-rating form alone without follow-up interview has not been validated. The M-CHAT has shown high levels of sensitivity and specificity in identifying children with ASD (Ventola et al. 2007). These features make the M-CHAT desirable for use in primary care and other settings where a brief screening measure is needed.

Autism Behavior Checklist

The Autism Behavior Checklist (ABC; Krug et al. 1980) is a screening checklist for ASD that is completed by the parent or a teacher familiar with the child. It is one component of the Autism Screening Instrument for Educational Planning (ASIEP), a more comprehensive system of ASD assessment, but it has frequently been used alone for screening. The scale includes a number of behaviors that are frequently seen in children with ASD, and the informant is asked to identify whether or not the child exhibits that behavior. The ABC was originally researched for use with school-age children but has effectively been used with children as young as 3 years. The greatest strength of the ABC is its demonstrated ability to discriminate children with ASD from those who exhibit other disorders (such as mental retardation) that are often confused with ASD (Eaves et al. 2000).

TABLE 8–4. Psychometric properties of scales assessing autism spectrum disorders

Scale (ages)	Type of scale, items, and factors	Availability of normative data and reliability data	Availability of validity data	Other
SCQ (4+ years) Rutter et al. 2003	Parent report (current and lifetime forms available) 40 items 0 subscales or factors identified	No normative data available IC: NR TR: NR IR: NR	CONV: Yes (clinical and nonclinical samples) DIVG: NR DISC: Yes (clinical and nonclinical samples) SENS and SPEC: Yes (clinical samples)	Administration time: <15 min to complete and score Spanish translation
ABC (3+ years) Krug et al. 1980	Parent report 57 items 5 subscales	No normative data available IC: Yes (clinical samples) TR: Yes (clinical samples) IR: NR	CONV: Yes (clinical samples) DIVG: NR DISC: Yes (autism spectrum disorders vs. mental retardation) SENS and SPEC: Yes (clinical samples)	Administration time: 15–20 min to complete and score Multiple translations
M-CHAT (18–24 months) Robins et al. 2001	Parent/teacher report: 23 items Clinical interview: variable number of items 0 subscales or factors identified	Normative data available IC: NR TR: NR IR: NR	CONV: Yes (clinical samples) DIVG: NR DISC: Yes (clinical samples) SENS and SPEC: Yes (clinical samples)	Administration time: variable dependent on items endorsed Multiple translations

Note. ABC=Autism Behavior Checklist; CONV=convergent validity; DISC=discriminant validity; DIVG=divergent validity; IC=internal consistency; IR=interrater reliability; M-CHAT=Modified Checklist for Autism in Toddlers; NR=not reported; SCQ=Social Communication Questionnaire; SENS=sensitivity; SPEC=specificity; TR=test-retest reliability.

Functional Impairment and Adaptive Functioning

These scales differ from the scales reviewed in the previous sections of this chapter, in that they are not keyed to specific psychiatric symptoms but tap deficits in functioning or adaptation (Winters et al. 2005). Impairment may result from the psychiatric illness or may have a shared etiology with the illness. The importance of impairment is attested by its coding on Axis V of DSM-IV to define "caseness." Both global scales and multidimensional scales are widely used. Global scales assign a summary score to describe the youth's overall impairment or adaptive functioning. The simplicity of a single score allows for easy comparison of impairment across diagnoses and time. However, global scales confound functioning with symptoms. Because they do not distinguish which domains of functioning are most impaired, they may not optimally assist treatment planning. Multidimensional scales are then more helpful. Psychometric properties of scales assessing functional impairment and adaptive functioning are included in Table 8–5.

Children's Global Assessment Scale

The Children's Global Assessment Scale (CGAS; Shaffer et al. 1983; see also Kutash et al. 2008) is a unidimensional clinician-rated scale adapted from the adult version, the Global Assessment Scale. During the diagnostic interview, the rater gathers a broad range of data regarding the youth's functioning in relation to history, symptomatology, and behavior across settings. This information is summarized into an overall score. The psychometric properties of the CGAS are sound. It has been used extensively in research and clinical work, domestically and internationally, to characterize psychosocial functioning in clinical samples, including medically ill youth. The CGAS has been used as an outcome variable to complement measures of syndromal improvement in both psychosocial (Vitiello et al. 2006) and pharmacological studies. Recently, a modified version of the CGAS has been developed to assess impairment in children with pervasive developmental disorders (DD-CGAS; Wagner et al. 2007). While the psychometric properties of the DD-CGAS appear to be sound, its utility in clinical and research samples has yet to be determined.

Vineland Adaptive Behavior Scales, 2nd Edition

Vineland Adaptive Behavior Scales, Second Edition (VABS-II; Sparrow et al. 2005), comprise the prototypical measure of functioning. The original version of the VABS has been used extensively, particularly with youth diagnosed with developmental impairments. The VABS-II has recently been released and includes a number of improvements, including current norms and a wider age range. It is completed as a semistructured interview with caregivers of individuals from birth through adulthood. Multiple forms are available. The Survey Form is most frequently used. The Expanded Form adds content to assess further problem areas and to assist with the development of individualized education and treatment programs. Parent and teacher rating forms are also available.

The VABS-II Survey Form is a lengthy but comprehensive scale whose items cover developmental skills in five clinically and empirically derived domains: Communication, Daily Living Skills, Socialization, Motor Skills, and an optional Maladaptive Behavior Domain. Rather than administering all items, estimated starting points are provided by age, and basal and ceiling rules are used to ensure that a youth's abilities are adequately represented.

The VABS-II has a good normative base, and its supplemental norms for selected developmental groups are a unique strength. Reliability and validity are robust. The VABS has a strong history of use in many diverse applications, including with very young developmentally impaired infants and preschoolers (Irwin et al. 2002) and with youth diagnosed with autism spectrum and other developmental disorders (Szatmari et al. 2002), as well as youth with psychiatric disorders. It is used to establish functional deficits in order to qualify children for school services and for disability insurance. The VABS-II is a comprehensive, versatile measure that can be used to assess youths' functioning over their life span. As such, it is the standard measure of adaptive behavior for children and adolescents with neurodevelopmental and other disorders.

Adaptive Behavior Assessment System, 2nd Edition

The Adaptive Behavior Assessment System, Second Edition (ABAS-II; Harrison and Oakland 2003) is another frequently used measure of adaptive function-

TABLE 8–5. Psychometric properties of scales assessing functional impairment and adaptive functioning

Scale (ages)	Type of scale, items, and factors	Availability of normative data and reliability data	Availability of validity data	Other
CGAS (4–16 years) American Psychiatric Association 2000; Shaffer et al. 1983	Parent report (current and lifetime forms available) 40 items 0 subscales or factors identified	No normative data available IC: NR TR: NR IR: NR	CONV: Yes (clinical and nonclinical samples) DIVG: NR DISC: Yes (clinical and nonclinical samples) SENS and SPEC: Yes (clinical sample)	Administration time: <15 min to complete and score Multiple translations
VABS-II (birth through adulthood) Sparrow et al. 2005	Clinician-administered scale 469 possible items (variable number of items given dependent on individual) Ages 0–6: 4 domains Ages 6–90: 3 domains	Normative data available IC: Yes (nonclinical sample) TR: Yes (both reporter and interviewer, nonclinical sample) IR: Yes (various reporters, nonclinical sample)	CONV: Yes (nonclinical sample) DIVG: NR DISC: NR	Administration time: 35–90 min to administer and score Available in Spanish
ABAS-II (birth to 89 years) Harrison and Oakland 2003	Parent/primary caregiver report (ages 0–5); 241 items Teacher/daycare provider (ages 2–5); 232 items Parent (ages 5–21); 239 items Teacher (ages 5–21); 193 items Adult form (ages 16–89); 239 items 10 subscales	Normative data available IC: Yes (clinical and nonclinical samples) TR: Yes (both reporter and interviewer) IR: Yes (various reporters, clinical and nonclinical samples)	CONV: Yes (clinical and nonclinical samples) DIVG: NR DISC: Yes (clinical vs. nonclinical samples)	Administration time: 20–30 min to complete and score Available in Spanish

Note. ABAS-II=Adaptive Behavior Assessment System, Second Edition; CGAS=Children's Global Assessment Scale; CONV=convergent validity; DISC=discriminative validity; DIVG=divergent validity; IC=internal consistency; IR=interrater reliability; NR=not reported; SENS=sensitivity; SPEC=specificity; TR=test-retest reliability; VABS-II=Vineland Adaptive Behavior Scales, Second Edition.

ing that provides information on the basis of age-related norms. The ABAS-II uses parents' or caregivers' reports of children's behaviors and abilities and assesses adaptive functioning in an individual from birth to age 89 years of age. The structure of the ABAS-II is based upon recommendations of the American Association on Intellectual and Developmental Disabilities and offers the following domain composite scores confirmed with factor analysis: Conceptual, Social, and Practical, as well as a General Adaptive Composite Score. There are 10 individual skill area scores, which are correlated but not so highly as to be redundant. The ABAS-II appears to be psychometrically sound with high internal consistency and concurrent validity, assessed in relation to the VABS (Rust and Wallace 2004). Overall, the ABAS-II offers a relatively comprehensive assessment of children's adaptive functioning in various domains using a simple and relatively short measure. Given its ease of use and the utility of the information it offers, the ABAS-II will likely be increasingly used in both research and clinical settings.

Summary Points

- Rating scales are adjunctive tools used to complement a diagnostic evaluation. They cannot be used alone to make a diagnosis.

- A rating scale's utility is highest when the scale is brief and easy to complete and has a single total score—or several subscale scores—that can be easily derived and interpreted.

- Rating scales must be geared to the youth's developmental abilities.

- Rating scales are best used with multiple informants to provide ecological validity. The low to moderate concordance among informants does not invalidate a scale's utility.

- For rating scales assessing externalizing behaviors, an adult report is most helpful.

- For rating scales assessing internalizing symptoms, a youth's self-report is most helpful.

- Rating scales for autism spectrum disorders can be helpful in identifying youth who require more extensive diagnostic evaluation.

- Rating scales assessing functional impairment or adaptive functioning help to define "caseness," establish treatment goals, and measure change in functioning with treatment.

References

Achenbach TM, Rescorla LA: Manual for the ASEBA School-age Forms and Profiles. Burlington, University of Vermont Research Center for Children, Youth, and Families, 2000

Achenbach TM, Rescorla LA: Manual for the ASEBA Preschool Forms and Profiles. Burlington, VT, University of Vermont Research Center for Children, Youth, and Families, 2001

Achenbach TM, Rescorla LA: Multicultural Supplement to the Manual for ASEBA School-Age Forms and Profiles. Burlington, University of Vermont, Research Center for Children, Youth, and Families, 2007

Aish AM, Wasserman D: Does Beck's Hopelessness Scale really measure several components? Psychol Med 31:367–372, 2001

American Psychiatric Association: Diagnostic and Statistical Manual of Mental Disorders, 3rd Edition. Washington, DC, American Psychiatric Association, 1980

American Psychiatric Association: Diagnostic and Statistical Manual of Mental Disorders, 4th Edition. Washington, DC, American Psychiatric Association, 1994

American Psychiatric Association: Diagnostic and Statistical Manual of Mental Disorders, 4th Edition, Text Revision. Washington, DC, American Psychiatric Association, 2000

Baldwin JS, Dadds ME: Reliability and validity of parent and child versions of the Multidimensional Anxiety Scale for Children in community samples. J Am Acad Child Adolesc Psychiatry 46:252–260, 2007

Beck AT: The Beck Hopelessness Scale (BHS) Manual. San Antonio, TX, Psychological Corporation, 1988

Beck AT: Beck Depression Inventory (BDI-II) Manual, 2nd Edition. San Antonio, TX, Psychological Corporation, 1996

Beck AT, Steer RA: Clinical predictors of eventual suicide: a 5- to 10-year prospective study of suicide attempters. J Affect Disord 17:203–209, 1989

Beidel DC, Turner SM, Morris TL: Social Phobia and Anxiety Inventory for Children (SPAI-C). North Tonawanda, NY, Multi-Health Systems, 1988

Birmaher B, Khetarpal S, Brent D, et al: The Screen for Child Anxiety Related Emotional Disorders (SCARED): scale construction and psychometric characteristics. J Am Acad Child Adolesc Psychiatry 36:545–553, 1997

Burns GL, Patterson DR: Normative data on the Eyberg Child Behavior Inventory and Sutter-Eyberg Student Behavior Inventory: parent and teacher rating scales of disruptive behavior problems in children and adolescents. Child Family Behav Ther 23:15–28, 2001

Cohen JA, Mannarino AP, Staron VR: A pilot study of modified Cognitive-Behavioral Therapy for Childhood Traumatic Grief (CBT-CTG). J Am Acad Child Adolesc Psychiatry 45:1465–1473, 2006

Compton SN, Grant PJ, Chrisman AK, et al: Sertraline in children and adolescents with social anxiety disorder: an open trial. J Am Acad Child Adolesc Psychiatry 40:564–571, 2001

Conners CK: Conners' Rating Scales—Revised. North Tonawanda, NY, Multi-Health Systems, 2002

Conners CK: Conners 3. North Tonawanda, NY, Multi-Health Systems, 2008

Dopfner M, Steinhausen HC, Coghill D, et al: Cross-cultural reliability and validity of ADHD assessed by the ADHD Rating Scale in a pan-European study. Eur Child Adolesc Psychiatry 15:46–55, 2006

DuPaul GJ, Power TJ, Anastopoulos AD, et al: ADHD Rating Scale-IV: Checklist, Norms, and Clinical Interpretation. New York, Guilford, 1998

Eaves RC, Campbell HA, Chambers D: Criterion-related and construct validity of the Pervasive Developmental Disorders Rating Scale and the Autism Behavior Checklist. Psychol Sch 37:311–321, 2000

Ellis BH, Lhewa D, Charney, et al: Screening for PTSD among Somali adolescent refugees: psychometric properties of the UCLA PTSD Index. J Trauma Stress 19:547–551, 2006

Eyberg S, Pincus D: Eyberg Child Behavior Inventory and Sutter-Eyberg Student Behavior Inventory—Revised Professional Manual. Odessa, FL, Psychological Assessment Resources, 1999

Feather JS, Ronan KR: Trauma-focused cognitive-behavioural therapy for abused children with posttraumatic stress disorder: a pilot study. NZ J Psychol 35:132–145, 2006

Gadow KD, Sprafkin J: Early Childhood Inventory-4: Norms Manual. Stony Brook, NY, Checkmate Plus, 1997

Gadow KD, Sprafkin J: Adolescent Symptom Inventory-4: Norms Manual. Stony Brook, NY, Checkmate Plus, 1998

Gadow KD, Sprafkin J: Childhood Symptom Inventory-4 Screening and Norms Manual. Stony Brook, NY, Checkmate Plus, 2002

Gracious BL, Youngstrom EA, Findling RL, et al: Discriminative validity of a parent version of the Young Mania Rating Scale. J Am Acad Child Adolesc Psychiatry 41:1350–1359, 2002

Harrison PL, Oakland T: Adaptive Behavior Assessment, 2nd Edition Manual (ABAS-II). San Antonio, TX, Harcourt Assessment, 2003

Higa CK, Fernandez SN, Nakamura BJ, et al: Parental assessment of childhood social phobia: psychometric properties of the Social Phobia and Anxiety Inventory for Children—Parent Report. J Clin Child Adolesc Psychol 35:590–597, 2006

Hutchings J, Bywater T, Davies C, et al: Do crime rates predict the outcome of parenting programmes for parents of "high-risk" preschool children? Educational Child Psychology 23:15–24, 2006

Inderbitzen-Nolan H, Davies CA, McKeon ND: Investigating the construct validity of the SPAI-C: comparing the sensitivity and specificity of the SPAI-C and the SAS-A. J Anxiety Disord 18:547–560, 2004

Irwin JR, Carter AS, Briggs-Gowan MJ: The social-emotional development of "late-talking" toddlers. J Am Acad Child Adolesc Psychiatry 41:1324–1332, 2002

Kamphaus RW, Frick PJ: Child and Adolescent Personality and Behavior, 2nd Edition. New York, Springer Science and Business Media, 2005

Kaplan S, Heiligenstein J, West S, et al: Efficacy and safety of atomoxetine in childhood attention-deficit/hyperactivity disorder with comorbid oppositional defiant disorder. J Atten Disord 8:45–52, 2004

Kazdin AE, Rodgers A, Colbus D: The Hopelessness Scale for Children: psychometric characteristics and concurrent validity. J Consult Clin Psychol 54:241–245, 1986

Kovacs M: Children's Depression Inventory Manual. North Tonawanda, NY, Multi-Health Systems, 1992

Krug DA, Arick JR, Almond PJ: Autism Screening Instrument for Educational Planning, ASIEP. Portland, OR, Pro-Ed Incorporated, 1980

Kutash K, Lynn N, Burns BJ: Children's Global Assessment Scale, in Handbook of Psychiatric Measures, 2nd Edition. Edited by Rush AJ, First MB, Blacker D. Washington, DC, American Psychiatric Publishing, 2008, pp 349–350

March JS: Manual for the Multidimensional Anxiety Scale for Children (MASC). North Tonawanda, NY, Multi-Health Systems, 1997

Masia CL, Klein RG, Storch EA, et al: School-based behavioral treatment for social anxiety disorder in adolescents: results of a pilot study. J Am Acad Child Adolesc Psychiatry 40:780–786, 2001

Myers K, Winters NC: Ten-year review of rating scales, I: overview of scale functioning, psychometric properties, and selection. J Am Acad Child Adolesc Psychiatry 41:114–122, 2002a

Myers K, Winters NC: Ten-year review of rating scales, II: scales for internalizing disorders. J Am Acad Child Adolesc Psychiatry 41:634–659, 2002b

Poznanski EO, Mokros HB: Children's Depression Rating Scale—Revised (CDRS-R). Los Angeles, CA, Western Psychological Services, 1999

Reynolds CR: Suicidal Ideation Questionnaire (SIQ): Professional Manual. Odessa, FL, Psychological Assessment Resources, 1987

Reynolds CR, Kamphaus RW: Behavior Assessment System for Children, 2nd Edition Manual. Circle Pines, MN, American Guidance Service Publishing, 2004

Reynolds WM: Reynolds Adolescent Depression Scale: Professional Manual. Odessa, FL, Psychological Assessment Resources, 1987

Reynolds WM: Reynolds Child Depression Scale: Professional Manual. Odessa, FL, Psychological Assessment Resources, 1989

Robins DL, Fein D, Barton ML, et al: The Modified Checklist for Autism in Toddlers: an initial study investigating the early detection of autism and pervasive developmental disorders. J Autism Dev Disord 31:131–144, 2001

Rodriguez N, Steinberg AM, Pynoos RS: UCLA PTSD Index for DSM-IV. Los Angeles, University of California at Los Angeles, Trauma Psychiatry Service, 1998

Rust JO, Wallace MA: Review of the Adaptive Behavior Assessment System, 2nd Edition. Journal of Psychoeducational Assessment 22:367–373, 2004

Rutter M, Bailey A, Lord C, et al: Social Communication Questionnaire. Los Angeles, CA, Western Psychological Services, 2003

Shaffer D, Gould MS, Brasic J, et al: A Children's Global Assessment Scale (CGAS). Arch Gen Psychiatry 40:1228–1231, 1983

Sparrow SS, Balla DA, Cicchetti DV: Interview Edition Survey Form Manual: Vineland Adaptive Behavior Scales. Minneapolis, MN, NCS Pearson Assessments, 2005

Swanson JM, Greenhill LL, Lopez FA, et al: Modafinil film coated tablets in children and adolescents with attention-deficit/hyperactivity disorder: results of a randomized, double-blind, placebo-controlled, fixed dose study followed by abrupt discontinuation. J Clin Psychiatry 67:137–147, 2006

Szatmari P, Merette C, Bryson SE, et al: Quantifying dimensions in autism: a factor-analytic study. J Am Acad Child Adolesc Psychiatry 41:467–474, 2002

Ventola P, Kleinman J, Pandey J, et al: Differentiating between autism spectrum disorders and other developmental disabilities in children who failed a screening instrument for ASD. J Autism Dev Disord 37:425–436, 2007

Verhulst FC, van der Ende J: Assessment Scales in Child and Adolescent Psychiatry. London, Informa Healthcare UK, 2006

Vitiello B, Rohde P, Silva S, et al: Functioning and quality of life in the Treatment for Adolescents with Depression Study (TADS). J Am Acad Child Adolesc Psychiatry 45:1419–1426, 2006

Voelz ZR, Haeffel GJ, Joiner TE Jr, et al: Reducing hopelessness: the interaction of enhancing and depressogenic attributional styles for positive and negative life events among youth psychiatric inpatients. Behav Res Ther 41:1183–1198, 2003

Wagner A, Lecavalier L, Arnold LE, et al: Developmental disabilities modification of the Children's Global Assessment Scale. Biol Psychiatry 61:504–511, 2007

Wagner KD, Jonas J, Findling RL, et al: A double-blind, randomized, placebo-controlled trial of escitalopram in the treatment of pediatric depression. J Am Acad Child Adolesc Psychiatry 45:280–288, 2006

Wijsbroek SAM, Hale WW, Raaijmakers Q, et al: Psychometric characteristics of the Screen for Child Anxiety Related Emotional Disorders (SCARED) in a Dutch population of adolescents. Ned Tijdschr Psychol 60:129–138, 2005

Winters NC, Myers K, Proud L: Ten-year review of rating scales, III: scales for suicidality, cognitive style, and self-esteem. J Am Acad Child Adolesc Psychiatry 41:1050–1181, 2002

Winters NC, Collett BR, Myers KM: Ten-year review of rating scales, VII: scales assessing functional impairment. J Am Acad Child Adolesc Psychiatry 44:309–338, 2005

Wolraich ML: Vanderbilt ADHD Parent Rating Scale (VADPRS). Cambridge, MA, American Academy of Pediatrics and The National Initiative for Children's Healthcare Quality, 2003a

Wolraich ML: Vanderbilt ADHD Teacher Rating Scale (VADTRS). Cambridge, MA, American Academy of Pediatrics and The National Initiative for Children's Healthcare Quality, 2003b

Wolraich ML, Feurer ID, Hannah JN, et al: Obtaining systematic teacher reports of disruptive behavior disorders utilizing DSM-IV. J Abnorm Child Psychol 26:141–152, 1998

Wolraich ML, Lambert W, Doffing MA, et al: Psychometric properties of the Vanderbilt ADHD diagnostic parent rating scale in a referred population. J Pediatr Psychol 28:559–567, 2003

Yonkers KA, Samson JA: Young Mania Rating Scale, in Handbook of Psychiatric Measures, 2nd Edition. Edited by Rush AJ, First MB, Blacker D. Washington, DC, American Psychiatric Publishing, 2008, pp 519–521

Young R, Biggs J, Ziegler V, et al: A rating scale for mania: reliability, validity and sensitivity. Br J Psychiatry 133:429–435, 1978

Youngstrom EA, Findling RL, Calabrese JR: Effects of adolescent manic symptoms on agreement between youth, parent, and teacher ratings of behavior problems. J Affect Disord 82(suppl):S5–S16, 2004

Chapter 9

Pediatric Evaluation and Laboratory Testing

Tami Benton, M.D.
Wanjiku Njoroge, M.D.
Amy Kim, M.D.

The initial comprehensive evaluation of a child or adolescent presenting with psychiatric symptoms provides an opportunity to gather information about the child's health status, health care providers, past or current medical illnesses, disabilities, hospitalizations, surgeries, allergies, and medications. It is imperative that physical ailments are investigated before assuming that the cause of concern is psychiatric in nature.

The assessment of children presenting with behavioral symptoms begins with identification of the child's primary care medical provider and clarification of the health supervision of the child, including regularly scheduled primary care visits that insure adequate nutrition, detect and immunize against infectious diseases, and monitor the child's development. The frequency and content of these visits are included in recommendations from the American Academy of Pediatrics (Hagan and Duncan 2007).

Medical Diagnostic Approach to the Patient Presenting With Psychiatric Symptoms

Essential Elements of the Medical History

A comprehensive medical history, the use of collateral informants, and close collaboration with the pediatric provider are essential in the evaluation of children and adolescents who present with psychiatric and behavioral symptoms.

For infants, toddlers, and preschoolers, the first questions should establish the presence of regular pediatric visits, well-child visits, and immunizations as scheduled. History gathering begins with the child's conception, gestation, and delivery. Questions about the circumstances of conception, prenatal care, and ease of pregnancy or complications and their treatments should be asked. A history of in-utero exposure to medications, substances, and environmental toxins should be obtained, as well as any history of travel that may have taken place outside of the country and associated immunizations that occurred during the pregnancy. A history of labor and delivery should be reviewed and should include gestational age, Apgar scores, nature of delivery, and complications such as hyperbilirubinemia, respiratory distress, infections, or congenital abnormalities (Thomas et al. 1997).

The history proceeds from birth until the present, focusing on physical concerns, illnesses, hospitalizations, and treatments. The history gathering should include the family pedigree and review of the family medical and psychiatric history from both parents, with emphasis on diseases or disorders that may manifest initially in very young children. Specific inquiries about a family history of sudden cardiac death and hypercholesterolemia are relevant in children who may be treated with psychotropic medications.

A detailed investigation of the child's development is an integral component of this assessment. (American Academy of Pediatrics Committee on Children With Disabilities 2001, 2006). One of the scales most commonly used by pediatricians is the Denver Developmental Screening Tool to screen for developmental problems in children up to 6 years of age (Frankenburg et al. 1975). The screen assesses gross and fine motor, personal-social, and language development. Corrections and allowance are made for prematurity until 2 years of age.

History for the 6- to 11-year-old child (middle childhood) focuses on growth, development, and skills acquisition. This phase is characterized by physical growth, episodic growth spurts lasting approximately 8 weeks, with final growth at an average rate of 3–3.5 kg and 6–7 cm per year. Head growth slows, reflecting a slowing of brain growth with head circumference increasing at only about 2–3 cm in circumference during this period. Myelinization is complete by 7 years of age, and the body habitus is more erect with longer legs when compared to torso (Feigelman 2007). The clinician should assess the early developmental history, ascertaining whether developmental milestones were achieved normally or if there were developmental de-

lays. If there were delays, were early intervention services used, and if services were used, were they effective? Information is gathered about temperament, sensory activities, feeding and sleep habits, and bowel and bladder control and when they were achieved. Eliciting information about medical illnesses or disabilities is especially important as medical and psychiatric symptoms are highly comorbid (Shaw and DeMaso 2006). Information about the child's current and past physical growth, including height, weight, head circumference, and pubertal status, should be obtained. Screening for hearing and vision should occur, with more detailed testing if abnormalities are noted. A detailed assessment of physical activities, including participation in organized sports or other activities, should be elicited (Boyce et al. 2002).

Adolescent physical development is characterized by physical growth and sexual development. Between 10–20 years of age, youth undergo rapid changes in body structure as well as changes in psychological and social development. Adolescent physical development is divided into three phases: early (10–13 years of age), middle (14–16 years), and late (17–20 years) adolescence. Puberty describes the process by which an adolescent becomes an adult, including the development of secondary sexual characteristics, growth to adult size, and the onset of reproductive ability (Marcel 2007). Hormonal interactions result in a complex and predictable pattern of sexual and physical development starting at approximately 10 years of age in girls and approximately 13 years of age in boys.

Growth acceleration for both sexes also occurs at this time, with increased growth velocity beginning in early adolescence and peaking at sexual maturity, with boys typically peaking 2–3 years after girls have stopped growing.

Review of Systems

The comprehensive review of systems in the pediatric population, organized by organ system or functional system, is especially important because parents are more likely to focus on one concrete concern while relegating other important symptoms to typical behavior. The clinician may gather seemingly unrelated threads and weave a complete picture regarding the child's health. Though parents may not understand the thoroughness of the review, it is important to assure them that the painstaking approach of gathering information will insure that their child receives the best care. Questionable findings, even in the face of clear psychiatric symptoms, should be thoroughly evaluated.

Preschool and school-age children who have genetic syndromes that were not discovered prenatally or postnatally may present for an initial assessment with social-emotional or behavioral concerns as their chief complaint. Some of these genetic disorders have recognizable behavioral phenotypes (King et al. 2005) and are noted in Table 9–1.

Brain Structure and Function

The assessment of brain structure and function is one of the cornerstones of the pediatric evaluation (see Chapter 10, "Neurological Examination, Electroencephalography, and Neuroimaging"). Important elements of this assessment should include

- Questions about head growth or abnormalities
- Questions about the child's temperament and changes in behavior (e.g., Has the child seemed more irritable? short-tempered?)
- Questions regarding balance with considerations for the child's level of development (e.g., Has the child learned to sit without support? Does he topple to one side or the other? Has his gait become increasingly unsteady, or has he not yet learned to ambulate, or does he have delayed motor development?)
- History of vomiting, loss of skills, or recently increased apathy
- History of recent febrile illness or any other signs of infection (If so, was the child treated by a pediatrician or treated with analgesics by parents?)
- History of head injury, loss of consciousness, seizures, child's falling from a surface such as a couch or bed, being hit in the head with an object or by another sibling, or any other occurrence that may have preceded the current concerns (Injuries sustained by a young child may lead to a disruption in behavior.)
- Headaches (If present, a detailed history should be obtained.)

Eye, Ear, Nose, Neck, and Throat

The clinician should inquire about the results of pediatric hearing and visual screening. Early identification of amblyopia and strabismus is important, because earlier intervention is associated with better outcomes. Furthermore, common childhood illnesses, such as recurrent otitis media, or the placement of myringotomy tubes may affect speech/language development or the child's perceived relatedness.

Symptoms of sleep apnea should be assessed in children who present with disruptive behavior, as well as other potential symptoms of sleep problems—such as snoring at night, having multiple nighttime arousals, experiencing increased irritability during the day, or having increased disruptive behaviors mimicking attention-deficit/hyperactivity (ADHD) symptoms.

Respiratory System

The evaluation of the respiratory system should include questions about dyspnea, cough, pain, wheezing, snoring, apnea, and cyanosis chronicity; the timing of these symptoms; diurnal variations; associations with activities such as exercise, meals, or stressors; and a history of environmental allergies. The family history should include information about respiratory illness in siblings or other family members presenting with similar symptoms or chronic diseases with respiratory symptoms.

Identifying a history of asthma is extremely important. In the United States, childhood asthma is the most common cause of childhood emergency department visits, hospitalizations, and missed school days (Centers for Disease Control and Prevention 2005). Children with asthma may present with increased irritability, decreased activity levels, or anxious behaviors related to the illness, its treatments, or sequelae of the interventions related to the illness, such as emergency room visits or intensive care admissions. Questions should focus on changes in the child's temperament, mood, or behavior. The review of systems should include medications taken by the child, as inhaled medications may cause behavioral symptoms. For example, inhaled albuterol and terbutaline may cause palpitations, tremor, and nervousness. Propranolol is contraindicated in individuals with asthma. Undertreatment or poor adherence to medication regimens may result in hypoxic episodes requiring consultation with the treating primary provider.

Cardiovascular System

Recent reports of sudden unexplained deaths in the presence of psychotropic medications and recommendations for cardiac monitoring with the use of stimulant medications underline the importance of this assessment (Villalaba 2006). Some studies suggest that certain psychiatric conditions, such as ADHD, may be more prevalent in children with heart disease than in the general population (Gothelf et al. 2003). Complicating this presentation is the fact that tachycardia, palpitations, and cardiac arrhythmias are among the most common signs of anxiety. The history should include details of the perinatal period, including respiratory distress, cyanosis, or prematurity. Maternal complications such as gestational diabetes, medications, sys-

TABLE 9–1.   Selected genetic syndromes with behavioral phenotypes

Syndrome	Behavioral phenotype
Angelman's syndrome	Developmental delay, hyperactivity diminishing with age, short attention span (Buntinx et al. 1995)
Cornelia de Lange's (Brachmann de Lange) syndrome	Developmental delay, hyperactivity, self-injury, aggression, sleep disturbance, diminished social relatedness, repetitive and stereotyped behaviors, "autistic-like" behaviors (Hyman et al. 2002)
Down syndrome	Developmental delay, stubbornness, inattention, opposition, depression and dementia (adults) (Collacott et al. 1998)
Fetal alcohol syndrome	Cognitive deficits, hyperactivity, short attention span, distractibility, impaired concentration, withdrawal (Kelly et al. 2000)
Fragile X syndrome	Cognitive deficits, inattention, hyperactivity, distractibility, disturbance in language/communication, social anxiety, social deficits, poor eye contact, cognitive abnormalities (Reiss and Hall 2007)
Lesch-Nyhan syndrome	Self-injurious behavior, self-biting, compulsive behaviors, coprolalia, copropraxia (Jinnah and Friedman 2000)
Neurofibromatosis I	Attentional problems, social withdrawal, hyperactivity, cognitive deficits (Lewis et al. 2004)
Noonan syndrome	Cognitive deficits, social problems, attention deficits, anxiety (Verhoeven et al. 2008).
Prader-Willi syndrome	Developmental delay, excessive food-seeking behaviors, oppositional behaviors, interpersonal problems, repetitive behaviors, affective dysregulation, and increased risk of ADHD, obsessive-compulsive disorder, and mood and psychotic symptoms (Benarroch et al. 2007)
Rett syndrome	Autistic symptoms, including loss of language and repetitive stereotypic behaviors (Ben Zeev Ghidoni 2007).
Rubenstein-Taybi syndrome	Developmental delay, short attention span, impulsivity, moodiness, hyperacusis, autistic behaviors (Stevens et al. 1999)
Smith-Lemli-Opitz syndrome	Self-stimulation, self-destructive behaviors, autism spectrum disorders (Sikora et al. 2006)
Smith-Magenis syndrome	Affective lability, temper tantrums, impulsivity, anxiety, physical aggression, destruction, argumentativeness, sleep difficulties (Shelley and Robertson 2005)
Sotos syndrome	Cognitive deficits, social deficits, peer difficulties (De Boer et al. 2006)
Tuberous sclerosis complex	Attention deficits, hyperactivity, impulsivity, learning disability, cognitive deficits (Lewis et al. 2004)
Turner syndrome	Uneven cognitive profile, increased risks of anxiety, low self-esteem, depression related to physical appearance (Kesler 2007)
Velocardiofacial syndrome (22q11 deletion)	Cognitive deficits; repetitive, stereotyped behaviors; higher rates of ADHD, anxiety disorders, affective disorders, and psychotic disorders; autistic spectrum disorders (Gothelf 2007)
Williams syndrome	Cognitive unevenness, hypersociability, social anxiety, anxiety, fears, inattention, hyperactivity, hyperacusis (Feinstein and Singh 2007)

Note.   ADHD=attention-deficit/hyperactivity disorder.

temic lupus erythematosus, or substance abuse can be associated with cardiac problems. When eliciting history, it is important to remember that symptoms of heart disease in infants and children are age specific.

For example, heart failure in infants may manifest as feeding difficulties, while heart failure in a school-age child might manifest as exercise intolerance, difficulty keeping up with peers in sports activities, or napping after school. The comprehensive cardiac history should include information about the following:

- History of fatigue during activities such as walking, bike riding, physical education class, or competitive sports
- Shortness of breath during exercise, at night, or during sleep
- Fainting or dizziness
- Rheumatic fever
- Change in exercise tolerance
- Palpitations, extra or skipped beats, or increased heart rates
- High blood pressure
- Heart murmurs
- Viral illness with chest pain or palpitations
- Prescribed or over-the-counter medications

The family history should include information about sudden death during exercise, arrhythmias, cardiomyopathies, cardiac conduction abnormalities, and Marfan syndrome and might reveal early coronary artery disease or stroke, generalized muscle disease, or congenital heart disease (Vetter et al. 2008). Chest pain is an uncommon symptom of cardiac disease in the pediatric population and is more commonly musculoskeletal or pulmonary in origin. Patients presenting with symptoms suggestive of heart disease should be referred for further cardiac evaluation.

Gastrointestinal System

This portion of the evaluation should focus on appetite; feeding practices, preferences, and behaviors; stool patterns such as diarrhea, constipation, and associated behaviors; vomiting; weight loss or gain; abdominal pain; anorexia; and overeating. For young children and school-age children, questions about growth, feeding behaviors (picky, poor, or restrictive eaters), excessive food intake, vomiting, and abdominal pain or abnormal stool patterns (constipation, diarrhea, or withheld stool) are appropriate. Gastrointestinal complaints, especially abdominal pain, are common. Pain perception and tolerance vary for each individual child, making the evaluation of abdominal pain challenging. A child with "functional" abdominal pain (no organic cause identified) can suffer as much as a child with an identified organic etiology. The more specific the description of the pain and the more consistent with a specific clinical condition, the more likely it will be that the pain will have an organic basis (Wylie 2007). All children presenting with abdominal pain should have a complete physical examination.

Gastrointestinal complaints in children vary significantly by age. Young children will present principally with pain, bowel abnormalities, or feeding difficulties. Adolescents will frequently present with excessive weight loss or gain. Excessive weight loss in adolescents may be related to pathologies such as ulcerative colitis or other gastrointestinal diseases; however, excessive weight loss is more likely to be related to eating disorders, laxative abuse, and induced vomiting, or to use of substances that may cause weight loss, such as amphetamines or cocaine. Patients who may have diabetes mellitus can also present with changes in appetite and weight, and the possibility of this diagnosis must be explored.

Genitourinary System

This review should include symptoms of urinary tract disorders as well as an assessment of menstrual (for females) and sexual functioning for the adolescent. Symptoms of changes in urinary patterns, frequency, urgency, pain, or infections should be elicited. History of trauma or abuse should be obtained, and an expert should evaluate any symptoms suggestive of abuse. Menstrual history, including age at onset, timing, regularity, cycle lengths, pain, or other associated difficulties such as changes in mood or irritability, should be obtained. Questions about sexual activity and exposures to sexually transmitted diseases should be asked, including questions about exposure to HIV. As some psychotropic medications affect these systems, questions about changes in urinary patterns (e.g., urinary hesitancy with anticholinergics) or patterns of sexual functioning (e.g., selective serotonin reuptake inhibitors and anorgasmia) should be specifically asked of adolescents.

Physical Assessment

Screening of hearing and vision, with further testing if indicated, might identify children with learning, language or social delays, or inattention and opposition due to deficits in these areas. Evaluation of major or minor physical anomalies, dysmorphic features, head circumference, or dermatologic abnormalities may provide clues to the etiologies of developmental disabilities. Effective collaboration between pediatric providers and child psychiatrists and other mental health clinicians will guide further medical evaluations or assessments.

Pediatric Vital Signs

There are age-dependent normative values for pediatric vital signs. In general, the resting heart rate in newborns and infants will be approximately 120 beats per minute, in toddlers and young school-age children 100–120 beats per minute, 70–80 beats per minute in latency-age children, and 70 beats per minute for adolescents. Normal respiratory rates can be as high as 30–40 breaths per minute in infants, with normal rates slowly decreasing to 12–25 breaths per minute in children and then averaging 12–15 breaths per minute in adolescents. Blood pressure normative values also change with age. In newborns, systolic blood pressure may range between 65 and 95 mmHg and the diastolic may range between 30 and 45 mmHg. Blood pressures in normal school-age children are in the range of 80–120 mmHg systolic and 40–80 mmHg diastolic. Normal systolic and diastolic blood pressures gradually increase as children grow until they reach adult values in adolescence.

Abnormal vital signs can occur as side effects from medications, in states of delirium, and from drug and alcohol intoxication and withdrawal. Blood pressure and heart rate should be monitored routinely in children who are on stimulants, atomoxetine, and venlafaxine, as these medications can be associated with increased pulse and blood pressure. One should also monitor blood pressure in children who are taking clonidine, which can be associated with hypotension.

Growth Measurements

The physical assessment of children and adolescents should always include measurements of somatic growth. This includes measuring height and weight; head circumference should be measured in infants and toddlers initially and then periodically as indicated until the age of 2 years. Inadequate growth may be associated with developmental disorders, genetic syndromes, feeding disorders, and nutritional and emotional deprivation, as well as several other medical conditions. Height, weight, and body mass index (BMI) should be monitored every 3–6 months in children who are on medications known to affect growth such as atypical antipsychotic medications, which can be associated with excessive weight gain and metabolic syndrome, and stimulants, which have been associated with weight loss and slowing of vertical growth.

Growth measurements should be plotted and tracked on standard growth charts noting the percentiles and trends over time. If there are discrepancies in percentiles for height, weight, or BMI or significant changes in the percentile due to weight gain, weight loss, or inadequate weight gain, the cause should be investigated further.

General Appearance

Note if the child's appearance, chronological age, behavior, developmental skills, and emotional level correspond with the stated age. Observe how the child and parent interact. Note whether the child appears well or ill and appropriately nourished. Is the child demonstrating distress emotionally or physically? Are there obvious dysmorphic features?

- *Skin:* One might observe the stigmata of neurofibromatosis, such as café au lait spots, neurofibromas, and axillary freckling. Unusual patterns of bruising or burns may be indicative of child abuse.
- *Head:* Note the size, shape, and symmetry of the skull and face or presence of atypical facial patterns. There are specific findings associated with various congenital syndromes or patterns or with specific abnormalities, such as with trichotillomania.
- *Neck:* Observe for goiter.
- *Eyes/vision:* Visual screening is part of a routine physical evaluation during the school-age years. After the child is age 3 years, the Snellen E can be used. When the child reaches 6–7 years of age, normal vision should be 20/20.
- *Ears/hearing:* Hearing evaluation and screening are also part of a routine pediatric physical evaluation. With younger children, the clinician can test hearing by whispering from 8 feet away or by using a tuning fork. Refer for more comprehensive hearing evaluation if there are abnormalities on exam, parent concerns, or speech/language delays.
- *Thorax/lungs:* Observe effort and work of breathing.
- *Musculoskeletal system:* Note muscle tone, gait, coordination, joint mobility, and range of motion.

Diagnostic Laboratory Assessments

Studies examining the utility of routine laboratory assessments for psychiatric disorders in the pediatric population have been limited. However, existing studies suggest that routine laboratory tests are not clinically useful in typical psychiatric settings, such as outpatient clinics and inpatient units (Adams et al. 1997;

Leo et al. 1997; Zametkin et al. 1998). One study examining laboratory screenings for 111 consecutively admitted adolescents with first-onset psychosis, who had normal physical examinations and unremarkable medical histories, found that 15.4% of the endocrine screening tests and 11% of the neuroimaging tests were identified as positive but that none provided diagnostic utility (Adams et al. 1997). Laboratory testing has produced higher yields in high-risk populations presenting with psychiatric symptoms, such as those presenting to emergency departments, treatment centers for substance abuse, and HIV treatment centers; in those with symptoms of physical illness; and in children with developmental disabilities and mental retardation (Guze and Love 2005).

Children and adolescents presenting with delirium, anxiety, depression, and hallucinations may have medical illnesses that produce these symptoms (Table 9–2) and should be evaluated for medical etiologies that can be treated.

Testing is also important in the monitoring of many psychotropic medications for therapeutic dosing or for monitoring parameters relevant to psychotropic treatments for adverse effects, such as metabolic abnormalities with antipsychotic medications or elevated prolactin levels with antipsychotic agents. These tests should occur in the context of the overall patient assessment to minimize discomfort to the patient, decrease risks of false positives requiring further testing, and lessen costs to families.

Hematological Functioning

Abnormalities of hematological functioning can produce psychiatric symptoms, and some psychiatric treatments may affect hematological functioning. Current recommendations are that a complete blood count (CBC) should be a part of a routine pediatric screen (Green 2004). The red blood cell indices, hemoglobin and hematocrit, can provide information about anemia and vitamin or mineral deficiencies, and the patterns of abnormalities can provide information about the etiologies of anemia. Asthenia, depression, and psychosis have been associated with anemia. Folate and vitamin B_{12} deficiencies have been associated with delirium and psychosis and can be found in adolescents who abuse alcohol, take phenytoin, or use estrogen-containing oral contraceptives. Individuals at risk for anemia—such as cow's milk–fed infants, as well as toddlers, adolescent girls, pregnant teens, and recent immigrants from foreign countries—should be selectively screened (Bertil 2007).

The white blood cell count may be elevated with infections or leukemias, or the counts may be lowered in response to certain psychotropic medications. Baseline white blood cell counts are indicated prior to the initiation of carbamazepine, lithium, clozapine, or lamotrigine and as recommended for treatment monitoring (Kowatch and DelBello 2007; Kranzler et al. 2006).

Serum Electrolytes

Abnormalities of the serum electrolytes, sodium, potassium, chloride, phosphorus, magnesium, and calcium can be found in patients presenting with a variety of psychiatric symptoms. They may occur as the result of a medical or psychiatric illness or may be induced by the use of psychotropic medications. Low levels of chloride, potassium, phosphorus, and calcium with elevated bicarbonate levels are commonly found in patients with eating disorders who purge or abuse laxatives or who have psychogenic vomiting. Phosphorus and bicarbonate levels may be low in anxious individuals who hyperventilate. Low levels of potassium are associated with weakness, fatigue, and electrocardiogram (ECG) changes that may be life-threatening. Low sodium levels can be found in the syndrome of inappropriate secretion of antidiuretic hormone, psychogenic water drinking, or carbamazepine use and can manifest as delirium. Abnormalities of serum calcium can manifest with psychosis, depression, delirium, irritability, and weakness (Guze and Love 2005).

Renal Function Tests

This assessment usually includes blood urea nitrogen, creatinine clearance, and urinalysis. Abnormalities of these indices are suggestive of renal impairment reflected in decreased capacity for clearance or concentration. Deficits in renal capacity can result in alterations of mental status. For individuals taking lithium, blood urea nitrogen, creatinine levels, and 24-hour urine creatinine clearance tests are used to determine renal function prior to medication initiation and follow-up treatment.

Liver Function Tests

Tests of liver function include alkaline phosphatase, alanine aminotransferase, aspartate aminotransferase, glutamyl transaminases, bilirubin, and amylase. Aminotransferase and alkaline phosphatase are nonspecific and can be elevated in other nonhepatic conditions. Alkaline phosphatase levels may be elevated

TABLE 9–2.   Medical conditions that may manifest with psychiatric symptoms

Neurological and cerebrovascular disorders	**Metabolic and systemic disorders**
Epilepsy	Fluid and electrolyte disturbances
Head trauma	Hepatic encephalopathy
Huntington's disease	Uremia
Idiopathic calcification of basal ganglia	Porphyria
Narcolepsy	Hepatolenticular degeneration (Wilson's disease)
Brain neoplasms	Chronic hypoxemia
Normal-pressure hydrocephalus	Hypotension
Multiple sclerosis	Hypertensive encephalopathy
Metachromatic leukodystrophy	**Infectious diseases**
Migraine	AIDS
Posttraumatic encephalopathy	Neurosyphilis
Postconcussion stroke	Viral meningitides and encephalitides
Stroke	Brain abscess
Endocrine disorders	Viral hepatitis
Hypothyroidism	Infectious mononucleosis
Hyperthyroidism	Tuberculosis
Hypoadrenalism	Bacteremia and viremia
Hyperadrenalism	Streptococcal infections
Hypoparathyroidism	PANDAS
Hyperparathyroidism	**Neoplastic disorders**
Hypoglycemia	CNS primary and metastatic tumors
Diabetes mellitus	Endocrine tumors
Panhypopituitarism	Paraneoplastic syndromes
Pheochromocytoma	**Toxic conditions**
Gonadotropic hormonal disturbances	Intoxication or withdrawal from substances
Autoimmune disorders	Over-the-counter or prescribed medications
Systemic lupus erythematosus	Environmental toxins (e.g., lead, carbon monoxide)
Nutritional deficiencies	
Vitamin B_{12} deficiency	
Nicotinic acid deficiency	
Thiamine deficiency	
Trace metal deficiency	
Folate deficiency	
Malnutrition/dehydration	

Note.   CNS=central nervous system; PANDAS=pediatric autoimmune neuropsychiatric disorders associated with streptococcal infection.

when phenothiazines are used. Glutamyl transaminases and bilirubin elevations are generally suggestive of liver disease and should be obtained prior to the initiation of psychotropic medications that are metabolized by the liver, specifically valproate and carbamazepine. Elevated amylase can be seen with pancreatic disease and in individuals with bulimia who engage in purging behaviors.

Endocrine Assessments

Endocrine testing is not a routine component of the baseline screening assessment in the pediatric patient presenting with psychiatric symptoms, with the exception of thyroid testing. Thyroid testing is used for the assessment of patients presenting with depression, anxiety, panic, and psychosis. The most common screening test for thyroid dysfunction is the measurement of thyroid-stimulating hormone (thyrotropin). Many clinicians also order serum thyroxine (T_4) and triiodothyronine (T_3). More than 90% of T_4 is bound to serum protein and is responsible for thyrotropin secretion and cellular metabolism. Other measures include T_4 radioimmunoassay, free T_4 index, and total serum T_3 measured by radioimmunoassay.

Evidence suggests that use of neuroendocrine testing for screening and diagnostic purposes in the child and adolescent psychiatric populations is not warranted and that the use of these tests should be guided by medical and family history and physical findings (Adams et al. 1997). ADHD-like symptoms have been reported to be associated with a variety of thyroid abnormalities. Routine thyroid screening should be done for children with a family history of thyroid disorders, goiter, low birth weight, growth retardation, and speech or hearing impairment (Zametkin et al. 1998) but should not be a part of the routine assessment of ADHD in nonfamilial ADHD (Elia et al. 1994). Tests for plasma cortisol, catecholamines, antidiuretic hormone, growth hormone, prolactin, testosterone, estrogen, gonadotropic-releasing hormones, and follicle-stimulating hormones should be obtained when indicated for evaluation of abnormal clinical findings suggestive of endocrine dysfunction.

Children and adolescents presenting with behavioral symptoms and whose history or physical findings suggest an organic etiology should receive baseline laboratory assessments (Table 9–3).

Cardiac Assessments

Current recommendations for the assessment of children and adolescents in psychiatric practice do not include routine ECGs for screening. A family or medical history of sudden cardiac death, symptoms of palpitations, fainting, exercise intolerance, chest pain, arrhythmias, syncope, and hypertension would suggest further cardiac evaluation and testing (Vetter et al. 2008). ECGs are most commonly used in psychiatric practice for monitoring the effects of medications known to adversely affect cardiac function or in those

TABLE 9–3. Baseline screening tests

Complete blood count
Serum electrolytes
Blood glucose
Renal function tests
Hepatic function tests
Thyroid function tests
Urinalysis
Drug screening (urine/serum)

individuals with psychiatric disorders known to occur with cardiac symptoms, such as individuals with eating disorders who purge (hypokalemia).

Medications used in psychiatric practice with cardiac effects include the tricyclic antidepressants (TCAs), the antipsychotic medications ziprasidone and thioridazine, and lithium. TCAs have been associated with prolongation of the PR, QT, and QRS intervals, along with ST-segment and T-wave abnormalities. They may exacerbate a preexisting atrioventricular or bundle branch block and have been associated with sudden cardiac death (Gutgesell et al. 1999). Agents associated with prolongation of the QTc interval have been associated with torsades de pointes, arrhythmias, and sudden death. Ziprasidone and thioridazine have been associated with prolongation of the QTc in adults and adolescents (Blair et al. 2005). Clinicians using these medications should obtain an ECG prior to initiation and use regular ECG monitoring, especially when used in high doses or when combined with other QTc-prolonging agents. Lithium therapy can cause benign reversible T-wave changes and impair SA nodal function, suggesting that an ECG should be obtained prior to initiation.

While screening ECGs have not routinely been recommended by the American Academy of Child and Adolescent Psychiatry (2007) for the treatment of ADHD in healthy children or by the American Heart Association (AHA; Gutgesell et al. 1999), recent concerns about cardiac safety with stimulant use have prompted a review of this issue. A recent statement issued by the American Academy of Pediatrics and the AHA regarding children and adolescents without known cardiac conditions recommends that clinicians carefully assess children for heart conditions when stimulant treatment is needed for ADHD, recognizing that certain heart conditions of childhood are difficult to detect (Perrin et al. 2008). Clinicians should obtain a patient and family health history and complete a physical examination focused on cardiovascular risk factors (Class I recommendations) before treatment with drugs for ADHD. The current policy recommendation is that healthy children do not need an ECG before initiating stimulant treatment (Perrin et al. 2008). Children with known cardiac conditions should be monitored by their physicians.

Indications for Specialized Testing

Certain pediatric presentations may suggest the need for more specialized diagnostic testing.

Developmental Disorders and Mental Retardation

The etiology of mental retardation remains unknown for most individuals, although severe disability is more likely due to a known genetic variation. Trisomy 21 (Down syndrome) or fragile X syndrome is present in approximately half of the individuals with mental retardation, indicating the need for genetic testing. Some congenital disorders are higher in individuals with autism or pervasive developmental disorders such as tuberous sclerosis, suggesting the utility of genetic testing to provide prognostic information, risk of recurrence, and life planning for families (Yeargen-Allsopp and Boyle 2002).

Disorders Manifesting With Psychotic Symptoms

Children and adolescents presenting with new-onset psychotic symptoms should be assessed for symptoms that may mimic psychosis, in addition to a thorough physical and neurological examination. However, most cases are not attributable to organic illness. Altered levels of consciousness, abnormal neurological findings, altered vital signs, or new-onset seizures should trigger an evaluation for acute intoxication, delirium, metabolic disorders, neurodegenerative processes, encephalopathies, seizure disorders, central nervous system lesions, tumors, infections, and trauma. In addition to the CBC, serum chemistries, and liver, renal, and thyroid function tests, additional examinations, including a toxicology screen looking for substances of abuse, neuroimaging, electroencephalography, and cerebrospinal fluid examination, and examinations for autoimmune diseases and metabolic studies should be done if suggested by physical findings.

Mood Disorders

Children and adolescents presenting with new-onset mood symptoms should be assessed for medical conditions contributing to this presentation as well. Infectious diseases such as Lyme disease, HIV, infectious mononucleosis, thyroid disease, systemic lupus erythematosus, diabetes, epilepsy, and illicit substance use may manifest as depressed mood, mood swings, or cognitive changes. Physical symptoms such as fever, headache, sore throat, nausea, fatigue, and loss of appetite with weight loss are suggestive of organic illness and should be evaluated (Shaw and DeMaso 2006).

Obsessive-Compulsive Disorder

In a minority of cases, acute onset of obsessive-compulsive disorder and tics may present following streptococcal infection. Current evidence suggests that acute cases associated with pharyngitis should receive a throat culture and serologic studies for group A beta hemolytic streptococcus infection, including antideoxyribonuclease B and antistreptolysin O antibody titers.

Substance Use and Abuse

Patients presenting with new-onset psychiatric or behavioral symptoms, particularly adolescents and those who are at risk due to previous substance abuse or involvement with the juvenile justice system, as well as youth with conduct disorder, should be screened for substance use (see Chapter 17, "Substance Abuse and Addictions").

Conclusion

Screening laboratory assessments for children and adolescents presenting with psychiatric symptoms have not been supported by empirical evidence. Both adult and child studies suggest that broad screening of healthy individuals with psychiatric symptoms may provide little useful information. The evidence suggests that testing for medical conditions occur based upon medical history, review of systems, and physical presentation. Groups at higher risk based upon age, illness, or environmental circumstances merit further testing. Understanding physical health and illness and close collaborations with our pediatric health partners are essential to our mission of promoting the health of children and families.

Summary Points

- A thorough and comprehensive medical history is an essential component of the evaluation of children and adolescents who present with psychiatric and behavioral symptoms.

- Eliciting information about medical illness or disabilities is especially important, as medical and psychiatric symptoms are highly comorbid.

- Close collaboration with pediatric health care providers is essential for the care of children with behavioral or emotional disturbances.

- Guided by the history, review of systems, psychiatric evaluation, and any physical findings, child and adolescent psychiatrists should use diagnostic testing, including neuroimaging and endocrine studies, to identify medical illnesses that could manifest with psychiatric symptoms. The psychiatric assessment remains the cornerstone for diagnosis of psychiatric disorders.

- Psychiatric and/or severe behavioral symptoms manifesting in very young children are more likely to have developmental, genetic, or organic etiologies and merit further evaluation.

- When stimulant medications are indicated for the treatment of ADHD, electrocardiograms are not routinely recommended for children and adolescents who do not have known cardiac conditions.

References

Adams M, Kutcher S, Antoniw E, et al: Diagnostic utility of endocrine and neuroimaging screening tests in first-onset adolescent psychosis. J Am Acad Child Adolesc Psychiatry 35:67–73, 1997

American Academy of Child and Adolescent Psychiatry: Practice parameter for the assessment and treatment of children and adolescents with attention-deficit/hyperactivity disorder. J Am Acad Child Adolesc Psychiatry 46:894–921, 2007

American Academy of Pediatrics Committee on Children With Disabilities: Developmental surveillance and screening of infants and young children. Pediatrics 108:192–196, 2001

American Academy of Pediatrics Committee on Children With Disabilities: Identifying infants and young children with developmental disorders in the medical home: an algorithm for developmental surveillance and screening. Pediatrics 118:405–420, 2006

Benarroch F, Hirsch HJ, Gentsil L, et al: Prader-Willi syndrome: medical prevention and behavioral challenges. Child Adolesc Psychiatr Clin N Am 16:695–708, 2007

Ben Zeev Ghidoni B: Rett syndrome. Child Adolesc Psychiatr Clin N Am 16:723–743, 2007

Bertil G: Anemias of inadequate production, in Nelson's Textbook of Pediatrics. Edited by Kleigman RM, Behrman RE, Jenson HB, et al. Philadelphia, PA, WB Saunders, 2007, pp 2006–2018

Blair J, Schahill L, State M, et al: Electrocardiographic changes in children and adolescents treated with ziprasidone: a prospective study. J Am Acad Child Adolesc Psychiatry 44:73–79, 2005

Boyce WT, Essex MJ, Woodward HR, et al: The confluence of mental, physical, social and academic difficulties in middle childhood, I: exploring the head waters of early life morbidities. J Am Acad Child Adolesc Psychiatry 41:580–587, 2002

Buntinx IM, Hennekam RL, Brouwer OF, et al: Clinical profile of Angelman syndrome at different ages. Am J Med Genet 56:176–183, 1995

Centers for Disease Control and Prevention: Reducing childhood asthma through community-based service delivery: New York City, 2001–2004. MMWR Morb Mortal Wkly Rep S4:11–14, 2005

Collacott RA, Cooper SA, Branford D, et al: Behavior phenotype for Down's syndrome. Br J Psychiatry 172:85–89, 1998

De Boer L, Roder I, Wit JM: Psychosocial, cognitive, and motor functioning in patients with suspected Sotos syndrome: a comparison between patients with and without NSD1 gene alterations. Dev Med Child Neurol 48:582–588, 2006

Elia J, Gullota C, Rose SR, et al: Thyroid function and attention-deficit/hyperactivity disorder. J Am Acad Child Adolesc Psychiatry 33:169–172, 1994

Feigelman S: Middle childhood, in Nelson Textbook of Pediatrics. Edited by Kleigman RM, Behrman RE, Jenson HB, et al. Philadelphia, PA, WB Saunders, 2007, pp 57–59

Feinstein C, Singh S: Social phenotypes in neurogenetic syndromes. Child Adolesc Psychiatr Clin N Am 16:631–647, 2007

Frankenburg WK, Dodds J, Fandal A: Denver Developmental Screening Test. Denver, CO, LADOCA, 1975

Gothelf D: Velocardiofacial syndrome. Child Adolesc Psychiatr Clin N Am 16:677–693, 2007

Gothelf D, Gruber R, Presburger G, et al: Methylphenidate treatment for attention-deficit hyperactivity disorder in children and adolescents with velocardiofacial syndrome: an open label study. J Clin Psychiatry 64:1163–1169, 2003

Green WH: Child and Adolescent Clinical Psychopharmacology, 3rd Edition. Philadelphia, PA, Lippincott Williams & Wilkins, 2004, pp 22–26

Gutgesell H, Atkins D, Barst R, et al: AHA Scientific Statement: cardiovascular monitoring of children and adolescents receiving psychotropic drugs. J Am Acad Child Adolesc Psychiatry 38:1047–1050, 1999

Guze BH, Love MJ: Medical assessment and laboratory testing in psychiatry, in Kaplan and Sadock's Comprehensive Textbook of Psychiatry, 8th Edition, Vol 1. Edited by Kaplan HI, Sadock BJ. Baltimore, MD, Lippincott, Williams & Wilkins, 2005, pp 916–928

Hagan JF, Duncan P: Maximizing children's health screening, anticipatory guidance and counseling, in Nelson Textbook of Pediatrics. Edited by Kleigman RM, Behrman RE, Jenson HB, et al. Philadelphia, PA, WB Saunders, 2007, pp 27–31

Hyman P, Oliver C, Hall S: Self-injurious behavior, self-restraint and compulsive behaviors in Cornelia de Lange syndrome. Am J Ment Retard 107:146–154, 2002

Jinnah GA, Friedman T: Lesch-Nyhan disease and its variants, in The Molecular and Metabolic Basis of Inherited Disease, 6th Edition. Edited by Scriver CR, Sly WS, Childs B, et al. New York, McGraw-Hill, 2000, pp 2537–2570

Kelly SJ, Day N, Streissguth AP: Effects of prenatal alcohol exposure on social behavior in humans and other species. Neurotoxicol Teratol 22:143–149, 2000

Kesler SR: Turner syndrome. Child Adolesc Psychiatr Clin N Am 16:709–722, 2007

King BH, Hodapp RM, Dykins EM: Mental retardation. Kaplan and Sadock's Comprehensive Textbook of Psychiatry, 8th Edition. Edited by Kaplan HI, Sadock BJ. Baltimore, MD, Lippincott, Williams & Wilkins, 2005, pp 3076–3106

Kowatch RA, DelBello MP: Pediatric bipolar disorder: emerging diagnostic and treatment approaches. Child Adolesc Psychiatr Clin N Am 15:73–108, 2007

Kranzler HN, Kester HM, Gerbino-Rosen G, et al: Treatment refractory schizophrenia in children and adolescents: an update on clozapine and other pharmacologic interventions. Child Adolesc Psychiatr Clin N Am 15:135–159, 2006

Leo RJ, Batterman-Faunce JM, Pickhardt D, et al: Utility of thyroid screening in adolescent psychiatric inpatients. J Am Acad Child Adolesc Psychiatry 36:103–111, 1997

Lewis JC, Thomas HV, Murphy KC, et al: Genotype and psychological phenotype in tuberous sclerosis. J Med Genet 41:203–207, 2004

Marcel AV: Adolescence, in Nelson Textbook of Pediatrics. Edited by Kleigman RM, Behrman RE, Jenson HB, et al. Philadelphia, PA, WB Saunders, 2007, pp 60–65

Perrin JM, Friedman RA, Knilans TK: Cardiovascular monitoring and stimulant drugs for attention-deficit/hyperactivity disorder. Pediatrics 122:451–453, 2008

Reiss AL, Hall SS: Fragile X syndrome: assessment and treatment implications. Child Adolesc Psychiatr Clin N Am 16:663–675, 2007

Shaw RJ, DeMaso DR: Mood disorders in medical illness, in Clinical Manual of Pediatric Psychosomatic Medicine. Washington, DC, American Psychiatric Publishing, 2006, pp 95–119

Shelley BP, Robertson MM: The neuropsychiatry and multisystem features of the Smith-Magenis syndrome: a review. J Neuropsychiatry Clin Neurosci 17:91–97, 2005

Sikora DM, Pettit-Kekel K, Penfield J, et al: Smith-Lemli Opitz (SLOS). Am J Med Genet A 140:1511–1518, 2006

Stevens CA, Schmitt C, Sperger S: Behavior in Rubenstein-Taybi syndrome. Proc Genet Ctr 18:144–145, 1999

Thomas JM, Benham AL, Gean M, et al: Practice parameters for the psychiatric assessment of infants and toddlers (0–36 months). J Am Acad Child Adolesc Psychiatry 36(suppl):21S–36S, 1997

Verhoeven W, Wingbermuhle E, Egger J, et al: Noonan syndrome: psychological and psychiatric aspects. Am J Med Genet A 146A:191–196, 2008

Vetter VL, Elia J, Erickson C, et al: Cardiovascular monitoring of children and adolescents with heart disease receiving medications for attention-deficit/hyperactivity disorder: a scientific statement from the American Heart Association Council on Cardiovascular Disease in the Young, Congenital Cardiac Defects Committee, and the Council on Cardiovascular Nursing. Circulation 117:2407–2426, 2008

Villalaba L: Follow up review of AERS search identifying cases of sudden death occurring with drugs used for the treatment of attention deficit hyperactivity disorder ADHD. Available at: http://www.fda.gov/ohrms/dockets/ac/06/briefing/2006-4210b_07_01_safetyreview.pdf. Accessed August 12, 2009.

Wylie R: Clinical manifestations of gastrointestinal disease, in Nelson Textbook of Pediatrics. Edited by Kleigman RM, Behrman RE, Jenson HB, et al. Philadelphia, PA, WB Saunders, 2007, pp 1521–1528

Yeargen-Allsopp M, Boyle C: Overview of the epidemiology of neurodevelopmental disorders. Ment Retard Dev Disabil Res Rev 8:113–116, 2002

Zametkin AJ, Ernst M, Silver R: Laboratory and diagnostic testing in child and adolescent psychiatry. J Am Acad Child Adolesc Psychiatry 37:464–472, 1998

Chapter 10

Neurological Examination, Electroencephalography, and Neuroimaging

Sigita Plioplys, M.D.
Miya R. Asato, M.D.

The Neurological Examination

Despite advances in neuroimaging, genetics, or biochemical assays, there is no substitution for the clinical art of history taking and thorough neurological examination.

Chief Complaint

While many patients and families may be able to articulate a specific symptom or problem(s), others may only be able to define a functional difficulty that may point to a neurological symptom, such as clumsiness in a child with hypotonia or ataxia, or inattention in a child with absence epilepsy. The clinician should elicit historical information to define the problem as

- Acute or chronic
- Static or progressive
- Focal or generalized/systemic.

The examination findings will point toward localization.

Case History

An 8-year-old boy with a history of premature birth and associated hypoxic ischemia resulting in spastic diplegia and mild mental retardation presents with a

TABLE 10–1. Elements of the neurological examination based on observation

Examination component	Observation questions
Mental status	How engaged and oriented is the patient to the presenting concern? Is he or she able to articulate and speak coherently? Does the speech have regular rate and prosody? Do there appear to be any language comprehension difficulties? What is the mood and affect of the patient? Does he or she make good eye contact?
Cranial nerves	Is the face symmetric, and is the patient able to demonstrate a good range of facial expression? Is there any eyelid or facial drooping?
Motor	What is the sitting posture of the patient? If the patient moves around during the interview, does there appear to be any asymmetry? Are there any extraneous movements, such as tics or choreiform movements? Can he or she get up and down from the chair without using the armrests (i.e., good proximal muscle strength)?
Sensory	Does the patient have a high-stepping gait, sometimes seen in sensory neuropathies (Friedrich's ataxia, vitamin B_{12} deficiency)?
Cerebellar	Are there any tremors or clumsiness noted during the interview?
Gait	Is there any toe walking (a potential sign of lower extremity spasticity) or asymmetry of arm swing while walking (a potential sign of mild limb paresis)?

4-week history of sudden jerking of the extremities. These events occur in the awake state only and involve a quick jerk of the arms and legs and a stiffening of the trunk without alteration in level of consciousness prior, during, or after the event. The events occur singly at random times. He is easily distractible and fidgety and has significant difficulties sustaining attention, following directions, and learning. The remainder of his history and review of systems is unremarkable.

Discussion: The events in question are episodic and may represent either an epileptic or nonepileptic phenomenon. Due to the seemingly symmetric nature of the event, bilateral cortical involvement in the motor cortex may be a possibility, as is involvement in the subcortical regions, such as the basal ganglia. Finally, bilateral signs may also point to lesions in the brainstem or the upper spinal cord. Relevant findings on the examination and diagnostic testing will be essential to finalize localization based on assessment of whether the events are tics, epileptic myoclonus, spinal myoclonus, and/or a sign of a more disseminated brain disease, such as paraneoplastic disease, infection, multiple sclerosis, or lupus.

General Guidelines and Developmental Aspects

A significant proportion of the neurological examination can be obtained by simply watching and speaking with the child or adolescent, and guidelines are included in Table 10–1. The younger the child, the less the neurological examination resembles the examination of an adult.

The *mental status examination* needs to assess level of consciousness and activity, speech and language, social skills, and affect. Depending on the age of the patient, assessments of specific cognitive skills (calculation, reading, recall) may be included.

Cranial nerve assessment is easily observed during the interview. Any asymmetry should be further evaluated during the extremity motor examination to elucidate whether this represents only facial involvement or the whole body and whether this would localize to the peripheral nerve, brainstem, or contralateral motor cortex. For a patient with suspected weakness in the oral or facial muscles, observing the patient chew or swallow is helpful. Muscle weakness due to dysfunction at the neuromuscular junction often can be assessed by testing eye muscle strength needed to maintain upgaze and watching for drooping eyelids.

The *sensory examination* can be challenging and is the least objective part of the examination in the nonverbal and/or young patient. The *motor examination* typically consists of assessment of muscle tone and strength. However, children younger than 4 years typically cannot understand directions adequately for a full muscular strength assessment. In such patients, having the patient perform different tasks will give at minimum an idea of how the muscles oppose gravity and whether they can withstand the resistance of their own body (e.g., getting up from the prone position without using furniture). Major motor developmental milestones in children include attainment of walking

TABLE 10–2. Patterns of weakness in upper motor neuron (UMN) versus lower motor neuron (LMN) lesions

	UMN	LMN
Character of weakness	Spastic paralysis with hypertonia	Flaccid paralysis with hypotonia
Mental status	Accompanying encephalopathy, developmental delay, intellectual disability, and seizures	Generally preserved
Distribution	Asymmetric if due to cortical lesion	Usually bilateral
DTRs	Increased	Decreased or absent
Other findings	Babinski reflex positive	Babinski reflex not present Fasciculations and fibrillations

Note.   DTR=deep tendon reflex.

around 12–17 months, running before age 2 years, and hopping on one foot by age 4 years. Hand dominance prior to 1 year of age can be a sign of weakness of the contralateral extremity. For evaluation of patients with chronic findings, documentation of functional abilities from one visit to the next can be a useful marker of clinical progression, such as increased difficulty getting up from a chair in a patient with muscular dystrophy who is having increased proximal muscle weakness.

For patients with motor limitations, localization of the presenting problem is necessary to differentiate whether the motor weakness is due to an upper or lower motor neuron weakness (Table 10–2). Since motor and muscle tone pathways share many of the same neuroanatomical pathways, weakness may often be accompanied by alterations in muscle tone. *Deep tendon reflexes* could point to either upper or lower motor neuron deficits, as noted on Table 10–2.

Coordination assessment may be accomplished by holding toys so the patient has to reach across the midline to reach them; any tremors, dysmetria, or dyscoordination may be noted. Having the patient kick an imaginary ball to assess gross motor lower extremity coordination or walk on imaginary tightropes to assess tandem gait is a nonthreatening way to perform this part of the examination. By the age of 3, children are able to stand on one foot; by the age of 4, children are able to hop on one foot, and by the age of 6, they can perform tandem gait.

Gait should be assessed in all patients as observation of the trunk and limbs is important. If the patient wears any splints or uses any assistive devices, he or she should ideally be observed with and without them. Note whether there is any asymmetry, particularly in shifting from leg to leg; how the foot makes contact with the walking surface (e.g., flat-footed, slapping, or walking on toes); and whether there are any associated unusual movements, such as posturing of the upper extremities in patients with hemiparesis and associated dystonia. These abnormalities can often be accentuated during running.

The *general physical examination* is also relevant, as many conditions can have multisystem effects. Starting with growth assessment, the patient's height, weight, and head circumference should be noted. Growth retardation affecting all parameters or just the head can be seen in genetic syndromes or congenital infections. Likewise, large head circumference (greater than the 98th percentile) should be investigated further to rule out whether there is an expansive process causing rapid head enlargement, such as hydrocephalus.

Dysmorphic features in conjunction with developmental or neurological problems may point to a clinical syndrome. Cleft lip and palate and aortic arch defects can signify midline brain structural abnormalities. The cardiac and renal systems can be involved in multisystem conditions such as myotonic dystrophy. Because the brain and skin have embryological origins in the ectoderm, clues to neurological disease can be found in the skin examination, such as café au lait spots and axillary freckling in neurofibromatosis type 1.

Neurological Differential Diagnosis Guided by the History and Examination

The initial differential diagnosis should be focused on broad etiologic categories, such as vascular, metabolic, epileptic, infectious, traumatic, toxic, congenital, or neoplastic. Knowledge of the full medical history and review of systems is essential to frame the chief complaint and the findings on the physical examination to determine whether they fall into a clinically recognizable syndrome.

Case History

A 3-year-old girl with autistic features and global developmental delay presents with staring spells, typically occurring at school and lasting 30 seconds to 1 minute. During this time, she is unresponsive, picks at her clothes, and seems tired afterwards. Her physical examination is otherwise unremarkable, except for a red papular rash on her cheeks and one hypopigmented macule on her back measuring 5 centimeters. Her neurological examination is notable only for limited verbal communication skills and eye contact and some clumsiness with rapidly alternating movements.

Discussion: The events under question are associated with alteration in consciousness, stereotypic movements, and fatigue after the event, suggestive of seizures. The examination findings are remarkable for possible neurocutaneous stigmata on the cheeks, possibly representing adenoma sebaceum, also known as facial angiofibromas. The hypopigmented macule could represent an ash leaf spot. Taken together, the two skin findings, preexisting autism, and events concerning for seizures may be representative of tuberous sclerosis. With this possible diagnosis in mind, localization of the paroxysmal events would most likely be central in origin, given that intracranial tubers can cause seizures that may be localized with electroencephalography and neuroimaging.

Electroencephalography

Electroencephalography (EEG) is an important part of the neurological evaluation of children and adolescents with suspected central nervous system (CNS) disorders. Electroencephalographic interpretation is optimally performed by a reader with experience in pediatric EEG who can provide interpretation in light of the patient's developmental and clinical status.

The electroencephalographic waves are recorded from surface electrodes and ideally document the patient in the awake, drowsy, and light sleep states. Each electroencephalographic channel measures the electrotential difference between the two points where the channel is applied on the scalp. (For more details, see Wylie et al. 2006.)

Indications for EEG include confirmation of the diagnosis of seizures, assessment of patients with altered mental status, or assessment of the adequacy of antiepileptic treatment. Electroencephalographic examination of the background and ongoing rhythm can offer insights into the baseline state of the patient. The waves are highly influenced by the state of the patient, whether the patient is alert and awake, drowsy, or asleep, and the child's age, medications, structural le-

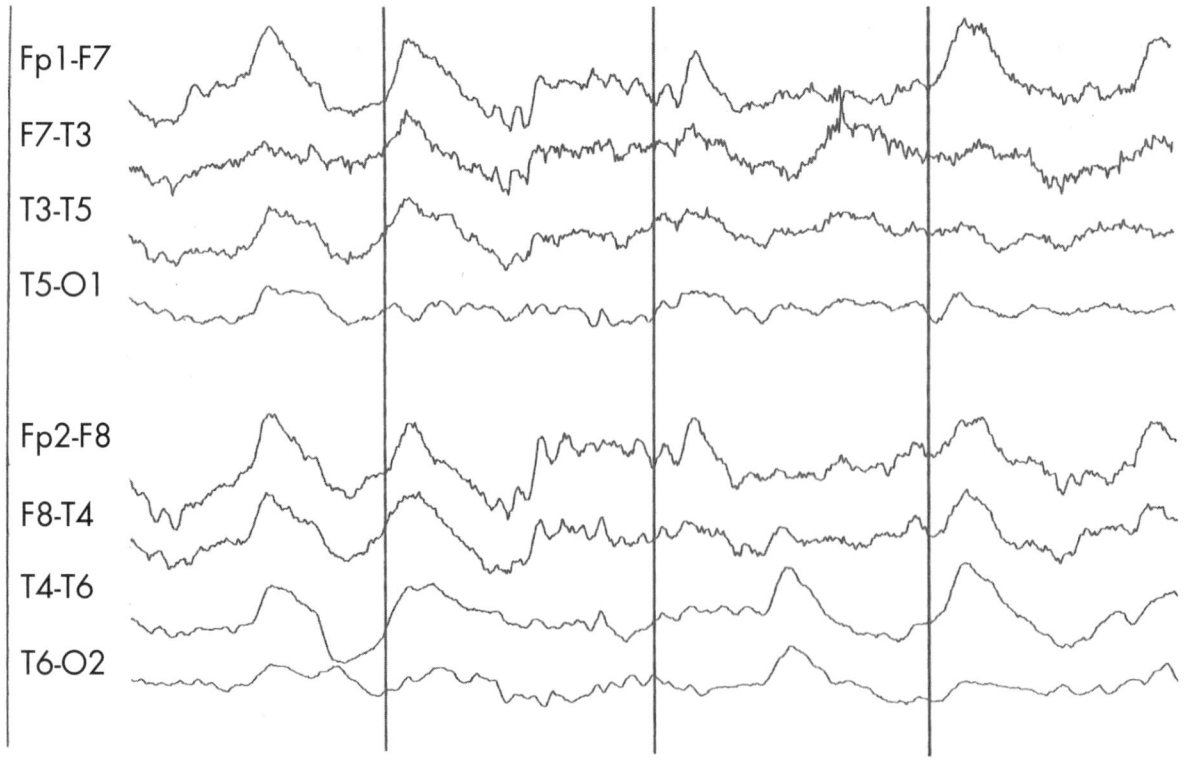

FIGURE 10–1.   Delta activity.

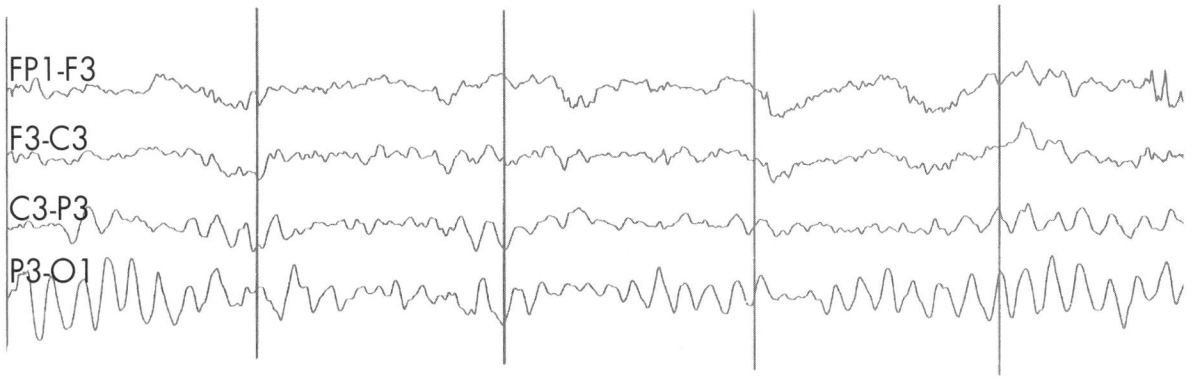

FIGURE 10–2. Alpha wave activity.

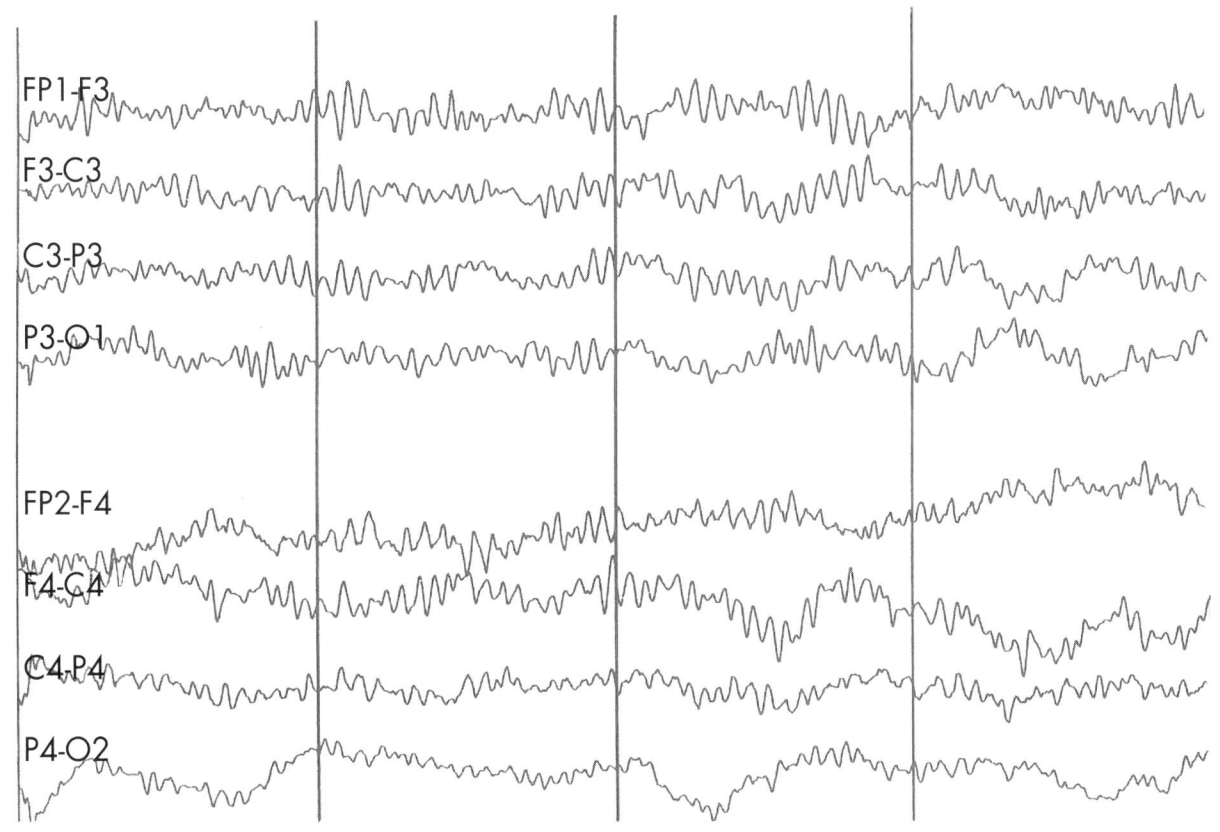

FIGURE 10–3. Beta activity.

sions, and disease states. Typical rhythms are classified according to their frequency as delta (1–3/sec; Figure 10–1), theta (4–7/sec), alpha (8–12/sec; Figure 10–2), and beta (13–20/sec; Figure 10–3). Delta can be seen in deeper stages of sleep and also in pathological states, such as encephalopathy. Alpha is the predominant pattern while awake with the eyes closed, best seen in the posterior head leads. Beta can be seen during sleep states, particularly in infants and children, and can also be seen in patients who have received medications such as benzodiazepines. Theta waves can be seen during awake states in children, although more commonly in drowsy states.

Patients with epilepsy may not consistently demonstrate seizures or epileptiform activity on electroencephalographic recordings, although with repeated and prolonged video electroencephalographic studies and under sleep deprivation, epileptiform interictal activity may be captured. Common electroencephalographic abnormalities are listed in Table 10–3.

TABLE 10–3. Summary of electroencephalographic findings and clinical implications

Electroencephalographic finding	Clinical implications
Background rhythm slowing	Brain lesion may be located in the region where background is slowed (if focal) and may reflect state of arousal if generalized, such as in certain coma states.
Rhythmic slowing	Polymorphic delta slowing may be related to structural lesions, a recent seizure, encephalopathy, migraine; rhythmic delta activity may be associated with structural lesions, metabolic disorders, trauma, encephalopathy.
Periodic lateralized epileptiform discharges	These reflect acute or subacute process such as infection, vascular insult, or trauma and may be an interictal phenomenon.
Spike and slow-wave discharges	These commonly reflect primary generalized epilepsy (e.g., absence and/or generalized tonic-clonic) and may be elicited by hyperventilation or photic stimulation in such patients.
Sharp and slow-wave complex discharges	These may be seen in patients with tonic seizures; patients may have accompanying developmental delay or mental retardation (as seen in Lennox-Gastaut syndrome).
Focal epileptiform discharges (e.g., spikes or sharp waves)	These may be seen in patients with partial-onset seizures and may also be an incidental and clinically nonsignificant finding in normal children.

On the other hand, not all epileptiform activity signifies epilepsy. In the event of documentation of epileptic discharges in an otherwise normal child, correlation of the EEG findings to the clinical scenario is crucial. For example, high amplitude slowing in school-age children is a normal phenomenon, whereas spike and slow-wave discharges induced by either hyperventilation or photic stimulation (Figure 10–4) are pathological and represent an increased tendency toward seizures.

Spikes are high-voltage, short-duration discharges (20–70 msec) that may emanate from one hemisphere in patients with focal epilepsy or multiple foci in patients with generalized seizures. Spikes may be followed by a slow-wave discharge, which may be single or repetitive. These often are associated with a generalized seizure disorder, such as in patients experiencing absence and/or generalized tonic-clonic seizures. Sharp waves are of longer duration than spikes (70–200 msec).

Compared with normal controls, patients with psychiatric diagnoses, such as attention-deficit/hyperactivity disorder (ADHD), have increased incidence of epileptiform abnormalities and risk for development of seizures (Hesdorffer et al. 2004). Patients with migraine also have been reported to have epileptiform abnormalities (Gronseth and Greenberg 1995), which may account in part for the common co-occurrence of both disorders (Andermann and Andermann 1987).

Clinical Indications for Electroencephalography Use in Child Psychiatry

Altered Mental Status

An EEG may be indicated to rule out nonconvulsive status epilepticus or frequent nonconvulsive seizures. CNS infections, such as herpes encephalitis manifesting with altered mental status, can have either generalized or lateralizing periodic epileptiform discharges that are not seizures but signify the ongoing disease process. Patients who are in the postictal state may present similarly and may demonstrate generalized or focal slowing on EEG. In general, the degree of slowing of the EEG correlates with the severity of the clinical state.

Loss of Language or Other Acquired Skills

Alterations of previously acquired skills may be due to epileptic processes, such as Landau-Kleffner syndrome or electrical status epilepticus of slow-wave sleep, in which continuous spike and slow-wave discharges predominate in at least 85% of slow-wave sleep time. In Landau-Kleffner syndrome, the child experiences acquired aphasia, which can be sudden or gradual, predominantly affecting receptive language. The EEG usually includes frequent, repetitive spike and sharp wave discharges that often originate bilaterally in the tempo-

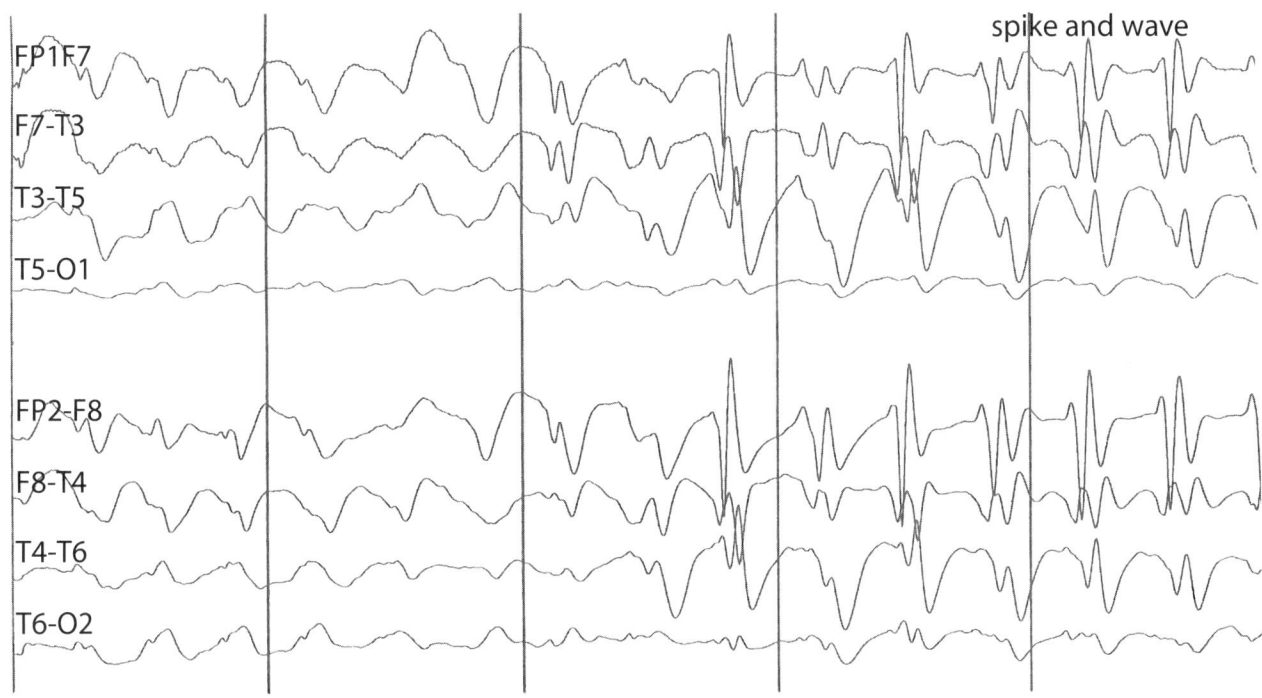

FIGURE 10–4. Generalized spike and slow-wave discharges elicited by hyperventilation in a patient with absence epilepsy.

ral or parietal-occipital regions, can be continuous in sleep, and may represent a clinical spectrum that includes electrical status epilepticus of slow-wave sleep. Seizure control is often attainable, although developmental recovery may be less likely (Besag 2004).

Paroxysmal Events

There is a broad spectrum of epileptic and nonepileptic events that occur in childhood and adolescence, listed by differential diagnosis in Table 10–4.

Events that may be concerning for seizures should be investigated with video EEG. Alternatively, an ambulatory EEG via a portable electroencephalographic recording device can offer extended monitoring for a patient with limited access to telemetry, and all clinical events in question should be noted and documented by the patient and/or family.

Neurodevelopmental Disabilities

Patients with mental retardation or autism pose the greatest diagnostic challenge, due to frequent baseline electroencephalographic abnormalities and limited cognitive and verbal abilities. The predictive value of epileptiform electroencephalographic findings and the higher risk for seizures in this clinical population continue to be studied; thus, electroencephalographic abnormalities may not actually represent seizures and do

not necessarily need to be treated. The improvement of the events under question with antiepileptic medications is not a reliable diagnostic test for seizures, as this type of treatment may represent a placebo effect or may be due to the drug's mood-stabilizing properties. However, nonepileptic events are also common in this population. Staring episodes, rage attacks, and repetitive movements should be investigated with EEG before a diagnosis of epilepsy is made and treatment with antiepileptic medications is started.

Neuroimaging

Significant progress in neuroimaging has advanced understanding of the structure and function of the brain and has further supported the neurodevelopmental model of pediatric psychiatric disorders (Castellanos et al. 2002; Gogtay et al. 2004; Lenroot and Giedd 2006).

Review of Neuroimaging Methods

In this section, we discuss basic theoretical and technical principles underlying neuroimaging methods. For detailed review of specific technological characteris-

TABLE 10–4. Paroxysmal nonepileptic events in children and adolescents

Altered responsiveness
  Syncope
  Migraine and equivalents
  Toxic ingestion
Falling with unresponsiveness
  Syncope (vasovagal or neurocardiogenic)
  Craniocervical junction disorders
  Chiari type I malformation
Organized repetitive movements
  Tics
  Stereotypic behaviors
  Paroxysmal torticollis
  Psychogenic myoclonus
  Psychogenic nonepileptic seizures
Disorganized movements
  Psychogenic nonepileptic seizures
  Chorea (Sydenham's, toxic, stroke related)
  Paroxysmal dyskinesia
  Dystonia
Staring
  Daydreaming
  Inattention
  Stereotypic behaviors
Nocturnal events
  Head banging, sleepwalking, and sleeptalking
  Night terrors and nightmares
  Narcolepsy and cataplexy
  Periodic leg movements

tics and interpretation of neuroimaging data, see Barkovich (2005) and Tortori-Donati et al. (2005).

Computed Tomography

Currently, the main indications for computed tomography (CT) are urgent evaluations of CNS trauma, acute brain hemorrhage, and increased intracranial pressure, or when magnetic resonance imaging (MRI) is not available or is contraindicated (for review, see Wycliffe et al. 2006). It may be superior to MRI in detecting small areas of calcification.

Magnetic Resonance Imaging

Contemporary MRI has an extremely high safety profile and does not expose patients to radiation. Thus, it is the first choice for neuroimaging in the pediatric population. MRI uses magnetic fields and radiofrequency pulses to obtain images of body organs (for review, see Barkovich 2005). MRI provides high resolution and discrimination of white and gray matter and cerebrospinal fluid, and it presents exquisite details of cortical and subcortical architecture and other brain structures (Durston et al. 2001; Giedd 2004).

Functional MRI (fMRI) measures perfusion changes and functional activity of the cortical gray matter during cognitive, sensory, and motor tasks (for review, see Ernst and Rumsey 2000). During an active task, neurons have higher metabolic demands, which result in increased cortical blood flow and oxygen concentration (for review, see Gaillard et al. 2001). Changes in oxygen concentration are detected within seconds after the initiation of the task. Clinically, fMRI is used to determine language dominance, evaluate hearing loss, and preoperatively evaluate patients with epilepsy and brain tumors (Cascio et al. 2007).

Magnetic Resonance Spectroscopy

Magnetic resonance spectroscopy (MRS) provides information on biochemical brain functions by measuring the concentration and distribution of several metabolites, such as creatine, choline, and N-acetyl aspartate (NAA) (for review, see Barkovich 2005). Creatine is an indicator of the brain's bioenergetic metabolism, choline is a marker of neuronal structural integrity, and NAA is a marker of neuronal functioning. In children, MRS is used for the assessment of metabolic, mitochondrial, and neurodegenerative disorders; identification of epileptic focus; and evaluation of brain functioning after traumatic and vascular injuries (Wycliffe et al. 2006). Although the exact relationship between the concentration of a particular metabolite and psychopathology is not clear, MRS has been extensively used as a research tool in ADHD and mood and anxiety disorders. MRS can measure concentrations of excitatory and inhibitory neurotransmitters, such as glutamate, glutamine, and γ-aminobutyric acid (GABA), as well as myo-inositol, a marker of the second-messenger system, involved in lithium's therapeutic mechanism.

Diffusion Tensor Imaging

Diffusion tensor imaging (DTI) measures the net movement (diffusion) of water molecules in the brain and is a fundamentally different MRI method for visualizing white matter (Cascio et al. 2007). DTI provides three-dimensional maps of the white matter microstructure and spatial organization in the hemispheres by showing local water diffusion along the tracts. Myelin sheets limit water diffusion and create "tubelike" directional patterns along the white matter axons (Cascio et al. 2007). Clinically, DTI is used for early assessment of ischemic and traumatic brain injury (Barkovich 2005). As a research tool, DTI is a primary method to investigate neural connectivity in normal and clinical conditions, such as language and learning disorders, working memory, autism, ADHD, and schizophrenia (Ashtari et al. 2007; Barnea-Goraly et al. 2005).

Positron Emission Tomography and Single Photon Emission Computed Tomography

Positron emission tomography (PET) and single photon emission computed tomography (SPECT) use radioactive isotopes to measure cerebral blood flow; metabolism of glucose, oxygen, and proteins; and neurotransmitters in the brain (Barkovich 2005). Clinically, PET and SPECT are most useful in identification of focal epileptogenic brain regions in patients with seizures and with or without structural MRI or electroencephalographic abnormalities (Wycliffe et al. 2006). Although modern radioactive isotopes have a very short radioactive half-life (2–20 minutes for 15O and carbon-11) and produce minimal radiation (Wycliffe et al. 2006), ethical considerations of potential patient exposure to radiation have limited use of PET and SPECT in clinical child psychiatry.

Insights Into Brain Development

Data on longitudinal brain development are available from the National Institute of Mental Health (NIMH) Pediatric Brain MRI project (Giedd et al. 1999, 2006). This study is an ongoing investigation of children and youth with normal development and those with psychopathology (Lenroot and Giedd 2006). Normative pediatric samples demonstrate that total brain volume reaches adult size by age 5–8 years and remains stable until about 20 years of age (Lenroot and Giedd 2006). Different brain structures mature at different times (Thompson et al. 2005). Phylogenetically older brain areas, such as the olfactory, visual, or somatosensory cortex, appear to mature first, followed by the temporal, parietal, and finally prefrontal cortex (Casey et al. 2000; Gogtay et al. 2004). Maturation of white matter is an intense process during the first 2 years of life (Zhang et al. 2005) but also continues throughout adolescence (Barnea-Goraly et al. 2005; Mukherjee et al. 2002; Schneider et al. 2004).

In the normal population, total cerebral volume, specifically the volume of prefrontal and subcortical gray matter, may explain variance in IQ (Shaw et al. 2006). However, the relationship between brain size and functions cannot be directly interpreted due to complex anatomical, chemical, and electrophysiological interactions in the distributed neural networks (Giedd 2001; Lenroot and Giedd 2006). For example, the total cerebral volume in patients with mental retardation due to genetic syndromes may be normal (fragile X, Turner syndromes); significantly smaller than normal (Down, Williams, velocardiofacial, Cohen's syndromes); or macrocephalic (Sotos syndrome) (Wycliffe et al. 2006).

New imaging data demonstrate the associations between brain maturation and improved cognitive abilities (Casey et al. 2000; Shaw et al. 2006; Zhang et al. 2005). For example, fMRI studies have shown that cortical activation changes from a more diffuse pattern in younger children to more focal in older subjects (Durston et al. 2006). The strength of hemispheric language lateralization continues to increase into adulthood, although primary language dominance is reached before 7 to 8 years of age (Holland et al. 2001; Lee et al. 1999). Increased white matter maturation in the frontostriatal and frontotemporal cortex is associated with improved language, semantic memory, and executive function performance (Ashtari et al. 2007). Developmental changes in the white and gray matter structures may be associated with enhanced neuronal connectivity and cortical differentiation.

Clinical Applications in Child Psychiatry

Neuroimaging has become an essential clinical diagnostic tool in pediatric neurology, but in today's child psychiatry, its primary use is in research. The use of imaging to diagnose or suggest treatment for a psychiatric disorders in children is unsupported by clinical and scientific data, as well as ethical considerations (Zametkin et al. 2005).

High-quality neuroimaging studies in children may be challenging to obtain. Young age and developmental delay often limit understanding and compliance with the procedures. Impulsivity, hyperactivity, anxiety, and phobia may also impair testing; thus, sedation is necessary for most MRI studies in children younger than 8 years, unless an audiovisual system is available for the child's entertainment during the procedure (Barkovich 2005). Sedation, however, impairs participation in the cognitive task; thus, it is not compatible with functional imaging. Sedation should be administered and monitored by a trained physician under the American Academy of Pediatrics Committee on Drugs (1992) guidelines for monitoring and

management of pediatric patients during and after sedation for diagnostic and therapeutic procedures.

In clinical child psychiatry practice, neuroimaging
is used for specific indications. Neurology consultation
and brain scanning are indicated for patients with new
neurological symptoms or deterioration of previously
stable neurological functioning and in cases of suspected child abuse or inconsistent history of a traumatic event. It is the child neurologist's role to determine the specific imaging modality. In psychiatric
patients, neuroimaging may be used to rule out systematic or CNS disorders that potentially contribute to
psychopathology. For example, MRI scans should be
ordered in the evaluation of movement disorders of
uncertain etiology, anorexia nervosa (to rule out a pituitary tumor), and severe treatment-resistant mood and
psychotic disorders (Giedd 2001).

Research Directions

To advance understanding of psychopathology, integrated multimodal imaging technologies should be
developed, with improved patient safety and comfort
during the imaging procedures. Longitudinal imaging
studies of normal and clinical populations are needed
to increase knowledge of structural and functional
changes in the developing brain and factors affecting
this process. Neuroimaging may become a valuable
tool in the early identification of psychiatric disorders
and determination of treatment modality and outcome, based on the unique structural and biochemical
profile of the individual brain.

Summary Points

- The three most important indications for a neurological evaluation in children with
  psychiatric problems:

    1. Focal signs and symptoms, suggestive of an acute or chronic (static or progres-
       sive) CNS lesion

    2. Episodic signs or symptoms suggestive of seizures

    3. Objective loss of previously well-developed skills (not just declining grades),
       suggesting a degenerative process

- The chief complaint, history, and physical examination all provide valuable clues for
  generating the differential diagnosis and guiding the neurological evaluation. The
  discerning clinician should try to fit constellations of findings into a clinical syndrome that encapsulates the presenting problem.

- Abnormal electroencephalographic patterns, such as generalized slowing or global
  suppression, often correlate with encephalopathic states. Specific electroencephalographic discharges, such as spikes, suggest an epileptogenic process.

- Epileptiform electroencephalographic discharges specify seizure localization; however, some epileptic discharges may not be detected by surface electrodes and may
  require more in-depth evaluation.

- Children and adolescents with psychiatric diagnoses and neurodevelopmental disorders, especially autism, often have electroencephalographic abnormalities that do
  not necessarily imply epilepsy. While epileptiform electroencephalographic findings
  may indicate an elevated risk for seizures, in the absence of clinical seizures, treatment of abnormal electroencephalographic findings with antiepileptic medications
  is not indicated. Electroencephalographic abnormalities should be considered in
  the context of the clinical neuropsychiatric picture.

- The relationship between brain size and function is complex due to anatomical,
  physiological, and functional interactions in the distributed neural networks.

- The use of neuroimaging to diagnose or suggest treatment for primary pediatric psychiatric disorders is unsupported by clinical and scientific data, in addition to ethical considerations.
- Brain abnormalities in youth with primary psychiatric disorders should be interpreted with consideration of comorbidities with other neurological and genetic disorders.

References

American Academy of Pediatrics Committee on Drugs: Guidelines for monitoring and management of pediatric patients during and after sedation for diagnostic and therapeutic procedures. Pediatrics 89:1110–1115, 1992

Andermann E, Andermann FA: Migraine-epilepsy relationships: epidemiological and genetic aspects, in Migraine and Epilepsy. Edited by Andermann FA, Lugaresi E. Boston, MA, Butterworths, 1987, pp 281–291

Ashtari M, Cervellione KL, Hasan KM, et al: White matter development during late adolescence in healthy males: a cross-sectional diffusion tensor imaging study. Neuroimage 35:501–510, 2007

Barkovich AJ: Techniques and methods in pediatric neuroimaging, in Pediatric Neuroimaging, 4th Edition. Philadelphia, PA, Lippincott Williams & Wilkins, 2005, pp 1–16

Barnea-Goraly N, Menon V, Eckert M, et al: White matter development during childhood and adolescence: a cross-sectional diffusion tensor imaging study. Cerebral Cortex 15:1848–1854, 2005

Besag FMC: Behavioral aspects of pediatric epilepsy syndromes. Epilepsy Behav 5:3–13, 2004

Cascio CJ, Gerig G, Piven J: Diffusion tensor imaging: application to the study of the developing brain. J Am Acad Child Adolesc Psychiatry 46:213–223, 2007

Casey BJ, Giedd JN, Thomas KM: Structural and functional brain development and its relation to cognitive development. Biol Psychol 54:241–257, 2000

Castellanos FX, Lee PP, Sharp W, et al: Developmental trajectories of brain volume abnormalities in children and adolescent with attention-deficit/hyperactivity disorder. JAMA 288:1740–1748, 2002

Durston S, Hulshoff HE, Casey BJ, et al: Anatomical MRI of the developing human brain: what have we learned? J Am Acad Child Adolesc Psychiatry 40:1012–1020, 2001

Durston S, Davidson MC, Tottenham N, et al: A shift from diffuse to focal cortical activity with development. Dev Sci 9:1–8, 2006

Ernst M, Rumsey J: Functional Neuroimaging in Child Psychiatry. Cambridge, England, Cambridge University Press, 2000

Gaillard WD, Grandin CB, Xu B: Developmental aspects of pediatric fMRI: considerations for image acquisition, analysis, and interpretation. Neuroimage 13:239–249, 2001

Giedd JN: Neuroimaging of pediatric neuropsychiatric disorders: is a picture really worth a thousand words? Arch Gen Psychiatry 58:443–444, 2001

Giedd JN: Structural magnetic resonance imaging of the adolescent brain. Ann NY Acad Sci 1021:77–85, 2004

Giedd JN, Blumenthal J, Jeffries NO, et al: Brain development during childhood and adolescence: a longitudinal MRI study. Nat Neurosci 2:861–863, 1999

Giedd JN, Clasen LS, Lenroot R, et al: Puberty-related influences on brain development. Mol Cell Endocrinol 254–255:154–162, 2006

Gogtay N, Giedd JN, Lusk L, et al: Dynamic mapping of human cortical development during childhood through early adulthood. Proc Natl Acad Sci USA 101:8174–8179, 2004

Gronseth GS, Greenberg MK: The utility of the electroencephalogram in the evaluation of patients presenting with headache: a review of the literature. Neurology 45:1263–1267, 1995

Hesdorffer DC, Ludvigsson P, Gudmundsson G, et al: ADHD as a risk factor for incident unprovoked seizures and epilepsy in children. Arch Gen Psychiatry 61:731–736, 2004

Holland SK, Plante E, Weber Byars A, et al: Normal fMRI brain activation patterns in children performing a verb generation task. Neuroimage 14:837–843, 2001

Lee BC, Kuppusamy K, Grueneich R, et al: Hemispheric language dominance in children demonstrated by functional magnetic resonance imaging. J Child Neurol 14:78–82, 1999

Lenroot RK, Giedd JN: Brain development in children and adolescents: insights from anatomical magnetic resonance imaging. Behav Cogn Neurosci Rev 30:718–729, 2006

Mukherjee P, Miller JH, Shimony JS, et al: Diffusion-tensor MR imaging of gray and white matter development during normal human brain maturation. Am J Neuroradiol 23:1445–1456, 2002

Schneider JFL, Ilyasov KA, Hennig J, et al: Fast quantitative diffusion-tensor imaging of cerebral white matter from the neonatal period to adolescence. Neuroradiology 46:258–266, 2004

Shaw P, Greenstein D, Lerch J, et al: Intellectual ability and cortical development in children and adolescents. Nature 440:676–679, 2006

Thompson PM, Sowell ER, Gogtay N, et al: Structural MRI and brain development. Int Rev Neurobiol 67:285–323, 2005

Tortori-Donati P, Rossi A, Biancheri R: Pediatric Neuroradiology. Berlin, Germany, Springer-Verlag, 2005

Wycliffe ND, Thompson JR, Holshouser BA, et al: Pediatric Neuroimaging in Pediatric Neurology: Principles and Practice, 4th Edition. Edited by Swaiman KF, Ashwal S, Ferriero DM. Philadelphia, PA, Mosby Elsevier, 2006

Wylie E, Gupta A, Lachhwani DK (eds): The Treatment of Epilepsy: Principles and Practice, 4th Edition. Philadelphia, PA, Lippincott Williams & Wilkins, 2006

Zametkin AJ, Schroth E, Faden D: The role of brain imaging in the diagnosis and management of ADHD. The ADHD Report 13:11–14, 2005

Zhang L, Thomas KM, Davidson MC, et al: MR quantitation of volume and diffusion changes in the developing brain. Am J Neuroradiol 26:45–49, 2005

Chapter 11

Psychological and Neuropsychological Testing

Ann J. Abramowitz, Ph.D.
Marcia L. Caron, M.A.

Psychological and Neuropsychological Testing

It is essential that mental health and pediatric clinicians serving children and adolescents have an understanding of psychological testing. They need to know when to refer a youngster for such testing, and they must be able to understand the results of testing when it has been performed for a youngster in their care. Typical questions that warrant a referral for psychological or neuropsychological testing include, but are not limited to, the following:

- What is this youngster's current level of intellectual and academic functioning?

- Is mental retardation or a learning disability present?
- Is there evidence of brain damage?
- Is the youngster intellectually gifted?
- Where does this youngster stand cognitively and academically as compared with some previous time?
- Are school-based accommodations or interventions indicated?
- How can the results of testing inform diagnosis and treatment planning?

What Are "Tests"?

A *test* is a "standardized procedure for sampling behavior and describing it with categories or scores"

(Gregory 2007, p. 2). Included in this definition are traditional tests such as those designed to measure intelligence, academic achievement, or personality and also standardized measures of such disparate areas as social skills, adaptive functioning, language development, and depression. The test battery of a psychological or neuropsychological evaluation always includes a number of tests, as well as observations, clinical interviews, and other procedures. Batteries are constructed to address the specific referral questions and vary considerably based on a person's age.

Most tests assess a variety of abilities, skills, or areas of functioning within some domain. Tests typically have several subtests, each of which measures some set of component skills of the broader instrument. Sometimes the broader instrument is referred to as a "battery," but to avoid confusion, in this chapter we refer to an instrument as a *test*, and we use the term *battery* to refer to a group of tests that are administered to a youngster in order to address a particular set of referral questions.

Standards for Tests and Testing Practices

It is important to be familiar with the psychometric concepts that underlie the construction and application of tests. Psychiatrists and other mental health clinicians should be familiar with the standards pertaining to testing, and they should expect that these standards are upheld. Widely accepted standards for psychological and educational testing, published in 1985 and revised in 1999, outline requirements for the ethical administration and interpretation of tests (American Educational Research Association et al. 1999). The following are clinically relevant highlights.

Test publishers have a number of responsibilities. Test manuals must describe the test's construction, reliability and validity studies, and normative data (these are explained later in this section). Tests must be marketed responsibly, including information regarding any potential for misuse and other limitations, such as the degree of appropriateness for nonnative English speakers, people from countries other than the United States, and people with various types of motor or sensory impairments.

Test users must be qualified in the areas in which they are conducting an assessment, including personality, neuropsychological functioning, intelligence, and so on. Typically, those qualified to perform testing are licensed, doctoral-level psychologists and their trainees and

employees who have been appropriately trained and are working under their supervision. Public schools have a separate certification for school psychologists, which allows them to test independently within the school setting. Neuropsychological testing requires expertise beyond that required to conduct other psychological testing.

Testing must be guided by the best interests of the patient. Parents must give consent in order for a child to be tested. When there are two parents, it is usually best if both consent to testing and understand its purpose. When parents are divorced and share custody, generally it is best if both parents consent and are involved in the process. Clinicians considering a referral for testing should consider the child's emotional adjustment at that time, and if testing could be too stressful, or even invalidated, by depression, other psychopathology, or a medical illness, delaying the testing process might be in the patient's best interest.

Decisions must be based on test data that are current. First, psychologists must use current tests. This can be challenging, as tests are regularly updated, and normative updates are sometimes provided for existing tests. Second, those who request and read psychological evaluations need to take into account the recency of the testing. There is no simple standard for this. Younger children tend to change more rapidly than older children, and those with more severe psychopathology are prone to exhibit instability in their test scores over time. As a general rule of thumb, testing conducted within the past year is considered current. A given instrument typically is not readministered within 1 year because of "practice effects," which may artificially raise scores (Hausknecht et al. 2007).

Standards for the tests themselves pertain to the *proper construction* of the instruments, as well as to their *psychometric properties*. Psychologists must be familiar with these standards and should select and interpret tests in accordance with the principles set forth by the American Educational Research Association et al. (1999).

First, *a psychological test must be appropriately constructed and standardized.* This means that scores must be based on norms from a sample of individuals representative of those for whom the test is intended. Raw scores, although sometimes reported, are not meaningful in the interpretation of test results. Interpretation instead is based on some type of *standardized score*, which in turn is based on the *standard deviation*, or dispersion, of test scores for the sample. Reported norms, then, generally are based on the *mean* (or average) score for a given age (and sometimes gender), as well as the standard deviation associated with that score. About 68% of scores fall within one standard deviation of the mean, and just over 95% of scores fall within two standard deviations of the mean. For many psychological tests, the standardized scores are constructed so that the mean is 100 and the standard deviation is 15 points. However, some tests are constructed where the mean is 50 and the standard deviation is 10 points (referred to as *t* scores), and some are constructed with a mean of 0 and a standard deviation of 1 (referred to as *z* scores). These variations are nothing more than differences in how scores are expressed. The standards state that the psychologist must report the mean and standard deviation for each test so that the scores can be understood. In addition, many tests provide qualitative descriptions of score ranges, such as "average," "below average," and "superior." While helpful, these are simply labels provided by the test developer, and they have no official meaning outside of that instrument.

A test must also have adequate *reliability*. This means that a test, if repeated or if administered by another examiner, would yield approximately the same score within acceptable measurement error. Several types of reliability are generally reported and include test-retest, interrater, and internal consistency. Without adequate reliability, the other psychometric properties of a test matter little.

A test also must have adequate *validity*. The generally accepted definition of validity is the degree to which the test measures what it claims to measure (Gregory 2007). Validity is a complex construct, and there are several key types, all of which are important. "A test is valid to the extent that inferences made from it are appropriate, meaningful, and useful" (Gregory 2007, p. 120).

Content validity is determined by "the degree to which the questions, tasks, or items on a test are representative of the universe of behavior the test was designed to sample" (Gregory 2007, p. 121). Content validity is based on appropriate sampling of test items from all possible items that could be used to assess a given construct. Generally, the judgment of experts with respect to items is essential to the statistical determination of content validity.

Criterion-related validity refers to the extent to which a test estimates a person's performance on some outcome measure, or criterion. There are two types of criterion-related validity. The first, *concurrent validity*, refers to the test's ability to predict performance on the criterion measure at the same point in time. The second, *predictive validity*, refers to the ability of the test to predict results on some outcome measure to be

obtained in the future. An example would be the predictive validity of IQ tests in relation to college graduation. Criterion-related validity is expressed as a correlation coefficient, which expresses the degree of association between two measures. A perfect correlation would be 1.0; the absence of any relationship would be expressed by a correlation coefficient of 0. While there is no single standard acceptable correlation coefficient, one might expect the correlation between two tests of the same construct to be at least 0.85, and higher in many cases. Sometimes, particularly in the case of predictive validity, many factors besides what is tested contribute to the criterion. For example, IQ is only one of many factors contributing to college graduation, so these correlation coefficients will be more modest.

Construct validity is the most complex type of validity. A construct is some theoretical, intangible quality or trait in which individuals differ (Messick 1995). Tests are designed to tap underlying constructs, which include such disparate characteristics as intelligence, verbal ability, expressive language skills, psychopathy, depression, social skills, adaptive functioning, and spatial reasoning skills, to name a few—some broad, some narrower. When psychological tests are designed to test such characteristics, determining their construct validity is an ongoing process that does not end at the point at which the test is published. Optimally, research continues that examines the test in question in relation to behaviors thought to characterize the trait in question, and in relation to other measures of that trait and of different traits. Perhaps the most clinically relevant aspect of construct validity is that there are multiple ways in which a test developer must demonstrate that the instrument can be trusted for its stated purpose and that many older instruments, and some newer ones as well, lack the necessary construct validation. Thus, in examining particular test results, it is always appropriate to ask to what extent, and in what ways, the construct validity has been demonstrated.

Psychologists are trained in assessing the appropriateness of an instrument's psychometric properties and are ethically required to use only those that meet rigorous standards and that are appropriate for the individual being tested. At times, this can be a difficult standard to meet, because the development (or revision) of a test with excellent psychometric properties takes a great deal of expertise and money. Many of these costs are borne, in turn, by test users. Additionally, until recently there was a lack of tests with satisfactory psychometric properties for many areas of psychological functioning. Fortunately, this is improving all the time, and well-constructed tests for more areas of functioning, and with current norms, are increasingly available.

Even for a test that has excellent psychometric properties, factors such as depression, sleeplessness, hunger, and inattention can contribute to a loss of validity for that person at that particular time. The psychologist will always include a description of the youngster's behavior during assessment and an impression of the overall validity of the testing, based on the presence of such factors. It is not uncommon for the psychologist to report that the results of a particular test must be interpreted cautiously, if at all, given the presence of mitigating factors.

The presentation of results generally should occur via both verbal feedback and a written report. It is essential that the results be presented in a manner that provides all necessary information and in a way that is appropriate to the level of training of the recipient. Best practice suggests that reports be written following the face-to-face feedback session rather than presented at the feedback session. This is so that the input of parents (and when appropriate, the input of the youngster) with respect to both the findings and the recommendations can be incorporated (Brenner 2003; Miller and Evans 2004). The report should be written in such a way that both parents and nonpsychologist professionals can understand the important information.

Overview of Psychological Tests

Tests of Intellectual Ability

Sometimes referred to as "IQ tests," these are individually administered tests that are designed to provide an overall appraisal of an individual's intellectual ability, as well as variability (strengths and weaknesses) in particular areas. Intelligence tests undergo revision approximately every 10–15 years to keep the norms current, update the item content, and reflect new scientific knowledge in the areas of cognitive development and functioning. Assessments must always involve the most recent version of a given test, and earlier results obtained with previous versions or results obtained with different intelligence tests should not be directly compared with results from a current assessment. Commonly used tests of intellectual abil-

ity include the Stanford-Binet Intelligence Scales, Fifth Edition (SB5; Roid 2003); Wechsler Intelligence Scale for Children, Fourth Edition (WISC-IV; Wechsler 2003); Differential Ability Scales, Second Edition (DAS-II; Elliott 2007); Kaufman Assessment Battery for Children, Second Edition (K-ABC-II; Kaufman and Kaufman 2004); and Woodcock-Johnson Tests of Cognitive Abilities and Achievement, Third Edition (WJ-III; Woodcock et al. 2001). The global score for each of these tests has a mean of 100 and a standard deviation of 15. That means that about 95% of youngsters obtain scores that fall between 70 and 130, and about 68% of youngsters obtain scores that fall between 85 and 115.

Over the years, intelligence tests have changed from largely atheoretical groups of diverse tasks tapping a variety of abilities to batteries with more theoretical coherence. One popular theory of the structure of intelligence is the Cattell-Horn-Carroll (CHC) theory, which postulates a three-level hierarchical organization of intellectual abilities (McGrew et al. 1997). At the broadest level, Stratum III, is g, or general intelligence, sometimes characterized by the overall composite score on an IQ test. The second level, Stratum II, includes broad abilities such as fluid intelligence (which involves diverse types of reasoning), crystallized intelligence (which heavily taps existing knowledge), visuospatial abilities, auditory processing, memory, and cognitive processing speed. Stratum I includes a large number of narrow abilities, the list of which is constantly being revised and expanded. Not all the abilities included within the comprehensive CHC theory are tapped by the subtests included in IQ tests, and most, if not all, subtests tap more than a single narrow ability. However, most current intelligence tests can be interpreted in accordance with this theoretical model, thereby providing a common theoretical framework for interpreting different instruments, revising them, and developing new ones.

Often, the IQ, or a similar composite score, is not a meaningful representation of a youngster's intellectual functioning due to the variability among the component (subtest or cluster) scores. In such cases, those scores should be viewed separately, as measuring different areas of the youngster's ability—for example, verbal reasoning, nonverbal reasoning, spatial reasoning, and quantitative reasoning. Similarly, cluster scores may not adequately reflect a youngster's abilities in the specified areas, again because of variability within the area. On the other hand, individual subtests are not extremely reliable; hence, any weaknesses found at the subtest level should be confirmed with other measures before inferences regarding cognitive functioning are drawn. All in all, the interpretation of intelligence test results requires considerable understanding of the specific instrument as well as any characteristics of the youngster that might have influenced his or her performance.

Tests of Academic Achievement and Assessment of Learning Disabilities

Assessment in the area of academic achievement is essential to gaining an understanding of a youngster's functioning. Youngsters having psychiatric problems almost invariably experience difficulty at school, and grades are almost always affected. For several reasons, grades are poor indicators of academic skills and at best can give only a rough appraisal of a youngster's school functioning. One reason for this is that even when academic achievement is at grade level or above, classroom performance and grades may suffer due to disorganization, failure to turn in assignments or homework (missing assignments often contribute grades of 0), inability to finish tests on time, careless errors, erratic attendance, and other factors. Conversely, a youngster who has learning difficulties but whose instruction is delivered at a slower pace and who is conscientious about completing assignments likely will receive satisfactory grades. Hence, objective assessment of achievement is warranted. Scores from recent group-administered achievement tests, such as the Iowa Tests of Basic Skills (Hoover et al. 1996) or the Stanford Achievement Test, Tenth Edition (Harcourt Assessment 2003), may be available. If scores on these instruments reveal satisfactory achievement, then in-depth achievement testing may not be necessary, with the exception of written expression, inasmuch as the group tests do not assess actual writing. From the clinical perspective, scores from group-administered or individually administered achievement tests or screens can be useful, as they can indicate if the youngster is functioning appropriately *in the areas tested*, and they can signal a need for a referral for in-depth assessment. It is critical to remember that none of these tests covers all the key academic areas and that none of the group-administered tests assesses the youngster's ability to write.

Learning Disabilities

Through either screening with standardized group achievement tests or individual achievement testing,

academic deficits often are confirmed or discovered. Often these deficits reflect learning disabilities, which are referred to in DSM-IV (American Psychiatric Association 1994) and its text revision, DSM-IV-TR (American Psychiatric Association 2000), as *learning disorders.* Assessing for possible learning disabilities may constitute the largest single reason for conducting psychological testing, particularly in elementary school children. DSM-IV states that learning disorders are diagnosed when the individual's academic achievement in reading, mathematics, or writing is substantially below what would be expected based on one's age, schooling, and intellectual ability. DSM-IV also provides a category, not otherwise specified (NOS), for which no criteria are given but where the example given is of an instance where all three areas are affected but none to the required degree. To meet DSM-IV criteria, learning problems must significantly interfere with achievement at school or the performance of activities in daily life that require reading, mathematics, or writing skills.

The DSM-IV definition goes on to state, albeit erroneously, that the usual discrepancy required between intellectual ability and achievement is more than two standard deviations. However, the measurement of discrepancy and the requirement that discrepancy be present are fraught with problems. From a purely psychometric standpoint, requiring a discrepancy of two standard deviations is an exceedingly stringent criterion and is seldom obtained on psychoeducational tests, even when assessing individuals with marked learning disabilities. In general, either one standard deviation, or slightly over one standard deviation, can be considered significant. However, research has failed to support IQ-achievement discrepancy as a valid or useful criterion for a diagnosis of learning disorder, and recent changes in federal law pertaining to eligibility for special education services for learning disabilities in the public schools have eliminated the discrepancy requirement (U.S. Department of Education 2006).

Rather than the description of learning disorders included in DSM-IV, the most commonly used definition of learning disabilities in the United States is that of the federal government, which specifies the categories of handicapping conditions that receive special education services in the public schools. In this law, a specific learning disability means "a disorder in one or more of the basic psychological processes involved in understanding or in using language, spoken or written, which may manifest itself in an imperfect ability to listen, think, speak, read, write, spell, or to do mathematical calculations" (U.S. Office of Education 1968, p. 34). Regardless, learning disabilities are diagnosed by means of a testing battery that includes a test of intellectual functioning, tests of academic achievement, and in-depth testing in any areas found to be lagging. Following is a description of the areas of potential learning disabilities and the methods for assessing each.

Reading Disorders (Learning Disabilities in Reading)

There are two primary areas of reading disabilities: basic reading (word recognition) and comprehension. Problems with basic reading can involve fluency as well as accuracy. While word recognition, fluency, and comprehension must be considered separately, they are interrelated, and each makes an essential contribution to reading competence. Problems with accuracy will limit comprehension. Difficulties in word recognition represent about 70%–80% of children identified with reading disorders (Lyon et al. 2003). The largest group with difficulties in word recognition are those children with problems in the phonological processes underlying decoding. These processes include understanding sound/symbol correspondence and the ability to segment spoken words into phonemes and syllables. Assessment of phonological processing can provide early identification of reading problems as well as identify prereaders likely to encounter difficulty.

Within the area of decoding, skills to be assessed include the ability to read words in isolation as well as in context and the ability to derive meaning from what is read. The reason for assessing the ability to read words out of context is that this evaluation is a purer measure of reading; the reason for assessing word reading within context is that this better approximates the demands of reading in the real world. The ability to sound out words by applying knowledge of letter sounds and blending must be assessed as well, as it underlies the ability to decode unfamiliar words and apply the rules of the language. Assessing this skill typically involves having the youngster read a series of nonsense words that can be read only via the application of phonetic principles. Reading rate should be assessed as well, because some readers are accurate but must expend extreme effort to decode, reducing their ability to derive meaning from what they have read. Such fluency problems can cause struggles with homework and failure to complete classwork.

There are a number of ways to assess comprehension, and more than one should be employed, since a youngster may have difficulty with some, but not all, aspects. For example, one method involves a *cloze procedure,* in which the child supplies a missing word to meaningfully complete a sentence. Another method involves asking the child to read a passage and answer questions that are read by the examiner. In general, however, tests of reading comprehension fail to assess how the youngster deals with the types of longer text that students encounter in actual reading.

Mathematics Disorders (Learning Disabilities in Mathematics)

Math disabilities can involve difficulties recognizing numbers and symbols, memorizing facts, grasping various aspects of mathematical reasoning to solve problems, or performing computations. Concepts such as place value, fractions, percentages, and square roots can be problematic for those with a mathematics disorder. Mathematics skills are involved in understanding time, money, and measurement; hence, these areas typically are affected by a math disorder.

Youngsters may exhibit disabilities in mathematics alone, or they may have more generalized difficulties that affect several academic areas, including mathematics. For example, memory weaknesses and deficits in ability to employ strategies are problematic for most basic skill areas. In mathematics, they can cause difficulty with conceptualization in performing math operations, recalling math facts, learning and understanding algorithms and formulas or solving word problems. Language and communication problems that underlie many children's reading disorders can impair mathematics achievement as well, most obviously in the performance of word problems. For some youngsters, deficiencies in processes and strategies affect acquisition of math skills and math performance, but not other curricular areas. It is important to assess the various skills involved in mathematics performance. Some achievement tests assess computational skills alone, but not mathematical reasoning ability or the understanding of concepts that underlie computation. Needless to say, mathematics performance comprises several separate skills that must be integrated, and youngsters may have problems with one or more of these. In addition, because of the important roles played by immediate, long-term, and working memory, these should be assessed as well (see the section "Neuropsychological Testing" later in this chapter). Competent performance of even rote computation requires adequate graphomotor skills and relies at least to some degree on processing speed. visuospatial skills are needed for performing written computation, for mastering concepts involving geometry, and for understanding algebraic relationships involving time and distance. In interpreting assessment results, it is essential to consider the broad picture of the youngster's achievement in other areas and his or her cognitive and graphomotor skills, as well as any possible relationships between mathematics deficits and those in other areas.

Disorders of Written Expression (Learning Disabilities in Written Expression)

Disorders of written expression can involve any of several aspects of written communication: graphomotor skills, grammar and usage, spelling, or limitations on the ability to put one's thoughts into words. Written language mechanics include punctuation, capitalization, and sentence structure. Putting one's thoughts into words involves many skills and processes, such as planning, revising, and using various self-regulation strategies (Graham et al. 1998). Problems with written expression may constitute a youngster's sole area of difficulty, or they may be secondary to reading problems and/or difficulties with spoken language. In general, youngsters with learning disabilities in this area produce very brief written products that contain little detail and lack organization. Students with learning disorders are less knowledgeable about writing and tend to think about it in its simplest terms (spelling, neatness) rather than in terms of the expression of ideas and as a way of communicating with others on a topic (Graham et al. 1998).

Unlike reading and mathematics, which are regularly assessed via nationally normed measures, such as the Iowa Tests of Basic Skills (Hoover et al. 1996) and the Stanford Achievement Test, Tenth Edition (Harcourt Assessment 2003), for all children attending public schools and most attending private schools, written expression is rarely and typically inadequately assessed. Thus, learning disorders in written expression frequently are missed until many years of schooling have passed, if they are identified at all. Youngsters who fail to complete written work or who turn in written work of poor quality often are dismissed as lazy and unmotivated, with no recognition of the underlying learning disability. It is therefore critical that any youngster exhibiting problems performing written work be promptly and thoroughly evaluated for a learning disorder in this area. Too often, other academic skills are screened as satisfactory based on group-administered multiple-choice tests, and no further assessment is performed.

Unfortunately, there is no single adequate test of written expression, and some of the most commonly used and best-normed individual tests of writing skills fail to comprehensively assess some of the most common areas affected by learning disabilities. Often, even when a youngster is being assessed for a learning disability in written expression, there is no task requiring him or her to write a composition of any length. Even on one of the most commonly used tests that does require the youngster to write a story for 15 minutes on a given topic (i.e., the Test of Written Language, Third Edition [TOWL-3; Hammill and Larsen 1996]), the scoring procedure, which relies in part on counting errors and in part on assessing the quality of the product, would barely penalize a youngster who managed to write only two or three sentences in that amount of time. As a result of these limitations in the available individual standardized tests, a qualitative assessment of writing skills has become an essential component of the evaluation in order to ensure that written expression disorders are not overlooked. A further caution is warranted: Because of the aforementioned limitations inherent in even the best tests available, obtained scores in the average or above-average range should not be interpreted as indicating that no learning disorder is present.

Communication Disorders (Learning Disabilities in Language)

Communication disorders (sometimes a possible category of learning disorder NOS) are conditions involving markedly delayed language not attributable to some other condition such as hearing impairment, autism, or mental retardation. The disorder may affect expressive language only, or it may affect both receptive and expressive language. Some characteristics of language disorders include improper use of words and their meanings, inability to express ideas, inappropriate grammatical patterns, reduced vocabulary, and difficulty following directions. The children often do not learn language incidentally and thus must be taught skills systematically. When a youngster undergoing a psychological evaluation appears to evidence any of the aforementioned difficulties, it is advisable to include language assessment in the psychological evaluation. A commonly used test for this purpose is the Clinical Evaluation of Language Fundamentals, Fourth Edition (CELF-4; Semel et al. 2003). Further assessment, when indicated, is conducted by a speech and language pathologist.

Academic Screening Versus In-Depth Testing

Sometimes a screen, as opposed to an in-depth assessment of academic achievement, is conducted. There are instruments with good psychometric properties that are available for this purpose. One commonly used test is the Wide Range Achievement Test, Fourth Edition (WRAT-4; Wilkinson and Robertson 2006). A screen may be as limited as having the youngster read a list of words of increasing difficulty, perform math computation, and spell a list of words. While such a screen can provide useful information, it cannot substitute for an in-depth academic assessment. In particular, a screen will fail to identify those youngsters who read accurately but very slowly, those who have difficulty deriving meaning from what they read, those who cannot put their ideas in writing for any of a variety of reasons, and those who can perform computation but not reason mathematically. Screening can be useful for determining when in-depth testing is needed; that is, if a youngster exhibits problems on a screen, further testing is warranted. A compromise can be adding to the screen subtests from an instrument such as the WJ-III (Woodcock et al. 2001) to cover areas (such as reading comprehension or math reasoning) that are not contained within the screening instrument.

Assessment of Individuals With Intellectual Deficiency

The interchangeable terms *intellectual deficiency* and *mental retardation* generally refer to intelligence test results two standard deviations below the mean, which would be a score of 70 on a test with a mean of 100 and a standard deviation of 15. However, the use of a full scale IQ or other similar test composite for this purpose often is not appropriate. When a youngster's subtest scores are widely distributed (this large amount of spread is referred to as *scatter*), the overall IQ score may not be a good representation of his or her ability. In fact, there often is no single score that can adequately describe that person's overall intellectual ability. However, when the majority of subtest scores, as well as the full scale IQ (when interpretable), are within the deficient range, a diagnosis of intellectual deficiency can be considered. In order to make that di-

agnosis, a standardized measure of *adaptive functioning* (i.e., personal and social skills used for everyday living) must similarly indicate that functioning is in the deficient range.

Assessment of Individuals With Sensory Impairment, Language Disorders, or Motor Disabilities

The assessment of youngsters whose disabilities limit their performance on standard psychological tests *for reasons other than the constructs that are being assessed* represents one of the greatest challenges of intellectual assessment, and assessment in general. First and foremost, the tests that are used to measure intellectual functioning must not rely on the skills that are affected by the disability. Thus, the intelligence of a youngster with expressive aphasia must be tested without requiring verbal expression, a deaf youngster must be tested with a nonauditory test, a youngster with fine motor difficulties cannot be given timed fine motor tasks, and so on. The affected areas (e.g., expressive language, hearing, or fine motor skills) certainly can be assessed, but tasks involving these skills cannot be part of the assessment of intelligence. Further, when the goal is assessment of something other than the affected skill itself, results must be interpreted accordingly. For example, it might be appropriate to give an oral reading test to a youngster who has hearing impairment, because oral reading is an important skill and also because the assessment of this skill yields information about the types of errors the youngster makes while reading, which would be crucial for intervention.

There are several excellent instruments that can be used selectively with individuals with various disabilities. One is the Leiter International Performance Scale—Revised, a nonlanguage test of intellectual functioning that often is used in assessing individuals with autism, hearing problems, and/or language problems (Roid and Miller 1998). Its tasks also are untimed, which makes it suitable for some youngsters with motor problems. Another approach to performing cognitive assessment is to give only those subtests of an intelligence test that do not require verbal responses (in the case of youngsters with language problems) or motor responses (in the case of youngsters with motor problems).

Assessment of Infants and Preschoolers

Testing infants and preschoolers carries some challenges. Identification of developmental delays and learning problems of all sorts is critical to early intervention efforts; thus, the very legitimate concerns about reliability and validity with the youngest age groups are offset to some degree by the importance of early identification. The predictive validity of infant intelligence tests is low (McCall 1979). For preschoolers, the predictive validity is generally adequate (Gregory 2007). For infants and toddlers, the Bayley Scales of Infant and Toddler Development, Third Edition (Bayley-III; Bayley 2005) is the most widely accepted instrument. The Bayley-III assesses development in the cognitive, language (receptive and expressive), motor (fine and gross), adaptive behavior, and social-emotional domains. The most widely used instruments with preschoolers are the K-ABC-II (Kaufman and Kaufman 2004), the DAS-II (Elliott 2007), the Wechsler Preschool and Primary Scale of Intelligence, Third Edition (WPPSI-III; Wechsler 2002), and the Stanford-Binet Intelligence Scales for Early Childhood, Fifth Edition (Early SB5; Roid 2005).

By their very nature, preschoolers may be reluctant or unready to participate in conventional, face-to-face testing sessions. Sessions usually must be brief, and flexibility is essential. This might include sitting on the floor with the child, using instruments that contain some parent-report items, testing in a familiar setting (such as the child's home or preschool), and using concrete rewards to sustain attention and cooperation. Psychologists always need to be careful to not attribute low results to low abilities when behavioral factors may be playing a large role.

Despite the existence of well-normed instruments for the purpose of cognitive assessment with this age group, often it is not necessary to administer an intelligence test per se when assessing a preschooler. In many cases, a broad developmental assessment that includes cognitive, language, motor, and adaptive skills is more appropriate for answering the most common referral question about a preschooler, whether he or she is developing normally. Several screening tools are available for this purpose, including the Developmental Indicators for the Assessment of Learning, Third Edition (DIAL-3; Mardell and Goldenberg 1998). The lengthier Mullen Scales of Early Learning (Mullen 1995) is an excellent tool for assessing language, motor, and perceptual skills.

Assessment of Behavioral and Emotional Functioning

Assessing a youth's behavioral and emotional functioning (including his or her personality and interpersonal relationships) is an essential component in any psychological evaluation. When considering the behavioral, emotional, and/or social problems that a youngster is experiencing, the psychologist is interested in identifying if they are clinically significant problems (often gauged in comparison to same-age peers), and if so, how extensive is the impact that they are having in this youngster's life. Might they be (at least in part) accounting for any areas of lower-than-expected academic performance? Moreover, might they be impairing, or even invalidating, the youngster's performance on tests from the evaluation at hand? Any significant psychomotor retardation or agitation that might accompany a youngster's depression would certainly affect his or her performance on tasks requiring motor or timed performance. In other examples, extreme shyness, anxiety, apathy, fatigue, inattentiveness, or impulsivity could also negatively affect a youngster's performance across a variety of tasks not designed to assess those particular constructs. Other questions raised by behavioral and emotional assessments are often related to cause-and-effect relationships: Is the youngster having trouble concentrating at school and elsewhere, thus causing anxiety about not doing well, or is the difficulty concentrating caused by anxiety at school and in other situations?

Components of Behavioral and Emotional Assessment

Questionnaires

There exists a wide variety of parent-, teacher-, and self-report measures designed to tap the behavioral and emotional functioning of infants, toddlers, preschoolers, school-age children, and adolescents. These are covered in Chapter 8, "Rating Scales."

Clinical and Informational Interviews

Clinical interviews with the youth and informational interviews with both parents (and sometimes with teachers, siblings, or others) are a crucial part of any proper behavioral and emotional assessment. These are covered in Chapter 1, "Assessing Infants and Toddlers"; Chapter 2, "Assessing the Preschool-Age Child"; Chapter 3, "Assessing the Elementary School–Age Child"; Chapter 4, "Assessing Adolescents"; Chapter 6, "The Process of Assessment and Diagnosis"; and Chapter 7, "Diagnostic Interviews." Information that is particularly important for the purposes of testing include the findings from any prior testing, medical information that could be relevant to test performance or the scheduling of testing, educational history (including academic performance and any behavioral problems), and the examinee's understanding of why he or she is being tested.

Behavioral Observations

Careful observation adds critical information to the assessment of the youngster's behavioral and emotional functioning. Sometimes formal behavioral observations are made by the psychologist during a classroom or home visit, and observations always occur in the one-on-one testing setting. This situation allows an examiner to assess a youngster's affect/mood, degree of relatedness to the examiner, interest in and motivation for testing, and language proficiency. Moreover, the examiner can personally observe indicators of inattention (e.g., careless mistakes, easily distracted), hyperactivity (e.g., fidgeting, excessive talking), impulsivity (e.g., blurting out of answers, interrupting), depression (e.g., low energy, difficulty concentrating), or anxiety (e.g., trembling, muscle tension, excessive requests for feedback, compulsive behaviors) during testing. However, behavioral observations during testing are limited by the extent to which a youngster's behavior within a unique one-on-one setting with an unfamiliar adult is representative of his or her behavior in other situations.

Limitations of Assessment With Projective Tests

Sometimes projective tests (i.e., those involving ambiguous stimuli intended to tap into a person's unconscious) such as the Rorschach (Rorschach 1921) or the Children's Apperception Test (CAT; Bellak and Bellak 1993) are used in an attempt to reveal a youngster's hidden emotions or internal conflicts. Such stimuli may involve pictures, abstract designs, or incomplete sentences. However, all of these projective instruments lack adequate psychometrics, so the information obtained from them should be used only to form clinical hypotheses that require further corroboration (Garb et al. 2004). Any inferences regarding behavioral and emotional functioning that rely exclusively or primarily on findings from projective instruments would at best be incomplete and at worst be entirely unacceptable.

Neuropsychological Testing

Neuropsychology is the study of brain-behavior relationships. Clinical neuropsychology seeks to understand how damaged, diseased, or poorly developed brain structures alter behavior and interfere with mental functioning. Neuropsychological testing is designed to be highly sensitive to the effects of brain dysfunction. As a result, neuropsychological assessments require more specialized training than do general psychological assessments, and they are also more often interpreted in conjunction with assessment from other sources, including brain imaging, physical examination, and laboratory information. Thus, neuropsychological testing is an extension of psychological testing, in that neuropsychological test batteries generally include additional areas of functioning that may be affected by a compromised central nervous system. Yet *all* psychological tests aim to determine the profile of an individual's strengths and weaknesses in order to inform treatment planning and set appropriate current and future behavioral expectations. In neuropsychological testing specifically, however, the treatment is sometimes framed as rehabilitation and the expectations stated in terms of the extent of functional recovery, in particular given any developmentally appropriate expectations for neural plasticity. Nevertheless, all psychological testing can be interpreted from a neuropsychological perspective, that is, one that seeks to link brain and behavior.

When Is Neuropsychological Testing Warranted?

A common question is when is it more appropriate to refer a youngster for neuropsychological rather than for general psychological testing? If one wishes to explore the functional impact of a known neurological condition or brain injury, then neuropsychological testing is the definitive choice. Longitudinal follow-ups with neuropsychological assessments conducted after baseline assessments can be important in tracking improvements/recovery or deterioration over time. If the presence of brain damage is at all part of the referral question, then neuropsychological testing is the obvious choice. It may also be fitting in the case of a youngster who is not achieving appropriate developmental milestones or one who experiences sudden, unexpected, and unaccounted changes in his or her personality or cognitive, physical, or sensory abilities.

Certain conditions have clear implications for brain function, such that they will most likely require neuropsychological testing: structural abnormalities such as microcephaly and hydrocephalus; infections such as cytomegalovirus and meningitis; toxic damage such as lead poisoning; traumatic brain injuries (including perinatal traumatic damage, closed head injuries, and the effects of severe child abuse); focal neurological disorders (including brain tumors, strokes, and aneurysms); cerebral palsy; convulsive disorders (including neonatal seizures, infantile spasms, and epilepsy); and hemispherectomy and other surgical interventions (Malik et al. 2006; Spreen et al. 1995). Certain other conditions whose effects *may* require neuropsychological testing include chromosomal and genetic disorders (including phenylketonuria, Turner syndrome, fragile X syndrome, and Williams syndrome); pervasive developmental disorders (including autism and Asperger's disorder); prematurity and low birth weight; infections (including maternally transmitted HIV and congenital rubella); toxic damage (including hyperbilirubinemia, prenatal intoxication, and childhood substance abuse); nutritional disorders (including kwashiorkor and marasmus); and anoxic episodes (Malik et al. 2006; Spreen et al. 1995). Neuropsychological testing is not warranted for the purpose of diagnosing attention-deficit/hyperactivity disorder.

Neuropsychological Systems

A variety of conceptual models of brain-behavior relationships have been proposed to organize the set of relatively independent functional domains that are controlled by brain systems and tapped by various neuropsychological tests. The following categories of neuropsychological systems are from Gregory (2007).

Sensory Input

Experiencing accurate sensory input provides a critical foundation for processing information at higher levels. Over- or understimulation by sensory input can otherwise interfere with daily living. A youngster's ability to detect and differentiate basic visual, auditory, and tactile sensations can be tested as part of a neuropsychological evaluation, although sometimes this can be provided through regular vision, hearing, and tactile testing by a pediatrician or child neurologist.

Learning and Memory

Learning and memory are intertwined processes that refer to how individuals encode, store, and retrieve information. Memory processes are often categorized into immediate (high-capacity, short-life perceptual records); short-term (limited-capacity, temporary information that can be manipulated); and long-term (prolonged retention of information) memory, and neuropsychological tests can detect deficits in each of these areas. In addition, neuropsychological tests typically assess learning and memory in both verbal/auditory and spatial/visual modalities. Two tests commonly used to assess these constructs in youngsters include the Children's Memory Scale (CMS, for ages 5 to 16; Cohen 1998) and the Wide Range Assessment of Memory and Learning, Second Edition (WRAML-2, for ages 5 and older; Sheslow and Adams 2003).

Language

In addition to helping assess for language disorders as discussed previously, neuropsychological testing is also employed to assess for *aphasias*, which are any of a variety of deviations in language performance caused by brain damage or dysfunction, generally to the left cerebral hemisphere (Gregory 2007). Aphasias can involve difficulties with verbal fluency, speech comprehension, articulation, repetition tasks, object naming, reading, spelling, writing, or computations. A variety of neuropsychological measures have been designed to assess across these diverse areas of potential impairment.

Spatial and Manipulatory Ability

Tests of spatial and manipulatory ability tap constructional performance on mostly drawing or assembly tasks, thus requiring both spatial analysis and motor performance. Ideally, these two components could be separated by a neuropsychological test, as with the Developmental Test of Visual-Motor Integration, Fourth Edition, Revised (VMI, for ages 3–17; Beery and Buktenica 1997). Weaknesses in these basic skills (including graphomotor coordination) can result in difficulty performing a variety of academic tasks (e.g., writing letters and numbers, doing well in geometry and art classes, or manipulating laboratory equipment).

Executive Function

Executive function is an umbrella term that subsumes various interconnected mental processes responsible for purposeful, goal-directed behavior (Anderson 2002). A review of this construct during childhood and adolescence identified four interrelated and interdependent domains of executive function: cognitive flexibility (including divided attention, working memory, conceptual transfer, and feedback utilization); goal setting (including initiative, conceptual reasoning, planning, and strategic organization); attentional control (including selective attention, self-regulation, self-monitoring, and inhibition); and information processing (including efficiency, fluency, and speed of processing) (Anderson 2002). Evidence suggests that the executive domains mature at different rates across different developmental stages, with attentional control emerging in infancy and developing rapidly in early childhood, with the other three domains maturing between ages 7 and 12 (Anderson 2002). As one might imagine, designing tests that uniquely tap any single domain or subcomponent of executive function has proven difficult, especially for youngsters whose functions are still developing.

Motor Output

Neuropsychological assessments of motor output are interested in the speed, strength, and accuracy components of both fine and gross motor performance. The right and left sides of the body are both typically assessed, as the findings could have important implications for lateralized brain damage. Neuropsychological testing in the motor domain can be used to help diagnose DSM-IV developmental coordination disorder. In addition, neuropsychological tests in this area are also designed to assess for a variety of motor impairments, such as *apraxias* (inability to perform a movement due to a neurological defect); *ataxias* (incoordination of movement); and tics ("sudden, rapid, recurrent, nonrhythmic, stereotyped motor movement or vocalization" [American Psychiatric Association 2000, p. 108]).

Neuropsychological Batteries

Several comprehensive neuropsychological batteries have been developed to assess across multiple neurological systems. These can be useful as screeners when later supplemented as appropriate with additional tests for corroborating evidence of suspected deficits. Some of the more widely used child and adolescent measures include the Bayley-III (for ages 1 to 42 months; Bayley 2005); the Halstead-Reitan Neuropsychological Test Battery, Second Edition (various versions for ages 5 and older; Reitan 1993); the Luria-Nebraska Neuropsychological Battery (various versions for ages 8 and older; Golden et al. 1986); and the NEPSY: A Developmental Neuropsychological Assessment, Second Edition (for ages 3–16; Korkman et al. 2007).

Summary Points

- Constructs measured by psychological tests include intelligence, academic achievement, social skills, adaptive functioning, executive function, memory, language development, anxiety, and depression.

- Standards for educational and psychological testing, published in 1999, address ethical responsibilities of test publishers and users and emphasize the importance of the psychometric properties.

- Crucial psychometric properties of tests include a current and appropriate standardization sample and adequate reliability and validity.

- Regardless of the referral question, behavioral observations are important, and testing should also include measures of behavior, emotional adjustment, and attention from multiple respondents in order to rule out difficulties in these areas.

- There are several excellent tests of intellectual ability, including the Stanford-Binet-5, Wechsler Intelligence Scale for Children–IV, Differential Ability Scales–II, Kaufman Assessment Battery for Children–II, and Woodcock-Johnson–III. The full scale or composite score is not necessarily a meaningful overall estimate of ability, and cluster or subtest scores may offer more meaningful information.

- Questions regarding learning disabilities in reading, mathematics, and written expression constitute a major reason for testing. These disorders can dramatically impact a youngster's functioning, and thorough testing is necessary for identifying them.
- Assessment of intellectual deficiency must include an assessment of adaptive functioning in addition to cognitive skills.
- Neuropsychological testing, an extension of psychological testing, is designed to be highly sensitive to the effects of brain dysfunction. Neuropsychological testing addresses questions relating to the functional impact of a known or suspected neurological condition or brain injury.

References

American Educational Research Association, American Psychological Association, National Council on Measurement in Education: Standards for Educational and Psychological Testing, 3rd Edition. Washington, DC, American Educational Research Association, 1999

American Psychiatric Association: Diagnostic and Statistical Manual of Mental Disorders, 4th Edition. Washington, DC, American Psychiatric Association, 1994

American Psychiatric Association: Diagnostic and Statistical Manual of Mental Disorders, 4th Edition, Text Revision. Washington, DC, American Psychiatric Association, 2000

Anderson P: Assessment and development of executive function (EF) during childhood. Child Neuropsychol 8: 71–82, 2002

Bayley N: Bayley Scales of Infant and Toddler Development, 3rd Edition. San Antonio, TX, Harcourt Assessment, 2005

Beery KE, Buktenica NA: Developmental Test of Visual-Motor Integration, 4th Edition, Revised. Parsippany, NJ, Modern Curriculum Press, 1997

Bellak L, Bellak SS: Children's Apperception Test. Lutz, FL, Psychological Assessment Resources, 1993

Brenner E: Consumer-focused psychological assessment. Prof Psychol Res Pr 34:240–247, 2003

Cohen MJ: Children's Memory Scale. San Antonio, TX, Psychological Corporation, 1998

Elliott CD: Differential Ability Scales, 2nd Edition. San Antonio, TX, Psychological Corporation, 2007

Garb HN, Lilienfeld SO, Wood JM: Projective techniques and behavioral assessment, in Comprehensive Handbook of Psychological Assessment, Vol. 3: Behavioral Assessment. Edited by Haynes SN, Heiby EM. Hoboken, NJ, Wiley, 2004, pp 453–469

Golden CJ, Purish AD, Hammeke TA: Luria-Nebraska Neuropsychological Battery: Forms I and II. Los Angeles, CA, Western Psychological Services, 1986

Graham S, Harris KR, Troia GA: Writing and self-regulation: cases from the self-regulated strategy development model, in Self-Regulated Learning: From Teaching to Self-Reflective Practice. Edited by Schunk DH, Zimmerman BJ. New York, Guilford, 1998, pp 20–41

Gregory RJ: Psychological Testing: History, Principles, and Applications, 5th Edition. Boston, MA, Allyn and Bacon, 2007

Hammill DD, Larsen SC: Test of Written Language, 3rd Edition. Austin, TX, Pro-Ed, 1996

Harcourt Assessment: Stanford Achievement Test, 10th Edition. San Antonio, TX, Harcourt Assessment, 2003

Hausknecht JP, Halpert JA, Di Paolo NT, et al: Retesting in selection: a meta-analysis of coaching and practice effects for tests of cognitive ability. J Appl Psychol 92:373–385, 2007

Hoover HD, Hieronymous AN, Frisbie DA, et al: Iowa Tests of Basic Skills, Forms K, L, and M. Chicago, IL, Riverside Publishing, 1996

Kaufman AS, Kaufman NL: Kaufman Assessment Battery for Children, 2nd Edition. Circle Pines, MN, American Guidance Service, 2004

Korkman M, Kirk U, Kemp S: NEPSY, 2nd Edition. San Antonio, TX, Harcourt Assessment, 2007

Lyon GR, Fletcher JM, Barnes MC: Learning disabilities, in Child Psychopathology, 2nd Edition. Edited by Mash EJ, Barkley RA. San Diego, CA, Academic Press, 2003, pp 529–575

Malik AB, Turner ME, Sadler C: Neuropsychological evaluation. June 20, 2006. Available online at: http://www.emedicine.com/pmr/topic149.htm. Accessed July 12, 2007.

Mardell CC, Goldenberg DS: Developmental Indicators for the Assessment of Learning, 3rd Edition. Circle Pines, MN, American Guidance Service, 1998

McCall RB: The development of intellectual functioning in infancy and the prediction of later IQ, in Handbook of Infant Development. Edited by Osofsky JD. New York, Wiley, 1979, pp 707–741

McGrew KS, Keith TZ, Flanagan DP, et al: Beyond "g": the impact of "Gf-Gc" specific cognitive abilities research on the future use and interpretation of intelligence test batteries in the schools. School Psych Rev 26:189–210, 1997

Messick S: Validity of psychological assessment: validation of inferences from persons' responses and performances as scientific inquiry into score meaning. Am Psychol 50:741–749, 1995

Miller C, Evans BB: Ethical issues in assessment, in Psychological Assessment in Clinical Practice: A Pragmatic Guide. Edited by Hersen M. New York, Brunner-Routledge, 2004, pp 21–32

Mullen EM: Mullen Scales of Early Learning: AGS Edition. Circle Pines, MN, American Guidance Service, 1995

Reitan RM: Halstead-Reitan Neuropsychological Test Battery, 2nd Edition. Tucson, AZ, Reitan Neuropsychology Laboratory/Press, 1993

Roid GH: Stanford-Binet Intelligence Scales, 5th Edition. Itasca, IL, Riverside Publishing, 2003

Roid GH: Stanford-Binet Intelligence Scales for Early Childhood, 5th Edition. Itasca, IL, Riverside Publishing, 2005

Roid GH, Miller LJ: Leiter International Performance Scale—Revised. Wood Dale, IL, Stoelting Company, 1998

Rorschach H: Psychodiagnostik. Bircher, Bern, Switzerland, 1921

Semel E, Wiig E, Secord WA: Clinical Evaluation of Language Fundamentals, 4th Edition. San Antonio, TX, Harcourt Assessment, 2003

Sheslow D, Adams W: Wide Range Assessment of Memory and Learning, 2nd Edition. Lutz, FL, Psychological Assessment Resources, 2003

Spreen O, Risser AH, Edgell D: Developmental Neuropsychology. New York, Oxford University Press, 1995

U.S. Department of Education: Assistance to states for the education of children with disabilities and preschool grants for children with disabilities: final rule. Fed Regist 71:46539–46845, 2006

U.S. Office of Education: First Annual Report of the National Advisory Committee on Handicapped Children. Washington, DC, U.S. Department of Health, Education, and Welfare, 1968

Wechsler D: Wechsler Preschool and Primary Scale of Intelligence, 3rd Edition. San Antonio, TX, Harcourt Assessment, 2002

Wechsler D: Wechsler Intelligence Scale for Children, 4th Edition. San Antonio, TX, Harcourt Assessment, 2003

Wilkinson GS, Robertson GJ: Wide Range Achievement Test, 4th Edition. Wilmington, DE, Jastak Associates, 2006

Woodcock WR, McGrew KS, Mather N, et al: Woodcock-Johnson Tests of Cognitive Abilities and Achievement, 3rd Edition. Itasca, IL, Riverside Publishing, 2001

PART III

DEVELOPMENTAL DISORDERS

Chapter 12

Intellectual Disability (Mental Retardation)

Karen Toth, Ph.D.
Bryan H. King, M.D.

In 1992, the American Association on Mental Retardation (AAMR), now the American Association on Intellectual Disability and Developmental Disabilities (AAIDD), proposed a new classification system for intellectual disability based on intensity of supports needed (intermittent, limited, extensive, and pervasive) as opposed to the traditional system of classification by IQ score (mild, moderate, severe, and profound). The current definition (not yet reflected in the current version of the *Diagnostic and Statistical Manual of Mental Disorders* [DSM-IV; American Psychiatric Association 1994] and its text revision, DSM-IV-TR [American Psychiatric Association 2000]) recognizes that intellectual disability is characterized by genuine impairments, but it also reflects the idea that these impairments are strongly influenced by the individual's interaction with the environment. The new definition emphasizes strengths rather than limitations.

Significant historical events impacting the lives of individuals with intellectual disabilities over the past two centuries (Trent 1994) include educational approaches developed by the French physician Jean-Marc-Gaspard Itard (1775–1838) and Edouard Seguin (1812–1880). Seguin's comprehensive treatment approach combined sensory training, development of self-care skills, and vocational education utilizing techniques of positive reinforcement, imitation, and generalization that are still in use today. Seguin went on to found the AAMR in 1876. Two other key events occurred early in the twentieth century in the United States: institutionalized care in the form of residential treatment schools (both state and privately operated), and, in 1910, the American version of the Binet test of intelligence was published by Henry Goddard. These developments allowed psychologists and educators to identify individuals with intellectual disabilities and

TABLE 12–1. Summary of DSM-IV-TR diagnostic criteria and severity classifications for mental retardation

Diagnostic criteria		
Significantly subaverage intellectual functioning: an IQ of approximately 70 or below (i.e., two standard deviations below the mean) on an individually administered IQ test. The diagnosis can also be made in individuals with IQ scores of 71–75 if significant adaptive deficits are present.	**Concurrent deficits in adaptive functioning in at least two of the following areas:** communication, self-care and home living, social/interpersonal skills, use of community resources, self-direction, functional academic skills, work, leisure, health issues, and safety.	**Onset is before age 18:** if the onset is after 18, the diagnosis is dementia.

Severity classification (% individuals with intellectual disabilities)	Level of functioning	IQ range
Mild (85%)	Develop social and communication skills during the preschool years, may not be identified until school age, and by adolescence have typically acquired academic success at about the sixth-grade level. As adults, these individuals, with proper supports, can usually live independently in the community or with some supervision.	50–55 to 70
Moderate (10%)	Acquire communication skills during the preschool and early school-age years, perform self-care activities with some supervision, and achieve academic skills of about a second-grade level. These individuals function very well in group homes and in the community, are employed (generally in unskilled or semiskilled jobs), and can take care of themselves with minimal supervision.	35–40 to 50–55
Severe (3%–4%)	Most do not acquire speech, learn only the most basic self-care skills, and demonstrate a limited ability to learn preacademic skills. They require supervision and assistance and often reside in group homes or with their families; some may live in specialized care facilities.	20–25 to 35–40
Profound (1%–2%)	Often have an identified genetic or neurological condition, and communication, adaptive skills, and motor development remain limited. They require full-time care and support and benefit from highly structured environments.	<20–25
Severity unspecified	This diagnosis is made when there is a "strong presumption" of intellectual disability, but the individual cannot be successfully assessed using standardized intelligence measures, or for very young children, for whom intelligence tests yielding IQ scores are not available.	Unknown, but presumed <70

Source. Adapted from American Psychiatric Association: *Diagnostic and Statistical Manual of Mental Disorders, 4th Edition, Text Revision.* Washington, DC, American Psychiatric Association, 2000. Used with permission.

then provide them with education and treatment through residential treatment schools (Biasini et al. 1999). The 1960s and 1970s, however, saw a growing disillusionment with institutional care that paralleled a rise in advocacy groups to promote more individualized treatment and education for individuals with intellectual and developmental disabilities.

Definition, Clinical Description, and Diagnosis

AAIDD and Developmental Disabilities Definition

The AAMR/AAIDD has been responsible for defining intellectual disability and providing diagnostic criteria since 1921. The 2002 definition describes five key assumptions essential to the application of the definition, including consideration of the individual's environment, diverse factors that affect valid assessment of strengths and challenges, the coexistence of strengths, and identification of needed supports to improve life functioning. The following is the proposed classification system for individuals with intellectual disabilities (American Association on Mental Retardation 1992, 2002):

- **Intermittent support**—Higher-functioning individuals who require little intervention in order to function, except during times of uncertainty or stress (mild intellectual disability under the old system of classification).
- **Limited support**—Individuals who may require additional support to navigate through everyday situations (moderate disability).
- **Extensive support**—Individuals who rely on around-the-clock daily support to function (severe disability).
- **Pervasive support**—Requiring daily interventions and lifelong support necessary to help the individual function in every aspect of daily routines (profound disability).

DSM-IV-TR Definition and Diagnostic Criteria

The current DSM-IV-TR definition of intellectual disability and current diagnostic criteria are summarized in Table 12–1.

Differential Diagnosis

Learning and communication disorders (see Chapter 14, "Developmental Disorders of Learning, Communication, and Motor Skills") are diagnosed (on Axis I) when there is impairment in a specific area but not general impairment in intellectual and adaptive functioning. Individuals with pervasive developmental disorders (i.e., autism spectrum disorders; see Chapter 13, "Autism Spectrum Disorders") also often have intellectual disability (historically, rates were 70%–75%; more recent epidemiological studies indicate a rate of 40%–55%; Chakrabarti and Fombonne 2001). When the onset of an intellectual disability occurs after a period of normal functioning, or after age 18 years, the diagnosis is often that of dementia, which captures the decline in memory and cognitive skills characteristic of these individuals. A diagnosis of borderline intellectual functioning (V code, on Axis II) describes individuals with IQ scores ranging from 71 to 84 with impairments in adaptive and academic functioning. Roughly 7% of the population falls within this range of intellectual functioning.

Assessment of Intellectual and Adaptive Functioning

A comprehensive assessment of functioning (see Chapter 11, "Psychological and Neuropsychological Testing")—cognitive, adaptive, sensory, motor, and other domains (such as sleep, mood, and self-injurious behavior) that may interfere with functioning—is critical to making an accurate diagnosis of intellectual disability and ensuring that the most appropriate, available treatments and supports are provided. Cytogenetics, metabolic testing, and neuroimaging also play a role in this evaluation and are useful in identifying underlying genetic syndromes and behavioral phenotypes (see the section "Evaluation" later in this chapter). The first step in establishing the diagnosis, however, is to obtain an appropriate and valid assessment of intellectual and adaptive functioning.

While intelligence tests are a necessary component of the diagnostic process, there are a number of potential problems in using standardized, norm-referenced tests with individuals with intellectual disabilities.

Standardized intelligence tests are of particularly limited value in assessing individuals with severe and profound intellectual disability. These individuals have difficulty following verbal directions and are often not able to display their knowledge within the parameters of most standardized tests, which have rigid administration and scoring procedures. Standardized tests also have a small number of items at the extreme ends of ability, further restricting the sampling of abilities of individuals with severe and profound intellectual disability. However, individual items on these tests may provide useful information about an individual's current abilities, and the test scores themselves provide a general index of the individual's current developmental level. It is important to recognize, however, that failure on an intelligence test should not be equated with an inability "to develop functionally useful skills or to progress in any meaningful way at all" (White and Haring 1978, p. 170).

Table 12–2 includes standardized instruments that are especially well suited for evaluating children with intellectual disabilities.

TABLE 12–2. Standardized tests of intelligence for use with children with intellectual disabilities

Test	Age range, years	Strengths	Limitations
Stanford-Binet Intelligence Scales, 5th Edition (SB5) Roid 2003	2.0–85+	Excellent standardization, reliability, and validity; clear scoring criteria.	Different batteries used at different age ranges; can be difficult to score; long administration time.
Wechsler Preschool and Primary Scale of Intelligence (WPPSI) Wechsler 2002	2.6–7.3	Excellent psychometric properties; useful diagnostic information; engaging for children.	Limited floor for children with significant delays; takes a long time to administer.
Wechsler Intelligence Scale for Children, 4th Edition (WISC-IV) Wechsler 2003	6.0–16.11	Excellent standardization, reliability, and validity.	Insufficient floor for the severely disabled; verbal responses can be difficult to score.
Kaufman Assessment Battery for Children, 2nd Edition (K-ABC-II) Kaufman and Kaufman 2004	3.0–18	Provides norms for children with developmental disabilities; provides a composite mental processing score for nonverbal children.	Heavy reliance on short-term memory and attention makes it less effective for children with difficulties in these areas; limited subtests for very young children.
Differential Ability Scales, 2nd Edition (DAS-II) Elliott 2006	2.6–17.11	The clinical samples were expanded in this edition to include children with a variety of special needs.	Certain subtests (e.g., early number concepts) rely heavily on complex verbal instructions, making it less useful for children with significant language delays.
Leiter International Performance Scale—Revised (Leiter-R) Roid and Miller 1997	2.0–20.11	Useful for nonverbal individuals and for treatment planning.	Measures only nonverbal problem-solving and reasoning abilities.
Universal Nonverbal Intelligence Test (UNIT) Bracken and McCallum 1998	5.0–17.11	Useful for nonverbal individuals and for treatment planning.	Measures only nonverbal problem-solving and reasoning abilities.

TABLE 12–3. Standardized measures of development for infants and toddlers

Test	Age range, years	Strengths	Limitations
Bayley Scales of Infant and Toddler Development, 3rd Edition (Bayley III) Bayley 2005	1.0–3.6	Provides separate indices for motor and cognitive abilities.	Valid administration requires considerable experience and practice to avoid under- or overestimating abilities; best for children without significant motor and language delays, and/or attentional difficulties.
Mullen Scales of Early Learning: AGS Edition Mullen 1995	0–5.8	Provides separate indices for receptive and expressive language.	Very few items at the lowest end of the age range, limiting usefulness with infants and toddlers with significant language and motor delays.

Table 12–3 provides information on psychometrically sound infant and toddler tests, which do not provide IQ scores but are useful for establishing the presence of early developmental delays, informing treatment approaches, and tracking progress over time.

Along with a measure of intellectual function, a valid assessment of adaptive behavior is required for the diagnosis of intellectual disability. A number of factors can influence the assessment of adaptive behavior (as well as the reliability and validity of scores obtained), including the scale used; the child's age and sex; the informant (expectancies, recall ability, response bias); the examiner; the setting (school, home, hospital); and the reasons for the evaluation (diagnosis, program placement). Table 12–4 provides a short list of reliable, standardized measures of adaptive behavior.

Epidemiology

Intellectual disability is one of the most common neuropsychiatric disorders in children and adolescents and has a male-female ratio of 1.3–1.9:1 (Kabra and Gulati 2003). Prevalence estimates vary from 1% (Croen et al. 2001) to 2%–3% (Kabra and Gulati 2003; Soto-Ares et al. 2003) to as high as 10% (Battaglia and Carey 2003), depending on the definition of intellectual disability, methods used to assess individuals, and population under consideration (Leonard and Wen 2002; Shapiro and Batshaw 2004). If the current DSM-IV-TR definition is used, the rates are 3% with mild intellectual disability, 0.4% with moderate intellectual disability, and 0.1% with severe disability (Greydanus and Pratt 2005).

Etiology, Mechanisms, and Risk Factors

Historically, only about 50% of all cases of intellectual disability were of known etiology (Curry et al. 1997), although more recent studies have suggested that a careful clinical evaluation can now determine etiology in as many as 70% of cases (Croen et al. 2001; Xu and Chen 2003). The most common known causes of intellectual disability are described in the next section, "Genetic Syndromes and Behavioral Phenotypes." Predisposing factors include chromosomal changes and exposure to toxins during prenatal development (e.g., Down syndrome, fetal alcohol spectrum disorder), which affect 30% of cases; heredity, which affects approximately 5% of cases and includes single-gene abnormalities (e.g., tuberous sclerosis complex), chromosomal defects (e.g., fragile X syndrome), and inborn errors of metabolism inherited through autosomal-recessive mechanisms (e.g., Tay-Sachs disease); pregnancy and perinatal complications (e.g., trauma, prematurity, hypoxia) affecting 10% of cases; acquired medical conditions (e.g., lead poisoning) affecting 5% of cases; and environmental influences (severe deprivation) and other predisposing disorders such as autism (15%–20% of cases; American Psychiatric Association 2000).

Risk factors for intellectual disability of unknown etiology continue to be studied. Croen et al. (2001) examined infant and maternal characteristics of over 11,000 children born between 1987 and 1994 in California with intellectual disability of unknown cause. The sample was further stratified into groups of children with mild, severe, and unspecified levels of disability.

TABLE 12–4. Measures of adaptive functioning

Measure	Age range, years	Strengths	Limitations
Adaptive Behavior Assessment System, 2nd Edition (ABAS-II); five rating forms Harrison and Oakland 2003	0–89	Incorporates current AAIDD guidelines for evaluating conceptual, social, and practical aspects of adaptive behavior, as well as all 10 adaptive skill areas specified in the DSM-IV-TR.	As with most caregiver-report measures, ratings depend heavily on informant's ability to accurately interpret items and provide information that adequately captures the individual's current level of functioning.
Vineland Adaptive Behavior Scales, 2nd Edition: Survey, Caregiver, and Expanded Forms Sparrow et al. 2005	0–18.11	Addition of early childhood items in this new edition improves classification of children with moderate to profound intellectual disability.	Versions are available only for child and adolescent functioning; some items rely on information the informant may not possess.
Vineland Adaptive Behavior Scales, 2nd Edition: Teacher Form Sparrow et al. 2005	3.0–21.11	Assesses adaptive behavior in school, preschool, or structured day care setting.	A birth to 3 years version is not available; ratings depend heavily on informant's ability to accurately interpret items.
Battelle Developmental Inventory, 2nd Edition (BDI-2) Newborg 2004	0–7.11	Combines structured test items with interview items and observational data, with provisions for assessing children with physical handicaps.	Available only for children under age 8; ratings depend heavily on informant's ability to provide accurate information.
Scales of Independent Behavior—Revised (SIB-R) Bruininks et al. 1996	0–80+	Expanded items for infant and geriatric populations. Support Score predicts level of support needed.	Ratings depend on informant's ability to accurately interpret items and provide information.
Supports Intensity Scale (SIS) Thompson et al. 2004	16–72	In line with current conceptualization of intellectual disability, assesses support needs in 85 life, behavioral, and medical areas.	Must be combined with a measure that assesses current level of adaptive skills; currently available only for individuals ages 16–72.

Note. AAIDD=American Association on Intellectual Disability and Developmental Disabilities.

Findings showed that low birth weight was the strongest predictor of disability, both mild and severe. Similar findings have been reported elsewhere (Trevathan et al. 1997). Males and children born to black women and older women were also at increased risk for both mild and severe intellectual disability. Lower level of maternal education was also associated with increased risk, independent of race, for severe disability in this sample. A lower level of maternal education is correlated with lower socioeconomic status (SES), which has been shown to be a strong and consistent predictor of mild but not severe forms of intellectual disability (Durkin et al. 1998). Additional risk factors for mild disability included multiple births and second or later born children; for severe disability, children born to Asian and Hispanic mothers. This large population-based study highlights the fact that both biological and social-environmental factors play a role in the etiology of intellectual disability of unknown cause. Moreover, these factors often interact. Thus, it is not uncommon to encounter a child with intellectual disability attributed to anoxia or some other well-documented complication at birth, only to later discover that the child has a chromosomal anomaly that may have predisposed to birth complications.

Genetic Syndromes and Behavioral Phenotypes

Genetic Advances

In the last decade, advances in the field of genetics have contributed greatly to our understanding of intellectual disability. The human genome mapping project and gene knockout animal studies have enabled scientists to map specific intracellular changes associated with gene mutations associated with cognitive deficits. Improved diagnostic methods, including high-resolution karyotyping, subtelomeric screening, chromosome microdissection, nuclear magnetic resonance spectroscopy (MRS), and fluorescence in situ hybridization (FISH) have made it possible to determine etiology in many more cases of intellectual disability, including milder forms of the disorder (Vasconcelos 2004). Further, specific genes have been identified, such as *MECP2,* responsible for over 80% of cases of Rett syndrome (Amir et al. 1999). Below, we review some common genetic syndromes associated with intellectual disability.

Angelman Syndrome

Angelman syndrome (AS) is a neurogenetic disorder that occurs at a rate of about 1 per 10,000 to 1 per 20,000 worldwide (Williams 2005). Prevalence in populations with severe intellectual disability is 1.4% (King et al. 2005). The clinical presentation is varied, with some features present in virtually all individuals with AS (severe developmental delays with severe speech impairment; ataxia of gait and/or tremulous movement of the limbs; frequent laughter/happy demeanor; excitable personality, often with hand flapping; and short attention span). Other signs and symptoms present in 20%–80% of individuals include delayed head growth resulting in microcephaly by age 2,

seizures, abnormal electroencephalography (EEG) with large amplitude slow-spike waves, protruding tongue, feeding problems, drooling, sleep disturbance, hypopigmented skin, strabismus, and prognathia (Williams 2005). Brain magnetic resonance imaging (MRI) or computed tomography scans are generally normal, although they may show mild cortical atrophy, and urine and blood tests including metabolic screening are also generally normal. In some cases a normal EEG is found in individuals proven to have AS by genetic testing. The diagnosis is much easier to make after age 3, when behavioral and movement patterns, seizures, and microcephaly are predominant.

In the 1980s, it was found that the majority of individuals with AS showed microdeletions on chromosome 15, specifically 15q11.2–15q13 (70% of cases), also implicated in Prader-Willi syndrome. However, it was soon determined that paternally derived 15q deletions cause Prader-Willi syndrome and maternally derived deletions cause AS. In the last 10 years, *UBE3A* (encodes for ubiquitin ligase enzyme) has been identified as responsible for 6% of cases (Kishino et al. 1997; Matsuura et al. 1997). Its expression in the AS brain with 15q deletion is only about 10% of normal (Rougeulle et al. 1997). There are then four genetic mechanisms known to cause AS (maternal deletion of chromosome 15q11–q13, paternal chromosome 15 uniparental disomy, *UBE3A* mutation, and imprinting defects. DNA testing can screen for three of these four. An additional 10%–15% of individuals with AS are negative for all four of these mechanisms.

Down Syndrome

Down syndrome is found in about 1 in every 800 newborns and is the most common genetic cause of intellectual disability. Down syndrome is caused by a triplication of chromosome 21. The phenotype is characterized by more than 80 features but the most common include cognitive impairments, muscle hypotonia, short stature, congenital heart disease, and facial dysmorphisms (Yahya-Graison et al. 2007). Individuals with Down syndrome are at increased risk for developing Alzheimer's dementia at an early age (Holland et al. 1998). Currently, the strongest hypothesis to explain the Down syndrome phenotype is a "gene-dosage effect" (Yahya-Graison et al. 2007), which posits that genes from chromosome 21 are overexpressed in individuals with segmental trisomies and thus contribute to abnormal phenotypic expression. A distinct cognitive profile in Down syndrome includes relative strengths in visual processing and significant language impairments (King et al. 2005). In adaptive functioning, strengths in social skills relative to communication and other adaptive behavior skill domains have been observed. Additionally, problems with attention, impulsivity, hyperactivity, and aggression are often reported (King et al. 2005).

Fetal Alcohol Spectrum Disorders

Now understood to be a spectrum disorder, with varying risk according to dose, timing, and pattern of alcohol exposure, fetal alcohol spectrum disorders occur at a rate of about 1% of live births, with the more narrowly defined fetal alcohol syndrome occurring in the United States at a rate of 0.5–2 per 1,000 births (May and Gossage 2001). Intellectual disability is a hallmark of fetal alcohol spectrum disorders. Other symptoms include a distinct pattern of facial anomalies (smooth philtrum, thin vermilion border of upper lip, short palpebral fissures), prenatal and/or postnatal growth retardation, and central nervous system abnormalities (May et al. 2004). Cardiovascular, renal, and orthopedic abnormalities may also be present (Manning and Hoyme 2007). Neuroimaging studies have revealed brain structural defects, such as abnormal brain size and shape, smaller cerebellar and ventricular size, and agenesis of the corpus callosum (Riley and McGee 2005; Stratton et al. 1996), suggesting that particular brain areas are especially vulnerable. Cognitive and behavioral abnormalities include verbal and nonverbal learning deficits, attention problems, and impairments in executive functioning (Hoyme et al. 2005). A six-category diagnostic classification system was developed to attempt to capture the various manifestations of this disorder (see Manning and Hoyme 2007). Several genetic syndromes share similar physical characteristics, including Williams syndrome, de Lange syndrome, and velocardiofacial syndrome, and must be excluded before making the fetal alcohol spectrum disorder diagnosis.

Fragile X Syndrome

Fragile X syndrome is a leading cause of intellectual disability. The incidence of fragile X syndrome is 1 per 4,000 males and 1 per 8,000 females (Crawford et al. 2001). As many as 25% of individuals with fragile X syndrome also meet criteria for autism (Rogers et al. 2001), but only 2.1% of individuals with autism have the syndrome (Kielinen et al. 2004). Fragile X syndrome is a result of a mutation in the X-linked gene (Xq27.3) known as *FMR1* (fragile X mental retardation 1). In families with fragile X syndrome, intellectual disability increases with each generation (Wittenberger et al. 2007). Most males with the full mutation also have intellectual disability compared to only about half of females with the full mutation. Females with average IQ scores show deficits in other areas of cognitive ability, such as executive functioning (Bennetto et al. 2001) and social affective abilities (Keysor and Mazzocco 2002). Fragile X syndrome is characterized by a specific neurocognitive profile of strengths and weaknesses and increased risk of psychopathology (see Dykens et al. 2000 for a review), but there is significant within-syndrome variability. Cognitive impairments include auditory short-term memory, sequential information processing, and sustaining attention, while relative strengths include long-term memory, processing simultaneous information, and theory of mind abilities. Behavioral characteristics include hyperarousal, hyperactivity, social anxiety, shyness, and gaze aversion. Individuals with fragile X syndrome, throughout the spectrum of intellectual disability, are also at increased risk for schizotypal disorders, attention-deficit/hyperactivity disorder (ADHD), and pervasive developmental disorders (King et al. 2005).

Prader-Willi Syndrome

Prader-Willi syndrome can be caused by either paternal deletion (about 70% of cases) or maternal uniparental disomy (about 29% of cases) on chromosome 15q11.13, the same region implicated in Angelman syndrome. Prader-Willi syndrome is found in 1 per 29,500 births and is characterized by hypotonia, intellectual disability, failure to thrive giving way to hyperphagia, early obesity, hypogonadism, short stature with small hands and feet, sleep apnea, and behavioral problems (Horsthemke and Buiting 2006). Compulsive food-seeking and hoarding behaviors are seen as early as 2 years of age and are lifelong challenges. Other compulsive behaviors are commonly observed, leading to an increased risk of developing obsessive-compulsive disorder (OCD). Impulse-control disorders and affective disorders that interfere with adaptive functioning are also often found (King et al. 2005).

Rett Syndrome

Rett syndrome (RS) affects primarily females (with reports of rare cases involving males; Zeev et al. 2002) and is one of the most common causes of severe intellectual disability in females, with an incidence of 1/10,000 by the age of 12 years (Leonard et al. 1997). Females with RS have a period of ostensibly normal development for the first 6–18 months of life (although more recent studies suggest the existence of subtle behavioral abnormalities in the first 6 months [Burford et al. 2003]) followed by a regression or loss of intellectual functioning and fine and gross motor skills, social withdrawal, the development of stereotypic hand-wringing movements, and a reduced life span. The progression and severity of this disorder vary across individuals, and there are now a number of identified atypical variants of RS. In the vast majority of cases (over 80%), RS is caused by mutations in the X-linked gene *MECP2* (Amir et al. 1999), with more recent discoveries of mutations in two other genes (*CDKL5* and *NTNG1*) in phenotypes that strongly overlap with RS (Borg et al. 2005; Tao et al. 2004).

The diagnosis is most often made based on clinical features. While the identification of a genetic mutation can support the diagnosis, it should not be used alone to diagnose RS (Williamson and Christodoulou 2006). Treatment approaches that are multidisciplinary and focused on optimizing the individual's abilities, and improving communication strategies in particular, are most effective. About 87% of RS females develop scoliosis by the age of 25 years (Kerr et al. 2003), which can severely limit mobility. Pharmacological treatment approaches typically target sleep and breathing disturbances, seizures, and stereotypic movements. Females with RS are at increased risk for developing arrhythmias associated with prolonged QT interval (Sekul et al. 1994), so care must be taken to avoid drugs such as prokinetic agents, antipsychotics, tricyclic antidepressants, certain antiarrhythmics, anesthetic agents, and certain antibiotics.

Velocardiofacial Syndrome (Chromosome 22q11 Deletion Syndrome)

Velocardiofacial syndrome (VCFS), as its name implies, is a disorder that typically involves abnormalities in the palate, heart, and face. The most common features are cleft palate; heart defects; characteristic facial features; and learning, speech, and feeding difficulties. VCFS is also known as Shprintzen syndrome, DiGeorge syndrome, and craniofacial syndrome. A myriad of physical anomalies can be associated with a deletion at 22q11.2 (more than 35 genes are present in the region most commonly affected), and increasingly these disorders are being grouped as 22q11 deletion syndromes. The gene that appears mainly responsible for the phenotypic features of VCFS is identified as

TBX1 (Kobrynski and Sullivan 2007). VCFS occurs in approximately 5%–8% of children born with a cleft palate, and estimates suggest that 130,000 persons in the United States have this syndrome (between 1 per 4,000 to 1 per 10,000 children; Sullivan 2007).

Speech difficulty, with defects in phonation, language acquisition, and comprehension, is a significant concern for children with chromosome 22q11.2 deletion syndrome. Expressive language skills are below that expected for cognitive development and generally are more delayed than receptive skills. Social language skills are even more problematic. Behavioral and psychiatric disturbances can be significant, particularly as children move into adolescence. A sizeable minority of persons with VCFS, up to 30%, develop major psychiatric illnesses including schizophrenia and bipolar disorder (Kobrynski and Sullivan 2007).

Williams Syndrome

Williams syndrome is caused by a microdeletion on chromosome 7q11.23, has a prevalence of 1/7,500, and is associated with a specific pattern of facial features, personality (excessively friendly, anxious), connective tissue abnormalities, heart disease, failure to thrive, and growth deficiency (Morris 2006). Individuals with Williams syndrome most often have mild to moderate intellectual and learning disabilities, although in some cases low-average to average intelligence has been reported (Mervis and Becerra 2007). A cognitive profile of relative strengths in verbal short-term memory and language, with significant weakness in visuospatial construction, characterizes the disorder (Mervis et al. 2000). Williams syndrome is also characterized by a distinct personality profile, including high levels of indiscriminate social initiation and empathy that may interfere with adaptive social functioning. ADHD behaviors are commonly seen, as well as anxiety disorders and phobias (King et al. 2005).

Developmental Course and Prognosis

The developmental course and prognosis for individuals with intellectual disabilities vary according to the etiology and severity of the disability, underlying genetic syndromes and medical conditions, and environmental and treatment factors. Outcomes range from severe impairment with need for constant supervision to less severe forms of intellectual disability and, with appropriate treatment opportunities, sufficient adaptive functioning such that the criteria for a diagnosis of intellectual disability are no longer met.

Sequence and Rate of Development

Some aspects of development in individuals with intellectual disabilities are similar to what we see in typical development, while others vary. In general, the sequence, or ordering, of developmental tasks is the same for all children, with or without a disability. The only exceptions appear to be children with autism spectrum disorders, who often show a disrupted sequence of development, primarily due to poor performance on social tasks, and some children with uncontrollable seizures (King et al. 2005). The rate of development is generally slowed in individuals with intellectual disability, with variation according to age and developmental tasks. For example, in fragile X syndrome, rates of development are steady to 9–10 years of age, after which they slow, while in Down syndrome development slows between 6 and 11 years (King et al. 2005). Children with particular genetic syndromes also show different patterns of development related to skill acquisition. Examples include particular impairments in certain aspects of language development (e.g., expressive vs. receptive language) in children with Down syndrome, or in particular skill domains, such as theory of mind skills in children with autism spectrum disorders.

Cognitive Profiles

In addition to differences in rate of development, there are also unique cognitive profiles, or patterns of strengths and weaknesses, associated with many genetic syndromes or organic forms of intellectual disability. Many of these have been delineated in the earlier section "Genetic Syndromes and Behavioral Phenotypes." Understanding of these cognitive profiles informs our understanding not only of the pathogenesis of such disorders but also the development of targeted treatment programs that can affect the course of development for individuals with intellectual disabilities.

Evaluation
Clinical History and Physical Examination

The comprehensive clinical evaluation should begin with a prenatal/birth history, family history, and three-generation pedigree (Curry et al. 1997). A thorough physical examination is also indicated, given that a number of genetic syndromes, such as tuberous sclerosis complex, are evidenced through skin changes and/or neuromotor impairments. Photographs and videos can be useful tools in documenting skin conditions, movement disorders, and behavioral characteristics (Battaglia and Carey 2003). Also useful for diagnosis are sequential evaluations of the patient over several years (Curry et al. 1997), as symptoms of many behavioral phenotypes emerge or become more evident over time.

Cytogenetics

The Consensus Conference of the American College of Medical Genetics (Curry et al. 1997) provided guidelines for cytogenetic analysis, which has become a standard component of the evaluation and diagnostic process, given that chromosomal abnormalities contribute to a significant number of cases of developmental and intellectual disabilities. In fact, many children originally thought to have a disability of unknown etiology were later found to have chromosomal abnormalities (Battaglia et al. 1999; Curry et al. 1996). Although these guidelines continue to be debated, the Consensus Conference recommended the following: a standard cytogenetic analysis at the 500-band level for individuals with an intellectual disability without a definite diagnosis, a focused FISH analysis for individuals with a provisional diagnosis of microdeletion syndrome, and a high-resolution chromosome analysis for individuals with a behavioral phenotype that is shared by chromosomal and nonchromosomal syndromes (Battaglia and Carey 2003). Subtelomeric analysis may also be useful in this last group, as high-resolution banding is not always sufficient to detect deletions (ASHG/ACMG Test and Technology Transfer Committee 1996). Due to the high cost of such testing and the lack of availability in some genetic centers, clinical preselection is suggested. de Vries et al. (2001) found five indicators of subtelomeric defects that can be used to select individuals for this testing: family history of intellectual disability, prenatal growth retardation, poor postnatal growth/overgrowth, two or more dysmorphic facial features, and one or more nonfacial dysmorphologies and/or congenital abnormalities.

Metabolic Testing

Because inborn errors of metabolism affect a low percentage of individuals with intellectual disabilities, the Consensus Conference of the American College of Medical Genetics (Curry et al. 1997) recommended that metabolic testing be used selectively. However, some metabolic conditions have discrete clinical presentations and would be missed without at least a general metabolic work-up for all children with intellectual disabilities.

Neuroimaging and Electroencephalography

Neuroimaging is most often performed in patients with micro- or macrocephaly, seizures, neurological signs, and/or loss of psychomotor skills (Curry et al. 1997). MRI has been useful in elucidating the neurobiology and pathogenesis of intellectual disability (Gothelf et al. 2005). MRI detected frequent cerebral and posterior fossa abnormalities in children with nonspecific intellectual disabilities ranging from mild to severe (Soto-Ares et al. 2003). There have also been published cases of normocephalic patients who were found to have neurological disorders through MRS, even when MRI and cytogenetic and metabolic work-ups were normal (Battaglia 2003; Bianchi et al. 2000). The diagnostic value of electroencephalographic investigations, such as waking/sleep video-EEG-polygraphic studies, has also been reported (Battaglia et al. 1999), both in patients with a clinical history of seizures and in patients with severe language deficits and/or specific genetic syndromes, such as Angelman and Wolf-Hirschborn syndromes.

For an overview of the diagnostic evaluation process and an algorithm to guide decision making regarding the most appropriate tests for the patient with intellectual disability, see Battaglia and Carey (2003).

Comorbid Psychopathology

Prevalence

Estimates of the prevalence of psychiatric disorders in individuals with intellectual impairments range from 10% to 39% (Borthwick-Duffy 1994; Bouras and Drummond 1992). In children and adolescents with intellectual disabilities, emotional and behavioral problems are 3–7 times higher than in typically developing youth (Dykens 2000). Symptoms of psychiatric disorders are often attributed to the intellectual disability rather than recognized as comorbid psychiatric symptomatology. Additionally, some mental health conditions manifest differently in individuals with intellectual disabilities than they do in the general population (e.g., psychotic features may be more frequent symptoms of depression in individuals with intellectual impairments). These difficulties are exacerbated in individuals with severe forms of intellectual disability because of their limited communication skills and bland symptomatology known as *psychosocial masking* (Kerker et al. 2004).

Risk Factors

There is general agreement that all of the common psychopathologies seen in children without intellectual impairment are also found in youth with intellectual disabilities but at significantly higher rates. These include ADHD, anxiety and mood disorders, eating disorders, impulse-control disorders, conduct problems, psychosis and schizophrenia, and other disorders, such as Tourette's disorder, enuresis, encopresis, somatoform disorders, and sleep disorders. Specific factors that increase risk include moderate (vs. mild) disability, lower adaptive behavior, language impairments, poor socialization, low SES, and families with only one biological parent in the home (Koskentausta et al. 2007). In addition, specific genetic syndromes are associated with increased rates of particular disorders, such as higher rates of depression in Down syndrome (Collacott et al. 1992) and increased risk for anxiety and ADHD in individuals with Williams syndrome. A recent study (de Ruiter et al. 2007) that examined developmental course of psychopathology in youth with and without intellectual disabilities found higher rates of psychopathology in youth with disabilities, but no differences in course between groups (i.e., normative trajectories—with decreases in externalizing behaviors and increases in internalizing problems between 6 and 18 years of age—were found for both groups).

Assessment

There are no standardized assessment tools specifically for use with youth with intellectual disabilities to assist with the diagnosis of psychiatric disorders (although some assessment tools do exist now for adults with developmental and intellectual disabilities). Assessment of psychiatric disorders in children and adolescents typically involves the child's own description of symptoms and experiences, descriptions from parents and teachers, and observations of behavior. In youth with intellectual impairments, limited linguistic and communication skills and symptom presentation that may differ from that observed in youth without intellectual impairments complicate this process. Therefore, interviews with family, teachers, and other caregivers regarding their observations, as well as assessment of nonverbal aspects of behavior, play a more critical role in evaluating mental disorders in this population. Additionally, the clinician must be careful to differentiate symptoms of mental illness from symptoms of underlying brain dysfunction. Finally, challenging behaviors (attention seeking, aggression, self-injurious behavior, inappropriate social or sexual behavior), which are common reasons for referral for psychiatric services in youth with disabilities, can be caused or exacerbated by psychiatric disorders but may also be the result of metabolic and/or brain dysfunction. Determining the cause of such behaviors —organic conditions, psychopathology, environment, or a combination of these— is often difficult, yet it has important implications for treatment.

Communication of the Diagnosis to Parents

The initial evaluation of the child for an intellectual disability is a stressful and emotionally significant experience for parents. This experience—from the initial referral, through the assessment process to receiving the results—can greatly influence the family's willingness to seek and use resources needed for optimal outcomes for their child. The clinician plays a critical role in this process and should remain mindful of the child's and family's experience throughout the assessment process. During the evaluation phase, the clinician should provide clear information about the type of testing that will take place and why, inquire about the family's expectations, and solicit their questions and reactions to the assessment process. In presenting results, candor and truthfulness are essential, and technical and diagnostic terms should be introduced and explained in terms the family can understand. Most importantly, communication of results should always reflect strengths as well as

challenges in the child's functioning. Finally, a written report of these results should contain additional sources of information, resource and referral information, and appropriate treatment recommendations (Mulick and Hale 1996).

Treatment

Prevention

Strategies to prevent intellectual disabilities include prenatal diagnostic testing; newborn metabolic screening, which has been highly successful in reducing the incidence and severity of certain syndromes; and folic acid supplementation during prenatal development to reduce neural tube defects (although adherence continues to be an issue). In some syndromes, however, prevalence rates appear unchanged in spite of advances in prevention and prenatal diagnostics (e.g., Down syndrome [King et al. 2005]).

Integrative Treatment Approaches

Response to treatment in children and adolescents with intellectual impairments varies based on level of severity of intellectual impairment, age at which interventions begin, family and environmental factors, comorbid psychopathology, and number and severity of problem behaviors being addressed. An integrative approach to treatment—one that considers the youth's developmental level, social and environmental factors, psychological factors influencing capacity to learn problem-solving skills, and biology—is likely to provide the most positive outcomes. Below is a summary of evidence-based psychotherapeutic and pharmacological treatments for youth with intellectual impairments.

Psychotherapeutic Approaches

Behavioral interventions, including treatments using principles of applied behavior analysis (ABA), have a large evidence base (Grey and Hastings 2005). Behavioral approaches begin with an analysis of the cause or function of the behavior (antecedent) and how it is being reinforced. Techniques such as functional communication training (e.g., learning how to request breaks), noncontingent reinforcement (i.e., on a fixed time schedule), and extinction are then used to reduce challenging behaviors (aggression, self-injury, task-avoidant behavior) and promote positive behaviors. Behavioral approaches target both skills deficits and modifications to the individual's environment and are most effective if applied across multiple settings to promote generalization of skills. Choice making as an intervention has also been shown to reduce problem behaviors and increase self-determination (Shogren et al. 2004).

Standard psychotherapeutic approaches, such as psychoeducation, behavioral activation, and cognitive-behavioral therapy (CBT) approaches to treating co-morbid mental health conditions, have been less well studied, particularly in children and adolescents. Barriers to implementing such treatments include the perception that such interventions will be ineffective due to the individual's limited cognitive and verbal abilities. Simplifying the delivery of cognitive approaches, as well as the CBT model itself, does appear to effect change in at least some individuals with intellectual disabilities, but the mechanism for change in these cases is less well understood (Sturmey 2004; Willner 2006).

Successful peer interactions can have significant benefits for youth with intellectual disabilities. Through social interactions, children and adolescents learn, practice, and refine social skills; develop friendships; and access support. Recent research on youth with intellectual disabilities has shown that increased social competence can also positively affect academic achievement and enhance quality of life (Carter and Hughes 2005; Goldstein et al. 2002; Hartup 1999). Specific interventions include social interaction skills instruction, peer-delivered training interventions, group training, and peer support (e.g., peer buddy) arrangements. Short- to moderate-length effects of such social skills interventions are clear, but long-term effects have been less well evaluated. A recommended approach combines skill-based and support-based strategies (see Carter and Hughes 2005).

Pharmacological Treatment

Prevalence of Psychotropic Medication Use

Reports of the prevalence of psychotropic medication use in persons with intellectual disability consistently demonstrate that upward of one-third of this population, both children and adults and across residential settings, is receiving at least one psychotropic drug. The general tone of these reports suggests alarm, for

example, that the population is "overmedicated" (Holden and Gitlesen 2004) and that drug use is imprecise and appears not to be specific to diagnosis (Shireman et al. 2005; Singh et al. 1997). Psychostimulants, antidepressants, antipsychotics, and anticonvulsants comprise the vast majority of psychotropic medication prescriptions in intellectual disability (Shireman et al. 2005). With respect to the perceived lack of specificity with which psychotropic medications are employed—for example, the off-label use of medications in intellectual disability for the treatment of target symptoms like aggression, hyperarousal, and behavioral disturbance (Haw and Stubbs 2005)—the picture is complicated. Moreover, risperidone, an atypical antipsychotic, has a U.S. Food and Drug Administration (FDA)–approved indication for the treatment of irritability, aggression, and self-injurious behavior in children with autism. As our knowledge of the underlying causes for specific intellectual disability syndromes grows, we are likely to see an even greater uncoupling of drug and mental disorder in favor of drug and disability syndrome.

Review of Drugs by Class

In the use of psychotropic agents in intellectual disability, it is worth underscoring that the usual rules generally apply. Although the literature tends to be sparse, perhaps because intellectual disability is an exclusionary criterion for most medication efficacy trials, expert consensus opinion uniformly holds that the starting place for the treatment of psychiatric disorders is the same regardless of the presence of intellectual disability. Thus, the pharmacological treatment of depression is with an antidepressant, for psychosis it is an antipsychotic, ADHD warrants a stimulant, and so on. What follows is a brief overview of special considerations, if any, that may be salient to intellectual disability.

Antipsychotic drugs.
This class of drug is commonly used, and recent surveys document a shift toward the newer, atypical agents. Bramble (2007) recently surveyed child and adolescent psychiatrists specializing in intellectual disability in the United Kingdom. These clinicians ranked risperidone as their most commonly prescribed antipsychotic drug. The evidence supporting expanded indications for risperidone, including behavioral disturbances in persons with intellectual disability, is now greater than that which exists for any other psychotropic drug. Thus, the presence of a pervasive developmental disorder and/or disruptive be-

havior is most predictive of antipsychotic drug use in children (de Bildt et al. 2006). In a randomized, placebo-controlled crossover trial of risperidone for disruptive behavior in 20 individuals with developmental disabilities of mixed etiology, with a response definition of a 50% reduction in mean Aberrant Behavior Checklist total scores, half of the subjects responded to active treatment (Zarcone et al. 2001). Weight gain (84% of subjects) and sedation (40% of subjects) were common side effects (Hellings et al. 2001). In a 48-week open-label extension study of children ages 5–12 years who were treated with liquid risperidone for disruptive behavior disorders in the context of borderline to moderate intellectual disability, Turgay et al. (2002) reported that average doses of 1.4 mg daily were associated with maintenance of improvement. An average of 4 kg of weight gain was attributed to the drug. Initially elevated prolactin levels retreated into the normal range (albeit significantly higher than at baseline) over the year of treatment.

Open-label studies exist in which the use of other atypical antipsychotic drugs has been described for similar indications, and at least one large, multisite trial of aripiprazole for the treatment of behavioral disturbance in autism is currently under way. Given the cumulative experience above, many clinicians would consider a trial of risperidone for the treatment of extreme irritability, aggression, or self-injury in the setting of intellectual disability. It would be reasonable to consider other drugs from the class of atypicals in the event that a response was inadequate or precluded by side effects. Relative doses appear to be much lower when used for this purpose than for the treatment of psychosis, consistent with the general axiom for this population of "start low, go slow."

Attempts to taper and discontinue antipsychotic drugs in persons long exposed to them continue to be justified in view of the experience of Ahmed et al. (2000) in an institutional setting. These investigators randomly assigned nonpsychotic subjects, most of whom had received antipsychotic drugs for over 5 years, to receive four 25% monthly drug reductions (leading to discontinuation) or no change (control). A third of the subjects assigned to discontinuation were able to tolerate the complete withdrawal of their medication. Another 20% were able to be maintained at a dose that was only half of their initial starting dose. Compared with the control group, drug reduction was not associated with an increase in maladaptive behavior. In addition to underscoring the importance of periodically testing the need for continued medication, this study is also helpful with respect to pace of reductions. It

demonstrates that some persons who have received medication for over 5 years may be completely withdrawn without incident in just 4 months. The study also showed that individuals who could not tolerate such a taper did not require higher doses for stabilization than had preceded the study—a concern that is occasionally raised in the context of discussions about whether to "fix something that isn't broken."

Anticonvulsants.

Anticonvulsants are also commonly used in persons with intellectual disability. In their survey, Robertson et al. (2000) observed that prevalence varied from 23% to 46% across residential settings. While in the majority of cases anticonvulsants are prescribed for seizure disorders, as for the general population, this class of medication is also being studied for potential behavioral stabilization.

Antidepressants.

Considerable interest exists for understanding the potential utility of selective serotonin reuptake inhibitors (SSRIs) in children and adolescents, particularly those with repetitive behaviors. Behavioral activation appears to be more common in children and in persons with intellectual disabilities, and recommendations to begin with extremely low doses in this population have been advanced.

Adrenergics.

Hyperactivity and related disorders are not uncommon in children with mental retardation, and problems of impulsivity and disinhibition, and behavioral difficulties often pose great problems for parents and teachers. Agarwal et al. (2001) conducted a small randomized controlled crossover trial of the alpha-2 agonist clonidine for symptoms of hyperactivity and impulsivity in children with intellectual disability. Ten children were treated with fixed doses of clonidine (4, 6, and 8 μg/day). Severity of intellectual disability ranged from mild to severe. Clonidine was associated with a significant, dose-related improvement in hyperactivity, impulsivity, and inattention. Half of the children became drowsy on the clonidine, but for most the effect dissipated over time. The investigators concluded that clonidine may have a place in the treatment of impulsive and hyperactive behaviors in children with intellectual disability and that longer-term studies of larger samples are warranted.

Psychostimulants.

Stimulant drugs are among the most commonly prescribed psychotropic medications for the treatment of disruptive behavior in children and adolescents with intellectual disability (de Bildt et al. 2006). Expert consensus supports the use of these agents, for example, methylphenidate, dextroamphetamine, and mixed amphetamine salts, as first-line treatments for ADHD symptoms in the setting of intellectual disability (American Journal of Mental Retardation 2000). One recent study compared the effects of methylphenidate and risperidone on ADHD symptoms in children with moderate intellectual disability. While risperidone seemed to have a greater effect in reducing total symptom burden, the investigators recommended that a trial of stimulants should generally precede a trial of an antipsychotic agent for this purpose (Correia Filho et al. 2005).

Opioid antagonists.

The opioid antagonist naltrexone has been explicitly studied for the treatment of repetitive self-injurious behavior. Symons et al. (2004) identified 27 independent studies involving 86 subjects who were treated with naltrexone for this indication. Doses range from 0.5 to 2 mg/kg, but the dosing schedule for many studies (e.g., three times per week) makes interpretation somewhat difficult. Moreover, while there are some spectacular successes reported in the literature, the largest controlled trials are negative. Naltrexone may indeed be an option worthy of consideration in treatment-refractory self-injurious behavior, but the overarching conclusion from the mixed literature on this drug is that there is a pressing need for studies that will help to identify potential responders from within the heterogeneous population of persons with intellectual disability who self-injure.

Other drugs.

Interest in piracetam, a putative nootropic or cognitive-enhancing agent, has been stoked by anecdotal reports of its positive effects on learning, memory, attention, and general well-being. Lobaugh et al. (2001) studied piracetam in children with Down syndrome. The investigators used a placebo-controlled, crossover design and assessed the effects of piracetam (80–100 mg daily) with a comprehensive neuropsychological battery. No benefits were found and piracetam was associated with a number of side effects including aggression, agitation, sexual arousal, poor sleep, and diminished appetite.

Sleep disturbance is a little-studied but often significant problem for some persons with intellectual disability. Melatonin has been evaluated for the treatment of insomnia in children with disabilities and in situations where its administration has led to sleep improvement, behavioral disturbances like self-injury have also been noted to improve (Jan and Freeman 2004).

M.M. Jan's (2000) experience with melatonin prescribed openly to children ages 1–11 years with moderate to severe intellectual disability of varied etiologies was positive. All but two of the children were described as dramatic responders to melatonin, using measures including hours of sleep, nocturnal awakenings, delayed sleep onset, and early morning awakening. In this case series, melatonin was administered as a single 3-mg dose, 1–2 hours before the target bedtime. Pillar et al. (2000) also administered a single 3-mg dose of melatonin and monitored sleep efficiency as well as activity using a wrist actigraph in their small sample of children with severe intellectual disability. Sleep was significantly improved in the subjects receiving melatonin, and two of the five subjects were still receiving melatonin up to 18 months following the completion of the study. The investigators concluded that melatonin deserves broader consideration for the treatment of children with intellectual disability and disturbed circadian rhythm of sleep. Although these studies support the consideration of melatonin for the treatment of insomnia in children and adolescents with multiple disabilities, the relative numbers of children studied to date remains extremely small and open trials are problematic (see Phillips and Appleton 2004 for review).

Educational and Community Services and Supports

Educational programs for youth with intellectual disabilities are often multidisciplinary and include behavior specialists, speech and occupational therapists, special education teachers, and case managers. These professionals collaborate with the individual's family and community to develop individualized treatment plans specific to the child's strengths and needs. Early intervention is essential for optimal development, and most states now offer programs for children from birth to 3 years of age. These programs provide services in multiple settings (home, center) and are designed to target communication, self-help, and social and cognitive development. Developmental preschool programs serve the same purpose for children ages 3–5.

Once the child reaches school age, an individualized education plan (IEP) is developed collaboratively by school staff, social services, and the child's family (see Chapter 63, "School-Based Interventions"). Specific placement decisions are determined based on level of functioning. Some children with mild impairments can be placed in a regular education classroom with time spent during the day in a learning support classroom (or "resource room") to address specific skills deficits. In a resource room, special educators work one-on-one or in small groups with students. Children with greater levels of impairment may be placed in a self-contained special education classroom, where they spend the entire day. Special education and learning support classrooms target both academic and independent living skills ("life skills") and also support social skills development and vocational training.

Support services for families of individuals with intellectual disabilities are available through each state's Division of Developmental Disabilities, as well as through organizations such as The Arc and through schools, churches, and other nonprofit groups (Table 12–5). Support services include respite care so that families caring for a child with a high level of need can take short-term breaks to relieve stress, get support, and restore energy; in-home behavioral interventions; and crisis intervention services to help families deal with extreme situations and to insure the safety of children with intellectual disabilities and their families.

TABLE 12–5. Resources for families and individuals with intellectual disabilities

Organization or agency	Mission	Contact information
American Association on Intellectual Disability and Developmental Disabilities (AAIDD)	Promotes policies, research, effective practices, and universal human rights for people with intellectual and developmental disabilities.	444 North Capitol Street NW, Suite 846 Washington, DC 20001-1512 (202) 387-1968; (800) 424-3688 Web: www.aamr.org
The ARC of the United States	Advocates for the rights and full participation of all children and adults with intellectual and developmental disabilities; works to improve systems of supports and services; connect families; and influence public policy.	1010 Wayne Avenue, Suite 650 Silver Spring, MD 20910 (301) 565-3842 Email: info@thearc.org Web: www.thearc.org www.thearcpub.com
Division on Developmental Disabilities of the Council for Exceptional Children	A professional organization of educators, family members, and others with goals of enhancing the competence of persons who work with individuals with intellectual disabilities; responding to critical issues in the field; and advocating on behalf of individuals with developmental disabilities.	The Council for Exceptional Children 1110 North Glebe Road, Suite 300 Arlington, VA 22201-5704 (888) 232-7733; (703) 620-3660 (866) 915-5000 TTY E-mail: cec@cec.sped.org Web: www.dddcec.org
National Dissemination Center for Children with Disabilities (NICHCY)	Central source of information on disabilities in infants, toddlers, children, and youth; Individuals With Disabilities Education Act (IDEA), which is the law authorizing special education; No Child Left Behind (as it relates to children with disabilities); and research-based information on effective educational practices.	P.O. Box 1492 Washington, DC 20013 (800) 695-0285 TTY www.nichcy.org www.nichcy.org/states.htm
Wrightslaw Special Education Law and Advocacy	Provides accurate, reliable information about special education law, education law, and advocacy for children with disabilities.	http://www.wrightslaw.com

Research Directions

It is difficult to highlight a singular area of focus for the field of intellectual disability research given the breadth of need. In recent years, policy-makers have focused upon the health care needs of this population (e.g., Krahn and Drum 2007). With respect to emotional and behavioral health, the population with intellectual disability would benefit tremendously from future research programs in the areas of intervention (treatment efficacy, syndrome-specific treatment approaches, language interventions for children, mental health interventions for youth); assessment and diagnosis of mental disorders (development and refinement of assessment tools and specific diagnostic criteria for diagnosing mental disorders in youth with intellectual disabilities); and efforts to increase the pace and effectiveness of translation of findings from advances in these areas of study to their implementation in real-world settings.

Summary Points

- The term *intellectual disability* is the preferred term, replacing the term "mental retardation." In 2007, the American Association on Mental Retardation changed its name to the American Association on Intellectual and Developmental Disabilities to reflect this preferred terminology.

- There are three diagnostic criteria for a diagnosis of intellectual disability: significant subaverage intellectual functioning; concurrent deficits in at least two areas of adaptive functioning; and onset before age 18.

- About 30%–50% of cases of intellectual disability are of unknown etiology. Known causes are the result of chromosomal changes and exposure to toxins during prenatal development; heredity, including single-gene abnormalities, chromosomal defects, and inborn errors of metabolism; pregnancy and perinatal complications; acquired medical conditions; and environmental influences.

- New diagnostic methods, including high-resolution karyotyping, subtelomeric screening, chromosome microdissection, nuclear magnetic resonance spectroscopy, and fluorescence in situ hybridization, have made it possible to determine etiology in many more cases of intellectual disability, including milder forms of the disorder.

- Development in children with intellectual disability occurs in the same sequence as in children with typical development, but at a different rate, with speeded or slowed development at various ages and/or related to various developmental tasks.

- Distinct cognitive profiles are associated with various genetic syndromes and should be taken into consideration when planning treatment programs for children with intellectual disability.

- The clinical evaluation for intellectual disability often includes: a clinical history and physical exam, cytogenetic analysis, metabolic testing, and neuroimaging and electroencephalography.

- Youth with intellectual disability are at increased risk of developing comorbid psychopathology as compared to youth without intellectual disability. Mental health disorders in this population are often unrecognized and remain undiagnosed and untreated.

- Treatment for intellectual disability should be integrative, taking into account the child's developmental level, social and environmental factors, psychological factors (capacity to learn problem-solving skills), and biology. Behavioral interventions and psychopharmacological approaches currently have the best evidence base.

References

Agarwal V, Sitholey P, Kumar S, et al: Double-blind, placebo-controlled trial of clonidine in hyperactive children with mental retardation. Ment Retard 39:259–267, 2001

Ahmed Z, Fraser W, Kerr MP, et al: Reducing antipsychotic medication in people with a learning disability. Br J Psychiatry 176:42–46, 2000

American Association on Mental Retardation: Mental Retardation: Definition, Classification and Systems of Supports, 9th Edition. Washington, DC, American Association on Mental Retardation, 1992

American Association on Mental Retardation: Mental Retardation: Definition, Classification and Systems of Supports, 10th Edition. Washington, DC, American Association on Mental Retardation, 2002

American Journal of Mental Retardation: Expert Consensus Guideline Series: treatment of psychiatric and behavioral problems in mental retardation. Am J Ment Retard 105:159–226, 2000

American Psychiatric Association: Diagnostic and Statistical Manual of Mental Disorders, 4th Edition. Washington, DC, American Psychiatric Association, 1994

American Psychiatric Association: Diagnostic and Statistical Manual of Mental Disorders, 4th Edition, Text Revision. Washington, DC, American Psychiatric Association, 2000

Amir RE, van den Veyver IB, Wan M, et al: Rett syndrome is caused by mutations in X-linked MECP2, encoding methyl-CpG-binding protein 2. Nat Genet 23:185–188, 1999

ASHG/ACMG Test and Technology Transfer Committee: Diagnostic testing for Prader-Willi and Angelman syndrome: report of the ASHG/ACMG Test and Technology Transfer Committee. Am J Hum Genet 58:1085–1088, 1996

Battaglia A: Neuroimaging studies in the evaluation of developmental delay/mental retardation. Am J Med Genet C Semin Med Genet 117C:25–30, 2003

Battaglia A, Carey JC: Diagnostic evaluation of developmental delay/mental retardation: an overview. Am J Med Genet C Semin Med Genet 117C:3–14, 2003

Battaglia A, Bianchini E, Carey JC: Diagnostic yield of the comprehensive assessment of developmental delay/mental retardation in an institute of child neuropsychiatry. Am J Med Genet 82:60–66, 1999

Bayley N: Bayley Scales of Infant and Toddler Development, 3rd Edition. San Antonio, TX, Psychological Corporation, 2005

Bennetto L, Pennington BF, Porter D, et al: Profile of cognitive functioning in women with the fragile X mutation. Neuropsychology 15:290–299, 2001

Bianchi MC, Tosetti M, Fornai F, et al: Reversible brain creatine deficiency in two sisters with normal blood creatine level. Ann Neurol 47:511–513, 2000

Biasini FJ, Grupe L, Huffman L, et al: Mental retardation: a symptom and a syndrome, in Child and Adolescent Psychological Disorders: A Comprehensive Textbook. Edited by Netherton SD, Holmes D, Walker CE. New York, Oxford University Press, 1999, pp 6–23

Borg I, Freude K, Kubart S, et al: Disruption of Netrin G1 by a balanced chromosome translocation in a girl with Rett syndrome. Eur J Hum Genet 13:921–927, 2005

Borthwick-Duffy SA: Epidemiology and prevalence of psychopathology in people with mental retardation. J Consult Clin Psychol 62:17–27, 1994

Bouras N, Drummond C: Behavior and psychiatric disorders of people with mental handicaps living in the community. J Intellect Disabil Res 36:349–357, 1992

Bracken BA, McCallum RS: Universal Nonverbal Intelligence Test (UNIT). Rolling Meadows, IL, Riverside Publishing, 1998

Bramble D: Psychotropic drug prescribing in child and adolescent learning disability psychiatry. J Psychopharmacol 21:486–491, 2007

Bruininks RH, Woodcock RW, Weatherman RF, et al: Scales of Independent Behavior—Revised (SIB-R). Rolling Meadows, IL, Riverside Publishing, 1996

Burford B, Kerr AM, Macleod HA: Nurse recognition of early deviation in development in home videos of infants with Rett disorder. J Intellect Disabil Res 47:588–596, 2003

Carter EW, Hughes C: Increasing social interaction among adolescents with intellectual disabilities and their general education peers: effective interventions. Research and Practice for Persons with Severe Disabilities: The Journal of TASH 30:179–193, 2005

Chakrabarti S, Fombonne E: Pervasive developmental disorders in preschool children. JAMA 285:3093–3099, 2001

Collacott R, Cooper JA, McGrother C: Differential rates of psychiatric disorders in adults with Down's syndrome compared with other mentally handicapped adults. Br J Psychiatry 161:671–674, 1992

Correia Filho AG, Bodanese R, Silva TL, et al: Comparison of risperidone and methylphenidate for reducing ADHD symptoms in children and adolescents with moderate mental retardation. J Am Acad Child Adolesc Psychiatry 44:748–755, 2005

Crawford DC, Acuna JM, Sherman SL: FMR1 and the fragile X syndrome: human genome epidemiology review. Genet Med 3:359–371, 2001

Croen LA, Grether JK, Selvin S: The epidemiology of mental retardation of unknown cause. Pediatrics 107:1410–1414, 2001

Curry CJ, Sandhu A, Frutos L, et al: Diagnostic yield of genetic evaluations in developmental delay/mental retardation. Clin Res 44:130A, 1996

Curry CJ, Stevenson RE, Aughton D, et al: Evaluation of mental retardation: recommendations of a Consensus Conference: American College of Medical Genetics. Am J Med Genet 72:468–477, 1997 de Bildt A, Mulder EJ, Scheers T, et al: Pervasive developmental disorder, behavior problems, and psychotropic drug use in children and adolescents with mental retardation. Pediatrics 118:e1860–e1866, 2006

de Ruiter KP, Dekker MC, Verhulst FC, et al: Developmental course of psychopathology in youths with and without intellectual disabilities. J Child Psychol Psychiatry 48:498–507, 2007

de Vries BB, White SM, Knight SJL, et al: Clinical studies on submicroscopic subtelomeric rearrangements: a checklist. J Med Genet 38:145–150, 2001

Durkin MS, Schupf N, Stein Z, et al: Mental retardation, in Public Health and Preventive Medicine. Edited by Wallace R. Stamford, CT, Appleton and Lange, 1998, pp 1049–1058

Dykens EM: Psychopathology in children with intellectual disability. J Child Psychol Psychiatry 41:407–417, 2000

Dykens EM, Hodapp RM, Finucane BM: Genetics and Mental Retardation Syndromes: A New Look at Behavior and Interventions. Baltimore, MD, Paul H. Brooks, 2000

Elliott CD: Differential Ability Scales, 2nd Edition. San Antonio, TX, Harcourt Assessment, 2006

Goldstein H, Kaczmarek LA, English KM (eds): Promoting Social Communication: Children With Developmental Disabilities From Birth to Adolescence. Baltimore, MD, Brookes Publishing, 2002

Gothelf D, Furfaro JA, Penniman LC, et al: The contribution of novel brain imaging techniques to understanding the neurobiology of mental retardation and developmental disabilities. Ment Retard Dev Disabil Res Rev 11:331–339, 2005

Grey IM, Hastings RP: Evidence-based practices in intellectual disability and behaviour disorders. Curr Opin Psychiatry 18:469–475, 2005

Greydanus DE, Pratt HD: Syndromes and disorders associated with mental retardation. Indian J Pediatr 72:859–864, 2005

Harrison P, Oakland T: Adaptive Behavior Assessment Scale, 2nd Edition. San Antonio, TX, Psychological Corporation, 2003

Hartup WW: Peer experience and its developmental significance, in Developmental Psychology: Achievements and Prospects. Philadelphia, PA, Psychology Press, 1999, pp 106–125

Haw C, Stubbs J: A survey of off-label prescribing for inpatients with mild intellectual disability and mental illness. J Intellect Disabil Res 49:858–864, 2005

Hellings JA, Zarcone JR, Crandall K, et al: Weight gain in a controlled study of risperidone in children, adolescents and adults with mental retardation and autism. J Child Adolesc Psychopharmacol 11:229–238, 2001

Holden B, Gitlesen JP: Psychotropic medication in adults with mental retardation: prevalence and prescription practices. Res Dev Disabil 25:509–521, 2004

Holland AJ, Hon J, Huppert FA, et al: Population-based study of the prevalence and presentation of dementia in adults with Down's syndrome. Br J Psychiatry 172:493–498, 1998

Horsthemke B, Buiting K: Imprinting defects on human chromosome 15. Cytogenet Genome Res 113:292–299, 2006

Hoyme HE, May PA, Kalberg WO, et al: A practical clinical approach to diagnosis of fetal alcohol spectrum disorders: clarification of the 1996 institute of medicine criteria. Pediatrics 115:39–47, 2005

Jan JE, Freeman RD: Melatonin therapy for circadian rhythm sleep disorders in children with multiple disabilities: what have we learned in the last decade? Dev Med Child Neurol 46:776–782, 2004

Jan MM: Melatonin for the treatment of handicapped children with severe sleep disorders. Pediatr Neurol 23:229–232, 2000

Kabra M, Gulati S: Mental retardation. Indian J Pediatr 70:153–158, 2003

Kaufman AS, Kaufman NL: Assessment Battery for Children, 2nd Edition (KABC-II). Los Angeles, CA, Western Psychological Services, 2004

Kerker BD, Owens PL, Zigler E, et al: Mental health disorders among individuals with mental retardation: challenges to accurate prevalence estimates. Public Health Rep 119:409–417, 2004

Kerr AM, Webb P, Prescott RJ, et al: Results of surgery for scoliosis in Rett syndrome. J Child Neurol 18:703–708, 2003

Keysor CS, Mazzocco MM: A developmental approach to understanding fragile X syndrome in females. Microsc Res Tech 57:179–186, 2002

Kielinen M, Rantala H, Timonen E, et al: Associated medical disorders and disabilities in children with autistic disorder: a population-based study. Autism 8:49–60, 2004

King BH, Hodapp RM, Dykens EM: Mental retardation, in Kaplan and Sadock's Comprehensive Textbook of Psychiatry, 8th Edition, Vol 2. Edited by Kaplan HI, Sadock BJ. Baltimore, MD, Lippincott Williams & Wilkins, 2005, pp 3076–3106

Kishino T, Lalande M, Wagstaff J: UBE3A/E6-AP mutations cause Angelman syndrome. Nat Genet 15:70–73, 1997 [published erratum appears in Nat Genet 15:411, 1997]

Kobrynski LJ, Sullivan KE: Velocardiofacial syndrome, DiGeorge syndrome: the chromosome 22q11.2 deletion syndromes. Lancet 370:1443–1452, 2007

Koskentausta T, Livanainen M, Almqvist F: Risk factors for psychiatric disturbance in children with intellectual disability. J Intellect Disabil Res 51:43–53, 2007

Krahn GL, Drum CE: Translating policy principles into practice to improve health care access for adults with intellectual disabilities: a research review of the past decade. Ment Retard Dev Disabil Res Rev 13:160–168, 2007

Leonard H, Wen X: The epidemiology of MR: challenges and opportunities in the new millennium. Ment Retard Dev Disabil Res Rev 8:117–134, 2002

Leonard H, Bower C, English D: The prevalence and incidence of Rett syndrome in Australia. Eur Child Adolesc Psychiatry 6(suppl):8–10, 1997

Lobaugh NJ, Karaskov V, Rombough V, et al: Piracetam therapy does not enhance cognitive functioning in children with down syndrome. Arch Pediatr Adolesc Med 155:442–448, 2001

Manning MA, Hoyme HE: Fetal alcohol spectrum disorders: a practical clinical approach to diagnosis. Neurosci Biobehav Rev 31:230–238, 2007

Matsuura T, Sutcliffe JS, Fang P, et al: De novo truncating mutations in E6-AP ubiquitin-protein ligase gene (UBE3A) in Angelman syndrome. Nat Genet 15:74–77, 1997

May PA, Gossage JP: Estimating the prevalence of fetal alcohol syndrome: a summary. Alcohol Res Health 25:159–167, 2001

May PA, Gossage JP, White-Country M, et al: Alcohol consumption and other maternal risk factors of fetal alcohol syndrome among three distinct samples of women before, during, and after pregnancy: the risk is relative. Am J Med Genet 127C:10–20, 2004

Mervis CB, Becerra AM: Language and communicative development in Williams syndrome. Ment Retard Dev Disabil Res Rev 13:3–15, 2007

Mervis CB, Robinson BF, Bertrand J, et al: The Williams syndrome cognitive profile. Brain Cogn 44:604–628, 2000

Morris CA: The dysmorphology, genetics, and natural history of Williams-Beuren syndrome, in Williams-Beuren Syndrome: Research, Evaluation, and Treatment. Edited by Morris CA, Lenhoff HM, Wang PP. Baltimore, MD, Johns Hopkins University Press, 2006, pp 3–17

Mulick JA, Hale JB: Communicating assessment results in mental retardation, in Manual of Diagnosis and Professional Practice in Mental Retardation. Edited by Jacobson JW, Mulick JA. Washington, DC, American Psychological Association, 1996, pp 257–263

Mullen EM: Mullen Scales of Early Learning. Circle Pines, MN, American Guidance Service, 1995

Newborg J: Battelle Developmental Inventory, 2nd Edition. Rolling Meadows, IL, Riverside Publishing, 2004

Phillips L, Appleton RE: Systematic review of melatonin treatment in children with neurodevelopmental disabilities and sleep impairment. Dev Med Child Neurol 46:771–775, 2004

Pillar G, Shahar E, Peled N, et al: Melatonin improves sleep-wake patterns in psychomotor retarded children. Pediatr Neurol 23:225–228, 2000

Riley EP, McGee CL: Fetal alcohol spectrum disorders: an overview with emphasis on changes in brain and behavior. Exp Biol Med 230:357–365, 2005

Robertson J, Emerson E, Gregory N, et al: Receipt of psychotropic medication by people with intellectual disability in residential settings. J Intellect Disabil Res 44:666–676, 2000

Rogers SJ, Wehner EA, Hagerman R: The behavioral phenotype in fragile X: symptoms of autism in very young children with fragile X syndrome, idiopathic autism, and other developmental disorders. J Dev Behav Pediatr 22:409–417, 2001

Roid GH: Stanford-Binet Intelligence Scales, 5th Edition. Rolling Meadows, IL, Riverside Publishing, 2003

Roid GH, Miller LJ: Leiter International Performance Scale—Revised (Leiter-R). Lutz, FL, Psychological Assessment Resources, 1997

Rougeulle C, Glatt H, Lalande M: The Angelman syndrome candidate gene, UBE3A/E6-AP, is imprinted in brain (letter). Nat Genet 17:14–15, 1997

Sekul EA, Moak JP, Schultz RJ, et al: Electrocardiographic findings in Rett syndrome: an explanation for sudden death? J Pediatr 125:80–82, 1994

Shapiro BK, Batshaw ML: "Mental Retardation," in Nelson Textbook of Pediatrics, 17th Edition. Edited by Behrman RE, Kliegman RM, Junson HS. Philadelphia, PA, WB Saunders, 2004, pp 138–143

Shireman TI, Reichard A, Rigler SK: Psychotropic medication use among Kansas Medicaid youths with disabilities. J Child Adolesc Psychopharmacol 15:107–115, 2005

Shogren KA, Faggella-Luby MN, Jik Bae S, et al: The effect of choice making as an intervention for problem behaviour: a meta analysis. J Positive Behav Interv 6:228–237, 2004

Singh NN, Ellis CR, Wechsler H: Psychopharmacoepidemiology of mental retardation: 1966 to 1995. J Child Adolesc Psychopharmacol 7:255–266, 1997

Soto-Ares G, Joyes B, Lemaître MP, et al: MRI in children with mental retardation. Pediatr Radiol 33:334–345, 2003

Sparrow S, Cicchetti D, Balla D: Vineland Adaptive Behavior Scales, 2nd Edition. Circle Pines, MN, American Guidance Service, 2005

Stratton KR, Howe CJ, Battaglia FC (eds): Fetal Alcohol Syndrome: Diagnosis, Epidemiology, Prevention, and Treatment. Washington, DC, National Academy Press, 1996

Sturmey P: Cognitive therapy with people with intellectual disabilities: a selective review and critique. Clin Psychol Psychother 11:222–232, 2004

Sullivan KE: DiGeorge syndrome/velocardiofacial syndrome: the chromosome 22q11.2 deletion syndrome. Adv Exp Med Biol 601:37–49, 2007

Symons FJ, Thompson A, Rodriguez MC: Self-injurious behavior and the efficacy of naltrexone treatment: a quantitative synthesis. Ment Retard Dev Disabil Res Rev 10:193–200, 2004

Tao J, Van Esch H, Hagedorn-Greiwe M, et al: Mutations in the X-linked cyclin-dependent kinase-like 5 (CDKL5/STK9) gene are associated with severe neurodevelopmental retardation. Am J Hum Genet 75:1149–1154, 2004

Thompson JR, Bryant B, Campbell EM: Supports Intensity Scale (SIS). Washington, DC, American Association on Intellectual and Developmental Disabilities, 2004

Trent JW Jr: Inventing the Feeble Mind: A History of Mental Retardation in the United States. Berkeley, University of California Press, 1994

Trevathan E, Murphy CC, Yeargin-Allsopp M: Prevalence and descriptive epidemiology of Lennox-Gastaut syndrome among Atlanta children. Epilepsia 38:1283–1288, 1997

Turgay A, Binder C, Snyder R, et al: Long-term safety and efficacy of risperidone for the treatment of disruptive behavior disorders in children with subaverage IQs. Pediatrics 110:e34, 2002

Vasconcelos MM: Mental retardation. J Pediatr (Rio J) 80(suppl):S71–S82, 2004

Wechsler D: Wechsler Preschool and Primary Scale of Intelligence. San Antonio, TX, Psychological Corporation, 2002

Wechsler D: Wechsler Intelligence Scale for Children, 4th Edition. San Antonio, TX, Psychological Corporation, 2003

White OR, Haring NG: Evaluating educational programs serving the severely and profoundly handicapped, in Teaching the Severely Handicapped, Vol 3. Edited by Haring NG, Bricker DD. Seattle, WA, American Association for the Education of the Severely/Profoundly Handicapped, 1978, pp 153–200

Williams CA: Neurological aspects of the Angelman syndrome. Brain Dev 27:88–94, 2005

Williamson SL, Christodoulou J: Rett syndrome: new clinical and molecular insights. Eur J Hum Genet 14:896–903, 2006

Willner P: Readiness for cognitive therapy in people with intellectual disabilities. J Appl Res Intellect Disabil 19:5–16, 2006

Wittenberger MD, Hagerman RJ, Sherman SL, et al: The FMR1 premutation and reproduction. Fertil Steril 87:456–465, 2007

Xu J, Chen Z: Advances in molecular cytogenetics for the evaluation of mental retardation. Am J Med Genet 117C:15–24, 2003

Yahya-Graison EA, Aubert J, Dauphinot L, et al: Classification of human chromosome 21 gene-expression variations in Down syndrome: impact on disease phenotypes. Am J Hum Genet 81:475–491, 2007

Zarcone JR, Hellings JA, Crandall K, et al: Effects of risperidone on aberrant behavior of persons with developmental disabilities, I: a double-blind crossover study using multiple measures. Am J Ment Retard 106:525–538, 2001

Zeev BB, Yaron Y, Schanen NC, et al: Rett syndrome: clinical manifestations in males with MECP2 mutations. J Child Neurol 17:20–24, 2002

Chapter 13

Autism Spectrum Disorders

Peter E. Tanguay, M.D.

In 1943, Leo Kanner, child psychiatrist and author of the first U.S. textbook on child psychiatry, published a paper in which he described 11 children "whose condition differs so markedly and uniquely from anything reported so far, that each case merits—and, I hope will eventually receive—a detailed review of its fascinating peculiarities" (Kanner 1943, p. 217). The following year, Hans Asperger described, in a German publication, a similar disorder (Asperger 1944/1991). Both reports had the word *autistic* in their title. Kanner's report was initially much better known in the West. Despite considerable interest, it was not until DSM-III (American Psychiatric Association 1980) was published that autism became an official and codified diagnosis. The DSM-III diagnostic criteria, which had been developed after numerous expert suggestions and field trials, were consistent with many, though not all, of Kanner's observations. Although the criteria have been adjusted through subsequent editions of DSM, the overall approach to the diagnosis of autism remains largely unchanged.

Key advances have been made in our understanding of one of the core symptoms of autism—the nature of the social deficits. Kanner believed that "these children have come into the world with innate inability to form the usual, biologically provided affective contact with people" (p. 250). Only when affordable and technically adequate audio- and video-recording devices were developed in the 1970s was it possible to observe and accurately quantify social responses in infants and children. Since then, studies have given us a rich understanding of how social interaction develops. Social communication research has afforded us an exciting new way to view autism (Kasari et al. 1990; Mundy 1995; Mundy and Crowson 1997; Sigman 1998).

The nature and development of human social communication are too complex to be adequately covered in this chapter (see Trevarthen and Aitken 2001 and Tuchman 2003 for reviews), but a brief summary is in order. Children are born with the behavioral propensity to emit social signals. By several months of age they are beginning to engage in a rich experience of communication using eye contact, social smile, social gesture, and body language. By 15 months of age, they appear to have a rudimentary understanding of "theory of mind"—that is, that others have minds that differ from their own, and that they can learn from watching the social signals of others. By 3 or 4 years of age, they begin to engage in to-and-fro conversation and to "mentalize"—that is, infer other's emotions and intent. In contrast, children who have autism appear to lack the behavioral propensity to interact with their caretakers, or they may begin to do so normally only to lose the ability by 12–15 months of age. They fail to develop joint interaction using eye contact, gesture, prosody, and body language; later they do not develop the capacity to mentalize (Tuchman 2003). Or they may develop some of these skills, but they remain deficient compared to the general population.

The social deficits in autism are now viewed as on a continuum, from severe to relatively mild, not necessarily correlated to the person's language skills and intellectual capacity (Constantino and Todd 2003; Constantino et al. 2000; Hoekstra et al. 2007; Posserud et al. 2006). Social communication skills may be continuously distributed in the general population, with people on the autism spectrum being at the most impaired end of the distribution. Constantino et al. (2000) have developed the Social Responsiveness Scale (SRS), comprising 65 items meant to assess a broad spectrum of social communication traits. The scale is capable of distinguishing between children with autism and children who have other psychiatric disorders. In populations of normal (neurotypical) schoolchildren (Constantino et al. 2000) or neurotypic twins (Constantino and Todd 2003), SRS scores were found to be continuously distributed, with a graph of the distribution resembling a bell-shaped curve. Posserud et al. (2006) have reported a similar continuous distribution of social communication skills in a population of 9,430 children ages 7–9 years, using the parent and teacher versions of the Autism Spectrum Screening Questionnaire (ASSQ). The authors found that 2.7% of children had scores in the extremely abnormal range, with males showing higher scores than females. Hoekstra et al. (2007) report finding a continuous distribution of Autism Spectrum Quotient scores in a population of 370 18-year-old twins, their 94 siblings, and 128 parents. Males had significantly higher autistic trait scores than females. These findings suggest that if proper social communication diagnostic instruments (not just screening questionnaires) could be developed, it might be possible to graph social communication skills as we do with height and weight. One might then define the social communication deficits in autism in terms of standard deviations from the mean in the normal population, much as we do now for general intellectual skill.

Definition, Clinical Description, and Diagnosis

Definition of Autistic Disorder

In DSM-IV (American Psychiatric Association 1994) and its text revision, DSM-IV-TR (American Psychiatric Association 2000), autism is defined by the presence of *severe* and *pervasive* impairments in reciprocal social interaction and in verbal and nonverbal communication skills. There must also be symptoms of restrictive and repetitive behaviors and/or stereotyped patterns of interest that are abnormal in their intensity or focus. The emphasis is on severe and pervasive. In the 1970s, when the DSM characteristics of autism were being defined, many of the persons with autism who came for assessment had moderate to severe retardation, major language impairments, and many repetitive and odd behaviors. Today, there is a wider spectrum of symptom severity in those referred as possibly autistic. Approximately 50% of persons with autism may have normal verbal expressions and IQ scores, despite having moderate to severe social skills deficits. And if there is a continuous distribution of social and communication skills in the general population, where do we draw the line to make a diagnosis? At present, one must use clinical experience to make the decision. Because services follow diagnosis, the issue can be contentious, with the service providers often opting for more stringent criteria and the parents for less stringent ones.

The specific DSM-IV-TR criteria for the diagnosis of autistic disorder are shown in Table 13–1.

Clinical Characteristics of Autism

Parents are acutely sensitive to delays in certain developmental milestones in their infants and toddlers. A child who is not standing by 15 months, not walking or using words by 20 months, or not using phrases in speech by 30 months will be noticed, leading to efforts to understand and remediate the delay. This is not nec-

TABLE 13–1. DSM-IV-TR diagnostic criteria for autistic disorder

A. A total of six (or more) items from (1), (2), and (3), with at least two from (1), and one each from (2) and (3):

    (1) qualitative impairment in social interaction, as manifested by at least two of the following:

        (a) marked impairment in the use of multiple nonverbal behaviors such as eye-to-eye gaze, facial expression, body postures, and gestures to regulate social interaction

        (b) failure to develop peer relationships appropriate to developmental level

        (c) a lack of spontaneous seeking to share enjoyment, interests, or achievements with other people (e.g., by a lack of showing, bringing, or pointing out objects of interest)

        (d) lack of social or emotional reciprocity

    (2) qualitative impairments in communication as manifested by at least one of the following:

        (a) delay in, or total lack of, the development of spoken language (not accompanied by an attempt to compensate through alternative modes of communication such as gesture or mime)

        (b) in individuals with adequate speech, marked impairment in the ability to initiate or sustain a conversation with others

        (c) stereotyped and repetitive use of language or idiosyncratic language

        (d) lack of varied, spontaneous make-believe play or social imitative play appropriate to developmental level

    (3) restricted repetitive and stereotyped patterns of behavior, interests, and activities, as manifested by at least one of the following:

        (a) encompassing preoccupation with one or more stereotyped and restricted patterns of interest that is abnormal either in intensity or focus

        (b) apparently inflexible adherence to specific, nonfunctional routines or rituals

        (c) stereotyped and repetitive motor mannerisms (e.g., hand or finger flapping or twisting, or complex whole-body movements)

        (d) persistent preoccupation with parts of objects

B. Delays or abnormal functioning in at least one of the following areas, with onset prior to age 3 years: (1) social interaction, (2) language as used in social communication, or (3) symbolic or imaginative play.

C. The disturbance is not better accounted for by Rett's disorder or childhood disintegrative disorder.

Source.   Reprinted from American Psychiatric Association: *Diagnostic and Statistical Manual of Mental Disorders, 4th Edition, Text Revision.* Washington, DC, American Psychiatric Association, 2000, p. 75. Used with permission. Copyright © 2000 American Psychiatric Association.

essarily so for the more subtle manifestations of the development of social communication, such as use of facial expressions or gestures, the degree of enthusiasm with which the child greets others, the amount of time the child spends in meaningful eye contact, or whether he or she uses gesture to direct another person's attention to things that interest the child or that the child wants. Parents are more likely to notice if their child uses stereotyped hand and finger mannerisms or becomes obsessively preoccupied with certain objects or activities, but not all autistic children behave in this way as infants or toddlers. Therefore, parents may not bring their autistic child for evaluation until 18 months of age or later. In addition, children with mild to moderate degrees of autism may show their least degree of handicap when interacting with their mothers, even while interacting less with their sib-

lings, and not at all with persons outside the family. Mothers may report that their child is affectionate to them but entirely aloof to others or that the child will preferentially show a desire to be with the mother while largely ignoring others.

Certain questions for parents are useful in the specific assessment for social communication disorders: Does your child talk to you or make sounds to you just to be friendly? Can you have a give-and-take conversation with your child, in which he says something, you reply, he replies in turn, and so on? Can your child choose topics of conversation that take into account your interests rather than just his own interests? Is it difficult to "catch" your child's eye? How has your child responded to others in distress? Does he even notice the distress, and if he notices, does he respond with appropriate empathy and comforting sounds and gestures? For children 3 and 4 years of age, play behaviors, both alone and with others, are crucial indicators of social communication deficits. One of the most important functions of play for children is to imitate and master the world in which they live. Even at a very young age, children imitate their parents: pretending to mow the lawn, to cook in the kitchen, to do the things they see their parents do. By 4 years of age (or earlier), they play out pretend scenarios of fantastic adventure but always ones that mirror what they know of the real world. Children who have a social communication deficit do not engage in this make-believe play. Their play is obsessive, unimaginative, and does not usually involve make-believe people. They may copy entire stories from television or books, but they play them out without embellishment or change. They do not engage in what is called *symbolic play*—for example, treating a toy car or doll as if it were a real car or a real person. In later years, when they interact with other people, they are severely handicapped because they are unable to fathom what the other person's intentions are or what his or her interests might be. The child with autism who has a fascination with and an encyclopedic knowledge of dinosaurs cannot understand why his obsessive dwelling on the topic with other children makes them scorn and reject him.

Many autistic children have associated deficits in addition to their DSM-IV symptoms. Approximately 50% have intellectual handicaps, reflected in IQ scores of less than 70. As a characteristic of autism, all have deficits in pragmatic communication (i.e., the social aspects of communication), but some have deficits in vocabulary and grammar as well. Up to 25% of autistic children and adolescents may have epilepsy (Fombonne et al. 1997), however the rate is less in those who have good intellectual function and good vocabulary and grammar. Some, perhaps 25%, have severe hypersensitivity to sounds, bright lights, touch, or taste. Some have gross and fine motor deficiencies. Only when one has cataloged these problems can the clinician have a sufficient understanding of the child to develop a program of remediation and treatment.

Evaluation Instruments

It is possible to diagnose autism by 18 months of age, if one knows what to look for, and to at least suspect autism at 12 months. Using naturalistic home movies of the birthday parties of 1-year-old children, raters who are trained to identify joint attention behaviors (pointing and showing), social communication affective

behaviors, and unusual autistic-like stereotyped behaviors are able to distinguish children later diagnosed with autism from typically developing children. The autistic children engaged in stereotyped inappropriate play, looked less at the camera, assumed unusual postures, and needed more adult prompting before they responded to their name (Baranek 1999; Osterling and Dawson 1994).

The Checklist for Autism in Toddlers (CHAT) was developed for use by pediatricians and nurses with children who are 18–24 months of age (Baron-Cohen et al. 1992). It takes less than 10 minutes to administer and uses information from the parent as well as observation of the child. Behaviors that are particularly deficient in toddlers with autism are protodeclarative pointing (calling parent's attention to an object of interest), protoimperative pointing (asking for something), and gaze monitoring (Baird et al. 2000). The original scoring of the CHAT was designed to minimize the risk of false positives that would needlessly alarm parents. Unfortunately, this led to a high rate of false negatives (failing to identify children who later were diagnosed autistic). The more recently developed M-CHAT (Robins et al. 2001) has improved diagnostic specificity. Because the M-CHAT uses only information derived from parental questionnaire, however, it may be less accurate than the CHAT.

For children 3 years of age and older, the Autism Diagnostic Interview—Revised (ADI-R) (Lord et al. 1994) and the Autism Diagnostic Observation Schedule—Generic (ADOS-G) (Lord et al. 2000) are universally recognized as the most comprehensive and valid diagnostic instruments available. The ADI-R is a semistructured interview of the child's primary caretaker that includes many items pertaining to social communication. The diagnosis is reached using an algorithm based on scores on clusters of items that correspond to social relationships; verbal and nonverbal communication; and restrictive, repetitive, and stereotyped patterns of behavior. In the method of interview, answers are not necessarily taken at face value but are further explored using probes to confirm that any reported unusual behaviors are truly due to impairment that is social in nature. The disadvantages of the ADI-R are that clinicians must be trained in its use and an interview takes 90 minutes or more to complete. It is an ideal research instrument, but it is likely impractical for routine clinical use. The ADOS-G, designed to be used for both children and adults, consists of a number of age-appropriate social "presses" in which the examiner uses his or her behavior to elicit social responses from the child. The interview is scored using a template designed to measure the same domains as does the ADI-R. Interviewers must be trained, but the interview usually takes 1 hour or less to administer. The ADI-R and the ADOS-G yield independent and additive diagnostic information (Risi et al. 2006), and both should be used in making a diagnosis.

Two instruments, the Childhood Autism Rating Scale (CARS; Schopler et al. 1988) and the Autism Behavior Checklist (ABC; Krug et al. 1980), were developed prior to our current understanding of social communication, but they are still popular. They are easy to administer, making them suitable for screening purposes. However, they may miss more nuanced symptoms of social communication deficits.

Two recently developed instruments appear very promising: the Autism Screening Questionnaire (ASQ; Berument et al. 1999) and the Developmental, Dimensional and Diagnostic Interview (3di; Skuse et al. 2004). The former is a screening questionnaire partly based on the ADI-R; it can be administered in a short time and is effective for screening persons on the autism spectrum. The latter attempts to combine the best features of structured and semistructured interviews, using the strengths of each. It is administered by raters whose scores are entered into a computer database, allowing for the rapid generation of a comprehensive diagnostic report. The 3di does not incorporate observation of the child's behavior, though one might achieve this by adding an observational interview such as the ADOS-G.

Although not a diagnostic interview for autism per se, the Vineland Adaptive Behavior Scales (VABS) have been used to evaluate the social skills of children who may have autism (Volkmar et al. 1993). The development of supplementary norms designed to enhance the use of the VABS in persons with autism (Carter et al. 1998) should add to its usefulness in evaluating individuals with social communication disorder.

Differential Diagnosis

Disorders Listed Under Pervasive Developmental Disorder in DSM-IV-TR

Asperger's Disorder

The criteria for Asperger's disorder are identical to those for autistic disorder (including the requirement that the symptoms be severe and pervasive) with the exception that there is no clinically significant delay in cognitive development or in the development of age-appropriate self-help skills, and no significant delay in language development. The former is often interpreted as having an IQ score above 70, and the latter is specified as having single word use by 2 years of age and communicative phrases by 3 years of age. There has been considerable controversy whether Asperger's disorder is justified as a separate diagnosis or whether it simply represents high-functioning autism (Macintosh and Dissanayake 2004). Also, of persons who meet the criteria for Asperger's at the time they are evaluated, often at age 5 years or later, few have a history of normal cognitive function and language early in life, as is required in DSM-IV (Mayes et al. 2001). Since Asperger's does exist as an official diagnosis, we suggest that the criteria of normal language and normal intelligence be judged at the time of evaluation rather than based on information about the child's first years of life.

Pervasive Developmental Disorder Not Otherwise Specified

DSM-IV states that this diagnosis should be used 1) when there is a severe and pervasive impairment in the development of reciprocal social interaction or verbal and nonverbal communication, or 2) when stereotyped behavior, interests, and activities are present, but the criteria for any of the more specific pervasive developmental disorder (PDD) diagnoses are not met. How this statement is to be interpreted in unclear. In practice, and especially in research projects, persons meeting the social and communication impairment criteria for autism but who may have few repetitive, restricted, and stereotyped behaviors (thus not meeting the full criteria for autistic disorder or Asperger's disorder), could be given a diagnosis of pervasive developmental disorder not otherwise specified (PDD-NOS).

Rett's Disorder

This syndrome is caused by mutations in X-linked *MECP2*, encoding methyl-CpG-binding protein 2. It is almost exclusively found in females, though rare cases of Rett's disorder have been reported in males who have a concomitant XXY abnormality. It is the second most important cause of mental retardation (after Down syndrome) in females. Characteristically, the infant develops as expected, with normal head circumference, for the first 5 months. This is followed by a deceleration in head growth between 6 months and 4 years of age, accompanied by loss of already developed skills, such as use of hands, gait and motor coordination, social engagement, and communication skills. In most cases the individual is left with profoundly impaired expressive and receptive language with severe psychomotor retardation. Epilepsy is a frequent complication. Rare cases of asymptomatic carriers have been reported, as well as several reports of a very rare preserved speech variant of the disorder, in which persons carrying the mutant gene have good communication skills with mild intellectual retardation (Huppke et al. 2006). They may have social communication deficits similar to those found in autism. Mutations in *MECP2* do not appear to play a role in autism (Beyer et al. 2002), thus autistic disorder and Rett's disorder with preserved speech variant are similar-appearing phenotypes that are genetically unrelated.

Childhood Disintegrative Disorder

In 1930, Theodore Heller described six children who had developed normally for several years only to undergo a catastrophic mental regression in which they lost language as well as intellectual and social skills. As currently described, the regression in childhood disintegrative disorder (CDD) begins no earlier than 2 years and no later than 10 years of age. The clinical features of CDD can be quite similar to autistic disorder, distinguished only by the age at onset. Seizures are common in CDD (Hendry 2000). For those children who have a more prolonged period of normal development, differentiation from autism may be fairly easy, but not so for those whose onset followed only 24 months of normal development. The most typical onset is between 2 and 4 years of age (Volkmar and Cohen 1989). A specific inborn error of metabolism or neurological disorder has not been identified. The prevalence of CDD is estimated as 1.7 per 100,000 (95% confidence interval of 0.6 to 3.8 per 100,000) (Fombonne 2002). Intervention methods for CDD are identical to those used for autism.

Disorders Not Listed Under Pervasive Developmental Disorder

Fragile X Syndrome

The cause of fragile X syndrome is a mutation in *FMR1* (including the occurrence of a greatly expanded trinucleotide repeat) at Xq27.3. The diagnosis is now easily made using Southern blotting and polymerase chain reaction testing of persons suspected of having the syndrome. Studies indicate that approximately 3%–5% of persons diagnosed as autistic have the *FMR1* mutation (Farzin et al. 2006; Fombonne et al. 1997; Wassink et al. 2001). While small, this prevalence rate is sufficient to warrant testing of all autistic persons for the mutation, if only because of the implication for family genetic counseling. Study of persons who have fragile X syndrome has revealed social and communicative handicaps that resemble the symptoms of autism (Loesch et al. 2007; Rogers et al. 2001). *FMR1* is known to play a role in many neurodevelopmental processes, and some of these may involve systems that are defective in autism (Feinstein and Reiss 1998).

Landau-Kleffner Syndrome (Acquired Epileptic Aphasia)

First described in 1957 (Landau and Kleffner 1957), this rare syndrome has a fairly uniform presentation: after a period of 3 to 7 years of normal development, a child loses receptive and expressive language, either precipitously (even within days) or gradually over a period of months. Electroencephalography reveals severe paroxysmal discharges over both hemispheres, centered over the temporal lobes and worse during non-REM sleep (Mouridsen 1995). At least initially, 30%–50% of the children do not have overt seizure activity. The language regression may affect social relationships, and the symptoms may be mistaken for autism. The course of the illness is variable. Antiepileptic medication may help, but a substantial number of children remain partially aphasic as adults.

Tuberous Sclerosis Complex

Tuberous sclerosis complex (TSC) is an autosomal-dominant disorder in which benign tumorlike masses grow in the brain, skin, heart, eye, and kidney. Both seizures and mental retardation are frequently present in persons with TSC (Gutierrez et al. 1998). Twenty-five percent of persons with TSC can be diagnosed as autistic, and as many as 50% may have milder symptoms of autism (Bolton et al. 2002; Curatolo et al. 2004). Conversely, the TSC gene abnormalities are found in only 1%–4% of persons with autism (Wiznitzer 2004).

Multiple Complex Developmental Disorder

Although first named and described in 1993 (Towbin et al. 1993), multiple complex developmental disorder has its roots in previous unofficial diagnoses, such as "borderline personality disorder of childhood" or "the borderline child." These children are described as intensely anxious, fearful, and even panic-stricken. They have an inability to initiate or maintain peer relationships and show profound limitations in empathy and in the ability to read or understand what others might be thinking. They also have impaired cognitive processing, manifested by irrational thinking, grandiose delusions, and thought intrusions. They do not have hallucinations. Children with multiple complex developmental disorder have much greater psychotic thinking, anxiety, suspiciousness, aggression, and social handicaps than do autistic children (Van der Gaag et al. 1995).

Epidemiology

The earliest epidemiological studies of autism, done in the mid-1960s, found a prevalence of 1 in 2,500 with a male-female ratio of approximately 4:1. More than 70% of affected individuals had IQs less than 70 (Lotter 1966). Large-scale epidemiological studies within the past decade have screened large populations within a specific catchment area using age-appropriate state-of-the-art instruments to identify persons within the autism spectrum. A study carried out in Staffordshire, England (Chakrabarti and Fombonne 2001), of 15,500 children ages 2.5–6.5 years found 97 children (79.4% male) confirmed to have a pervasive developmental disorder (PDD). The prevalence of PDDs was estimated to be 62.6 per 10,000 children, or approximately 1 in 160 children. Prevalences were 16.8 per 10,000 for autistic disorder and 45.8 per 10,000 for other PDDs. Of the 97 children with a PDD, 25.8% had some degree of mental retardation and 9.3% had an associated medical condition.

A study (Yeargin-Allsopp et al. 2003) examined the prevalence of autism among children ages 3–10 years in the five counties of metropolitan Atlanta, Georgia. Children were identified and diagnosed only from their medical and educational records, with case status determined by expert review. A total of 987 children displayed behaviors consistent with autism, Asperger's disorder, or PDD-NOS. The prevalence of autism was 3.4 per 1,000, and the male-female ratio was 4:1. Overall, the prevalence was comparable for black and white children. Sixty-eight percent of children with IQ or developmental test results had cognitive impairment. As severity of cognitive impairment increased from mild to profound, the male-female ratio decreased from 4.4:1 to 1.3:1.

In a Japanese epidemiological survey of childhood autism defined using ICD-10 research criteria (World Health Organization 1992) in 18- and 36-month-old children, the prevalence of autism was 21.1 per 10,000, or approximately 1 in 475 (Honda et al. 1996). Half of the children had IQs over 70, with most of these scoring above 85. The findings are limited in that they did not use standardized instruments, and some children who have milder degrees of autism might be missed at 36 months of age.

We have learned from these and other epidemiological studies that IQ in the normal range is more common in persons with autism than was thought to be the case 30 years ago. This is likely due to our now identifying people as having social communication disorders despite their having normal syntactic language and intellectual skills. We have also discovered that the prevalence of autism is higher than we once thought, although the increase may be less than it initially appears. Though Lotter (1966) reported a prevalence of 1 in 2,500 in 1966, he noted that there was a group of children who, while they were not autistic, showed many autistic features. If this group was added to those whom he diagnosed as autistic, the prevalence would be approximately 1 in 1,400. Current prevalence studies estimate the rate is 30–60 per 10,000 (approximately 1 in 330 to 1 in 170), an increase in prevalence of between four-fold and sevenfold. It is difficult to determine if this is greater than one would expect given our broadening diagnostic criteria and the greater familiarity of the public with the symptoms of autism and Asperger's disorder.

One pernicious result of concern regarding a perceived increased prevalence of autism has played out over the past decade around the issue of vaccination. Based on an inadequate study of the effects of the measles-mumps-rubella (MMR) vaccine (Wakefield et al. 1998), it was alleged that the MMR vaccine led to gastrointestinal disease and an encephalitis resulting in developmental regression into autism. This was taken up as a cause célèbre by antivaccination advocates and some parents, to the point at which parents questioned whether they should vaccinate their children. This was similar to what had happened in the United Kingdom in the early 1970s, when anecdotal reports linked pertussis vaccination with infant brain damage. A national study later showed that these reports were untrue (except for a very few children), but parental and professional anxiety soared, and the national immunization rate for pertussis fell from 80% to 30%. Twelve years after the initial scare, three major pertussis epidemics occurred, resulting in 300,000 cases and 70 deaths. Many large studies, some involving hundreds of thousands of children, have examined the effects of the MMR vaccine; 11 are listed in a major review (Madsen and Vestergard 2004), and none support the MMR autism hypothesis. On the heels of the MMR vaccine controversy, it was alleged that the mercury preservative (thimerosal) in vaccines could cause autism. Again, numerous studies (see Rutter 2005) have refuted this claim. In particular, in some countries thimerosal was withdrawn as a preservative in vaccines, with no change in the incidence of autism in the population. Offit (2008) has chronicled the vaccination-mercury story quite well, revealing the hidden financial motives of some of its most vociferous supporters.

Comorbidity

Clinicians who work with autistic persons have long observed the additional presence of symptoms of other psychiatric disorders. Indeed, Kanner (1943) noted in his original paper that anxiety was a prominent feature of the syndrome. In a study by Simonoff et al. (2008), a sample of children drawn from the community, who had been identified as having PDD or as having special school needs, were surveyed using the Social Communication Questionnaire (SCQ). Children with the highest SCQ scores ($n=112$) were further evaluated using a variety of standardized assessment tools, including the ADOS, the ADI-R, and the Child and Adolescent Psychiatric Assessment (CAPA)—Parent Version. Ninety-eight children were male (male-female ratio of 7:1). The mean IQ in the sample was 73, with a range of 19–124. Fifty-seven percent of the group had one or two psychiatric disorders in addition to autism spectrum disorder (ASD), and 24% had three or more disorders. The most common disorders were social anxiety disorder (29%), attention-deficit/hyperactivity disorder (ADHD; 28%), and oppositional defiant disorder (28%). Other disorders occurring in greater than 10% of the children were generalized anxiety disorder (13%), panic disorder (10%), and enuresis (11%). The rates of major depressive disorder, dysthymic disorder, and conduct disorder were low (1%–3%). The authors note that there were relatively few females in the sample, which may limit the generalizability of the findings to females. They also suggested that had the children been questioned directly about symptoms, the prevalence of psychiatric disorders might have been higher.

Although only 8.2% of the children in the Simonoff et al. (2008) study were diagnosed as having obsessive-compulsive disorder (OCD), two studies of adults with autism (McDougle et al. 1995; Russell et al. 2005) have reported higher prevalence of OCD. McDougle et al. (1995) reported that the patients with autistic disorder could be distinguished from nonautistic subjects with OCD by the types of repetitive thoughts and behavior. Compared to the OCD group, the autistic patients were significantly less likely to experience thoughts with aggressive, contamination, sexual, religious, symmetry, and somatic content. Repetitive ordering; hoarding; telling or asking (trend toward significance); touching, tapping, or rubbing; and self-damaging or self-mutilating behavior occurred significantly more frequently in the autistic patients, whereas cleaning, checking, and counting behavior were less common in the autistic group than in the patients with OCD. Russell et al. (2005) reported that their ASD and OCD groups had similar frequencies of obsessive-compulsive symptoms, with only somatic obsessions and repeating rituals being more common in the OCD group. The OCD group had higher obsessive-compulsive symptom severity ratings, but up to 50% of the ASD group reported at least moderate levels of interference from their symptoms. The autistic persons in Russell's study had considerably higher IQ scores than did those in the McDougle group. It was argued that having a higher IQ score allowed for subjects to more accurately report their symptoms. It is possible that children with autism may experience fewer symptoms of OCD than adults but are at risk for developing them in adolescence or adulthood.

Etiology
Genetic Risk Factors

Autism is the most highly heritable of all mental disorders, exceeding that of schizophrenia or bipolar disorder. Twin and family studies have convincingly demonstrated that genetic factors play a role in disorders throughout the autism spectrum (for a review, see Lauritsen and Ewald 2001). Recent studies have shown that the concordance rates in monozygotic twins is between 60% and 90%. In those instances where the twins were discordant for autism, the nonautistic twin often had impairments in communication and social interaction as well as stereotypic behaviors, though not at a sufficient level to merit a diagnosis.

The likelihood that the parents of a child with autism will have another child with autism has been estimated at 3%–5%. This is likely to be an underestimation, since parents may elect to have no more children after the autistic child is diagnosed.

Family studies have found that what has been called the "broader phenotype"—encompassing impairments in communication and reciprocal social interaction and stereotypic behaviors milder than those required for the diagnosis of autism—is common in the siblings and parents of persons with autism. They may be isolated, show little spontaneous affection, be seen as odd, and have few friends. In contrast, intellectual abilities have generally not been shown to be impaired in the first-degree relatives, suggesting that subnormal intellectual functioning may not be strongly linked to autism per se—that is, the genetic factors influencing subnormal intellectual functioning in autism may differ from those in nonautistic persons with subnormal intellectual functioning.

The past two decades have seen a burgeoning interest in identifying what gene abnormalities might lead to susceptibility to develop autism. Results were negative for fragile X syndrome, tuberous sclerosis, Williams syndrome, and other rare disorders where symptoms of autism may occasionally be seen. Multiple consortiums of research investigators have pursued molecular genetic studies (Lauritsen and Ewald 2001). There were few significant findings, and those were not replicated. One recent linkage study (Autism Genome Project Consortium et al. 2007) has sought to overcome previous shortcomings in genetic research with autistic subjects. Investigators used Affymetrix 10K single-nucleotide polymorphism (SNP) arrays to study 1,168 multiplex families. Linkage and copy-number variation analyses implicated an abnormality at chromosome 11p12-p13, highlighting glutamate-related genes as promising candidates for contributing to ASDs.

A study by Weiss et al. (2008) of 751 multiplex families recruited by the Autistic Genetic Resource Exchange (AGRE) sought to identify copy-number variants that could influence susceptibility to autism. Copy-number variants are either deletions or duplications of genetic material that can exist at some point on a chromosome. Control subjects were all parents of the multiplex families as well as 2,814 individuals with bipolar disorder. A region on chromosome 16p11.2 carried a deletion in five children (four boys and one girl). These were de novo deletions, not found in their parents, but three subjects in the bipolar control group were also found to have the deletion. There was also a reciprocal duplication of the 593-kb deleted segment in seven children from three families. The duplication was inherited in two families. The findings were replicated in two additional cohorts of autistic children and their parents: 512 children from Children's Hospital in Boston, and 299 subjects with ASD recruited by DeCode Genetics in Iceland. Suitable controls were also studied at each site. Five 593-kb deletions at 16p11.2 (all in boys) were found in the sample of children from Boston Children's Hospital. One was inherited from a mother who had mild mental retardation; the others were de novo. Four duplications were identified in the autistic group, and no deletions or duplications in the control group. Three subjects in the DeCode group had the deletion; none had the duplication. Among the 18,234 subjects in the DeCode control group, two had the deletion and five had the duplication. Deletions or duplications were found in 1% of the subjects with autism. This is small, but the finding lends hope that future genetic research, using this or other novel techniques, may begin to be productive.

Neurobiological Factors

Since the late 1960s, investigators have been pursuing a myriad of neurobiological studies of persons with autism (see DiCicco-Bloom et al. 2006 for an overview). These "fishing expeditions" have for the most part not been successful. Lately there have been some very promising new developments in studies based on the normative neurobiology of facial recognition and of the possible circuitry of what has been termed the "social brain network." The relevance of facial recognition as a probe to understand brain function in autism has been given its impetus by studies of the differences in eye tracking of social scenes by autistic as compared to control subjects (Klin et al. 2002). While viewing social scenes, visual fixations on four regions were coded: mouth, eyes, body, and objects. Significant between-group differences in autistic versus control subjects were obtained for all four regions. The best predictor of autism was reduced eye region fixation time. Fixation on mouths and objects was significantly correlated with social functioning: increased focus on mouths predicted better social adjustment and less autistic social impairment, whereas more time on objects predicted the opposite relationship. It was concluded that fixation times on mouths and objects but not on eyes are strong predictors of a lack of social competence.

Previous work in neurotypical subjects had demonstrated that facial recognition activates the fusiform gyrus (more specifically the fusiform face area [FFA]), and it does so in a more pronounced way on the right as compared to the left side of the brain. This observation has led to a number of studies of the fusiform gyrus and FFA activation to facial expression in persons with autism (Pierce et al. 2001). Using functional magnetic resonance imaging (fMRI), Pierce et al. (2001) compared brain responses in autistic subjects with those in control subjects during a face perception task. Control subjects activated several brain regions (fusiform gyrus, inferior temporal gyrus, middle temporal gyrus, and amygdala) in a fairly uniform way. In contrast, although autistic subjects could perform the task, they activated brain areas markedly different from those activated in the control subjects. The activated areas differed among the autistic subjects themselves. This does not mean that the fusiform gyrus and associated FFA are congenitally abnormal in autism. As Schultz et al. (2003) point out, these areas of the brain are quite plastic and can be molded by early experience. Inadequate attention to faces during critical periods of development should affect the maturation of these areas and lead to underreactivity of the FFA during face perception.

Social neuroscience has recently used ingenious methods to study social cognitive processes (Cacioppo et al. 2006). Schultz et al. (2003) describe one of these, the social attribution task, which has recently been adapted for fMRI studies. Subjects view short movies of interacting geometric shapes. Humans find that these activities evoke strong social responses, leading to interpretations such as: the circles are fighting the squares, these triangles are hiding from the squares. Using this technique it has been possible to begin mapping the social neural network in humans, which may in the future lead to studies of the activity of social neural nets in autism.

As originally observed by Kanner (1943), there is a highly replicated finding that many autistic persons have increased head circumference. In fact, there is evidence that growth in head circumference accelerates and decelerates over time (Courchesne et al. 2003). Compared with normative data of healthy infants, birth head circumference in infants with ASD was significantly smaller ($P<0.001$); after birth, head circumference increased 1.67 SDs and mean head circumference was at the 84th percentile by ages 6–14 months. Only 6% of the healthy infants in the longitudinal data showed accelerated head circumference growth trajectories (>2.0 SDs) from birth to 6–14 months; 59% of infants with autistic disorder showed these accelerated growth trajectories. They concluded that the clinical

onset of autism appears to be preceded by two phases of brain growth abnormality: a smaller than typical head size at birth and a sudden and excessive increase in head size between 1–2 months and 6–14 months. There is as yet no explanation for this phenomenon.

Psychological Theories
Theory of Mind

This concept originally began many years ago in nonhuman primate research with the question: Does one chimpanzee understand that another chimpanzee has a mind different than his own, capable of having different thoughts and intentions? The answer, for chimps, appears largely to be no. The question was then raised in regard to persons with autism. Numerous studies using a "false belief" paradigm have reported that autistic children may fail the task but that less socially handicapped autistic persons will not. The latter finding may be due to the tasks being relatively easy to solve. While it has been useful in making specific predictions about the impairments in socialization, imagination, and communication shown by people with autism, it does not provide an explanation of why this might be so.

Folk Psychology Versus Folk Physics

A concept developed by Simon Baron-Cohen (Baron-Cohen et al. 2001) postulates that based on our evolutionary history, we have evolved two neurocognitive adaptations. One is "folk psychology," for inferring social causality, understanding others' intentions, and predicting their social responses. The other is "folk physics," for inferring physical causality and for understanding and being fascinated with factual information (lineages of dinosaurs, the solar system). Baron-Cohen et al. (2001) have postulated that each adaptation is under genetic control. It has been amply demonstrated that people with Asperger's disorder can have very good "folk physics" skills and very poor "folk psychology" skills. The concept may be helpful as an organizing principal to understand behaviors seen in verbal autistic persons with good intellectual skills. It is possible that genetic and neurobiological research will someday provide a framework for expanding our understanding of these concepts.

Executive Function Deficits in Autism

Executive function is a term used to describe a set of mental processes that helps us connect past experience with present action. Executive function is called into action when a person performs such activities as planning, organizing, strategizing, and paying attention to and remembering details. People with executive functioning problems may also show weakness with working memory, which is needed to guide one's actions. There have been many studies that have documented that persons with autism have deficits in the various components of executive functioning (Pennington and Ozonoff 1996); however, such deficits (differing perhaps in degree and profile) have also been reported in many other psychiatric disorders, including schizophrenia. The concept needs to be refined and studied in greater detail in normal populations before it can be fruitfully applied to understanding the manifestations of various mental illnesses.

Parental Age

Two studies suggest that maternal and paternal age may influence the likelihood that offspring will develop ASD. In a study done in Israel (Reichenberg et al. 2006), there was a significant monotonic association between advancing paternal age and risk of ASD. Offspring of men 40 years or older were 5.75 times ($P<0.001$) more likely to have ASD compared with offspring of men younger than 30 years. Advancing maternal age showed no association with ASD after adjusting for paternal age. A second study (Croen et al. 2007) found risk of ASDs increased significantly with each 10-year increase in maternal age and paternal age. Adjusted relative risks for both maternal and paternal age were elevated for children with autistic disorder and for children with Asperger's disorder or PDD-NOS. Although neither of the above studies used standardized diagnostic instruments, the large sample sizes and the systematic and comprehensive way in which data were gathered lend some credence to the results. Neither study addressed the question of whether late marriage played a role in determining the outcome. Men or women who themselves might have Asperger's disorder, or the wider variant of autism disorder, might marry later because of their social limitations or overall "oddity." Such individuals would be at greater risk of having a child with ASD than would other parents in the cohort.

Treatment
General Principles

This section will focus on those topics most relevant to child psychiatrists, child psychologists, pediatricians, and family practitioners. Because persons on the autism spectrum can be affected with many diverse behavioral, cognitive, and emotional difficulties, treatment must be both broad and tailored to the needs of each person. The initial evaluation should provide information not only about the specific symptoms of autism but also about the person's level of intellectual functioning; basic vocabulary and grammar skills; fine and gross motor skills; the presence of hypersensitivity to auditory, tactile, or visual sensory input; and the presence of other psychiatric diagnoses, in particular anxiety disorder and symptoms of attention-deficit disorder with or without hyperactivity (DSM-IV does not allow a diagnosis of ADHD in the presence of a PDD). A treatment plan must be developed that addresses that particular person's needs. Other specialists must be consulted by the family: speech pathologists, occupational and recreational therapists, behavioral specialists with expertise in autism, a sleep medicine specialist for children with serious sleep problems, and special education teachers who can design a suitable curriculum and who know how to deal with the specific problems that may interfere with the child's learning in school. Autistic persons may not understand that if they follow the teacher's instruction that the teacher will be pleased, they may not know why "fitting in" to the school routines is important, and they may, of course, have moderate to severe intellectual handicap as well.

And are such resources available? The National Academy of Sciences funded a project of the National Research Council to study this question (National Academy of Sciences 2001). In their report, the committee members recommended that educational services begin as soon as a child is suspected of having an ASD. These services should include a "minimum of 25 hours a week, 12 months a year, in which the child is engaged in systematically planned and developmentally appropriate educational activity toward identified objectives" (p. 6). They recommended that interventions should focus on education in six areas: 1) functional spontaneous communication, 2) social skills, 3) play skills, 4) cognitive development taught in a natural setting to facilitate generalization, 5) reduction of problem behaviors, and 6) functional academic skills.

In an interview with the *New York Times* shortly after the report was published, Catherine Lord, the chair of the committee, stated, "Fewer than 10% of children are getting the recommended level of therapy. Almost everywhere schools will say kids are getting services, but what they are getting varies enormously" (New York Times, February 8, 2002). While we have effective methods of treatment, we lack the public (federal and state government) interest to train therapists (including teachers and parents) and fund the adequate delivery of the services to all children with developmental disabilities, from infancy to adulthood.

Behavioral Interventions

Interventions can be classified along several dimensions. Does the therapist determine what the child should learn (such as a teacher in the classroom who has a specific curriculum), or does the therapist encourage the child to choose the activity and determine how the interaction will proceed? In severely autistic children, who may not be motivated to attend to others, the therapist has to identify what the child enjoys, join in the activity, and by varying the parameters of the activity, hope to kindle a nascent relationship with the child. Is the intervention given 1:1, or is it in a group setting, such as a classroom or a social coaching group? For very handicapped children, a one-on-one engagement, even in the classroom, may be necessary at times. And lastly, Are the parents involved, either as cotherapists or as primary therapists in their own right, guided by a consultant on a weekly or biweekly basis?

A number of specific therapies are outlined below. Many have overlapping approaches, and not all are suitable for all children, given the large variability among autistic persons in severity of autistic symptoms and differences in intellectual ability and use of language.

Applied Behavior Analysis

Applied Behavior Analysis (ABA) is one of the oldest of the behavioral therapies, having been developed by Lovaas at UCLA in the 1970s. As its use expanded, it has been adapted by many therapists to suit children with different needs. ABA, in a form that came to be called Discrete Trial Training, relied on the principles of operant conditioning, which comprise the presentation of a stimulus (a question or a command) to evoke a specific response. If necessary, physical prompts would be given to encourage the response. Reinforcers (such as small candies or other desired objects) were provided as a reward. In some versions of ABA, incorrect responses might be followed by an aversive stimulus, such as a verbal reprimand. An innovative feature of ABA was that therapists worked in the home with the parents as cotherapists. As many as 35 hours a week of ABA therapy has been recommended by some

of its proponents. A caveat: Therapists should be well versed in normal development so that they can choose goals that are within the range of a child's developmental capabilities. ABA is one of the few therapies that has had some empirical validation (McEachin et al. 1993). After intensive behavioral intervention, an experimental group of 19 preschool-age children with autism achieved less restrictive school placements and higher measured IQs than did an age-matched control group of 19 similar children. Follow-up study of the subjects at 11.5 years of age showed that the experimental group preserved its gains over the control group. Critics have contended that for some children, the pure Discrete Trial Training method is not effective. A subsequent ABA approach, Pivotal Response Training, was developed by Koegel (Koegel et al. 2001), with the goal of finding ways to the child's motivation, responsiveness to multiple cues, engagement in self-management, and self-initiation of social interactions that were identified as pivotal factors in determining the success of behavioral interventions. To increase motivation, the child may be encouraged to incorporate self-chosen materials, activities, topics, and toys into the learning situation. Although the clinician follows the child's lead, the environment remains structured, such that the target behaviors are incorporated into the activities, while maintaining the child's attention and decreasing the likelihood that the child will engage in disruptive behavior. Self-management is increased by teaching individuals to discriminate between appropriate and inappropriate behavior. The child is encouraged to actively record how many correct responses he makes and to administer self-rewards. Similar approaches are used to help the child learn other pivotal factors, which in turn enhance learning of social skills. Studies of Pivotal Response Training have shown that it can be successful in enhancing adaptive behaviors in persons with autism.

Floor Time

Developed by Greenspan and Wieder (1998), floor time has been renamed as the Developmental, Individual-Difference (DIR) approach to intervention. Like Pivotal Response Training, DIR is child centered. The goal of DIR is to build increasingly larger "circles of interaction" between the therapist and the child in a developmentally appropriate way. Emphasis is on two-way interactions that are gratifying to the child, working up to more sophisticated symbolic interactions. The approach consists of three parts: 1) parents do "floor time" with their child, creating experiences that promote mastery of the milestones in social development; 2) other therapists and educators work with the child, using techniques informed by floor time to deal with the child's specific challenges and to facilitate development; and 3) parents work to improve their own responses and styles of relating with regard to the social milestones to create a family pattern that supports emotional and intellectual growth in all family members. A national network of therapists expert in floor time has been developed to work with parents in implementing DIR. Although the therapy seems reasonable, no empirical studies with control groups have been published. This same criticism could be made for several other behavioral treatments.

Relationship Development Intervention

Relationship Development Intervention (RDI) is a parent-based, cognitive-developmental approach, in which primary caregivers are trained to provide daily opportunities for successful functioning in increasingly challenging dynamic systems. It targets behaviors that follow the developmental model of social communication, starting with affective reciprocity and joint attention and culminating in theory of mind and the acquisition of intuitive social knowledge (social mentation). The exercises are designed to catch and hold the child's attention. Parents learn the basics of the treatment at 4-day workshops with Steven Gutstein, the developer of RDI. Regional consultants act as local advisors to the parents. A small outcome study (Gutstein et al. 2007) without control groups but with good diagnostic and measurement instruments indicated that the method has promise. (For more information, visit the Web site at: www.RDIconnect.com.)

Social Communication, Emotional Regulation, and Transactional Support Treatment

Developed by Barry Prizant and Amy Wetherby, Social Communication, Emotional Regulation and Transactional Support Treatment (SCERTS) is a child-centered multidisciplinary approach that focuses on the development of the capacity to regulate attention, arousal, and emotional state. Transactional activities are designed and implemented across settings to foster more successful interpersonal interactions and relationships at home, in the school, and in the community. The SCERTS model includes a well-coordinated assessment process that helps a team measure the child's progress and determine the necessary supports

to be used by the child's social partners (educators, peers, and family members). (For more information, visit the Web site at: www.barryprizant.com.)

Picture Exchange Communication System

Picture Exchange Communication System is a modified ABA program designed for early nonverbal symbolic communication. It is not designed to teach speech, although the latter is indirectly encouraged. Using a trainer and a facilitator (who models the target behaviors for the child) the child is led to understand that requests for objects (using picture cards) can lead to one's receiving the object as a reward. Later iterations of the exercises are designed to teach the child to use cards to express more elaborated requests and to express thanks for the rewards. The program is popular in classrooms for nonverbal autistic children. (For more information, visit the Web site at: www.pecs.com.)

Social Stories

Developed by teacher Carol Gray, a Social Story describes a situation, skill, or concept in terms of relevant social cues, perspectives, and common responses in a specifically defined style and format. The goal of a Social Story is to share accurate social information in a patient and reassuring manner that is easily understood by its audience. Half of all Social Stories developed should affirm something that an individual does well. Although the goal of a Social Story should never be to solely change the individual's behavior, that individual's improved understanding of events and expectations may lead to more effective responses. Social Stories may be used with children, adolescents, and adults. (For more information, visit the Web site at: www.thegraycenter.org.)

Sensory Integration Therapy

Developed by Jean Ayres many years ago, Sensory Integration Therapy is a popular treatment with occupational and recreational therapists. Although Ayres postulated a complex neurobiological hypothesis as rationale for the therapy, few accept this highly speculative model as accurate. Sensory Integration Therapy is a child-centered approach that provides the child with a variety of controlled sensory experiences. Because it usually entails one-on-one interaction, there is an opportunity to foster relationship building. It may be useful for lessening oversensitivity to auditory and tactile stimuli and for improving fine and gross motor skills. There have been no controlled studies of its effectiveness.

Psychopharmacological Treatment

A substantial body of literature describes trials of psychopharmacological agents in autism. Unfortunately, much of it consists of small open trials, some done for a brief period of time, with little long-term follow-up (Broadstock et al. 2007). Many studies lacked adequate diagnostic or symptom measurement instruments. A listing of most salient drug trials of antipsychotic drugs in autism is summarized in Chapter 49, "Antipsychotic Medications," Table 49–6 and related text. No medications have been found effective in ameliorating the social, language, or cognitive deficits in autism. Medications that reduce anxiety may lead to a slight increase in social spontaneity, but this is likely to be due to the fact that anxious individuals tend to withdraw from social interaction. There is evidence, some from placebo-controlled studies, that the selective serotonin reuptake inhibitors and the atypical antipsychotics can be effective in reducing aggression, temper outbursts, and self-injurious behavior. They can also reduce stereotyped behaviors. A reduction in these behaviors can allow an autistic person to participate more fully in treatment, which can lead to better adaptation and learning. To date, the methodologically best investigation has been the Research Unit in Pediatric Psychopharmacology study of risperidone treatment of autism (McDougle et al. 2005). The study comprised an 8-week double-blind, placebo-controlled trial ($N=101$) and a 16-week open-label continuation study ($N=63$) of risperidone for children and adolescents with autism. Gold standard instruments were used throughout. Risperidone resulted in signif-icantly greater reductions in scores on the Children's Yale-Brown Obsessive Compulsive Scale and Vineland Maladaptive Behavior domain. This pattern of treatment response was maintained for 6 months. The investigators concluded that risperidone led to significant improvements in the restricted, repetitive, and stereotyped patterns of behavior, interests, and activities of autistic children but did not significantly change their deficits in social interaction and communication. Although in the past, stimulant medications were believed to be contraindicated in persons with autism, there is some evidence that symptoms of inattention that interfere with learning may be improved with stimulant medication.

Prognosis

Some young children with a diagnosis of autism can show a surprising increase in language and intellectual level by ages 6–10 years (Harris et al. 1991; Sigman et al. 1999). Some will also develop better affective reciprocity and joint attention as they mature. But even in the relatively lesser handicapped persons with Asperger's disorder, the impaired ability to engage in the give-and-take of social interactions and to understand and respond to the social signals of others remains a serious problem. There comes a time, especially in adolescence, when it may be important to not focus solely on what the person cannot do but on the skills in which the child excels. I have heard heart-warming stories of computer gurus who had Asperger's disorder who found a place in Internet companies, where they became the identified expert at some obscure but quite profitable line of work. As one mother told me: "He's famous now. He's still socially awkward, but now people don't seem to care about that. He even has a girlfriend."

Summary Points

- Children come into the world with a behavioral propensity to interact socially with others and to learn complex social skills and knowledge, even before they learn language. Children with autism fail to learn such skills and knowledge.

- DSM-IV is a categorical system of diagnosis. It appears, however, that the various categories of disorder listed under pervasive developmental disorders may be better conceived as a spectrum of social communication skills and knowledge, perhaps as an extreme end of the normal distribution of such skills in the general population.

- Using available screening instruments, autism may be suspected at least as early as 18 months of age. The screening can be carried out in the office of most pediatricians or family practitioners.

- There is solid epidemiological evidence that approximately 1 in 200 persons have a disorder on the autism spectrum. This is higher than was described three decades ago. Broader diagnostic criteria and better public knowledge about autism may explain this increase.

- Autism is not caused by the measles-mumps-rubella vaccine nor by thimerosal, the vaccine preservative.

- The most frequent comorbid disorders in autism are anxiety disorders, symptoms of attention-deficit disorder with or without hyperactivity, and to a lesser extent, obsessive-compulsive disorder.

- Genetic factors play an important role in autism, more than in any other psychiatric disorder studied so far. The nature of the genetic factors are unknown, but they are likely to be numerous and to interact with each other and with as-yet-unknown environmental factors.

- We possess a number of reasonable psychosocial treatments, but we lack the public will to demand that teachers and therapists be trained and that their work be financially supported. Fewer than 10% of persons on the autism spectrum are receiving adequate therapy.

- Certain medications, primarily selective serotonin reuptake inhibitors and atypical antipsychotics, have shown promise in alleviating aggressive outbursts, repetitive and stereotyped behaviors, and self-injurious behaviors in persons with autism. No medication has been shown to be effective in improving the social, language, or cognitive deficits in autism.

- It is important to focus on what persons with autism spectrum disorders do well, rather than solely on their impairments. Playing to their strengths may enhance the likelihood that they will find some satisfaction in life.

References

American Psychiatric Association: Diagnostic and Statistical Manual of Mental Disorders, 3rd Edition. Washington, DC, American Psychiatric Association, 1980

American Psychiatric Association: Diagnostic and Statistical Manual of Mental Disorders, 4th Edition. Washington, DC, American Psychiatric Association, 1994

American Psychiatric Association: Diagnostic and Statistical Manual of Mental Disorders, 4th Edition, Text Revision. Washington, DC, American Psychiatric Association, 2000

Asperger H: "Autistic psychopathology" in childhood (1944), in Autism and Asperger Syndrome. Edited by Frith U. Cambridge, UK, Cambridge University Press, 1991, pp 37–92

Autism Genome Project Consortium, Szatmari P, Paterson AD, et al: Mapping autism risk loci using genetic linkage and chromosomal rearrangements. Nat Genet 39:319–328, 2007

Baird G, Charman T, Baron-Cohen S, et al: A screening instrument for autism at 18 months of age: a six-year follow-up study. J Am Acad Child Adolesc Psychiatry 39:694–702, 2000

Baranek GT: Autism during infancy: a retrospective video analysis of sensory-motor and social behaviors at 9–12 months of age. J Autism Dev Disord 29:213–224, 1999

Baron-Cohen S, Allen J, Gillberg C: Can autism be detected at 18 months? The needle, the haystack, and the CHAT. Br J Psychiatry 161:839–843, 1992

Baron-Cohen S, Wheelwright S, Spong A, et al: Studies of theory of mind: are intuitive physics and intuitive psychology independent? Journal of Developmental and Learning Disorders 5:47–78, 2001

Berument SK, Rutter M, Lord C, et al: Autism Screening Questionnaire: diagnostic validity. Br J Psychiatry 175:444–451, 1999

Beyer KS, Blasi F, Bacchelli E, et al: Mutation analysis of the coding sequence of the MECP2 gene in infantile autism. Hum Genet 111:305–309, 2002

Bolton PF, Park RJ, Higgins JN, et al: Neuroepileptic determinants of autism spectrum disorders in tuberous sclerosis complex. Brain 125:1247–1255, 2002

Broadstock M, Doughty C, Eggleston M: Systematic review of the effectiveness of pharmacological treatments for adolescents and adults with autism spectrum disorder. Autism 11:335–348, 2007

Cacioppo JT, Visser PS, Pickett CL, et al: Social Neuroscience: People Thinking About Thinking People. Cambridge, MA, MIT Press, 2006

Carter AS, Volkmar FR, Sparrow SS, et al: The Vineland Adaptive Behavior Scales: supplementary norms for individuals with autism. J Autism Dev Disord 28:287–302, 1998

Chakrabarti S, Fombonne E: Pervasive developmental disorders in preschool children (comments). JAMA 285: 3093–3099, 2001

Constantino JN, Todd RD: Autistic traits in the general population: a twin study. Arch Gen Psychiatry 60:524–530, 2003

Constantino JN, Przybeck T, Friesen D, et al: Reciprocal social behavior in children with and without pervasive developmental disorders. J Dev Behav Pediatr 21:2–11, 2000

Courchesne E, Carper R, Akshoomoff N: Evidence of brain overgrowth in the first year of life in autism (comment). JAMA 290:337–344, 2003

Croen LA, Najjar DV, Fireman B, et al: Maternal and paternal age and risk of autism spectrum disorders. Arch Pediatr Adolesc Med 161:334–340, 2007

Curatolo P, Porfirio MC, Manzi B, et al: Autism in tuberous sclerosis. Eur J Paediatr Neurol 8:327–332, 2004

DiCicco-Bloom E, Lord C, Zwaigenbaum L, et al: The developmental neurobiology of autism spectrum disorder. J Neurosci 26:6987–6906, 2006

Farzin F, Perry H, Hessl D, et al: Autism spectrum disorders and attention-deficit/hyperactivity disorder in boys with fragile X permutation. J Dev Behav Pediatr 27(suppl): S137–S144, 2006

Feinstein C, Reiss AL: Autism: the point of view from fragile X studies. J Autism Dev Disord 28:393–405, 1998

Fombonne E: Prevalence of childhood disintegrative disorder. Autism 6:149–157, 2002

Fombonne E, Du MC, Cans C, et al: Autism and associated medical disorders in a French epidemiological survey. J Am Acad Child Adolesc Psychiatry 36:1561–1569, 1997

Greenspan SI, Wieder S: The Child With Special Needs. New York, Pereus Books, 1998

Gutierrez GC, Smalley SL, Tanguay PE: Autism in tuberous sclerosis complex. J Autism Dev Disord 28:97–103, 1998

Gutstein SE, Burgess AF, Montfort K: Evaluation of the Relationship Development Intervention Program. Autism 11:397–411, 2007

Harris SL, Handleman JS, Gordon R, et al: Changes in cognitive and language functioning of preschool children with autism. J Autism Dev Disord 21:281–290, 1991

Heller T: Über dementia infantalis (1930), in Modern Perspectives in International Child Psychiatry. Edited by Howells JG. Edinburgh, Oliver & Boyd, 1969

Hendry CN: Childhood disintegrative disorder: should it be considered a distinct diagnosis? Clin Psychol Rev 20:77–90, 2000

Hoekstra RA, Bartels M, Verweij CJ, et al: Heritability of autistic traits in the general population. Arch Pediatr Adolesc Med 161:372–377, 2007

Honda H, Shimizu Y, Misumi K, et al: Cumulative incidence and prevalence of childhood autism in children in Japan (comments). Br J Psychiatry 169:228–235, 1996

Huppke P, Maier EM, Warnke A, et al: Very mild cases of Rett syndrome with skewed X inactivation. J Med Genet 43:814–816, 2006

Kanner L: Autistic disturbances of affective contact. Nerv Child 2:217–250, 1943

Kasari C, Sigman M, Mundy P, et al: Affective sharing in the context of joint attention interactions of normal, autistic, and mentally retarded children. J Autism Dev Disord 20:87–100, 1990

Klin A, Jones W, Schultz R, et al: Visual fixation patterns during viewing of naturalistic social situations as predictors of social competence in individuals with autism. Arch Gen Psychiatry 59:809–816, 2002

Koegel RL, Koegel LK, McNerney EK: Pivotal areas in intervention for autism. J Clin Child Psychol 30:19–32, 2001

Krug DA, Arick JR, Almond PG: Behavior checklist for identifying severely handicapped individuals with high levels of autistic behavior. J Child Psychol Psychiatry 21: 221–229, 1980

Landau WM, Kleffner FR: Syndrome of acquired aphasia with convulsive disorder. Neurology 7:523–530, 1957

Lauritsen M, Ewald H: The genetics of autism. Acta Psychiatr Scand 103:411–427, 2001

Loesch DZ, Bui QM, Dissanayake C: Molecular and cognitive predictors of the continuum of autistic behaviours in fragile X. Neurosci Biobehav Rev 31:315–326, 2007

Lord C, Rutter M, Le Couteur A: Autism Diagnostic Interview—Revised: a revised version of a diagnostic interview for caregivers of individuals with possible pervasive developmental disorders. J Autism Dev Disord 24:659–685, 1994

Lord C, Risi S, Lambrecht L, et al: The Autism Diagnostic Observation Schedule—Generic: a standard measure of social and communication deficits associated with the spectrum of autism. J Autism Dev Disord 30:205–223, 2000

Lotter V: Epidemiology of autistic conditions in young children, 1: prevalence. Soc Psychiatry 1:124–137, 1966

Macintosh KE, Dissanayake C: Annotation: the similarities and differences between autistic disorder and Asperger's disorder: a review of the empirical evidence. J Child Psychol Psychiatry 45:421–434, 2004

Madsen KM, Vestergard M: MMR vaccination and autism. Drug Saf 27:831–840, 2004

Mayes SD, Calhoun SL, Crites DI: Does DSM-IV Asperger's disorder exist? J Abnorm Child Psychol 29:263–271, 2001

McDougle CJ, Kresch LE, Goodman WK, et al: A case-controlled study of repetitive thoughts and behavior in adults with autistic disorder and obsessive-compulsive disorder. Am J Psychiatry 152:772–777, 1995

McDougle CJ, Scahill L, Aman MG, et al: Risperidone for the core symptom domains of autism: results from the study by the autism network of the research units on pediatric psychopharmacology (comment). Am J Psychiatry 162:1142–1148, 2005

McEachin JJ, Smith T, Lovaas OI: Long-term outcome for children with autism who received early intensive behavioral treatment. Am J Ment Retard 97:359–372, 1993

Mouridsen SE: The Landau-Kleffner syndrome: a review. Eur J Child Adolesc Psychiatry 4:223–228, 1995

Mundy P: Joint attention and social-emotional approach behavior in children with autism. Dev Psychopathol 7:63–82, 1995

Mundy P, Crowson M: Joint attention and early social communication: implications for research on intervention with autism. J Autism Dev Disord 27:653–676, 1997

National Academy of Sciences: Educating Children With Autism. Washington, DC, National Academy Press, 2001

Offit PA: Autism's False Prophets. New York, Columbia University Press, 2008

Osterling J, Dawson G: Early recognition of children with autism: a study of first birthday home videotapes. J Autism Dev Disord 24:247–257, 1994

Pennington BF, Ozonoff S: Executive functions and developmental psychopathology. J Child Psychol Psychiatry 37:51–87, 1996

Pierce K, Muller RA, Ambrose J, et al: Face processing occurs outside the fusiform "face area" in autism: evidence from functional MRI. Brain 124:2059–2073, 2001

Posserud MB, Lundervold AJ, Gillberg C: Autistic features in a total population of 7–9-year-old children assessed by the ASSQ (Autism Spectrum Screening Questionnaire). J Child Psychol Psychiatry 47:167–175, 2006

Reichenberg A, Gross R, Weiser M, et al: Advancing paternal age and autism. Arch Gen Psychiatry 63:1026–1032, 2006

Risi S, Lord C, Gotham K, et al: Combining information from multiple sources in the diagnosis of autism spectrum disorders. J Am Acad Child Adolesc Psychiatry 45:1094–1103, 2006

Robins DL, Fein D, Barton ML, et al: The Modified Checklist for Autism in Toddlers: an initial study investigating the early detection of autism and pervasive developmental disorders (comments). J Autism Dev Disord 31:131–144, 2001

Rogers SJ, Wehner DE, Hagerman R: The behavioral phenotype in fragile X: symptom of autism in very young children with fragile X syndrome, idiopathic autism, and other developmental disorders. J Dev Behav Pediatr 22:409–417, 2001

Russell AJ, Mataix-Cols D, Anson M, et al: Obsessions and compulsions in Asperger syndrome and high-functioning autism. Br J Psychiatry 186:525–528, 2005

Rutter M: Incidence of autism spectrum disorders: changes over time and their meaning. Acta Paediatr 94:2–15, 2005

Schopler E, Reichler R, Renner BR: The Childhood Autism Rating Scale (CARS). Los Angeles, CA, Western Psychological Services, 1988

Schultz RT, Grelotti DJ, Klin A, et al: The role of the fusiform face area in social cognition: implications for the pathobiology of autism. Philos Trans R Soc Lond B Biol Sci 358:415–427, 2003

Sigman M: The Emanuel Miller Memorial Lecture 1997: change and continuity in the development of children with autism. J Child Psychol Psychiatry 39:817–827, 1998

Sigman M, Ruskin E, Arbeile S, et al: Continuity and change in the social competence of children with autism, Down syndrome, and developmental delays (comments). J Child Psychol Psychiatry 64:1–114, 1999

Simonoff E, Pickles A, Charman T, et al: Psychiatric disorders in children with autism spectrum disorders: prevalence, comorbidity, and associated factors in a population-derived sample. J Am Acad Child Adolesc Psychiatry 47:921–928, 2008

Skuse D, Warrington R, Bishop D, et al: The Developmental Dimensional and Diagnostic Interview (3di): a novel computerized assessment for autism spectrum disorders. J Am Acad Child Adolesc Psychiatry 43:548–558, 2004

Towbin KE, Dykens EM, Pearson GS, et al: Conceptualizing "borderline syndrome of childhood" and "childhood schizophrenia" as a developmental disorder. J Am Acad Child Adolesc Psychiatry 32:775–782, 1993

Trevarthen C, Aitken KJ: Infant intersubjectivity: research, theory, and clinical applications. J Child Psychol Psychiatry 42:3–48, 2001

Tuchman R: Autism. Neurol Clin 21:915–932, 2003

Van der Gaag RJ, Buitelaar J, Van den Ban E, et al: A controlled multivariate chart review of multiple complex developmental disorder. J Am Acad Child Adolesc Psychiatry 34:1096–1106, 1995

Volkmar FR, Cohen DJ: Disintegrative disorder or "late onset" autism. J Child Psychol Psychiatry 30:717–724, 1989

Volkmar FR, Carter A, Sparrow SS, et al: Quantifying social development in autism. J Am Acad Child Adolesc Psychiatry 32:627–632, 1993

Wakefield AJ, Murch SH, Anthony A, et al: Ileal-lymphoid-nodular hyperplasia, nonspecific colitis, and pervasive developmental disorder in children (comments). Lancet 351:637–641, 1998

Wassink TH, Piven J, Patil SR: Chromosomal abnormalities in a clinic sample of individuals with autistic disorder. Psychiatr Genet 11:57–63, 2001

Weiss LA, Shen Y, Korn JM, et al: Association between microdeletion and microduplication at 16p11.2 and autism (comment). N Engl J Med 358:667–675, 2008

Wiznitzer M: Autism and tuberous sclerosis. J Child Neurol 19:675–679, 2004

World Health Organization: International Statistical Classification of Diseases and Related Health Problems, 10th Revision. Geneva, Switzerland, World Health Organization, 1992

Yeargin-Allsopp M, Rice C, Karapurkar T, et al: Prevalence of autism in a US metropolitan area (comment). JAMA 289:49–55, 2003

Chapter 14

Developmental Disorders of Learning, Communication, and Motor Skills

Karen Pierce, M.D.

Developmental learning, communication, and motor problems affect children throughout development, influencing their lives and personalities. These disorders have long-term implications in a child's emotional and regulatory development and affect their move into adulthood. Some of these disorders, when detected and treated early, can be remediated successfully. Others are chronic, and compensatory skills must be taught. All children should be screened and treated early to prevent long-term sequelae. Many children referred for psychiatric assessment have language impairments, processing deficits, or problem with cognition that for some of them remains unsuspected unless the clinician is thinking about cognition as well as psychiatric symptoms.

Children who struggle academically are subject to chronic stress. This chronic stress on the hypothalamic pituitary axis and the autonomic nervous system affects metabolism, cardiovascular, and immune system functioning, and even brain development (Kaufman et al. 2006). Recent meta-analyses on the prevalence of depression in children with learning disabilities show a higher than normal rate of depression (Sideridis 2006). Disruptive and aggressive behavior occurring in school may be the result of poor cognitive skills rather than a psychiatric disorder. Early detection of cognitive disabilities leads to smoother developmental progression and treatment.

In defining learning disability (LD) or communication disorders, the various categorical systems often do not agree or define the same disorder. DSM-IV

(American Psychiatric Association 1994) and its text revision, DSM-IV-TR (American Psychiatric Association 2000), describe these as Axis I disorders. The federal government definition that is used by classroom teachers classifies these disorders somewhat differently. However, processing styles (i.e., a visual or a verbal strength) impact behavior and learning and may not make the threshold to diagnosis as a formal learning disorder but may impact functioning profoundly. Clinicians will need to define these disorders one way when using the DSM system but be prepared to adapt for educational recommendations. Knowledge of both sets of definitions is essential to advocate for and to give comprehensive care to the child patient.

Rarely do learning, communication, and motor disorders occur alone; rather, they co-occur with other learning and psychiatric problems. These disorders may or may not be apparent to the clinician when evaluating psychiatric diagnosis and maladaptive behavior. Since communication is the key to relationships and ultimately most adaptive functioning, clinicians must be alert to the possibility that there are neurocognitive deficits in this arena. As an example, if a child with an expressive language difficulty answers in one-word sentences or shakes his head, the clinician might mistake this shyness as mutism or even a serious thought disorder rather than a communication disorder. If a child routinely loses behavioral or emotional control during the school day, the clinician must determine what class is being taught during that time, since poor frustration tolerance may be related to a learning issue rather than a mood disorder. A child with poor handwriting secondary to poor fine motor control may get disruptive when writing is required. School subjects that can be difficult for the child, such as math or writing, may reveal poor visual processing. Both visuospatial and visual memory deficits can be silent learning issues that may manifest only as behavior problems. The clinician is urged to become familiar with these disorders and their effect on communication and behavior.

Learning Disorders

The specific LD category assumes that these are brain-based processes that interfere with learning. LDs are heterogeneous, persistent, and inherent to each individual. Learning disabilities were federally classified as "handicapping conditions" in the United States in the 1960s. Since then, the research into learning's origin and its treatment has blossomed. Special education

classrooms contain one-half of all students with LDs (U.S. Department of Education Office of Special Education and Rehabilitative Services 2002). The average expense to educate a student with a LD is $10,588 per year, 1.6 times the cost for a regular education student. Yet LDs are poorly understood and the definition is applied differently among schools, states, and on a federal level. Because LDs are both an unobservable construct and dimensional, definitions are ambiguous.

Why is an understanding of LD important? Forty percent of children with LDs drop out of school or enter the juvenile justice system (Lichtenstein and Blackorby 1995). As more children receive instruction in regular education classes with mainstreaming, the risk of psychiatric symptoms grows as a child faces frustration and limited mastery of academic material. Research in adult psychiatric illness demonstrates cognitive impairments in all of the major psychiatric disorders: schizophrenia (Cervellione et al. 2007; Schretlen 2007), bipolar disorder (Dickstein et al. 2007), anxiety disorders (Goldston et al. 2007), and the personality disorder clusters. Cognitive deficits appear to be an important determinant of functional outcomes (Bromley 2007). Euthymic adult bipolar patients perform significantly poorer than controls on measures of verbal learning and memory (Martinez-Aran et al. 2004). The link between reading disorder and attention-deficit/hyperactivity disorder (ADHD) is well established (Hinshaw 1992). White adolescents with reading problems were more likely to have substance use disorders than minority youth (Goldston et al. 2007). Most cognitive impairments start in childhood and create subtle issues in personality formation. Not all processing deficits meet the threshold of a diagnosed LD but may still affect development.

This section reviews the varying definitions of LD, the current federal guidelines, the DSM-IV LD diagnoses, and then, briefly, subthreshold processing deficits.

Definition

Perhaps the greatest obstacle in discussing LDs is that of definition. The lack of clarity has impeded recognition and treatment. Even with special education mandates from the federal government, the threshold for positive identification of LDs and definition and categories of special education vary from state to state, causing widely discrepant prevalence rates. By definition, in order to have an LD one must have normal intelligence, hearing, and vision. An aptitude-achievement discrepancy criterion was used initially but was found to be unsatisfactory at appropriately identifying children.

TABLE 14–1. Comparison of DSM-IV and federal categories of learning disability

DSM-IV-TR diagnosis	Federal categories
Reading disorder (315.00)	Basic reading skills
Reading disorder (315.00)	Reading fluency skills
Reading disorder (315.00)	Reading comprehension
Mathematics disorder (315.1)	Mathematics calculation
Mathematics disorder (315.1)	Mathematics problem solving
Disorder of written expression (315.2)	Written expression
Expressive language disorder (315.31)	Oral expression
Receptive language disorder (315.31)	Listening comprehension

LDs are a group of chronic, heterogeneous disorders that have a negative impact on learning, achievement, and self-esteem. Although there is a strong genetic component, some learning disabilities have environmental causes, such as prenatal exposure to drugs or alcohol, lead toxicity, and brain injury. Whatever the origin, early identification is essential.

In 2004, the Office of Special Education and Rehabilitative Services (through the Individuals with Disabilities Education Act [IDEA]) reauthorized the criteria for learning difficulties (for more information, see http://idea.ed.gov). If a child does not achieve adequately or meet state-approved, grade-level standards in one or more of the following areas listed below, then further intervention is needed. The basic standards are as follows:

- Basic reading skills
- Reading fluency skills
- Reading comprehension
- Mathematics calculation
- Mathematics problem solving
- Written expression
- Oral expression
- Listening comprehension

Since these are the categories as defined by federal mandates, they will be placed in **boldface** type as they are discussed below. As noted, these are very different definitions of LD from those in DSM-IV-TR (Table 14–1).

Identification of a Learning Disability

There are several ways to assess a disability depending on the theory of classification and local standards that are used.

In the past, a discrepancy model was used until the reauthorization of IDEA required a response-to-intervention definition. The most consistent procedure for identification was based on an aptitude-achievement discrepancy model. Achievement is a dimensional trait that has varying boundaries, depending on context and definition. When an LD diagnosis is based on a cutoff point of achievement, it can be arbitrary and doesn't account for measurement error.

Another classification, based on intra-individual differences in processing information, would use psychological tests that measure cognition. Categories such as poor phonological awareness or weak visual processing would result, but the relationship to education and achievement would not be clear. Though children have these learning weaknesses, the translation to the classroom can be problematic.

Types of evaluations, like neuropsychological or educational-psychological, provide different and more comprehensive data (see Chapter 11, "Psychological and Neuropsychological Testing"). It is important to assess a child's learning strengths in any evaluation, as these will be the resources that a child will use to help him through any areas of weakness. Astute clinicians can begin to look for possible neuropsychological patterns in the testing data as well as do some screening as part of their clinical exam. Often missed are struggling learners who did not meet criteria for an LD or other disabilities. With schools using an age-based assessment, clinicians must be ready to recommend further psychological testing if it is clinically indicated. Laboratory constructs of learning are not equivalent to cognitive skills and behaviors seen in the clinic.

The discrepancy model of diagnosing LDs changed with the new authorization of IDEA. When IDEA was finalized in 2006, states were mandated not to require the use of a model of a severe discrepancy between intellectual ability and achievement for the identification of students for the category of LD. Recommended is the use of a process-based evaluation of the child's response to scientific- and research-based intervention. This classroom-based evaluation may permit the use of alternative research-based procedures for determining whether a child has a specific LD. The new law added an exclusion for determining a learning need if a student is receiving poor instruction or has limited English proficiency.

The new special education law mandates screening all children by measuring the Response to Intervention (RTI; Fuchs et al. 2003). RTI is based on the dual-discrepancy model. The student must be both below the same-grade peers and have poor response to carefully planned and precisely delivered instruction. This requires all classroom teachers to develop benchmark- or curriculum-based measures (data norms) for the classroom, grade level, school, and district. If a skill deficit is noted, then an accountability plan is developed to intervene. The plan must describe the intervention, where it is being done, for how long, the people responsible, and the measurement of progress. These data are compared and shared with the team. Curriculum-based measures determine both the need and the ongoing progress (Fletcher et al. 2007, p. 64).

The goal of any evaluation would be early intervention to those at risk. Requesting an LD evaluation in the schools is no longer the first step; rather, the clinician asks how the child is functioning as related to his peers and the curricula and how he is responding to intervention. As in the DSM-IV system, an LD is diagnosed only when there is both a skill deficit and a resulting functional impairment. The definition of LD automatically excludes children with a visual, hearing, or motor disability; mental retardation; emotional disturbance; or limited English proficiency; or when cultural factors, environmental factors, or economic disadvantage are involved. The change in language that defines LD makes communication with schools harder, since as clinicians, we are taught to make a diagnosis first and then an intervention, but schools intervene when a student's performance lags before doing a comprehensive assessment.

In general, reading recognition and fluency are easily measured and highly correlated. Reading comprehension and mathematics are a bit more difficult to measure, since there are many brain processes that help performance in these areas. Written expression assessment is difficult, as what defines a disorder is not well established (Fletcher et al. 2007). Speech and language skills assessment is well researched, but higher-level language skills like pragmatics are just beginning to be researched.

Reading Disorder

The DSM-IV definition of **reading disorder** uses a broader classification system for the complicated pro-

cess often called "dyslexia." The prevalence of dyslexia has been estimated to be as high as 17.4% in the school-age population (Shaywitz 2003). Dyslexia is the most common LD and the most common diagnosis of children receiving special education services. With more sophisticated testing, no longer is there a greater prevalence of dyslexia in boys (Rutter et al. 2004). The proportions of sex differences in developmental reading disability are estimated to be at about 1.5–2.1 in favor of males.

According to DSM-IV, any reading difficulty would be labeled under reading disorder not otherwise specified because our diagnostic system does not specify the different reading processes that impair reading. Although this label is helpful for psychiatric diagnosis, it lends little specificity and guidance for the school in order to remediate a child's reading skills. For the clinician, knowing the type of reading difficulty weakness can help clinically. Often, children with poor reading fluency show fluency deficits in other areas, such as listening, speaking, and writing, thus giving a clinician a broader understanding of the frustrations the child is enduring. Since reading disorders have been well researched, further elaboration of the reading processes as defined by research and education categories are basic reading skills disability, reading fluency problems, and reading comprehension difficulties.

Basic Reading Skills or Reading Disability

Basic reading skills or reading disability is a common complex condition that is assumed to be based on linguistic or phonological impairment. It is dimensional rather than categorical and persistent over time (Shaywitz and Shaywitz 2005). Functional brain imaging shows the neurological underpinnings of dyslexia. The four areas of the brain involved in reading processing include the fusiform gyrus, the posterior portion of the middle temporal gyrus, the angular gyrus, and the posterior portion of the superior temporal gyrus. Evidence suggests that reading disorder is located in the language system of the left hemisphere posterior brain systems (Shaywitz 2003).

It is well established that dyslexia is a heritable condition. Research studies to clarify this concept include twin, family, and sib-pair designs (Coch et al. 2007a). These studies demonstrate genetic similarities in families with members with reading difficulties as the main source of familiality of dyslexia. Based on review, Grigorenko (2005) identified eight loci including sites on chromosomes 1, 2, 3, 6, 11, 15, and 18. There have been no specific genes identified since the complexity and the heterogeneity of this disorder preclude a single genetic deficit. It is also important to recognize that genetic factors do not account for all of the variability; rather, environmental risks also contribute.

The core cognitive processes that make reading difficult for many comprise two theories. The most popular and researched theory demonstrates that deficits in reading result from phonological awareness and fluency difficulties (Fletcher et al. 2007). The other theory considers multiple factors, not only phonological awareness, that give rise to many subtypes of reading disorders (Pennington, cited in Coch et al. 2007a, p. 127). Any theory needs to consider the basic building blocks of reading, defined below:

- *Phonological awareness* is the metacognitive ability to understand the words we hear and read that have basic structure related to sound. Speech sounds, or phonemes, are patterns that make up words. Spoken language is done rapidly without the listener deciphering each sound. English has 44 phonemes; Spanish has 24. To read, one must break letters into a sound-symbol relationship. How quickly the child does this determines his fluency. The best predictor of reading is a child's ability to detect these phonemes. This is true across all languages including Chinese, Greek, Turkish, French, and English (Coch et al. 2007b). There is a universal sequence of phonological development from awareness of large units (syllables) to awareness of small units (phonemes).
- *Rapid naming* is the rapid automatized naming of letters and digits. This usually predicts reading skills over time (Schatschneider et al. 2004). Although some authors disagree, most would say the ability to name quickly enhances reading fluency.
- *Phonological memory* is the ability to use working memory to retain sounds and then words. The relationship to poor reading is still not conclusive.
- *Word recognition.* Word-level reading disability or "dyslexia" is characterized by difficulty in single-word decoding. Without the ability to read a word, fluency and understanding are limited. This is the area where most research has been done. The inability to decode interferes with reading comprehension, recognizing words, and reading fluently.
- *Spelling* is the ability to encode words either in isolation or in context and is difficult without word recognition. Some children can spell but not decode. Spelling is a multidimensional skill that is related to both phonological processing and memory.

Since problems can occur in any of these processes, schools need to evaluate each one before intervention is begun. A deficit in any of these processes would manifest as a reading disability. Intervention would vary depending on the deficit. Psychologically, children with reading problems will avoid reading or procrastinate this task. Poor reading impacts many areas in a child's life, including reading directions, knowing signs, or reading notes. Even many social networks on the computer or computer games require reading skills. A clinician can suspect a reading problem if there has been a history of delayed language; problems with the sounds of words, such as rhyming words and pairing sound with symbol; and a family history of reading disorders.

Reading Fluency

Reading speed is the ability to read connected text rapidly, smoothly, and automatically with little attention to decoding (Meyer and Felton 1999). In order to be fluent, a child must recognize words quickly. Children with **reading fluency** problems read slower, have a harder time keeping ideas in short-term working memory, and use more energy to read. Most people have a constant reading rate that increases with age. Fluency is easily measured by having a child read a list of words or short passages and dividing the number of words read correctly by the total amount of time reading. Fluency interventions expose children to repeated words and word phrases. The reading material is then scaffolded to the instructional level in reading.

Psychologically, fluency disorders can be very embarrassing when a child is asked to read aloud. Stumbling over words, losing one's place, and having trouble with decoding is easily noticed by peers and can have a profound impact on a child's self-esteem as well as a child's avoidance of reading aloud. Fluency deficiencies make reading slower, interfering with the efficiency of reading long passages (Paul et al. 2006).

Reading Comprehension

Reading comprehension refers to the ability to understand information in written form. It is a way to connect ideas on the page to what one knows. One needs to be motivated, hold ideas, concentrate, and have good study techniques. There are many places where this process can be derailed, not only with cognitive problems but with behavior, attention, and emotional difficulties. Active readers will monitor how well they understand what they are reading (Swanson 1999). A good assessment requires the reading of a complex text, not usually seen in standard reading tests. A child who reads adequately for a standardized test may fail to read and understand the more complicated ideas in a textbook. Core cognitive processes for comprehension include language skills, listening comprehension, working memory, and the higher-order processing of inference, prior knowledge, comprehension monitoring, and structure sensitivity. A deficit here affects all academic subject areas where reading is required. Reading comprehension is difficult to assess, as there are many aspects of reading for understanding.

Intervention is important since poor reading impairs educational, social, and occupational functioning. Early intervention can protect children at risk from later failure. It is clear that both classroom and small-group tutorial programs are effective and not all children need individualized one-on-one instruction (Fletcher et al. 2007). Studies of remediation show that there are effective methods of improving word recognition. There are many programs (with a good evidence base) to remediate these disorders. In general, reading programs that are explicit, oriented to academic content, teach to mastery with scaffolding and emotional support, and monitor progress can be effective (Fletcher et al. 2007). Treatment that includes asking children to ask themselves questions about what they read, predict what will happen next, or retell a story can improve their understanding. Many children can ultimately decode words but their rate of reading may be slow, making reading less automatic and more effortful. These children should have extended time to decode and read.

Children with reading problems can present to a clinician with avoidance of schoolwork, disruption in class, and oppositional behavior. Children with fluency problems take more mental energy and time to complete tasks and may present with fatigue, poor time management, or slow response to questions. Often children who don't like school have trouble with the basic skills of reading. It is important to determine the child's reading skills, as depression or severe anxiety can impair a child's academic functioning. In a child with low energy, sad mood, and poor concentration, the hallmarks of depression can masquerade as a reading disorder, but history could reveal no earlier problems with reading, so both must be screened. Psychiatric disorders often interfere here, as a child with depression or poor attention would have trouble reading because of the psychiatric disorder rather than an LD.

Mathematics Disorder

DSM-IV does not break down mathematics disability into the ability to do calculations and the ability of problem solving, as do the federal guidelines. The difficulty with defining a math disability is that mathematics is a broad term without consistent standards (Mazzocco and Myers 2003). Research in dyscalculia lag behind dyslexia. No core deficits or processes have been identified in the mathematics arena. If a child has trouble in reading, then it follows that certain of the language-based math problems will also be difficult. The prevalence of a math disability is estimated to be 5%–6% (Shalev et al. 2005). Neurobiological studies reveal different neural systems involved with learning mathematics. These systems are best studied in the brain-injured population, and the correlation with the child with a math LD is not yet available. There is a strong evidence for the heritability of math difficulties.

To do math, one must use language, nonverbal problem solving, concept formation, working and long-term memory, processing speed, phonological decoding, attention, and sight word recognition. Research suggests that "number sense," or the ability to represent, discriminate, and operate on a limited degree of precision, develops early (Feigenson 2005), between ages 2 and 4 years. Clinicians can screen for this by asking children to count objects and do simple calculations.

The federal government breaks down math difficulties as follows:

- **Mathematics calculations**—Processes that can be problematic include memory, processing issues in visual memory, and visuospatial problems that make lining up columns and understanding base 10 systems difficult.
- **Mathematics problem solving**—Many areas of brain functioning go into solving a math word problem. Reading, understanding language, finding the salient point, doing multiple steps, and using working memory all are needed to solve a math problem. There are many avenues for a disability to arise in this arena.

Although these are the federal categories, there is no support in research of math difficulties in neurologically normal or brain-injured children (Jordan et al. 2006) Intervention for students with LDs in math includes the need to teach the foundational skills and higher-order skills in problem solving. No clear research-based interventions have been thoroughly studied, though interventions can be helpful.

Children with math disabilities with weaknesses in visualization may present to the clinician with socialization problems, such as poor social judgment, poor spatial awareness, and troubles on the playground. Often children with poor visualization have trouble self-soothing or falling asleep. Children that cannot memorize math facts should be screened for working memory deficits that may impact other areas of learning.

Disorder of Written Expression

Written expression is the last and most complex skill to develop. Here the DSM-IV definition reflects the education system's definition. Deficits in this area are usually not noticed until fourth or fifth grade, when the curriculum requires higher-level language and written organization skills. When children present to the clinician in the late fall of fifth grade with sudden onset of behavior issues in school, a query of their writing abilities should be explored. Writing includes the basic writing skills of spelling, punctuation, and legible writing and more complex skills such as detection of writing errors and planning. Writing requires simultaneous integration of motor skills, memory, language, and organizational strategies. Deficits in fine motor planning, as affecting legibility, spelling, and spacing, can be easily spotted. Messy handwriting is often called *dysgraphia*, defined as a neurological disorder where a person's writing is distorted or incorrect. Often children with oral language organization difficulties also have trouble in written language. (See Chapter 11, "Psychological and Neuropsychological Testing," for tests used to evaluate written expression.)

Remediation strategies include both the mechanics of writing and pencil grip. Occupational therapy can be helpful. Computer keyboarding can help those with illegible writing or poor spacing, but the same skill it takes to write with a pencil is required to learn keyboarding. When written organization is a problem, graphic organizers can be helpful and a variety of types are available. There are computer programs that teach outlining and then turning words into narrative form. Rarely, some children may not be able to master the difficult task of written language and may need oral exams or be permitted to use main ideas rather than a narrative.

Communication Disorders

Speech is a complicated process with input from many parts of the brain (Levelt 1999). For every spoken word, one first must choose and access the semantically correct word and then retrieve the phonological or sound

structure of the word. Finally, the word must be encoded in context and planned, produced, and articulated. This complicated process has a strong neurogenetic basis (Barry et al. 2006). Adults are more likely to refer a child for evaluation services with a language impairment based on speech production skills (articulation) rather than the child's language (vocabulary and syntax) (Tomlin 2006). Clinicians must be alert to language skills since an interview relies on oral communication as well as nonverbal cues.

Disorders of speech and language are highly comorbid and possibly related to each other. There is growing evidence of the associations between speech-sound disorders and reading disability, as well as specific language impairment and reading disability (Grigorenko 2007). The overall estimated prevalence of speech and language disorders is about 5% of school-age children. This includes voice disorders (3%), stuttering (1%), and developmental disorders (2%–3%). Estimates of hearing impairments vary considerably. It is widely accepted that all forms of speech and language difficulties occur in families as seen in studies of first-degree relatives, twin studies, and adoptive studies (Grigorenko 2009). Two broad categories of communication disorders have been distinguished: speech disorders and language disorders. Speech disorders refer to the motor production of speech sounds, and language disorders refer to problems with understanding and/or producing a narrative for understanding (Verhoeven and van Balkom 2004).

Speech Disorders

Phonological speech disorders refer to the motor production of speech; *sound skills* refer to the ability to perceive and understand speech sounds that make up words. First one must detect the individual sounds (phonological awareness), then retrieve and access the use and name of sounds, and then remember the sounds.

Phonological disorder is the inability to use expected speech sounds appropriate for the child's age and dialect. Voice pitch, loudness, quality, nasal resonance, and vocal hygiene are important to assess, as they impact the listener. Fluency (stuttering) is the unexpected disturbance in the normal patterns and flow of speech. The nature and severity of dysfluency may vary at different levels of pragmatic complexity. More typical fluency disorders are hesitations, interjections, phrase revisions, unfinished words, and word repetitions. Less typical fluency problems such as syllable repetitions, sound repetition, prolongations, or blocks usually are visible or audible tension with disfluency. There is some relationship between speech disfluency and competency in language and phonology.

Language Disorders

DSM-IV separates language disorders into expressive language disorder and mixed receptive-expressive disorder. An expressive disorder identifies the delays and difficulties in producing speech, and mixed receptive-expressive disorder includes the former along with problems understanding spoken language.

Receptive language is the comprehension of single words, language concepts, directions, grammar, concrete/abstract language, auditory memory, inferential reasoning, phonological processing (reading readiness), and combined linguistic skills. *Expressive language* uses vocabulary, word retrieval by context, semantic association skills, grammar, narrative skills, and pragmatic/social language skills (Rhea 2007). The federal guidelines list the disability as problems in **listening comprehension,** though one needs both understanding of the input and output of language to comprehend the spoken word. *Auditory processing* is a term used to describe what happens when the brain recognizes and interprets the sound (American Speech-Language-Hearing Association 1993). Children with auditory processing disorder often do not recognize subtle differences between sounds in words, even though the sounds themselves are loud and clear. It is not a sensory or hearing impairment. *Auditory processing disorder* is an umbrella term that describes a variety of problems with the brain that can interfere with processing auditory information. Shaywitz et al. (2002) describe children with auditory processing disorder as having difficulty reading. If a reading difficulty is suspected, referral to a speech and language specialist is important.

Oral expression is the ability to convey information and ideas through speech. DSM-IV puts this under expressive language disorder. The child usually understands language better than he can communicate. Later this deficit will impact written language. Oral expression requires pragmatic skills. Pragmatics is the application of language in social or learning situations, for problem solving, or in expressing affect. Although there is no formal LD category for pragmatic language, this is vital for a child's communication. Language is used to communicate information, participate in community, and learn. Turn taking, language organization, and expression of meaning and content

are needed for human interaction. These skills include the following (Bishop 2000):

- Knowing that one has to answer when a question has been asked
- Being able to participate in a conversation by taking turns with the other speaker
- The ability to notice and respond to the nonverbal aspects of language (reacting appropriately to the other person's body language and perceived mood, as well as his words)
- Awareness that one has to introduce a topic of conversation in order for the listener to fully understand
- Knowing which words or what sort of sentence type to use when initiating a conversation or responding to something someone has said
- The ability to maintain a topic (or change topic appropriately or interrupt politely)
- The ability to maintain appropriate eye contact (not too much staring and not too much looking away) during a conversation
- The ability to distinguish how to talk and behave toward different communicative partners (formal with some, informal with others)

Pragmatic disorders occur when there are difficulties in using language in a social, situational, or communication context. Children with ADHD have been shown to have a variety of pragmatic deficits (Haynes et al. 2006). Children with thought disorder also have confused language that can be mistaken for a pragmatic deficit, and children with pragmatic deficits can be confused with those having a thought disorder. A good screening in a psychiatric interview is asking a child to tell a story orally and seeing how the ideas connect, noting the fluency and organization. Often as clinicians, we structure an interview asking a series of questions, which possibly can lead to missing this problem that impacts the child's friendships and written language.

Learning Disorders Not Otherwise Specified

Neither DSM-IV nor the federal regulations currently have a category for nonverbal communication deficits. These disorders involve a group of developmentally based skills that include motor planning (dyspraxia), visuospatial processing, mathematics, memory, and executive functioning. Children with these disorders have strong verbal reasoning abilities, vocabulary, factual knowledge, auditory memory, receptive and expressive language, and reading skills. These disorders can have a profound impact on communication, learning, and relationships. Nonverbal communication makes up so much of our communication. Children who have trouble reading these nonverbal cues may have profound impairment in their ability to socialize. A wave can be interpreted as a threat, or a facial expression can be missed. Perspectives on a social group can be lacking, and this makes it difficult for a child with nonverbal learning disability (NLD) to enter the group—by standing too close, interrupting, missing the gist of the conversation, and causing awkwardness for all involved.

NLD deficits include those in visuospatial-organizational skills, leading to poor visual recall, inability or difficulty forming a visual image, faulty spatial perceptions, difficulties with executive functioning, and problems with spatial relationships. These children have difficulty adapting to novel situations, adjusting to transitions, and accurately reading nonverbal signals and cues. They have difficulty generalizing previously learned information. Children with NLD will have difficulty following multistep instructions, make very literal translations, and impart the illusion of competence because of their strong verbal skills.

Rourke (1995) describes a subset of nonverbal learning issues with deficits in small motor skills, complex conceptual skills involving understanding cause-effect relationships, seeing the big picture rather than focusing on details, poor visuospatial-organizational skills, and poor social skills. There is controversy about this syndrome, and its impact on school adaptation and performance has not been systematically studied. These deficits have been described as part of the higher-functioning autism spectrum disorders with problems in social relationships (Palombo 2006). These children may have trouble judging a face or a social situation or understanding the nuance of jokes, metaphors, or nonverbal signals. Prognosis is based on the success of these children to learn appropriate social behaviors and to develop close relationships with peers, teachers, or clinicians. Strategies that are helpful include the need to verbally label everything that happens to comprehend circumstances, spatial orientation, directional concepts, and coordination. Do not assume a child understands something because he or she can repeat what was just said, but offer added verbal explanations when the child seems lost or registers confusion.

Persons with NLD are particularly inclined toward developing secondary internalizing disorders such as stress, anxiety, and panic. Recent work at the National Institute of Mental Health (McClure et al. 2005) reveals children with bipolar disorder having an increased chance of having this learning profile. Without appropriate intervention, the cumulative effect of ongoing stress can advance to an unmanageable state of anxiety for an NLD person, who is already predisposed to internalizing disorders.

Executive functioning is a poorly agreed-upon set of symptoms that is felt to be part of the prefrontal cortex to direct behavior to a goal and to sustain that behavior over time (Pennington and Ozonoff 1996). There is general agreement that executive functioning is an umbrella term for functions that help provide goal-directed behaviors (Meltzer 2007). Three areas with neuroanatomical correlation have been described: 1) dorsolateral circuit for working memory, organization, planning, problem solving, environmental monitoring, attention, and mental flexibility; 2) orbitofrontal cortex with connection to the basal ganglia for behavioral regulation to delay gratification, anticipate the future, and sustain the behavior; and 3) medial cortex with links to the limbic system to modulate emotion (Ochsner and Gross 2005). Executive functioning progresses with development (Anderson et al. 2001). Deficits in working memory and recall, activation, arousal and effort (getting started, paying attention, completing work), emotion control (tolerating frustration, thinking before acting or speaking), internalizing language (using self-talk to control one's behavior and direct future actions), and complex problem solving (taking an issue apart, analyzing the pieces, and reconstituting and organizing them into new ideas) impact all areas of a person's engagement with the world.

Executive functioning has been examined in children with ADHD, but research in other psychiatric disorders or in executive functioning deficits as an LD alone is lacking. Its specificity to ADHD is not determined (Sergeant et al. 2002), and executive functioning deficits may be present in other children with profound impacts on learning. The ability to devise and react to goal-directed plans is important to function. Patients with poor executive functioning have difficulties in many areas of living. Clinicians should be alert to these disorders even in patients without ADHD. Depression, severe obsessive-compulsive disorder (OCD), and anxiety can produce poor executive skills, such as a patient with a hand-washing ritual who does not get ready for school in the morning or go to bed on time. Addressing the OCD or psychiatric disorder should improve executive functioning deficits if they are secondary. Treatment of primary executive functioning disorders is not well researched. There may be a role for cognitive-behavioral skills for improvement, but this has not been studied.

Motor Skills Deficits

Motor disorders and poor coordination are also known as clumsiness or dyspraxia. DSM-IV uses the term *developmental coordination disorder* (DCD) and broadens the terms to both fine and gross motor problems that interfere with academic achievement. There is no consensus if these disorders are developmental or multisensory. Often children with motor skills deficits have co-occurring disorders in the area of learning, congenital issues, or other psychiatric disorders. Few data exist as to the prevalence, severity, or comorbidity of DCD. Martin et al. (2006), reporting the results of a survey of 1,285 twin pairs ages 5–16 years, showed that DCD with fine motor problems and ADHD-inattentive subtypes were most strongly linked. Not only do gross and fine motor skills need tone, strength, and planning, but movements must be sequenced and done at a certain speed (Barnhart et al. 2003).

Children with movement difficulties may avoid physical activities, and this low level of activity puts them at risk for later life problems in motor skills, cardiopulmonary fitness, and weight control. Difficulties with writing and keyboarding prevent a child from demonstrating what they learn and interfere with note taking and academic performance.

No universal treatment is recommended for these disorders since they are often heterogeneous. These children can be referred to occupational or physical therapists (Watenberg et al. 2007) for further treatment. There are many approaches: cognitive motor intervention with feedback and measurable goals, sensory integration therapy, kinesthetic training, and a variety of others (Wilson 2005).

The Clinical Evaluation

Clinicians need to pay attention to the type of LD in the child whom they are evaluating. A reading disorder may impact only school performance, but if a child's

reading weakness includes visual processing or fluency deficits, it can have profound impact on a child's daily functioning. Knowing how a child processes information and his cognitive communication style will make it easier to assess the emotional and behavior style that a child uses. Cognitive deficits are not accurately assessed through the patient self-report or by the clinical exam (Moritz et al. 2004). Children with poor oral expression will take longer to interview, and their pauses and word retrieval can be misunderstood as depression or preoccupation of thought. Children with math problem-solving issues may have trouble with visual sequencing and social problem solving, since the parietal lobe is used in social situations and in assessing a problem. Children with fluency issues may be delayed in answering questions, and the interviewer will need to wait for the child both to process the answer and to respond fully. Children with expressive language deficits may use physical responses to solve problems, since they do not get to their words quickly to diffuse the situation. Doing therapy with a child with poor language skills can be difficult and not helpful. A shy child may have difficulties with language or trouble reading the social situation. A good-enough parent often compensates for a child's cognitive weakness, making early identification more difficult. Astute clinicians can begin to look for possible neuropsychological patterns from their clinical exam.

In addition, the clinician may be called on to write a letter and be part of the individualized education program process. Communication needs to be clear, accurate, in the school's language, and indicate why there might be a learning issue in addition to the emotional or behavioral issues.

Conclusion

Disorders of learning, communication, and motor skills are common and impair development of academic skills, social skills, emotional regulation, problem-solving skills, and behavior. Cognitive impairment negatively affects activities of daily living, level of care or schooling, required prognosis outcomes, and adherence to treatment. Being alert to how a child is processing information leads to a better understanding of the child, his or her diagnosis, and the most appropriate treatment plan.

Summary Points

- Learning disabilities (LDs) are common and comorbid, affecting communication and behavior.

- LDs are neurobiological, with a strong genetic component.

- Definitions of learning disorders in DSM-IV-TR vary from those in the federal guidelines.

- Response to Intervention is the federal government's model of guidelines for identifying children that need educational intervention based on a dual-discrepancy model of learning as related to same-age peers and poor response to instruction.

- Reading disorder is the most common, best-studied, and most complex learning disorder, with difficulties in word recognition, phonological awareness, rapid naming, phonological memory, fluency, spelling, and comprehension.

- Communication disorders—both articulation difficulties and language problems—are highly correlated with psychiatric disorders.

- Although not federally described, problems with pragmatic language, nonverbal learning, and executive function have profound impact on development.

- Early intervention is imperative and preventative.

References

American Psychiatric Association: Diagnostic and Statistical Manual of Mental Disorders, 4th Edition. Washington, DC, American Psychiatric Association, 1994

American Psychiatric Association: Diagnostic and Statistical Manual of Mental Disorders, 4th Edition, Text Revision. Washington, DC, American Psychiatric Association, 2000

American Speech-Language-Hearing Association: Definition of communication disorders. ASHA 35(suppl):40–41, 1993

Anderson VA, Enderson P, Northam E, et al: Development of executive functions through late childhood and adolescence in an Australian sample. Dev Neuropsychol 20:385–406, 2001

Barnhart RC, Davenport MJ, Epps SB, et al: Developmental coordination disorder. Phys Ther 83:722–731, 2003

Barry JG, Yasin I, Bishop DV: Heritable risk factors associated with language impairments. Genes Brain Behav 6:66–76, 2006

Bishop DVM: Pragmatic language impairment: a correlate of SLI, a distinct subgroup, or part of the autistic continuum? in Speech and Language Impairments in Children: Causes, Characteristics, Intervention and Outcome. Edited by Bishop DVM, Leonard LB. Hove, UK, Psychology Press, 2000, pp 99–113

Bromley E: Barriers to appropriate clinical use of medications that improve the cognitive deficits of schizophrenia. Psychiatr Serv 58:475–481, 2007

Cervellione K, Burdick K, Cottone J, et al: Neurocognitive deficits in adolescents with schizophrenia: longitudinal stability and predictive utility for short-term functional outcome. J Am Acad Child Adolesc Psychiatry 46:867–878, 2007

Coch D, Dawson G, Fischer KW: Human Behavior, Learning, and the Developing Brain: Atypical Development. New York, Guilford, 2007a

Coch D, Dawson G, Fischer KW: Human Behavior, Learning, and the Developing Brain: Typical Development. New York, Guilford, 2007b

Dickstein D, Nelson E, McClure E, et al: Cognitive flexibility in phenotypes of pediatric bipolar disorder. J Am Acad Child Adolesc Psychiatry 4:341–353, 2007

Feigenson L: A double-dissociation in infants' representations of object arrays. Cognition 95:B37–B48, 2005

Fletcher JM, Lyon GR, Fuchs LS, et al: Learning Disabilities: From Intervention to Intervention. New York, Guilford, 2007

Fuchs D, Mock D, Margan PL, et al: Responsiveness-to-intervention: definitions, evidence, and implications for the learning disabilities construct. Learn Disabil Res Pract 18:157–171, 2003

Goldston D, Walsh A, Arnold E, et al: Reading problems, psychiatric disorders, and functional impairment from mid to late adolescence. J Am Acad Child Adolesc Psychiatry 46:25–32, 2007

Grigorenko EL: A conservative meta-analysis of linkage and linking-association studies of developmental dyslexia. Scientific Studies of Reading 9:285–316, 2005

Grigorenko EL: Rethinking disorders of spoken and written language: generating working hypotheses. J Dev Behav Pediatr 28:478–486, 2007

Grigorenko EL: Behavior-genetic and molecular studies of disorders of speech and language: an overview, in Handbooks of Genetics. Edited by Kim Y-K. New York, Springer, 2009, 300–310

Haynes WO, Pindzola R, Moran M: Communication Disorders in the Classroom: An Introduction for Professionals in School Settings. Boston, MA, Jones and Bartlett Publishers, 2006

Hinshaw S: Externalizing behavior problems and academic underachievement in childhood and adolescents: causal relationships and underlying mechanism. Psychol Bull 1111:127–155, 1992

Jordan NC, Kaplan D, Olah LN, et al: Number sense growth in kindergarten: a longitudinal investigation. Child Dev 77:153–175, 2006

Kaufman J, Yang BZ, Douglas-Palumberi H, et al: Brain-derived neurotrophic factor- 5-HTTLPR gene interactions and environmental modifiers of depression in children. Biol Psychiatry 59:673–680, 2006

Levelt WJ: Models of word production. Trends Cogn Sci 3:223–232, 1999

Lichtenstein S, Blackorby J: Who drops out and what happens to them? Journal for Vocational Special Needs Education 18:6–11, 1995

Martin NC, Piek JP, Hay D: DCD and ADHD: a genetic study of their shared etiology. Hum Mov Sci 25:110–124, 2006

Martinez-Aran A, Vieta E, Colom F, et al: Cognitive impairment in euthymic bipolar patients: implications for clinical and functional outcomes. Bipolar Disord 6:233–244, 2004

Mazzocco MM, Myers GF: Complexities in identifying and defining mathematics learning disability in the primary school age years. Annals of Dyslexia 53:218–253, 2003

McClure EB, Treland JE, Snow J, et al: Deficits in social cognition and response flexibility in pediatric bipolar disorder. Am J Psychiatry 162:1644–1651, 2005

Meltzer L: Executive Function in Education: From Theory to Practice. New York, Guilford, 2007

Meyer MS, Felton RH: Repeated reading to enhance fluency: old approaches and new directions. Ann Dyslexia 49: 283–306, 1999

Moritz S, Ferahli S, Naber D: Memory and attention performance in psychiatric patients: lack of correspondence between clinician-rated and patient-rated functioning with neuropsychological test results. J Int Neuropsychiatry 10:623–633, 2004

Ochsner KN, Gross JJ: The cognitive control of emotion. Trends Cogn Sci 9:242–249, 2005

Palombo J: Nonverbal Learning Disabilities: A Clinical Perspective. New York, WW Norton, 2006

Paul LM, Georgios D, Sideridis GD: Contrasting the effectiveness of fluency interventions for students with or at risk for learning disabilities: a multilevel random coefficient modeling meta-analysis. Learn Disabil Res Pract 21:191–210, 2006

Pennington BF, Ozonoff S: Executive functions and developmental psychopathology. J Child Psychol Psychiatry 37: 51–87, 1996

Rhea P: Language Disorders From Infancy Through Adolescence. St. Louis, MO, Mosby, 2007

Rourke BP: Syndrome of Nonverbal Learning Disabilities, Neurodevelopmental Manifestations. New York, Guilford, 1995

Rutter M, Caspi A, Fergusson D, et al: Sex differences in developmental reading disability: new findings from four epidemiological studies. JAMA 291:2007–2012, 2004

Schatschneider C, Fletcher JM, Francis DJ, et al: Kindergarten prediction of reading skills: a longitudinal comparative analysis. J Educ Psychol 96:265–282, 2004

Schretlen D: The nature and significance of cognitive impairment in schizophrenia. Johns Hopkins Advanced Studies in Medicine 7:72–78, 2007

Sergeant JA, Geurts H, Oosterlaan J: How specific is a deficit of executive functioning for attention-deficit-hyperactivity disorder. Behav Brain Res 130:3–28, 2002

Shalev RS, Manor O, Gross-Tsur V: Developmental dyscalculia: a prospective six-year follow-up. Dev Med Child Neurol 47:121–125, 2005

Shaywitz BA, Shaywitz SE, Pugh KR, et al: Disruption of posterior brain systems for reading in children with developmental dyslexia. Biol Psychiatry 52:101–110, 2002

Shaywitz SE: Overcoming Dyslexia. New York, Knopf, 2003

Shaywitz SE, Shaywitz BA: Dyslexia. Biol Psychiatry 57: 1301–1309, 2005

Sideridis GD: Understanding low achievement and depression in children with learning disabilities: a goal orientation approach. Int Rev Res Ment Retard 31:163–203, 2006

Swanson HL: Reading research for students with LD: a meta-analysis of intervention outcome. J Learn Disabil 32:504–532, 1999

Tomlin JB: A normativist account of language-based learning disabilities. Learn Disabil Res Pract 21:8–18, 2006

U.S. Department of Education Office of Special Education and Rehabilitative Services: A New Era: Revitalizing Special Education for Children and Their Families. Washington, DC, 2002

Verhoeven L, van Balkom H (eds): Classification of Developmental Language Disorders. Mahwah, NJ, Lawrence Erlbaum, 2004

Watenberg N, Waiserberg N, Zuk L, et al: Developmental coordination disorder with attention deficit hyperactivity disorder and physical therapy intervention, Dev Med Child Neurol 49:920–925, 2007

Wilson PH: Practitioner review: approaches to assessment and treatment of children with DCD: an evaluative review. J Child Psychol Psychiatry 46:806–823, 2005

PART IV

AXIS I PSYCHIATRIC DISORDERS OF BEHAVIOR

Chapter 15

Attention-Deficit/Hyperactivity Disorder

Steven R. Pliszka, M.D.

While attention-deficit/hyperactivity disorder (ADHD) is sometimes portrayed as a "modern" condition, George Still (1902) is now credited with the first clinical description of what today would be recognized as ADHD. The first treatment of impulsive, hyperactive, and disruptive behavior with stimulant medication was reported in the 1930s (Bradley 1937). Virginia Douglas (Douglas and Peters 1979) first critically examined the psychological data emerging from the study of "hyperactive" children and laid out the cardinal symptoms of the disorder as inattention, impulsivity, and hyperactivity; it was further noted that a subset of children with "hyperactivity" were inattentive without being hyperactive. Such data led to introduction of the term *attention deficit disorder* (ADD) with and without hyperactivity. Since then, the criteria have undergone refinements, leading to the current terminology of ADHD with its inattentive, hyperactiv-

ity-impulsive, and combined subtypes in DSM-IV (American Psychiatric Association 1994) and its text revision, DSM-IV-TR (American Psychiatric Association 2000; see Table 15–1).

Definition, Clinical Description, and Diagnosis

ADHD is a neurodevelopmental disorder in which a child's ability to attend to and control impulses (including inhibiting motor activity when appropriate) 1) is significantly less than that of a typically developing child, 2) causes impairment in the child's academic or social functioning, and 3) is not accounted for by some other medical or psychiatric condition. Table 15–1 pre-

TABLE 15–1. DSM-IV-TR diagnostic criteria for attention-deficit/hyperactivity disorder

A. Either (1) or (2):

  (1) six (or more) of the following symptoms of **inattention** have persisted for at least 6 months to a degree that is maladaptive and inconsistent with developmental level:

  Inattention

  (a) often fails to give close attention to details or makes careless mistakes in schoolwork, work, or other activities

  (b) often has difficulty sustaining attention in tasks or play activities

  (c) often does not seem to listen when spoken to directly

  (d) often does not follow through on instructions and fails to finish schoolwork, chores, or duties in the workplace (not due to oppositional behavior or failure to understand instructions)

  (e) often has difficulty organizing tasks and activities

  (f) often avoids, dislikes, or is reluctant to engage in tasks that require sustained mental effort (such as schoolwork or homework)

  (g) often loses things necessary for tasks or activities (e.g., toys, school assignments, pencils, books, or tools)

  (h) is often easily distracted by extraneous stimuli

  (i) is often forgetful in daily activities

  (2) six (or more) of the following symptoms of **hyperactivity-impulsivity** have persisted for at least 6 months to a degree that is maladaptive and inconsistent with developmental level:

  Hyperactivity

  (a) often fidgets with hands or feet or squirms in seat

  (b) often leaves seat in classroom or in other situations in which remaining seated is expected

  (c) often runs about or climbs excessively in situations in which it is inappropriate (in adolescents or adults, may be limited to subjective feelings of restlessness)

  (d) often has difficulty playing or engaging in leisure activities quietly

  (e) is often "on the go" or often acts as if "driven by a motor"

  (f) often talks excessively

  Impulsivity

  (g) often blurts out answers before questions have been completed

  (h) often has difficulty awaiting turn

  (i) often interrupts or intrudes on others (e.g., butts into conversations or games)

B. Some hyperactive-impulsive or inattentive symptoms that caused impairment were present before age 7 years.

C. Some impairment from the symptoms is present in two or more settings (e.g., at school [or work] and at home).

D. There must be clear evidence of clinically significant impairment in social, academic, or occupational functioning.

E. The symptoms do not occur exclusively during the course of a pervasive developmental disorder, schizophrenia, or other psychotic disorder and are not better accounted for by another mental disorder (e.g., mood disorder, anxiety disorder, dissociative disorder, or a personality disorder).

TABLE 15–1. DSM-IV-TR diagnostic criteria for attention-deficit/hyperactivity disorder *(continued)*

Code based on type:

314.01 Attention-deficit/hyperactivity disorder, combined type: if both Criteria A1 and A2 are met for the past 6 months

314.00 Attention-deficit/hyperactivity disorder, predominantly inattentive type: if Criterion A1 is met but Criterion A2 is not met for the past 6 months

314.01 Attention-deficit/hyperactivity disorder, predominantly hyperactive-impulsive type: if Criterion A2 is met but Criterion A1 is not met for the past 6 months

Coding note: For individuals (especially adolescents and adults) who currently have symptoms that no longer meet full criteria, "In Partial Remission" should be specified.

Source. Reprinted from American Psychiatric Association: *Diagnostic and Statistical Manual of Mental Disorders*, 4th Edition, Text Revision. Washington, DC, American Psychiatric Association, 2000, pp. 92–93. Used with permission. Copyright © 2000 American Psychiatric Association.

sents the specific criteria, including the definition of the three subtypes of ADHD: inattentive, hyperactive-impulsive, and combined.

Epidemiology

ADHD is among the most common of childhood disorders. The U.S. National Health Interview Survey found the prevalence of ADHD for the period 1997–2000 to be 6.7% (Woodruff et al. 2004), while the Centers for Disease Control and Prevention (2005) asked parents of over 100,000 children ages 4–17 years whether their child had *ever* been diagnosed with ADHD or received medication treatment (as opposed to currently being treated). The rate of lifetime childhood diagnosis of ADHD was 7.8%, while 4.3% (or only 55% of those diagnosed with ADHD) had ever been treated with medication for the disorder. A review and meta-analysis suggested a worldwide prevalence rate of 5.3% (Polanczyk et al. 2007). In community-based studies, boys are found to have ADHD three to five times more often than girls (Barkley 2006b). For the most part, the clinical picture of ADHD is similar in both genders (Gaub and Carlson 1997; Gershon 2002), although boys with ADHD are more likely to show the comorbidity of oppositional defiant disorder (ODD) or conduct disorder (CD), while girls may show higher levels of comorbid internalizing disorders.

Comorbidity

As in other psychiatric disorders, comorbidity is common in ADHD (Barkley 2006a; Biederman 2005; Biederman et al. 1991, 1993; Pliszka et al. 1999). Figure 15–1

summarizes the overlap of the most common comorbid conditions and illustrates the complexity of that overlap. Both ODD and CD as well as anxiety disorders are present in 25%–33% of children with ADHD, while learning and language disorders affect another quarter. As noted in the figure, many children with ADHD will have two or more comorbid disorders, complicating both research into comorbidity and clinical management. The overlap of ADHD and ODD/CD has been best studied. Compared to children with ADHD alone, those with ODD/CD show more severe symptoms of impulsivity, higher rates of aggression, a greater prevalence of learning disorders, and a greater propensity to develop both antisocial personality and substance abuse during their adolescent years (Pliszka et al. 1999). Family studies suggest that ADHD with ODD/CD is a separate genetic subtype than ADHD alone (Biederman et al. 1992).

Compared to those with ADHD alone, those with comorbid anxiety (without ODD/CD) show lower levels of impulsivity on laboratory measures of attention and a greater tendency to respond to psychosocial interventions (Jensen et al. 2001a; March et al. 2000; Newcorn et al. 2001). Of interest, it is the parent report of anxiety rather than the child report that predicts such response. ADHD and anxiety appear to arise from independent genetic contributions (Biederman et al. 1992). When children with ADHD have the "double" comorbidity of both anxiety and ODD/CD, they tend to resemble children with ADHD and ODD/CD in their cognitive profile (Newcorn et al. 2001) yet show an enhanced response to combined medication and psychosocial intervention (Jensen et al. 2001a).

The overlap of ADHD with mood disorders (both unipolar depression and bipolar disorder) is less well studied. In the Multimodal Treatment Study of Children With ADHD (MTA) study, 11% of the sample

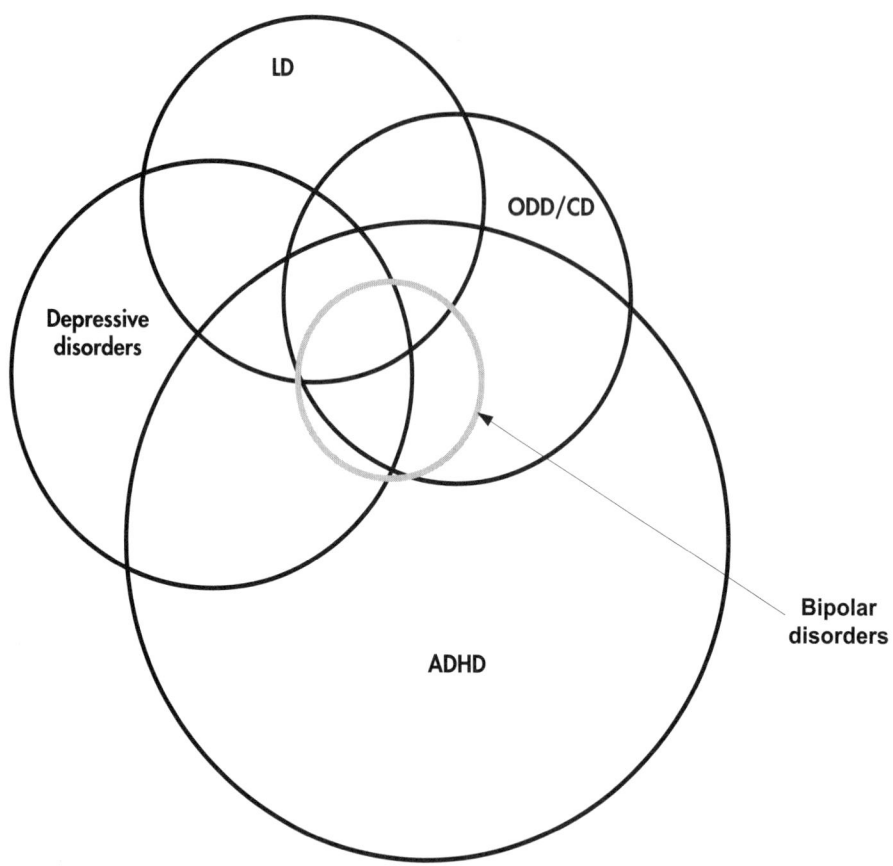

FIGURE 15–1.   Comorbidity of psychiatric disorders with attention-deficit/hyperactivity disorder (ADHD).
LD=learning disorder; ODD/CD=oppositional defiant disorder/conduct disorder.

also met criteria for major depressive disorder (MDD). Other studies have shown a wide variety of rates of comorbidity, up to 75% (Barkley 2006b; Pliszka et al. 1999). How depression affects the clinical expression of ADHD has not been explored; family studies suggest that ADHD and MDD might share genetic factors (Biederman et al. 1992). Since treatment of depression rarely leads to remission of ADHD symptoms, it seems unlikely that MDD masquerades as ADHD to any significant degree. If the full DSM-IV-TR criteria for MDD are met in a child with ADHD, this most likely represents the full syndrome of MDD and not a state of demoralization due to the ADHD symptoms (Biederman et al. 1998). The current clinical consensus is that ADHD and MDD represent separate conditions, each requiring its own treatment (Pliszka et al. 2006a).

More contentious is the overlap of ADHD and bipolar disorder (Biederman 1998; Klein et al. 1998). The MTA study (Jensen et al. 2001a) did not find it necessary to exclude any child with ADHD because of a diagnosis of bipolar disorder (although a small subset [n=13] did show signs of "hypomania"), but Bieder-

man and colleagues (Biederman et al. 1996a; Wozniak et al. 1995) found that 16% of a sample of ADHD patients met criteria for mania. In preadolescents, nearly all children diagnosed with bipolar disorder also meet criteria for ADHD, as do 68% of adolescents diagnosed with bipolar disorder (Geller et al. 1998a, 1998b).

Etiology and Risk Factors

Genetics

The genetics of ADHD have been explored via three types of studies—family/adoption studies, twin studies, and, more recently, molecular genetic studies. Family studies have consistently shown that if a child has ADHD, 10%–35% of first-degree relatives are likely to have the disorder as well (Biederman et al. 1992). If a parent has ADHD, the risk to the child of developing ADHD is as high as 57% (Biederman et al. 1995a). Sprich et al. (2000) examined the rates of ADHD in the relatives of both adopted (i.e., nonbiological) and nonadopted children with ADHD. The rate of ADHD in biological relatives of children with ADHD was 18% compared to only 6% in the adopted relatives, suggesting a strong genetic effect.

Twin studies compare concordance rates for ADHD in monozygotic and dizygotic twins to determine the relative influence of genes and environment on the variance in symptoms of ADHD. About 75% of the variance in ADHD traits is found to be attributable

to genetics (Faraone et al. 2005; see Table 15–2). If the risk of ADHD in the general population is about 5%, then carrying one of these alleles will increase the person's risk of ADHD by a factor of about 1.5—that is, to 7.5%. ADHD is likely to be a polygenetic disorder, and further study is needed to determine how these polymorphisms might be associated with functional changes in the gene output and related brain function.

TABLE 15–2. Genes suspected to be related to attention-deficit/hyperactivity disorder (ADHD)

Gene	Odds ratio (increased risk for ADHD if patient carries risk allele)	Functional implication/comment
DRD4 7-repeat allele Dopamine D_4 receptor	1.45 (95% CI, 1.27–1.65)	D_4 receptor is prevalent in frontal-subcortical regions. In vitro studies of a repeat polymorphism in exon III of *DRD4* have shown that the 7-repeat allele produces a blunted response to dopamine
DRD5 Dopamine D_5 receptor, a dinucleotide repeat near the transcription start site	1.20 (95% CI, 1.1–1.4)	Unknown
SLC6A3 Dopamine transporter— most studies have examined a 10-repeat sequence in the 3′ untranslated region	1.13 (95% CI, 1.03–1.24)	No known functional significance of 10-repeat sequence; 10-repeat allele makes transporter gene more susceptible to neurotoxins?
Synaptosomal-associated protein (SNAP)–25 gene	1.19 (95% CI, 1.03–1.38)	Coloboma mice with SNAP deletion are hyperactive; show dopamine and serotonin deficiencies
Catecholamine-*O*-methyl transferase (COMT) gene	Pooled studies do not show association with ADHD	Met allele is associated with more errors of commission on continuous performance test
Dopamine beta-hydroxylase gene	1.33 (95% CI, 1.11–1.59)	Enzyme converts dopamine to norepinephrine 5′ *Taq*1 polymorphism is associated with ADHD; functional significance not known
SLC6A4 Serotonin transporter	1.31 (95% CI, 1.09–1.59)	S allele is associated with less transcription of transporter gene; interacts with life stress to predict depression, but serotonergic agents are ineffective in ADHD
HTR1B Serotonin$_{1B}$ receptor	1.44 (95% CI, 1.14–1.83)	Unknown Serotonergic agents are ineffective in ADHD

Note. CI=confidence interval.

Environmental Risk Factors

A number of nongenetic risk factors for ADHD have been established (Nigg 2006). These include perinatal stress and low birth weight (Mick et al. 2002b), traumatic brain injury (Max et al. 1998), maternal smoking during pregnancy (Mick et al. 2002a), and very severe early deprivation (Kreppner et al. 2001). Interestingly, the 20% of the variance that twin studies attribute to environment appears to be related primarily to *nonshared* environmental effects (Barkley 2007). For instance, Sharp et al. (2003) found that in identical twins discordant for ADHD, the twin with ADHD was more likely to have suffered problematic perinatal events and had a lower birth weight. Greater levels of environmental adversity (low social class, maternal psychopathology, family conflict) are associated with an increasing risk for ADHD and other comorbidities in a dose-dependent fashion (Biederman et al. 1995b, 1995c). It would be incorrect, however, to conclude that the presence of such psychosocial risk factors contributes to the *etiology* of ADHD. Risk may in fact be mediated via genetic effects—that is, parental ADHD results in a father or mother who does poorly on the job and disciplines erratically; these behaviors of parents with ADHD can negatively affect the entire family (Barkley 2006a).

Genes and environment combine to produce endophenotypes such as poor inhibitory control or motor timing problems, as well as difficulties delaying reward or with higher executive function (Barkley 1997; Castellanos and Tannock 2002).

Pathophysiology

ADHD has been associated with poor inhibitory control, assessed principally with go/no-go and stop signal tasks (Barkley 1997). A meta-analysis of 17 studies involving the Stop Signal task showed that only 45%–50% of children with ADHD had a performance level more impaired than the 90th percentile of the control sample (Nigg et al. 2005). On any given measure of executive function, only 16%–50% of ADHD children are found to be impaired (Nigg et al. 2005; Willcutt et al. 2005). Other deficits must play a role in ADHD and include inability to delay response to reward (Solanto et al. 2001; Sonuga-Barke 2002), greater intra-individual variability of reaction time (Castellanos et al. 2005), cerebellar-related problems with motor timing (Durston et al. 2007), and possible alterations in "default-

mode" resting brain states (Castellanos et al. 2008; Clare Kelly et al. 2008).

Neuroanatomical Findings

In a recent meta-analysis, identified regions of the brain showed a significant difference in volume between ADHD and controls in at least three different studies (Valera et al. 2007). These regions included (in order of the magnitude of the difference) posterior inferior vermis of the cerebellum, cerebellar vermis, splenium, total cerebral volume, right cerebellum, left cerebellum, and caudate. Studies varied in the degree of comorbidity in the sample, as well as in the imaging technique. Other studies have been consistent with this meta-analysis, with ADHD subjects showing less volume than controls in the dorsolateral prefrontal cortex, anterior cingulate, and caudate (Casey et al. 2007; Makris et al. 2007; Pliszka et al. 2006b; Seidman et al. 2006; van't Ent et al. 2007). The limbic areas have not been a major focus of study in ADHD, though recently hippocampal volume was found to be increased bilaterally in a large sample of children with ADHD relative to controls, but 27% of the children with ADHD had depressive disorders (Plessen et al. 2006). Amygdala volume bilaterally correlated positively with orbitofrontal cortex volume in controls, but there was no such correlation in subjects with ADHD, suggesting less ability of the cortex to modulate amygdala activity in ADHD.

Functional Neuroimaging

A recent activation likelihood estimation meta-analysis of 16 neuroimaging studies contrasting subjects with ADHD and controls has been performed (Dickstein et al. 2006). In studies using response inhibition tasks, an increased likelihood of activation was seen for controls in the prefrontal cortex bilaterally, anterior cingulate cortex, left parietal lobe, and right caudate. Examining parent-child dyads, child subjects with ADHD showed less activation on a go/no-go task in the middle frontal gyrus, inferior frontal gyrus, anterior cingulate cortex, and caudate (Epstein et al. 2007). The parents of ADHD children (who had ADHD themselves) also showed decreased activity in the frontostriatal areas and anterior cingulate cortex, but adults with ADHD had greater activation of the precuneus and inferior parietal lobule than controls.

Motor timing tasks that engage the cerebellum have recently been shown to differentiate children with ADHD from controls (Durston et al. 2007; Mulder et al. 2008). These studies use a variation of the go/no-go task in which stimuli can appear unexpectedly; these unexpected presentation trials strongly activate the cerebellar hemispheres relative to expected trials. Children with ADHD and their unaffected siblings showed decreased activation of the cerebellum during the timing manipulation and decreased activation of the anterior cingulate cortex during the expected presentation trials. Thus ADHD may be seen as a disorder of both frontostriatal and frontocerebellar circuitry.

Course and Prognosis

Very significant numbers (60%–85%) of children with ADHD continue to meet criteria for the disorder during the teenage years (Barkley et al. 1990; Biederman et al. 1996b; Claude and Firestone 1995). Barkley and colleagues (Barkley et al. 1990; Fischer et al. 1990) followed up 158 children with ADHD 8–10 years after diagnosis and, using a large number of functional measures, compared them with a control group of 81 children. Not only did 83% of the ADHD children still meet criteria for the disorder in their late teen years, but they were more likely than controls to have car accidents (Barkley et al. 1993), smoke cigarettes (Barkley et al. 1990), and fail a grade or be suspended (Fischer et al. 1990). At a 3-year follow-up, the MTA study found that 40% of the sample no longer met criteria for ADHD and that the children fell into three trajectories of outcome: those who improved acutely and maintained improvement, a second group that showed very gradual improvement and "caught up" to the first group, while a third group improved initially but then showed a deteriorating course (Jensen et al. 2007; Swanson et al. 2007).

Four studies have followed fairly large samples of children with hyperactivity or ADHD into adulthood: the Montreal study (Weiss and Hechtman 2003), the New York study (Mannuzza et al. 1998), the Milwaukee study (Barkley et al. 2006), and, most recently, the Massachusetts General study (Biederman et al. 2006a). These studies vary in the rates of ADHD found in adulthood as well as comorbidity of adult disorders. In general, studies tracking children with ADHD only (and no ODD/CD) or that use patient self-report find that under 10% of children with ADHD still have it as adults (the New York study), while those studies including ADHD children with comorbidity and that use parent informants find rates of 49%–67% of ADHD at follow-up.

Adults with a childhood history of ADHD have higher than expected rates of antisocial behavior (Barkley et al. 2004), injuries and accidents (Barkley 2004), employment and marital difficulties, health problems, teen pregnancies (Barkley et al. 2006), and children out of wedlock (Johnston 2002). Biederman et al. (2006a) found that adults with a childhood history of ADHD had higher rates of major psychopathology and substance use disorders than controls. Thus ADHD, particularly when it is comorbid with other disorders, is a precursor to adult psychopathology.

Clinical Evaluation

The clinician should perform a detailed interview with the parent about each of the 18 ADHD symptoms listed in DSM-IV-TR, and if a symptom is present, the clinician should inquire about its duration, severity, and frequency. The patient must have a chronic course (symptoms do not remit for weeks or months at a time) and onset of symptoms during childhood. After all the symptoms are assessed, the clinician should determine in which settings (school, work, home) impairment occurs. The interview with the parent is most critical, but it is important to gather data from the child's school, via teacher rating scales (see below) and/or review of schoolwork. Preschool children or young school-age children (ages 5–8 years) can be interviewed with the parent present, but all children over age 8 should be interviewed individually.

A variety of rating scales for quantifying ADHD symptoms are available (see Chapter 8, "Rating Scales"). While rating scales cannot make a diagnosis, they allow the clinician to assess symptoms and impairments in multiple domains (e.g., school, home) and establish baseline severity. Follow-up rating scales can then be used to more precisely assess the degree of improvement.

Differential Diagnosis and Comorbidity

The first differential diagnosis is with "normality," that is, the child has developmentally appropriate levels of attention, activity, and impulse control. Lack of any problems in school or symptoms that are not witnessed outside the home are inconsistent with ADHD. On the other hand, lack of evidence of symptoms during the office visit itself should not be used to rule out

ADHD. Children with ADHD regularly engage in "fun" activities (video games, sports) without difficulty, so the clinician should inquire about behavior in cognitively demanding situations. Teacher reports of inattention or impulse-control problems should generally be accepted unless there is strong evidence to contradict such reports.

The clinician should, in an organized manner, ask the parent about oppositional behavior, conduct and aggression problems, depression, anxiety, and tic disorders. If the child is over 10 years of age, queries should be made about substance and alcohol abuse. The clinician should ask if the child has severe rage outbursts or mood lability. In general, ODD and CD comorbid with ADHD may improve with treatment of the child's ADHD (Klein et al. 1997; Newcorn et al. 2005; Spencer et al. 2006). The clinician should determine the presence or absence of depressive symptoms in the child. Intermittent dysphoria over difficulties at home or school is not uncommon in children and adolescents with ADHD, but pervasive depression, neurovegetative signs, or suicidal ideation is strongly suggestive of comorbid MDD. If the attentional symptoms had onset after the depressive symptoms (and full criteria for ADHD are not met), then the clinician should consider whether the depressive symptoms might be causing problems with concentration.

Mania should never be diagnosed on the basis of severe hyperactivity or aggression alone, but the clinician should question the parent regarding any periods of the child's intense irritability, rage outbursts, or euphoria. If these periods last for hours a day, several days a week, then a diagnosis of mania should be entertained, but the clinician should see evidence of associated symptoms, such as decreased need for sleep, grandiosity, hypersexuality, or pathological risk taking (see Chapter 19, "Bipolar Disorder").

Low scores on standardized testing of academic achievement frequently characterize ADHD patients (Tannock 2002). Academic impairment is commonly due to the ADHD itself. Many months or years of not listening in class, not mastering material in an organized fashion, and not practicing academic skills (e.g., not doing homework) lead to a decline in achievement relative to the patient's intellectual ability. If the parent and teacher report that the patient performs at (or even above) grade level on subjects when given one-to-one supervision, then a formal learning disorder is less likely. If learning problems are secondary to ADHD, they should begin to resolve within 2–3 months of successful treatment of the ADHD.

In other cases, symptoms of comorbid learning and language disorders are present that cannot be accounted for by ADHD. These include deficits in expressive and receptive language, poor phonological processing, poor motor coordination, or difficulty grasping fundamental mathematical concepts.

Clinical Examination and Mental Status Findings

The primary purpose of the interview with the child or adolescent is not to confirm or refute the diagnosis of ADHD. Young children are often unaware of their symptoms of ADHD, and older children and adolescents may be aware of symptoms but will minimize their significance. The interview with the child or adolescent allows the clinician to identify signs or symptoms inconsistent with ADHD or suggestive of comorbid disorders. Careful assessment of mood, anxiety, and symptoms of thought disorder should be performed, as parents may not be aware of such symptoms in their child. In cases of primary ADHD without comorbidity, the mental status examination is within normal limits. The child's speech should be assessed for evidence of language delay or articulation problems. Because overt hyperactivity during the one-on-one clinical interview occurs only in the most severe cases, normal attention and activity while alone with the examiner should not be used to rule out ADHD. If the child reports pervasive depression or anxiety, flight of ideas, thought disorder, or suicidal ideation, these are inconsistent with a sole diagnosis of ADHD and may represent either a comorbid disorder or a primary disorder that is impairing attention and impulse control.

Psychological Testing

IQ and achievement testing to rule out learning disabilities are not mandatory prior to making a diagnosis of ADHD. Such testing may yield the most valid results after the symptoms of inattention have been controlled. If a child's academic performance does not improve with control of ADHD symptoms or if the developmental history or mental status examination yields evidence of language or motor delays, then IQ and achievement testing should be performed, as the child most likely has a comorbid language or learning disorder (see Chapter 11, "Psychological and Neuropsychological Testing").

Pediatric Evaluation and Laboratory Tests

The child's medical history should be obtained, as well as a physical examination within the past year. Rarely, ADHD may be secondary to severe head injury (Max et al. 1998), early exposure to lead (Lidsky and Schneider 2003), or fetal alcohol syndrome (O'Malley and Nanson 2002). There are no medical conditions that masquerade as ADHD without any other medical signs or symptoms. Children with ADHD have a higher than expected rate of sleep problems, but there is no evidence of a causative relationship between sleep disorders and ADHD (Cohen-Zion and Ancoli-Israel 2004). While children with a history of cardiovascular disease or significant cardiac symptoms (severe palpitations; fainting; exercise intolerance not accounted for by obesity; strong family history of sudden death; unexplained chest pain; or family history of arrhythmias, hypertension, or syncope) should have consultation with a pediatric cardiologist prior to starting stimulant medication, there is no need for cardiac screening (i.e., electrocardiogram) in otherwise healthy children and adolescents (Biederman et al. 2006b).

A neurological examination is not contributory to the diagnosis of ADHD. Children with ADHD may have more nonfocal "soft signs" on their neurological exam than children without ADHD, but such signs are not diagnostic and do not have relevance for selection of treatment (Pine et al. 1993). Neuroimaging studies are not indicated for the assessment of ADHD (http://archive.psych.org/edu/other_res/lib_archives/archives/200501.pdf). In the absence of specific indicators elicited in the medical history, laboratory testing is not required.

Treatment

Pharmacological treatment of ADHD is the best studied intervention in child and adolescent psychiatry. Psychosocial interventions (particularly behavior therapy) also have been extensively studied in the treatment of ADHD (Pelham et al. 1998). Over the last decade, research has focused on whether behavioral interventions can achieve the same degree of effectiveness as medication treatment or if combined medication and psychosocial interventions are superior to medication alone. Jadad et al. (1999) reviewed six studies that compared pharmacological to non-pharmacological interventions in the treatment of ADHD; superiority of stimulant over nondrug treatment was consistently found. Twenty studies compared combination therapy with a stimulant or psychosocial intervention, but no evidence of an additive benefit of combination therapy was found.

In the MTA study (Richters et al. 1995), children with ADHD were randomized to four groups: algorithmic medication treatment alone, intensive psychosocial treatment alone, a combination of algorithmic medication management and psychosocial treatment, and community treatment as usual. Algorithmic medication treatment consisted of monthly supportive appointments in which the dose of medication was carefully titrated according to parent and teacher rating scales. Children in all four treatment groups showed reduced symptoms of ADHD at 14 months relative to baseline. The two groups of children who received algorithmic medication management showed a superior outcome with regard to ADHD symptoms compared with those who received intensive behavioral treatment alone or community treatment (MTA Cooperative Group 1999). Those who received behavioral treatment alone were not significantly more improved than the group of community controls who received community treatment (two-thirds of the subjects in this group received stimulant treatment). Thus, a pharmacological intervention for ADHD is more effective than a behavioral treatment alone.

Both the MTA and Multimodal Psychosocial Treatment studies (Klein et al. 2004) examined whether adding psychosocial interventions to stimulant treatment yields a superior outcome to medication alone. The studies randomized children with ADHD alone (no significant comorbidities) to treatment with methylphenidate alone, methylphenidate plus an intensive psychosocial intervention, or methylphenidate plus an attention control. After 2 years of treatment, children who received the psychosocial intervention were no different from those treated with medication alone in terms of ADHD symptoms (Abikoff et al. 2004b), academics (Hechtman et al. 2004), or social skills (Abikoff et al. 2004a). Results in the MTA were more complex. Patients with ADHD *and* comorbid disorders and/or psychosocial stressors showed greater benefit from a combined pharmacological-psychosocial intervention relative to medication alone. Comorbid anxiety (as reported by the child's parent) predicted a better response to behavioral treatment relative to those without comorbidity (March et al. 2000), particularly when the ADHD patient had both an anxiety and a disruptive behavior disorder (ODD or CD) (Jensen et al. 2001b). Children receiving public assistance and ethnic minorities also showed a better outcome with combined treatment (Hinshaw 2007). The most recent findings of the MTA have shown that the four treatment groups continued to converge in outcome, suggesting a lack of a long-term effect of the early intensive interventions (Jensen et al. 2007; Swanson et al. 2007). At this point, the choice of treatment should be individualized to the patient, but further, very-long-term interventions (3–5 years) need to be studied to determine the best way to improve long-term outcomes for children with ADHD, particularly those with severe comorbidity.

Pharmacological Treatments

Specific information regarding the dosing, titration, and side effects of the agents reviewed below can be found in Chapter 46, "Medications Used for Attention-Deficit/Hyperactivity Disorder," and Chapter 50, "Alpha-Adrenergics, Beta-Blockers, Benzodiazepines, Buspirone, and Desmopressin."

Algorithms

Both the American Academy of Child and Adolescent Psychiatry (2007) and the Texas Children's Medication Algorithm Project (CMAP; Pliszka et al. 2006a) have issued guidelines on the selection of appropriate agents for the pharmacological treatment of ADHD. These guidelines can be found on the Internet (www.aacap.org; www.dshs.state.tx.us/mhprograms/CMAP.shtm) and are summarized in Figure 15–2. Briefly, a U.S. Food and Drug Administration (FDA)–approved agent (stimulant or atomoxetine) should be the initial choice; the CMAP algorithm recommends a stimulant treatment as the first stage. If one class of stimulant (methylphenidate or amphetamine) does not yield satisfactory results, then the other class of stimulant should be used. If a long-acting guanfacine is approved by the FDA for the treatment of ADHD, it might warrant inclusion among the agents used initially, although clinical experience with the safety and effectiveness of the agent would need to be obtained, as well as comparative studies with the stimulants and atomoxetine. Bupropion and tricyclic antidepressants should be used only when the above agents have failed.

Comorbidity influences the order of agents used for the treatment of ADHD as well as possible supplementary medications (Pliszka et al. 2006a). As shown in Figure 15–2, when anxiety is present, atomoxetine may be more likely to treat symptoms of both disorders (Geller et al. 2007). Or treatment may be initiated with a stimulant for ADHD symptoms, and a specific serotonin reuptake inhibitor (SSRI) may be added in order to control anxiety. When faced with the comorbidity of ADHD and MDD, the clinician should determine which of the two disorders is more severe; the MDD CMAP algorithm (Hughes et al. 2007) should be initiated if the depressive disorder is causing more impairment. In contrast, if the ADHD is clearly more problematic, then pharmacological intervention for it should take precedence. Whichever disorder is treated first, treatment for the comorbid disorder should be added if monotherapy does not lead to remission of both ADHD and depressive symptoms. Finally, the presence of tics is not a contraindication to the use of stimulants for treatment of ADHD (Gadow and Sverd 2006). The clinician should go stepwise through the various agents until one is found that reduces ADHD symptoms without worsening tics. Atomoxetine may reduce tics (Allen et al. 2005). In some cases, the ADHD can be controlled only by a stimulant that worsens the child's tics; in such cases an alpha-agonist can be added to the stimulant (Tourette's Syndrome Study Group 2002).

Stimulants

There are voluminous data regarding the efficacy and safety of stimulant treatment for ADHD. In a review of reviews, Swanson (1993) reported over 3,000 citations and 250 reviews of stimulant treatment, principally methylphenidate. Similar efficacy was later found for mixed amphetamine salts (Biederman et al. 2002). In more recent years, long-acting forms of methylphenidate (Concerta, Focalin XR, Metadate CD, Ritalin LA, Daytrana transdermal system) and amphetamine (Adderall XR, Vyvanse) have been widely studied and extensively reviewed (American Academy of Child and Adolescent Psychiatry 2007; Greenhill 2002); the long-acting agents are similar in efficacy and safety to the immediate-release forms. Stimulants are as effective in adolescents as in school-age children (Spencer et al. 2006; Wilens et al. 2006). Use of methylphenidate in preschoolers has been the focus of recent study. In the National Institute of Mental Health (NIMH)–funded Preschool ADHD Treatment Study (PATS), 183 children ages 3–5 years underwent an open-label trial of methylphenidate; 165 of these subjects were then randomized into a double-blind, placebo-controlled crossover trial of methylphenidate lasting 6 weeks (Greenhill et al. 2006). Methylphenidate was found to be highly effective in preschoolers, though at a lower optimal dose (0.7 mg/kg/day) than was used in the MTA school-age study; a higher rate of emotional adverse events was also noted (Wigal et al. 2006), leading to the conclusion that stimulant dose should be titrated more cautiously in preschoolers relative to older children.

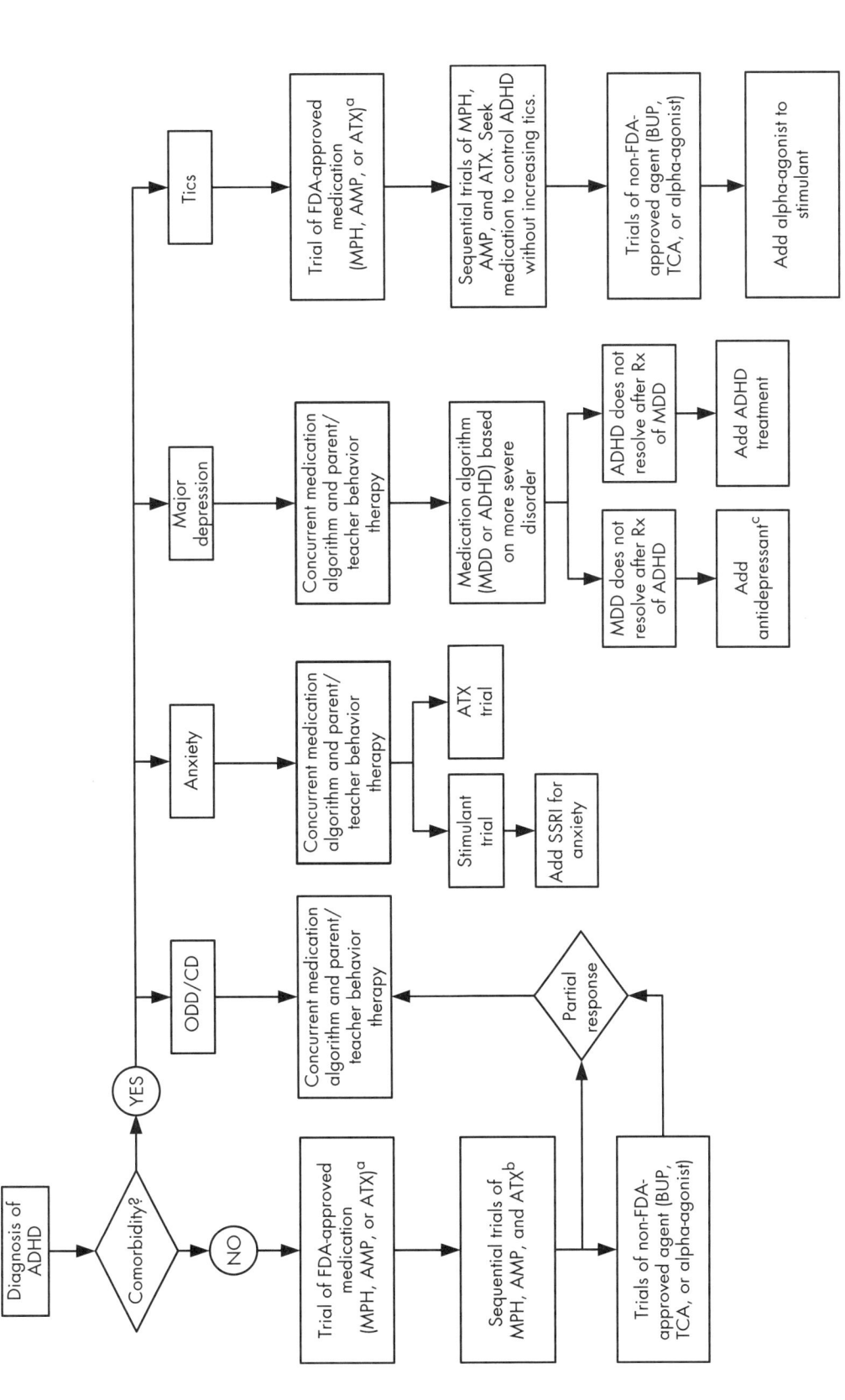

FIGURE 15–2. **Algorithm for the treatment of attention-deficit/hyperactivity disorder (ADHD) and its common comorbid disorders.**

AMP=amphetamine; ATX=atomoxetine; BUP=bupropion; FDA=U.S. Food and Drug Administration; MDD=major depressive disorder; MPH=methylphenidate; ODD/CD=oppositional defiant disorder/conduct disorder; Rx=treatment; SSRI=selective serotonin reuptake inhibitor; TCA=tricyclic antidepressants.

[a]Children's Medication Algorithm Project (CMAP) recommends stimulants as stage 1.

[b]CMAP also suggests low-dose ATX can be combined with stimulants in the event of a partial response to one agent alone.

[c]TCA and BUP have efficacy in ADHD but not childhood depression.

Arnold (2000) reviewed studies in which subjects underwent a trial of both amphetamine and methylphenidate. This review suggested that approximately 41% of subjects with ADHD responded equally to both methylphenidate and amphetamine, while 44% responded preferentially to one of the classes of stimulants. This suggests the initial response rate to stimulants may be as high as 85% if *both* stimulants are tried (in contrast to the finding of 65%–75% response when only one stimulant is tried). There is at present, however, no method to predict which stimulant will produce the best response in a given patient.

Atomoxetine

This nonstimulant agent is a noradrenergic reuptake blocker that has some indirect agonism on dopamine. Numerous studies (Michelson et al. 2001, 2002, 2003, 2004; Newcorn et al. 2005) show that it is superior to placebo in the treatment of ADHD in children and adolescents (and adults), although its effect size (0.62) appears smaller than that of stimulants (~1.0) (Faraone et al. 2003). Its full therapeutic effect may not be seen in some patients until after a month of treatment (Michelson et al. 2002).

Alpha-Agonists

The alpha-2 receptor agonists clonidine and guanfacine have varied effects on noradrenergic function (see Chapter 50, "Alpha-Adrenergics, Beta-Blockers, Benzodiazepines, Buspirone, and Desmopressin"). A meta-analysis of 11 studies of clonidine in the treatment of ADHD found variability in both method and outcome, with open-label studies showing a larger effect than controlled studies. The conclusion was that clonidine did show efficacy (Connor et al. 1999). A long-acting form of guanfacine has been shown to be efficacious in a large-scale, phase-III, double-blind, placebo-controlled study. All doses of guanfacine (1–3 mg/day) were superior to placebo at week 3, with maximal effect at week 6 (Melmed et al. 2006). The medication was well tolerated (the most common side effect was sedation); serious cardiovascular effects were not reported.

Other Agents

Antidepressants that have noradrenergic effects (bupropion, tricyclic antidepressants) have been shown to be superior to placebo in the treatment of ADHD (Conners et al. 1996; Daly and Wilens 1998). Like alpha-agonists, these medications are used when a child has not responded to stimulants or atomoxetine. Use of tri-

cyclic antidepressants has declined due to the need for monitoring with electrocardiograms and reports of a small number of cases of sudden death associated with desipramine (Riddle et al. 1991, 1993).

Psychosocial Interventions

Behavior therapy (implemented by parents and teachers) is the only psychosocial intervention validated in the treatment of ADHD (Smith et al. 2006). The principles of behavior therapy are covered in Chapter 55, "Behavioral Parent Training." Key principles of parent (or teacher) behavior therapy in the treatment of ADHD are as follows (Smith et al. 2006): 1) learning information about the nature of ADHD, 2) learning to attend more carefully to the child's misbehavior and to when the child complies, 3) establishing a home token economy, 4) using time-out effectively, 5) managing noncompliant behaviors in public settings, 6) using a daily school report card, and 7) anticipating future misconduct. Occasional booster sessions are often recommended. Importantly, parental ADHD may interfere with the success of such programs (Sonuga-Barke et al. 2002), suggesting that treatment of an affected parent may be an important part of the child's treatment. Generalized family dysfunction (parental depression, substance abuse, marital problems) may also need to be addressed for psychosocial or medication treatment to be fully effective for the child with ADHD (Chronis et al. 2004).

These procedures can be adapted for the classroom. A meta-analysis of 70 studies of behaviorally based school interventions found an effect size of 0.60 for designs comparing the active intervention to control groups (DuPaul and Eckert 1997). In contrast, cognitive-behavioral therapy for children with ADHD has not been shown to be effective (Abikoff et al. 1988) and social skills training has had mixed results (Mayhew 2003) with two recent studies showing no effects and even some evidence of peer deviancy training (Antshel and Remer 2003). Thus, behavior training done directly with the child's parent and teacher (rather than in group settings) is the most justified approach.

Practice parameters of the American Academy of Child and Adolescent Psychiatry (2007) recommend that psychosocial interventions (behavior therapy) should be added to pharmacological treatment if the child exhibits a comorbid condition or if remission of symptoms is not obtained with medication treatment alone. Figure 15–2 shows how psychosocial interventions can be used in conjunction with pharmacological intervention.

Other Treatment Modalities

There has been a long history of attempting to treat ADHD via alternative methods that do not involve the use of medication, including restrictive diets and supplements. There is, however, no therapeutic effect of removing either sugar (Milich and Pelham 1986) or food additives (Gross et al. 1987) from the child's diet. No herbal supplement has been scientifically tested for efficacy in the treatment of ADHD and any benefit of electroencephalographic "neurofeedback" remains unproven (Loo and Barkley 2005).

Research Directions

Despite six decades of research and many advances in our understanding of ADHD, much remains to be learned regarding its etiology, life course, and treatment. Further studies of candidate genes in ADHD need to determine if these polymorphisms are associated with changes in brain function leading to the clinical presentation. Genetic and neuroimaging research must come together as it is likely that genetic differences in individuals lead to alterations in brain activation during functional brain studies. It remains to be seen if neuroimaging will prove clinically useful. More longitudinal studies of the effects of treatment are needed, particularly those that follow a single cohort of children with ADHD from preschool to the middle adult years, ideally combined with neuroimaging and genetic studies. Better treatments for those with comorbid disorders, particularly learning and mood disorders, and for those who are unresponsive to first-line agents are sorely needed.

Summary Points

- Attention-deficit/hyperactivity disorder (ADHD) is a neurobiological disorder of mostly genetic origin affecting 5%–8% of children and 4% of adults. It most likely involves dysfunction in frontostriatal, cingulate, and cerebellar circuits that underlie inhibitory control, response variability, motor timing, and response to reward.

- ADHD is associated with significant morbidity. While some children have remission of symptoms as they age, others begin to develop serious adult sequelae, including antisocial behavior, academic underachievement, teen pregnancy, substance abuse, and poor employment records.

- ADHD is associated with comorbid disorders including anxiety (~33%), depression (~11%), oppositional defiant disorder, and conduct disorder (up to 50%), learning disorders (~20%), and controversially, bipolar disorder (4%–16%). Comorbid disorders complicate treatment.

- The principal treatment of ADHD is pharmacological, proceeding from the FDA-approved agents (stimulants or atomoxetine) to second-line agents (bupropion, tricyclic antidepressants, alpha-agonists).

- Psychosocial intervention (primarily behavior therapy) for ADHD should be added when comorbid disorders are present or when response to pharmacological intervention does not result in remission of symptoms.

References

Abikoff H, Ganeles D, Reiter G, et al: Cognitive training in academically deficient ADHD boys receiving stimulant medication. J Abnorm Child Psychol 16:411–432, 1988

Abikoff H, Hechtman L, Klein RG, et al: Social functioning in children with ADHD treated with long-term methylphenidate and multimodal psychosocial treatment. J Am Acad Child Adolesc Psychiatry 43:820–829, 2004a

Abikoff H, Hechtman L, Klein RG, et al: Symptomatic improvement in children with ADHD treated with long-term methylphenidate and multimodal psychosocial treatment. J Am Acad Child Adolesc Psychiatry 43:802–811, 2004b

Allen AJ, Kurlan RM, Gilbert DL, et al: Atomoxetine treatment in children and adolescents with ADHD and comorbid tic disorders. Neurology 65:1941–1949, 2005

American Academy of Child and Adolescent Psychiatry: Practice parameter for the assessment and treatment of children and adolescents with attention-deficit/hyperactivity disorder. J Am Acad Child Adolesc Psychiatry 46:894–921, 2007

American Psychiatric Association: Diagnostic and Statistical Manual of Mental Disorders, 4th Edition. Washington, DC, American Psychiatric Association, 1994

American Psychiatric Association: Diagnostic and Statistical Manual of Mental Disorders, 4th Edition, Text Revision. Washington, DC, American Psychiatric Association, 2000

Antshel KM, Remer R: Social skills training in children with attention deficit hyperactivity disorder: a randomized-controlled clinical trial. J Clin Child Adolesc Psychol 32:153–165, 2003

Arnold LE: Methylphenidate vs. amphetamine: comparative review. J Atten Disord 3:200–211, 2000

Barkley RA: Behavioral inhibition, sustained attention, and executive functions: constructing a unifying theory of ADHD. Psychol Bull 121:65–94, 1997

Barkley RA: Driving impairments in teens and adults with attention-deficit/hyperactivity disorder. Psychiatr Clin North Am 27:233–260, 2004

Barkley RA: Comorbid disorders, social and family adjustment, and subtyping, in Attention Deficit Hyperactivity Disorder. Edited by Barkley RA. New York, Guilford, 2006a, pp 184–218

Barkley RA: Primary symptoms, diagnostic criteria, prevalence and gender differences, in Attention Deficit Hyperactivity Disorder: A Handbook of Diagnosis and Treatment. Edited by Barkley RA. New York, Guilford, 2006b, pp 76–121

Barkley RA: Etiologies, in Attention-Deficit Hyperactivity Disorder. Edited by Barkley RA. New York, Guilford, 2007, pp 219–247

Barkley RA, Fischer M, Edelbrock CS, et al: The adolescent outcome of hyperactive children diagnosed by research criteria, I: an 8-year prospective follow-up study. J Am Acad Child Adolesc Psychiatry 29:546–557, 1990

Barkley RA, Guevremont DC, Anastopoulos AD, et al: Driving-related risks and outcomes of attention deficit hyperactivity disorder in adolescents and young adults: a 3- to 5-year follow-up survey. Pediatrics 92:212–218, 1993

Barkley RA, Fischer M, Smallish L, et al: Young adult follow-up of hyperactive children: antisocial activities and drug use. J Child Psychol Psychiatry 45:195–211, 2004

Barkley RA, Fischer M, Smallish L, et al: Young adult outcome of hyperactive children: adaptive functioning in major life activities. J Am Acad Child Adolesc Psychiatry 45:192–202, 2006

Biederman J: Resolved: mania is mistaken for ADHD in prepubertal children, affirmative. J Am Acad Child Adolesc Psychiatry 37:1091–1093, 1998

Biederman J: Attention-deficit/hyperactivity disorder: a selective overview. Biol Psychiatry 57:1215–1220, 2005

Biederman J, Newcorn J, Sprich S: Comorbidity of attention deficit hyperactivity disorder with conduct, depressive, anxiety, and other disorders. Am J Psychiatry 148:564–577, 1991

Biederman J, Faraone SV, Keenan K, et al: Further evidence for family genetic risk factors in attention deficit hyperactivity disorder: patterns of comorbidity in probands and relatives psychiatrically and pediatrically referred samples. Arch Gen Psychiatry 49:728–738, 1992

Biederman J, Faraone SV, Spencer T, et al: Patterns of psychiatric comorbidity, cognition, and psychosocial functioning in adults with attention deficit hyperactivity disorder. Am J Psychiatry 150:1792–1798, 1993

Biederman J, Faraone SV, Mick E, et al: High risk for attention deficit hyperactivity disorder among children of parents with childhood onset of the disorder: a pilot study. Am J Psychiatry 152:431–435, 1995a

Biederman J, Milberger S, Faraone SV, et al: Family environment risk factors for attention-deficit hyperactivity disorder: a test of Rutter's indicators of adversity. Arch Gen Psychiatry 52:464–470, 1995b

Biederman J, Milberger S, Faraone SV, et al: Impact of adversity on functioning and comorbidity in children with attention-deficit hyperactivity disorder. J Am Acad Child Adolesc Psychiatry 34:1495–1503, 1995c

Biederman J, Faraone SV, Mick E, et al: Attention deficit hyperactivity disorder and juvenile mania: an overlooked comorbidity? J Am Acad Child Adolesc Psychiatry 35:997–1008, 1996a

Biederman J, Faraone S, Milberger S, et al: A prospective 4-year follow-up study of attention-deficit hyperactivity and related disorders. Arch Gen Psychiatry 53:437–446, 1996b

Biederman J, Mick E, Faraone SV: Depression in attention deficit hyperactivity disorder (ADHD) children: "true" depression or demoralization? J Affect Disord 47:113–122, 1998

Biederman J, Lopez FA, Boellner SW, et al: A randomized, double-blind, placebo-controlled, parallel-group study of SLI381 (Adderall XR) in children with attention-deficit/hyperactivity disorder. Pediatrics 110:258–266, 2002

Biederman J, Monuteaux MC, Mick E, et al: Young adult outcome of attention deficit hyperactivity disorder: a controlled 10-year follow-up study. Psychol Med 36:167–179, 2006a

Biederman J, Spencer TJ, Wilens TE, et al: Treatment of ADHD with stimulant medications: response to Nissen perspective in the New England Journal of Medicine. J Am Acad Child Adolesc Psychiatry 45:1147–1150, 2006b

Bradley C: The behavior of children receiving benzedrine. Am J Psychiatry 94:577–585, 1937

Casey BJ, Epstein JN, Buhle J, et al: Frontostriatal connectivity and its role in cognitive control in parent-child dyads with ADHD. Am J Psychiatry 164:1729–1736, 2007

Castellanos FX, Tannock R: Neuroscience of attention deficit/hyperactivity disorder: the search for endophenotypes. Nat Rev Neurosci 3:617–628, 2002

Castellanos FX, Sonuga-Barke EJ, Scheres A, et al: Varieties of attention-deficit/hyperactivity disorder-related intra-individual variability. Biol Psychiatry 57:1416–1423, 2005

Castellanos FX, Margulies DS, Kelly C, et al: Cingulate-precuneus interactions: a new locus of dysfunction in adult attention-deficit/hyperactivity disorder. Biol Psychiatry 63:332–337, 2008

Centers for Disease Control and Prevention: Prevalence of diagnosis and medication treatment for attention deficit/hyperactivity disorder—United States 2003. MMWR Morb Mortal Wkly Rep 54:842–847, 2005

Chronis AM, Chacko A, Fabiano GA, et al: Enhancements to the behavioral parent training paradigm for families of children with ADHD: review and future directions. Clin Child Fam Psychol Rev 7:1–27, 2004

Clare Kelly AM, Uddin LQ, Biswal BB, et al: Competition between functional brain networks mediates behavioral variability. Neuroimage 39:527–537, 2008

Claude D, Firestone P: The development of ADHD boys: a 12 year follow up. Can J Behav Sci 27:226–249, 1995

Cohen-Zion M, Ancoli-Israel S: Sleep in children with attention-deficit hyperactivity disorder (ADHD): a review of naturalistic and stimulant intervention studies. Sleep Med Rev 8:379–402, 2004

Conners CK, Casat CD, Gualtieri CT, et al: Bupropion hydrochloride in attention deficit disorder with hyperactivity. J Am Acad Child Adolesc Psychiatry 35:1314–1321, 1996

Connor DF, Fletcher KE, Swanson JM: A meta-analysis of clonidine for symptoms of attention-deficit hyperactivity disorder. J Am Acad Child Adolesc Psychiatry 38:1551–1559, 1999

Daly JM, Wilens T: The use of tricyclics antidepressants in children and adolescents. Pediatr Clin North Am 45:1123–1135, 1998

Dickstein SG, Bannon K, Castellanos FX, et al: The neural correlates of attention deficit hyperactivity disorder: an ALE meta-analysis. J Child Psychol Psychiatry 47:1051–1062, 2006

Douglas VI, Peters KG: Toward a clearer definition of the attentional deficit of hyperactive children, in Attention and Cognitive Development. Edited by Hale GA, Lewis M. New York, Plenum, 1979, pp 173–248

DuPaul GJ, Eckert TL: The effects of school-based interventions for attention deficit hyperactivity disorder: a meta-analysis. Sch Psychol Dig 26:5–27, 1997

Durston S, Davidson MC, Mulder MJ, et al: Neural and behavioral correlates of expectancy violations in attention-deficit hyperactivity disorder. J Child Psychol Psychiatry 48:881–889, 2007

Epstein JN, Casey BJ, Tonev ST, et al: ADHD- and medication-related brain activation effects in concordantly affected parent-child dyads with ADHD. J Child Psychol Psychiatry 48:899–913, 2007

Faraone SV, Spencer TJ, Aleadri M, et al: Comparing the efficacy of medications used for ADHD using meta-analysis. Presented at the 156th Annual Meeting of the American Psychiatric Association, San Francisco, CA, May 2003

Faraone SV, Perlis RH, Doyle AE, et al: Molecular genetics of attention-deficit/hyperactivity disorder. Biol Psychiatry 57:1313–1323, 2005

Fischer M, Barkley RA, Edelbrock CS, et al: The adolescent outcome of hyperactive children diagnosed by research criteria, II: academic, attentional, and neuropsychological status. J Consult Clin Psychol 58:580–588, 1990

Gadow KD, Sverd J: Attention deficit hyperactivity disorder, chronic tic disorder, and methylphenidate. Adv Neurol 99:197–207, 2006

Gaub M, Carlson CL: Gender differences in ADHD: a meta-analysis and critical review. J Am Acad Child Adolesc Psychiatry 36:1036–1045, 1997

Geller B, Warner K, Williams M, et al: Prepubertal and young adolescent bipolarity versus ADHD: assessment and validity using the WASH-U-KSADS, CBCL and TRF. J Affect Disord 51:93–100, 1998a

Geller B, Williams M, Zimerman B, et al: Prepubertal and early adolescent bipolarity differentiate from ADHD by manic symptoms, grandiose delusion, ultra-rapid or ultradian cycling. J Affect Disord 51:81–91, 1998b

Geller D, Donnelly C, Lopez F, et al: Atomoxetine treatment for pediatric patients with attention-deficit/hyperactivity disorder with comorbid anxiety disorder. J Am Acad Child Adolesc Psychiatry 46:1119–1127, 2007

Gershon J: A meta-analytic review of gender differences in ADHD. J Atten Disord 5:143–154, 2002

Greenhill LL: Stimulant medication treatment of children with attention deficit hyperactivity disorder, in Attention Deficit Hyperactivity Disorder: State of Science, Best Practices. Edited by Jensen PS, Cooper JR. Kingston, NJ, Civic Research Institute, 2002, pp 9-1–9-27

Greenhill LL, Kollins S, Abikoff H, et al: Efficacy and safety of immediate-release methylphenidate treatment for preschoolers with ADHD. J Am Acad Child Adolesc Psychiatry 45:1284–1293, 2006

Gross MD, Tofanelli RA, Butzirus SM, et al: The effects of diets rich in and free from additives on the behavior of children with hyperkinetic and learning disorders. J Am Acad Child Adolesc Psychiatry 26:53–55, 1987

Hechtman L, Abikoff H, Klein RG, et al: Academic achievement and emotional status of children with ADHD treated with long-term methylphenidate and multimodal psychosocial treatment. J Am Acad Child Adolesc Psychiatry 43:812–819, 2004

Hinshaw SP: Moderators and mediators of treatment outcome for youth with ADHD: understanding for whom and how interventions work. Ambul Pediatr 7:91–100, 2007

Hughes CW, Emslie GJ, Crismon ML, et al: Texas Children's Medication Algorithm Project: update from Texas Consensus Conference Panel on Medication Treatment of Childhood Major Depressive Disorder. J Am Acad Child Adolesc Psychiatry 46:667–686, 2007

Jadad AR, Boyle M, Cunningham C, et al: Treatment of attention-deficit/hyperactivity disorder. Evid Rep Technol Assess (Summ) Nov:i–viii, 1–341, 1999

Jensen PS, Hinshaw SP, Kraemer HC, et al: ADHD comorbidity findings from the MTA study: comparing comorbid subgroups. J Am Acad Child Adolesc Psychiatry 40:147–158, 2001a

Jensen PS, Hinshaw SP, Swanson JM, et al: Findings from the NIMH Multimodal Treatment Study of ADHD (MTA): implications and applications for primary care providers. J Dev Behav Pediatr 22:60–73, 2001b

Jensen PS, Arnold LE, Swanson JM, et al: 3-year follow-up of the NIMH MTA Study. J Am Acad Child Adolesc Psychiatry 46:989–1002, 2007

Johnston C: The impact of attention deficit hyperactivity disorder on social and vocational functioning in adults, in Attention Deficit Hyperactivity Disorder: State of the Science, Best Practices. Edited by Jensen PS, Cooper JR. Kingston, NJ, Civic Research Institute, 2002, pp 6-2–6-21

Klein RG, Abikoff H, Klass E, et al: Clinical efficacy of methylphenidate in conduct disorder with and without attention deficit hyperactivity disorder. Arch Gen Psychiatry 54:1073–1080, 1997

Klein RG, Pine DS, Klein DF: Resolved: mania is mistaken for ADHD in prepubertal children, negative. J Am Acad Child Adolesc Psychiatry 37:1093–1096, 1998

Klein RG, Abikoff H, Hechtman L, et al: Design and rationale of controlled study of long-term methylphenidate and Multimodal Psychosocial Treatment in children with ADHD. J Am Acad Child Adolesc Psychiatry 43:792–801, 2004

Kreppner JM, O'Connor TG, Rutter M: Can inattention/overactivity be an institutional deprivation syndrome? J Abnorm Child Psychol 29:513–528, 2001

Lidsky TI, Schneider JS: Lead neurotoxicity in children: basic mechanisms and clinical correlates. Brain 126:5–19, 2003

Loo SK, Barkley RA: Clinical utility of EEG in attention deficit hyperactivity disorder. Appl Neuropsychol 12:64–76, 2005

Makris N, Biederman J, Valera EM, et al: Cortical thinning of the attention and executive function networks in adults with attention-deficit/hyperactivity disorder. Cereb Cortex 17:1364–1375, 2007

Mannuzza S, Klein RG, Bessler A, et al: Adult psychiatric status of hyperactive boys grown up. Am J Psychiatry 155:493–498, 1998

March JS, Swanson JM, Arnold LE, et al: Anxiety as a predictor and outcome variable in the multimodal treatment study of children with ADHD (MTA). J Abnorm Child Psychol 28:527–541, 2000

Max JE, Arndt S, Castillo CS, et al: Attention-deficit hyperactivity symptomatology after traumatic brain injury: a prospective study. J Am Acad Child Adolesc Psychiatry 37:841–847, 1998

Mayhew JE: Neuroscience: a measured look at neuronal oxygen consumption. Science 299:1023–1024, 2003

Melmed RD, Patel A, Konow J, et al: Efficacy and safety of guanfacine extended release for ADHD treatment. Presented at the 53rd Annual Meeting of the American Academy of Child and Adolescent Psychiatry, San Diego, CA, October 2006

Michelson D, Faries D, Wernicke J, et al: Atomoxetine in the treatment of children and adolescents with attention-deficit/hyperactivity disorder: a randomized, placebo-controlled, dose-response study. Pediatrics 108:1–9, 2001

Michelson D, Allen AJ, Busner J, et al: Once-daily atomoxetine treatment for children and adolescents with attention deficit hyperactivity disorder: a randomized, placebo-controlled study. Am J Psychiatry 159:1896–1901, 2002

Michelson D, Adler L, Spencer T, et al: Atomoxetine in adults with ADHD: two randomized, placebo-controlled studies. Biol Psychiatry 53:112–120, 2003

Michelson D, Buitelaar JK, Danckaerts M, et al: Relapse prevention in pediatric patients with ADHD treated with atomoxetine: a randomized, double-blind, placebo-controlled study. J Am Acad Child Adolesc Psychiatry 43:896–904, 2004

Mick E, Biederman J, Faraone SV, et al: Case-control study of attention-deficit hyperactivity disorder and maternal smoking, alcohol use, and drug use during pregnancy. J Am Acad Child Adolesc Psychiatry 41:378–385, 2002a

Mick E, Biederman J, Prince J, et al: Impact of low birth weight on attention-deficit hyperactivity disorder. J Dev Behav Pediatr 23:16–22, 2002b

Milich R, Pelham WE: Effects of sugar ingestion on the classroom and playground behavior of attention deficit disordered boys. J Consult Clin Psychol 54:714–718, 1986

MTA Cooperative Group: 14-Month randomized clinical trial of treatment strategies for children with attention deficit hyperactivity disorder. Arch Gen Psychiatry 56:1073–1086, 1999

Mulder MJ, Baeyens D, Davidson MC, et al: Familial vulnerability to ADHD affects activity in the cerebellum in addition to the prefrontal systems. J Am Acad Child Adolesc Psychiatry 47:68–75, 2008

Newcorn JH, Halperin JM, Jensen PS, et al: Symptom profiles in children with ADHD: effects of comorbidity and gender. J Am Acad Child Adolesc Psychiatry 40:137–146, 2001

Newcorn JH, Spencer TJ, Biederman J, et al: Atomoxetine treatment in children and adolescents with attention-deficit/hyperactivity disorder and comorbid oppositional defiant disorder. J Am Acad Child Adolesc Psychiatry 44:240–248, 2005

Nigg JT: What Causes ADHD? New York, Guilford, 2006

Nigg JT, Willcutt EG, Doyle AE, et al: Causal heterogeneity in attention-deficit/hyperactivity disorder: do we need neuropsychologically impaired subtypes? Biol Psychiatry 57:1224–1230, 2005

O'Malley KD, Nanson J: Clinical implications of a link between fetal alcohol spectrum disorder and attention-deficit hyperactivity disorder. Can J Psychiatry 47:349–354, 2002

Pelham WE, Wheeler T, Chronis A: Empirically supported psychosocial treatments for attention deficit hyperactivity disorder. J Clin Child Psychol 27:190–205, 1998

Pine D, Shaffer D, Schonfeld IS: Persistent emotional disorder in children with neurological soft signs. J Am Acad Child Adolesc Psychiatry 32:1229–1236, 1993

Plessen KJ, Bansal R, Zhu H, et al: Hippocampus and amygdala morphology in attention-deficit/hyperactivity disorder. Arch Gen Psychiatry 63:795–807, 2006

Pliszka SR, Carlson CL, Swanson JM: ADHD With Comorbid Disorders: Clinical Assessment and Management. New York, Guilford, 1999

Pliszka SR, Crismon ML, Hughes CW, et al: The Texas Children's Medication Algorithm Project: revision of the algorithm for pharmacotherapy of attention-deficit/hyperactivity disorder. J Am Acad Child Adolesc Psychiatry 45:642–657, 2006a

Pliszka SR, Lancaster J, Liotti M, et al: Volumetric MRI differences in treatment-naive vs chronically treated children with ADHD. Neurology 67:1023–1027, 2006b

Polanczyk G, de Lima MS, Horta BL, et al: The worldwide prevalence of ADHD: a systematic review and metaregression analysis. Am J Psychiatry 164:942–948, 2007

Richters JE, Arnold LE, Jensen PS, et al: NIMH collaborative multisite multimodal treatment study of children with ADHD, I: background and rationale. J Am Acad Child Adolesc Psychiatry 34:987–1000, 1995

Riddle MA, Nelson JC, Kleinman CS, et al: Sudden death in children receiving Norpramin: a review of three reported cases and commentary. J Am Acad Child Adolesc Psychiatry 30:104–108, 1991

Riddle MA, Geller B, Ryan N: Another sudden death in a child treated with desipramine. J Am Acad Child Adolesc Psychiatry 32:792–797, 1993

Seidman LJ, Valera EM, Makris N, et al: Dorsolateral prefrontal and anterior cingulate cortex volumetric abnormalities in adults with attention-deficit/hyperactivity disorder identified by magnetic resonance imaging. Biol Psychiatry 60:1071–1080, 2006

Sharp WS, Gottesman RF, Greenstein DK, et al: Monozygotic twins discordant for attention-deficit/hyperactivity disorder: ascertainment and clinical characteristics. J Am Acad Child Adolesc Psychiatry 42:93–97, 2003

Smith BH, Barkley RA, Shapiro CJ: Attention deficit hyperactivity disorder, in Treatment of Childhood Disorders. Edited by Mash EJ, Barkley RA. New York, Guilford, 2006, pp 65–136

Solanto MV, Abikoff H, Sonuga-Barke E, et al: The ecological validity of delay aversion and response inhibition as measures of impulsivity in AD/HD: a supplement to the NIMH multimodal treatment study of AD/HD. J Abnorm Child Psychol 29:215–228, 2001

Sonuga-Barke EJ: Psychological heterogeneity in AD/HD: a dual pathway model of behaviour and cognition. Behav Brain Res 130:29–36, 2002

Sonuga-Barke EJ, Daley D, Thompson M: Does maternal ADHD reduce the effectiveness of parent training for preschool children's ADHD? J Am Acad Child Adolesc Psychiatry 41:696–702, 2002

Spencer TJ, Abikoff HB, Connor DF, et al: Efficacy and safety of mixed amphetamine salts extended release (Adderall XR) in the management of oppositional defiant disorder with or without comorbid attention-deficit/hyperactivity disorder in school-aged children and adolescents: a 4-week, multicenter, randomized, double-blind, parallel-group, placebo-controlled, forced-dose-escalation study. Clin Ther 28:402–418, 2006

Sprich S, Biederman J, Crawford MH, et al: Adoptive and biological families of children and adolescents with ADHD. J Am Acad Child Adolesc Psychiatry 39:1432–1437, 2000

Still GF: Some abnormal psychical conditions in children. Lancet i:1008–1012, 1007–1082, 1163–1168, 1902

Swanson JM: Effect of stimulant medication on children with attention deficit disorder: a "review of reviews." Except Child 60:154–162, 1993

Swanson JM, Hinshaw SP, Arnold LE, et al: Secondary evaluations of MTA 36-month outcomes: propensity score and growth mixture model analyses. J Am Acad Child Adolesc Psychiatry 46:1003–1014, 2007

Tannock R: Cognitive correlates of ADHD, in Attention Deficit Hyperactivity Disorder: State of the Science, Best Practices. Edited by Jensen PS, Cooper JR. Kingston, NJ, Civic Research Institute, 2002, pp 8-1–8-27

Tourette's Syndrome Study Group: Treatment of ADHD in children with tics: a randomized controlled trial. Neurology 58:527–536, 2002

Valera EM, Faraone SV, Murray KE, et al: Meta-analysis of structural imaging findings in attention-deficit/hyperactivity disorder. Biol Psychiatry 61:1361–1369, 2007

van't Ent D, Lehn H, Derks EM, et al: A structural MRI study in monozygotic twins concordant or discordant for attention/hyperactivity problems: evidence for genetic and environmental heterogeneity in the developing brain. Neuroimage 35:1004–1020, 2007

Weiss G, Hechtman L: Hyperactive Children Grown Up. New York, Guilford, 2003

Wigal T, Greenhill LL, Chuang S, et al: Safety and tolerability of methylphenidate in preschool children with ADHD. J Am Acad Child Adolesc Psychiatry 45:1294–1303, 2006

Wilens TE, McBurnett K, Bukstein O, et al: Multisite controlled study of OROS methylphenidate in the treatment of adolescents with attention-deficit/hyperactivity disorder. Arch Pediatr Adolesc Med 160:82–90, 2006

Willcutt EG, Doyle AE, Nigg JT, et al: Validity of the executive function theory of attention-deficit/hyperactivity disorder: a meta-analytic review. Biol Psychiatry 57:1336–1346, 2005

Woodruff TJ, Axelrad DA, Kyle AD, et al: Trends in environmentally related childhood illnesses. Pediatrics 113:1133–1140, 2004

Wozniak J, Biederman J, Kiely K, et al: Mania-like symptoms suggestive of childhood onset bipolar disorder in clinically referred children. J Am Acad Child Adolesc Psychiatry 34:867–876, 1995

Chapter 16

Oppositional Defiant Disorder and Conduct Disorder

Christopher R. Thomas, M.D.

Disruptive and antisocial behavior in youth is the longest and most heavily studied syndrome in child and adolescent mental disorders. This interest is understandable as externalizing behaviors are more alarming and easily noticed by caregivers, resulting in the disruptive behavior disorders being the most frequent referral problem for youth and accounting for one-third to half of all cases seen in mental health clinics. This focus also reflects the recognition that adult sociopathy is almost always preceded by disruptive behavior in childhood, and our current understanding of antisocial behavior development is the most detailed description of the course of any psychopathology over the life span. The study of and intervention efforts with antisocial youth had a direct impact on the development of child mental health care in the United States. The founding of juvenile court clinics in 1899 to deal with delinquents directly resulted in the creation

of the child guidance movement and the establishment of child and adolescent psychiatry as a subspecialty.

Differences in patterns and outcomes in antisocial youth prompted Richard Jenkins and Lester Hewitt (1944) to propose specific subtypes of disruptive behavior based on study of clinic-referred youth, including the unsocialized aggressive, socialized delinquent, and overinhibited child. This led to longitudinal studies to determine which features of disruptive children were most predictive of adult outcome, most notably Lee Robins' (1966) *Deviant Children Grown Up.* Environmental factors were the mainstay of scientific inquiry until the groundbreaking studies on temperament by Thomas and Chess (1977) in the 1950s. Understanding criminal behavior as a biological or physiological phenomenon has continued with advances made in the fields of genetics and neuroscience in understanding behavior, and current studies are focusing on the complex interaction between constitutional and environmental factors.

The diagnoses of oppositional defiant disorder (ODD) and conduct disorder (CD) currently comprise the disruptive behavior disorders in the *Diagnostic and Statistical Manual of Mental Disorders* (DSM-IV [American Psychiatric Association 1994] and its text revision, DSM-IV-TR [American Psychiatric Association 2000]).

Oppositional Defiant Disorder

Definition, Clinical Description, and Diagnosis

The behaviors characteristic of ODD (Table 16–1) can lead to difficulties in all realms of social, academic, or occupational functioning. The central feature is conflict with authority, and problem behaviors are most frequently seen in interactions with those in charge. Requests or limits on behavior typically elicit a sharp reaction, and confrontations quickly degenerate into control struggles. The disputes and conflicts may be over seemingly trivial matters, but perceived threats to control and autonomy are critical issues for children with this disorder. Although negative and disobedient behavior can be normative at certain stages of development or in special circumstances, this disorder is characterized by behaviors that are more severe and frequent than normally expected and result in significant functional impairment.

Epidemiology

Prevalence of ODD in community samples varies among studies, ranging from 2% to 16%. The National Comorbidity Survey Replication, a retrospective study of 3,199 adults using DSM-IV criteria, reported a lifetime prevalence of 10.2%: 11.2% for males and 9.2% for females (Nock et al. 2007). Changes in diagnostic criteria account for some of the variation in reports. One study found a 25% reduction in prevalence in the same population using the DSM-III-R criteria instead of DSM-III (American Psychiatric Association 1980, 1987; Boyle et al. 1996). A comparison of DSM-III-R and DSM-IV (American Psychiatric Association 1994) criteria found no overall difference in community prevalence, but children diagnosed with the DSM-IV

criteria were described as more disturbed (Angold and Costello 1996). Prevalence can also be influenced by social and economic characteristics of the community, as the diagnosis is more often found in children from low-socioeconomic-status families. ODD is only slightly more common among boys than girls before age 13, and there is no apparent gender difference among teenagers (Loeber et al. 2000).

Comorbidity

Attention-deficit/hyperactivity disorder (ADHD) is the most common comorbid condition found with ODD (Speltz et al. 1999), and many children diagnosed with ADHD also have ODD (Lahey et al. 1999). It can be difficult at times to distinguish the behaviors between these two disorders and determine the root cause. Children with ADHD may be described as disobedient when actually their poor compliance is due to inattention and forgetfulness rather than willful defiance. Another important consideration is the possible presence of an anxiety disorder. Separation anxiety disorder and obsessive-compulsive disorder may initially manifest with complaints of severe tantrums. Children with ODD appear to be at higher risk for developing an anxiety disorder (Lavigne et al. 2001). Similar consideration should be given for the mood disorders, as antagonistic and disobedient behaviors are often associated features for children with mood disorders, and studies indicate children with ODD are at similar increased risk for a comorbid mood disorder (Lavigne et al. 2001).

Etiology, Mechanisms, and Risk Factors

Biological Factors

The frequent clustering of disruptive behaviors in siblings and biological relatives supports the impression that genetic factors may play a role in these disorders, but genetic studies on ODD have reported mixed findings. A twin study suggested genetic vulnerability for comorbid ODD, CD, and ADHD (Nadder et al. 2002). Separate research on 42 candidate genes for ADHD suggested association with ODD (Comings et al. 2000). Other genetic studies have associated ODD with the androgen receptor gene (Comings et al. 1996) and three dopaminergic genes (dopamine D_2 receptor, *DRD2*; dopamine-beta-hydroxylase, *DBH*; and dopamine transporter, *DAT1*; Comings et al. 1999), but some of these samples included participants with Tourette's disorder, suggesting that the

TABLE 16–1. DSM-IV-TR diagnostic criteria for oppositional defiant disorder

A. A pattern of negativistic, hostile, and defiant behavior lasting at least 6 months, during which four (or more) of the following are present:

(1) often loses temper

(2) often argues with adults

(3) often actively defies or refuses to comply with adults' requests or rules

(4) often deliberately annoys people

(5) often blames others for his or her mistakes or misbehavior

(6) is often touchy or easily annoyed by others

(7) is often angry and resentful

(8) is often spiteful or vindictive

 Note: Consider a criterion met only if the behavior occurs more frequently than is typically observed in individuals of comparable age and developmental level.

B. The disturbance in behavior causes clinically significant impairment in social, academic, or occupational functioning.

C. The behaviors do not occur exclusively during the course of a psychotic or mood disorder.

D. Criteria are not met for conduct disorder, and if the individual is age 18 years or older, criteria are not met for antisocial personality disorder.

Source. Reprinted from American Psychiatric Association: *Diagnostic and Statistical Manual of Mental Disorders,* 4th Edition, Text Revision. Washington, DC, American Psychiatric Association, 2000, p. 102. Used with permission. Copyright © 2000 American Psychiatric Association.

oppositional defiant behavior is dependent on the presence of other concurrent psychopathology.

Most investigations consider the full range of aggressive behaviors rather than ODD alone. Findings must be interpreted carefully as the samples may include participants with more severe CD or other comorbid conditions, such as ADHD. One study that looked at such distinctions found elevated levels of dehydroepiandrosterone sulfate (DHEAS) in children with ODD in comparison to children with ADHD and normal controls (van Goozen et al. 2000). Elevated DHEAS levels distinguished between children with ODD and children with ADHD while reports from their parents on the Child Behavior Checklist did not. The study authors speculate that the elevated adrenal androgen functioning in children with ODD indicates a shift in ACTH [adrenocorticotropic hormone]–beta-endorphin functioning in the hypothalamic-pituitary-adrenal axis due to early stress or genetic factors. Further investigation is needed focusing on ODD apart from other conditions in order to elucidate any underlying biological features.

Psychological Factors

Temperament is often used to explain difficult behaviors in children, but the evidence of a relationship between temperament and later behavior problems is mixed. Most of the longitudinal studies considering temperament generally support the view that the associated risk for development of later oppositional behaviors depends on the presence of other environmental factors (Frick and Morris 2004). ODD is associated with overreactive response or difficulty calming down. Attachment theory offers a plausible explanation for the development of oppositional behaviors since they typically involve control struggles with caregivers and issues of autonomy (Guttmann-Steinmetz and Crowell 2006). ODD has been associated with insecure attachment, but only in school-age children, not preschool children. While this might indicate that a secure attachment serves as a protective factor in the face of other risks for the development of the disorder, it may also reflect that early ODD behaviors in children adversely affect child-parent attachment. Research in cognitive processing has focused on how defiant children develop a hostile perspective based on early negative experiences. In comparison to other children, those with ODD are more vigilant for hostile cues from others and twice as likely to generate aggressive responses to problems (Coy et al. 2001). Additional research shows how they have other deficits in social problem solving, using less pertinent social information and generating fewer alternative reactions. Studies focusing on information processing outside of relationships have found that children with ODD have difficulty with response preservation and motivational inhibition tasks. In one study (van Goozen et al. 2004), the motivational inhibition task correctly discriminated 77% of children as normal controls or youth with ODD. The investigators concluded that when oppositional children are stimulated by possible reward, they are less sensitive to the possibility of punishment.

Sociological Factors

Various environmental factors are correlated with increased risk for ODD. Lower socioeconomic status is associated with risk, but this is probably mediated by family stresses and resulting dysfunction. Many other family attributes are correlated with higher rates of oppositional behaviors and include poor parenting practices, parental discord, domestic violence, low family cohesion, child abuse, and parental mental disorder, especially substance abuse and antisocial personality disorder (Greene et al. 2002). Mothers of children at increased risk for oppositional and disruptive behaviors report feeling less competent as parents, having fewer solutions for child behavior problems, and being less assertive in management of child misbehavior (Cunningham and Boyle 2002). Studies also support that harsh or inconsistent limit setting is predictive of later oppositional and antisocial behaviors (Burke et al. 2002). Most developmental theories propose that parental response to normal oppositional behavior in toddlers is central in shaping either adaptive social skills or increased defiance. Patterson's coercion model describes how deviant behavior may be reinforced in parent-child interactions when a parent drops a demand or limit in response to a negative reaction by the child (Patterson et al. 1992). While this dynamic occurs in all families, it becomes critical when it is the predominant parental reaction. It must be remembered that the influences in parent-child interactions go both ways and that the extreme negative behaviors of a child can add to family conflict and parental stress.

Prevention

While some prevention efforts focus specifically on ODD behaviors, most have included all CD behaviors in concentrating on the entire range of disruptive behaviors and long-term outcomes. Prevention efforts for ODD should then include for consideration all of the programs that target the age groups younger than the usual onset of the disorder: infants, toddlers, and preschoolers. Given the target age group, most of these efforts work on improving parenting skills or the parent-child relationship (Webster-Stratton and Taylor 2001). Nurse home-visitation programs for at-risk mothers have shown outcome differences in randomized controlled studies for lower rates of child abuse and neglect and delinquency (Olds et al. 1998). One of the more extensively studied prevention programs is The Incredible Years parenting program (Webster-Stratton et al. 2008), a parent group training approach, which is effective in reducing disruptive behaviors among at-risk children or those with emerging problems. There are now two versions of this program, one for preschool children ages 2–6 years and one for school-age children ages 5–10 years. Both programs train parents in behavioral management techniques and foster better parenting practices and involvement in their child's education and development. Two additional programs with evidence for preventing oppositional behaviors in at-risk children that use parent group training are the Coping Skills Parenting Program (Cunningham et al. 1995) and the DARE to Be You program (not associated with the Drug Abuse Resistance Education [DARE] program) (Miller-Heyl et al. 1998).

Course and Prognosis

The typical age at onset appears to be around age 6 years, when most children have outgrown earlier, normative oppositional behaviors. ODD demonstrates high stability over time, and stability correlates to the severity of the symptoms (Loeber et al. 2000). Longitudinal studies have shown that children diagnosed with the disorder are at significant risk for continued disruptive behavior symptoms. While most children with ODD will not go on to develop CD, they are at greater risk for later development of it. Among boys with ODD, those who developed CD had higher numbers of ODD symptoms than those who did not, and the symptoms of ODD typically persisted after the onset of CD (Loeber et al. 1993). In boys with ODD, atypical family structure appears to increase the risk of progression to CD (Rowe et al. 2002). Just as CD is an associated and predictive condition for later development of antisocial personality disorder, so ODD appears to be associated and predictive of CD. In preschool-age children, the presence of ODD is also predictive of later diagnosis of ADHD (Lavigne et al. 2001).

Evaluation

Interview

Determination of a diagnosis of ODD requires a thorough and complete examination following the general principles of child psychiatric evaluation (see Chapter 6, "The Process of Assessment and Diagnosis"). Interviews should be conducted with both the child and the parent or guardian. Information should be collected regarding the manifesting problems and any ODD criterion behaviors that are not volunteered by the family (American Academy of Child and Adolescent Psychiatry 2007). Particular attention should also be given to signs and symptoms for differential diagnoses and comorbid diagnoses. The onset, frequency, and severity of each problem behavior can be helpful in distinguishing ODD from other conditions with defiant behaviors. It is best to conduct separate interviews of the parent and child, as a long litany of parental complaints can be humiliating to the child and potentially provoke a confrontation during the examination. It can be misleading to take at face value a parent's complaint that a child won't listen or follow directions, since this could reflect inattention, receptive language problems, or hearing loss, as opposed to defiance. It is better to ask caregivers to describe a recent example or incident. Oppositional youth will typically view their defiance as a justified and appropriate response and readily tell their side of the story. They are less likely to cooperate if interviewed in a way that implies they are to blame, so it is important to maintain a neutral stance in asking about their behaviors and avoid using pejorative terms. A thorough developmental, family, and social history is critical in distinguishing between ODD, normative behavior, and behaviors due to situational stress. Information should also be collected on parenting practices and expectations, especially how the behaviors are handled and any previous attempts to deal with them, such as time-outs or star charts. Careful attention should be given to the potential for physical or sexual abuse and neglect as these are known risk factors. In addition, disruptive behavior can elicit harsh, physical punishment. Collateral information from other sources, like teachers and other caregivers, is particularly useful in determining if the defiant behavior is seen only in the parent-child relationship or also occurs in other settings.

Rating Scales

A number of rating scales exist that can help in distinguishing deviant oppositional and disruptive behavior from normative development or other conditions. One of the most commonly used is the Child Behavior Checklist (Achenbach and Rescorla 2000) and related Teacher Report Form, with an Aggressive subscale consisting of primarily disruptive and oppositional behaviors. The Eyberg Child Behavior Inventory and Sutter-Eyberg Student Behavior Inventory—Revised (Eyberg and Pincus 1999) are more extensive parent and teacher reports of disruptive behaviors in children and adolescents associated with ODD, CD, and ADHD and are helpful in discriminating among the different disorders and nonclinical conditions (Burns and Patterson 2000). A different approach to assessment of disruptive behaviors is taken with the Home and School Situations Questionnaires (Barkley 1997). These instruments assess the context of the problem behaviors and provide information about potential intervention opportunities based on specific precipitants, settings, or time of day in designing treatment plans and tracking results.

Differential Diagnosis

It is critical to distinguish ODD from developmentally appropriate oppositional behaviors, but studies have shown that the diagnosis can reliably be made in both preschool children and adolescents. Oppositional behaviors may occur as a transient reaction to a specific stressor and are therefore more appropriately diagnosed as an adjustment disorder with disturbance of conduct. The presence of more severe antisocial behaviors should indicate the possibility of CD. ODD behaviors do not include physical aggression or violations of the law. As previously noted, many youth with CD will also have symptoms of ODD, but the DSM-IV-TR rule is to diagnose only CD in those situations. The inattentive, impulsive behaviors of ADHD can often appear to be oppositional but are not usually willful defiance. ODD and ADHD frequently co-occur, and both diagnoses should be given in those patients meeting criteria for both disorders. Transient oppositional behaviors and irritability can be seen in reaction to stress, such as a family move, divorce, physical illness, or sleep deprivation. Because youth with mood and psychotic disorders can exhibit oppositional behavior, ODD should not be diagnosed if the disruptive behaviors are seen only during an episode of a mood or psychotic disorder. Oppositional behaviors can also be seen in children with mental retardation but should not be diagnosed as ODD unless those behaviors are in excess of what is developmentally appropriate. Failure to follow instructions may also result from impaired hearing or language comprehension problems.

While psychotic and pervasive developmental disorders can also exhibit hostile and negativistic behaviors, the presence of more bizarre symptoms usually distinguishes these disorders from ODD.

Other Evaluations

A pediatric physical exam can help in screening for illness that might underlie disruptive behaviors as well as signs of abuse or neglect. A hearing exam can also rule out the possibility of hearing impairment or loss. Speech and language evaluation can clarify if there are language processing difficulties. Associated learning impairments can be identified with appropriate intelligence and achievement testing.

Treatment

Pharmacological Treatments

No evidence exists to support an indication for specific medication use in treatment of ODD, per se. There are reports of reduction in oppositional behaviors with indicated pharmacological treatment of concurrent disorders (American Academy of Child and Adolescent Psychiatry 2007), such as ADHD. Medications for ADHD, including stimulants and clonidine, have been noted to reduce comorbid oppositional behaviors along with the primary symptoms of inattention, hyperactivity, and impulsivity (see Chapter 15, "Attention-Deficit/Hyperactivity Disorder"). There are clinical reports that atomoxetine (Bangs et al. 2008) and buspirone (Gross 1995) can reduce ODD behaviors in children with comorbid ADHD. Other symptoms of ODD are reduced with medication treatment of more severe physical aggression in youth (see the discussion of CD in the subsection "Treatment" later in this chapter; see also Chapter 37, "Aggression and Violence"), including the neuroleptics and mood stabilizers, but these medications have not been systematically studied in cases with only ODD.

Psychotherapeutic Treatments

Numerous interventions have been developed and tried, usually based on associated parental risk factors and individual social skills deficits that contribute to oppositional and defiant behavior. Several reviews and meta-analytic studies have identified promising evidence-based treatment approaches. Of these, parent management training and child problem-solving skills training have demonstrated the greatest efficacy with ODD. Parent management training indirectly af-

fects child behavior by improving parent skills in dealing with negative acts and promoting desired behaviors (Kazdin 2005; see Chapter 55, "Behavioral Parent Training"). Child problem-solving skills training derives from cognitive-behavioral therapy techniques in correcting dysfunctional social interactions and focuses on delaying impulsive responses, increasing reflection on alternative solutions, anticipating consequences, and practicing self-assessment of behaviors (Kazdin 2000). Parent management and child problem-solving skills training can be combined, and reports indicate significant additional improvement when used together as opposed to using just one approach (Kazdin et al. 1992). As with most conditions, early intervention appears to increase the chances for improvement.

Conduct Disorder

Definition, Clinical Description, and Diagnosis

The central feature of CD (Table 16–2) is a repetitive pattern of behavior that violates the rights of others or major societal rules. There is no one required or pathognomonic behavior for diagnosis but rather a range of acts that by their number, severity, and persistence for at least 12 months define the condition. Although some of the behaviors may be chargeable offenses and result in arrest, the diagnosis of CD should not be confused with the legal term of *delinquency*. In contrast to the diagnosis of adult antisocial personality disorder, all of the diagnostic criteria for CD are observable, objective behaviors rather than inferred, internal constructs, such as lack of remorse or deceitfulness. Repeated studies have found the CD behaviors to be reliable and valid criteria in identifying those youth at greatest risk for continued antisocial behavior (Loeber et al. 2000). Studies have considered the association of interpersonal callousness and CD and compared their ability to predict later psychopathy, but the relationships are complicated and require further study (Burke et al. 2007).

Related to the issue of outcome, various subtypes of CD have been proposed in the past, usually in an attempt to better identify those individuals at greatest risk for continuation onto antisocial personality disorder. DSM-IV-TR classifies CD into three subtypes based on age at onset: childhood, adolescent, or unspecified. Research indicates that those with child-

TABLE 16–2. DSM-IV-TR diagnostic criteria for conduct disorder

A. A repetitive and persistent pattern of behavior in which the basic rights of others or major age-appropriate societal norms or rules are violated, as manifested by the presence of three (or more) of the following criteria in the past 12 months, with at least one criterion present in the past 6 months:

Aggression to people and animals

(1) often bullies, threatens, or intimidates others

(2) often initiates physical fights

(3) has used a weapon that can cause serious physical harm to others (e.g., a bat, brick, broken bottle, knife, gun)

(4) has been physically cruel to people

(5) has been physically cruel to animals

(6) has stolen while confronting a victim (e.g., mugging, purse snatching, extortion, armed robbery)

(7) has forced someone into sexual activity

Destruction of property

(8) has deliberately engaged in fire setting with the intention of causing serious damage

(9) has deliberately destroyed others' property (other than by fire setting)

Deceitfulness or theft

(10) has broken into someone else's house, building, or car

(11) often lies to obtain goods or favors or to avoid obligations (i.e., "cons" others)

(12) has stolen items of nontrivial value without confronting a victim (e.g., shoplifting, but without breaking and entering; forgery)

Serious violations of rules

(13) often stays out at night despite parental prohibitions, beginning before age 13 years

(14) has run away from home overnight at least twice while living in parental or parental surrogate home (or once without returning for a lengthy period)

(15) is often truant from school, beginning before age 13 years

B. The disturbance in behavior causes clinically significant impairment in social, academic, or occupational functioning.

C. If the individual is age 18 years or older, criteria are not met for antisocial personality disorder.

Code based on age at onset:

312.81 Conduct disorder, childhood-onset type: onset of at least one criterion characteristic of conduct disorder prior to age 10 years

312.82 Conduct disorder, adolescent-onset type: absence of any criteria characteristic of conduct disorder prior to age 10 years

312.89 Conduct disorder, unspecified onset: age at onset is not known

Specify severity:

Mild: few if any conduct problems in excess of those required to make the diagnosis **and** conduct problems cause only minor harm to others

Moderate: number of conduct problems and effect on others intermediate between "mild" and "severe"

Severe: many conduct problems in excess of those required to make the diagnosis **or** conduct problems cause considerable harm to others hood onset are at greater risk than adolescent onset for continued and more severe disruptive and antisocial behaviors (Loeber et al. 1998). Childhood onset is defined as the appearance of at least one criterion CD behavior prior to age 10. Those with childhood onset are typically male, exhibit physically aggressive behaviors, previously had ODD, and have concurrent ADHD. Further qualification is given to the subtype classification with description of the symptoms as being mild, moderate, or severe, based on the variety and seriousness of the antisocial behaviors, as these features are also predictive of continued disruptive behavior.

Epidemiology

Prevalence of CD has ranged from 1% to 16% in community studies, with most indicating a rate of 5%. As with ODD, prevalence rates for CD vary depending on which DSM edition criteria were used, as well as other characteristics of the sample. The National Comorbidity Survey Replication reported a lifetime prevalence of 9.5%: 12% for males and 7.1% for females (Nock et al. 2006). It and some other studies found a slight increase in prevalence with age, while others report no differences in prevalence from childhood to adolescence. The specific CD behaviors show great variation in prevalence by age. For example, the overall prevalence of any physical fighting decreases from childhood to adolescence, but more serious physical assaults tend to increase.

A striking and consistent finding is that CD is more prevalent among boys than girls, with rates three to four times higher (Loeber et al. 2000). This feature has prompted discussion that the diagnostic criteria be modified for girls, since their antisocial behaviors tend to be less aggressive than boys. CD is also more common among children and adolescents from low-socioeconomic-status families and from neighborhoods with high rates of crime and social disorganization (Burke et al. 2002). Although CD is typically perceived as a problem of inner-city youth, studies comparing prevalence between urban and rural populations have found conflicting results.

Comorbidity

ODD is not diagnosed if criteria for CD are met by the DSM-IV-TR rule, although ODD symptoms may be present. The relationship between the two disorders is the focus of extensive research in view of the frequent co-occurrence. Some argue that ODD and CD represent a single disorder (Rowe et al. 2005), but other epidemiological studies support the DSM-IV-TR position that they represent two separate but related disorders (Loeber et al. 1998). ADHD is a common current or prior diagnosis in CD youth, especially those with childhood onset. Longitudinal research on the risk associated with ADHD for later development of CD has been less clear, although retrospective reports in the National Comorbidity Survey Replication indicated impulse problems preceded conduct problems (Nock et al. 2006). When CD does appear in children with ADHD, the antisocial behaviors are more severe and appear earlier than in children without ADHD. Substance use is also strongly associated with CD and vice versa. CD typically precedes or coincides with the onset of substance use. Perhaps surprisingly, CD appears to co-occur with the anxiety disorders. Studies conflict as to whether the onset of anxiety disorder precedes or follows CD. Symptoms of depression and antisocial behaviors frequently co-occur in adolescence, but studies on the association between major depression and CD have conflicting results. The National Comorbidity Survey Replication found that CD typically preceded the onset of mood disorders. When they do occur together, resolution of depressive symptoms is correlated with reduction in antisocial behaviors. While bipolar disorder frequently manifests with disruptive behaviors, there is little information on its relationship with CD. Studies have found in adolescents with their first bipolar episode that if there was a prior childhood psychiatric diagnosis, it was usually a disruptive behavior disorder or ADHD. The risk for development of comorbid disorders is not uniform across all youth with CD (Loeber et al. 2000). Those with childhood onset appear to have a different risk profile than those with adolescent onset, including higher rates of ADHD, low IQ, and other neuropsychiatric disorders. The difference by gender for comorbid disorder is most striking, as girls with CD are at far greater risk for concurrent psychiatric illness, including ADHD, anxiety disorders, mood disorders, and substance use.

Etiology, Mechanisms, and Risk Factors

It is no surprise any specific etiology has yet to be identified that accounts for all cases of CD, since it is a syndrome defined by a combination of various antisocial acts. Researchers have described an impressive number of factors that identify increased risk for onset and further development of the condition. Many of these risk factors may be associated with or prove to be causal mechanisms. Several models have been proposed that include many of the factors associated with disruptive behaviors, but there is no agreement on a single etiology, and further research is likely to identify several mechanisms. It is generally agreed that this heterogeneous syndrome is developmental in nature and results from the action of adverse environmental influences on a vulnerable individual at critical stages of growth (Loeber and Hay 1994).

Biological Factors

The occurrence of cases within families and differences in risk by gender support the view of possible genetic influences on the disorder. Antisocial behavior is likely a polygenetic phenomenon, with different genes being expressed at different stages of development, although certain genes may be associated with specific behaviors (Burt and Mikolajewski 2008; Moffitt 2005). Studies report a moderate degree of heritability for aggression, delinquency, and antisocial behavior from childhood to adulthood (Eley et al. 1999; Taylor et al. 2000). Behavioral genetics research also indicates heritability for other factors associated with increased risk of CD, such as impulsivity, temperament, and attention deficits (Cadoret et al. 1995; Miles and Carey 1997). Twin studies suggest that the relative importance of genetic and environmental influences may vary for different components of the disorder (Eley et al. 1999; Rowe 1985). Adoption studies demonstrate significant interactions between genetic heritage and adverse environment, although less than that reported in twin studies. The risk for CD and aggression in the children of biological parents with antisocial behaviors was a function of the relative adverse environment in the adoptive home.

One obvious piece of evidence in support of a genetic contribution to CD is the gender difference in prevalence, but gender differences also are not solely genetic and include social attitudes and conditions. High testosterone levels are associated with aggression and the early onset of aggressive behaviors (Pliszka 1999). Curiously, twin and adoption studies have not revealed any differences by sex in the extent or type of influence for either genetic or environmental influences. Attention has recently focused on the association of antisocial behaviors and the gene for monoamine oxidase A (MAOA), an enzyme involved in the metabolism of several neurotransmitters. Among abused boys, those with a variant gene for low MAOA activity appear to be twice as likely to develop CD compared to those with normal MAOA activity (Caspi et al. 2002). Environmental influences on this possible genetic vulnerability are critical, as when there is no history of abuse, boys with the low-activity MAOA gene seem to be at no greater risk than other nonabused boys for the later development of antisocial behavior.

Other neurotransmitter differences—especially those involved in sympathetic arousal—appear to play a role in antisocial and aggressive behaviors, but the reports are inconsistent. There are contrary findings on activity of both norepinephrine and dopamine metabolites in association with CD, but these inconsistencies may be the result of the differences in age groups sampled or the small numbers of study participants. While low cerebrospinal fluid levels of 5-hydroxyindoleacetic acid, a serotonin metabolite, are found in CD children (Kruesi et al. 1990), high peripheral blood levels of serotonin are correlated with childhood-onset CD (Unis et al. 1997). A related area of research is with physiological markers that have associated low sympathetic arousal to CD. Low resting heart rate is predictive of adolescent antisocial behavior (Mezzacappa et al. 1996) and later criminal behavior (Ortiz and Raine 2004). Skin conductance in response to arousing stimuli was found to be inversely correlated in children with CD (Herpertz et al. 2003), but there are conflicting reports. Low-level salivary cortisol is predictive of boys who progress from CD to antisocial personality disorder (Vanyukow et al. 1993). Just as with the genetic studies, many of the physiological differences reported may represent alterations brought about by adverse events or influences at specific stages of development. There is growing evidence from animal and human studies of lasting physical and metabolic changes in the brain as a result of severe stress or insult, which is of particular relevance in our understanding of biological factors affecting antisocial behavior.

Development of antisocial behaviors is associated with early toxic exposures, such as lead (Needleman et al. 1996), and with opiate and methadone exposure (prenatal) (De Cubas and Field 1993). Maternal smoking during pregnancy also increases risk for CD (Wakschlag et al. 2002), independent of whether there is comorbid ADHD or not (Wakschlag et al. 2006). Children exposed to prenatal maternal smoking were also more likely to have an earlier onset of delinquent behavior.

Psychological Factors

Several areas of psychological impairment are associated with increased risk for CD. Poor academic achievement is consistently noted, but this association may be reciprocal with antisocial behaviors disrupting academic performance, as well as academic frustration prompting acting-out behaviors. Just as complicated is the association of low IQ and antisocial behaviors. A meta-analytic review of studies conducted by Hogan (1999) found that comorbid ADHD accounted for any relationship between CD and low intelligence, but a more recent study (Simonoff et al. 2004) indicated that low intelligence was significantly correlated with conduct problems. Impaired verbal ability is significantly associated with antisocial behaviors even after controlling for other possible confounds, including race, socioeconomic status, and academic achievement (Moffitt et al. 1993). A key factor in the association between deficits in verbal abilities and antisocial behaviors may be the additional presence of attention problems (Lahey et al. 1995). CD is correlated with other problems in executive functions, including anticipation and planning, inhibition of impulsive behaviors, and abstract reasoning, especially in those with comorbid ADHD. Longitudinal studies have found that the presence of these deficits appears to be related to the early onset as well as subsequent persistence of antisocial behaviors. As in ODD, CD is associated with deficits in social cognition and essential skills in dealing with confrontations with others (Dodge 1993). These youth perceive others as hostile, miss important social cues, generate fewer alternative responses, and react impulsively in social interactions. Temperament traits of negative emotionality (such as overreactivity) are associated with antisocial behaviors, and there is evidence that fearlessness and stimulation seeking in early childhood are predictive of later aggression (Sanson and Prior 1999). Children with chronic illness or disability are three times more likely to have conduct misbehaviors, and the risk increases to five times more likely if the illness involves the central nervous system (Cadman et al. 1987).

Sociological Factors

Numerous environmental factors, such as family and neighborhood characteristics, are correlated with increased risk of CD (Burke et al. 2002). Harshly disciplined and physically or sexually abused youth are at greater risk for developing antisocial behaviors. One study reported that sexually abused children were 12 times more likely to develop CD even when controlling for other factors, although further research in this area is needed (Trickett and Putnam 1998). Physical abuse and neglect are particularly associated with later aggressive and violent behavior (Widom and

Maxfield 1996). As described above, physical abuse may be a necessary trigger for aggressive and antisocial behaviors in specifically vulnerable children with low MAOA activity. Parental rejection, neglect, and lack of involvement with their children also contribute to antisocial outcomes (McFayden-Ketchum et al. 1996). Other family problems associated with increased occurrence of CD include poverty, marital discord, domestic violence, parental alcohol or substance abuse, parental criminality, and parental mental illness. Higher rates of CD are found in disadvantaged neighborhoods characterized by poor housing, crime, substance abuse, and community disorganization. These influences may act by both placing the family under greater stress and presenting negative role models. Exposure to physical violence is consistently found to be a contributing factor in the development of later aggression and other antisocial behaviors, whether it is in the family, in the neighborhood, or through the media. Repeated viewing of violent acts leads to direct imitation and generally increased aggressive behavior. Association with deviant peers is a significant factor in the onset of delinquency and escalation of violence (Dishion et al. 1995; Henry et al. 2001). In addition to serving as role models, peers and their activities can directly promote antisocial behavior, with two-thirds of all delinquent acts committed by adolescents occurring in groups of two or more (Aultman 1980). The presence of a delinquent adolescent in a peer group can influence the entire group, resulting in delinquent behavior even if the other adolescents had few prior conduct problems (Patterson et al. 1992). The influence of youth gangs on delinquent and aggressive behavior of members is even greater than associating with antisocial peers (Battin et al. 1998; Thomas et al. 2003).

The best theoretical and empirical models propose cumulative risk, with increasing likelihood of CD with each additional negative influence. Longitudinal studies suggest that certain risks exert more or less influence depending upon the age of the child, the stage of the disorder, or the presence of some other factor. This might explain contradictory findings of studies focusing on the same risk factor, because their samples differed in key aspects. It is also important to consider that risk factors are not static and can interact with or mediate the influence of other risks, such as marital discord leading to inconsistent discipline. The importance of the various risks is in the accrual and progression of influences over the unfolding development of antisocial behaviors.

Prevention

The emotional and physical costs of this disorder for individuals, their families, and society have prompted numerous attempts in prevention for both the general and at-risk populations (Offord and Bennett 1994). Many prevention efforts are an extension of treatments, such as parent management or individual skills training, in an attempt to improve outcomes by earlier intervention and reduced interference with normal development (Greenberg 2006). Head Start is an example of an enrichment program for academic performance that, as an indirect benefit, reduces adolescent rates of delinquency and antisocial behaviors for high-risk groups of children. Other programs have been developed to target specific early or pathway entry behaviors, such as truancy or bullying (Smith et al. 2003). Preliminary studies indicate that some of the school-based skills programs can lead to reduced rates of disruptive behavior in comparison (Mytton et al. 2006).

Protective factors identified as improving resilience (often the converse of specific risk factors) include being female, having a high IQ, or having an easy temperament. Others appear to counterbalance certain risk factors, as in having a positive relationship with at least one parent or adult that can compensate for other negative relationships. Other protective factors include having areas of competence outside of school, good academic skills, and the ability to plan ahead or use other coping strategies (Dishion and Connell 2006). One important area of protection appears to be good interpersonal skills, such as being able to relate to others. Further study is necessary to confirm the exact nature of protective factors within high-risk groups and if they offer new means for prevention programs.

Course and Prognosis

CD is a very stable diagnosis over time, with 45%–90% still meeting criteria for diagnosis after 3–4 years. While the diverse and individual clustering of antisocial behaviors seems to be random, their appearance and development typically follow a predictable course. Initial problems are minor, with less severe acts that progress over time to include new and more severe behaviors. Based on multifactorial analysis and longitudinal studies, Rolf Loeber and colleagues have proposed a model that describes the developmental progression of three types of antisocial behaviors (Loeber and Hay 1994).

The three groups of highly associated behaviors are termed overt, authority conflict, and covert behaviors. *Overt behaviors* include physically aggressive acts and develop from bullying to physical fighting and then on to more severe assaults. *Authority conflict* starts with stubbornness that then leads to more defiant acts, such as running away or truancy. *Covert behaviors* often begin with lying or shoplifting and then progress to vandalism and burglary. Each group of behaviors appears to have a typical age at onset, with authority conflict the earliest of the three. While many youth will exhibit early and minor behaviors, fewer and fewer advance to each successive stage of more severe antisocial acts. The further a youth develops in a particular pathway cluster, the more likely it is that behavior from the other pathways will appear. Youth with the most severe behaviors will then often exhibit the widest variety of antisocial acts. This model may explain some of the differences in findings and difficulties with previous attempts in defining subcategories of CD. About 40% of individuals diagnosed with CD go on to have antisocial personality disorder. Among those who do not, most will manifest significant functional impairment in relationships and work. CD has also been linked to other adverse adult outcomes, including substance use and other psychiatric disorders (Hechtman and Offord 1994). Retrospective reports indicate that a history of CD increases the risk for subsequent psychiatric disorder, but remission of CD is associated with significantly lower risk. It remains to be shown whether the adult problems with functioning and mental disorders are a direct result of CD, a consequence of associated conditions and impairments (such as academic failure and incarceration), or both.

Evaluation

Interview

The examination of complaints of antisocial behaviors should follow the same steps and techniques as described for evaluation of oppositional behaviors above. The hostile and often suspicious nature of antisocial youth can present problems in establishing rapport. This is also often true for their parent or guardian, since many of these evaluations have not been initiated by the family but were required by other agencies. It is best to make clear to both the parent and the child the purpose of and what will happen during the interview and that it is very important to hear both sides of the story. A matter-of-fact approach that avoids making judgmental observations or placing blame is most productive. Research has found self-report of antisocial behavior to be quite accurate, although multiple sources are the most helpful in obtaining a complete picture. It is often mistakenly assumed that antisocial youth will deny or not report their misdeeds. In fact, they usually consider their antisocial behaviors to be justified and appropriate and sometimes are even boastful. Antisocial youth may conceal or lie about their activities if they believe that revealing information will result in consequences or punishment. When confronted with inconsistencies in their explanations for an incident, they will often offer another excuse without hesitation. Physical agitation and threats should be taken seriously and responded to quickly, and the interview should be terminated if there is any question as to the physical safety of those involved. The onset, frequency, and severity of each antisocial behavior are important in determining the specific subtype and overall severity classification of CD. Presence of risk factors, including history of physical and sexual abuse and family violence and criminality, should be determined (American Academy of Child and Adolescent Psychiatry 1997). Information about gang membership and peer antisocial behavior, as well as positive peer relationships, is important in determining adverse influences and potential opportunities for change. School information is extremely helpful in assessing academic difficulties and behavior outside the home. Inquiries should be made about any involvement of child protective services and juvenile justice. Legal charges and court history should be collected for any delinquency. Frequently associated behaviors and problems, including substance abuse and risk taking behaviors, should be assessed.

Rating Scales

The rating scales described for ODD are useful in assessment of the range and intensity of antisocial behaviors. In addition, there are scales that specifically appraise aggression, delinquency, and sociopathic traits. The Overt Aggression Scale was originally developed to measure verbal and physical aggression among child and adult psychiatric inpatients (Yudofsky et al. 1986). It has proved to be a useful tool in tracking changes in aggressive behaviors in response to treatment. The Children's Aggression scale is another measure of aggression, specifically developed for children ages 6–11 based on parent or teacher report (Halperin et al. 2002), but it is relatively new and there is less information regarding its use. The Antisocial Process Screening Device (Frick and Hare 2001) is a parent and teacher report based on the adult Hare

Psychopathy Checklist—Revised that seeks to measure callousness, narcissism, and impulsivity, all of which are considered features of sociopathy.

Differential Diagnosis

Antisocial behaviors can be part of many different conditions that merit careful consideration. A single occurrence of deviant behavior or minor incidents of misbehavior may represent isolated antisocial acts or normative risk-taking behaviors. Conduct misbehavior that appears following a significant stressor should merit consideration as an adjustment disorder with disturbance of conduct, but this would not cover preexisting antisocial behaviors exacerbated by stressors. As previously noted, youth with ODD will not have antisocial behaviors, but appearance of antisocial acts that do not yet meet criteria for diagnosis may indicate the onset of CD. ADHD can be marked by extremely disruptive behaviors that do not conform to rules or expectations but by itself does not represent a violation of age-appropriate societal norms. ADHD and CD are both diagnosed when found together. Conduct problems and irritability are frequently encountered in youth with mood disorders and usually can be distinguished by the occurrence of behavior problems only during episodes of the mood disorder. Psychotic disorders can sometimes mimic the appearance of CD with symptoms of physical aggression or other antisocial acts. Antisocial personality disorder should be considered as the diagnosis for individuals older than age 18 years.

Other Evaluations

A physical exam and medical history are important to assess any concurrent medical problems, as well as to screen for signs of abuse. Health issues associated with risk-taking behavior, such as head trauma, pregnancy, sexually transmitted diseases, and hepatitis serum, should be screened, and urine drug screens can detect and monitor substance abuse. Educational testing is important in screening for and addressing any related learning difficulties in dealing with academic problems.

Treatment

Many of the difficulties in youth with CD require the involvement of multiple social agencies, including education, mental health, juvenile justice, and child protection, and interventions must deal with various system issues and coordination of care. There are also comorbid conditions to contend with, such as substance abuse, which confound and interfere with treatment. Many treatments have shown efficacy in one demonstration only to have replication efforts fail in a different population. The heterogeneous nature of CD is the greatest challenge in developing treatments, where even specific types of symptoms may have multiple origins that require different approaches for intervention. Despite these difficulties, effective and promising treatments for CD do exist.

Pharmacological Treatments

No evidence currently supports the use of medication alone to treat the symptoms of CD. Medications indicated for the treatment of any comorbid disorder that is present should be considered and may result in the reduction of antisocial behaviors as well. Successful treatment of ADHD with stimulants can result in reduction of impulsive, aggressive, antisocial behaviors (see Chapter 46, "Medications Used for Attention-Deficit/ Hyperactivity Disorder"). Medications have been reported to be successfully used to treat physical aggression in CD, but most of these reports are from uncontrolled studies (Steiner et al. 2003). Medications that have been shown to reduce aggressive behaviors in youth with CD include lithium, neuroleptics, anticonvulsants, clonidine, and propranolol (Schur et al. 2003).

Psychotherapeutic Treatments

Most reported psychotherapies for CD have not been properly studied. A wide variety of treatments have been evaluated, and several meta-analytic studies of those reports have indicated promising interventions demonstrating significant, if modest, effect. Those treatments with the strongest findings include behavioral, skills training, and family-based programs or combinations of these techniques (Woolfenden et al. 2002). Studies have also revealed that certain treatments, such as shock (i.e., Scared Straight programs) or brief, one-time interventions, are not only ineffective but also may actually exacerbate antisocial behaviors (Lilienfeld 2005). Two of the most effective treatments for CD are parent management and problem-solving skills training. Parent management training with CD is typically longer in duration than with ODD, ranging from 12 to 25 weeks. It is also modified in some versions to include video modeling to assist in educating parents on problems and techniques. Parent management training is most effective with school-age children or less severe cases, as the results with adolescents are mixed. Problem-solving skills training for CD is similar to that with ODD. Treatment effect appears to be less with problem-solving skills training for children with comorbid disorders, intellectual impairments, or extreme family dysfunction.

Functional family therapy and multisystemic therapy are additional treatments with substantial evidence of efficacy in CD. Functional family therapy focuses on understanding and altering problematic interactions and communications between family members that contribute to the family's inability to effectively deal with the child's antisocial behavior (Alexander et al. 1998). All family members attend, and the therapist concentrates on improving family communication patterns. Evaluations of functional family therapy with severe delinquents in comparison to other traditional interventions have demonstrated clear and sustained improvements in behavior. Multisystemic therapy, as the name implies, considers antisocial behavior as a result of the various systems with which the adolescent interacts, including peers, school, neighborhood, and family, and seeks to alter the influences of those systems through the family (Henggeler et al. 1998). It is intensive, home-based, and typically 3 months in duration. Studies have found it superior and cost-effective in comparison to traditional services and a viable alternative to residential placement.

Research Directions

The heterogeneous nature of the disruptive disorders and differences in conceptualization will continue to fuel debate as to the best way to identify and subcategorize the syndrome. A central question is how best to understand and designate the relationships among ODD, CD, and antisocial personality disorder. DSM-IV-TR and ICD-10 (World Health Organization 1992) take different approaches to ODD and CD, with the former treating them as related but separate and the latter lumping the two together. The relationship between CD and antisocial personality disorder is also questioned in the planning for DSM-V (Pine et al. 2002), with the obvious incongruity of CD being on Axis I while antisocial personality disorder is on Axis II. There is also debate about whether sociopathy is important in CD and if it should be included as part of the diagnostic criteria. These debates may seem remote from clinical experience but will have profound impact on which children are diagnosed with disruptive behavior disorders and how they will be viewed, as well as the direction of future research into treatment and prevention.

The majority of research in the disruptive behavior disorders has been conducted with boys. The limited research on girls with oppositional and antisocial behaviors indicates that there may be key differences and that it cannot be assumed that findings with boys can be generalized to girls.

In risk factor research, studies are beginning to bridge the molecular to the nervous system to the social system by considering the interaction of factors in the progressive stages and pathways of development of oppositional and antisocial behaviors. New techniques in molecular genetics and neuroimaging, coupled with longitudinal prospective studies, will provide a more accurate understanding of the specific mechanisms and psychopathology of these disorders. This knowledge will open new avenues for prevention and treatment.

Summary Points

- Disruptive behavior disorders are the most frequent referral problem for youth, accounting for one-third to half of all cases seen in mental health clinics.

- Multiple risk factors appear to contribute to the onset and influence the course of the disruptive behavior disorders and represent the critical interaction of vulnerable individuals with their surroundings.

- Negative and disobedient behavior can be normal in certain stages of development or in special circumstances, but oppositional defiant disorder differs in that the behaviors are more severe and frequent than normally expected and result in significant functional impairment.

- The central feature of CD is a repetitive pattern of behavior that violates the rights of others or major societal rules.

- All adults with antisocial personality disorder have a history of CD, but only about 40% of youth with CD will become adults with antisocial personality disorder.

- Girls with disruptive behavior disorders have higher rates of comorbid psychiatric disorders than boys with disruptive behavior disorders.

- Careful screening for comorbid disorders is very important as appropriate treatment of concurrent psychiatric illness may reduce disruptive behaviors as well.

- Effective prevention and treatment programs exist for the disruptive behavior disorders and include parent and child skills training, family therapy, and medication for impulsive aggression.

References

Achenbach TM, Rescorla LA: Manual for the ASEBA School-Age Forms and Profiles. Burlington, University of Vermont, Department of Psychiatry, 2000

Alexander J, Barton C, Gordon D, et al: Functional Family Therapy: Blueprints for Violence Prevention, Book Three: Blueprints for Violence Prevention Series (D.S. Elliott, series editor). Boulder, Center for the Study and Prevention of Violence, Institute of Behavioral Science, University of Colorado, 1998

American Academy of Child and Adolescent Psychiatry: Practice parameters for the assessment and treatment of children and adolescents with conduct disorder. J Am Acad Child Adolesc Psychiatry 36(suppl):122S–139S, 1997

American Academy of Child and Adolescent Psychiatry: Practice parameter for the assessment and treatment of children and adolescents with oppositional defiant disorder. J Am Acad Child Adolesc Psychiatry 46:126–141, 2007

American Psychiatric Association: Diagnostic and Statistical Manual of Mental Disorders, 3rd Edition. Washington, DC, American Psychiatric Association, 1980

American Psychiatric Association: Diagnostic and Statistical Manual of Mental Disorders, 3rd Edition Revised. Washington, DC, American Psychiatric Association, 1987

American Psychiatric Association: Diagnostic and Statistical Manual of Mental Disorders, 4th Edition. Washington, DC, American Psychiatric Association, 1994

American Psychiatric Association: Diagnostic and Statistical Manual of Mental Disorders, 4th Edition, Text Revision. Washington, DC, American Psychiatric Association, 2000

Angold A, Costello EJ: Toward establishing an empirical basis for the diagnosis of oppositional defiant disorder. J Am Acad Child Adolesc Psychiatry 35:1205–1212, 1996

Aultman M: Group involvement in delinquent acts: A study of offense type and male-female participation. Crim Justice Behav 7:185–192, 1980

Bangs ME, Hazell P, Danckaerts M, et al: Atomoxetine for the treatment of attention-deficit/hyperactivity disorder and oppositional defiant disorder. Pediatrics 121:e314–e320, 2008

Barkley RA: Defiant Children: A Clinician's Manual for Assessment and Parent Training, 2nd Edition. New York, Guilford, 1997

Battin S, Hill K, Abbott R, et al: The contribution of gang membership to delinquency beyond delinquent friends. Criminology 36:93–115, 1998

Boyle MH, Offord DR, Racine Y, et al: Identifying thresholds for classifying psychiatric disorder: issues and prospects. J Am Acad Child Adolesc Psychiatry 35:1440–1448, 1996

Burke JD, Loeber R, Birmaher B: Oppositional defiant disorder and conduct disorder: a review of the past 10 years, part II. J Am Acad Child Adolesc Psychiatry 41:1275–1293, 2002

Burke JD, Loeber R, Lahey BB: Adolescent conduct disorder and interpersonal callousness as predictors of psychopathy in young adults. J Clin Child Adolesc Psychol 36:334–346, 2007

Burns G, Patterson DR: Factor structure of the Eyberg Child Behavior Inventory: a parent rating scale of oppositional defiant behavior toward adults, inattentive behavior, and conduct problem behavior. J Clin Child Psychol 29:569–577, 2000

Burt SA, Mikolajewski AJ: Preliminary evidence that specific candidate genes are associated with adolescent-onset antisocial behavior. Aggress Behav 34:437–445, 2008

Cadman D, Boyle M, Szatmari P, et al: Chronic illness, disability, and mental and social well-being: findings of the Ontario Child Health Study. Pediatrics 79:805–813, 1987

Cadoret RJ, Yates WR, Troughton E, et al: Genetic-environment interaction in the genesis of aggressivity and conduct disorders. Arch Gen Psychiatry 52:916–924, 1995

Caspi A, McClay J, Moffitt TE, et al: Role of genotype in the cycle of violence in maltreated children. Science 297:851–854, 2002

Comings DE, Wu S, Chiu C, et al: Polygenic inheritance of Tourette syndrome, stuttering, attention deficit hyperactivity, conduct, and oppositional defiant disorder: the additive and subtractive effect of the three dopaminergic genes—DRD2, D beta H, and DAT1. Am J Med Genet 67:264–88, 1996

Comings DE, Chen C, Wu S, et al: Association of the androgen receptor gene (AR) with ADHD and conduct disorder. Neuroreport 10:1589–1592, 1999

Comings DE, Gade-Andavolu R, Gonzalez N, et al: Multivariate analysis of associations of 42 genes in ADHD, ODD and conduct disorder. Clin Genet 58:31–40, 2000

Coy K, Speltz ML, DeKlyen M, et al: Social-cognitive processes in preschool boys with and without oppositional defiant disorder. J Abnorm Child Psychol 29:107–119, 2001

Cunningham CE, Boyle MH: Preschoolers at risk for attention-deficit hyperactivity disorder and oppositional defiant disorder: family, parenting, and behavioral correlates. J Abnorm Child Psychol 30:555–569, 2002

Cunningham CE, Bremner R, Boyle M: Large group community-based parenting programs for families of preschoolers at risk for disruptive behaviour disorders: utilization, cost effectiveness, and outcome. J Child Psychol Psychiatry 36:1141–1159, 1995

De Cubas MM, Field T: Children of methadone-dependent women: developmental outcomes. Am J Orthopsychiatry 63:266–276, 1993

Dishion TJ, Connell A: Adolescents' resilience as a self-regulatory process: promising themes for linking intervention with developmental science. Ann NY Acad Sci 1094:125–138, 2006

Dishion TJ, Andrews DW, Crosby L: Antisocial boys and their friends in early adolescence: relationship characteristics, quality, and interactional processes. Child Dev 66:139–151, 1995

Dodge KA: Social-cognitive mechanisms in the development of conduct disorder and depression. Annu Rev Psychol 44:559–584, 1993

Eley TC, Lichenstein P, Stevenson J: Sex differences in the etiology of aggressive and nonaggressive antisocial behavior: results for two twin studies. Child Dev 70:155–168, 1999

Eyberg SM, Pincus D: Eyberg Child Behavior Inventory and Sutter-Eyberg Student Behavior Inventory—Revised, Professional Manual. Odessa, FL, Psychological Assessment Resources, 1999

Frick PJ, Hare RD: Antisocial Process Screening Device (APSD) Technical Manual. North Tonawanda, NY, Multi-Health Systems, 2001

Frick PJ, Morris AS: Temperament and developmental pathways to conduct problems. J Clin Child Adolesc Psychol 33:54–68, 2004

Greenberg MT: Promoting resilience in children and youth: preventive interventions and their interface with neuroscience. Ann NY Acad Sci 1094:139–150, 2006

Greene RW, Biederman J, Zerwas S, et al: Psychiatric comorbidity, family dysfunction, and social impairment in referred youth with oppositional defiant disorder. Am J Psychiatry 159:1214–1224, 2002

Gross MD: Buspirone in ADHD with ODD. J Am Acad Child Adolesc Psychiatry 34:1260, 1995

Guttmann-Steinmetz S, Crowell JA: Attachment and externalizing disorders: a developmental psychopathology perspective. J Am Acad Child Adolesc Psychiatry 45:440–451, 2006

Halperin JM, McKay KE, Newcorn JH: Development, reliability, and validity of the Children's Aggression Scale—Parent Version. J Am Acad Child Adolesc Psychiatry 41:245–252, 2002

Hechtman L, Offord DR: Long-term outcome of disruptive disorders. Child Adolesc Psychiatr Clin N Am 3:379–403, 1994

Henggeler SW, Schoenwald SK, Borduin CM, et al: Multisystemic Treatment of Antisocial Behavior in Children and Adolescents. New York, Guilford, 1998

Henry DB, Tolan PH, Gorman-Smith D: Longitudinal family and peer group effects on violence and nonviolent delinquency. J Clin Child Psychol 30:172–186, 2001

Herpertz SC, Wenning B, Mueller B, et al: Psychophysiologic responses in ADHD boys with and without conduct disorder: implications for adult antisocial behavior. J Am Acad Child Adolesc Psychiatry 40:1222–1230, 2003

Hogan AE: Cognitive functioning in children with oppositional defiant disorder and conduct disorder in Handbook of Disruptive Behavior Disorders. Edited by Quay HC, Hogan AE. New York, Kluwer Academic/Plenum, 1999, pp 317–335

Jenkins RL, Hewitt LE: Types of personality structure encountered in child guidance clinics. Am J Orthopsychiatry 14:84–94, 1944

Kazdin AE: Treatments for aggressive and antisocial children. Child Adolesc Psychiatr Clin N Am 9:841–858, 2000

Kazdin AE: Parent Management Training: Treatment for Oppositional, Aggressive, and Antisocial Behavior in Children and Adolescents. New York, Oxford University Press, 2005

Kazdin AE, Bass D, Siegel T: Cognitive problem-solving skills training and parent management training in the treatment of antisocial behavior in children. J Consult Clin Psychol 60:733–747, 1992

Kruesi MJ, Rapoport JL, Hamburger S, et al: Cerebrospinal fluid monoamine metabolites, aggression, and impulsivity in disruptive behavior of children and adolescents. Arch Gen Psychiatry 47:419–426, 1990

Lahey BB, Loeber R, Hart EL, et al: Four-year longitudinal study of conduct disorder in boys: patterns and predictors of persistence. J Abnorm Psychol 104:83–93, 1995

Lahey BB, Miller TL, Gordon RA, et al: Developmental epidemiology of the disruptive behavior disorders, in Handbook of the Disruptive Behavior Disorders. Edited by Quay HC, Hogan A. New York, Plenum, 1999, pp 23–48

Lavigne JV, Cicchetti C, Gibbons RD, et al: Oppositional defiant disorder with onset in preschool years: longitudinal stability and pathways to other disorders. J Am Acad Child Adolesc Psychiatry 40:1393–1400, 2001

Lilienfeld SO: Scientifically unsupported and supported interventions for childhood psychopathology: a summary. Pediatrics 115:761–764, 2005

Loeber R, Hay DF: Developmental approaches to aggression and conduct problems, in Development Through Life: A Handbook for Clinicians. Edited by Rutter M, Hay DF. London, Blackwell, 1994, pp 488–515

Loeber R, Keenan K, Lahey BB, et al: Evidence for developmentally based diagnoses of oppositional defiant disorder and conduct disorder. J Abnorm Child Psychol 21:377–410, 1993

Loeber R, Keenan KE, Russo MF, et al: Secondary data analyses for DSM-IV on the symptoms of oppositional defiant disorder and conduct disorder, in DSM-IV Sourcebook, Vol 4. Edited by Widiger TA, Frances AJ, Pincus HA, et al. Washington, DC, American Psychiatric Association, 1998, pp 465–489

Loeber R, Burke JD, Lahey BB, et al: Oppositional defiant and conduct disorder: a review of the past 10 years, part I. J Am Acad Child Adolesc Psychiatry 39:1468–1484, 2000

McFayden-Ketchum SA, Bates JE, Dodge KA, et al: Patterns of change in early child aggressive-disruptive behavior: gender differences in predictors from early coercive and affectionate mother-child interactions. Child Dev 67:2417–2433, 1996

Mezzacappa E, Tremblay RE, Kindlon D, et al: Relationship of aggression and anxiety to autonomic regulation of heart rate variability in adolescent males. Ann NY Acad Sci 20:376–379, 1996

Miles DR, Carey G: Genetic and environmental architecture of human aggression. J Pers Soc Psychol 72:207–217, 1997

Miller-Heyl J, MacPhee D, Fritz JJ: DARE to Be You: a family support, early prevention program. J Prim Prev 18:257–285, 1998

Moffitt TE: Genetic and environmental influences on antisocial behaviors: evidence from behavioral-genetic research. Adv Genet 55:41–104, 2005

Moffitt TE, Caspi A, Harkness AR, et al: The natural history of change in intellectual performance. Who changes? How much? Is it meaningful? J Child Psychol Psychiatry 34:455–506, 1993

Mytton J, DiGuiseppi C, Gough D, et al: School-based secondary prevention programmes for preventing violence. Cochrane Database Syst Rev 3:CD004606, 2006

Nadder TS, Rutter M, Silberg JL, et al: Genetic effects on the variation and covariation of attention deficit-hyperactivity disorder (ADHD) and oppositional-defiant disorder/conduct disorder (Odd/CD) symptomatologies across informant and occasion of measurement. Psychol Med 32:39–53, 2002 [Erratum in: Psychol Med 32:378, 2002]

Needleman HL, Reiss J, Tobin M, et al: Bone lead levels and delinquent behavior. JAMA 275:363–369, 1996

Nock MK, Kazdin AE, Hiripi E, et al: Prevalence, subtypes, and correlates of DSM-IV conduct disorder in the National Comorbidity Survey Replication. Psychol Med 36:699–710, 2006

Nock MK, Kazdin AE, Hiripi E, et al: Lifetime prevalence, correlates, and persistence of oppositional defiant disorder: results from the National Comorbidity Survey Replication. J Child Psychol Psychiatry 48:703–713, 2007

Offord DR, Bennett KJ: Conduct disorder: long-term outcomes and intervention effectiveness. J Am Acad Child Adolesc Psychiatry 33:1069–1078, 1994

Olds D, Henderson CR Jr, Cole R, et al: Long-term effects of nurse home visitation on children's criminal and antisocial behavior: 15-year follow-up of a randomized controlled trial. JAMA 280:1238–1244, 1998

Ortiz J, Raine A: Heart rate level and antisocial behavior in children and adolescents: a meta-analysis. J Am Acad Child Adolesc Psychiatry 43:154–162, 2004

Patterson GR, Reid JB, Dishion TJ: A Social Learning Approach, Vol 4: Antisocial Boys. Eugene, OR, Castalia, 1992

Pine DS, Alegria M, Cook EH, et al: Advances in developmental science and DSM-V, in A Research Agenda for DSM-V. Edited by Kupfer DJ, First MB, Regier DA. Washington, DC, 2002, American Psychiatric Association, pp 85–122

Pliszka SR: The psychobiology of oppositional defiant disorder and conduct disorder, in Handbook of Disruptive Behavior Disorders. Edited by Quay HC, Hogan AE. New York, Kluwer Academic/Plenum, 1999, pp 371–395

Robins LN: Deviant Children Grown Up. Baltimore, MD, Williams & Wilkins, 1966

Rowe DC: Sibling interaction and self-reported delinquent behavior: a study of 265 twin pairs. Criminology 23:223–240, 1985

Rowe R, Maughan B, Pickles A, et al: The relationship between DSM-IV oppositional defiant disorder and conduct disorder: findings from the Great Smoky Mountains Study. J Child Psychol Psychiatry 43:365–373, 2002

Rowe R, Maughan B, Costello EJ, et al: Defining oppositional defiant disorder. J Child Psychol Psychiatry 46:1309–1316, 2005

Sanson A, Prior M: Temperament and behavioral precursors to oppositional defiant disorder and conduct disorder, in Handbook of Disruptive Behavior Disorders. Edited by Quay HC, Hogan AE. New York, Kluwer Academic/ Plenum, 1999, pp 397–417

Schur SB, Sikich L, Findling RL, et al: Treatment recommendations for the use of antipsychotics for aggressive youth (TRAAY), part I: a review. J Am Acad Child Adolesc Psychiatry 42:132–144, 2003

Simonoff E, Elander J, Holmshaw J, et al: Predictors of antisocial personality: continuities from childhood to adult life. Br J Psychiatry 184:118–127, 2004

Smith PK, Ananiadou K, Cowie H: Interventions to reduce school bullying. Can J Psychiatry 48:591–599, 2003

Speltz ML, McClellan J, Deklyen M, et al: Preschool boys with oppositional defiant disorder: clinical presentation and diagnostic change. J Am Acad Child Adolesc Psychiatry 38:838–845, 1999

Steiner H, Saxena K, Chang K: Psychopharmacologic strategies for the treatment of aggression in juveniles. CNS Spectr 8:298–308, 2003

Taylor J, Iacono WG, McGue M: Evidence for a genetic etiology of early onset delinquency. J Abnorm Psychol 109: 634–643, 2000

Thomas A, Chess S: Temperament and Development. New York, Brunner Mazel, 1977

Thomas C, Holzer C, Wall J: Serious delinquency and gang membership. Adolesc Psychiatry 27:61–81, 2003

Trickett PK, Putnam FW: Developmental consequences of child sexual abuse, in Violence Against Children in the Family and the Community. Edited by Trickett PK, Schellenbach CJ. Washington, DC, American Psychological Association, 1998, pp 39–56

Unis AS, Cook EH, Vincent JG, et al: Platelet serotonin measures in adolescents with conduct disorder. Biol Psychiatry 42:553–559, 1997

van Goozen SHM, van den Ban E, Matthys W, et al: Increased adrenal androgen functioning in children with oppositional defiant disorder: a comparison with psychiatric and normal controls. J Am Acad Child Adolesc Psychiatry 39:1446–1455, 2000

van Goozen SH, Cohen-Kettenis PT, Snoek H, et al: Executive functioning in children: a comparison of hospitalised ODD and ODD/ADHD children and normal controls. J Child Psychol Psychiatry 45:284–292, 2004

Vanyukow MM, Moss HB, Plial JA, et al: Antisocial symptoms in preadolescent boys and in their parents: associations with cortisol. Psychiatry Res 46:9–17, 1993

Wakschlag L, Pickett K, Cook E, et al: Maternal smoking during pregnancy and severe antisocial behavior in offspring: a review. Am J Public Health 92:969–974, 2002

Wakschlag L, Pickett K, Kasza KE, et al: Is prenatal smoking associated with a developmental pattern of conduct problems in young boys? J Am Acad Child Adolesc Psychiatry 45:461–467, 2006

Webster-Stratton C, Taylor T: Nipping early risk factors in the bud: preventing substance abuse, delinquency, and violence in adolescence through interventions targeted at young children (0–8 years). Prev Sci 2:165–192, 2001

Webster-Stratton C, Jamila Reid M, Stoolmiller M: Preventing conduct problems and improving school readiness: evaluation of the Incredible Years Teacher and Child Training Programs in high-risk schools. J Child Psychol Psychiatry 49:471–488, 2008

Widom CS, Maxfield MG: A prospective examination of risk for violence among abused and neglected children. Ann NY Acad Sci 20:224–237, 1996

Woolfenden SR, Williams K, Peat JK: Family and parenting interventions for conduct disorder and delinquency: a meta-analysis of randomised controlled trials. Arch Dis Child 86:251–256, 2002

World Health Organization: International Statistical Classification of Diseases and Related Health Problems, 10th Revision. Geneva, Switzerland, World Health Organization, 1992

Yudofsky SC, Silver JM, Jackson W, et al: The Overt Aggression Scale for the objective rating of verbal and physical aggression. Am J Psychiatry 143:35–39, 1986

Chapter 17

Substance Abuse and Addictions

Oscar G. Bukstein, M.D., M.P.H.
Deborah Deas, M.D., M.P.H.

Substance use and abuse by adolescents remain critical problems because of the common use of psychoactive substances by youth, the ensuing consequences, and the persistence into adulthood of pathology related to substance use. Clinicians seeking to understand the risk for substance use and abuse, the acquisition of use behaviors, and their development into substance use disorders (SUDs) should consider neurobiology, all aspects of development, and the adolescent. The treatment should focus on specific substance use behaviors as well as risk factors that have a role in the onset and maintenance of SUDs.

Definitions, Clinical Description, and Diagnosis

Substance Use

There is a range of use behaviors and patterns of use. At one end of the use spectrum lies *abstinence*. Sub-

stance *use* (often without significant consequences or impairment) comprises the largest group of adolescents. DSM-IV (American Psychiatric Association 1994), and its text revision, DSM-IV-TR (American Psychiatric Association 2000), contain two substance-related diagnoses, *abuse* and *dependence*. Substance use per se is not sufficient for a diagnosis of abuse or dependence, even in adolescents. There are three distinct concepts to consider: abuse and dependence, misuse (which includes use), and diversion. Although not an official term, *misuse* can be defined as use for a purpose not consistent with medical guidelines (e.g., modifying dose, using to achieve euphoria, and/or using with other nonprescribed psychoactive substances [World Health Organization 2007]). The term *diversion* is the transfer of medication from the individual for whom it was prescribed to one for whom it was not prescribed. While *abuse* and *dependence* are terms that connote psychopathology related to substance use, diversion and misuse are not.

The diagnosis of *substance abuse* requires evidence of a maladaptive pattern of substance use with clinically significant levels of impairment or distress. Recurrent use in adolescents results in an inability to meet major role obligations, leading to impaired functioning in one or more major areas of their life and an increase in the likelihood of legal problems due to possession, risk-taking behavior, and exposure to hazardous situations. *Substance dependence* requires that the adolescent meet at least three criteria, including such symptoms as withdrawal, tolerance, and loss of control over use. For example, for alcohol use disorders (AUDs), adolescents commonly exhibit tolerance (i.e., requiring increasing amounts of a substance to achieve the same effect) but less frequently show withdrawal or other symptoms of physiological dependence (Martin et al. 1995). Many adolescents do manifest withdrawal symptoms with cannabis and opiate use disorders (Crowley et al. 2001). Preoccupation with use is often demonstrated by giving up previously important activities, increasing the time spent in activities related to substance use, and using more frequently or for longer amounts of time than planned. The adolescent may use despite the continued existence or worsening of problems caused by substance use. For adolescents, it is important to include criteria such as alcohol-related blackouts, craving, and impulsive sexual behavior when determining if criteria are met. Polysubstance use by adolescents appears to be the rule rather than the exception; therefore, adolescents often present with multiple SUD diagnoses (Martin et al. 1995). Adolescents' alcohol and drug symptom profiles appear to vary along a severity dimension rather than fitting into DSM-IV's abuse and dependence categories (Chung and Martin 2001, 2005).

Gambling and Internet Addiction

Pathological gambling is listed in DSM-IV under impulse-control disorders not elsewhere classified and is characterized by recurrent and persistent maladaptive gambling behavior. The specific criteria are similar to those for substance dependence and abuse with the addition of typical but specific gambling behavior, such as "chasing" one's losses or relying on others to relieve a desperate financial situation caused by gambling.

Even less is known about Internet addiction. Preoccupation with the Internet is usually focused on a specific area, not generalized across different activities, and there is evidence that individuals should be classified according to their involvement in specific online activities, such as gambling, shopping, or pornography, which have a more robust basis as "addictions"

(Yellowlees and Marks 2007). Individuals with a history of impulse control and other addictive disorders with other SUD risk factors may be at increased risk of using the Internet in a problematic way.

Epidemiology

Data on alcohol and other drug use in the United States come from two major sources: 1) the Monitoring the Future (MTF; Johnston et al. 2008) survey of 48,000 eighth, tenth, and twelfth graders in more than 400 schools nationwide; and 2) the National Survey on Drug Use and Health (NSDUH; Substance Abuse and Mental Health Services Administration 2007), an annual survey of the noninstitutionalized civilian population of the United States ages 12 years and older.

Substance Use

A large minority of youth use psychoactive substances. According to the 2007 MTF survey (Johnston et al. 2008), the percentage of U.S. adolescents who use illicit drugs or drink alcohol continued a decade-long drop in 2006, revealing that a fifth (19%) of eighth graders, over a third (36%) of tenth graders, and about half (47%) of all twelfth graders had taken an illicit drug (other than alcohol) during their lifetime. According to the NSDUH (Substance Abuse and Mental Health Services Administration 2007), the rate of current illicit drug use among youth ages 12–17 was 11.6% in 2002 and 9.9% in 2005. In 2005, 9.9% of youth ages 12–17 were current illicit drug users: 6.8% used marijuana, 3.3% used prescription-type drugs nonmedically, 1.2% used inhalants, 0.8% used hallucinogens, and 0.6% used cocaine (Substance Abuse and Mental Health Services Administration 2007). In 2005, among adults age 18 or older who first tried marijuana at age 14 or younger, 13.3% were classified with illicit drug dependence or abuse versus the 2.4% of adults who had first used marijuana at age 18 or older.

In 2007, after a long period of steadily increasing narcotic drug use among twelfth graders, the MTF study reported that use of narcotic drugs (e.g., OxyContin and Vicodin) other than heroin reached a peak in 2004, with relatively little change since then. OxyContin use increased steadily among twelfth graders from 2002 until 2005, with annual prevalence (in the last 12 months) rising from 4% to 5.5%, before dropping back to 5.2% in 2007.

Sedatives (including barbiturate sedatives and benzodiazepines) showed a substantial, if gradual, increase over a period of years. In the MTF study, use for twelfth graders rose from 2.8% in 1993 to 7.2% in 2005 before decreasing to 6.6% in 2006. In the 2006 survey, most of the illegal drugs like LSD, ecstasy, cocaine, and heroin had shown considerable decline in recent years, while the misuse of prescription-type drugs has been growing. Amphetamines constitute the only class of prescribed psychotropic drugs used outside of a medical regimen that have not been showing a recent increase in use. Annual prevalence of use today is about one-half of its peak in 1996 for eighth graders, about two-thirds what it was in 1996 among tenth graders, and about three-quarters of the more recent peak level (in 2002) for twelfth graders. The use of over-the-counter cough or cold medicines (usually containing dextromethorphan, a cough suppressant) was reported by 4%, 5%, and 7% in eighth, tenth, and twelfth grades, respectively. For steroid use, high school students report a drop of 40%–50% since peak levels in the later 1990s. In 2006 and 2007 the pattern of changes was mixed, with the increase in use continuing at tenth grade, but with some decline occurring at eighth and twelfth grades. Finally, in the MTF study, inhalant use showed a mixed picture. After 1995, inhalant use had been declining in all three grades before a period of increased use among the eighth graders in 2003. Since then, prevalence data have been mixed, with a decline in perceived risk among younger students.

Alcohol Use

Among eighth graders, the MTF study reported that 30-day prevalence of alcohol use has declined by more than one-third since its peak level in 1996. In 2007, among twelfth graders, the 30-day prevalence of alcohol use was 44%, and the prevalence of being drunk at least once in the prior month stood at 5.5% of eighth graders, 18.1% of tenth graders, and 28.7% of twelfth graders. In the NSDUH, the rate of current alcohol use among youth ages 12–17 declined from 17.6% in 2004 to 16.5% in 2005 (Substance Abuse and Mental Health Services Administration 2007). Youth binge drinking also declined during that period, from 11.1% to 9.9%, but heavy drinking did not change significantly (2.7% in 2004 and 2.4% in 2005). Although from 2004 and 2005 there were declines in past-month and binge alcohol use among youth ages 12–17, overall underage (persons ages 12–20) past-month and binge drinking

rates have remained essentially unchanged since 2002, with 28.2% of this age group reporting drinking alcohol in the past month, 18.8% reporting binge drinking, and 6.0% reporting heavy drinking. The NSDUH reported that most (88.9%) of the 4.3 million recent alcohol initiates were younger than 21 at the time of initiation of use (Substance Abuse and Mental Health Services Administration 2007).

Tobacco Use

Following a decade of substantial improvement, the MTF study found that daily smoking among adolescents plateaued. Since the mid-1990s, current daily smoking has fallen by half among twelfth graders and by more than half among those in eighth and tenth grades. Daily smoking was 12.2% in 2006, and half-pack-a-day smoking, 5.9% (Substance Abuse and Mental Health Services Administration 2007). Like rates for cigarettes, the 30-day prevalence of using smokeless tobacco reached a peak in the mid-1990s and then began to decline, with 2006 prevalence rates for any use in the prior 30 days at 3.7%, 5.7%, and 6.1% in eighth, tenth, and twelfth grades, respectively. Similar data from the NSDUH found that the rate of past-month cigarette use among 12- to 17-year-olds declined from 13.0% in 2002 to 10.8% in 2005. Past-month smokeless tobacco use was reported by 2.1% of youth in 2005, similar to estimates since 2002. According to the NSDUH, most new smokers in 2005 were under age 18 when they first smoked cigarettes (63.4%).

Diversion and misuse are widespread, especially among high school and college students (Wilens et al. 2008). In a study of 1,086 public school students, opioid analgesics were the most widely prescribed and the most widely abused (Boyd et al. 2006). Stimulant and sedative or anxiety medications had the highest illicit-to-medical-use ratios. Diversion of prescription medication was common; within the previous year, 29%–62% of 390 students with legal prescriptions were approached to divert their medications. In a survey of junior and senior high school students in Canada ($N=13,549$; 5.3% of whom were prescribed stimulants), 15% of those prescribed stimulants reported having given away some of their medication, 7% having sold some of their medication, 4% having experienced theft of their medication, and 3% having been forced to give up some of their medication in the 12 months before the survey (Poulin 2001).

Substance Use Disorders

The prevalence of SUDs increases with age through young adulthood. National survey data indicate that very few youth (less than 3%) met criteria for any past-year SUD before age 14. SUD increased steadily from age 14 (7%) to age 21 (25%), with peak prevalence occurring in the 20s (Substance Abuse and Mental Health Services Administration 2005). Among 12- to 17-year-olds, 9% met criteria for a past-year DSM-IV SUD abuse or dependence diagnosis; 6% had an alcohol diagnosis, and 4% had a cannabis diagnosis (2% met criteria for both alcohol and at least one illicit substance) (Substance Abuse and Mental Health Services Administration 2005). In addition, subthreshold cases, termed *diagnostic orphans,* account for up to an additional 17% of adolescents who reported alcohol-related problems in community surveys (Chung et al. 2002).

National survey data indicate little to no difference in rates of past-year SUD prevalence by gender for alcohol or illicit drugs (Substance Abuse and Mental Health Services Administration 2005). Similar to ethnic differences in substance use prevalence, larger proportions of white and Hispanic youth ages 12–17 years met criteria for a past-year DSM-IV alcohol or drug diagnosis than African Americans (10%, 10%, and 6%, respectively), although American Indian adolescents had the highest proportion of alcohol or other drug diagnoses (20%) (Substance Abuse and Mental Health Services Administration 2005).

Gambling

Between 60% and 80% of adolescents report having engaged in some form of gambling during the past year (Derevensky 2007), with most described as social, recreational, and occasional gamblers, although 3%–8% of adolescents may have a very serious gambling problem, with another 10%–15% at risk for the development of a gambling problem.

Internet Addiction

Almost all of the limited literature describing Internet addiction comes from Taiwan. However, in a survey of Italian adolescents, 5.4% were found to be Internet addicted, similar to rates in other countries (Pallanti et al. 2006).

Comorbidity

In both community surveys of adolescents with SUD and samples of adolescents in addictions treatment, the majority have a co-occurring non-substance-related

mental disorder (Hser et al. 2001). More than half of those adolescents in addictions treatment who have a co-occurring mental illness have three or more co-occurring psychiatric disorders (Dennis et al. 2003). The most commonly comorbid psychiatric disorders among youth in addictions treatment include conduct problems, attention-deficit/hyperactivity disorder (ADHD), mood disorders (e.g., depression), and trauma-related symptoms (Grella et al. 2001). Some studies of youth with SUD (e.g., Clark et al. 1997) have found that females are more likely to exhibit internalizing (e.g., depression, anxiety) symptoms and trauma syndromes compared to males.

Comorbid psychopathology may precede, exacerbate, or follow the onset of heavy substance use. A review of adolescent community surveys found that childhood mental illness generally predicted earlier initiation of substance use and SUD onset, particularly in relation to conduct disorder (Armstrong and Costello 2002). The early symptoms of most psychiatric disorders, excluding depression, generally emerged prior to the onset of substance use; full criteria for a nonsubstance psychiatric disorder were typically met prior to SUD onset in adolescence (Costello et al. 1999). Among treated adolescents, comorbid psychopathology generally predicted early return to substance use, particularly conduct problems (Brown et al. 1996) and major depression (Cornelius et al. 2004). Co-occurring psychopathology also generally predicted a more persistent course of substance involvement over 1-year follow-up (Grella et al. 2001). Rather than type of diagnosis, the total number of psychiatric symptoms may predict relapse risk (McCarthy et al. 2005). With regard to conduct problems, a 4-year study of treated youth found that the majority (61%) of adolescents with conduct disorder at the time of treatment met criteria for antisocial personality disorder at follow-up and that these individuals had higher levels of drug involvement over follow-up compared to those without antisocial personality disorder (Myers et al. 1998). In a 5-year pilot study of adolescents treated for both AUD and major depression, substance involvement declined overall; however, a more chronic course of depression was observed into young adulthood (Cornelius et al. 2005).

Etiology, Mechanisms, and Risk Factors

First experiences with substance use most often take place in a social context with the use of "gateway" substances, such as alcohol and cigarettes, which are legal for adults and readily available to minors (Kandel and Yamaguchi 2002). Initial use may occur because of adolescent curiosity or the availability of a substance. Progressively fewer adolescents advance to later and more serious levels of substance use. Although drug consumption frequently follows a predictable sequence referred to as the "gateway hypothesis" (Kandel and Yamaguchi 2002), the risk for and rate of progression to SUD are the same whether consumption begins with a legal or illegal drug (Tarter et al. 2006). The early onset of substance use and a more rapid progression through the stages of substance use are among the risk factors for the development of SUDs (Grant and Dawson 1997). The literature on the development of substance use and SUDs in adolescents has identified an assortment of individual, peer, family, and community risk factors. Within a developmental context, genetic predispositions to affective, cognitive, and behavioral dysregulation are exacerbated by family and peer factors and the developmental issues of puberty, leading to substance use and pathological use (Tarter et al. 1999). Both temperament and social interactions (e.g., family, peer relations) have a critical role in adolescent SUD outcomes. Many family factors have been implicated in increasing SUD risk in children and adolescents. The most widely recognized factors involve affectional bonding, parental supervision, discipline style, and adherence to religious practices (Clark et al. 1998). Affiliation with socially deviant peers has been shown in many studies to promote substance use (Oetting and Beauvais 1987). Affiliation with older peers may be especially hazardous because of premature exposure to risky situations, including drugs, sex, automobile travel, and social settings without adult supervision. Negative affect, irritability, and "difficult" temperament have been documented in children at high risk for SUD (Chassin et al. 2004).

In twin studies, heritability varies for different SUDs, reaching as high as 0.8 in both males and females (Kendler et al. 2003). Finally, it is important to note that liabilities associated with use and abuse of different categories of drugs, alcohol, and tobacco share as much as 50%–85% of their genetic variance (Tsuang et al. 1998). Common factors have been shown to virtually completely account for heritability for SUD related to different categories of illicit drugs (Kendler et al. 2003), thus indicating the common genetic factors that largely underlie the genetic risk for most or all of the DSM-IV SUDs. Recent research supports an etiologic model for individual differences in substance use, in which initiation and early patterns of use are strongly influenced by social and familial environmental factors, while later levels of use are strongly influenced by genetic factors (Kendler et al. 2008). The correlations seen in levels of use across substances appear to be the result of social and environmental factors in adolescence, with genetic factors becoming progressively more important through early and middle adulthood.

The substantial genetic commonality between highly heritable disinhibitory/externalizing behavioral traits and SUD liability (Krueger et al. 2002) is consistent with behavior dysregulation as a major component of SUD liability (Tarter et al. 1999). ADHD symptoms as traits are well known to be early indicators of SUD risk (Molina and Pelham 2003). A relationship, possibly genetically mediated, has been shown between childhood disruptive behavior and adult antisociality and SUD (Vanyukov et al. 2000). While there is no single "substance abuse personality," a certain proportion of variation in the liability to SUD is shared in common with personality/behavior phenotypic variation that predates the initiation of substance use and is related to the concept of self-regulation (dysregulation/disinhibition).

Prevention

Most prevention interventions are based on social learning models, including educational approaches, family-based interventions, and community-based projects. Empirically based prevention interventions primarily involve strengthening resilience factors and reducing risk factors for the development of SUDs (National Institute on Drug Abuse 2003; see Table 17–1). School-based and some community-based prevention methods can be effective in reducing substance use (Substance Abuse and Mental Health Services Administration 2007). In 2005 almost four-fifths (77.9%) of youth ages 12–17 years who were enrolled in school reported that they had seen or heard drug or alcohol prevention messages at school in the past year. Self-reported past-month use of an illicit drug was lower for youth exposed to such messages in school (9.2%) than for youth not reporting such exposure (13.2%). Approximately one in eight (11.7%) youth ages 12–17 years reported in 2005 that they had participated in drug, tobacco, or alcohol prevention programs outside of school in the past year. The prevalence of self-reported past-month alcohol use was lower among youth who reported participating in these programs (14.0%) than among youth who did not (16.9%). There were no differences in marijuana or cigarette use in the

TABLE 17–1. Principles for effective prevention programs

Principle 1—Prevention programs should enhance protective factors and reverse or reduce risk factors.

Principle 2—Prevention programs should address all forms of drug abuse, alone or in combination, including the underage use of legal drugs (e.g., tobacco or alcohol); the use of illegal drugs (e.g., marijuana or heroin); and the inappropriate use of legally obtained substances (e.g., inhalants), prescription medications, or over-the-counter drugs.

Principle 3—Prevention programs should address the type of drug abuse problem in the local community, target modifiable risk factors, and strengthen identified protective factors.

Principle 4—Prevention programs should be tailored to address risks specific to population or audience characteristics, such as age, gender, and ethnicity, to improve program effectiveness.

Principle 5—Family-based prevention programs should enhance family bonding and relationships and include parenting skills; practice in developing, discussing, and enforcing family policies on substance abuse; and training in drug education and information.

Principle 6—Prevention programs can be designed to intervene as early as preschool to address risk factors for drug abuse, such as aggressive behavior, poor social skills, and academic difficulties.

Principle 7—Prevention programs for elementary school children should target improving academic and social-emotional learning to address risk factors for drug abuse, such as early aggression, academic failure, and school dropout. Education should focus on the following skills:
- Self-control
- Emotional awareness
- Communication
- Social problem-solving
- Academic support, especially in reading

Principle 8—Prevention programs for middle or junior high and high school students should increase academic and social competence with the following skills:
- Study habits and academic support
- Communication
- Peer relationships
- Self-efficacy and assertiveness
- Drug-resistance skills
- Reinforcement of antidrug attitudes
- Strengthening of personal commitments against drug abuse

Principle 9—Prevention programs aimed at general populations at key transition points, such as the transition to middle school, can produce beneficial effects even among high-risk families and children. Such interventions do not single out risk populations and, therefore, reduce labeling and promote bonding to school and community.

Principle 10—Community prevention programs that combine two or more effective programs, such as family- and school-based programs, can be more effective than a single program.

Principle 11—Community prevention programs reaching populations in multiple settings—for example, schools, clubs, faith-based organizations, and the media—are most effective when they present consistent community-wide messages in each setting.

Principle 12—When communities adapt programs to match their needs, community norms, or differing cultural requirements, they should retain core elements of the original research-based intervention that include
- Structure (how the program is organized and constructed)
- Content (what the information, skills, and strategies of the program are)
- Delivery (how the program is adapted, implemented, and evaluated)

Principle 13—Prevention programs should be long term, with repeated interventions (i.e., booster programs) to reinforce the original prevention goals. Research shows that the benefits from middle school prevention programs diminish without follow-up programs in high school.

TABLE 17–1. Principles for effective prevention programs *(continued)*

Principle 14—Prevention programs should include teacher training on good classroom management practices, such as rewarding appropriate student behavior. Such techniques help to foster students' positive behavior, achievement, academic motivation, and school bonding.

Principle 15—Prevention programs are most effective when they employ interactive techniques, such as peer discussion groups and parent role-playing, that allow for active involvement in learning about drug abuse and reinforcing skills.

Principle 16—Research-based prevention programs can be cost-effective.

Source. Adapted from National Institute on Drug Abuse 2003.

two groups. Past-month rates of use of any substance (including any illicit drug, marijuana, any illicit drug other than marijuana, alcohol, and binge alcohol) among those reporting no exposure to drug or alcohol prevention messages outside of school were similar to rates among those who reported that they had seen prevention messages outside of school. Only past-month cigarette use showed a significant difference (12.6% among those who had not been exposed vs. 10.3% among those who had seen such messages).

Course

In examining the clinical course of alcohol use disorders (AUDs) in community samples, among adolescents with an AUD, 55% had an AUD at young adult follow-up (Rohde et al. 2001), suggesting some remission with maturation, as well as a more chronic course of adolescent-onset AUD for certain individuals. Although the majority of treated adolescents return to some substance use following treatment (Winters 1999), treated adolescents generally show reductions in substance use and problems over both short- and longer-term follow-up (e.g., Chung et al. 2003).

Changes in different domains of psychosocial functioning occurred at different rates: school functioning generally improved within the first year of follow-up, but improvements in family functioning emerged only after 2 years (Chung et al. 2003). Despite significant reductions in substance involvement and improvements in school performance, interpersonal relations, and other areas, treated adolescents continued to show greater problem severity across multiple domains compared to a community comparison sample (Chung 2007). Thus, adolescent-onset SUD, likely in combination with co-occurring psychopathology and other risk factors (e.g., negative environmental influences), interferes with the achievement of normative adolescent developmental tasks.

Evaluation

Perhaps the most critical skill for clinicians is evaluation, which includes screening, baseline assessment, and ongoing assessment of progress. For more detailed guidelines to both evaluation and treatment, the reader is referred to the "Practice Parameters for the Assessment and Treatment of Children and Adolescents with Substance Use Disorders" (American Academy of Child and Adolescent Psychiatry 2005; see Table 17–2).

Validity of Adolescent Report

Although the clinician should always question whether any self-report about substance use is truthful, the majority of adolescents in drug clinics or schools give temporally consistent reports of substance use (Winters et al. 1991). Most youth in drug treatment settings admit to use of substances; few treatment-seeking adolescents endorse questions that indicate blatant faking of responses (e.g., admit to the use of a fictitious drug). Specific populations, especially extremely antisocial youth, have much higher responses of "faking good" than clinical samples (Winters et al. 1991).

Both clinicians and investigators have noted an "intake-discharge effect" in which level of use reported at discharge and problems as well as SUDs are higher than those endorsed at admission to a treatment program (Stinchfield 1997). The possible causes of the intake-discharge effect include factors at intake such as denial, reluctance to self-disclose due to embarrassment, and wish to avoid sanctions for use, as well as ability of the adolescent in treatment to more carefully examine the extent of substance use.

The use of structured interviews or standardized questionnaires may also serve to support or validate the self-report. The adolescent may feel less threat-

TABLE 17–2. American Academy of Child and Adolescent Psychiatry practice parameter for the assessment and treatment of children and adolescents with substance use disorders (SUDs): recommendations

1. The clinician should observe an appropriate level of confidentiality for the adolescent during the assessment and treatment.

2. The mental health assessment of older children and adolescents requires screening questions about the use of alcohol and other substances of abuse.

3. If the screening raises concerns about substance use, the clinician should conduct a more formal evaluation to determine the quantity and frequency of use and consequences of use for each substance used and whether the youth meets criteria for SUD(s).

4. Toxicology, through the collection of bodily fluids or specimens, should be a routine part of the formal evaluation and the ongoing assessment of substance use both during and after treatment.

5. Adolescents with SUDs should receive specific treatment for their substance use.

6. Adolescents with SUDs should be treated in the least restrictive setting that is safe and effective.

7. Family therapy or significant family/parental involvement in treatment should be a component of treatment of SUDs.

8. Treatment programs and interventions should develop procedures to minimize treatment dropout and to maximize motivation, compliance, and treatment completion.

9. Medication can be used when indicated for the management of craving and withdrawal and for aversion therapy.

10. Treatment should encourage and develop peer support, especially regarding the nonuse of substances.

11. Twelve-step approaches may be used as a basis for treatment. Attendance at Alcoholics Anonymous and Narcotics Anonymous groups comprises an adjunct to professional treatment of SUDs and should be encouraged.

12. Programs and interventions should attempt to provide comprehensive services in other domains (e.g., vocational, recreational, medical, family, and legal).

13. Adolescents with SUDs should receive thorough evaluation for comorbid psychiatric disorders.

14. Comorbid conditions should be appropriately treated.

15. Programs and interventions should provide or arrange for posttreatment aftercare.

Source. National Institute on Drug Abuse 2003.

ened by self-report questionnaires, many of which have questions to ascertain response bias. The use of toxicological methods such as urine drug screens can validate self-report by testing for the use of a specific agent. The use of urine or other toxicology screens has been associated with greater drug-use disclosures (Wish et al. 1997). Finally, the attitude and skill of the assessment interviewer are often the best promoter of the validity of self-report, with engagement with the adolescent predicting more valid responses.

Levels of Assessment

There are two levels of assessment: screening and the comprehensive assessment. Screening is a process in which adolescents are identified according to characteristics that indicate that they possibly have a problem with substance use. Screening does not inform the

clinician of the severity of the adolescent's substance use or the presence of SUDs. Screening identifies the *need* for a comprehensive assessment and is not a substitute for an assessment. The comprehensive assessment is a thorough process that includes variables or factors contributing to and maintaining substance abuse, the severity of the problems, and the variety of consequences associated with the adolescent's substance use.

Screening

In order to screen large numbers of youth, clinicians and others such as school professionals, mental health professionals, and primary health care professionals often rely on the use of screening instruments.

The two alternative approaches to screening involve 1) specific screen of substance use and related behaviors, focusing on this behavior alone; or 2) screen-

TABLE 17–3. Selected instruments for screening of substance use problems in adolescents

Instrument	Reference	Comments
CRAFFT	Knight et al. 2002	6 items; is a brief screen for primary care professionals
Drug Use Screening Inventory—Adolescents (DUSI-A)	Tarter 1990	159 items; documents the level of involvement with a variety of drugs and quantifies severity of consequences associated with drug use
Problem Oriented Screening Instrument for Teenagers (POSIT)	Dembo et al. 1997	139 items; is designed to identify problems and potential need for service in 10 functional areas, including substance use and abuse
Personal Experience Screening Questionnaire (PESQ)	Winters 1992	40 items; screens for the need for further assessment of drug use disorders
Substance Abuse Subtle Screening Inventory (SASSI)	Feldstein and Miller 2007	81 items; has scales that include face-valid alcohol, face-valid other drug, obvious attributes, subtle attributes, and defensiveness
Adolescent Alcohol and Drug Involvement Scale (AADIS)	Moberg 2003	30 items; measures problem severity for alcohol, illicit substances
Drug Abuse Screening Test for Adolescents (DAST-A)	Martino et al. 2000	27 items; predicts DSM-IV substance-related disorders

ing for SUD as part of a multidomain screen that includes mental health problems and high-risk behaviors. Primary health care staff (e.g., physicians and nurses) typically use a brief series of questions to screen for substance use problems (e.g., CRAFFT, Knight et al. 2002; see Table 17–3), while mental health professionals use one of a variety of available screening instruments. In a primary care setting, questions for all youth about substance use follow a general inquiry about health behaviors and should include questions about cigarette, alcohol, and other substance use. In settings such as child welfare, mental health, or juvenile justice, the high-risk status is sufficient to require screening of each adolescent. Although specific interview questions with established validity such as the CRAFFT are often sufficient, many clinicians or other relevant professionals use specific screening instruments (see Table 17–3).

Professionals need to decide what screening threshold will trigger a comprehensive assessment. Generally, an adolescent report of regular substance use (e.g., greater than two times a month for several consecutive months) and/or consequences of use is sufficient for referral for a comprehensive assessment. Other factors, such as past history of substance use, high-risk behaviors, or moderate to severe high-risk status, may prompt such a referral even in the absence of an adolescent report of regular use or consequences.

Comprehensive Assessment

The assessment process is used to identify those individuals who have an SUD (see Table 17–4) and whether they meet criteria for a DSM-IV diagnosis. Substance use behaviors, the pattern of use, and any consequences of use are also discussed. The results of the comprehensive assessment will usually identify which individuals require treatment, what level of treatment, and other problems as well as strengths of the adolescent that may be helpful.

The domain model of assessment (Tarter 1990) recognizes that evaluation of many domains of functioning in the adolescent's life and possible psychopathology is required. These domains include substance use behaviors, psychiatric and behavioral problems, school and occupational functioning, family functioning, social competency and peer relations, and leisure/recreation.

The Interview

A comprehensive substance use history includes age at onset, duration, frequency, and route of ingestion for each individual drug, including alcohol, tobacco, illicit drugs, inhalants, over-the-counter medications, and prescription drugs such as benzodiazepines, opiates, and stimulants. Additional inquiry should cover negative consequences as well as attempts and moti-

TABLE 17–4. Selected instruments for evaluation of substance use problems in adolescents

Instrument	Reference	Comments
Adolescent Drug Abuse Diagnosis (ADAD)	Friedman and Utada 1989	Provides severity ratings on multiple domains of functioning
Adolescent Problem Severity Index (APSI)	Metzger et al. 1991	Provides severity ratings on multiple domains of functioning
Teen Addiction Severity Index (T-ASI)	Kaminer et al. 1993	Provides severity ratings on multiple domains of functioning
Comprehensive Addiction Severity Inventory for Adolescents (CASI-A)	Meyers et al. 1995	Provides severity ratings on multiple domains of functioning
Global Appraisal of Individual Needs (GAIN)	Dennis 1998	Documents SUD and other psychiatric diagnoses; placement criteria; health, mental distress, and environment; and service utilization outcomes (a brief version allows for screening and an outcome version provides information about critical outcome variables)
Customary Drinking and Drug Use Record (CDDR)	Brown et al. 1998	Contains current and lifetime measures of four alcohol- and other drug-related domains
Adolescent Diagnostic Interview (ADI)	Winters and Henly 1993	Assesses symptoms associated with SUDs; obtains diagnoses, substance use history, and psychosocial functioning
Modified Structured Clinical Interview for DSM-IV (SCID)	Martin et al. 1995	Is a semistructured interview to assess DSM-IV SUDs
Personal Experience Inventory (PEI)	Winters et al. 1996	Is self-administered; has scales that measure substance use, severity, psychosocial risk, and response distortion

Note. SUD=substance use disorder.

vation to control use or quit. Areas covered by questions detailing the context of use include the setting of use (time and place), whether the adolescent uses alone or with peers, and the attitudes of these peers about substance use. Variability in quantity and frequency of adolescent substance use is often great. The adolescent may report periods of abstinence as well as periods of rapid acceleration of use and heavy use of particular agents. A timeline drug chart or calendar is often useful to allow the adolescent to report quantity, frequency, and variability data across time with important dates, holidays, and other time cues as a guide. Additional substance use–related information includes attitudes and/or expectancies of use, and motivation(s) or perceived benefits to use. Assessment of substance use behavior may follow a functional analysis of use to determine usual antecedents to use and consequences of use. Such an analysis may allow a more specific targeting of relevant antecedents during treatment. Along with specific attitudes and beliefs

about substance use, the clinician should also inquire about the adolescent's values and attitudes in general.

Although substance use may be the target domain for the assessment, the other domains are also very important. In choosing the level of inquiry into psychopathology, the clinician is guided by the setting and the purpose of the assessment. Screening questions about depression, suicidality, aggression, psychosis, and treatment history may be sufficient in order to augment other information in determining when an adolescent should be referred for a more detailed, comprehensive psychiatric evaluation. The medical history and possible physical exam search for symptoms and illnesses that may be related to SUDs and behaviors, including trauma, pregnancies, HIV/AIDS, sexually transmitted diseases, infections or wounds, and possible liver diseases. School/vocational, peer, and family domains would emphasize family and peer substance use and attitudes toward use, parental monitoring and supervision, family history of SUDs and psychiatric disorders, and the effect of substance use on academic and/or vocational functioning. Inquiry into recreational or prosocial activities such as sports, interests, and hobbies will provide the clinician with information about the adolescent's social repertoire and whether this will have to be targeted for change.

Confidentiality

Adolescents are more likely to provide truthful information if they believe that their information, at least the details, will not be shared. Prior to the adolescent interview, the clinician should review exactly what information the clinician is obliged to share and with whom. Typically, a clinician should inform the adolescent that a threat of danger to self or others will force the clinician to inform a responsible adult, usually the parents. Information about physical or sexual abuse must be reported to the authorities. The clinician should be knowledgeable about state and federal laws that limit what information may be released from drug and alcohol treatment programs. Confidentiality statutes include information about illegal behavior such as selling drugs, who sells the adolescent drugs, and peer behaviors. In order for the assessment team to speak with the adolescent's family, school, or legal staff members, the adolescent must sign a consent form. In some states, parents must also sign a consent form. The clinician should encourage and support the adolescent's revealing to parents the extent of substance use and other problems. The clinician should discuss what information the adolescent will allow the clinician to reveal, such as a general recommendation for treatment or impressions rather than a detailed report of specific behaviors.

Toxicology

Toxicological tests—of bodily fluids (usually urine but also saliva) and of hair samples—to detect the presence of specific substances should be part of the formal evaluation and the ongoing assessment of substance use (Jaffee et al. 2008; see Table 17–5). The optimal use of urine screening requires proper collection techniques, including monitoring of obtaining the sample, evaluation of positive results, and specific plan(s) of action should the specimen be positive or negative for the presence of substance(s) (Casavant 2002). Prior to testing, the clinician should establish rules regarding the confidentiality of the results. Because of the limited time a drug will remain in the urine and possible adulteration, a negative urine screen does not indicate that

TABLE 17–5. Urine toxicology

Substance	Half-life, hrs	Detection after last use, days
Amphetamines	10–15	1–2
Barbiturates	20–96	3–21
Benzodiazepines	20–90	2–9
Cocaine	0.8–6.0	0.2–4 (metabolites)
Methaqualone	20–60	7–24
Opiates	2–4	1–2
Phencyclidine	7–16	2–8
Cannabinoids	10–40	2–8 (acute); 14–42 (chronic)
Alcohol		12 hours
Heroin	2–3	1–3
Methadone	15–60	7–10

Note. Drugs not usually tested: lysergic acid diethylamide (LSD); psilocybin; methylenedioxymethamphetamine (MDMA); 3,4-methylenedioxyamphetamine (MDA); and other designer drugs. These drugs may be tested by chromatography methods.

the youngster does not use drugs. A positive specimen indicates only the presence of specific drug(s) and not necessarily the presence of an SUD or a specific pattern of use.

Outcome Assessment

Ongoing evaluation of the effects of treatment on relevant variables is critical to planning treatment and determining whether existing treatment is working. Ongoing assessment generally consists of toxicology in addition to questioning the adolescent about the extent of his or her recent or interim substance use. In addition to substance use, clinicians should monitor the effects of treatment on other domains of functioning.

Treatment

Reviews of studies of adolescent treatment outcome have concluded that treatment is better than no treatment (Deas and Thomas 2001; Williams et al. 2000). In the year following treatment, adolescents report decreased heavy drinking, marijuana and other illicit drug use, and criminal involvement, as well as improved psychological adjustment and school performance (Grella et al. 2001; Hser et al. 2001). Longer duration of treatment is associated with several favorable outcomes. Pretreatment factors associated with poorer outcomes (usually substance use and relapse to use) are co-occurring psychopathology, nonwhite race, higher severity of substance use, criminality, and lower educational status. The in-treatment factors predictive of outcome are greater readiness to change, time in treatment, involvement of family, use of practical problem solving, and provision of comprehensive services such as housing, academic assistance, and recreation. Posttreatment variables that are thought to be the most important determinants of outcome include association with nonusing peers and involvement in leisure time activities, work, and school. Variables reported to be most consistently related to successful outcome are treatment completion, low pretreatment use, and peer and parent social support and nonuse of substances (Grella et al. 2001; Tomlinson et al. 2004). However, posttreatment factors account for more of the variance in outcome over 1-year follow-up than do pre- and during-treatment factors (Hsieh et al. 1998).

The primary goal for the treatment of adolescents with SUDs is achieving and maintaining abstinence from substance use. While abstinence should remain the explicit long-term goal for treatment, a realistic view recognizes both the chronicity of SUDs in some populations of adolescents and the self-limited nature of substance use and substance use–related problems in others. Given these considerations, harm reduction may be an interim, implicit, acceptable outcome, if not goal, of treatment. Included in the concept of harm reduction is a reduction in the use and negative consequences of substances, a reduction in the severity and frequency of relapses, and an improvement in one or more domains of the adolescent's functioning (e.g., academic performance or family functioning). While adolescents may not initially be motivated to stop substance use in treatment, the attainment of skills to deal with substance use may provide the adolescent with greater self-efficacy to not only reduce use but also ultimately move toward the future goal of abstinence. "Controlled use" of any nonprescribed substance of abuse should never be an explicit goal in the treatment of adolescents. In addition, control of substance use should not be the only goal of treatment. A broad concept of rehabilitation involves targeting associated problems and domains of functioning for treatment. Integrated interventions that concurrently deal with coexisting psychiatric and behavioral problems, family functioning, peer and interpersonal relationships,

and academic or vocational functioning not only will produce general improvements in psychosocial functioning but most likely will yield improved outcomes in the primary treatment goal of achieving and maintaining abstinence.

Based on the combination of empirical research and current clinical consensus, the clinician dealing with adolescents with SUDs should develop a treatment plan that uses modalities that target 1) motivation and engagement; 2) family involvement to improve supervision, monitoring, and communication between parents and adolescent; 3) improved problem solving, social skills, and relapse prevention; 4) comorbid psychiatric disorders through psychosocial and/or medication treatments; 5) social ecology in terms of increasing prosocial behaviors, peer relationships, and academic functioning; and 6) adequate duration of treatment and follow-up care. Self-support groups can be encouraged as adjuncts to the modalities above.

Only a small percentage of adolescents with SUDs actually receive treatment. Among youth ages 12–17, there were 1.3 million (4.9%) who needed treatment for an illicit drug use problem in 2005. Of this group, only 142,000 received treatment at a specialty facility (11.3% of youth ages 12–17 who needed treatment), leaving 1.1 million youth who needed treatment at a specialty facility but did not receive it (Substance Abuse and Mental Health Services Administration 2007). Among 12- to 17-year-olds in publicly funded addictions treatment, most were referred by the criminal justice system, with smaller proportions referred by schools or family; rates of self-referral to treatment begin to increase only in young adulthood (Dennis et al. 2003).

Pharmacological Treatments

Although there are few data on pharmacological treatment for adolescents with SUD, the use of pharmacotherapy is very prevalent, reaching 55% of adolescents seen in SUD treatment (Clark et al. 2003). The majority of the research in pharmacotherapy of adolescents with SUD relates to the treatment of comorbid psychiatric disorders, such as depression and ADHD. Strategies in pharmacological interventions for SUDs include substitution therapies, detoxification, blocking therapies, craving reduction, and aversion therapies (Waxmonsky and Wilens 2005).

Substitution therapies, which are used to prevent withdrawal, eliminate drug craving, and block the euphoric effects of illicit opiate use, use an agonist (e.g., nicotine replacement therapy [NRT] for nicotine dependence, methadone maintenance for opioid dependence) or a partial agonist (e.g., buprenorphine for opioid dependence) that acts on the same receptors that mediate the psychotropic effects of a substance.

Detoxification strategies generally use agonists or medications that provide symptomatic relief (e.g., clonidine for opioid withdrawal; benzodiazepines for alcohol withdrawal). In the absence of data, it is reasonable to use for adolescents the pharmacotherapy protocols similar to those used in adults, when needed. Since adolescents may not use substances in the same amount, frequency, or duration as adults, they may be less likely to have withdrawal symptoms as compared to adults (e.g., alcohol) (Brown et al. 2001).

Aversive interventions, such as disulfiram (Antabuse), blocking strategies (e.g., naltrexone for opiate dependence), and anticraving medications (naltrexone, acamprosate, and ondansetron for alcohol; bupropion for nicotine; and buprenorphine for opioids), require medication adherence and are likely most effective among patients with high motivation. With the possible exception of bupropion and buprenorphine, there is very modest evidence supporting their use in adolescents. These agents should be prescribed to youth only after a thorough consideration of previous treatment attempts.

Nicotine dependence or cigarette smoking is commonly present in adolescents with SUDs and/or psychiatric disorders, but few are diagnosed with nicotine dependence and offered smoking cessation treatment (Upadhyaya et al. 2002). NRTs (transdermal patch, gum, inhaler, and lozenge), varenicline, and bupropion sustained-release (SR) are currently approved by the U.S. Food and Drug Administration for smoking cessation in adults. NRT and bupropion SR are the agents most studied for adolescent smokers, with most studies of NRT using the transdermal nicotine patch. The efficacy of the transdermal nicotine patch has been modest among adolescents, with resulting abstinence rates ranging from 5% to 18% (Moolchan et al. 2004). Nicotine withdrawal symptoms may be a significant problem in situations where adolescents with nicotine dependence cannot smoke, such as psychiatric hospitals, and NRT may need to be provided to counter nicotine withdrawal symptoms, even to non-treatment-seeking adolescent smokers (Upadhyaya et al. 2005). Bupropion has also shown promise in an open study in the treatment of adolescent smokers (Upadhyaya et al. 2004).

Buprenorphine is a partial agonist. It is difficult to overdose on buprenorphine, and its combination with naloxone (opiate antagonist) makes it difficult to abuse intravenously. Naloxone is not absorbed orally and hence is not active if the combination is taken sublingually (e.g., buprenorphine is taken sublingually). In case someone tries to inject the medication, naloxone blocks the opiate receptors and hence no euphoric effects of buprenorphine are experienced. In a recent double-blind, double-dummy trial of buprenorphine versus clonidine detoxification in a 28-day outpatient clinic with 36 adolescents with opiate dependence, buprenorphine had almost double the retention and half the number of positive urine tests for opiates compared to clonidine (Marsch et al. 2005). Current evidence does not support use of pharmacotherapy of any other SUDs or other drug use (e.g., cocaine, stimulants, sedative/hypnotics, or club drugs) in adolescents.

Comorbid Psychiatric Disorders

Recent emerging research and experience suggest that pharmacotherapy can be used safely and effectively in adolescents with SUDs (Waxmonsky and Wilens 2005). A double-blind, placebo-controlled trial with cognitive-behavioral therapy (CBT) for SUDs plus fluoxetine or placebo for adolescents with major depressive disorder and SUD showed greater improvement for the active medication for depressive symptoms while there were no significant group differences for substance use (Riggs et al. 2007). A double-blind, placebo-controlled trial of a stimulant medication (pemoline) demonstrated the efficacy of medication improving ADHD symptoms in adolescents with comorbid ADHD and SUD, although there were no differences between groups on substance use (Riggs et al. 2004). In a randomized controlled trial including adolescents with SUDs and comorbid bipolar disorder (Geller et al. 1988), lithium showed significant improvements over placebo on both mood and substance use variables.

Some commonly used pharmacological agents, such as psychostimulants and benzodiazepines, have inherent abuse potential. The risk of diversion or misuse of a therapeutic agent by the adolescent, his or her peer group, or family members should prompt a thorough assessment of the risk of this outcome (e.g., history of abuse of the specific or other potentially abusable agents, family/parental history of substance abuse or antisocial behavior). Often, parental or adult supervision of medication administration can alleviate concerns about potential abuse. The clinician should also consider alternative agents to psychostimulants, such as atomoxetine or bupropion, which do not have abuse potential. The long-acting stimulant preparations may offer less potential for abuse or diversion due to their form of administration, reduced level of reinforcement due to more gradual and longer time to maximum plasma concentration, and ability to more easily monitor and supervise once-a-day dosing. For example, both OROS methylphenidate and lisdexamfetamine have minimal, if any, effects if snorted or injected. Many anxiety symptoms or disorders in adolescents can be treated successfully with psychosocial methods such as behavior therapy. If pharmacotherapy is required, the use of selective serotonin reuptake inhibitors, tricyclic antidepressants, or buspirone is preferred over the use of benzodiazepines.

Psychotherapeutic Treatments

Substance Use

Family therapy approaches have the most empirical support (Stanton and Shadish 1997; Williams et al. 2000). Family interventions for substance abuse treatment have common goals: providing psychoeducation about SUDs, which decreases familial resistance to treatment and increases motivation and engagement; assisting parents and family to initiate and maintain efforts to get the adolescent into appropriate treatment and achieve abstinence; assisting parents and family to establish or reestablish structure with consistent limit setting and careful monitoring of the adolescent's activities and behavior; improving communication among family members; and getting other family members into treatment and/or support programs. Specific engagement procedures have been incorporated as part of many family-based interventions. Other family-based treatments such as multidimensional family therapy (Rowe et al. 2002) and multisystemic therapy (Randall et al. 2001) also have strong engagement goals and components.

Although not ideal, treatment can be effective without participation of the adolescent (Waldron et al. 2001). Similarly, interventions with the adolescent alone (e.g., CBT or CBT plus motivational enhancement therapy) are also effective (Kaminer and Burleson 1999). Individual approaches such as CBT, both alone and with motivational enhancement have been shown to be efficacious (Azrin et al. 2001; Kaminer and Burleson 1999; Waldron et al. 2001). Community reinforcement approaches using contingency contracting and vouchers also appear to be promising (Henggeler et al. 2007). Modifications of motivational interviewing or enhancement techniques for adolescents (see Chapter 60, "Motivational Interviewing") have shown promise for both evaluation and treatment, based on limited treatment studies (Monti et al. 2001).

Twelve-step approaches, using Alcoholics Anonymous (AA) and Narcotics Anonymous (NA) as a basis for treatment, are perhaps the most common approaches for treatment in the United States. Naturalistic studies of adolescent SUD treatment find that attendance in aftercare treatment or self-support groups (e.g., AA or NA) is related to positive outcomes (Alford et al. 1991; Winters et al. 2000) and higher rates of abstinence and other measures of improved outcome, when compared with adolescents not participating in such groups following treatment (Kelly et al. 2000).

In 12-step programs, adolescents work on specific steps toward recovery, attend self-support groups (AA or NA), and obtain the assistance of a sponsor (another person in recovery from substance use problems) (Jaffe 2001). Specific developmentally appropriate 12-step programs and self-support groups offer several benefits including a recovering (i.e., nonsubstance-using) peer group, available sponsors, and other types of support. Although 12-step programs may be effective for many adolescents, they have not been subject to controlled clinical trials.

SUDs are often chronic disorders requiring ongoing intervention. Participation in aftercare services following treatment in a program is related to improved outcomes (Williams et al. 2000). Adolescents attending more intensive aftercare programs involving case management and community reinforcement were more likely than those who did not receive these services to be abstinent from marijuana and to reduce their alcohol use at 3 months postdischarge (Godley et al. 2002). After the acute treatment for substance use, ongoing attention should be paid to comorbid psychopathology and other comprehensive needs of the adolescent and his or her family.

Treatment of Gambling and Internet Addiction

There are few controlled studies to guide treatment planning for gambling and Internet addiction. Based on the similarities of these problems with SUDs, similar approaches appear reasonable pending future studies. Some investigators have proposed modified CBT for adolescent gambling (Derevensky 2007). As motivation to desist may be an issue among youth, motivational interviewing or enhancement (Chapter 60, "Motivational Interviewing") may be useful as a lead-in or adjunct to specific treatment for these problems. Although the intervention approaches may be similar, such youth should not be treated in SUD programs.

Research Directions

Despite the many recent advances in understanding the etiology of SUDs in adolescents, better defining the relevant phenomenology, and conducting intervention trials, further research is necessary. Many interventions that have demonstrated efficacy and effectiveness in adult SUD populations, such as motivational interviewing, need to have additional trials in adolescent populations. Given the extent and influence of psychiatric comorbidity on the presentation and course of SUDS, researchers need to see how the psychosocial and pharmacological treatment of psychiatric comorbidity affects the course of SUDs in adolescents.

Summary Points

- Clinicians should distinguish among substance use, misuse, abuse, dependence, and diversion.

- Some illicit substance use is normative for adolescents; however, preoccupation, compulsive use, and/or negative consequences of use indicate potential pathology.

- Risk factors for the development of SUDs include individual, peer, and family factors; risk factors are likely not specific for a particular substance but are common across substances.

- While most adolescents start with gateway drugs that are legal for older individuals (e.g., tobacco and alcohol), they may start with other drugs such as marijuana and bypass gateway drugs.

- Comorbidity with other psychiatric disorders is the rule rather than the exception in adolescents with SUDs.

- Comorbid psychiatric disorders should be treated concurrently with SUDs.

- Evidence-based practices for SUDs include specific family therapies, CBT, and motivational interviewing/enhancement.

- Aftercare and involvement in prosocial activities with nondeviant peers are critical following an acute treatment episode.

- Empirically based prevention interventions primarily involve strengthening resilience factors and reducing risk factors for the development of SUDs.

References

Alford GS, Koehler RA, Leonard J: Alcoholics Anonymous–Narcotics Anonymous model inpatient treatment of chemically dependent adolescents: a 2-year outcome study. J Stud Alcohol 52:118–126, 1991

American Academy of Child and Adolescent Psychiatry: Practice parameters for the assessment and treatment of children and adolescents with substance use disorders. J Am Acad Child Adolesc Psychiatry 44:609–621, 2005

American Psychiatric Association: Diagnostic and Statistic Manual of Mental Disorders, 4th Edition. Washington, DC, American Psychiatric Association, 1994

American Psychiatric Association: Diagnostic and Statistic Manual of Mental Disorders, 4th Edition, Text Revision. Washington, DC, American Psychiatric Association, 2000

Armstrong TD, Costello EJ: Community studies of adolescent substance use, abuse, or dependence and psychiatric comorbidity. J Consult Clin Psychol 70:1224–1239, 2002

Azrin NH, Donohue B, Teichner GA, et al: A controlled evaluation and description of individual-cognitive problem solving and family behavior therapies in dually diagnosed conduct-disordered and substance-dependent youth. J Child Adolesc Subst Abuse 11:1–43, 2001

Boyd CJ, McCabe SE, Teter CJ: Medical and nonmedical use of prescription pain medication by youth in a Detroit-area public school district. Drug Alcohol Depend 81:37–45, 2006

Brown SA, Gleghorn A, Schuckit MA, et al: Conduct disorder among adolescent alcohol and drug abusers. J Stud Alcohol 57:314–324, 1996

Brown SA, Myers MG, Lippke L, et al: Psychometric Evaluation of the Customary Drinking and Drug Use Record (CDDR): a measure of adolescent alcohol and drug involvement. J Stud Alcohol 59:427–438, 1998

Brown SA, D'Amico EJ, McCarthy DM, et al: Four-year outcomes from adolescent alcohol and drug treatment. J Stud Alcohol Suppl 62:381–388, 2001

Casavant MJ: Urine drug screening in adolescents. Pediatr Clin North Am 49:317–327, 2002

Chassin L, Flora D, King K: Trajectories of alcohol and drug use and dependence from adolescence to adulthood: the effects of familial alcoholism and personality. J Abnorm Psychol 113:483–498, 2004

Chung T: Adolescent substance use, abuse, and dependence: prevalence, course, and outcomes, in Adolescent Substance Abuse: Psychiatric Comorbidity and High Risk Behaviors. Edited by Kaminer Y, Bukstein OG. New York, Haworth Press, 2007, pp 29–52

Chung T, Martin CS: Classification and course of alcohol problems among adolescents in addictions treatment programs. Alcohol Clin Exp Res 25:1734–1742, 2001

Chung T, Martin C: Classification and short-term course of DSM-IV cannabis, hallucinogen, cocaine, and opioid disorders in treated adolescents. J Consult Clin Psychol 73:995–1004, 2005

Chung T, Martin CS, Armstrong TD, et al: Prevalence of DSM-IV alcohol diagnoses and symptoms in adolescent community and clinical samples. J Am Acad Child Adolesc Psychiatry 41:546–554, 2002

Chung T, Martin CS, Grella C, et al: Course of alcohol problems in treated adolescents: symposium proceedings of 2002 Research Society on Alcoholism Meeting. Alcohol Clin Exp Res 27:253–261, 2003

Clark DB, Pollock N, Bukstein OG, et al: Gender and comorbid psychopathology in adolescents with alcohol dependence. J Am Acad Child Adolesc Psychiatry 36: 1195–1203, 1997

Clark DB, Neighbors BD, Lesnick LA, et al: Family functioning and adolescent alcohol use disorders. J Fam Psychol 12:81–92, 1998

Clark DB, Wood DS, Cornelius JR, et al: Clinical practices in the pharmacological treatment of comorbid psychopathology in adolescents with alcohol use disorders. J Subst Abuse Treat 25:293–295, 2003

Cornelius JR, Maisto SA, Martin CS, et al: Major depression associated with earlier alcohol relapse in treated teens with AUD. Addict Behav 29:1035–1038, 2004

Cornelius JR, Clark DB, Bukstein OG, et al: Acute phase and five-year follow-up study of fluoxetine in adolescents with major depression and comorbid substance use disorder: a review. Addict Behav 30:1824–1833, 2005

Costello EJ, Erkanli A, Federman E, et al: Development of psychiatric comorbidity with substance abuse in adolescents: effects of timing and sex. J Clin Child Psychol 28:298–311, 1999

Crowley TJ, Mikulich SK, Ehlers KM, et al: Validity of structured clinical evaluations in adolescents with conduct and substance problems. J Am Acad Child Adolesc Psychiatry 40:265–273, 2001

Deas D, Thomas SE: An overview of controlled studies of adolescent substance abuse treatment. Am J Addict 10:178–189, 2001

Dembo R, Schmeidler J, Borden P, et al: Use of the POSIT among arrested youths entering a juvenile detention center: a replication and update. J Child Adolesc Subst Abuse 6:19–42, 1997

Dennis ML: Global Appraisal of Individual Needs (GAIN): Administration Guide for the GAIN and Related Measures. Bloomington, IL, Lighthouse Publications, 1998

Dennis ML, Dawud-Noursi S, Muck RD, et al: The need for developing and evaluating adolescent treatment models, in Adolescent Substance Abuse Treatment in the United States: Exemplary Models From a National Evaluation Study. Edited by Stevens SJ, Morral AR. Binghamton, NY, Haworth Press, 2003, pp 3–34

Derevensky JL: Gambling behaviors, in Adolescent Substance Abuse: Psychiatric Comorbidity and High Risk Behaviors. Edited by Kaminer Y, Bukstein OG. New York, Haworth Press, 2007, pp 403–433

Feldstein SW, Miller R: Does subtle screening for substance abuse work? A review of the Substance Abuse Subtle Screening Inventory (SASSI). Addiction 102:41–50, 2007

Friedman AS, Utada A: A method for diagnosing and planning the treatment of adolescent drug abusers: Adolescent Drug Abuse Diagnosis instrument. J Drug Educ 19:285–312, 1989

Geller B, Cooper TB, Sun K, et al: Double-blind and placebo-controlled study of lithium for adolescent bipolar disorders with secondary substance dependency. J Am Acad Child Adolesc Psychiatry 37:171–178, 1988

Godley MD, Godley SH, Dennis ML, et al: Preliminary outcomes from the Assertive continuing care experiment for adolescents discharged from residential treatment. J Subst Abuse Treat 23:21–32, 2002

Grant B, Dawson D: Age at onset of alcohol use and its associated DSM-IV alcohol abuse and dependence: results from the National Longitudinal Alcohol Epidemiologic Survey. J Subst Abuse Treat 9:103–110, 1997

Grella C, Hser YI, Joshi V, et al: Drug treatment outcomes for adolescents with comorbid mental and substance use disorders. J Nerv Ment Dis 189:384–392, 2001

Henggeler SW, Chapman JE, Rowland MD, et al: If you build it, they will come: statewide practitioner interest in contingency management for youths. J Subst Abuse Treat 32: 121–131, 2007

Hser YI, Grella CE, Hubbard RL, et al: An evaluation of drug treatments for adolescents in four U.S. cities. Arch Gen Psychiatry 58:689–695, 2001

Hsieh S, Hoffman NG, Hollister CD: The relationship between pre-, during-, and posttreatment factors and adolescent substance abuse behaviors. Addict Behav 23:477–488, 1998

Jaffe S: Adolescent Substance Abuse Intervention Workbook: Taking a First Step. Washington, DC, American Psychiatric Press, 2001

Jaffee WB, Trucco E, Teter C, et al: Focus on alcohol and drug abuse: ensuring validity in urine drug testing. Psychiatr Serv 59:140–142, 2008

Johnston LD, O'Malley PM, Bachman JG, et al: Monitoring the Future: National Results on Adolescent Drug Use. Overview of Key Findings, 2007 (NIH Publication No. 08–6418). Bethesda, MD, National Institute on Drug Abuse, 2008. Available at: http://monitoringthefuture.org/pubs/monographs/overview2007.pdf. Accessed May 5, 2008.

Kaminer Y, Burleson JA: Psychotherapies for adolescent substance abusers: 15-month follow-up of a pilot study. Am J Addict 8:114–119, 1999

Kaminer Y, Wagner E, Plummer B, et al: Validation of the Teen Addiction Severity Index (T-ASI): preliminary findings. Am J Addict 2:221–224, 1993

Kandel D, Yamaguchi K: Stages of drug involvement in the U.S. population, in Stages and Pathways of Drug Involvement: Examining the Gateway Hypothesis. Edited by Kandel D. New York, Cambridge University Press, 2002, pp 65–89

Kelly JF, Myers MG, Brown SA: A multivariate process model of adolescent 12-step attendance and substance use outcome following inpatient treatment. Psychol Addict Behav 4:376–389, 2000

Kendler KS, Jacobson KC, Prescott CA, et al: Specificity of genetic and environmental risk factors for use and abuse/dependence of cannabis, cocaine, hallucinogens, sedatives, stimulants, and opiates in male twins. Am J Psychiatry 160:687–695, 2003

Kendler KS, Schmitt E, Aggen SH, et al: Genetic and environmental influences on alcohol, caffeine, cannabis, and nicotine use from early adolescence to middle adulthood. Arch Gen Psychiatry 65:674–682, 2008

Knight JR, Sherritt L, Shrier LA, et al: Validity of the CRAFFT substance abuse screening test among adolescent clinic patients. Arch Pediatr Adolesc Med 156:607–614, 2002

Krueger RF, Hicks BM, Patrick CJ, et al: Etiologic connections among substance dependence, antisocial behavior, and personality: modeling the externalizing spectrum. J Abnorm Psychol 111:411–424, 2002

Marsch LA, Bickel WK, Badger GJ, et al: Comparison of pharmacological treatments for opioid-dependent adolescents: a randomized controlled trial. Arch Gen Psychiatry 62:1157–1164, 2005

Martin CS, Kaczynski NA, Maisto SA, et al: Patterns of DSM-IV alcohol abuse and dependence symptoms in adolescent drinkers. J Stud Alcohol 56:672–680, 1995

Martino S, Grilo CM, Fehon DC: The development of the Drug Abuse Screening Test for Adolescents (DAST-A). Addict Behav 25:57–70, 2000

McCarthy DM, Tomlinson KL, Anderson KG, et al: Relapse in alcohol- and drug-disordered adolescents with comorbid psychopathology: changes in psychiatric symptoms. Psychol Addict Behav 19:28–34, 2005

Metzger D, Kushner H, McLellan AT: Adolescent Problem Severity Index. Philadelphia, University of Pennsylvania, 1991

Meyers K, McLellan AT, Jaeger JL, et al: The development of the Comprehensive Addiction Severity Index for Adolescents (CASI-A): an interview for assessing multiple problems of adolescents. J Subst Abuse Treat 12:181–193, 1995

Moberg DP: Screening for Alcohol and Other Drug Problems Using the Adolescent Alcohol and Drug Involvement Scale (AADIS). Madison, Center for Health Policy and Program Evaluation, University of Wisconsin, 2003

Molina BS, Pelham WE: Childhood predictors of adolescent substance use in a longitudinal study of children with ADHD. J Abnorm Psychol 112:497–507, 2003

Monti PM, Barnett NP, O'Leary TA, et al: Motivational enhancement for alcohol-involved adolescents, in Adolescents, Alcohol, and Substance Abuse: Reaching Teens Through Brief Interventions. Edited by Monti PM, Colby SM, O'Leary TA. New York, Guilford, 2001, pp 145–182

Moolchan ET, Robinson ML, Ernst M, et al: Safety and efficacy of the nicotine patch and gum for the treatment of adolescent tobacco addiction. Pediatrics 115:407–414, 2004

Myers MG, Stewart DG, Brown SA: Progression from conduct disorder to antisocial personality disorder following treatment for adolescent substance abuse. Am J Psychiatry 155:479–485, 1998

National Institute on Drug Abuse: Preventing Drug Use Among Children and Adolescents: A Research-Based Guide for Parents, Educators, and Community Leaders, 2nd Edition. Rockville, MD, National Institute on Drug Abuse/National Institutes of Health, 2003

Oetting E, Beauvais F: Peer cluster theory, socialization, characteristics, and adolescent drug use: a path analysis. J Consult Clin Psychol 58:385–394, 1987

Pallanti S, Bernardi S, Quercioli L: The shorter PROMIS questionnaire and the Internet Addiction Scale in the assessment of multiple addictions in a high-school population: prevalence and related disability. CNS Spectr 11:966–974, 2006

Poulin C: Medical and nonmedical stimulant use among adolescents: from sanctioned to unsanctioned use. CMAJ 165:1039–1044, 2001

Randall J, Henggeler SW, Cunningham PB, et al: Adapting multisystemic therapy to treat adolescent substance abuse more effectively. Cogn Behav Pract 8:359–366, 2001

Riggs PD, Hall SK, Mikulich-Gilbertson SK, et al: A randomized controlled trial of pemoline for attention-deficit/hyperactivity disorder in substance-abusing adolescents. J Am Acad Child Adolesc Psychiatry 43:420–429, 2004

Riggs PD, Mikulich-Gilbertson SK, Davies RD, et al: A randomized controlled trial of fluoxetine and cognitive behavioral therapy in adolescents with major depression, behavior problems, and substance use disorders. Arch Pediatr Adolesc Med 161:1026–1034, 2007

Rohde P, Lewinsohn PM, Kahler CW, et al: Natural course of alcohol use disorders from adolescence to young adulthood. J Am Acad Child Adolesc Psychiatry 40:83–90, 2001

Rowe CL, Liddle HA, McClintic K, et al: Integrative treatment development: multidimensional family therapy for adolescent substance abuse, in Comprehensive Handbook of Psychotherapy. Edited by Kaslow F, Lebow J. New York, Wiley, 2002, pp 133–161

Stanton MD, Shadish WR: Outcome, attrition, and family couples treatment for drug abuse: a meta-analysis and review of the controlled, comparative studies. Psychol Bull 122:170–191, 1997

Stinchfield RD: Reliability of adolescent self-reported pretreatment alcohol and other drug use. Subst Use Misuse 32:63–76, 1997

Substance Abuse and Mental Health Services Administration: Results from the 2004 National Household Survey on Drug Use and Health: National Findings (NSDUH) Series H-28 (DHHS Publ No SMA-05–4062). Rockville, MD, Office of Applied Studies, 2005

Substance Abuse and Mental Health Services Administration: Results from the 2005 National Household Survey on Drug Use and Health: National Findings. Rockville, MD, Office of Applied Studies. Available at: http://www.oas.samhsa.gov/nsduh/2k5nsduh/2k5Results.htm#TOC. Accessed July 15, 2007.

Tarter R: Evaluation and treatment of adolescent substance abuse: a decision tree method. Am J Drug Alcohol Abuse 16:1–46, 1990

Tarter R, Vanyukov M, Giancola P, et al: Etiology of early age onset substance use disorder: a maturational perspective. Dev Psychopathol 11:657–683, 1999

Tarter R, Vanyukov M, Kirisci L, et al: Predictors of marijuana use in adolescent before and after illicit drug use: examination of the gateway hypothesis. Am J Psychiatry 163:2134–2140, 2006

Tomlinson KL, Brown SA, Abrantes A: Psychiatric comorbidity and substance use treatment outcomes of adolescents. Psychol Addict Behav 18:160–169, 2004

Tsuang MT, Lyons MJ, Meyer JM, et al: Co-occurrence of abuse of different drugs in men: the role of drug-specific and shared vulnerabilities. Arch Gen Psychiatry 55:967–972, 1998

Upadhyaya HP, Deas D, Brady KT, et al: Cigarette smoking and psychiatric comorbidity in children and adolescents. J Am Acad Child Adolesc Psychiatry 41:1294–1305, 2002

Upadhyaya HP, Brady KT, Wang W: Bupropion SR in adolescents with comorbid ADHD and nicotine dependence: a pilot study. J Am Acad Child Adolesc Psychiatry 43:199–205, 2004

Upadhyaya HP, Deas D, Brady KT: A practical clinical approach to the treatment of nicotine dependence in adolescents. J Am Acad Child Adoles Psychiatry 44:942–946, 2005

Vanyukov MM, Moss HB, Kaplan BB, et al: Antisociality, substance dependence, and the DRD5 gene: a preliminary study. Am J Med Genet 96:654–658, 2000

Waldron HR, Slesnick N, Brody JL, et al: Treatment outcomes for adolescent substance abuse at 4- and 7-month assessments. J Consult Clin Psychol 69:802–813, 2001

Waxmonsky JG, Wilens TE: Pharmacotherapy of adolescent substance use disorders: a review of the literature. J Child Adolesc Psychopharmacol 15:810–825, 2005

Wilens TW, Adler LA, Adams J, et al: Misuse and diversion of stimulants prescribed for ADHD: a systematic review of the literature. J Am Acad Child Adolesc Psychiatry 47:21–31, 2008

Williams RJ, Chang SY, Addiction Centre Adolescent Research Group: A comprehensive and comparative review of adolescent substance abuse treatment outcome. Clin Psychol Sci Pract 7:138–166, 2000

Winters KC: Development of an adolescent alcohol and drug abuse screening scale: Personal Experiences Screening Questionnaire. Addict Behav 17:479–490, 1992

Winters KC: Treating adolescents with substance use disorders: an overview of practice issues and treatment outcome. Subst Abuse 20:203–225, 1999

Winters KC, Henly GA: Adolescent Diagnostic Interview Schedule and Manual. Los Angeles, CA, Western Psychological Services, 1993

Winters KC, Stinchfield RD, Henly GA, et al: Validity of adolescent self-report of alcohol and other drug involvement. Int J Addict 25:1379–1395, 1991

Winters KC, Stinchfield RD, Henly GA: Convergent and predictive validity of the Personal Experience Inventory. J Child Adolesc Subst Abuse 5:37–55, 1996

Winters KC, Stinchfield RD, Opland E, et al: The effectiveness of the Minnesota Model approach in the treatment of adolescent drug abusers. Addiction 95:601–612, 2000

Wish E, Hoffman A, Nemes S: The validity of self-reports of drug use at treatment admission and at follow-up: comparisons with urinalysis and hair analysis. NIDA Res Monogr 167:200–226, 1997

World Health Organization: Lexicon of Alcohol and Drug Terms Published by the World Health Organization. Geneva, Switzerland, World Health Organization. Available at: http://www.who.int/substance_abuse/terminology/who_lexicon/en/index.html. Accessed July 15, 2007.

Yellowlees PM, Marks S: Problematic Internet use or Internet addiction? Comput Human Behav 23:1447–1450, 2007

PART V

AXIS I MOOD AND ANXIETY DISORDERS

Chapter 18

Depression and Dysthymia

Boris Birmaher, M.D.
David A. Brent, M.D.

Definition, Clinical Description, and Diagnosis

Depressive disorders are familial recurrent illnesses associated with significant morbidity and mortality. Early identification and effective treatment may reduce the impact of depression on the child's normal development and psychosocial functioning and reduce the risk for suicide and other conditions such as substance abuse.

The criteria for major depressive disorder (MDD) and dysthymic disorder (DD) used in this chapter are consistent with the *Diagnostic and Statistical Manual of Mental Disorders,* Fourth Edition (DSM-IV; American Psychiatric Association 1994), and its text revision (DSM-IV-TR; American Psychiatric Association 2000). Unless specified, the term *depression* encompasses both MDD and DD. Also, unless specified, the term *youth* refers to both children and adolescents.

Since there are few clinical studies and no controlled trials for the treatment of DD in youth, the information included in this chapter, particularly regarding treatment, pertains mainly to MDD.

Epidemiology

The prevalence of MDD is approximately 2% in children and 4%–8% in adolescents, with a male-female ratio of 1:1 during childhood and 1:2 during adolescence (Birmaher et al. 1996). The risk for depression increases by a factor of two to four after puberty, particularly in females, and the cumulative prevalence by age 18 is approximately 20% in community samples. Approximately 5%–10% of children and adolescents have subsyndromal symptoms of MDD. These youth have considerable psychosocial impairment and high family loading for depression, and are at increased risk for suicide and developing full symptoms of depression (Birmaher et al. 1996).

The few epidemiological studies that include DD report a prevalence of 0.6%–1.7% in children and 1.6%–8.0% in adolescents (Birmaher et al. 1996).

Clinical Description

Currently, the diagnosis of MDD in youth is made according to the DSM-IV-TR criteria (Table 18–1) or the ICD-10 (World Health Organization 1992).

Overall, the clinical picture of MDD in children and adolescents is similar to the clinical picture in adults, but there are some differences that can be attributed to the child's psychosocial developmental stage (Birmaher et al. 1996; Lewinsohn et al. 2003a; Luby et al. 2004; Yorbik et al. 2004). For example, children tend to be more irritable and have more low frustration tolerance, temper tantrums, somatic complaints, hallucinations, and/or social withdrawal instead of verbalizing feelings of depression when compared to adolescents. In contrast, adolescents usually have more melancholic symptoms and suicide attempts.

Subtypes of MDD have prognostic and treatment implications (Birmaher et al. 1996; Hughes et al. 2007). Psychotic depression has been associated with family history of bipolar and psychotic depression, more severe depression, greater long-term morbidity, resistance to antidepressant monotherapy, and, most notably, increased risk of bipolar disorder. MDD can be manifested with atypical symptoms such as increased reactivity to rejection, lethargy (leaden paralysis), increased appetite, craving for carbohydrates, and hypersomnia. Youth with seasonal affective disorder mainly have symptoms of depression during the season with less daylight. However, seasonal affective disorder should be differentiated from depression triggered by school stress, because both usually coincide with the school calendar.

The DSM-IV-TR criteria for DD are enumerated in Table 18–2. Since DD consists of a long-term change in mood that generally is less intense but more chronic than in MDD, it is often overlooked or misdiagnosed. However, although the symptoms of dysthymia are not as severe as in MDD, they cause as much, or more, psychosocial impairment (Kovacs et al. 1994; Masi et al. 2001).

Comorbidity

Depending on the setting, source of referral, and methodology used to ascertain comorbid disorders, 40%–90% of youth with depressive disorders also have other psychiatric disorders, with up to 50% having two or more comorbid diagnoses. The most frequent comorbid diagnoses are anxiety disorders, followed by disruptive disorders, attention-deficit/hyperactivity disorder (ADHD), and, in adolescents, substance use disorders. MDD and DD usually manifest after the onset of other psychiatric disorders (e.g., anxiety), but depression also increases the risk for the development of nonmood psychiatric problems such as conduct and substance abuse disorders (Angold et al. 1999; Birmaher et al. 1996; Fombonne et al. 2001; Lewinsohn et al. 2003a). MDD and DD may occur together (the so-called "double depression"), and either can be accompanied by medical or neurological illness.

Etiology, Mechanisms, and Risk Factors

As evidenced by high-risk, bottom-up (families of depressed youth), adoption, and twin studies, MDD runs in families (Birmaher et al. 1996; Caspi et al. 2003; Kendler et al. 2005; Pilowsky et al. 2006; Weissman et al. 2006b). In fact, the single most predictive factor associated with the risk of developing MDD is high family loading for this disorder (Birmaher et al. 1996). The heritability of MDD is about 40%–60% (Craddock et al. 2005), but it appears that genes only predispose a person to react to ongoing stressful situations with depressive symptoms. People who are homozygous or heterozygous for the less functional allele for the neuronal serotonin presynaptic reuptake site are most likely to develop MDD when they are also exposed to recurrent negative life events (Caspi et al. 2003; Kendler et al. 2005). Thus, the onset and recurrences of major depression may be precipitated by the presence of stressors such as losses, abuse, neglect, ongoing conflicts, exposure to violence, and frustrations. The effects of these stressors also depend on the child's cognitive and coping styles with stress, IQ, socioeconomic status, family and social support, and perhaps other genetic factors. For example, subjects who have negative cognitive styles and tendency toward rumination and hopelessness are at high risk to become depressed when exposed to negative life events (the cognitive

TABLE 18–1. DSM-IV-TR diagnostic criteria for major depressive episode

A. Five (or more) of the following symptoms have been present during the same 2-week period and represent a change from previous functioning; at least one of the symptoms is either (1) depressed mood or (2) loss of interest or pleasure.

Note: Do not include symptoms that are clearly due to a general medical condition, or mood-incongruent delusions or hallucinations.

(1) depressed mood most of the day, nearly every day, as indicated by either subjective report (e.g., feels sad or empty) or observation made by others (e.g., appears tearful). **Note:** In children and adolescents, can be irritable mood.

(2) markedly diminished interest or pleasure in all, or almost all, activities most of the day, nearly every day (as indicated by either subjective account or observation made by others)

(3) significant weight loss when not dieting or weight gain (e.g., a change of more than 5% of body weight in a month), or decrease or increase in appetite nearly every day. **Note:** In children, consider failure to make expected weight gains.

(4) insomnia or hypersomnia nearly every day

(5) psychomotor agitation or retardation nearly every day (observable by others, not merely subjective feelings of restlessness or being slowed down)

(6) fatigue or loss of energy nearly every day

(7) feelings of worthlessness or excessive or inappropriate guilt (which may be delusional) nearly every day (not merely self-reproach or guilt about being sick)

(8) diminished ability to think or concentrate, or indecisiveness, nearly every day (either by subjective account or as observed by others)

(9) recurrent thoughts of death (not just fear of dying), recurrent suicidal ideation without a specific plan, or a suicide attempt or a specific plan for committing suicide

B. The symptoms do not meet criteria for a mixed episode.

C. The symptoms cause clinically significant distress or impairment in social, occupational, or other important areas of functioning.

D. The symptoms are not due to the direct physiological effects of a substance (e.g., a drug of abuse, a medication) or a general medical condition (e.g., hypothyroidism).

E. The symptoms are not better accounted for by bereavement, i.e., after the loss of a loved one, the symptoms persist for longer than 2 months or are characterized by marked functional impairment, morbid preoccupation with worthlessness, suicidal ideation, psychotic symptoms, or psychomotor retardation.

Source. Reprinted from American Psychiatric Association: *Diagnostic and Statistical Manual of Mental Disorders,* 4th Edition, Text Revision. Washington, DC, American Psychiatric Association, 2000, p. 356. Used with permission. Copyright © 2000 American Psychiatric Association.

vulnerability-transactional stress model) (Alloy and Abramson 2007).

Family history of other disorders such as anxiety and substance abuse and the youth's factors such as prior history of depression, subsyndromal depressive symptoms, presence of other psychiatric disorders (e.g., anxiety, substance abuse, ADHD, eating disorders), medical illness (e.g., diabetes), medications (e.g., corticosteroids), and sociocultural factors have also been related to the development and maintenance of depressive symptomatology (Alloy and Abramson 2007; Birmaher et al. 1996; Caspi et al. 2003; Costello et

al. 2002; Kendler et al. 2005; Pine et al. 1998; Reinherz et al. 2003; Weissman et al. 2006a, 2006b).

Neurochemical, neuroimaging, and genetic studies are promising but not yet relevant to clinical practice (Birmaher et al. 1996; Zalsman et al. 2006).

Prevention

Strategies for the prevention of onset or recurrence of depression include the amelioration of risk factors

TABLE 18–2. DSM-IV-TR diagnostic criteria for dysthymic disorder

A. Depressed mood for most of the day, for more days than not, as indicated either by subjective account or observation by others, for at least 2 years.   **Note:** In children and adolescents, mood can be irritable and duration must be at least 1 year.

B. Presence, while depressed, of two (or more) of the following:

(1) poor appetite or overeating

(2) insomnia or hypersomnia

(3) low energy or fatigue

(4) low self-esteem

(5) poor concentration or difficulty making decisions

(6) feelings of hopelessness

C. During the 2-year period (1 year for children or adolescents) of the disturbance, the person has never been without the symptoms in Criteria A and B for more than 2 months at a time.

D. No major depressive episode has been present during the first 2 years of the disturbance (1 year for children and adolescents); i.e., the disturbance is not better accounted for by chronic major depressive disorder, or major depressive disorder, in partial remission.

Note: There may have been a previous major depressive episode provided there was a full remission (no significant signs or symptoms for 2 months) before development of the dysthymic disorder. In addition, after the initial 2 years (1 year in children or adolescents) of dysthymic disorder, there may be superimposed episodes of major depressive disorder, in which case both diagnoses may be given when the criteria are met for a major depressive episode.

E. There has never been a manic episode, a mixed episode, or a hypomanic episode, and criteria have never been met for cyclothymic disorder.

F. The disturbance does not occur exclusively during the course of a chronic psychotic disorder, such as schizophrenia or delusional disorder.

G. The symptoms are not due to the direct physiological effects of a substance (e.g., a drug of abuse, a medication) or a general medical condition (e.g., hypothyroidism).

H. The symptoms cause clinically significant distress or impairment in social, occupational, or other important areas of functioning.

Specify if:

Early Onset: if onset is before age 21 years

Late Onset: if onset is age 21 years or older

Specify (for most recent 2 years of dysthymic disorder):

With Atypical Features

Source.   Reprinted from American Psychiatric Association: *Diagnostic and Statistical Manual of Mental Disorders,* 4th Edition, Text Revision. Washington, DC, American Psychiatric Association, 2000, pp. 380–381. Used with permission. Copyright © 2000 American Psychiatric Association.

such as subsyndromal symptoms of depression, underlying psychiatric disorders (e.g., anxiety disorders), ongoing stressful situations, and parental psychopathology (Birmaher et al. 1996). The relationship between stress or conflict and depression is often bidirectional because depression can make a person more irritable, which then increases interpersonal tension, causing others to distance themselves from the depressed person, which then leads the patient to experience loneliness and lack of support. Involvement in deviant peer groups may lead to antisocial behavior,

generating more stressful life events and increasing the likelihood of depression (Fergusson et al. 2003). Thus, for those with recurrent depression, a proactive plan to avoid and/or cope with ongoing or anticipated difficulties may be helpful to diminish or prevent the risk for relapse and recurrence. Also, early identification of signs and symptoms of depression may help to abort relapses or new episodes of depression.

Successful treatment of mothers with depression was associated with significantly fewer new psychiatric diagnoses and higher remission rates of existing disorders in their children (Weissman et al. 2006a). Maternal depression has also been associated with less response to cognitive-behavioral therapy (CBT) for depression (Brent et al. 1998). These findings support the importance of early identification and vigorous treatment for depressed mothers in primary care or psychiatric clinics (Gunlicks and Weissman 2008).

Meta-analysis evaluated 30 studies of psychoeducation; cognitive, coping, and social skills; and family therapy to assess efficacy of the prevention of new onset or worsening of depressive symptomatology in general populations (universal studies) or youth at high risk to develop MDD because of parental depression or subsyndromal depression (Horovitz and Garber 2006). Programs for populations at risk were more effective than those targeting general populations, particularly for females and older subjects. However, the effects of these treatments were small to modest, both immediately postintervention and at an average follow-up of 6 months.

Early-onset dysthymia is associated with an increased risk of MDD (Kovacs et al. 1994), indicating the need for early treatment. Also, there is evidence that anxiety disorder is a precursor of depression (Birmaher et al. 1996; Pine et al. 1998; Weissman et al. 2006b), and treatment of this anxiety may reduce the onset and recurrences of depression (Dadds et al. 1999; Hayward et al. 2000). Since selective serotonin reuptake inhibitors (SSRIs) appear to have much greater efficacy for anxiety than for depression, vigorous detection and treatment of anxiety disorders may reduce the risk for subsequent depression.

Finally, although less or not well studied, prevention may include lifestyle modifications—regular and adequate sleep, exercise, a coping plan for stress (e.g., meditation, yoga, exercise, or social activities), pursuit of enjoyable and meaningful activities, and avoidance of situations that are predictably stressful and nonproductive.

Clinical Course and Outcome

The median duration of a major depressive episode in clinically referred youth is about 8 months, and in community samples, about 1–2 months. Although most children and adolescents recover from their first depressive episode, longitudinal studies of both clinical and community samples of depressed youth have

shown that the probability of recurrence reaches 20%–60% by 1–2 years after remission and climbs to 70% after 5 years (Birmaher et al. 2002; Costello et al. 2002). Recurrences can persist throughout life, and a substantial proportion of children and adolescents with MDD will continue to have MDD episodes as adults. For the most part, the predictors of recovery, relapse, and recurrence overlap. In general, greater severity, chronicity or multiple recurrent episodes, comorbidity, hopelessness, presence of residual subsyndromal symptoms, negative cognitive style, family problems, low socioeconomic status, and exposure to ongoing negative events (e.g., abuse, family conflict) are associated with poor outcome (Birmaher et al. 2002).

Childhood depression, compared with adolescent-onset depression, appears to be more heterogeneous. Some children have a strong family history of mood disorders and high risk for recurrences, whereas others are more likely to develop behavior problems and substance abuse than depression (Birmaher et al. 2002). About 20%-40% of depressed youth develop bipolar disorder. Those with high risk to develop bipolar disorder seem to have more psychotic depression, family history of depression, and pharmacological-induced manias or hypomanias (Birmaher et al. 2002; see Chapter 19, "Bipolar Disorder").

Childhood DD has a protracted course, with a mean episode length of approximately 3–4 years for clinical and community samples, and is associated with an increased risk for subsequent MDD and substance use disorders (Birmaher et al. 2002; Kovacs et al. 1994).

If untreated, depressive disorders affect the development of a child's emotional, cognitive, and social skills and interfere considerably with family relationships (Birmaher et al. 1996, 2002; Lewinsohn et al. 2003b). Suicide attempts and completion are among the most significant and devastating sequelae of MDD, with approximately 60% reporting having thought about suicide and 30% actually attempting suicide (Brent et al. 1999; see Chapter 35, "Youth Suicide"). The risk for suicidal behavior increases if there is a history of suicide attempts, comorbid psychiatric disorders (e.g., disruptive disorders, substance abuse), impulsivity and aggression, availability of lethal agents (e.g., firearms), exposure to negative events (e.g., physical or sexual abuse, violence), or family history of suicidal behavior.

Youth with depressive disorders are also at high risk for substance abuse (including nicotine dependence), legal problems, exposure to negative life events, physical illness, early pregnancy, and poor work, academic, and psychosocial functioning. After an acute episode of depression, a slow and gradual improvement in psychosocial functioning may occur unless there are relapses or recurrences. However, psychosocial difficulties and subsyndromal depressive symptoms frequently persist after the remission of the depressive episode, underscoring the need for continuing treatment for the depression as well as treatment that addresses associated psychosocial and contextual issues (Fergusson and Woodward 2002; Fergusson et al. 2005; Hammen et al. 2004; Lewinsohn et al. 2003b).

Evaluation

The most useful tool to diagnose depressive disorders is a comprehensive psychiatric diagnostic evaluation that is sensitive to the child's developmental stage, sex, race, environmental conditions, and cultural and religious background. No biological or imaging tests are clinically useful for the diagnosis of depression.

The evaluation should ascertain information from both the child and the parents regarding DSM-IV-TR or ICD-10 (World Health Organization 1992) symptoms and subtypes of depressive disorders (e.g., seasonal, psychotic), bipolar depression, other psychiatric and medical disorders, current and past treatments (types, dose, response, side effects), the child's current and past psychosocial functioning (e.g., school, family, social), the child's and family's strengths, exposure to acute and ongoing stressful life events (e.g., conflicts, abuse, exposure to violence), and family psychiatric and medical history (Chapter 3, "Assessing the Elementary School–Age Child," and Chapter 4, "Assessing Adolescents").

In the first episode of depression, it is difficult to differentiate unipolar major depression from the depressive phase of bipolar disorder. Certain indicators such as high family loading for bipolar disorder, psychosis, and history of pharmacologically induced mania or hypomania may herald the development of bipolar disorder (Birmaher et al. 1996). It is important to evaluate carefully for the presence of subtle or short-duration hypomanic symptoms because these symptoms often are overlooked, and these children and adolescents may be more likely to become manic when treated with antidepressant medications (Martin et al. 2004). However, it is also important to note that not all children who become activated or hypomanic while receiving antidepressants have bipolar disorder (Wilens et al. 1998).

MDD and DD need to be differentiated from other psychiatric (e.g., anxiety, ADHD, oppositional defiant disorder, pervasive developmental disorder, substance abuse) and medical (e.g., hypothyroidism, mononucleosis, anemia, certain cancers, autoimmune diseases, premenstrual dysphoric disorder, chronic fatigue syndrome) disorders, as well as conditions such as bereavement and depressive reactions to stressors (adjustment disorder). These conditions may also mimic or induce symptoms of depression such as poor self-esteem, demoralization, tiredness, sleep disturbances, and poor concentration. However, youth with these conditions should not be diagnosed with MDD or DD unless they meet the criteria for these disorders. Also, medications (e.g., stimulants, corticosteroids, and contraceptives) can induce depression-like symptomatology. The diagnosis of MDD or DD can be made if depressive symptoms are not due solely to the illnesses or the medications and if the youth fulfill the criteria for these depressive disorders.

Suicidal ideation and behaviors are very common in youth with depressive disorders. Thus, it is crucial to evaluate their presence before, during, and after treatment as well as the risks (e.g., age, sex, stressors, comorbid conditions, hopelessness, impulsivity) and protective factors (e.g., religious belief, concern not to hurt family) that might influence the desire to attempt suicide (see Chapter 35, "Youth Suicide"). The presence of guns or other potential suicidal (or homicidal) methods in the home should be ascertained, and the clinician should recommend that the parents secure or remove them (Brent et al. 1993a). Clinicians should also differentiate suicidal behavior from other types of self-harm behaviors, the goal of which is to relieve negative affect. This type of behavior most commonly involves repetitive self-cutting, with clear motivation to relieve anger, sadness, or loneliness rather than to end one's life.

Homicidal ideation and behaviors may occur in youth with depressive symptoms and co-occur with suicidal ideation in the same individuals. About one-third of adolescent suicide victims in one study had homicidal ideation in the week before their suicide (Brent et al. 1993b). Thus, clinicians must conduct an assessment similar to that described for suicidal ideation with regard to what factors are influencing, either positively or negatively, the degree of likelihood the patient will carry out a homicidal act.

Finally, the clinician, together with the child and parents, should evaluate the appropriate intensity and restrictiveness of care (e.g., hospitalization). The decision for the level of care will depend primarily on levels of function and safety to self and others, which in turn are determined by the severity of depression, presence of suicidal and/or homicidal symptoms, psychosis, substance dependence, agitation, child's and parents' adherence to treatment, parental psychopathology, and family environment.

Instruments

Standardized structured and semistructured interviews are available for the evaluation of psychiatric symptoms in children older than 7 years old and more recently in younger children (see Chapter 7, "Diagnostic Interviews"). The interviews are typically too long to be carried out in nonresearch settings and require special training.

In the assessment of the onset and course of mood disorders, it is helpful to use a mood diary and a mood timeline that use school years, birthdays, and so forth as anchors. Mood is rated from very happy to very sad and/or as very irritable to nonirritable. Normative and nonnormative stressors as well as treatments are noted. The mood timeline can help children and their parents to visualize the course of their mood and comorbid conditions, identify events that may have triggered the depression, and examine the relationship between treatment and response.

Clinician-based scales such as the Children's Depression Rating Scale (CDRS) (Poznanski and Mokros 1995) and parent and child self-report instruments such as the Mood and Feelings Questionnaire (Daviss et al. 2006) may be useful to assess the severity of the depressive symptoms before, during, and after treatment (Chapter 8, "Rating Scales").

Treatment

The treatment of depression is usually divided into three phases: acute, continuation, and maintenance. The main goal of the acute phase is to achieve response and ultimately *full* symptomatic remission. (For definitions of outcome, see Table 18–3.) Continuation treatment is required for all depressed youth to consolidate the response to treatment and avoid relapses. Finally, maintenance treatment is used to avoid recurrences or new episodes. The choice of treatment at each phase should be governed by factors such as age and cognitive development; severity and subtype of depression; chronicity; comorbid conditions; family psychiatric history; family and social environment; family and patient treatment preference and expectations; ethnical, cultural, and religious issues; and availability of expertise in pharmacotherapy and/or psychotherapy. During all treatment phases, clinicians should arrange frequent follow-up contacts that allow sufficient time to monitor the subject's clinical status (e.g., symptoms of depression, development of mania or hypomania, comorbid disorders, functioning) and environmental conditions.

Treatment response is usually defined as the absence of MDD criteria (e.g., no more than one DSM symptom) or a significant reduction (e.g., 50%) in symptom severity. However, using the latter criterion, patients deemed "responders" may still have considerable residual symptoms. Therefore, an absolute final score on the CDRS (Poznanski and Mokros 1995) ≤28 together with persistent improvement in the patient's functioning for at least 2 weeks or longer may better reflect a satisfactory response. Overall improvement has also been measured using the Clinical Global Impression Scale, Improvement subscale (Guy 1976).

Since the goal is to restore function and not just reduce symptoms, a lack of progress in functional status is an important clue that the depression is incompletely treated or that impaired functional status is due to a comorbid psychiatric or medical disorder or environmental factors. Functional improvement can be tracked using a score ≥70 on the Global Assessment of Functioning (GAF; American Psychiatric Association 2000) or the Children's Global Assessment Scale (Shaffer et al. 1983).

TABLE 18–3. Definitions of outcome

Response	No symptoms or a significant reduction in depressive symptoms for at least 2 weeks
Remission	A period of at least 2 weeks and less than 2 months with no or very few depressive symptoms
Recovery	Absence of significant symptoms of depression (e.g., no more than one to two symptoms) for ≥2 months
Relapse	A DSM episode of depression during the period of remission
Recurrence	Emergence of symptoms of depression during the period of recovery (a new episode)

If a patient is being treated with medication, it is important to evaluate adherence to medication treatment, presence of side effects, and youth and parent beliefs about the medication benefits and its side effects that may contribute to poor adherence or premature discontinuation of treatment. History of suicidality, homicidal ideation, or somatic symptoms should be evaluated before starting the pharmacological treatment, to assist in differentiating from symptoms of mood and other psychiatric or medical conditions or medication side effects during treatment.

Psychoeducation and Supportive Management

Each phase of treatment should include psychoeducation, supportive management for the family and patient, and school involvement (American Academy of Child and Adolescent Psychiatry 2007; see also Chapter 54, "Parent Counseling, Psychoeducation, and Parent Support Groups"). Parents and patient (and sometimes teachers) should be enlisted as collaborators in the diagnosis and treatment plan. Family members, patient, and, if appropriate, school personnel should be educated about the causes, symptoms, course, and treatments of depression and the risks associated with these treatments as well as of no treatment. Also, written material and reliable Web sites about depression and its treatment can be provided. Psychoeducation improves adherence to treatment and reduces the symptoms of depression (Ackerson et al. 1998; Brent et al. 1993c; Goodyer et al. 2007; Renaud et al. 1998; Sanford et al. 2006). For families with depressed parents, psychoeducation with or without further interventions improves the ability of families to solve problems around parental illness and children's behavior and attitudes.

The clinician and the family may need to advocate for school accommodations (e.g., schedule, workload) until recovery has been achieved. However, if after recovery the child continues to have academic difficulties, then the clinician should suspect subsyndromal depression or comorbid conditions (e.g., developmental learning disorders, ADHD, anxiety, substance abuse) or environmental factors that might explain the child's persistent difficulties. Students with a depressive disorder may qualify for the emotional disturbance disability categorization under the Individuals With Disabilities Education Act and therefore be eligible to receive school-based services (e.g., counseling) and accommodations that enable them to continue to learn (see Chapter 63, "School-Based Interventions").

It is crucial to involve the family to ascertain symptoms, assure that the youth is safe and adherent to treatment, and monitor progress and possible pharmacological side effects. Interventions with the family must take into account the family's cultural and religious background and focus on strengthening the relationship between the identified patient and caregiver(s), provide parenting guidance (e.g., management of conflicts), reduce family dysfunction, and facilitate treatment referral for caregivers or siblings with psychiatric disorders and for marital conflict (Birmaher et al. 2000; Garber et al. 2002; Hammen et al. 2004; Nomura et al. 2002).

Evidence that supportive management may help comes from pharmacotherapy and psychotherapy randomized controlled trials (RCTs), which have shown that up to an average of 50%–60% of children and adolescents with MDD respond to "placebo" (Bridge et al. 2007). Moreover, 15%–30% respond to very brief nonspecific treatments (Goodyer et al. 2007; Renaud et al. 1998). Thus it is reasonable, for a patient with a mild or brief depression, mild psychosocial impairment, and the absence of clinically significant suicidality or psychosis, to begin treatment with education, support, and case management related to environmental stressors in the family and school. Response is expected after 4–6 weeks of supportive therapy. However, when patients do not respond to supportive management, are more severely depressed, and have significant melancholic symptoms, hopelessness, or suicidal ideation/behaviors, supportive treatment is insufficient (Barbe et al. 2004b; Mufson et al. 1999; Renaud et al. 1998; Treatment of Adolescent Depression Study Team 2004) and these youth need a trial of specific psychotherapy and/or antidepressants.

Acute Treatment

Although it is still not clear which treatment is best for a particular youth with acute MDD, the choice of treatment may be dictated by availability, patient and family preference, or clinical presentation (e.g., a psychotic depressed child will not be able to engage in psychotherapy).

Psychotherapy

Several types of psychotherapy are being used for the treatment of youth with depression. However, only CBT and interpersonal psychotherapy (IPT) have evidence of efficacy from RCTs, particularly for depressed adolescents (Weisz et al. 2006; see also Chapter 57, "Interpersonal Psychotherapy for Depressed Adolescents," and Chapter 59, "Cognitive-Behavioral Therapy for Depression"). Psychodynamic therapy is widely used in clinical practice despite lack of evidence for efficacy. Because family interaction is related to the onset and course of adolescent depression (Birmaher et al. 2000; Nomura et al. 2002; Pilowsky et al. 2006), the improvement of family interactions is a logical treatment target in adolescent depression. However, only one RCT has examined the impact of family therapy and found that CBT was superior to a systemic behavioral family therapy in the short-term reduction of adolescent depression (Brent et al. 1997).

In general, the overall effects of psychotherapy for the acute treatment of depressed youth are modest (Weisz et al. 2006). The few psychotherapy studies that included follow-up after the acute treatment showed that the beneficial effects of psychotherapy appear durable for the initial months, but not for 1 year. Thus, more studies are needed to evaluate the effects of "boosters" and continuation therapy. Also, few studies have assessed suicidality as an outcome. On average, these studies showed a small reduction in suicidality without clear specific treatment effects, emphasizing the need for more targeted techniques to address this worrisome symptom (Weisz et al. 2006). Finally, the effects of the psychotherapy for depressed youth also improved anxiety but not externalizing symptoms, indicating the need for modified psychotherapy techniques to manage comorbid disruptive disorders.

The most widely studied type of psychotherapy for the treatment of youth with MDD is CBT. This psychotherapy is effective and appears to be more efficacious even in the face of comorbidity, suicidal ideation, and hopelessness. However, when there is a history of sexual abuse or when one of the parents is depressed, CBT does not appear to perform as well (Barbe et al. 2004a). Clinical trials conducted in primary care settings also suggest that CBT can be delivered effectively in primary care settings to depressed children and adolescents and results in better outcomes than treatment as usual (Asarnow et al. 2005; Weersing et al. 2006).

In contrast with most CBT studies, a recent large RCT did not find differences between CBT and placebo for adolescents with MDD (Treatment of Adolescent Depression Study Team 2004). Moreover, while the combination of CBT and fluoxetine showed a more rapid decline in depressive symptoms (Kratochvil et al. 2006), rates of clinical improvement and baseline-adjusted symptom ratings at endpoint were not different between combination treatment and medication alone. Also, the combined treatment was better than

fluoxetine alone mainly for mild to moderate depression and for depression with high levels of cognitive distortion, but not for severe depression (Curry et al. 2006). The combination treatment did result in a greater rate of remission than in any of the other treatments, but the effects were modest (remission rate 37% in combined treatment) (Kennard et al. 2006). It is unclear why CBT did not differ from placebo in this study with regard to acute treatment. Possible explanations include that the adolescents were not blind to medication assignment in the two CBT cells and that treatment delivered a "low dose" of a large number of skills and techniques, whereas some of the more successful treatment studies with CBT used a flexible protocol that focused mainly on cognitive restructuring and behavior activation (Weisz et al. 2006). Other RCTs examining the effects of combined treatment versus medication alone have also been disappointing. Goodyer et al. (2007) found that in moderate to severely depressed adolescents who did not respond to a brief psychosocial treatment, the combination of CBT plus an SSRI was no better than the SSRI alone in relief of depressive symptoms or improvement in overall outcome. Melvin et al. (2006) were unable to demonstrate the superiority of combined sertraline and CBT over either treatment alone for adolescents with mild to moderate depression. After acute treatment, CBT was found to be superior to sertraline alone, which may suggest an advantage to CBT but might also be explained by the relatively low sertraline dose. Finally, Clarke et al. (2005) compared the addition of CBT to SSRI management in primary care and found some modest improvement on quality of life but not on the primary outcome. Moreover, an unexpected result of the combined treatment was that those patients were more likely to discontinue their SSRIs.

IPT is emerging as another efficacious psychotherapy for adolescent depression, especially in patients who were moderately or severely depressed and in older teens (Mufson et al. 2004; see also Chapter 57, "Interpersonal Psychotherapy for Depressed Adolescents"). IPT has been shown to be at least as efficacious as CBT for adolescent depression (Rossello and Bernal 1999). IPT appears to be relatively easy to disseminate, insofar as therapists in school-based health clinics with brief training and supervision were able to improve depression using IPT compared with treatment as usual (Mufson et al. 2004).

Most of the above-noted clinical trials were carried out with adolescents rather than in younger children. However, randomized CBT trials for symptomatic volunteers have suggested that this therapy may be useful for younger children (Weisz et al. 2006). Most clinicians recommend the adaptation of cognitive, interpersonal, and psychodynamic techniques for younger children. In addition, because of the prominent role of family issues in early-onset depression and the greater dependency of the child on parents, some form of family intervention is recommended. However, no RCTs have been conducted in clinically referred depressed children.

Pharmacotherapy

Efficacy.

A meta-analysis of all published and unpublished pharmacological RCTs for MDD in youth showed an average response of 61% (95% confidence interval [CI], 58%–63%) for the SSRI antidepressants and 50% (95% CI, 47%–53%) for placebo, yielding a risk difference of 11%–95% CI, 7–15) (Bridge et al. 2007). Using these data, the number needed to treat to get one response that is attributable to active treatment was 10 overall (95% CI, 7–15). Several studies showed small or no differences between the SSRI and placebo, in part because the rates of placebo response were high. This was more obvious in depressed children than adolescents. Thus, it is possible that depressive symptoms in youth may be highly responsive to supportive management, that these studies included subjects with mild depression, or that other methodological issues, such as low medication doses, are responsible for the lack of difference between medication and placebo. Interestingly, the difference between the response to SSRIs and placebo was inversely related to the number of sites involved in the study (Bridge et al. 2007).

Fluoxetine showed a larger difference between medication and placebo than other antidepressants. This may be due to actual differences in the effect of the fluoxetine or other related properties of this medication (e.g., long half-life may lessen the effect of poor adherence to treatment) or because the studies involving fluoxetine were better designed and conducted or included more severely depressed patients.

The rate of remission, usually defined as a CDRS score of 28, ranged between 30% and 40% (Bridge et al. 2005). Possible explanations for this low rate are that it may take longer to observe higher rates of remission after response, optimal pharmacological treatment may involve a higher dose or longer duration of treatment, the lack of treatment of comorbid conditions might affect depressive symptoms, and/or some children and adolescents need to receive a combination of pharmacological and psychosocial interventions.

Few trials have evaluated the effects of other classes of antidepressants for the treatment of depressed youth (Hughes et al. 2007). RCTs have shown no differences between venlafaxine or mirtazapine and placebo (Bridge et al. 2007). Secondary analysis of the venlafaxine trials showed an age effect, with drug being better than placebo for depressed adolescents but not depressed children. However, children were treated with low doses (Emslie et al. 2007). One study showed better response in most measurements between nefazodone and placebo for adolescents with MDD, but a second study including depressed children and adolescents was negative. Finally, RCTs as well as a meta-analysis have shown that tricyclic antidepressants (TCAs) are no more efficacious than placebo for the treatment of child and adolescent depression (Hazell et al. 2002). For this reason, as well as side-effect profile and fatality after an overdose, TCAs should be far down the list of choices for treatment of youth depression.

Side effects.

The side effects of antidepressants are described in Chapter 47, "Antidepressants." Of these side effects, in addition to the rare risk to trigger hypomania in disposed children, the most serious side effect of the antidepressants is the small but statistically significant risk of onset or worsening of suicidal ideation and, more rarely, suicide attempts. A meta-analysis that reanalyzed the U.S. Food and Drug Administration (FDA) analyses (Hammad et al. 2006), including more published and unpublished antidepressant RCTs and using more appropriate statistical analyses (Bridge et al. 2007), found that for MDD, obsessive-compulsive disorder (OCD), and non-OCD anxiety disorders, the pooled risk difference for new or increased *spontaneously reported* suicidal ideation or suicidal behaviors for all antidepressants (SSRIs, venlafaxine, and bupropion) to be 0.7% (95% CI, 0.1%–1.3%). Thus, about 1 in 100 youth exposed to antidepressants had a new or worsening spontaneously reported suicidal ideation or behavior. There were very few suicide attempts and *no completions*. Interestingly, when the analyses were done for each disorder separately, there were no significant differences between the antidepressants and placebo. For example, for MDD the rates of suicidal ideation/attempts were 3% (95% CI, 2%–4%) for those taking the antidepressants and 2% (95% CI, 1%–2%) for those receiving placebo, yielding a risk difference of 1% (95% CI, –0.1%–2%). Using these data, the number of depressed subjects needed to treat to observe one adverse event (number needed to "harm") that can be attributed to the active treatment for antidepressants was 112 (Bridge et al. 2007).

In contrast to the analyses of *spontaneously* suicidal reported adverse events, evaluation of suicidal ideation and attempts ascertained through rating scales in 17 studies did not show significant onset or worsening of suicidality (risk ratios approximately 0.90) (Hammad et al. 2006).

As stated by the FDA (Hammad et al. 2006), the implications and clinical significance regarding the above-noted findings are uncertain, since with the increase in use of SSRIs there has been a dramatic decline in adolescent suicide (Olfson et al. 2003). In contrast, after the black box warning for all antidepressants was imposed by the FDA, the prescription of antidepressants diminished (Libby et al. 2007), and although not clearly due to the reduction of antidepressants, the rates of suicide increased (Hamilton et al. 2007). Pharmacoepidemiological studies, while correlative rather than causal, support a positive relationship between SSRI use and the reduction in the adolescent and young adult suicide rate (Gibbons et al. 2006; Valuck et al. 2004). Also, one recent study showed increased suicide attempts only immediately before the SSRIs were administered (Simon and Savarino 2007) and, as in the Treatment for Adolescents With Depression Study, a decreased rate of attempts after treatment was initiated.

In summary, in acute RCTs, the SSRIs and venlafaxine minimally but significantly increase *spontaneously* reported suicidal ideation and, to a lesser extent, suicide attempts. Nevertheless, given the greater number of patients who benefit from SSRIs than those who experience these side effects, the lack of any completed suicides in the RCTs, and the decline in overall suicidality on rating scales, the risk-benefit ratio for SSRI use in pediatric depression appears to be favorable, with careful monitoring.

Continuation Treatment

The few continuation pharmacotherapy and psychotherapy studies suggest that the relapse rate is higher in youth who do not continue treatment, particularly in those with residual symptoms (Brent et al. 2001; Emslie et al. 2008). Given these data, together with the fact that the rate of relapse is very high even after successful acute treatment, it is recommended that after acute response every child and adolescent should continue treatment for at least 6–12 months (American Academy of Child and Adolescent Psychiatry 2007).

When indicated, discontinuation can be tried during the summer so that a relapse would be less disruptive to school function. However, it is important to note that the treatment for depression can also be helping other disorders (e.g., anxiety) and that discontinuation may accelerate the symptoms of these other conditions. During the continuation phase, patients typically are seen at least monthly, depending on clinical status, functioning, support systems, environmental stressors, motivation for treatment, and presence of comorbid psychiatric or medical disorders. In this phase, psychotherapy consolidates the skills learned during the acute phase and helps patients cope with the psychosocial sequelae of the depression but also addresses the antecedents, contextual factors, environmental stressors, and internal as well as external conflicts that may contribute to a relapse. Moreover, if the patient is taking antidepressants, follow-up sessions should continue to foster medication adherence, optimize the dose, and evaluate for the presence of side effects.

Maintenance Treatment

Although there are no maintenance studies in youth with depression, once a youth has been asymptomatic for approximately 6–12 months, the clinician must decide whether maintenance therapy is indicated, which therapy, and for how long (American Academy of Child and Adolescent Psychiatry 2007). Extrapolation from adult studies would suggest that youth with more than two episodes of depression or severe or chronic depression should have maintenance treatment for 1 year or longer. Also, youth with double depression (depression with comorbid DD), subsyndromal symptoms of depression, other psychiatric or medical conditions, psychosis, suicidality, past or ongoing stressors (e.g., abuse, divorce, and conflicts), family psychopathology, or lack of community support may also need maintenance treatment. During the maintenance phase, visits may be monthly to quarterly or more frequent, depending on the patient's clinical status, functioning, support systems, environmental stressors, motivation for treatment, existence of comorbid psychiatric/medical disorders, and availability of the clinician.

Use of Antidepressants

The general use of antidepressants is described in Chapter 47 ("Antidepressants"). This section briefly focuses on the use of antidepressants for youth with MDD. Overall, it appears that the dosages of the antidepressants in children and adolescents are similar to those used for adult patients. However, the half-lives of sertraline, citalopram, paroxetine, and sustained-release bupropion are shorter than reported in adults

(Axelson et al. 2002; Findling et al. 2006). Therefore, psychiatrists should be alert for the possibility of withdrawal side effects when these medications are prescribed once a day. Also, to avoid side effects and improve adherence to treatment, it is recommended to start with a low dosage and increase it slowly until appropriate dosages have been achieved. Clinical response should be assessed at 4- to 6-week intervals, and if the child has tolerated the antidepressant, the dosage may be increased if a complete response has not been obtained (Hughes et al. 2007). At each step, adequate time should be allowed for clinical response, and frequent, early dose adjustments should be avoided. By about 12 weeks of treatment, the goal should be remission of symptoms, and in youth who are not remitted by that time, alternative treatment options may be warranted (American Academy of Child and Adolescent Psychiatry 2007).

All patients receiving antidepressants should be monitored for the minimal but plausible possibility of worsening or de novo suicidal thoughts and behavior, as well as other side effects. The FDA recommends that depressed youth should be seen every week for the first 4 weeks and biweekly thereafter. However, it is not always possible to schedule weekly face-to-face appointments. In this case, evaluations should be briefly carried out by phone. It is important to emphasize that there are no data to suggest that either the monitoring schedule proposed by the FDA or telephone calls have any impact on the risk of suicide. Monitoring is important for all patients, but patients at increased risk for suicide (e.g., those with current or prior suicidality, impulsivity, substance abuse, history of sexual abuse, family history of suicide) should be scrutinized particularly closely (American Academy of Child and Adolescent Psychiatry 2007). Those with a family history of bipolar disorder should be carefully monitored for onset of mania or mixed state. After the continuation and maintenance phases are over, or when the antidepressants need to be discontinued, all antidepressants, except for fluoxetine, should be discontinued slowly. Abrupt discontinuation of antidepressants may induce withdrawal symptoms, some of which may mimic a relapse or recurrence of a depressive episode (e.g., tiredness, irritability, and severe somatic symptoms). Sometimes withdrawal symptoms can be accompanied by worsening or emergent suicidal symptoms. The withdrawal symptoms can appear after as few as 6–8 weeks on the antidepressants and within 24–48 hours of discontinuation.

Careful attention to possible medication interactions is recommended because most antidepressants are metabolized by hepatic cytochrome P450 isoenzymes. In addition, interactions of antidepressants with other serotonergic and/or noradrenergic medications, in particular monoamine oxidase inhibitors (MAOIs), may induce the serotonergic syndrome, marked by agitation, confusion, and hyperthermia.

Treatment of Subtypes of Depression

Psychotic depression.

Extrapolating from adult studies suggests the atypical antipsychotic medications combined with SSRIs as the treatment of choice for depressed youth who are psychotic (Hughes et al. 2007). Vague or mild psychotic symptoms in a depressed youth may respond to antidepressants alone. How long the antipsychotic should be continued after the psychotic symptoms have improved is unclear, but the recommendation is to slowly taper these medications, with the eventual goal of keeping the child on monotherapy with an antidepressant. If the child is going to be maintained for long periods of time on both medications, side effects associated with the use of atypical antipsychotics and possible interactions with the antidepressants need to be monitored. Noncontrolled reports suggest that electroconvulsive therapy (ECT) may be useful for depressed psychotic adolescents.

Seasonal affective disorder.

A small RCT showed that bright light therapy is efficacious for youth with seasonal affective disorder (Swedo et al. 1997). Morning sessions are recommended, but morning hours may be difficult on school days and for youth who refuse to wake up early in the morning. Bright light therapy has been associated with some side effects, such as headaches and eye strain. Some authors have recommended an ophthalmological evaluation before initiating light therapy, but the need for this practice is not established unless the patient has a history of eye illness. Treatment with light may induce episodes of hypomania or mania in vulnerable patients.

Bipolar depression.

Early in the course of illness, it is difficult to determine whether a patient has unipolar depression or bipolar depression. If a depressed youth has indicators of risk for bipolar disorder such as psychosis or family history for bipolar disorder, the clinician should discuss with the patient and family the pros and cons of initiating mood stabilizers. For mild to moderate unipolar depression in patients with a bipolar diathesis, it may be best to start with psychotherapy because the risk for manic conversion with the use of antidepressants is substantial (Martin et al. 2004). (For further discussion, see Chapter 19, "Bipolar Disorder.")

Treatment-Resistant Depression

Each of the above-noted strategies requires implementation in a systematic fashion, education of the patient and family, and support and education to reduce the potential for the patient to become hopeless.

Many factors can account for a depressed youth's failure to respond to treatment, including misdiagnosis, unrecognized or untreated comorbid psychiatric or medical disorders (e.g., anxiety, dysthymia, eating disorders, substance use, personality disorders, hypothyroidism), undetected bipolar disorder, inappropriate pharmacotherapy or psychotherapy, inadequate length of treatment or dosage, lack of adherence to treatment, medication side effects, exposure to chronic or severe life events (such as sexual abuse or ongoing family conflicts), personal identity issues (such as concern about same-sex attraction), cultural/ethnic factors, and inadequate fit with or skill level of psychotherapist (Birmaher et al. 1996; Hughes et al. 2007).

Results of the National Institute of Mental Health (NIMH) multicenter study, the Treatment of Resistant Depression in Adolescents, showed that in depressed adolescents who have failed to respond to an adequate trial with an SSRI, a switch to another antidepressant plus CBT resulted in a better response than a switch to another antidepressant without additional psychotherapy (Brent et al. 2008).

Several psychopharmacological strategies that have been recommended for adults with resistant depression may be applicable to youth: optimization (extending the initial medication trial and/or adjusting the dose; adding CBT or IPT), switching to another agent in the same or a different class of medications, augmentation, or a combination (e.g., lithium, triiodothyronine) (Hughes et al. 2007). Optimization and augmentation strategies are usually used when patients have shown a partial response to the current regimen, and switching is usually used when patients have not responded to or cannot tolerate the medications, but no studies have validated these practices in children.

Finally, the use of somatic therapies that have not been well studied in children, such as transcranial magnetic stimulation, or more intensive somatic therapies for depressed teens, such as ECT, should be considered (see Chapter 52, "Electroconvulsive Therapy, Transcranial Magnetic Stimulation, and Deep Brain Stimulation").

Management of Comorbid Conditions

There are very few studies to guide the clinician in how to sequence the treatment of depression and other comorbid disorders (Hughes et al. 2007). Usually, clinicians make a determination of which condition is causing the greatest distress and functional impairment and begin treatment with that disorder. Also, if recovery from depression is unlikely until a comorbid condition is addressed (e.g., severe malnutrition in anorexia, or severe substance dependence, such as cocaine or intravenous drug dependence), then the comorbid condition must be addressed first.

Several psychosocial and pharmacological treatments used to treat depression may also be useful for the treatment of comorbid conditions (e.g., anxiety and substance abuse disorders, and ADHD) (see respective chapters in this book). For depressed youth with comorbid substance abuse, it is important to treat both disorders because depressive symptomatology increases the risk of persistent substance abuse and vice versa: substance abuse worsens the prognosis of the depression, and depression comorbid with substance abuse is a potent risk factor for completed suicide. One RCT suggested that 16 weeks of CBT plus fluoxetine was better than CBT plus placebo for the treatment of MDD symptoms in adolescents with substance abuse and conduct disorders (Riggs et al. 2007). Further studies regarding the use of psychosocial and pharmacological treatments for depressed youth with comorbid substance abuse are necessary.

There are few published studies examining the efficacy of psychopharmacological or psychotherapeutic treatments for depression in medically ill children and adolescents. Studies are necessary, however, because diagnosable depression may occur frequently in children and adolescents with medical diseases, and medical illness and its treatment may change the natural course of depression (Lewinsohn et al. 1996). Furthermore, the pharmacokinetics, pharmacodynamics, and side effects of the antidepressants may be affected by both the medical illnesses and the medications used to treat these illnesses. Psychotherapy is useful not only for treating depression in these children but for helping these patients and their families cope with the medical illness (Kovacs et al. 1996; Szigethy et al. 2007).

Research Directions

Further studies are needed in the areas of etiology, prevention, and treatment of MDD and DD in youth. Also, phenomenological as well as treatment studies in minorities and youth of different ethnicities and cultures are warranted.

The availability of the human genome and advances in the field of genetics and neuroimaging may shed light on the etiology of depression. These studies, in conjunction with the study of the environmental, emotional, and cognitive factors associated with the onset and maintenance of depression, may help to prevent the onset and recurrence of depression as well develop new treatments.

It is important to develop pharmacological and psychotherapy treatments that will achieve remission and not only good response. These treatments need to be practical and transportable to the community. Also, RCTs are needed to guide clinicians in how, for whom, and for how long treatment should be administered during the continuation and maintenance phases. Also, studies regarding the management of depression comorbid with other psychiatric and medical conditions are warranted. Finally, studies using other treatment modalities such as exercise, yoga, transcranial magnetic stimulation, and omega-3 fatty acids for depressed youth are warranted.

Summary Points

- Major depression and dysthymia are familial recurrent illnesses associated with significant psychosocial morbidity and mortality.
- MDD onsets during early childhood and equally affects males and females. Its prevalence increases after puberty, affecting twice as many females as males.
- The etiology of MDD seems to be determined by the interaction of certain genes with the environment and supportive systems and the youth's cognitive and coping style.
- There are no biological tests that guide the diagnosis and treatment of depressed youth. The diagnosis is based on a comprehensive evaluation with a youth and other informants, such as parents and teachers.
- The goal of treatment is to achieve remission and good psychosocial functioning.
- During all phases of treatments, depressed youth and their families should be offered education and support. Some mildly depressed youth may respond well to a short course of management with education and support.
- There is evidence that CBT, IPT, and the SSRI antidepressants, and in particular, fluoxetine, are efficacious for the treatment of depressed youth. These medications may induce side effects (e.g., agitation, mania, gastrointestinal symptoms), and about 1 in 100 children and adolescents treated with these medications may show onset or worsening of suicidal ideation and, more rarely, suicide attempts.
- Depending on the severity and chronicity of the depression and other factors (e.g., environment, child and parental motivation, IQ), treatment during the acute phase should include antidepressants and/or psychotherapy. Moderate depression may respond to CBT or IPT alone. More severe depressive episodes will generally require treatment with antidepressants. Treatment with antidepressants may be administered alone until the child is amenable to psychotherapy, or if appropriate, it can be combined with psychotherapy from the beginning of treatment.
- After successful acute treatment, all youth should be offered continuation treatment with SSRIs and/or psychotherapy for at least 6–12 months to prevent relapses.
- Depressed youth who do not respond to prior monotherapy treatment, either psychotherapy or antidepressants, require a combination of these two treatment modalities.

- After the continuation phase, some depressed youth, especially those with severe depression or frequent recurrences, should have maintenance treatment with SSRIs and/or psychotherapy for at least 1 year or more to prevent recurrences.
- Treatment of subtypes of depression, including seasonal, psychotic, and bipolar depression, may require special treatments such as light therapy, antipsychotics, and mood stabilizers, respectively.
- Management of comorbid disorders, ongoing conflicts, and family psychopathology is necessary to achieve remission.
- Management of resistant depression should consider factors associated with poor response to treatment such as poor adherence to treatment, misdiagnoses, ongoing negative life events, and presence of comorbid disorders.

References

Ackerson J, Scogin F, McKendree-Smith N, et al: Cognitive bibliotherapy for mild and moderate adolescent depressive symptomatology. J Consult Clin Psychol 66:685–690, 1998

Alloy LB, Abramson LY: The adolescent surge of depression and emergence of gender differences: a biocognitive vulnerability-stress model in developmental context, in Adolescent Psychopathology and Developing Brain. Edited by Romer D, Walker EF. New York, Oxford University Press, 2007

American Academy of Child and Adolescent Psychiatry: Practice parameter for the assessment and treatment of children and adolescents with depressive disorders. J Am Acad Child Adolesc Psychiatry 46:1503–1526, 2007

American Psychiatric Association: Diagnostic and Statistical Manual of Mental Disorders, 4th Edition. Washington, DC, American Psychiatric Association, 1994

American Psychiatric Association: Diagnostic and Statistical Manual of Mental Disorders, 4th Edition, Text Revision. Washington, DC, American Psychiatric Association, 2000

Angold A, Costello EJ, Erkanli A: Comorbidity. J Child Psychol Psychiatry 40:57–87, 1999

Asarnow JR, Jaycox LH, Duan N, et al: Effectiveness of a quality improvement intervention for adolescent depression in primary care clinics: a randomized controlled trial. JAMA 293:311–319, 2005

Axelson DA, Perel JM, Birmaher B, et al: Sertraline pharmacokinetics and dynamics in adolescents. J Am Acad Child Adolesc Psychiatry 41:1037–1044, 2002

Barbe RP, Bridge J, Birmaher B, et al: Lifetime history of sexual abuse, clinical presentation, and outcome in a clinical trial for adolescent depression. J Clin Psychiatry 65:77–83, 2004a

Barbe RP, Bridge J, Birmaher B, et al: Suicidality and its relationship to treatment outcome in depressed adolescents. Suicide Life Threat Behav 34:44–55, 2004b

Birmaher B, Ryan ND, Williamson DE, et al: Childhood and adolescent depression: a review of the past ten years, Part I. J Am Acad Child Adolesc Psychiatry 35:1427–1439, 1996

Birmaher B, Brent DA, Kolko D, et al: Clinical outcome after short-term psychotherapy for adolescents with major depressive disorder. Arch Gen Psychiatry 57:29–36, 2000

Birmaher B, Arbelaez C, Brent D: Course and outcome of child and adolescent major depressive disorder. Child Adolesc Psychiatr Clin N Am 11:619–637, 2002

Brent DA, Johnson B, Bartle S, et al: Personality disorder, tendency to impulsive violence, and suicidal behavior in adolescents. J Am Acad Child Adolesc Psychiatry 32:69–75, 1993a

Brent DA, Perper JA, Moritz G, et al: Firearms and adolescent suicide: a community case-control study. Am J Dis Child 147:1066–1071, 1993b

Brent DA, Poling K, McKain B, et al: A psychoeducational program for families of affectively ill children and adolescents. J Am Acad Child Adolesc Psychiatry 32:770–774, 1993c

Brent DA, Holder D, Kolko D, et al: A clinical psychotherapy trial for adolescent depression comparing cognitive, family, and supportive treatments. Arch Gen Psychiatry 54:877–885, 1997

Brent DA, Kolko D, Birmaher B, et al: Predictors of treatment efficacy in a clinical trial of three psychosocial treatments for adolescent depression. J Am Acad Child Adolesc Psychiatry 37:906–914, 1998

Brent DA, Baugher M, Bridge J, et al: Age- and sex-related risk factors for adolescent suicide. J Am Acad Child Adolesc Psychiatry 38:1497–1505, 1999

Brent DA, Birmaher B, Kolko D, et al: Subsyndromal depression in adolescents after a brief psychotherapy trial: course and outcome. J Affect Disord 63:51–58, 2001

Brent DA, Emslie G, Clarke G, et al: Switching to another SSRI or to venlafaxine with or without cognitive behavioral therapy for adolescents with SSRI-resistant depression: the TORDIA randomized controlled trial. JAMA 299:901–913, 2008

Bridge JA, Salary CR, Birmaher B, et al: The risks and benefits of antidepressant treatment for youth depression. Ann Med 37:404–412, 2005

Bridge JA, Iyengar S, Salary CB, et al: Clinical response and risk for reported suicidal ideation and suicide attempts in pediatric antidepressant treatment: a meta-analysis of randomized controlled trials. JAMA 297:1683–1696, 2007

Caspi A, Sugden K, Moffitt T, et al: Influence of life stress on depression: moderation by a polymorphism in the 5-HTT gene. Science 301:386–389, 2003

Clarke G, Debar L, Lynch F, et al: A randomized effectiveness trial of brief cognitive-behavioral therapy for depressed adolescents receiving antidepressant medication. J Am Acad Child Adolesc Psychiatry 44:888–898, 2005

Costello EJ, Pine DS, Hammen C, et al: Development and natural history of mood disorders. Biol Psychiatry 52:529–542, 2002

Craddock N, O'Donovan MD, Owen MJ: The genetics of schizophrenia and bipolar disorder: dissecting psychosis. J Med Genet 42:193–204, 2005

Curry J, Rohde P, Simons A, et al: Predictors and moderators of acute outcome in the Treatment for Adolescents with Depression Study (TADS). J Am Acad Child Adolesc Psychiatry 45:1427–1439, 2006

Dadds MR, Holland DE, Laurens KR, et al: Early intervention and prevention of anxiety disorders in children: results at 2-year follow-up. J Consult Clin Psychol 67:145–150, 1999

Daviss WB, Birmaher B, Melhem NA, et al: Criterion validity of the Mood and Feelings Questionnaire for depressive episodes in clinic and nonclinic subjects. J Child Psychol Psychiatry 47:927–934, 2006

Emslie GJ, Findling RL, Yeung PP, et al: Venlafaxine ER for the treatment of pediatric subjects with depression: results of two placebo-controlled trials. J Am Acad Child Adolesc Psychiatry 46:479–488, 2007

Emslie GJ, Kennard BD, Mayes TL, et al: Fluoxetine versus placebo in preventing relapse of major depression in children and adolescents. Am J Psychiatry 165:459–467, 2008

Fergusson DM, Woodward LJ: Mental health, educational, and social role outcomes of adolescents with depression. Arch Gen Psychiatry 59:225–231, 2002

Fergusson DM, Wanner B, Vitaro F, et al: Deviant peer affiliations and depression: confounding or causation. J Abnorm Child Psychol 31:605–618, 2003

Fergusson DM, Horwood LJ, Ridder EM, et al: Subthreshold depression in adolescence and mental health outcomes in adulthood. Arch Gen Psychiatry 62:66–72, 2005

Findling RL, McNamara NK, Stansbrey RJ, et al: The relevance of pharmacokinetic studies in designing efficacy trials in juvenile major depression. J Child Adolesc Psychopharmacol 16:131–145, 2006

Fombonne E, Wostear G, Cooper V, et al: The Maudsley long-term follow-up of child and adolescent depression, 1: psychiatric outcomes in adulthood. Br J Psychiatry 179:210–217, 2001

Garber J, Keiley MK, Martin NC: Developmental trajectories of adolescents' depressive symptoms: predictors of change. J Consult Clin Psychol 70:79–95, 2002

Gibbons RD, Hur K, Bhaumik DK, et al: The relationship between antidepressant prescription rates and rate of early adolescent suicide. Am J Psychiatry 163:1898–1904, 2006

Goodyer IM, Harrington R, Breen S, et al: Selective serotonin reuptake inhibitors (SSRIs) and routine specialist care with and without cognitive behavior therapy in adolescents with major depression: randomized controlled trial. BMJ 335:142–146, 2007

Gunlicks ML, Weissman MM: Change in child psychopathology with improvement in parental depression: a systematic review. J Am Acad Child Adolesc Psychiatry 47:379–389, 2008

Guy W: ECDEU Assessment Manual of Psychopharmacology. U.S. Department of Health, Education, and Welfare Publication (ADM). Rockville, MD, National Institute of Mental Health, Psychopharmacology Research Branch, 1976, pp 76–338

Hamilton BE, Minino AM, Martin JA, et al: Annual summary of vital statistics: 2005. Pediatrics 119:345–360, 2007

Hammad TA, Laughren T, Racoosin J: Suicidality in pediatric patients treated with antidepressant drugs. Arch Gen Psychiatry 63:332–339, 2006

Hammen C, Brennan PA, Shih JH, et al: Family discord and stress predictors of depression and other disorders in adolescent children of depressed and nondepressed women. J Am Acad Child Adolesc Psychiatry 43:994–1002, 2004

Hayward C, Varady S, Albano AM, et al: Cognitive-behavioral group therapy for social phobia in female adolescents: results of a pilot study. J Am Acad Child Adolesc Psychiatry 39:721–726, 2000

Hazell P, O'Connell D, Heathcote D, et al: Tricyclic drugs for depression in children and adolescents. Cochrane Database of Systematic Reviews 2002, Issue 2. Art. No.: CD002317. DOI: 10.1002/14651858.CD002317

Horovitz J, Garber J: The prevention of depressive symptoms in children and adolescents: a meta-analytic review. J Consult Clin Psychol 74:401–415, 2006

Hughes CW, Emslie GJ, Crismon ML, et al: Texas Consensus Conference Panel on Medication Treatment of Childhood Major Depressive Disorder. Texas Children's Medication Algorithm Project: update from Texas Consensus Conference Panel on Medication Treatment of Childhood Major Depressive Disorder. J Am Acad Child Adolesc Psychiatry 46:667–686, 2007

Kendler KS, Kuhn JW, Vittum J, et al: The interaction of stressful life events and a serotonin transporter polymorphism in the prediction of episodes of major depression: a replication. Arch Gen Psychiatry 62:529–535, 2005

Kennard B, Silva S, Vitiello B, et al: Remission and residual symptoms after short-term treatment in the Treatment of Adolescents with Depression Study (TADS). J Am Acad Child Adolesc Psychiatry 45:1404–1411, 2006

Kovacs M, Akiskal S, Gatsonis C, et al: Childhood-onset dysthymic disorder. Arch Gen Psychiatry 51:365–374, 1994

Kovacs M, Mukerji P, Iyengar S, et al: Psychiatric disorder and metabolic control among youths with IDDM: a longitudinal study. Diabetes Care 19:318–323, 1996

Kratochvil C, Emslie G, Silva S, et al: Acute time to response in the Treatment for Adolescents with Depression Study (TADS). J Am Acad Child Adolesc Psychiatry 45:1412–1418, 2006

Lewinsohn PM, Seeley JR, Hibbard J, et al: Cross-sectional and prospective relationships between physical morbidity and depression in older adolescents. J Am Acad Child Adolesc Psychiatry 35:1120–1129, 1996

Lewinsohn PM, Pettit JW, Joiner TE Jr, et al: The symptomatic expression of major depressive disorder in adolescents and young adults. J Abnorm Psychol 112:244–252, 2003a

Lewinsohn PM, Rohde P, Seeley JR, et al: Psychosocial functioning of young adults who have experienced and recovered from major depressive disorder during adolescence. J Abnorm Psychol 112:353–363, 2003b

Libby AM, Brent DA, Morrato EH, et al: Decline in treatment of pediatric depression after FDA advisory on risk of suicidality with SSRIs. Am J Psychiatry 164:884–891, 2007

Luby JL, Mrakotsky C, Heffelfinger A, et al: Characteristics of depressed preschoolers with and without anhedonia: evidence for a melancholic depressive subtype in young children. Am J Psychiatry 161:1998–2004, 2004

Martin A, Young C, Leckman JF, et al: Age effects on antidepressant-induced manic conversion. Arch Pediatr Adolesc Med 158:773–780, 2004

Masi G, Favilla L, Mucci M, et al: Depressive symptoms in children and adolescents with dysthymic disorder. Psychopathology 34:29–35, 2001

Melvin GA, Tonge BJ, King NJ, et al: A comparison of cognitive-behavioral therapy, sertraline, and their combination for adolescent depression. J Am Acad Child Adolesc Psychiatry 45:1151–1161, 2006

Mufson L, Weissman MM, Moreau D, et al: Efficacy of interpersonal psychotherapy for depressed adolescents. Arch Gen Psychiatry 56:573–579, 1999

Mufson L, Dorta KP, Wickramaratne P, et al: A randomized effectiveness trial of interpersonal psychotherapy for depressed adolescents. Arch Gen Psychiatry 61:577–584, 2004

Nomura Y, Wickramaratne PJ, Warner V, et al: Family discord, parental depression, and psychopathology in offspring: ten-year follow-up. J Am Acad Child Psychiatry 41:402–409, 2002

Olfson M, Shaffer D, Marcus SC, et al: Relationship between antidepressant medication treatment and suicide in adolescents. Arch Gen Psychiatry 60:978–982, 2003

Pilowsky DJ, Wickramaratne P, Nomura Y, et al: Family discord, parental depression, and psychopathology in offspring: 20-year follow-up. J Am Acad Child Psychiatry 45:452–460, 2006

Pine DS, Cohen P, Gurley D, et al: The risk for early adulthood anxiety and depressive disorders in adolescents with anxiety and depressive disorders. Arch Gen Psychiatry 55:56–64, 1998

Poznanski EO, Mokros HB: Children's Depression Rating Scale, Revised (CDRS-R) Manual. Los Angeles, CA, Western Psychological Services, 1995

Reinherz HZ, Paradis AD, Giaconia RM, et al: Childhood and adolescent predictors of major depression in the transition to adulthood. Am J Psychiatry 160:2141–2147, 2003

Renaud J, Brent DA, Baugher M, et al: Rapid response to psychosocial treatment for adolescent depression: a two-year follow-up. J Am Acad Child Adolesc Psychiatry 37:1184–1190, 1998

Riggs PD, Mikulich-Gilbertson SK, Davies RD, et al: A randomized controlled trial of fluoxetine and cognitive behavior therapy in adolescents with major depression, behavior problems, and substance use disorders. Arch Pediatr Adolesc Med 161:1026–1034, 2007

Rossello J, Bernal G: The efficacy of cognitive-behavioral and interpersonal treatments for depression in Puerto Rican adolescents. J Consult Clin Psychol 67:734–745, 1999

Sanford M, Boyle M, McCleary L, et al: A pilot study of adjunctive family psychoeducation in adolescent major depression: feasibility and treatment effect. J Am Acad Child Adolesc Psychiatry 45:386–495, 2006

Shaffer D, Gould MS, Brasic J, et al: A children's global assessment scale (CGAS). Arch Gen Psychiatry 40:1228–1231, 1983

Simon GE, Savarino J: Suicide attempts among patients starting depression treatment with medications or psychotherapy. Am J Psychiatry 164:1029–1034, 2007

Swedo SE, Allen AJ, Glod CA, et al: A controlled trial of light therapy for the treatment of pediatric seasonal affective disorder. J Am Acad Child Adolesc Psychiatry 36:816–821, 1997

Szigethy E, Whitton SW, Levy-Warren A, et al: Cognitive-behavioral therapy for adolescents with inflammatory bowel disease and subsyndromal depression. J Am Acad Child Adolesc Psychiatry 46:1290–1298, 2007

Treatment of Adolescent Depression Study (TADS) Team: Fluoxetine, cognitive-behavioral therapy, and their combination for adolescents with depression: Treatment for Adolescents with Depression Study (TADS) randomized controlled trial. JAMA 292:807–820, 2004

Valuck RJ, Libby AM, Sills MR, et al: Antidepressant treatment and risk of suicide attempt by adolescents with major depressive disorder: a propensity-adjusted retrospective cohort study. CNS Drugs 18:1119–1132, 2004

Weersing VR, Iyengar S, Kolko DJ, et al: Effectiveness of cognitive-behavioral therapy for adolescent depression: a benchmarking investigation. Behav Ther 37:36–48, 2006

Weissman MM, Pilowsky PA, Wickramaratne P, et al: Remissions in maternal depression and child psychopathology: a STAR*D-child report. JAMA 22:1389–1399, 2006a

Weissman MM, Wickramaratne P, Nomura Y, et al: Offspring of depressed parents: 20 years later. Am J Psychiatry 163:1001–1008, 2006b

Weisz JR, McCarty CA, Valeri SM: Effects of psychotherapy for depression in children and adolescents: a meta-analysis. Psychol Bull 132:132–149, 2006

Wilens TE, Wyatt D, Spencer TJ: Disentangling disinhibition. J Am Acad Child Adolesc Psychiatry 37:1225–1227, 1998

World Health Organization: International Classification of Diseases, 10th Revision (ICD-10). Geneva, Switzerland, World Health Organization, 1992

Yorbik O, Birmaher B, Axelson D, et al: Clinical characteristics of depressive symptoms in children and adolescents with major depressive disorder. J Clin Psychiatry 65: 1654–1659, 2004

Zalsman G, Oquendo M A, Greenhill L, et al: Neurobiology of depression in children and adolescents. Child Adolesc Psychiatr Clin N Am 15:843–868, 2006

Chapter 19

Bipolar Disorder

Gabrielle A. Carlson, M.D.
Stephanie E. Meyer, Ph.D.

Bipolar disorder (BP) clearly exists in children and adolescents (Pavuluri et al. 2005). The relevant issues concern its prevalence, continuity between the various conceptualizations of BP in youth and adult BP (this is important insofar as treatment in youth has been extrapolated from treatment in adults), and the treatment and research implications of missing the diagnosis of BP, versus implications when another condition is mistakenly identified as BP.

Definition

BP is defined by episodes of mania (bipolar I disorder; BP-I); hypomania (bipolar II disorder; BP-II)—that is, briefer duration of manic symptoms with less impairment; or manic symptoms of insufficient number and/ or duration to meet mania or hypomania criteria (bipo-

lar disorder not otherwise specified; BP-NOS). Depressive episodes, at all levels of severity and duration, need not occur in BP-I, but usually do. In BP-II, full major depression occurs with hypomania. Cyclothymia refers to cycles of subsyndromal mania and depression. Tables 19–1, 19–2, and 19–3 outline current DSM-IV-TR (American Psychiatric Association 2000) criteria for manic, hypomanic, and depressive episodes. Mood symptoms, then, appear to exist as spectrums.

According to DSM-IV (American Psychiatric Association 1994) and its text revision, DSM-IV-TR, BP is further classified by how the manic and depressive symptoms and episodes relate to each other. When episodes of mania and depression follow each other without a well interval, the type is said to be "circular." The presence of four or more episodes per year defines "rapid cycling." If manic and depressive symptoms occur simultaneously during an episode, the episode is called "mixed."

Finally, there is a severity spectrum with increasing psychosis including mood-congruent symptoms (those that are consistent with an elevated or depressed mood), mood-incongruent symptoms (most often paranoia but other delusions and hallucinations that are less understandably part of a mood), and probably schizoaffective mania, where more prominent symptoms of schizophrenia occur. Schizoaffective, depressive type may be closer to schizophrenia than to a mood disorder.

Clinical Description

According to Goodwin and Jamison (2007), classic mania has an acute onset and lasts several months during which the person experiences a roller coaster of feelings. Even in predominantly euphoric mania, a labile mood with highs and lows, irritability, and anxiety co-occur. Simultaneously, energy, activity level, speech, and flow of ideas are on "overdrive." Patience is short and anger can intrude quickly. Sleep is unnecessary and time is filled with extravagant plans. Delusional thinking and sometimes hallucinations are present about half the time, though psychosis is not usually sustained. Patients can cycle out gradually or quickly and can return to a euthymic state or plunge immediately into a depressive episode, which is as bleak, despairing, and anergic as mania is ebullient, optimistic, and activated. However, depressive episodes are longer, taking up to a year to remit.

TABLE 19–1.   DSM-IV-TR diagnostic criteria for manic episode

A.   A distinct period of abnormally and persistently elevated, expansive, or irritable mood, lasting at least 1 week (or any duration if hospitalization is necessary).

B.   During the period of mood disturbance, three (or more) of the following symptoms have persisted (four if the mood is only irritable) and have been present to a significant degree:

   (1)   inflated self-esteem or grandiosity

   (2)   decreased need for sleep (e.g., feels rested after only 3 hours of sleep)

   (3)   more talkative than usual or pressure to keep talking

   (4)   flight of ideas or subjective experience that thoughts are racing

   (5)   distractibility (i.e., attention too easily drawn to unimportant or irrelevant external stimuli)

   (6)   increase in goal-directed activity (either socially, at work or school, or sexually) or psychomotor agitation

   (7)   excessive involvement in pleasurable activities that have a high potential for painful consequences (e.g., engaging in unrestrained buying sprees, sexual indiscretions, or foolish business investments)

C.   The symptoms do not meet criteria for a mixed episode.

D.   The mood disturbance is sufficiently severe to cause marked impairment in occupational functioning or in usual social activities or relationships with others, or to necessitate hospitalization to prevent harm to self or others, or there are psychotic features.

E.   The symptoms are not due to the direct physiological effects of a substance (e.g., a drug of abuse, a medication, or other treatment) or a general medical condition (e.g., hyperthyroidism).

   Note: Manic-like episodes that are clearly caused by somatic antidepressant treatment (e.g., medication, electroconvulsive therapy, light therapy) should not count toward a diagnosis of bipolar I disorder.

Source.   Reprinted from American Psychiatric Association: *Diagnostic and Statistical Manual of Mental Disorders,* 4th Edition, Text Revision. Washington, DC, American Psychiatric Association, 2000, p. 362. Used with permission. Copyright © 2000 American Psychiatric Association.

TABLE 19–2. DSM-IV-TR diagnostic criteria for hypomanic episode

A. A distinct period of persistently elevated, expansive, or irritable mood, lasting throughout at least 4 days, that is clearly different from the usual nondepressed mood.

B. During the period of mood disturbance, three (or more) of the following symptoms have persisted (four if the mood is only irritable) and have been present to a significant degree:

(1) inflated self-esteem or grandiosity

(2) decreased need for sleep (e.g., feels rested after only 3 hours of sleep)

(3) more talkative than usual or pressure to keep talking

(4) flight of ideas or subjective experience that thoughts are racing

(5) distractibility (i.e., attention too easily drawn to unimportant or irrelevant external stimuli)

(6) increase in goal-directed activity (either socially, at work or school, or sexually) or psychomotor agitation

(7) excessive involvement in pleasurable activities that have a high potential for painful consequences (e.g., the person engages in unrestrained buying sprees, sexual indiscretions, or foolish business investments)

C. The episode is associated with an unequivocal change in functioning that is uncharacteristic of the person when not symptomatic.

D. The disturbance in mood and the change in functioning are observable by others.

E. The episode is not severe enough to cause marked impairment in social or occupational functioning, or to necessitate hospitalization, and there are no psychotic features.

F. The symptoms are not due to the direct physiological effects of a substance (e.g., a drug of abuse, a medication, or other treatment) or a general medical condition (e.g., hyperthyroidism).

Note: Hypomanic-like episodes that are clearly caused by somatic antidepressant treatment (e.g., medication, electroconvulsive therapy, light therapy) should not count toward a diagnosis of bipolar II disorder.

Source. Reprinted from American Psychiatric Association: *Diagnostic and Statistical Manual of Mental Disorders,* 4th Edition, Text Revision. Washington, DC, American Psychiatric Association, 2000, p. 368. Used with permission. Copyright © 2000 American Psychiatric Association.

Diagnosis

Case Example 1: Child With "Classic" Early-Onset BP ("Narrow Phenotype")

Background and Referral Information

Nicola, a girl age 12 years and 9 months, who was previously shy, helpful, and academically normal, presented with a sudden onset of behavior change over 2–3 weeks consisting of a change in dress to very revealing clothes, uninhibited talking to strangers by phone and Internet, increased energy around the clock, and extreme mood changes from laughing hysterically one minute to swearing and smashing things the next to crying uncontrollably, all without much provocation.

Nicola's only prior mental health problem had been an apparent depression at age 10 with the death of her grandmother. She recovered with brief psychotherapy. She had menarche at age 12 and started middle school the same year.

Nicola could be heard in the waiting room talking with everyone loudly and rapidly, bragging about waiting for a cell phone call from a famous actor. She frantically tried to organize playroom toys, becoming furious when another parent told her to calm down. She was suspicious about letting her parents be interviewed alone and furious when asked about drug and alcohol use (which she denied).

Nicola's father was a Wall Street broker who had become depressed with stock reversals in the past. He also drank heavily. Her mother had had a postpartum depression.

Case Example 2: Possible "Broad Phenotype" or "Severe Mood Dysregulation" BP

Background and Referral Information

Lynda, an 11-year-old girl, had been hyperactive, disinhibited, and impulsive since preschool. Increasing problems academically and with peers prompted medication treatment. Stimulant treatments since age 8 resulted in only partially controlled symptoms. She was not learning disabled. At school she couldn't sit still

TABLE 19–3. DSM-IV-TR diagnostic criteria for major depressive episode

A. Five (or more) of the following symptoms have been present during the same 2-week period and represent a change from previous functioning; at least one of the symptoms is either (1) depressed mood or (2) loss of interest or pleasure.

   Note: Do not include symptoms that are clearly due to a general medical condition, or mood-incongruent delusions or hallucinations.

   (1) depressed mood most of the day, nearly every day, as indicated by either subjective report (e.g., feels sad or empty) or observation made by others (e.g., appears tearful).   **Note:** In children and adolescents, can be irritable mood.

   (2) markedly diminished interest or pleasure in all, or almost all, activities most of the day, nearly every day (as indicated by either subjective account or observation made by others)

   (3) significant weight loss when not dieting or weight gain (e.g., a change of more than 5% of body weight in a month), or decrease or increase in appetite nearly every day.   **Note:** In children, consider failure to make expected weight gains.

   (4) insomnia or hypersomnia nearly every day

   (5) psychomotor agitation or retardation nearly every day (observable by others, not merely subjective feelings of restlessness or being slowed down)

   (6) fatigue or loss of energy nearly every day

   (7) feelings of worthlessness or excessive or inappropriate guilt (which may be delusional) nearly every day (not merely self-reproach or guilt about being sick)

   (8) diminished ability to think or concentrate, or indecisiveness, nearly every day (either by subjective account or as observed by others)

   (9) recurrent thoughts of death (not just fear of dying), recurrent suicidal ideation without a specific plan, or a suicide attempt or a specific plan for committing suicide

B. The symptoms do not meet criteria for a mixed episode.

C. The symptoms cause clinically significant distress or impairment in social, occupational, or other important areas of functioning.

D. The symptoms are not due to the direct physiological effects of a substance (e.g., a drug of abuse, a medication) or a general medical condition (e.g., hypothyroidism).

E. The symptoms are not better accounted for by bereavement, i.e., after the loss of a loved one, the symptoms persist for longer than 2 months or are characterized by marked functional impairment, morbid preoccupation with worthlessness, suicidal ideation, psychotic symptoms, or psychomotor retardation.

and talked too much and often about topics unrelated to task. Social skills were poor because she was bossy and intrusive. She was oppositional, sometimes insubordinate, but basically manageable in class.

Over the year prior to referral, Lynda had become increasingly angry, irritable, provocative, destructive, and capricious. She bullied smaller children and expressed interest in lewd material on the Internet. She was often a show-off, and when lots of people were around, she would act silly and repeat jokes long past the time they were funny. In spite of poor grades, she told her family that she planned to be a doctor, a record producer, a professional wrestler, or an acrobat. Her rages when she didn't get her way, or when a demand was made on her, were severe and could last for several hours. She would scream, curse, throw dishware, and occasionally threatened with a knife. This behavior got her sent to a psychiatric emergency room for an overnight stay.

On interview, Lynda was calm but disrespectful to her parents, and tried to be a "femme fatale" with the young male resident who was interviewing her. She could focus on what she wanted but would ask irrelevant questions trying to control the direction of conversation.

Alone, Lynda admitted to being distractible, forgetful, and restless. She often felt sad, was suicidal when angry, and admitted to flying off the handle easily. She had many complaints about her parents and unfair treatment by the girls in school. She denied euphoria but said her speech was rapid though we did not observe this. She described insomnia (i.e., doesn't get to sleep until 1 A.M. but slept until 3 P.M. the following afternoon). She was starting to smoke and experiment with marijuana and sex. In terms of the future, she thought she could go to law school if she brought up her grades.

There is a history in first-degree relatives of depression, hypomania, and attention-deficit/hyperactivity disorder (ADHD).

There are three competing approaches to diagnosing mania (and thus pediatric BP) in children:

1. Mania/hypomania should be narrowly defined to fit unmodified adult criteria. Leibenluft et al. (2003) call this condition "narrow phenotype" BP-I and require clear episodes, euphoria, and grandiosity to make the diagnosis. A pattern of severe irritability, anger, and aggressive, explosive episodes without euphoria or grandiosity is defined as "severe mood dysregulation." By this definition, Nicola would have BP and Lynda would have "severe mood dysregulation."
2. Criteria may be modified for children with strict operational guidelines in the Washington University Schedule for Affective Disorders and Schizophrenia for School-Aged Children (Geller et al. 2001). Nicola would still be manic. Parents' history made Lynda sound manic, possibly with rapid cycles, though the child herself disagreed.
3. Severe, explosive irritability and other symptoms of mania define a specific prepubertal mania phenotype. Euphoria and grandiosity are not required, though other manic symptoms are. Both cases would meet mania criteria by this definition (e.g., Biederman et al. 2000).

In all three approaches, parents are virtually the only source of information, although in some studies children are interviewed. Shortcomings common to all approaches are lack of requirement for impairment in two or more settings (as is true for ADHD), absence of ascertaining developmental information and learning, language, and pervasive developmental disorders. In both cases, parents agreed on mania symptoms. In case 2, disagreement occurred between parent and child. In school, Lynda appeared to have ADHD with oppositional defiant symptoms.

The two cases described above were rated by child psychiatrists in the United States and United Kingdom (Dubicka et al. 2008), and 96% of the U.S. clinicians and 92% of the U.K. clinicians thought the patient in case 1 had mania (NS). For case 2, however, 75% of U.S. child psychiatrists diagnosed mania, usually with comorbid ADHD, versus 33% of U.K. child psychiatrists

($P<0.001$), where clinicians conceptualized her as having ADHD and/or a behavior disorder only.

Family history of BP has been used to validate all three positions. Where parent and child psychopathology are defined similarly, the child is likely to manifest what is present at a high rate in his family (cosegregation). Neurobiological and treatment validators are being examined. At this point, none of the studies has followed samples into adulthood.

Epidemiology

In the United States, among adults, rates of lifetime BP-I disorder vary between 0.8 and 1.6%, while the rate of lifetime BP-II is about 1.1%; the lifetime rate of subthreshold manic symptoms ranges from 2.4% to about 6%. In teens, rates of lifetime mania (0.1%) and BP-II and cyclothymia (0.85%) are lower, and the rate for "subthreshold BP" is about 6% (Lewinsohn et al. 1995). Five-year follow-up of the "subthreshold cases" did not reveal any conversion to BP-I, however (Lewinsohn et al. 2000). Children under age 9 have not been studied in community samples. No children were found to have had a manic episode in the Great Smoky Mountains epidemiological study of children ages 9–13 (Costello et al. 1996), though a 3-month prevalence rate, and not a lifetime rate, was used.

Examination of hospital discharge diagnoses using the National Hospital Discharge Survey revealed a rate jump from 1.4 in 10,000 to 7.3 in 10,000 in 9- to 13-year-olds and from 5.1 in 10,000 to 20.4 in 10,000 in 14- to 19-year-olds (Blader and Carlson 2007), but in a clinic using the same methodology over the past 15 years, no true increase in rate was found (Biederman et al. 2004).

Comorbidity

People who meet criteria for mania almost invariably meet criteria for at least one other disorder. The most common simultaneous comorbidities (ADHD, oppositional defiant disorder [ODD], conduct disorder [CD], anxiety) occur during mania and are difficult to distinguish from it without a good history. They may represent a halo effect of a manic or depressive episode, subsiding when the mood disorder is treated. The comorbid disorder often has its own comorbidities. Thus, ADHD is often comorbid with ODD and CD, anxiety, and learning disabilities. Anxiety disorders are often comorbid with each other.

ADHD, which begins prior to BP and may co-occur with it, may be found in up to 90% of prepubertal children and about half of adolescents with BP (Faraone et al. 1997; Tillman et al. 2003).

CD may precede or co-occur with BP. The combination of externalizing disorders and BP may represent a phenotype specific to prepubertal children (Biederman et al. 2000). Adults with BP-I and co-occurring substance abuse have significantly higher rates of adolescent CD compared to those without. Substance abuse or dependence in adolescents is also a significant comorbidity, one which often perpetuates mood cycles.

Anxiety disorders occur with surprising frequency though rates vary widely depending on whether the disorder is diagnosed when the patient is euthymic (Dickstein et al. 2005).

BP in children with developmental disorders is less well studied (see Gutkovich and Carlson 2008 for review). About 20% of children diagnosed with mania also had comorbid pervasive developmental disorder but up to 60% of patients with mood disorders obtained parent ratings of autism spectrum behaviors in the "likely autism spectrum disorders" range.

Substance and alcohol abuse are common comorbidities in adolescents with BP. ADHD and CD which may be co-occurring in early-onset BP are both risk factors for the development of Substance and alcohol abuse. However, early-onset BP itself appears to increase rates of substance abuse over and above other externalizing disorders. Cannabis abuse increases rates of psychosis in general. Substance and alcohol abuse also complicates BP by increasing both the severity and number of episodes. Finally, DSM-IV-TR recognizes that many people will develop mania or depression secondary to substance abuse and that the episode may remit when the patient stops abusing drugs. Disentangling these entities is next to impossible while drug and alcohol abuse continue.

Etiology, Mechanisms, and Risk Factors

Genetic Factors

Adult twin studies suggest that genetic influences explain approximately 60%–93% of the variance in BP, while shared and unique environmental factors account for 30%–40% and 10%–21%, respectively (reviewed in Althoff et al. 2005). There are no "narrow phenotype" twin studies of early-onset BP. BP-I rates are elevated in relatives of children with narrow-phenotype BP but not in broad phenotype/severe mood dysregulation (Brotman et al. 2007) though they may cosegregate in certain families.

Findings from top-down studies over the past 30 years, summarized in Table 19–4, have reported elevated rates of affective disorder (mainly depression), anxiety, and behavioral disorders (especially ADHD) among offspring of parents with BP (Hirshfeld-Becker et al. 2006; Lapalme et al. 1997).

Environmental risk factors like physical and sexual abuse (Leverich et al. 2002), irritable and negative parenting styles (Geller et al. 2004; Meyer et al. 2006), poor social support, and prenatal alcohol exposure (O'Connor et al. 2002) may interact with genetic vulnerability to enhance early age at onset of BP, as well as a variety of negative course indicators, including rapid cycling, substance use, elevated risk of suicidal behavior, and high comorbidity rates (Alloy et al. 2005).

Brain Structure and Function

Similar to studies of adults, preliminary results from structural magnetic resonance imaging (MRI) studies suggest that early-onset BP is associated with abnormalities in cortical and subcortical brain regions thought to be involved in the regulation of emotion (Frazier et al. 2005), including the presence of white matter hyperintensities (Frazier et al. 2005) and decreased amygdala volume (Blumberg et al. 2005).

Recent functional MRI studies suggest perturbations in prefrontal-limbic circuitry (Pavuluri et al. 2007): bipolar children detected greater hostility in emotionally neutral faces (Rich et al. 2006), as well as elevated levels of fear when viewing them, and exhibited increased activation of the left amygdala-striatal-ventral prefrontal circuit when rating face hostility. Heightened activation of the amygdala during emotional challenges may interfere with attentional capacities among children with BP, thus increasing the probability that they will misinterpret the nature of incoming stimuli (facial expression) and respond in an inappropriate manner.

Studies employing magnetic resonance spectroscopy are very preliminary and provide further support for the presence of cortical and subcortical abnormalities in pediatric BP.

TABLE 19–4. Reports of offspring studies in parents with bipolar disorder (BP)

Sample	Parent sample	Age of child at assessment, years	Rate BP-I/ any BP	Rate any disorder
Meta-analysis Lapalme et al. 1997	Literature review	Children and adolescents	5.4% 26.5%	52%
National Institute of Mental Health Meyer et al. 2004	31 BP mothers	18–26	6.0% 18.8%	65%
Dutch Reichart et al. 2004	BP-I from manic depressive association N=132	16–26	4%	59%
Amish Shaw et al. 2005	14 BP-I parents	>13 years, n=69 <13 years, n=40	2 w/BP-I (2%) 2 w/BP-II	N/A
Canada Duffy et al. 2007	137 (lithium responders=67; lithium nonresponders=60)	10–25; mean age=20	2.2% 20%	70%
Mood disorders clinics				
Cincinnati Singh et al. 2007	Adult mood clinic N=37	10.2 (SD=2.5)	16% 38%	78%
Stanford Chang et al. 2000	Adult mood clinic N=60	11.1 (SD=3.5)	N/A 15%	55%
Massachusetts General Hospital Henin et al. 2005	Research clinic N=117	8, 12, and 18[a]	10%≤12 years 33% 18 years	N/A

Note. BP-I=bipolar I disorder; BP-II=bipolar II disorder; N/A=not applicable; SD=standard deviation.
[a]Morbidity risk assessed at these ages.

Age at Onset, Course, and Prognosis

Age at onset varies by whether it is dated from the age at which the person meets criteria for a full mood episode or displays behavioral or emotional symptoms that are felt to be harbingers of the disorder. BP often begins with depression or dysthymia. If broad phenotype BP is included in age at onset data, it is possible that onset could be dated to preschool.

Over a 2- to 4-year follow-up in U.S. samples, early-onset BP (both broad and narrow phenotypes) is characterized by slow response to treatment, persistent mood fluctuations, elevated risk for suicide attempts, and severe psychosocial impairment. Rates of remission are variable, but even when high, they are followed by high rates of recurrence (see Table 19–5).

Children with BP-NOS suffer from a more chronic course of illness than youth with BP-I or II, with persistent subthreshold symptoms and slower response to acute treatment. Within 2 years of follow-up, one-quarter of individuals initially diagnosed with BP-NOS converted to BP-I or II (Birmaher et al. 2006).

Impairment is most profound among the youngest bipolar patients. Fewer than half of child samples experienced remission at 6- and 12-month follow-up, and subthreshold symptoms, mania, depression, and comorbid conditions often persist between episodes (Birmaher and Axelson 2006; Birmaher et al. 2006; Strober et al. 1995).

Nonadherence with pharmacologic treatment, low socioeconomic status, low maternal warmth, psychosis, comorbid anxiety, and rapid cycling are poor prognosis indicators (Birmaher et al. 2006; DelBello et al. 2007b; Geller et al. 2004).

TABLE 19–5. Naturalistic follow-up of samples of children and adolescents with bipolar I disorder (BP-I)

Study	BP diagnoses	Origin of most of the sample; sample size	Mean age, years	Frequency and duration of follow-up	% Remission/ recovery	% Relapse/ recurrence
Lewinsohn et al. 2000	BP-I, BP-II, BP-NOS	Community N=17	17	Once at age 24	65% by age 19 88% by age 24	27%
Srinath et al. 1998	BP-I	Outpatients N=30	14	Once after 4–5 years	100%	67%
Geller et al. 2004	BP-I	Outpatients N=86	11	Every 6 months for 3 years and then at 1 year for 48 months	87%	70%
Jairam et al. 2004	BP-I	Outpatients N=25	14	Every 6 months for 52 months	100%	64%
Strober et al. 1995	BP-I	Inpatients N=54	16	Every 6 months for 60 months	98%	44%
Birmaher and Axelson 2006	BP-I (BP-II and BP-NOS not included here)	Inpatients and outpatients N=152	13	Every 6 months for 24 months	68%	45%
Carlson et al. 2000	BP-I with psychosis	Inpatient N=23	18	Every 6 months for 24 months	36.4% complete remission	64.7% mania recurrence 17.6% depression recurrence
DelBello et al. 2007b	BP-I	Inpatient N=71		1, 4, 8, 12 months	86% syndromal, 43% symptomatic, 41% functional recovery; 20% with all three types of recovery	54% recurrence

Note. BP-I=bipolar I disorder; BP-II=bipolar II disorder; BP-NOS=bipolar disorder not otherwise specified.

Rates of conversion from subsyndromal mania to BP-I were 0.1% per year in a community sample. A community study of severe mood dysregulation found an elevated risk for depressive disorders at young adult follow-up compared to unaffected children (Brotman et al. 2006).

Evaluation

An efficient, thorough evaluation of a serious psychiatric disorder includes screening, an interview of parents and child, and other diagnostic information as needed. This is difficult to accomplish in less than 2 hours, even with articulate parents.

Screening

The Child Behavior Checklist (CBCL) and the Child Symptom Inventory, 4th Edition (CSI-4) are efficient screening instruments for acute mania and depression because they assess both mood symptoms and other psychiatric behaviors and disorders that are confused with, or may co-occur with, BP. Elevated anxiety/depression, aggression, and attention subscale scores on the CBCL (T scores >67) have been called the CBCL-JBD (juvenile bipolar disorder) phenotype and may suggest acute mania but do not make the diagnosis. That is also true for high scores on the mania items on the CSI-4. Screening instruments directed more specifically at mania/hypomania include parent-completed versions of the General Behavior Inventory (P-GBI), Child Mania Rating Scale (P-CMRS), and Young Mania Rating Scale (P-YMRS) (Youngstrom et al. 2006). As with most other conditions in child psychiatry, cross-informant agreement is low.

Parent Interview

Parents are the most useful source of information, and they should be interviewed first, regardless of the patient's age. After the clinician elicits parent concerns and a general psychiatric history, details about the child's mood and activity level should be elicited. Antecedents to "mood swings" or aggressive, agitated, explosive behavior (rages) and how or if they differ from the child's "usual self" must be established. Fatigue, hunger, and sedating medications may increase such behaviors. This information is necessary for planning interventions.

Family History

Family history of mood disorders (bipolar and unipolar) and other psychiatric disorders must be solicited. Descriptions of behavior to ensure the accuracy of the diagnostic label are important to determine if the condition is lithium-responsive, has been mostly depressed, or is significantly comorbid. Adults are sometimes incorrectly given a BP diagnosis in lieu of more pessimistic or stigmatizing diagnoses (e.g., schizophrenia, substance abuse, personality disorder).

Child Interview

Besides ascertaining the presence of manic and depressive symptoms germane to the diagnosis of BP, it is necessary to directly assess the child's language; presence of thought disorder, psychosis, anxiety, suicidal behavior, physical/sexual abuse, and illicit substance use; and evidence of racing thoughts and flight of ideas.

It is important to reconcile parent and child information. If child information does not jibe with parent information, the child should be told what his or her parent has said and be asked for clarification. Parents sometimes misinterpret; children sometimes deny. Keeping the information separate unnecessarily complicates the evaluation unless there are true confidentiality or research reasons for doing so.

Other Evaluations

Teacher information is important to establish the pervasiveness of mania or depression. A child with rages at home who is completely asymptomatic at school is likely to have a different condition from one who is similarly symptomatic in both places. Also, children with BP may require specific school interventions. This requires information from school. For a child having scholastic difficulties, a psychoeducational evaluation (IQ and achievement tests) is needed. For children with communication problems, a language examination with a speech sample is needed. If there is a question of reading disorder, certain reading tests are helpful. In addition to a good medical history (or information from the primary care doctor), polysomnography (for sleep apnea), a thorough neurological assessment, or laboratory tests may be needed. The complex nature of early-onset BP requires an assessment beyond ascertainment of mania and depression criteria alone.

Systematic Interviews

Structured and semistructured interviews are the cornerstones of most clinical research. In clinical settings, these should be used to confirm diagnosis after the clinician himself or herself has obtained a good history, or enough information to know that the diagnoses of interest are covered by the systematic interview. Structured and semistructured interviews are discussed in Chapter 7, "Diagnostic Interviews."

Rating Scales

Rating scales may guide treatment response and track mania (including mood lability), depression, anxiety, ADHD, aggression, and psychosis. The Young Mania Rating Scale (YMRS) has been used in drug studies to assess significant severity (a cutoff score of 20). Ironically, the YMRS does not assess all the symptoms of mania. The Children's Depression Rating Scale—Revised was developed for children and is used to rate the severity of depression. Scores over 40 are indicative of moderately severe depression. Neither instrument replaces a history. See Chapter 8, "Rating Scales."

Differential Diagnosis

Differential diagnosis and comorbidity are two sides of the same coin. For instance, if "severe mood dysregulation" is a specific variant of early-onset BP, then other disorders that co-occur with it are considered comorbidities. If not, one considers the mood dysregulation as nonspecific and part of the primary disorder, and it is important to identify the primary disorder. Severe tantrums occur in ADHD and ODD/CD, autism spectrum disorders, in children with a history of prior severe abuse or domestic violence, and in children having panic attacks who are responding to the fear stimulus with "fight" rather than "flight or freeze." The clinical relevance is whether one treats the mood dysregulation first, because it represents mania, or treats the other disorder first, because it is considered to be the reason for the mood dysregulation (Kowatch et al. 2005).

Clearly defined mood episodes with durations longer than a week, and which are clearly distinguishable from premorbid personality, are more easily diagnosed. Depression is often the reason for which children and teens seek treatment. It is important to look for hints of mania or hypomania in their past, recognizing there may be none, and that it may take a number of years for a manic episode to occur as was seen in case 1. Postpubertal mania and depression can occur with very severe psychosis. Schizophrenia and substance-induced psychosis are part of the differential diagnosis of severe psychosis.

The following are areas in which careful history and symptom ascertainment are necessary to make distinctions (see Carlson and Meyer 2006 for a review):

Symptoms

- The silly, disinhibited behavior of a child with ADHD trying to be funny and not knowing when to quit versus someone with an elated mood
- Impulsivity versus pleasure seeking without heeding consequences
- A child's resistance to bedtime versus a reduced need for sleep

Onset of illness

- The exacerbation of subthreshold ADHD symptoms because of increased late elementary or middle school demands versus the start of a mood disorder
- The progression of ADHD symptoms to include more oppositional/explosive/conduct disordered behavior in the context of family, school, and/or peer difficulties

Mental status

- The pragmatic, distracted, or odd language seen in children who have language disorders as part of ADHD or an autism spectrum disorder versus the flight of ideas and thought disorder of mania
- The "hallucinations" seen in a very anxious child versus mood-incongruent symptoms of a mood disorder
- The mood-incongruent psychotic symptoms of mania or depression versus symptoms of early schizophrenia

Finally, teens who are abusing marijuana, alcohol, or other drugs may have psychosis and/or mood symptoms. While a positive toxicology screen helps document the involvement of drugs, negative drug screens do not rule out substance abuse, and symptoms of mania may continue for a number of weeks even if the patient is drug-free.

Treatment

Although medication treatment of BP is vital, adequate preparation for treatment is more likely to insure its success.

Psychoeducation and Psychosocial Management

1. Educate patient and family members about BP (including any comorbidities).
2. Include in the treatment recommendations the advantages, limitations, and risks of medication use, as well as consequences of no use.
3. Remind parents to keep medications secure and to administer them reliably.
4. Try to obtain baseline labs: complete blood count, platelets, fasting blood sugar, tests of liver and renal functioning, cholesterol, lipids, and thyroid test (specifically, thyroid-stimulating hormone).
5. To separate psychiatric adverse events from baseline disorder and to evaluate medication benefit, obtain baseline ratings for the major symptom areas being addressed (e.g., aggression/irritability, psychosis, hyperactivity, inattention, anxiety, depression, episode shifts). For children with rages/outbursts, establish their frequency, intensity, number, and duration.
6. Discuss medication risks. If side effects are minimal and treatment efficacy is clear, continue treatment. If adverse events appear to be worse than the condition being treated, change treatment. If there is no improvement after several months, there is no reason to continue that treatment. It is necessary to establish a clear baseline of symptoms and functional impairment in order to be able to clearly. The decision to try another (similar or different) medication or that same medication at a different dose must be made on a case-by-case basis.
7. Prepare patient and family for the fact that different strategies may be needed, but tell parents to give each dose adequate time to work.
8. Address educational aspects of the disorder with necessary teacher rating scales, psychoeducational testing, classroom observation, and development of an individualized educational plan.
9. If the child has comorbid ADHD, autism spectrum disorder, anxiety, or ODD/CD, address these conditions.
10. Recommend treatment for parents so that they can effectively manage their child. The family impact of BP is profound and reciprocal, and rates of family mental illness are quite high.

Specific Psychosocial Interventions

Psychosocial interventions are discussed more fully in Chapter 54, "Parent Counseling, Psychoeducation, and Parent Support Groups."

Pharmacological Treatment

The American Academy of Child and Adolescent Psychiatry (2007) has recently updated its practice parameter for treatment of BP. It confirms the primacy of medication treatment for BP and clarifies that medication choice should be based on evidence of effectiveness, phase of illness, subtype of disorder (psychosis, mixed episode, rapid cycling), the side-effect profile with respect to the particular patient, the patient's history of medication response, and possibly a family member's history of medication response. This is a rapidly changing area, so clinicians must keep abreast of the evidence and the literature (see also Chapter 48, "Mood Stabilizers," and Chapter 49, "Antipsychotic Medication").

As of 2007, eight medications (lithium, divalproex, extended-release carbamazepine, olanzapine, quetiapine, risperidone, aripiprazole, ziprasidone) have U.S. Food and Drug Administration (FDA) approval in adults for the treatment of acute mania, and two (olanzapine plus fluoxetine combined [OFC] and quetiapine) have approval for bipolar depression. Two medications have approval for maintenance treatment; lithium is approved for prevention of mania, and lamotrigine for bipolar depression. In young people, lithium has been approved for adolescent mania, and risperidone and aripiprazole have been approved to treat mania in children as young as age 10.

Although it may make more sense to address treatment in children and adolescents by whether the condition is the broad or narrow phenotype, published treatment algorithms only distinguish manic episodes by the presence or absence of psychotic symptoms. If psychosis is absent, the first-line treatment may include a single antimanic drug, including lithium, valproate, carbamazepine, or any of the atypical or even typical antipsychotic medications. If psychosis is present, or mania is severe, lithium or the aforementioned anticonvulsants are combined with an antipsychotic medication from the outset. If response is poor, combinations other than the one that hasn't worked are used. Electroconvulsive therapy or clozapine is reserved for the most treatment-resistant cases.

Mania trials are usually short-term, 3–8 weeks depending on the medication. Efficacy has been measured in three ways: 1) change from baseline on the YMRS score; 2) response, which is usually a 50% reduction in YMRS entry score (which averages about 30), and 3) remission, which is variously defined as a YMRS score ≤12, a Clinical Global Improvement score on manic symptoms rating the child as improved or very much improved, or both. Completion rates for studies conducted with children and adolescents to date are 60%–80%.

The results from placebo-controlled trials are summarized in Table 19–6. Lithium response has been modest; divalproex was better than placebo in one 8-week study (Kowatch et al. 2007), but not in a 4-week industry-sponsored study (Wagner et al. 2007). Other anticonvulsants, topiramate and oxcarbazepine, have not been significantly better than placebo (Delbello et al. 2005; Wagner et al. 2006). Four atypical antipsychotic medication trials have been completed for pediatric BP (Chang et al. 2007; DelBello et al. 2007a; Pandina et al. 2007; Tohen et al. 2007). Using response as measured by a 50% reduction in YMRS entry score, 50%–70% of subjects improved on active medication versus 20%–37% on placebo. The absolute treatment benefit (percent of drug responders minus placebo responders) averaged 20%–25%, and the number needed to treat (NNT) in successful trials (1 divided by the absolute treatment benefit), where drug was better than placebo, varied from 3.8 to 5.3.

Open trials of lithium for mania have usually been done with psychiatrically hospitalized youth and have demonstrated medication utility, but there has been no control for the actual intervention of hospitalization itself. Nor is it possible to determine whether the bipolar youth had "classic" or "mood dysregulated" forms of BP. There is some suggestion that adjunctive antipsychotic medication adds additional protection. It did not appear that lithium protected against mania relapse after hospital discharge (see Kowatch et al. 2005 for a review).

Divalproex has been studied in non-placebo-controlled trials as well as those described in Table 19–6 (Kowatch et al. 2000). Under those circumstances, about 50% of children and adolescents improved.

Given the level of severity and impairment with which most children and teens begin a bipolar treat-

ment study, the improvement, when it occurs, is noteworthy but often is not sufficient. Little data are available to predict treatment response. Using more than one medication has increasingly become acceptable for treating mania/BP in both adults and young people. In youth, there are three types of studies: 1) comparing two medications to one, such as combined divalproex and quetiapine versus quetiapine alone (Delbello et al. 2002); 2) adding one medication to another if the first drug doesn't work, for example, adding risperidone to lithium or divalproex (Pavuluri et al. 2004); 3) starting two together, for instance, lithium and divalproex and discontinuing one (Findling et al. 2006). This last study was designed as a maintenance treatment study and suggested that a child stabilized on two medications needs to be maintained as such since the relapse rate on one drug alone was high. These data suggest that at least these medication combinations are additive, both in effectiveness and in side effects.

Mania and/or ADHD

ADHD can frequently complicate the treatment of BP. A meta-analysis, albeit using only five studies and 273 patients, found a reduction in relative risk that favored treatment response in children and adolescents having BP-I only without comorbid ADHD (Consoli et al. 2007).

Consensus documents recommend stabilizing the mood disorder symptoms and then treating the comorbid disorder (American Academy of Child and Adolescent Psychiatry 2007; Kowatch et al. 2005). ADHD is the only condition that has been systematically studied in children with mania or BP-NOS. Although there have been concerns about treating ADHD in children with definite or possible mania, an increasing number of studies are substantiating the utility of doing so either with or without prior mood stabilization (Galanter et al. 2003; Scheffer et al. 2005; Tillman and Geller 2006).

In cases where clinicians cannot decide between possible mania and ADHD, we advise discussing with parents the risks and benefits of using atypical antipsychotics or mood stabilizers first versus ADHD treatment first. If the child becomes more irritable or aggressive with ADHD treatment, it makes most sense to use an atypical antipsychotic or a mood stabilizer, perhaps followed by retrying the ADHD treatment. Keep in mind that "rebound," the apparent return of worse ADHD symptoms at the end of the day, has no diagnostic implications and sometimes subsides or diminishes over time (Carlson and Kelly 2003).

TABLE 19–6. Controlled trials for the treatment of acute mania in children and adolescents

Study	Age group, years/Origin of sample	Drug/Sample size	Dose	Trial status/duration	Outcome: change from baseline YMRS	Outcome: % response	Other clinical response criteria
Kowatch et al. 2005[+]	Children and teens Hospitalized + outpatient	Lithium N=<20	~900–1,500 mg 0.9–1.1 mEq/L	Small placebo-controlled trials	Mixed results	Mixed results	
Kowatch et al. 2007	Ages 7–17 Mean age=10 Outpatient	Lithium n=66 DVP n=56 Placebo n=31	Started at 20 mg/kg/day; increased to 30 mg/kg/day 0.8–1.2 µg/L Started at 15 mg/kg; increased to 20 mg/kg 85–110 µg/L	DBPC 8-week trial	No information	YMRS[a] Lithium=42%, NS[b] DVP=53%, P=0.05[b] Placebo=29%	No information
Wagner et al. 2007	Ages 10–17 67% 10–13 Mostly outpatient	DVP, extended release N=150	15–35 mg/kg/day Mean dose=1,457 mg FDA written request	DBPC 4-week trial	DVP=–8.8 Placebo=–7.9 NS	YMRS[a] DVP=24%, NS[b] Placebo=23%	Remission: YMRS[c] DVP=19%, NS[b] Placebo=16%
DelBello et al. 2006	Ages 13–17 Mean age=15 Inpatient only	DVP and QUE N=50	DVP level >100 QUE 400–600 mg No control for hospitalization	Double-blind, randomized 6-week trial	Mean entry YMRS=35 DVP=–19 QUE=–22 P=0.0001 from baseline; no drug difference	YMRS[c] DVP=28% QUE=60% P=0.02 between drugs	CGI≤2 DVP=40% QUE=72% P=0.02 between drugs
Delbello et al. 2005	Teens Mean age=13.8 Mostly outpatient	TOP n=56	200–400 mg/day Mean=278 mg/day	DBPC, part of adult trial 4 weeks' duration	Mean entry YMRS=~31 Drug=–11.7 Placebo=–5.1 P=0.064	CGI-I≤2 Drug=34.5%, NS[b] Placebo=22.2%	Study underpowered; might have shown significance with larger sample
Wagner et al. 2006	Ages 7–17 Mean age=11.1 (SD=2.9)	OXC n=116	Up to 2,400 mg/day Mean dose=1,515 mg/day	DBPC 6-week trial	Change in entry YMRS=30.5 Drug=–10.9 Placebo=–9.79	YMRS[a] Drug 42%, NS[b] Placebo=26%	Child response: 41% vs. 17% Teen response: 43% vs. 40%

TABLE 19–6. Controlled trials for the treatment of acute mania in children and adolescents (*continued*)

Study	Age group, years/Origin of sample	Drug/ Sample size	Dose	Trial status/ duration	Outcome: change from baseline YMRS	Outcome: % response	Other clinical response criteria
Tohen et al. 2007	Ages 13–17 Mean age=15 Mostly outpatient	OLA N=161	2.5–20 mg Mean dose= 8.9 mg	DBPC 3-week trial	Mean entry YMRS=33 Drug=–17.65 Placebo=–9.99 P=0.001	YMRS[a] Drug=48.6%, P=0.002[b] Placebo=22.2%	YMRS[c] Drug=35.2% Placebo=11.1%
Pandina et al. 2007	Ages 10–17 Mean age=10.9 (SD=3.3) 40%≤12 Mostly outpatient	RIS N=169	Low dose= 0.5–2.5 mg High dose= 3–6 mg	DBPC 3-week trial	Mean entry YMRS=~31 Low dose=–18.5 High dose=–16.5 Placebo=–9.1	YMRS[a] Low dose=59%, P=0.002[b] High dose=63%, P=0.001[b] Placebo=26%	YMRS[c] Low dose=51% High dose=50% Placebo=20%
Chang et al. 2007	Ages 10–17 Mean age=13.4 22%≤11	ARI N=302	Low dose=10 mg High dose=30 mg	DBPC 4-week trial	Mean entry YMRS=30 Low dose=–14.2 High dose=–16.5 Placebo=–8.2	YMRS[a] Low dose=44.8%, P=0.05[b] High dose=63.6%, P=0.001[b] Placebo=26.1%	Remission: YMRS[c], CGI-BP≤2 Low dose=25.0%, P=0.05[b] High dose=47.5%, P=0.001[b] Placebo=5.4%
DelBello et al. 2007a	Ages 10–17 43%≤12	QUE N=277	Low dose= 400 mg High dose= 600 mg	DBPC 3-week trial	Mean entry YMRS=~29 Low dose=14.25 High dose=15.60 Placebo=9.04	YMRS[a] Low dose=63%, P=0.003[b] High dose=58%, P=0.01[b] Placebo=37%	Remission: YMRS[c] Low dose=53% High dose=54% Placebo=30%

Note. ARI=aripiprazole; CGI-BP=Clinical Global Impression ratings for Bipolar Disorder; CGI-I=Clinical Global Improvement–Improvement score; DBPC=double-blind placebo-controlled; DVP=divalproex; FDA=U.S. Food and Drug Administration; NS=not significant; OLA=olanzapine; OXC=oxcarbazepine; QUE=quetiapine; RIS=risperidone; TOP=topiramate; YMRS=Young Mania Rating Scale.
[†]Review.
[a]≥50% drop in YMRS.
[b]Compared with placebo.
[c]YMRS score≤12.

Bipolar Depression

There are no placebo-controlled or otherwise randomized data for children and adolescents in the depressive phase of BP. In the absence of any data for youth, data for bipolar depression in adults shows the greatest utility for OFC, quetiapine, and lamotrigine as judged by FDA approval for those medications. The use of antidepressants alone or in combination with lithium/divalproex appears to be less useful in adults. Moreover, the risk of "switching" or developing mood elevation as a result of most medications used to improve mood is a contentious topic. Extrapolating from information about activation in studies of selective serotonin reuptake inhibitors, rates are higher in children than in adolescents and adults but may average about 10% (Ostacher 2006; Safer and Zito 2006).

Of particular relevance to youth is a first episode of depression with a bipolar family history. Here, the risks of precipitating a mania/hypomania/bipolar course with an antidepressant must be weighed against treating with medications for which there are either minimal or no data regarding effectiveness in children or adolescents. Any history suggestive of a bipolar diathesis (including clear bipolar history in first-degree relatives), the reliability of parent observation and child adherence to treatment, and family preference should be carefully considered in the decision-making process.

Maintenance

Young people with BP have higher relapse rates than adults. Lithium alone has not been successful in this age group as a maintenance medication. Six-month extension data from recent studies of atypical antipsychotics are not yet available. However, both the available data and clinical experience suggest that if remission is achieved on a particular regimen, it should be continued as long as possible, and at least until the child or adolescent has navigated his or her most important developmental, academic, and social milestones.

Treatment Implications for Broad and Narrow Phenotypes

At this time, no definitive recommendations can be made regarding the relative efficacy of treatment response in youth with narrow versus broad phenotype/severe mood dysregulation. However, insofar as early-onset BP resembles classic adult BP, we can speculate that medication efficacy might well be similar. Lithium, divalproex, and atypical antipsychotics appear to have considerable effectiveness. If youth with severe mood dysregulation/broad phenotype have a condition that is continuous with mixed, rapid cycling, then strategies aimed at these subtypes are warranted. Many medications are the same, though treatment response is less impressive. Insofar as rapid cycles are often between bipolar depression and hypomania, and depressive symptoms are prominent in mixed episodes, medications aimed at bipolar depression are recommended in adults. Unfortunately, there are no data in children or adolescents for those medications.

When severe mood dysregulation meets criteria for ADHD and particularly fulminant ODD (Carlson 2007), a treatment algorithm for ADHD and aggression might be a reasonable course of action. Interestingly, the same medications that are labeled as antimanic drugs also have efficacy as antiaggression medications. The differences in the two approaches, then, is the addition of a medication aimed at ADHD (not used to treat mania) and psychosocial strategies that consist of behavior modification in children with ADHD/ODD versus bipolar-based strategies aimed at mood regulation.

Nicola, for instance, responded well to lithium, though she developed a sufficiently severe postmanic depression such that she needed to be placed in a special education program for the following year. Lynda was in and out of hospitals, tried on various medications, responding well while hospitalized and relapsing when she returned home. She was sent to live with a relative out of state and appeared most stable on mixed amphetamine salts and a low-dose atypical antipsychotic.

BP in children and at least young adolescents has been overlooked for too long. It is an important condition to recognize and treat. However, it is also important not to overlook other conditions in which mood dysregulation can figure prominently because the treatment implications can be quite different, although certain medication treatments are often interchangeable. The differences have to do with not treating other aspects of the child's symptomatology or treating it incorrectly. Table 19–7 outlines some of the differences in treatment that should be considered.

Research Directions

Despite significant progress in our understanding of mania in youth, there remain unanswered questions that warrant further investigation.

TABLE 19–7. Treatments for mania and conditions confused with mania

Treatment type	Mania/BP	MDD	PDD	Abuse	Aggression	ADHD
Lithium	×				×	
Divalproex	×		×		×	
Antipsychotics	×		×		×	
Antidepressants		×	×		×	
ADHD medications			×		×	×
Specific IEP			×			
Language therapy			×			
Psychotherapy	Family-focused therapy, cognitive-behavioral strategies, BP psychoeducation	CBT	Social skills, social stories; collaborative problem solving	CBT, other therapy	Behavior modification	Behavior modification, ADHD, psychoeducation
Protective services				×		

Note. ADHD=attention-deficit/hyperactivity disorder; BP=bipolar disorder; CBT=cognitive-behavioral therapy; IEP=individualized education plan; MDD=major depressive disorder; PDD=pervasive developmental disorder.

It will be important to clarify the definition of BP and measures used to assess it. Depending on the focus of research, it may be important to distinguish current from lifetime mania, BP-I from BP spectrum disorder, explosive outbursts from rapid cycles, and the different components of irritability/affective aggression. Future research will need to elucidate the ways in which narrow versus broad phenotype, developmentally altered criteria definitions, and specific prepubertal-onset BP map onto adult BP versus other psychopathology.

Treatment progress will be enhanced with better understanding of the implications of varying temporal relationships between mania and its comorbid conditions. In other words, is a 15-year-old with mania who had separation anxiety at age 5 different from a 15-year-old with mania who has concurrent panic attacks, and does that teen differ from an adult who is euthymic but who reported episodes of mania and anxiety in his or her past?

Longitudinal studies will be critical for identifying children at risk for BP versus those who will develop other psychopathology. Additional clinical studies are needed to determine why early-onset BP is associated with seemingly poor prognosis and to improve treatment efficacy for children with early-onset BP and their families.

Future genetics studies will clarify how, if at all, the genetics of early-onset BP differ from those of adult-onset BP. Given that BP is partly genetic, it will be important to identify what exactly is inherited and whether there are endophenotypes or neurobiological markers that can be found.

Summary Points

- BP in general, and mania in particular, is identified somewhat differently by different investigators and methods of investigation. The difference is not whether DSM criteria are used, but how they are applied. The degree to which they identify the same children and predict a course consistent with what has been called bipolar in adults is the subject of ongoing study.

- Simultaneous comorbidity of mania and externalizing disorders is high in prepubertal children and somewhat lower in adolescents. Anxiety and developmental disorders are other important comorbidities. Substance abuse is both a complication and comorbidity of BP in teens.

- Neurobiological validators are being sought, but studies have a number of methodological problems. Nevertheless, there is some consistency to the finding of decreased amygdala volume and abnormalities in the prefrontal cortex.

- BP in youth is a heritable condition though there are also environmental contributions. Complex comorbidity in parents may confer higher rates of psychopathology onto offspring. Candidate genes are being sought.

- Age at onset varies by how bipolar conditions are defined (first behavior disorder symptoms, first mood episode, first manic episode). Early onset appears to be associated with worse outcome, both in terms of episode recurrence and functional outcome.

- Evaluation requires interview of parent, child, and if possible, confirmatory information from another source. Comorbidities need to be assessed.

- The differential diagnosis of BP includes ADHD, anxiety disorders, schizophrenia, substance abuse disorder, and conditions in which there are problems with emotion regulation. There are no quick tips for establishing the diagnosis definitively.

- Treatment modalities for early-onset mania are evolving. At this time, there is more evidence for the efficacy of atypical antipsychotics from industry-sponsored studies than for lithium or anticonvulsants. There are no placebo-controlled studies of treatment for bipolar depression in youth. Maintenance and prophylactic studies are also needed.

References

Alloy LB, Abramson LY, Urosevic S, et al: The psychosocial context of bipolar disorder: environmental, cognitive, and developmental risk factors. Clin Psychol Rev 25:1043–1075, 2005

Althoff RR, Faraone SV, Rettew DC, et al: Family, twin, adoption, and molecular genetic studies of juvenile bipolar disorder. Bipolar Disord 7:598–609, 2005

American Academy of Child and Adolescent Psychiatry: Practice parameter for the assessment and treatment of children and adolescents with bipolar disorder. J Am Acad Child Adolesc Psychiatry 46:107–125, 2007

American Psychiatric Association: Diagnostic and Statistical Manual of Mental Disorders, 4th Edition. Washington, DC, American Psychiatric Association, 1994

American Psychiatric Association: Diagnostic and Statistical Manual of Mental Disorders, 4th Edition, Text Revision. Washington, DC, American Psychiatric Association, 2000

Biederman J, Mick E, Faraone SV, et al: Pediatric mania: a developmental subtype of bipolar disorder? Biol Psychiatry 48:458–466, 2000

Biederman J, Faraone SV, Wozniak J, et al: Further evidence of unique developmental phenotypic correlates of pediatric bipolar disorder: findings from a large sample of clinically referred preadolescent children assessed over the last 7 years. J Affect Disord 82:S45–S58, 2004

Birmaher B, Axelson D: Course and outcome of bipolar spectrum disorder in children and adolescents: a review of the existing literature. Dev Psychopathol 18:1023–1035, 2006

Birmaher B, Axelson D, Strober M, et al: Clinical course of children and adolescents with bipolar spectrum disorders. Arch Gen Psychiatry 63:175–183, 2006

Blader J, Carlson GA: Increased rates of bipolar disorder diagnoses among U.S. child, adolescent, and adult inpatients, 1996–2004. Biol Psychiatry 62:104–106, 2007

Blumberg HP, Fredericks C, Wang F, et al: Preliminary evidence for persistent abnormalities in amygdala volumes in adolescents and young adults with bipolar disorder. Bipolar Disord 7:570–576, 2005

Brotman MA, Schmajuk M, Rich BA, et al: Prevalence, clinical correlates, and longitudinal course of severe mood dysregulation in children. Biol Psychiatry 60:991–997, 2006

Brotman MA, Kassem L, Reising MM, et al: Parental diagnoses in youth with narrow phenotype bipolar disorder or severe mood dysregulation. Am J Psychiatry 164:1238–1241, 2007

Carlson GA: Who are the children with severe mood dysregulation, a.k.a. "rages"? Am J Psychiatry 164:1140–1142, 2007

Carlson GA, Kelly KL: Stimulant rebound: how common is it and what does it mean? J Child Adolesc Psychopharmacol 13:137–142, 2003

Carlson GA, Meyer SE: Diagnosis of bipolar disorder across the lifespan: complexities and developmental issues. Dev Psychopathol 18:939–969, 2006

Carlson GA, Bromet EJ, Sievers S: Phenomenology and outcome of subjects with early and adult-onset psychotic mania. Am J Psychiatry 157:213–219, 2000

Chang KD, Steiner H, Ketter TA: Psychiatric phenomenology of child and adolescent bipolar offspring. J Am Acad Child Adolesc Psychiatry 39:453–460, 2000

Chang KD, Nyilas M, Aurang C, et al: Efficacy of aripiprazole in children (10–17 years old) with mania. Presented at the American Academy of Child and Adolescent Psychiatry Annual Meeting, Boston, MA, October 2007

Consoli A, Bouzamondo A, Guilé JM, et al: Comorbidity with ADHD decreases response to pharmacotherapy in children and adolescents with acute mania: evidence from a meta-analysis. Can J Psychiatry 52:323–328, 2007

Costello EJ, Angold A, Burns BJ, et al: The Great Smoky Mountains Study of Youth: goals, design, methods, and the prevalence of DSM-III-R disorders. Arch Gen Psychiatry 53:1129–1136, 1996

DelBello MP, Schwiers ML, Rosenberg HL, et al: A double-blind, randomized, placebo-controlled study of quetiapine as adjunctive treatment for adolescent mania. J Am Acad Child Adolesc Psychiatry 41:1216–1223, 2002

DelBello MP, Findling RL, Kushner S, et al: A pilot controlled trial of topiramate for mania in children and adolescents with bipolar disorder. J Am Acad Child Adolesc Psychiatry 44:539–547, 2005

DelBello MP, Kowatch RA, Adler CM, et al: A double-blind randomized pilot study comparing quetiapine and divalproex for adolescent mania. J Am Acad Child Adolesc Psychiatry 45:305–313, 2006

DelBello MP, Findling RL, Earley WR, et al: Efficacy of quetiapine in children and adolescents with bipolar mania: a 3 week, double-blind, randomized, placebo-controlled trial. Presented at the American Academy of Child and Adolescent Psychiatry Annual Meeting, Boston, MA, October 2007a

DelBello MP, Hanseman D, Adler CM, et al: Twelve-month outcome of adolescents with bipolar disorder following first hospitalization for a manic or mixed episode. Am J Psychiatry 164:582–590, 2007b

Dickstein DP, Rich BA, Binstock AB, et al: Comorbid anxiety in phenotypes of pediatric bipolar disorder. J Child Adolesc Psychopharmacol 15:534–548, 2005

Dubicka B, Carlson G, Vail A, et al: Prepubertal mania: diagnostic differences between US and UK clinicians. Eur Child Adolesc Psychiatry 17(suppl):153–161, 2008

Duffy A, Alda M, Kutcher S, et al: A prospective study of the offspring of bipolar parents responsive and nonresponsive to lithium treatment. J Clin Psychiatry 63:1171–1178, 2002

Duffy A, Alda M, Crawford L, et al: The early manifestations of bipolar disorder: a longitudinal prospective study of the offspring of bipolar parents. Bipolar Disord 9:828–838, 2007

Faraone SV, Biederman J, Wozniak J, et al: Is comorbidity with ADHD a marker for juvenile-onset mania? J Am Acad Child Adolesc Psychiatry 36:1046–1055, 1997

Findling RL, McNamara NK, Stansbrey R, et al: Combination lithium and divalproex sodium in pediatric bipolar symptom restabilization. J Am Acad Child Adolesc Psychiatry 45:142–148, 2006

Frazier JA, Ahn MS, DeJong S, et al: Magnetic resonance imaging studies in early-onset bipolar disorder: a critical review. Harv Rev Psychiatry 13(suppl):125–140, 2005

Galanter CA, Carlson GA, Jensen PS, et al: Response to methylphenidate in children with attention deficit hyperactivity disorder and manic symptoms in the multimodal treatment study of children with attention deficit hyperactivity disorder titration trial. J Child Adolesc Psychopharmacol 13:123–136, 2003

Geller B, Zimerman B, Williams M, et al: Reliability of the Washington University in St. Louis Kiddie Schedule for Affective Disorders and Schizophrenia (WASH-U-K-SADS) mania and rapid cycling sections. J Am Acad Child Adolesc Psychiatry 40:450–455, 2001

Geller B, Tillman R, Craney JL, et al: Four-year prospective outcome and natural history of mania in children with a prepubertal and early adolescent bipolar disorder phenotype. Arch Gen Psychiatry 61:459–467, 2004

Goodwin FK, Jamison KR: Manic-Depressive Illness Bipolar Disorders and Recurrent Depression. New York, Oxford University Press, 2007

Gutkovich ZA, Carlson GA: Medication treatment of bipolar disorder in developmentally disabled children and adolescents. Minerva Pediatr 60:69–85, 2008

Henin A, Biederman J, Mick E, et al: Psychopathology in the offspring of parents with bipolar disorder: a controlled study. Biol Psychiatry 58:554–561, 2005

Hirshfeld-Becker DR, Biederman J, Henin A, et al: Psychopathology in the young offspring of parents with bipolar disorder: a controlled pilot study. Psychiatry Res 145: 155–167, 2006

Jairam R, Srinath S, Girimaji SC, et al: A prospective 4–5 year follow-up of juvenile-onset bipolar disorder. Bipolar Disord 6:386–394, 2004

Kowatch RA, Suppes T, Carmody TJ, et al: Effect size of lithium, divalproex sodium, and carbamazepine in children and adolescents with bipolar disorder. J Am Acad Child Adolesc Psychiatry 39:713–720, 2000

Kowatch RA, Fristad M, Birmaher B, et al: Treatment guidelines for children and adolescents with bipolar disorder. J Am Acad Child Adolesc Psychiatry 44:213–235, 2005

Kowatch RA, Scheffer R, Findling RL: Placebo controlled trial of divalproex versus lithium for bipolar disorder. Presented at the American Academy of Child and Adolescent Psychiatry Annual Meeting, Boston, MA, October 2007

Lapalme M, Hodgins S, LaRoche C: Children of parents with bipolar disorder: a meta-analysis of risk for mental disorders. Can J Psychiatry 42:623–631, 1997

Leibenluft E, Charney DS, Towbin KE, et al: Defining clinical phenotypes of juvenile mania. Am J Psychiatry 160:430–437, 2003

Leverich GS, McElroy SL, Suppes T, et al: Early physical and sexual abuse associated with an adverse course of bipolar illness. Biol Psychiatry 51:288–297, 2002

Lewinsohn P, Klein DN, Seeley JR: Bipolar disorders in a community sample of older adolescents: prevalence, phenomenology, comorbidity, and course. J Am Acad Child Adolesc Psychiatry 34:454–463, 1995

Lewinsohn P, Klein D, Seeley J: Bipolar disorder during adolescence and young adulthood in a community sample. Bipolar Disord 2:281–293, 2000

Meyer SE, Carlson GA, Wiggs EA, et al: A prospective study of the association among impaired executive functioning, childhood attentional problems, and the development of bipolar disorder. Dev Psychopathol 16:461–476, 2004

Meyer SE, Carlson GA, Wiggs EA, et al: A prospective high-risk study of the association among maternal negativity, apparent frontal lobe dysfunction, and the development of bipolar disorder. Dev Psychopathol 18:573–589, 2006

O'Connor MJ, Shah B, Whaley S, et al: Psychiatric illness in a clinical sample of children with prenatal alcohol exposure. Am J Drug Alcohol Abuse 28:743–754, 2002

Ostacher MJ: The evidence for antidepressant use in bipolar depression. J Clin Psychiatry 67:18–21, 2006

Pandina G, DelBello M, Kushner S, et al: Risperidone for the treatment of acute mania in bipolar youth. Presented at the American Academy of Child and Adolescent Psychiatry Annual Meeting, Boston, MA, October 2007

Pavuluri MN, Henry DB, Carbray JA, et al: Open-label prospective trial of risperidone in combination with lithium or divalproex sodium in pediatric mania. J Affect Disord 82(suppl):S103–S111, 2004

Pavuluri MN, Birmaher B, Naylor M: Pediatric bipolar disorder: a review of the past 10 years. J Am Acad Child Adolesc Psychiatry 44:846–871, 2005

Pavuluri MN, O'Connor MM, Harral E, et al: Affective neural circuitry during facial emotion processing in pediatric bipolar disorder. Biol Psychiatry 62:158–167, 2007

Reichart CG, Wals M, Hillegers MH, et al: Psychopathology in the adolescent offspring of bipolar parents. J Affect Disord 78:67–71, 2004

Rich BA, Vinton DT, Roberson-Nay R, et al: Limbic hyperactivation during processing of neutral facial expressions in children with bipolar disorder. Proc Natl Acad Sci U S A 103:8900–8905, 2006

Safer DJ, Zito JM: Treatment-emergent adverse events from selective serotonin reuptake inhibitors by age group: children versus adolescents. J Child Adolesc Psychopharmacol 16:159–169, 2006

Scheffer RE, Kowatch RA, Carmody T, et al: Randomized, placebo-controlled trial of mixed amphetamine salts for symptoms of comorbid ADHD in pediatric bipolar disorder after mood stabilization with divalproex sodium. Am J Psychiatry 162:58–64, 2005

Shaw JA, Egeland JA, Endicott J, et al: A 10-year prospective study of prodromal patterns for bipolar disorder among Amish youth. J Am Acad Child Adolesc Psychiatry 44:1104–1111, 2005

Singh MK, DelBello MP, Stanford KE, et al: Psychopathology in children of bipolar parents. J Affect Disord 102:131–136, 2007

Srinath S, Janardhan Reddy YC, Girimaji SR, et al: A prospective study of bipolar disorder in children and adolescents from India. Acta Psychiatr Scand 98:437–442, 1998

Strober M, Schmidt-Lackner S, Freeman R, et al: Recovery and relapse in adolescents with bipolar affective illness: a five-year naturalistic, prospective follow-up. J Am Acad Child Adolesc Psychiatry 34:724–731, 1995

Tillman R, Geller B: Controlled study of switching from attention-deficit/hyperactivity disorder to a prepubertal and early adolescent bipolar I disorder phenotype during 6-year prospective follow-up: rate, risk, and predictors. Dev Psychopathol 18:1037–1053, 2006

Tillman R, Geller B, Bolhofner K, et al: Ages of onset and rates of syndromal and subsyndromal comorbid DSM-IV diagnoses in a prepubertal and early adolescent bipolar disorder phenotype. J Am Acad Child Adolesc Psychiatry 42:1486–1493, 2003

Tohen M, Kryzhanovskaya L, Carlson G, et al: Olanzapine versus placebo in the treatment of adolescents with bipolar mania. Am J Psychiatry 164:1547–1556, 2007

Wagner KD, Kowatch RA, Emslie GJ, et al: A double-blind, randomized, placebo-controlled trial of oxcarbazepine in the treatment of bipolar disorder in children and adolescents. Am J Psychiatry 163:1179–1186, 2006

Wagner KD, Redden L, Kowatch RA, et al: Safety and efficacy of divalproex ER in youth with mania. Presented at the American Academy of Child and Adolescent Psychiatry Annual Meeting, Boston, MA, October 2007

Youngstrom E, Meyers O, Youngstrom JK, et al: Diagnostic and measurement issues in the assessment of pediatric bipolar disorder: implications for understanding mood disorder across the life cycle. Dev Psychopathol 18:989–1021, 2006

Generalized Anxiety Disorder, Specific Phobia, Panic Disorder, Social Phobia, and Selective Mutism

Sucheta D. Connolly, M.D.
Liza M. Suárez, Ph.D.

When providing care to anxious youth, clinicians must distinguish normal, transient, developmentally appropriate worries and fears, as well as responses to the stressors of daily life, from anxiety disorders. Worries and fears are distinct concepts: *worry* involves anxious apprehension and thoughts focused on the possibility of negative future events, while *fear* is related to the response to threat or danger that is perceived as actual or impending. Occasional worry is normative in children (Muris et al. 1998). The fears reported by children tend to decline with increasing age and change over time from immediate and tangible concerns to

anticipatory and less tangible ones, whereas the content and complexity of worries increase with age and cognitive ability (Craske 1997).

Common fears among infants include loud noises, someone dropping them, and later normal separation anxiety. Toddlers typically experience fears of imaginary creatures or monsters and darkness. These normative fears diminish after age 6. From age 5 to 6, worries about physical well-being (e.g., injury or kidnapping) emerge, and later fears of natural events (storms) develop. The most commonly reported fears in children ages 8–13 include concerns about the dark, spiders, and thunderstorms (Muris et al. 1999). From age 8, worries about school performance, behavioral competence, rejection by peers, and health and illness emerge, and by age 12 and into adolescence, worries about social competence, social evaluation, and psychological well-being become prominent (Albano and Hayward 2004; Muris et al. 1998).

This chapter will cover information about diagnosis, epidemiology, assessment, and treatment of five childhood anxiety disorders: generalized anxiety disorder (GAD), specific phobia, panic disorder, social phobia, and selective mutism (SM). Separation anxiety disorder (SAD) and school refusal behavior are covered in Chapter 21, "Separation Anxiety Disorder and School Refusal," and obsessive-compulsive disorder (OCD) is covered in Chapter 23, "Obsessive-Compulsive Disorder."

Diagnostic Criteria and Additional Features

In order for patients to receive a diagnosis, the symptoms described below must cause significant interference in functioning or marked distress for the child. Tables 20–1 through 20–8 summarize the diagnostic criteria and additional features associated with the clinical disorders covered in this chapter.

Epidemiology and Comorbidity

Prevalence, Course, and Prognosis

Current or 3-month prevalence rates for any anxiety disorder in youth range from 2% to 4%, with median 6-month and 12-month estimates between 10% to 20%, and lifetime estimates only slightly higher. Table 20–9 summarizes research findings on prevalence, course, and prognosis for GAD, specific phobia, panic disorder, social phobia, and SM in children. Costello et al. (2004) provide a more extensive review of prevalence rates and developmental trends in epidemiological studies using DSM-III-R (American Psychiatric Association 1987), DSM-IV (American Psychiatric Association 1994), and ICD-10 (World Health Organization

1992) criteria for childhood anxiety disorders. Anxiety disorders are common in preschool children, and they follow similar patterns as those of older children (Egger and Angold 2006).

Prospective longitudinal data from the Great Smoky Mountain Study showed that anxiety disorders in childhood are predictors of a range of psychiatric disorders in adolescence (Bittner et al. 2007). More specifically, SAD in childhood predicted SAD in adolescence; overanxious disorder (OAD) was associated with later OAD, panic attacks, depression, and conduct disorder; childhood social phobia was associated with adolescent OAD, social phobia, and attention-deficit/hyperactivity disorder (ADHD); and GAD was only related to conduct disorder.

Anxiety disorders in childhood often precede the onset of other disorders commonly experienced in childhood, such as disruptive behavior disorders (emerging in mid childhood) and depression (emerging in late childhood; Kovacs and Devlin 1998). Children with anxiety disorders are at greater risk of developing substance abuse and conduct problems and have increased use of long-term psychiatric and medical services and greater overall functional impairment (Marquenie et al. 2007; Weissman et al. 1999). A childhood diagnosis of anxiety disorders is associated with greater severity and impairment, familial risk, and greater risk of developing a range of disorders across the life span (Egger and Angold 2006).

Comorbidity

Anxiety disorders are highly comorbid with other anxiety disorders (Verduin and Kendall 2003) and with other psychiatric disorders, including depression (Angold and Costello 1993; Lewinsohn et al. 1997) and ADHD (Kendall et al. 2001). Approximately one-third of children in the Multimodal Treatment Study of Children with ADHD had co-occurring anxiety disorders (MTA Cooperative Group 2001). Other conditions that frequently co-occur with anxiety include oppositional defiant disorder, learning disorders, and language disorders (Manassis and Monga 2001). The co-occurrence of anxiety and depression increases with age and is associated with greater impairment and severity (Bernstein 1991; Manassis and Menna 1999). Accurate diagnosis is made difficult by the frequency of overlapping symptoms between anxiety disorders and comorbid conditions (American Academy of Child and Adolescent Psychiatry 2007). Symptoms of inattention, for example, may be indicative of anxiety, ADHD, depression, learning disorders, and

TABLE 20–1. Generalized anxiety disorder: diagnostic criteria and additional features

DSM-IV-TR diagnostic criteria for generalized anxiety disorder

A. Excessive anxiety and worry (apprehensive expectation), occurring more days than not for at least 6 months, about a number of events or activities (such as work or school performance).

B. The person finds it difficult to control the worry.

C. The anxiety and worry are associated with three (or more) of the following six symptoms (with at least some symptoms present for more days than not for the past 6 months).   **Note:** Only one item is required in children.

   (1) restlessness or feeling keyed up or on edge

   (2) being easily fatigued

   (3) difficulty concentrating or mind going blank

   (4) irritability

   (5) muscle tension

   (6) sleep disturbance (difficulty falling or staying asleep, or restless unsatisfying sleep)

D. The focus of the anxiety and worry is not confined to features of an Axis I disorder, e.g., the anxiety or worry is not about having a panic attack (as in panic disorder), being embarrassed in public (as in social phobia), being contaminated (as in obsessive-compulsive disorder), being away from home or close relatives (as in separation anxiety disorder), gaining weight (as in anorexia nervosa), having multiple physical complaints (as in somatization disorder), or having a serious illness (as in hypochondriasis), and the anxiety and worry do not occur exclusively during posttraumatic stress disorder.

E. The anxiety, worry, or physical symptoms cause clinically significant distress or impairment in social, occupational, or other important areas of functioning.

F. The disturbance is not due to the direct physiological effects of a substance (e.g., a drug of abuse, a medication) or a general medical condition (e.g., hyperthyroidism) and does not occur exclusively during a mood disorder, a psychotic disorder, or a pervasive developmental disorder.

Additional features[a]

- Anxiety and worry occur in a number of areas (school, interpersonal relationships, health/safety of self, health/safety of others, family, natural disasters, and future events) and the types of worries exhibited by children with generalized anxiety disorder are more typical of adults (Kendall et al. 2004a).

- Excessive self-consciousness; frequent reassurance-seeking from parents, peers, and teachers; cognitive distortions; and persistent worry about negative consequences are characteristic.

- Youth with generalized anxiety disorder are perfectionistic, display unreasonable expectations regarding their own performance, and are excessively critical of themselves when they cannot meet these expectations; worries persist in the absence of any real concerns (Albano et al. 2003).

- Additional common somatic complaints include gastrointestinal distress, headaches, frequent urination, sweating, and tremor.

- Prior to DSM-IV, children with excessive worry were diagnosed with overanxious disorder.

[a]Additional features not included in DSM-IV-TR and presented by the authors for purposes of this textbook.
Source. DSM-IV-TR criteria reprinted from American Psychiatric Association: *Diagnostic and Statistical Manual of Mental Disorders,* 4th Edition, Text Revision. Washington, DC, American Psychiatric Association, 2000, p. 476. Used with permission. Copyright © 2000 American Psychiatric Association.

TABLE 20–2. Specific phobia: diagnostic criteria and additional features

DSM-IV-TR diagnostic criteria for specific phobia

A. Marked and persistent fear that is excessive or unreasonable, cued by the presence or anticipation of a specific object or situation (e.g., flying, heights, animals, receiving an injection, seeing blood).

B. Exposure to the phobic stimulus almost invariably provokes an immediate anxiety response, which may take the form of a situationally bound or situationally predisposed panic attack. **Note:** In children, the anxiety may be expressed by crying, tantrums, freezing, or clinging.

C. The person recognizes that the fear is excessive or unreasonable. **Note:** In children, this feature may be absent.

D. The phobic situation(s) is avoided or else is endured with intense anxiety or distress.

E. The avoidance, anxious anticipation, or distress in the feared situation(s) interferes significantly with the person's normal routine, occupational (or academic) functioning, or social activities or relationships, or there is marked distress about having the phobia.

F. In individuals under age 18 years, the duration is at least 6 months.

G. The anxiety, panic attacks, or phobic avoidance associated with the specific object or situation is not better accounted for by another mental disorder, such as obsessive-compulsive disorder (e.g., fear of dirt in someone with an obsession about contamination), posttraumatic stress disorder (e.g., avoidance of stimuli associated with a severe stressor), separation anxiety disorder (e.g., avoidance of school), social phobia (e.g., avoidance of social situations because of fear of embarrassment), panic disorder with agoraphobia, or agoraphobia without history of panic disorder.

Specify type:

Animal Type

Natural Environment Type (e.g., heights, storms, water)

Blood-Injection-Injury Type

Situational Type (e.g., airplanes, elevators, enclosed places)

Other Type (e.g., fear of choking, vomiting, or contracting an illness; in children, fear of loud sounds or costumed characters)

Additional features[a]

- In children, the anxiety may be expressed by crying, tantrums, freezing, or clinging rather than a recognizable anxiety response.

- Specific phobia symptoms can be clustered into three intercorrelated factors, each associated with different psychological and cognitive symptoms (Antony et al. 1997; Muris et al. 1999):

  1. Animal phobias: More likely to experience tachycardia (evidence of sympathetic activation)

  2. Blood-injection-injury phobias: Commonly experience bradycardia (evidence of parasympathetic activation)

  3. Environmental or situational phobia: Commonly experience cognitive symptoms, such as fear of going crazy or misinterpretation of body symptoms

[a]Additional features not included in DSM-IV-TR and presented by the authors for purposes of this textbook.
Source. DSM-IV-TR criteria reprinted from American Psychiatric Association: *Diagnostic and Statistical Manual of Mental Disorders*, 4th Edition, Text Revision. Washington, DC, American Psychiatric Association, 2000, pp. 449–450. Used with permission. Copyright © 2000 American Psychiatric Association.

TABLE 20–3. DSM-IV-TR diagnostic criteria for panic attack

Note: A panic attack is not a codable disorder. Code the specific diagnosis in which the panic attack occurs (e.g., 300.21 panic disorder with agoraphobia).

A discrete period of intense fear or discomfort, in which four (or more) of the following symptoms developed abruptly and reached a peak within 10 minutes:

    (1) palpitations, pounding heart, or accelerated heart rate

    (2) sweating

    (3) trembling or shaking

    (4) sensations of shortness of breath or smothering

    (5) feeling of choking

    (6) chest pain or discomfort

    (7) nausea or abdominal distress

    (8) feeling dizzy, unsteady, light-headed, or faint

    (9) derealization (feelings of unreality) or depersonalization (being detached from oneself)

    (10) fear of losing control or going crazy

    (11) fear of dying

    (12) paresthesias (numbness or tingling sensations)

    (13) chills or hot flushes

Source. Reprinted from American Psychiatric Association: *Diagnostic and Statistical Manual of Mental Disorders,* 4th Edition, Text Revision. Washington, DC, American Psychiatric Association, 2000, p. 432. Used with permission. Copyright © 2000 American Psychiatric Association.

TABLE 20–4. DSM-IV-TR diagnostic criteria for agoraphobia

Note: Agoraphobia is not a codable disorder. Code the specific disorder in which the agoraphobia occurs (e.g., 300.21 panic disorder with agoraphobia or 300.22 agoraphobia without history of panic disorder).

A. Anxiety about being in places or situations from which escape might be difficult (or embarrassing) or in which help may not be available in the event of having an unexpected or situationally predisposed panic attack or panic-like symptoms. Agoraphobic fears typically involve characteristic clusters of situations that include being outside the home alone; being in a crowd or standing in a line; being on a bridge; and traveling in a bus, train, or automobile.

    Note: Consider the diagnosis of specific phobia if the avoidance is limited to one or only a few specific situations, or social phobia if the avoidance is limited to social situations.

B. The situations are avoided (e.g., travel is restricted) or else are endured with marked distress or with anxiety about having a panic attack or panic-like symptoms or require the presence of a companion.

C. The anxiety or phobic avoidance is not better accounted for by another mental disorder, such as social phobia (e.g., avoidance limited to social situations because of fear of embarrassment), specific phobia (e.g., avoidance limited to a single situation like elevators), obsessive-compulsive disorder (e.g., avoidance of dirt in someone with an obsession about contamination), posttraumatic stress disorder (e.g., avoidance of stimuli associated with a severe stressor), or separation anxiety disorder (e.g., avoidance of leaving home or relatives).

Source. Reprinted from American Psychiatric Association: *Diagnostic and Statistical Manual of Mental Disorders,* 4th Edition, Text Revision. Washington, DC, American Psychiatric Association, 2000, p. 433. Used with permission. Copyright © 2000 American Psychiatric Association.

TABLE 20–5. DSM-IV-TR diagnostic criteria for panic disorder without agoraphobia

A. Both (1) and (2):

(1) recurrent unexpected panic attacks

(2) at least one of the attacks has been followed by 1 month (or more) of one (or more) of the following:

(a) persistent concern about having additional attacks

(b) worry about the implications of the attack or its consequences (e.g., losing control, having a heart attack, "going crazy")

(c) a significant change in behavior related to the attacks

B. Absence of agoraphobia.

C. The panic attacks are not due to the direct physiological effects of a substance (e.g., a drug of abuse, a medication) or a general medical condition (e.g., hyperthyroidism).

D. The panic attacks are not better accounted for by another mental disorder, such as social phobia (e.g., occurring on exposure to feared social situations), specific phobia (e.g., on exposure to a specific phobic situation), obsessive-compulsive disorder (e.g., on exposure to dirt in someone with an obsession about contamination), posttraumatic stress disorder (e.g., in response to stimuli associated with a severe stressor), or separation anxiety disorder (e.g., in response to being away from home or close relatives).

Source. Reprinted from American Psychiatric Association: *Diagnostic and Statistical Manual of Mental Disorders,* 4th Edition, Text Revision. Washington, DC, American Psychiatric Association, 2000, p. 440. Used with permission. Copyright © 2000 American Psychiatric Association.

TABLE 20–6. Panic disorder with agoraphobia: diagnostic criteria and additional features

DSM-IV-TR diagnostic criteria for panic disorder with agoraphobia

A. Both (1) and (2):

(1) recurrent unexpected panic attacks

(2) at least one of the attacks has been followed by 1 month (or more) of one (or more) of the following:

(a) persistent concern about having additional attacks

(b) worry about the implications of the attack or its consequences (e.g., losing control, having a heart attack, "going crazy")

(c) a significant change in behavior related to the attacks

B. The presence of agoraphobia.

C. The panic attacks are not due to the direct physiological effects of a substance (e.g., a drug of abuse, a medication) or a general medical condition (e.g., hyperthyroidism).

D. The panic attacks are not better accounted for by another mental disorder, such as social phobia (e.g., occurring on exposure to feared social situations), specific phobia (e.g., on exposure to a specific phobic situation), obsessive-compulsive disorder (e.g., on exposure to dirt in someone with an obsession about contamination), posttraumatic stress disorder (e.g., in response to stimuli associated with a severe stressor), or separation anxiety disorder (e.g., in response to being away from home or close relatives).

Additional features[a]

• Although the presence of panic disorder in children and adolescents has been debated over the years, many studies have documented the presence of panic attacks and full panic disorder in adolescents (Ollendick 1998).

• While panic disorder is present in children and adolescents, it is less common in younger children, and the presentation of symptoms is slightly different (Ollendick 1998). For example, panic attacks experienced by younger children are usually cued or triggered by a specific event or stressor, while the experience of out-of-the-blue panic attacks is rare.

[a]Additional features not included in DSM-IV-TR and presented by the authors for purposes of this textbook.
Source. DSM-IV-TR criteria reprinted from American Psychiatric Association: *Diagnostic and Statistical Manual of Mental Disorders,* 4th Edition, Text Revision. Washington, DC, American Psychiatric Association, 2000, p. 441. Used with permission. Copyright © 2000 American Psychiatric Association.

TABLE 20–7. Social phobia: diagnostic criteria and additional features

DSM-IV-TR diagnostic criteria for social phobia

A. A marked and persistent fear of one or more social or performance situations in which the person is exposed to unfamiliar people or to possible scrutiny by others. The individual fears that he or she will act in a way (or show anxiety symptoms) that will be humiliating or embarrassing.   **Note:** In children, there must be evidence of the capacity for age-appropriate social relationships with familiar people and the anxiety must occur in peer settings, not just in interactions with adults.

B. Exposure to the feared social situation almost invariably provokes anxiety, which may take the form of a situationally bound or situationally predisposed panic attack.   **Note:** In children, the anxiety may be expressed by crying, tantrums, freezing, or shrinking from social situations with unfamiliar people.

C. The person recognizes that the fear is excessive or unreasonable.   **Note:** In children, this feature may be absent.

D. The feared social or performance situations are avoided or else are endured with intense anxiety or distress.

E. The avoidance, anxious anticipation, or distress in the feared social or performance situation(s) interferes significantly with the person's normal routine, occupational (academic) functioning, or social activities or relationships, or there is marked distress about having the phobia.

F. In individuals under age 18 years, the duration is at least 6 months.

G. The fear or avoidance is not due to the direct physiological effects of a substance (e.g., a drug of abuse, a medication) or a general medical condition and is not better accounted for by another mental disorder (e.g., panic disorder with or without agoraphobia, separation anxiety disorder, body dysmorphic disorder, a pervasive developmental disorder, or schizoid personality disorder).

H. If a general medical condition or another mental disorder is present, the fear in Criterion A is unrelated to it, e.g., the fear is not of stuttering, trembling in Parkinson's disease, or exhibiting abnormal eating behavior in anorexia nervosa or bulimia nervosa.

Specify if:

  Generalized: if the fears include most social situations (also consider the additional diagnosis of avoidant personality disorder)

Additional features[a]

• Commonly feared social situations include giving public performances (reading aloud in front of the class, music or athletic performances), being in ordinary social situations (starting conversations, joining in on conversations, speaking to adults), ordering food in a restaurant, attending dances or parties, taking tests, working or playing with other children, and asking the teacher for help (Beidel et al. 1999).

• Characteristics include diminished social skills, longer speech latencies (Beidel et al. 1999), few or no friends, limited involvement in extracurricular or peer activities, and school refusal.

[a]Additional features not included in DSM-IV-TR and presented by the authors for purposes of this textbook.
Source.   DSM-IV-TR criteria reprinted from American Psychiatric Association: *Diagnostic and Statistical Manual of Mental Disorders,* 4th Edition, Text Revision. Washington, DC, American Psychiatric Association, 2000, p. 456. Used with permission. Copyright © 2000 American Psychiatric Association.

TABLE 20–8. Selective mutism: diagnostic criteria and additional features

DSM-IV-TR diagnostic criteria for selective mutism

A. Consistent failure to speak in specific social situations (in which there is an expectation for speaking, e.g., at school) despite speaking in other situations.

B. The disturbance interferes with educational or occupational achievement or with social communication.

C. The duration of the disturbance is at least 1 month (not limited to the first month of school).

D. The failure to speak is not due to a lack of knowledge of, or comfort with, the spoken language required in the social situation.

E. The disturbance is not better accounted for by a communication disorder (e.g., stuttering) and does not occur exclusively during the course of a pervasive developmental disorder, schizophrenia, or other psychotic disorder.[a]

Additional features[a]

• Transient mutism may occur during transitional periods or stressors, such as the first month of school or a move to a new home.

• Associated features may include "excessive shyness, fear of social embarrassment, social isolation and withdrawal, clinging, compulsive traits, negativism, temper tantrums, or controlling or oppositional behavior, particularly at home" (American Psychiatric Association 2000, p. 126).

• Research increasingly supports the relationship of selective mutism to social phobia (Vecchio and Kearney 2005; Yeganeh et al. 2003).

[a]Additional features not included in DSM-IV-TR and presented by the authors for purposes of this textbook.
Source. DSM-IV-TR criteria reprinted from American Psychiatric Association: *Diagnostic and Statistical Manual of Mental Disorders*, 4th Edition, Text Revision. Washington, DC, American Psychiatric Association, 2000, p. 127. Used with permission. Copyright © 2000 American Psychiatric Association.

substance abuse. Childhood anxiety disorders increase the risk of developing alcohol abuse in adolescence (Schuckit and Hesselbrock 1994).

The high degree of comorbidity may have implications for level of functional impairment and treatment outcomes. Several studies have demonstrated, for example, a greater severity of internalizing symptoms among highly comorbid children (Manassis and Menna 1999; Nottelmann and Jensen 1995). In studies of children with SM, nearly all children also met criteria for social phobia (Vecchio and Kearney 2005). Developmental disorders/delay, communication disorders, and elimination disorders were also common in some studies of SM (Kristensen 2000).

Etiology, Mechanisms, and Risk Factors

Genetic predisposition can lead to the development of specific anxiety disorders as a result of the interplay with environmental influences (Gar et al. 2005). While genetic factors are associated with a propensity toward fearfulness, environmental factors may determine the presence of specific fears, and therefore specific anxiety disorders (Ollendick et al. 2002). Table 20–10 summarizes common biological and environmental influences on the development of childhood anxiety.

As described in Table 20–10, several characteristics within the family and specific parenting behaviors have been identified as playing a key role in childhood anxiety. However, it is important to consider the interaction between parent and child variables. For example, Whaley et al. (1999) examined parent-child communication among mothers with and without anxiety. Clinically anxious mothers had higher levels of criticism and tendencies to catastrophize compared to nonclinically anxious mothers, and these behaviors, in turn, predicted childhood anxiety. Moore et al. (2004) added a comparison group of children without anxiety and found less warmth and less granting of autonomy among mothers of anxious children. Some of these parenting behaviors may develop in reaction to the characteristics of the child. Behavioral inhibition, attachment, and parenting proved to have additive effects on child anxiety symptoms (van Brakel et al. 2006).

Two parenting dimensions can facilitate or inhibit a sense of control in children: 1) warmth, consistency, and contingency; and 2) encouragement of autonomy (Barlow 2002). A sense of uncontrollability and inabil-

TABLE 20–9. Prevalence, course, and prognosis for specific anxiety disorders

Prevalence	Course and prognosis
Generalized anxiety disorder (GAD)	
Community samples (ages 15–54 years) Prevalence across ages at least 3% Lifetime prevalence 4%–6% Female-male ratio of 2:1 (Costello et al. 2004) *Children and adolescents with overanxious disorder* Prevalence rates 2.9%–4.6% Mean age at onset in children 8.8 years (Costello et al. 2004)	Chronic condition Waxing and waning course One-third of lifetime cases with spontaneous remission (Wittchen et al. 1994)
Specific phobias	
Children and adolescents Prevalence rates 2.6%–9.1% Average 5% across studies (Ollendick et al. 2002) More common among girls and younger children	Childhood phobias relatively stable over time (Ollendick et al. 2002) Symptoms tend to decline with age (Muris et al. 1999)
Panic disorder	
Community samples Panic attacks: 16%–63% of adolescents; panic disorder: 0.6%–5% of adolescents (see Ollendick 1998 for review)	The age at onset for panic disorder is late adolescence and early adulthood (American Psychiatric Association 2000) Less common in younger children
Social phobia	
Community samples Lifetime prevalence rates 8.7%–16% (Lipsitz and Schneier 2000) 12-month prevalence rates were 4% and 3%, respectively, for adolescents ages 14–17; nongeneralized subtype predominates (Wittchen et al. 1999) Rates higher for females in community samples *Clinical samples* Youth and adults have reported equal or higher prevalence rates for social phobia in males (Beidel et al. 1999; Compton et al. 2000; Lipsitz and Schneier 2000) Generalized subtype predominates in clinical samples in adults, adolescents, and children (Beidel et al. 1999; Rao et al. 2007)	*Children and adults* Relatively stable problem, likely to persist over time if left untreated Usually begins between early and midadolescence, but occurs in children as young as age 8 (Beidel et al. 1999) Generalized subtype shows earlier age at onset, greater functional impairment, and association with higher risk for comorbid conditions relative to the nongeneralized subtype (Velting and Albano 2001)
Selective mutism (SM)	
Community samples Prevalence rates 0.3%–0.76% (Bergman et al. 2002) Prevalence rates high for immigrant preschool children (Elizur and Perednik 2003) Prevalence rate of 2% for teacher-rated SM, including with milder symptoms (Kumpulainen et al. 1998) Equally common in boys and girls: male-female ratio 1:1 to 1:1.6 (Bergman et al. 2002; Elizur and Perednik 2003)	Onset between 3–5 years of age Persistent difficulty in speaking situations and a chronic course of mutism Children who do not improve prior to adolescence may have a more persistent form of SM (reviewed in Cohan et al. 2006b)

TABLE 20–10. Common biological and environmental influences on the development of childhood anxiety

Biological influences

Heredity

Strong familial aggregation and high heritability are found among anxiety disorders (Bolton et al. 2006).

Trait anxiety (a more stable personality characteristic guiding responses to anxiety-provoking situations) has demonstrated more evidence for genetic influences when compared to state anxiety (a transitory pattern of anxiety symptoms in response to stressors) (Lau et al. 2006).

Temperament

Behavioral inhibition in children (e.g., tendency toward being shy, timid, quiet, and initially avoidant of novel and uncertain stimuli) is associated with the development of anxiety (Kagan 1988).

Autonomic reactivity

Children with anxiety disorders show greater autonomic reactivity in response to stress (Kagan 1988) and have different patterns of cortisol dysregulation (Feder et al. 2004).

Children at risk for anxiety disorders display gastrointestinal distress in response to stressors (Campo et al. 2003) and are more likely to have irregularities in sleeping and eating patterns (Ong et al. 2006).

Anxiety sensitivity

Anxiety sensitivity, a tendency to ascribe negative consequences to physiological responses typically associated with anxiety (e.g., shortness of breath, increased heart rate, trembling), is common among children at risk for anxiety disorders (Reiss 1991).

Longitudinal studies show specific link between anxiety sensitivity and the development of panic disorder (e.g., Weems et al. 2002).

Environmental influences

Attachment styles

Parents of anxious children are likely to display insecure attachment styles (Shamir-Essakow et al. 2005).

Early insecure attachment styles have been associated with subsequent development of anxiety disorders (Warren et al. 1997).

Parenting behaviors

Control: High levels of parental control (overprotective/overcontrolling parenting) are thought to encourage children's dependence on parents, lower their sense of mastery and control in difficult situations, and thus contribute to higher levels of anxiety (Chorpita and Barlow 1998).

Acceptance: Low levels of parental warmth and sensitivity and higher levels of parental rejection and criticism are thought to influence children's ability to regulate their own emotions and tolerate negative affect, including their experiences of anxiety (Lieb et al. 2000).

Anxious parenting: By modeling anxious responses to potentially threatening situations, parents may reinforce the child's own anxious coping responses, reducing the likelihood of learning effective strategies to reduce anxiety.

Peer/social problems

Children with anxiety disorders report

* Early peer victimization experiences (bullying) (Gladstone et al. 2006).
* Rejection and neglect by peers (Strauss et al. 1988).
* Social skills deficits and a greater tendency toward negative self-evaluations in social situations (Spence et al. 2000).

Negative/stressful life events

Anxiety disorders are common in children who have experienced

* Negative life events (losing a family member, experiencing parental separation, moving to another school, or experiencing a natural disaster) (Boer et al. 2002).
* Exposure to community violence (Berman et al. 1996).

ity to cope lies at the core of the experience of anxious individuals when faced with challenging situations and unpredictable events, leading to more negative emotional responses (Suárez et al. 2008). A diminished sense of personal control (external locus of control) mediates the relationship between environmental family characteristics and the development of anxiety (Chorpita et al. 1998).

In a recent review of the literature, Gunnar and Fisher (2006) summarize social influences in the regulation of cortisol levels early in human development. High cortisol responsivity, associated with higher levels of anxiety, diminishes with responsive caregiving. Children learn that they can count on their parents for support when in distress and therefore respond more confidently in the face of threat. This is particularly true among children who are anxious and fearful or easily angered and frustrated. This review links early parenting behaviors (overcontrolling and lack of warmth) with child coping responses and the expression of neurobiological processes associated with anxiety.

Evidence for the interaction between biological and environmental influences can also be found when examining child characteristics and school experiences. In a recent study, anxious solitude (tendency for children to be shy and socially anxious and to prefer to play alone) assessed at preschool predicted peer rejection and victimization in first grade, while classroom climate (teacher and peer interactions that contribute to positive and negative experiences) was associated with subsequent emotional adjustment (Gazelle 2006). Taken together, these findings point to the importance of understanding the complex nature of childhood anxiety and the interplay between various known biological and environmental risk factors.

Barlow (2002) has described an interacting set of three vulnerabilities or diatheses leading to the development of anxiety disorders and related conditions. These include 1) a generalized (heritable) biological vulnerability contributing to the development of anxiety and negative affect; 2) a generalized psychological vulnerability related to early developmental experiences that lead to a diminished sense of control (e.g., low levels of parental warmth, consistency, and contingency and lack of encouragement of autonomy); and 3) specific psychological vulnerabilities relating to early learning experiences that seem to focus anxiety on specific life circumstances that can lead to the development of specific anxiety disorders. For example, a child with a biological predisposition for anxiety (as indicated by a history of anxiety disorders in the family) who is also reared by overcontrolling parents (limiting

the child's sense of controllability in his or her environment) is likely to develop anxiety symptoms. The specific type of anxiety disorder that this child could develop, however, may be determined by various types of learning experiences, such as being in a dangerous or threatening situation (e.g., a dog attack leading to specific phobia of dogs) or experiencing a false alarm within a specific context (e.g., a panic attack during a speech could mark the beginning of social phobia), or vicarious conditioning such as by observing or being told that a situation is dangerous (e.g., observing parents become alarmed by their own physiological responses to fear could lead to the development of panic disorder) (Suárez et al. 2008).

Screening and Assessment

Anxiety disorders in children and adolescents remain underrecognized and undertreated. Recommendations to increase the likelihood of identification and early and appropriate treatment (American Academy of Child and Adolescent Psychiatry 2007) include the following:

- Routine screening for anxiety symptoms should be done during the initial mental health assessment.
- If the screening indicates significant anxiety, then further evaluation should follow to determine which anxiety disorders are present, along with the severity of the anxiety symptoms and functional impairment.
- The psychiatric assessment should include differential diagnosis of other physical conditions and psychiatric disorders that may mimic anxiety symptoms.
- Comorbid conditions should be assessed.

Screening and Clinical Interview

Obtaining information about anxiety symptoms from multiple informants, including the child, parents, teacher, and other care providers is important because of variable agreement between informants (Choudhury et al. 2003). Young children may lack the understanding and vocabulary needed to communicate anxiety symptoms or related distress directly, and parental report is essential. Alternatively, the child's anxiety may cause significant internal distress but be behaviorally less evident to others (e.g., GAD). Teachers may be more readily aware of anxiety symptoms that affect academic or social functioning (e.g., social phobia). An anxious child's desire to please adults and concerns about performance during the assessment can also affect the child's report.

The clinician needs to be sensitive to the severity of the child's anxiety and monitor the child's physical and emotional cues from the beginning of the evaluation process. In their efforts to please the clinician and their parents, some children with anxiety may attempt to do what is asked of them despite experiencing internal distress or feeling overwhelmed and then acutely shut down. Just discussing anxiety symptoms during the evaluation may be too much for some children, and they may want parents to give details initially.

There are several child self-report measures for anxiety that may assist the clinician with screening of youth 8 years and older and monitoring response to treatment (please refer to Chapter 8, "Rating Scales"). The Multidimensional Anxiety Scale for Children (MASC) and the Screen for Child Anxiety Related Emotional Disorders (SCARED) were developed to be sensitive and specific to assessing clinical levels of anxiety in youth, are sensitive to change, and are of utility in clinical practice (Langley et al. 2002; Velting et al. 2004). Self-report measures for assessment and follow-up of specific anxiety disorders, such as social phobia in youth, are discussed in Chapter 8 and Chapter 58, "Cognitive-Behavioral Treatment for Anxiety Disorders." The Selective Mutism Questionnaire has parent- and teacher-report forms that can assist with baseline assessment and clinical monitoring of SM (Bergman et al. 2008).

Differentiating and diagnosing the specific anxiety disorders can be challenging. Structured interviews lead to more reliable anxiety diagnoses than unstructured interviews (Silverman and Ollendick 2005; Velting et al. 2004). The Anxiety Disorders Interview Schedule for DSM-IV: Child Version (ADIS-IV-C; Silverman and Albano 1996), Child and Parent Interview Schedules, is well studied and the most commonly used semistructured interview for anxiety disorders in youth ages 6–17 years. It is also sensitive to treatment effects and outcome (Silverman and Ollendick 2005). The ADIS-IV-C may be used in its entirety, or sections corresponding to various disorders may be used to supplement the clinical interview, confirm an anxiety diagnosis, or assist in discriminating between childhood anxiety disorders. It uses language and situations that are developmentally appropriate for children and adolescents and evaluates the presence and severity of anxiety disorders along with comorbid de-

pressive disorders and externalizing disorders. Children with anxiety symptoms who do not meet full criteria for anxiety disorders may still have significant functional impairment and distress and be at risk for development of anxiety disorders in the future (Dadds et al. 1997). The ADIS-IV-C has a Feelings Thermometer (ratings from 0 to 8) that allows the child and parents to quantify the severity of anxiety symptoms and interference with the child's functioning. The ratings can be used to make a diagnosis, structure self-monitoring and parent monitoring of anxiety, and assess treatment progress over time.

Family assessment can determine possible environmental reinforcements, parenting styles (controlling, critical, overprotective), family responses to child's anxiety symptoms, expectations, and coping approaches modeled by parents. Additionally, whether a parent has an anxiety disorder should be considered during treatment planning.

Physical Examination, Mental Status Findings, and Laboratory Tests

It is common for children with anxiety disorders to present with physical symptoms such as muscle tension, headaches, abdominal complaints, restlessness, and difficulty sleeping, which they may not relate to anxiety symptoms. It is important to inquire about and document somatic symptoms during the evaluation to help the child and parents understand these symptoms and the relationship to the anxiety disorder. Documenting physical symptoms before initiation of treatment with medications can decrease the likelihood of mistaking baseline somatic complaints for medication side effects (American Academy of Child and Adolescent Psychiatry 2007).

There are no standard laboratory tests for children or adolescents with anxiety disorders, and the clinician needs to consider family history of medical illness and physical symptoms in each child that may warrant further work-up. However, a thyroid panel (thyroid-stimulating hormone, T_3, T_4), especially if there is a family history of thyroid disease or comorbid depressive symptoms, should be considered.

Developmental Considerations

The evaluation should include differentiating anxiety disorders from developmentally appropriate worries

TABLE 20–11. Differential diagnosis of psychiatric and physical conditions that may manifest with symptoms similar to those of anxiety disorders

Psychiatric disorders and symptoms	
Attention-deficit/hyperactivity disorder	Motor restlessness, fidgeting, inattention
Depression	Poor concentration, insomnia, somatic complaints
Pervasive developmental disorders (especially Asperger's disorder)	Social awkwardness, withdrawal, social skills deficits, communication deficits, repetitive behaviors, adherence to routines
Learning disorders	Persistent worries focused on school performance; school refusal
Bipolar disorder	Restlessness, irritability, insomnia
Psychotic disorders	Restlessness, agitation, social withdrawal
Physical conditions	
More common	Hyperthyroidism, caffeinism (including carbonated beverages, energy drinks), migraine, asthma, seizure disorder, lead intoxication
Less common	Hypoglycemic episodes, pheochromocytoma, central nervous system disorders (e.g., delirium, brain tumors), cardiac arrythmias
Medication side effects	
Prescription medications	Antiasthmatics, sympathomimetics, steroids, selective serotonin reuptake inhibitors, antipsychotics (akathisia), haloperidol, pimozide (neuroleptic-induced separation anxiety disorder), and atypical antipsychotics
Nonprescription medications	Diet pills, antihistamines, cold medicines

Source. American Academy of Child and Adolescent Psychiatry 2007.

or fears and normal responses to stressors. Significant psychosocial stressors or traumas should be carefully considered to determine how they may be contributing to the development or maintenance of anxiety symptoms. Anxiety disorders in children may manifest with behavioral symptoms such as crying, irritability, angry outbursts or tantrums, and argumentativeness. These behaviors may be misunderstood by adults as oppositionality or disobedience, when in fact they could represent the child's expression of overwhelming fear or effort to avoid the anxiety-provoking object or situation. Children with anxiety disorders may not recognize their fears or worry as unreasonable or excessive, even when it is evident to others that their anxiety and avoidance impair their functioning and judgment.

Differential Diagnosis

Assessment of anxiety disorders in youth should include a differential diagnosis of psychiatric conditions and physical conditions that may mimic anxiety symptoms (Table 20–11).

Treatment

Treatment Planning

Treatment planning for childhood anxiety disorders should consider both severity and impairment (American Academy of Child and Adolescent Psychiatry 2007). For children with anxiety disorders of mild severity and associated with minimal impairment, it is recommended that treatment begin with psychotherapy. However, combination treatment with medication and psychotherapy may be necessary for acute symptom reduction in a severely anxious child, concurrent treatment of a comorbid disorder, or partial response to psychotherapy and potential for improved outcome with combined treatment (March and Ollendick 2004). Residual symptoms of an anxiety disorder can increase the risk for persistence or relapse of the same or another anxiety disorder (Birmaher et al. 2003; Dadds et al. 1997). Functional impairment, not just reduction of anxiety symptoms, needs to be monitored during the treatment process.

To investigate monotherapies versus combined treatment in childhood anxiety disorders, the Child-Adolescent Anxiety Multimodal Study (CAMS) was a randomized controlled trial that was designed to evaluate the relative and combined efficacy of CBT and SSRIs in youth (Walkup et al. 2008). Children and adolescents (N=488) with moderate to severe SAD, GAD, and/or social phobia participated in CBT (14 sessions) or received sertraline (up to 200 mg/day), placebo drug, or a combination of sertraline and CBT for 12 weeks. At posttreatment, 60% of the children with CBT alone, 55% with sertraline alone, 81% with combination treatment, and 24% with placebo were much improved or very much improved on the Clinical Global Impression–Improvement scale. Both CBT and sertraline showed relatively equal efficacy and were significantly superior to placebo for the treatment of childhood anxiety disorders, and a combination of CBT and sertraline yielded a significantly superior response rate than either alone. All three of these active treatments may be recommended with consideration of the availability of the specific treatment and the individual preferences of the family regarding type of treatment, time involved, and cost factors (Walkup et al. 2008).

Psychotherapeutic Treatments

Among the psychotherapies, exposure-based cognitive-behavioral therapy (CBT) has received the most empirical support from randomized controlled studies for the treatment of anxiety disorders in children and adolescents and is currently the psychotherapy of choice for this population (reviewed in Compton et al. 2004; In-Albon and Schneider 2007). CBT has been shown to reduce anxiety symptoms and is superior to waitlist control; however, relative efficacy and effectiveness versus alternative psychotherapeutic interventions have not been investigated.

Cognitive-Behavioral Therapy

CBT is a diverse group of interventions that are administered by trained clinicians in a flexible manner for the patient presenting with one disorder or comorbid disorders (Compton et al. 2004). Behavioral therapies are grounded in conditioning and social learning models and have guided interventions used to treat specific phobias and social phobia (Graczyk et al. 2005). CBT for childhood anxiety disorders consists of several components: psychoeducation, somatic management, cognitive restructuring, problem solving, exposure, and relapse prevention (Velting et al. 2004).

(For further details of CBT for anxiety disorders, see Chapter 58, "Cognitive-Behavioral Treatment for Anxiety Disorders.")

Educational support showed efficacy comparable to CBT in youth with anxiety disorders in two studies when it included psychoeducation about anxiety disorders (Last et al. 1998; Silverman et al. 1999). In these studies, psychoeducation and supportive therapy alone may have led to self-directed exposure that in turn reduced anxiety. The child and family may also be encouraged to read about anxiety disorders and treatment with CBT and medications (Connolly et al. 2006; Rapee et al. 2000). Further research comparing CBT to alternative psychosocial interventions is needed for children with anxiety disorders.

The current evidence base supports the short-term efficacy and long-term effectiveness (Barrett et al. 2001; Kendall et al. 2004b) of child-focused, individual, and group CBT for youth with anxiety disorders. However, these studies indicate that 20%–50% of children may continue to meet criteria for an anxiety disorder after treatment with child-focused CBT. Additional psychosocial interventions and multimodal treatments need to be flexibly considered as well in the treatment of youth with anxiety disorders. The Child-Adolescent Anxiety Multimodal Study demonstrated that combining treatment with sertraline and CBT significantly increased the global improvement rating for moderate to severe anxiety disorders in children and adolescents than either treatment alone (Walkup et al. 2008).

Applications of CBT for Specific Anxiety Disorders

Generalized anxiety disorder.

Children with GAD may benefit from some modifications to standard CBT to target core symptoms of uncontrollable worry and physical signs of anxiety (Grover et al. 2006). Relaxation skills such as diaphragmatic breathing and progressive muscle techniques can be introduced early and practiced often to target physical symptoms. Cognitive restructuring is a vital component for GAD to identify and challenge persistent worries in a range of situations. Problem solving is a useful technique to generate possible solutions and then develop a realistic action plan ahead of time to respond to various challenging situations.

Specific phobias.

Systematic desensitization procedures have accumulated much research support and usually involve three components: 1) induction of muscle relaxation, 2) development of a fear-producing stimulus hierarchy, and 3) systematic, graduated pairing of items in the hierarchy with relaxation. Developmentally appropriate adaptations of systematic desensitization procedures for children with specific phobias may include use of real-life desensitization programs (in vivo), emotive imagery (narrative stories), live modeling (demonstration of nonphobic response), participant modeling (the child has physical contact with the model-therapist and the phobic object), and contingency management (shaping, positive reinforcement, extinction) (King et al. 2005). Different types of specific phobias may warrant specific treatment modifications. For example, patients with blood/injection/injury phobias should use applied tension strategies to prevent fainting, and patients with environmental/situational phobias with faulty expectancies and misinterpretations will benefit from cognitive interventions (Muris et al. 1999).

Panic disorder.

CBT strategies employed with panic disorder patients include psychoeducation about physiological processes that lead to physical sensations, progressive muscle relaxation, breathing retraining, cue-controlled relaxation, cognitive coping, and gradual exposure to agoraphobic situations (Barlow and Craske 2007). Additionally, interoceptive exposure (gradual exposure to somatic sensations such as dizziness, shortness of breath, and sweating by using exercise that induces these sensations) has been used effectively to manage worry about future panic attacks (Barlow and Craske 2007). Developmental adaptations from adult models of panic control treatment have been developed specifically for adolescents (Hoffman and Mattis 2000). Modifications include 1) the use of clear, simple language with verbal and visual examples; 2) parental participation; 3) and reframing exposures as "hypothesis testing" activities.

Social phobia.

Programs for social phobia have included exposure-based CBT with an emphasis on social skills training. Cognitive Behavioral Group Treatment for Adolescents for social phobia in adolescents that involved skills training and exposure-based CBT with a parent component showed significant improvement in self-report measures of anxiety and depression throughout treatment and at 1-year follow-up in a preliminary study (Albano et al. 1995). Social Effectiveness Therapy for Children (SET-C) includes a peer generalization component in which children join a group of nonanxious peers in a group activity. Children treated with SET-C

showed maintenance of a majority of posttreatment gains at 3-year follow-up, with 72% of treated children free of a social phobia diagnosis (Beidel et al. 2005).

Selective mutism.

The majority of recent treatment reviews of SM have concluded that there is good evidence to support behavioral interventions for SM (Cohan et al. 2006a). Most behavioral interventions evaluated have not targeted communication deficits, developmental delays, or second-language acquisition, and addressing these comorbidities may be promising (Cohan et al. 2006b).

A multimodal psychosocial treatment approach has been proposed for SM with comorbid social phobia and mutism at school (Cohan et al. 2006a). Psychotherapy focused on verbal and nonverbal communication skills and anxiety management is combined with a behavioral program in the school to shape appropriate communication. Social interactions and communication in all settings are rewarded along a hierarchy of feared speaking situations. Adults, siblings, and classmates are encouraged not to speak for the child. Efforts at nonverbal communication (pointing and participating in activities) are reinforced, and over time verbal behaviors (mouthing words, whispering, speaking in soft voice) are rewarded as the child learns to manage anxiety through standard CBT strategies. Stimulus fading (gradual removal of people or objects that increase the child's comfort level) can be used initially to develop comfort with the therapist and later to develop comfort with individuals and areas in the school setting in order to generalize speech. This may involve inviting peers to settings where the child is comfortable (home) and then moving playdates to the child's classroom over time. In the classroom, teachers or classmates can be faded in and out systematically from the periphery of the classroom while a comfortable person such as a parent is present, and when comfort develops, the parent can be faded out.

Parent-Child and Family Interventions

Parents and families have an important role in the development and maintenance of childhood anxiety disorders. Child-focused interventions may not address risk factors such as parental anxiety, insecure attachment, and parenting styles. Interventions that improve parent-child relationships, strengthen family problem-solving and communication skills, reduce parental anxiety, and foster parenting skills that reinforce healthy coping and autonomy in the child are often integrated into treatment with anxious children in clinical settings (American Academy of Child and Adolescent Psychiatry 2007).

The benefits of adding a parental component to established child-focused CBT for childhood anxiety, in addition to standard psychoeducation and coaching, need further study. Parental involvement has been shown to be most critical when the parent is anxious (Cobham et al. 1998). (See Chapter 58, "Cognitive-Behavioral Treatment for Anxiety Disorders," for further details.)

Parental overinvolvement, criticism, and control are some of the variables felt to contribute to development and maintenance of childhood anxiety (Ginsburg and Schlossberg 2002). Integrative models for family treatment of anxious children have been proposed and are being tested that consider the interaction between attachment, parent-child learning processes, and behavioral and temperamental characteristics of both the child and parent (Dadds and Roth 2001).

Other Psychotherapeutic Treatments

Psychoanalysis and psychodynamic psychotherapy have been used in the clinical treatment of anxiety disorders in children and adolescents, but empirical evidence regarding efficacy or effectiveness is very limited (In-Albon and Schneider 2007; King et al. 2005). A 2-year follow-up study of a time-limited (11-week) psychodynamic psychotherapy intervention for children with depressive or anxiety disorders (mainly dysthymia, SAD, or phobias) used community services as usual as the comparison group (Muratori et al. 2003). Significant improvement relative to that of the comparison group was demonstrated on the Children's Global Assessment Scale at 6-month follow-up and Child Behavior Checklist at 2-year follow-up.

Other Treatment Modalities

Clinical treatment of anxiety disorders in children often requires coordination of psychoeducation, CBT interventions, and a positive reinforcement schedule between the home and school setting. Adolescents with anxiety disorders had elevated rates of academic underachievement as young adults (Woodward and Fergusson 2001). Also, first graders who reported high levels of anxiety were at significant risk for persistent anxiety and low achievement scores in reading and math in fifth grade (Ialongo et al. 1995). The clinician can consider classroom-based accommodations when anxiety disorders interfere with school functioning. It is helpful to identify an adult other than the teacher in the school setting to assist the child with problem-solving or anxiety management strategies when needed. If performance or test anxiety is present, then testing in a quiet, private environment and increased testing time

may reduce excess anxiety. For speeches or performances, the child may practice in a stepwise fashion on a tape recorder or videotape, then in the classroom without others present, and gradually with familiar students and then the teacher. Specific recommendations for the anxiety disorder can be written into the student's 504 Plan or individualized education plan.

Pharmacological Treatments

Selective Serotonin Reuptake Inhibitors

Medications are considered when the severity of anxiety symptoms or related impairment makes participation in psychotherapy difficult or treatment with psychotherapy alone results in a partial response. Anxious children and anxious parents may be very sensitive to any worsening of the children's somatic symptoms or development of even mild or transient side effects of medications. Carefully assessing somatic symptoms at baseline prior to starting medication trials is important. A developing evidence base suggests that the selective serotonin reuptake inhibitors (SSRIs) should be considered the first-line pharmacological treatment for pediatric anxiety disorders (Seidel and Walkup 2006). Several randomized, placebo-controlled trials with SSRIs have established the short-term efficacy of SSRIs for the treatment of childhood anxiety disorders (Table 20–12). SAD, GAD, and social phobia often occur together; are treated with similar pharmacological strategies; and are often studied together in medication trials as they have been in CBT trials (Birmaher et al. 2003; Research Units on Pediatric Psychopharmacology Anxiety Study Group 2001; Walkup et al. 2008). Specific anxiety disorders with controlled trials include SM with social phobia (Black and Uhde 1994), social phobia alone (Wagner et al. 2004), and GAD (Rynn et al. 2001).

The U.S. Food and Drug Administration issued a black box warning for use of any antidepressant medication in the pediatric population, including SSRIs. Clinicians need to carefully monitor for worsening depression, agitation, or suicidality, particularly at the beginning of medication treatment or at dosage changes. This small but significant increased relative risk for suicidality did not seem to be elevated in the pediatric anxiety versus depression trials. This along with the larger effect size of SSRIs for childhood anxiety disorders compared to depression suggests the risk-benefit ratio for anxiety disorders may be more favorable than that for depression (Seidel and Walkup 2006).

TABLE 20–12. Placebo-controlled pharmacological treatment studies[a]

Author	Treatment	Demographics	Diagnoses	Results
Serotonin reuptake inhibitors				
Black and Uhde 1994 [rdb]	Fluoxetine (12–27 mg/day), 12 weeks	N=15, ages 6–11	SM plus SoP or AD	Fluoxetine>Pbo
Research Units on Pediatric Psychopharmacology Anxiety Study Group 2001 [rct]	Fluvoxamine (50–250 mg/day child, max 300 mg/day adolescent), 8 weeks	N=128, ages 6–17	SoP, SAD, GAD	Fluvoxamine>Pbo
Rynn et al. 2001 [rdb]	Sertraline (50 mg/day), 9 weeks	N=22, ages 5–17	GAD	Sertraline>Pbo
Birmaher et al. 2003 [rdb]	Fluoxetine (20 mg/day), 12 weeks	N=74, ages 7–17	GAD, SoP, SAD	Fluoxetine>Pbo; Fluoxetine=Pbo
Wagner et al. 2004 [rdb]	Paroxetine (10–50 mg/day), 16 weeks	N=322, ages 8–17	SoP	Paroxetine>Pbo
Walkup et al. 2008 [rdb]	Sertraline (25–200 mg/day), 12 weeks	N=209, ages 7–17	SoP, SAD, GAD	Sertraline>Pbo
Other antidepressants				
Gittelman-Klein and Klein 1971 [rdb]	Imipramine (100–200 mg/day)	N=35, ages 6–14	School phobia with anxiety disorders	Imipramine>Pbo
Berney et al. 1981 [rdb]	Clomipramine (40–75 mg/day)	N=51, ages 9–14	School refusal	Clomipramine=Pbo
Klein et al. 1992 [rdb]	Imipramine (75–275 mg/day)	N=21, ages 6–15	SAD with or without school phobia	Imipramine=Pbo
Rynn et al. 2007 [rdb]	Venlafaxine ER (37.5–225 mg/day), 8 weeks	N=320, ages 6–17 (two studies combined)	GAD	Venlafaxine ER>Pbo (study 1); Venlafaxine ER=Pbo (study 2)
Benzodiazepines				
Bernstein et al. 1990 [rdb]	Alprazolam (0.75–4.0 mg/day) vs. imipramine (50–175 mg/day)	N=24, ages 7–18	School refusal, SAD	Alprazolam=imipramine=Pbo
Simeon et al. 1992 [rdb]	Alprazolam (0.5–3.5 mg/day)	N=30, ages 8–17	OAD, AD	Alprazolam=Pbo
Graae et al. 1994 [rdb]	Clonazepam (0.5–2.0 mg/day)	N=15, ages 7–13	SAD	Clonazepam=Pbo

Note.   AD=avoidant disorder; ER=extended release; GAD=generalized anxiety disorder; OAD=overanxious disorder; OCD=obsessive-compulsive disorder; Pbo=placebo; rct=randomized controlled trial; rdb=randomized double-blind trial; SAD=separation anxiety disorder; SM=selective mutism; SoP=social phobia.
[a]Data reported in this table reflect medication arm of multimodal study only.

SSRIs have generally been well tolerated for children with anxiety disorders. Common side effects reported in clinical trials include gastrointestinal symptoms, headache, increased motor activity, and insomnia. Often these side effects are mild and transient, and medication treatment can continue. Less common side effects such as disinhibition and more severe forms of behavioral activation, such as agitation or reactive aggression, need to be monitored as well. Motor and behavioral activation often improves by reducing the dose of the SSRI. Acute changes in level of active defiance, "mouthiness," or heightened emotional reactivity that can be part of disinhibition need to be distinguished from improvements in spontaneity and assertiveness that are positive effects of SSRIs in anxious children.

The clinician should routinely screen for symptoms of bipolar disorder or family history of bipolar disorder prior to initiating an SSRI or other antidepressant. In addition, it is important to obtain a family history, including previous medication trials, and evaluation of psychosocial factors that may predispose a patient to risk for aggression or suicide (Seidel and Walkup 2006).

The presence of social phobia (Research Units on Pediatric Psychopharmacology Anxiety Group 2001), a family history of anxiety disorders (Birmaher et al. 2003), and greater severity of illness in both studies predicted a less favorable outcome for the SSRI medication group versus placebo. Also, improvement on medication did not result in full resolution in symptoms in 50% of the fluoxetine treatment group (Birmaher et al. 2003), and it was suggested that higher doses of medication or a combination of treatments may have been beneficial. Both of these studies indicated that clinicians should consider increasing the SSRI dose by the fourth week of treatment if significant improvement in anxiety symptoms or impairment is not achieved by then.

A paroxetine study in social phobia showed some significant adverse effects in the treatment group, such as vomiting, decreased appetite, and insomnia (Wagner et al. 2004). Also the relative suicide risk in this trial was elevated, though not statistically significant.

Children with SM and comorbid social phobia showed greater improvement on fluoxetine than placebo on parent rating of mutism and global change, but not on clinician and teacher ratings (Black and Uhde 1994). Also, the medication and placebo groups remained very symptomatic at the end of the trial. A controlled case series with sertraline (Carlson et al. 1999) showed positive response in children with SM.

There are currently no controlled studies in youth for medication treatment of panic disorder. Clinically, SSRIs are considered first-line treatment in youth with panic disorder and may be combined with benzodiazepines (clonazepam or lorazepam) when severe panic disorder is present (Reinblatt and Riddle 2007; Renaud et al. 1999).

Controlled medication trials have established the safety and efficacy of short-term treatment with SSRIs for youth with anxiety disorders, but studies of long-term risks and benefits are limited. Pine (2002) recommended that clinicians consider a medication-free trial for children who achieve marked improvement in anxiety or depressive symptoms and impairment. The medication-free trial can occur during the first low-stress period (such as vacations) after 1 year of SSRI treatment. Children who exhibit signs of relapse during the trial off medication should be restarted promptly on the SSRI.

There is no evidence that a particular SSRI is more effective than another SSRI for the treatment of childhood anxiety disorders. The clinician can consider side-effect profile, duration of action and patient compliance, and positive response to one of the SSRIs in a first-degree relative with anxiety. Currently there are no specific dosing guidelines for use of SSRIs in youth with anxiety disorder. However, some differences in effects and side effects by age group are emerging. Activation and vomiting were more prevalent in children than adolescents on SSRIs (Safer and Zito 2006), and children (especially females) showed a higher exposure to fluvoxamine (higher peak plasma concentration) than adolescents at similar doses (Labellarte et al. 2004). Clinicians can start at low doses, monitor side effects closely, and then increase the dose slowly on the basis of treatment response and tolerability. Side effects were low overall, but the adverse effect of behavioral disinhibition was noted in some studies with SM (Carlson et al. 1999; Sharkey and McNicholas 2006). Especially for young children with SM, using the liquid form of SSRI medications and starting at very low doses may reduce the likelihood of side effects.

Other Medications

The safety and efficacy of medications other than SSRIs for the treatment of childhood anxiety disorders have not been well established. Venlafaxine, tricyclic antidepressants (TCAs), buspirone, and benzodiazepines have been suggested as clinical alternatives to be used alone or in combination with the SSRIs; however, research is limited or not conclusive. Data to guide treatment for use of combinations of medications when a single medication is not effective or there is a partial response are even more limited, and no controlled studies exist. Based on the literature in OCD, it is important to make sure that the diagnosis is accurate, the medication trial was of adequate length, and dosing was maximized (Reinblatt and Riddle 2007; Seidel and Walkup 2006). For more complex patients, combination or intensive treatment with CBT and other psychotherapies along with medication may lead to better results. Switching SSRIs to treat resistant anxiety has been shown to be a useful treatment strategy (Research Units on Pediatric Psychopharmacology Anxiety Group 2002), and adding a second medication may be useful when there is a partial response. Comorbid diagnoses are strongly considered in selection of medication (American Academy of Child and Adolescent Psychiatry 2007; Compton et al. 2004; Reinblatt and Riddle 2007).

The response rate for extended-release venlafaxine was significantly greater than for placebo (69% vs. 48%) in youth with GAD when results from two medication trials were combined (Rynn et al. 2007). However only one of the trials showed significant improvements relative to placebo in primary outcome measures, and it is unclear why the two trials differed in their outcomes (Table 20-12). Based on significant changes in blood pressure, pulse, and cholesterol levels during treatment, venlafaxine is considered for treatment of GAD in youth only if several trials of SSRIs have failed and vital signs are monitored carefully. Preliminary findings from a placebo-controlled study of extended-release venlafaxine also suggests efficacy for treatment of youth with social phobia (Tourian et al. 2004). Relative risk for suicidality with venlafaxine may be higher than with other SSRIs.

TCAs are used less often due to the need for close cardiac monitoring and greater medical risks with overdose. Controlled trials of TCAs for youth with anxiety disorders have demonstrated conflicting results, and efficacy for their use in this population has not been established (see Table 20–12). Clomipramine is a TCA with serotonergic properties that can be used alone or combined with an SSRI to boost the effect of the SSRI when there is a partial response. It has shown efficacy in a number of controlled trials for childhood OCD but has not been examined for treatment of non-OCD anxiety disorders (Reinblatt and Riddle 2007). Side effects such as tremor, constipation, dry mouth, fatigue, and dizziness make it difficult for patients to tolerate higher doses of clomipramine. Clomipramine may be considered at a low dose with close monitoring

of anticholinergic and cardiac side effects, electrocardiogram, and blood level.

Buspirone may be used as an alternative to SSRIs for GAD in children and adolescents or as an adjunct medication when there is a partial result, but there are no published controlled trials in youth with anxiety disorders. An industry-sponsored clinical trial showed buspirone may be tolerated at doses of 5–30 mg twice daily in anxious adolescents and at lower doses of 5–7.5 mg twice daily in anxious children (Salazar et al. 2001). The most common side effects were light-headedness, headache, and dyspepsia.

Benzodiazepines have not shown efficacy in controlled trials in childhood anxiety disorders (see Table 20–12), despite established efficacy in adult trials. Clinically they can be used as an adjunctive short-term treatment to achieve acute reduction in severe anxiety symptoms while an SSRI dose is maximized. They may reduce anxiety symptoms enough to permit initiation of the exposure phase of CBT for school refusal behavior, panic disorder, or specific phobias (Renaud et al. 1999). Benzodiazepines should be used cautiously in youth because of the possibility of developing physical and psychological dependency (American Academy of Child and Adolescent Psychiatry 2007; Reinblatt and Riddle 2007). They are contraindicated in youth with a history of substance abuse. Possible side effects include sedation, disinhibition (aggressivity and irritability), behavioral dyscontrol in adolescents, and cognitive impairments. Withdrawal symptoms may be severe, especially if the medication is stopped abruptly, and include insomnia, anxiety, gastrointestinal upset, and seizures. Gradual tapering off the benzodiazepine is needed to reduce the severity of withdrawal symptoms.

Early Intervention and Prevention

Early intervention can alleviate some of the difficulties experienced by youth with anxiety. Severity and impairment increase with age, with older anxious children experiencing the greatest anxiety (Hirshfeld-Becker and Biederman 2002). Effective prevention efforts should target known risk factors that can be treated with evidence-based interventions (Spence 2001). Efforts for early intervention and prevention of anxiety disorders in children should include screening and early assessments, interventions in community settings, psychoeducational programming, and parent skills training (American Academy of Child and Adolescent Psychiatry 2007).

Although anxiety disorders are common in children, only a small proportion of those affected receive care. Prevention efforts targeting youth at risk, and even universal interventions directed at schools, should be considered in order to maximize benefits to overall youth functioning (Farrell and Barrett 2007). The FRIENDS program (Barrett 2004) is a CBT approach for children that has been proven effective in clinical samples, among youth identified at risk and in settings where the program was delivered to entire classrooms of youth not yet identified with anxiety disorders. The FRIENDS program teaches youth skills to manage stress, anxiety, and depression and has been found to reduce symptoms of anxiety (Farrell and Barrett 2007).

Research Directions

Research suggests that anxiety disorders in childhood are predictive of greater impairment and comorbidity later in life (Bittner et al. 2007). However, more studies are needed to determine the developmental continuity among the anxiety disorders and between specific anxiety disorders and other diagnoses. Efforts should be devoted to raising awareness about the needs of anxious youth among parents, teachers, pediatricians, and other adults in contact with youth in order to increase early identification.

There is overwhelming evidence suggesting that CBT treatments are efficacious for some children with anxiety. However, many of these studies have taken place in academic research settings with populations that are not representative of those seen in community settings (Weisz et al. 2005). More research on the transportability of CBT in community settings and with diverse populations (Ginsburg and Drake 2002) is needed. Additionally, although CBT has been deemed superior to waitlist control conditions, more research is needed to determine the relative efficacy and effectiveness of CBT versus alternative psychotherapeutic interventions (In-Albon and Schneider 2007). In order to increase applications to real-world practice, controlled studies of CBT for anxiety disorders in youth should include patients on medication (who may have more severe illness) and patients with common comorbid diagnoses (Baer and Garland 2005) and should consider impairment in addition to symptom reduction as a measure of treatment response. Combining treatments and considering optimal multimodal treatment approaches for children who have a partial response or those who are nonresponders to one type of intervention also need further investigation. The Child-Adolescent Anxiety Multimodal Study addressed several of these gaps in the research by including youth with moderate to severe anxiety disorders and comparing treatment with CBT or medication alone to combined treatment (Walkup et al. 2008).

Summary Points

- Anxiety disorders are common, and routine screening during assessment is recommended.
- ADHD and depression are common comorbid disorders.
- To understand the etiology of anxiety disorders, it is important to consider the interplay between key biological (e.g., heredity, behavioral inhibition) and environmental (e.g., parenting styles, negative life experiences, peer/social problems) risk factors.
- A comprehensive assessment and treatment planning should consider severity of the anxiety disorder, functional impairment, comorbid conditions, and information from several sources.
- The presence of parental anxiety disorders needs to be considered in the treatment process.
- Exposure-based CBT and medication with SSRIs are evidence-based treatment interventions for childhood anxiety disorders.
- Prevention and early intervention efforts have been successful in clinical and school settings.

References

Albano AM, Hayward C: Social anxiety disorder, in Phobic and Anxiety Disorders in Children and Adolescents. Edited by Ollendick TH, March JS. New York, Oxford University Press, 2004, pp 198–235

Albano AM, Marten PA, Holt CS, et al: Cognitive-behavioral group treatment for social phobia in adolescents. J Nerv Ment Dis 183:649–656, 1995

Albano AM, Chorpita BF, Barlow DH: Childhood anxiety disorders, in Child Psychopathology, 2nd Edition. Edited by Mash EJ, Barkley RA. New York, Guilford, 2003, pp 279–329

American Academy of Child and Adolescent Psychiatry: Practice parameter for the assessment and treatment of children and adolescents with anxiety disorders. J Am Acad Child Adolesc Psychiatry 46:267–283, 2007

American Psychiatric Association: Diagnostic and Statistical Manual of Mental Disorders, 3rd Edition, Revised. Washington, DC, American Psychiatric Association, 1987

American Psychiatric Association: Diagnostic and Statistical Manual of Mental Disorders, 4th Edition. Washington, DC, American Psychiatric Association, 1994

American Psychiatric Association: Diagnostic and Statistical Manual of Mental Disorders, 4th Edition, Text Revision. Washington, DC, American Psychiatric Association, 2000

Angold A, Costello EJ: Depressive comorbidity in children and adolescents: empirical, theoretical, and methodological issues. Am J Psychiatry 150:1779–1791, 1993

Antony MM, Brown TA, Barlow DH: Heterogeneity among specific phobia types in DSM-IV. Behav Res Ther 35:1089–1100, 1997

Baer S, Garland JE: Pilot study of community-based cognitive behavioral group therapy for adolescents with social phobia. J Am Acad Child Adolesc Psychiatry 44:258–264, 2005

Barlow DH: The origins of anxious apprehension, anxiety disorders, and related emotional disorders: triple vulnerabilities, in Anxiety and Its Disorders: The Nature and Treatment of Anxiety and Panic, 2nd Edition. Edited by Barlow DH. New York, Guilford, 2002, pp 252–291

Barlow DH, Craske MG: Mastery of Your Anxiety and Panic: Therapist Guide. New York, Oxford University Press, 2007

Barrett PM: Friends for Life! For Children. Participant Workbook and Leader's Manual. Brisbane, Australia, Australian Academic Press, 2004

Barrett PM, Duffy AL, Dadds MR, et al: Cognitive-behavioral treatment of anxiety disorders in children: long-term (6-year) follow-up. J Consult Clin Psychol 69:135–141, 2001

Beidel DC, Turner SM, Morris TL: Psychopathology of childhood social phobia. J Am Acad Child Adolesc Psychiatry 38:643–650, 1999

Beidel DC, Turner SM, Young B, et al: Social Effectiveness Therapy for Children: three-year follow-up. J Consult Clin Psychol 73:721–725, 2005

Bergman RL, Piacentini J, McCracken JT: Prevalence and description of selective mutism in a school-based sample. J Am Acad Child Adolesc Psychiatry 41:938–946, 2002

Bergman RL, Keller ML, Piacentini J, et al: The development and psychometric properties of the Selective Mutism Questionnaire. J Clin Child Adolesc Psychology 37:456–464, 2008

Berman SL, Kurtines WM, Silverman WK, et al: The impact of exposure to crime and violence on urban youth. Am J Orthopsychiatry 66:329–336, 1996

Berney T, Kolvin I, Bhate SR, et al: School phobia: a therapeutic trial with clomipramine and short-term outcome. Br J Psychiatry 138:110–118, 1981

Bernstein GA: Comorbidity and severity of anxiety and depressive disorders in a clinical sample. J Am Acad Child Adolesc Psychiatry 30:43–50, 1991

Bernstein GA, Garfinkel BD, Borchardt CM: Comparative studies of pharmacotherapy for school refusal. J Am Acad Child Adolesc Psychiatry 29:773–781, 1990

Birmaher B, Axelson DA, Monk K, et al: Fluoxetine for the treatment of childhood anxiety disorders. J Am Acad Child Adolesc Psychiatry 42:415–423, 2003

Bittner A, Egger HL, Erkanli A, et al: What do childhood anxiety disorders predict? J Child Psychol Psychiatry 48:1174–1183, 2007

Black B, Uhde TW: Treatment of elective mutism with fluoxetine: a double-blind, placebo-controlled study. J Am Acad Child Adolesc Psychiatry 33:1000–1006, 1994

Boer R, Markus M, Maingay R, et al: Negative life events of anxiety disordered children: bad fortune, vulnerability, or reporter bias. Child Psychiatry Hum Dev 32:187–199, 2002

Bolton D, Eley TC, O'Connor TG, et al: Prevalence and genetic and environmental differences on anxiety disorders in 6-year-old twins. Psychol Med 36:335–344, 2006

Campo JV, Dahl RE, Williamson DE, et al: Gastrointestinal distress to serotonergic challenge: a risk marker for emotional disorder. J Am Acad Child Adolesc Psychiatry 42:1221–1226, 2003

Carlson JS, Kratochwill TR, Johnston HF: Sertraline treatment of 5 children diagnosed with selective mutism: a single-case research trial. J Child Adolesc Psychopharmacol 9:293–306, 1999

Chorpita BF, Barlow DH: The development of anxiety: the role of control in the early environment. Psychol Bull 124:3–21, 1998

Chorpita BF, Brown TA, Barlow DH: Perceived control as a mediator of family environment in etiological models of childhood anxiety. Behav Ther 29:457–476, 1998

Choudhury MS, Pimentel SS, Kendall PC: Childhood anxiety disorders: parent-child (dis)agreement using a structured interview for the DSM-IV. J Am Acad Child Adolesc Psychiatry 42:957–964, 2003

Cobham VE, Dadds MR, Spence SH: The role of parental anxiety in the treatment of childhood anxiety. J Consult Clin Psychol 66:893–905, 1998

Cohan SL, Chavira DA, Stein MB: Practitioner review: psychosocial interventions for children with selective mutism: a critical evaluation of the literature from 1990–2005. J Child Psychol Psychiatry 47:1085–1097, 2006a

Cohan SL, Price JM, Stein MB: Suffering in silence: why a developmental psychopathology perspective on selective mutism is needed. J Dev Behav Pediatr 27:341–355, 2006b

Compton SN, Nelson AH, March JS: Social phobia and separation anxiety symptoms in community and clinical samples of children and adolescents. J Am Acad Child Adolesc Psychiatry 39:1040–1046, 2000

Compton SN, March JS, Brent D, et al: Cognitive-behavioral psychotherapy for anxiety and depressive disorders in children and adolescents: an evidence-based medicine review. J Am Acad Child Adolesc Psychiatry 43:930–959, 2004

Connolly S, Simpson D, Petty C: Anxiety Disorders. New York, Chelsea House, 2006

Costello EJ, Egger HL, Angold A: Developmental epidemiology of anxiety disorders, in Phobic and Anxiety Disorders in Children and Adolescents. Edited by Ollendick TH, March JS. New York, Oxford University Press, 2004, pp 334–380

Craske MG: Fear and anxiety in children and adolescents. Bull Menninger Clin 61(suppl):A4–A36, 1997

Dadds MR, Spence SH, Holland D, et al: Early intervention and prevention of anxiety disorders: a controlled trial. J Consult Clin Psychol 65:627–635, 1997

Dadds MR, Roth JH: Family processes in the development of anxiety problems, in The Developmental Psychopathology of Anxiety. Edited by Vasey MW, Dadds MR. New York, Oxford University Press, 2001, pp 278–303

Egger HL, Angold A: Common emotional and behavioral disorders in preschool children: presentation, nosology, and epidemiology. J Child Psychol Psychiatry 47:313–337, 2006

Elizur Y, Perednik R: Prevalence and description of selective mutism in immigrant and native families: a controlled study. J Am Acad Child Adolesc Psychiatry 42:1451–1459, 2003

Farrell LJ, Barrett PM: Prevention of childhood emotional disorders: reducing the burden of suffering associated with anxiety and depression. Child Adolesc Ment Health 12:58–65, 2007

Feder A, Coplan JD, Goetz RR, et al: Twenty-four hour cortisol secretion patterns in prepubertal children with anxiety or depressive disorders. Biol Psychiatry 53:198–204, 2004

Gar NS, Hudson JL, Rapee RN: Family factors and the development of anxiety disorders, in Psychopathology and the Family. Edited by Hudson JL, Rapee RM. Oxford, United Kingdom, Elsevier LTD, 2005

Gazelle H: Class climate moderates peer relations and emotional adjustment in children with an early history of anxious solitude: a child x environment model. Dev Psychol 42:1179–1192, 2006

Ginsburg GS, Drake KL: Anxiety sensitivity and panic attack symptomatology among low-income African-American adolescents. Anxiety Disord 16:83–96, 2002

Ginsburg GS, Schlossberg MC: Family-based treatment of childhood anxiety disorders. Int Rev Psychiatry 14:143–154, 2002

Gittelman-Klein R, Klein DF: Social phobia: controlled imipramine treatment. Calif Med 115(3):42–54, 1971

Gladstone GL, Parker GB, Malhi GS: Do bullied children become anxious and depressed adults? A cross-sectional investigation of the correlates of bullying and anxious depression. J Nerv Ment Dis 194:201–208, 2006

Graae F, Milner J, Rizzotto L, et al: Clonazepam in childhood anxiety disorders. J Am Acad Child Adolesc Psychiatry 33:372–376, 1994

Graczyk PA, Connolly SD, Corapci F: Anxiety disorders in children and adolescents: theory, treatment, and prevention, in Handbook of Adolescent Behavior Problems: Evidence-Based Approaches to Prevention and Treatment. Edited by Gullotta TP, Adams GR. New York, Springer, 2005, pp 131–157

Grover RL, Hughes AA, Bergman RL, et al: Treatment modifications based on childhood anxiety diagnosis: demonstrating the flexibility in manualized treatment. Journal of Cognitive Psychotherapy: An International Quarterly 20:275–286, 2006

Gunnar MR, Fisher PA: Bringing basic research on early experience and stress neurobiology to bear on preventive interventions for neglected and maltreated children. Dev Psychopathol 18:651–677, 2006

Hirshfeld-Becker DR, Biederman J: Rationale and principles for early interventions with young children at risk for anxiety disorders. Clin Child Fam Psychol Rev 5:161–172, 2002

Hoffman EC, Mattis SG: A developmental adaptation of panic control treatment for panic disorder in adolescence. Cogn Behav Pract 7:253–261, 2000

Ialongo N, Edelsohn G, Werthamer-Larsson L, et al: The significance of self-reported anxious symptoms in first grade children: prediction to anxious symptoms and adaptive functioning in fifth grade. J Child Psychol Psychiatry 36:427–437, 1995

In-Albon T, Schneider S: Psychotherapy of childhood anxiety disorders: a meta-analysis. Psychother Psychosom 76:15–24, 2007

Kagan J: Biological bases of childhood shyness. Science 240:167–171, 1988

Kendall PC, Brady EU, Verduin TL: Comorbidity in childhood anxiety disorders and treatment outcome. J Am Acad Child Adolesc Psychiatry 40:787–794, 2001

Kendall PC, Pimentel S, Rynn MA, et al: Generalized anxiety disorder, in Phobic and Anxiety Disorders in Children and Adolescents. Edited by Ollendick TH, March JS. New York, Oxford University Press, 2004a, pp 334–380

Kendall PC, Safford S, Flannery-Schroeder E, et al: Child anxiety treatment: outcomes in adolescence and impact on substance use and depression at 7.4-year follow-up. J Consult Clin Psychol 72:276–287, 2004b

King NJ, Muris P, Ollendick TH: Childhood fears and phobias: assessment and treatment. Child Adolesc Mental Health 10:50–56, 2005

Klein RG, Koplewicz HS, Kanner A: Imipramine treatment in children with separation anxiety disorder. J Am Acad Child Adolesc Psychiatry 31:21–28, 1992

Kovacs M, Devlin B: Internalizing disorders in childhood. J Child Psychol Psychiatry 39:47–63, 1998

Kristensen H: Selective mutism and comorbidity with developmental disorder/delay, anxiety disorder, and elimination disorder. J Am Acad Child Adolesc Psychiatry 39:249–256, 2000

Kumpulainen K, Räsänen E, Raaska H, et al: Selective mutism among second-graders in elementary school. Eur Child Adolesc Psychiatry 7:24–29, 1998

Labellarte M, Biederman J, Emslie G, et al: Multiple-dose pharmacokinetics of fluvoxamine in children and adolescents. J Am Acad Child Adolesc Psychiatry 43:1497–1505, 2004

Langley AK, Bergman RL, Piacentini JC: Assessment of childhood anxiety. Int Rev Psychiatry 14:102–113, 2002

Last CG, Hansen C, Franco N: Cognitive-behavioral treatment of school phobia. J Am Acad Child Adolesc Psychiatry 37:404–411, 1998

Lau JY, Eley TC, Stevenson J: Examining the state-trait anxiety relationship: a behavioural genetic approach. J Abnorm Child Psychol 34:19–27, 2006

Lewinsohn PM, Zinbarg R, Seeley JR, et al: Lifetime comorbidity among anxiety disorders and between anxiety disorders and other mental disorders in adolescents. J Anxiety Disord 11:377–394, 1997

Lieb R, Wittchen HU, Höfler M, et al: Parental psychopathology, parenting styles, and the risk of social phobia in offspring: a prospective-longitudinal community study. Arch Gen Psychiatry 57:859–866, 2000

Lipsitz JD, Schneier FR: Social phobia, epidemiology and cost of illness. Pharmacoeconomics 18:23–32, 2000

Manassis K, Menna R: Depression in anxious children: possible factors in comorbidity. Depress Anxiety 10:18–24, 1999

Manassis K, Monga S: A therapeutic approach to children and adolescents with anxiety disorders and associated comorbid conditions. J Am Acad Child Adolesc Psychiatry 40:115–117, 2001

Marquenie LA, Schade A, van Balkom AJ, et al: Origin of the comorbidity of anxiety disorders and alcohol dependence: findings from a general population study. Eur Addict Res 13:39–49, 2007

March JS, Ollendick TH: Integrated psychosocial and pharmacological treatment, in Phobic and Anxiety Disorders in Children and Adolescents. Edited by Ollendick TH, March JS. New York, Oxford University Press, 2004, pp 141–172

MTA Cooperative Group: ADHD comorbidity findings from the MTA study: comparing comorbid subgroups. J Am Acad Child Adolesc Psychiatry 40:147–158, 2001

Moore PS, Whaley SE, Sigman M: Interactions between mothers and children: impacts of maternal and child anxiety. J Abnorm Psychol 113:471–476, 2004

Muratori F, Picchi L, Bruni G, et al: A two-year follow-up of psychodynamic psychotherapy for internalizing disorders in children. J Am Acad Child Adolesc Psychiatry 42:331–339, 2003

Muris P, Meesters C, Merckelbach H, et al: Worry in normal children. J Am Acad Child Adolesc Psychiatry 37:703–710, 1998

Muris P, Schmidt H, Merckelbach H: The structure of specific phobia symptoms among children and adolescents. Behav Res Ther 37:863–868, 1999

Nottelmann ED, Jensen PS: Comorbidity of disorders in children and adolescents: developmental perspectives. Advances in Clinical Child Psychology 17:109–155, 1995

Ollendick TH: Panic disorder in children and adolescents: new developments, new directions. J Clin Child Psychol 27:234–245, 1998

Ollendick TH, King NJ, Muris P: Fears and phobias in children: phenomenology, epidemiology and aetiology. Child and Adolescent Mental Health 7:98–106, 2002

Ong SH, Wickramaratne P, Tang M, et al: Early childhood sleep and eating problems as predictors of adolescent and adult mood and anxiety disorders. J Affect Disord 96:1–8, 2006

Pine DS: Treating children and adolescents with selective serotonin reuptake inhibitors: how long is appropriate? J Child Adolesc Psychopharmacol 12:189–203, 2002

Rao PA, Beidel DC, Turner SM, et al: Social anxiety disorder in childhood and adolescence: descriptive psychopathology. Behav Res Ther 45:1181–1191, 2007

Rapee RM, Spence SH, Cobham V, et al: Helping Your Anxious Child. Oakland, CA, New Harbinger, 2000

Reinblatt SP, Riddle MA: The pharmacological management of childhood anxiety disorders: a review. Psychopharmacology 191:67–86, 2007

Reiss S: Expectancy model of fear, anxiety, and panic. Clin Psychol Rev 11:141–153, 1991

Renaud J, Birmaher B, Wassick SC, et al: Use of selective serotonin reuptake inhibitors for the treatment of childhood panic disorder: a pilot study. J Child Adolesc Psychopharmacol 9:73–83, 1999

Research Units on Pediatric Psychopharmacology Anxiety Study Group: Fluvoxamine for the treatment of anxiety disorders in children and adolescents. N Engl J Med 344:1279–1285, 2001

Research Units on Pediatric Psychopharmacology Anxiety Study Group: Treatment of pediatric anxiety disorders: an open-label extension of the research units on pediatric psychopharmacology anxiety study. J Child Adolesc Psychopharmacology 3:175, 2002

Rynn MA, Siqueland L, Rickels K: Placebo-controlled trial of sertraline in the treatment of children with generalized anxiety disorder. Am J Psychiatry 158:2008–2014, 2001

Rynn MA, Riddle MA, Yeung PP, et al: Efficacy and safety of extended-release venlafaxine in the treatment of generalized anxiety disorder in children and adolescents: two placebo-controlled trials. Am J Psychiatry 164:290–300, 2007

Safer DJ, Zito JM: Treatment-emergent adverse events from selective serotonin reuptake inhibitors by age group: children versus adolescents. J Child Adolesc Psychopharmacol 16:159–169, 2006

Salazar DE, Frackiewicz EJ, Dockens R, et al: Pharmacokinetics and tolerability of buspirone during oral administration to children and adolescents with anxiety disorder and normal healthy adults. J Clin Pharmacol 41:1351–1358, 2001

Schuckit MA, Hesselbrock V: Alcohol dependence and anxiety disorders: what is the relationship? Am J Psychiatry 151:1723–1734, 1994

Seidel L, Walkup JT: Selective serotonin reuptake inhibitor use in the treatment of pediatric non-obsessive-compulsive disorder anxiety disorders. J Child Adolesc Psychopharmacol 16:171–179, 2006

Shamir-Essakow G, Ungerer JA, Rapee RM: Attachment, Behavioral inhibition, and anxiety in preschool children. J Abnorm Child Psychol 33:131–143, 2005

Sharkey L, McNicholas F: Female monozygotic twins with selective mutism-a case report. J Dev Behav Pediatr 27:129–133, 2006

Silverman WK, Albano AM: Anxiety Disorders Interview Schedule for DSM-IV: Child Version, Child and Parent Interview Schedules. San Antonio, TX, Psychological Corporation, 1996

Silverman WK, Ollendick TH: Evidence-based assessment of anxiety and its disorders in children and adolescents. J Clin Child Adolesc Psychol 34:380–411, 2005

Silverman WK, Kurtines WM, Ginsburg GS, et al: Contingency management, self-control, and education support in the treatment of childhood phobic disorders: a randomized clinical trial. J Consult Clin Psychol 67:675–687, 1999

Simeon JG, Ferguson HB, Knott V, et al: Clinical, cognitive, and neurophysiological effects of alprazolam in children and adolescents with overanxious and avoidant disorders. J Am Acad Child Adolesc Psychiatry 31:29–33, 1992

Spence SH: Prevention strategies, in The Developmental Psychopathology of Anxiety. Edited by Vasey MW, Dadds MR. New York, Oxford University Press, 2001

Spence SH, Donovan C, Brechman-Toussaint M: The treatment of childhood social phobia: the effectiveness of a social skills training-based, cognitive-behavioural intervention, with and without parental involvement. J Child Psychol Psychiatry 41:713–726, 2000

Strauss CC, Lahey BB, Frick P, et al: Peer social status of children with anxiety disorders. J Consult Clin Psychol 56:137–141, 1988

Suárez L, Barlow D, Bennett S, et al: Understanding anxiety disorders from a "triple vulnerabilities" framework, in Handbook of Anxiety and the Anxiety Disorders. Edited by Anthony M, Stein M. Oxford University Press, New York, 2008

Tourian KA, March JS, Mangano RM: Venlafaxine ER in children and adolescents with social anxiety disorder. Poster presented at the annual meeting of the American Psychiatric Association, New York, May 2004

van Brakel AML, Muris P, Bögels SM, et al: A multifactorial model for the etiology of anxiety in nonclinical adolescents: main and interactive effects of behavioral inhibition, attachment and parental rearing. J Child Fam Stud 15:569–579, 2006

Vecchio JL, Kearney CA: Selective mutism in children: comparison to youths with and without anxiety disorders. J Psychopathol Behav Assess 27:31–37, 2005

Velting ON, Albano AM: Current trends in the understanding and treatment of social phobia in youth. J Child Psychol Psychiatry 42:127–140, 2001

Velting ON, Setzer NJ, Albano AM: Update on and advances in assessment and cognitive-behavioral treatment of anxiety disorders in children and adolescents. Prof Psychol Res Pr 35:42–54, 2004

Verduin TL, Kendall PC: Differential occurrence of comorbidity within childhood anxiety disorders. J Clin Child Adolesc Psychol 32:290–295, 2003

Wagner KD, Berard R, Stein MB, et al: A multicenter, randomized, double-blind, placebo-controlled trial of paroxetine in children and adolescents with social anxiety. Arch Gen Psychiatry 61:1153–1162, 2004

Walkup JT, Albano AM, Piacentini J, et al: Cognitive-behavioral therapy, sertraline, or a combination in childhood anxiety. N Engl J Med 359:2753–2766, 2008

Warren SL, Huston L, Egeland B, et al: Child and adolescent anxiety disorders and early attachment. J Am Acad Child Adoles Psychiatry 36:637–644, 1997

Weems CF, Hayward C, Killen JD, et al: A longitudinal investigation of anxiety sensitivity in adolescence. J Abnorm Psychol 111:471–477, 2002

Weissman MM, Wokk S, Wickramaratne P, et al: Children with prepubertal-onset major depressive disorder and anxiety group up. Arch Gen Psychiatry 56:794–801, 1999

Weisz JR, Dos AJ, Hawley KM: Youth psychotherapy outcome research: a review and critique of the evidence base. Annu Rev Psychol 56:337–363, 2005

Whaley SE, Pinto A, Sigman M: Characterizing interactions between anxious mothers and their children. J Consult Clin Psychol 67:826–836, 1999

Wittchen H-U, Zhao S, Kessler RC, et al: DSM-III-R generalized anxiety disorder in the National Comorbidity Survey. Arch Gen Psychiatry 51:355–364, 1994

Wittchen H-U, Stein MB, Kessler RC: Social fears and social phobia in a community sample of adolescents and young adults. Psychol Med 29:309–323, 1999

Woodward LJ, Fergusson DM: Life course outcomes of young people with anxiety disorders in adolescence. J Am Acad Child Adolesc Psychiatry 40:1086–1093, 2001

World Health Organization: International Statistical Classification of Diseases and Related Health Problems, 10th Revision. Geneva, Switzerland, World Health Organization, 1992

Yeganeh R, Beidel DC, Turner SM, et al: Clinical distinctions between selective mutism and social phobia: an investigation of childhood psychopathology. J Am Acad Child Adolesc Psychiatry 42:1069–1075, 2003

Chapter 21

Separation Anxiety Disorder and School Refusal

Gail A. Bernstein, M.D.
Andrea M. Victor, Ph.D.

Separation anxiety disorder (SAD) is the only anxiety disorder in DSM-IV (American Psychiatric Association 1994) and its text revision, DSM-IV-TR (American Psychiatric Association 2000), that is included under the category of disorders usually first diagnosed in infancy, childhood, or adolescence. The onset of the disorder is prior to 18 years of age, and it is not typically diagnosed in adulthood. School refusal is a symptom, not a diagnosis, in DSM-IV but is often associated with anxiety and/or mood disorders. It is also restricted to childhood and adolescence.

Separation Anxiety Disorder

Definition, Clinical Description, and Diagnosis

Separation anxiety is a developmentally appropriate response in young children upon separation from their primary caregivers. This is normal for infants from 6 to 30 months of age and usually intensifies between 13 and 18 months of age (Kearney et al. 2003). Separation anxiety typically declines between 3 and 5 years of age as a result of the child's cognitive maturation that allows the child to comprehend that separation from a caregiver is temporary. SAD occurs when the child demonstrates developmentally inappropriate distress associated with separation from a primary caregiver (American Psychiatric Association 2000). The DSM-IV-TR diagnostic criteria for SAD are presented in Table 21–1.

The key feature of SAD is the child's excessive worry or fear about being separated from his or her primary attachment figures or being away from home. The child's anxiety may be present prior to, during, and/or in anticipation of the separation. When separation is about to occur, children often resist by crying or hiding from parents. Children with SAD fear that harm will come to themselves or their parents, which will result in permanent separation. Oftentimes, these

TABLE 21–1. DSM-IV-TR diagnostic criteria for separation anxiety disorder

A. Developmentally inappropriate and excessive anxiety concerning separation from home or from those to whom the individual is attached, as evidenced by three (or more) of the following:

(1) recurrent excessive distress when separation from home or major attachment figures occurs or is anticipated

(2) persistent and excessive worry about losing, or about possible harm befalling, major attachment figures

(3) persistent and excessive worry that an untoward event will lead to separation from a major attachment figure (e.g., getting lost or being kidnapped)

(4) persistent reluctance or refusal to go to school or elsewhere because of fear of separation

(5) persistently and excessively fearful or reluctant to be alone or without major attachment figures at home or without significant adults in other settings

(6) persistent reluctance or refusal to go to sleep without being near a major attachment figure or to sleep away from home

(7) repeated nightmares involving the theme of separation

(8) repeated complaints of physical symptoms (such as headaches, stomachaches, nausea, or vomiting) when separation from major attachment figures occurs or is anticipated

B. The duration of the disturbance is at least 4 weeks.

C. The onset is before age 18 years.

D. The disturbance causes clinically significant distress or impairment in social, academic (occupational), or other important areas of functioning.

E. The disturbance does not occur exclusively during the course of a pervasive developmental disorder, schizophrenia, or other psychotic disorder and, in adolescents and adults, is not better accounted for by panic disorder with agoraphobia.

Specify if:

Early Onset: if onset occurs before age 6 years

Source. Reprinted from American Psychiatric Association: *Diagnostic and Statistical Manual of Mental Disorders*, 4th Edition, Text Revision. Washington, DC, American Psychiatric Association, 2000, p. 125. Used with permission. Copyright © 2000 American Psychiatric Association.

children shadow their parents and have difficulty going places without their parents (e.g., friends' houses, school) because they are afraid to be away from them. Children with SAD often have nightmares that they will get kidnapped or taken away from their parents. In order to avoid separation, children also complain of headaches or stomachaches when they have to leave home or separate from their parents.

Epidemiology

The prevalence rate of SAD in youth typically ranges between 3% and 5% (Black 1995; Shear et al. 2006). SAD is more prevalent in children compared to adolescents (Breton et al. 1999). Several studies have demonstrated higher prevalence rates of SAD in females compared to males (e.g., Ehringer et al. 2006); however, other studies have not found significant gender differences (e.g., Costello et al. 1996; Last et al. 1992). Many youth ex-

hibit subclinical levels of separation anxiety but do not meet diagnostic criteria for SAD. Kashani and Orvaschel (1990) found a prevalence rate of approximately 50% for subclinical symptoms of SAD among a community sample of 8-year-old children.

Comorbidity

Table 21–2 presents the comorbidity rates for SAD based on the following two studies. Verduin and Kendall (2003) compared comorbidity rates in 199 children (8–13 years) with a primary diagnosis of generalized anxiety disorder (GAD), SAD, or social phobia (SP). Children with SAD had a higher mean number of comorbid diagnoses compared to children with GAD or SP. Furthermore, children with SAD were the least likely to have a comorbid mood disorder and most likely to be diagnosed with sleep terror disorder. Children with SAD had a higher rate of specific phobia

TABLE 21–2. Comorbidity rates in separation anxiety disorder

Comorbid diagnosis	Verduin and Kendall (2003)	Last et al. (1987)
GAD/OAD	74%	33%
Specific phobia	58%	13%
ADHD	22%	17%
Social phobia	20%	8%
ODD	12%	17%
Enuresis	8%	8%
Sleep terror disorder	8%	—
OCD	4%	4%
Dysthymic disorder	2%	13%
MDD	0%	8%
Panic disorder	2%	4%

Note. ADHD=attention-deficit/hyperactivity disorder; GAD=generalized anxiety disorder; MDD=major depressive disorder; OAD=overanxious disorder; OCD = obsessive-compulsive disorder; ODD=oppositional defiant disorder.

compared to children with SP and a similar rate as children with GAD. Oppositional defiant disorder (ODD) was determined to occur relatively evenly among the three anxiety disorders (12% in SAD, 10% in GAD, 5% in SP).

Last et al. (1987) found contrasting results compared to the above findings when they evaluated a sample of 73 youth (5–18 years). No significant differences were found for the mean number of comorbid diagnoses among the diagnostic groups of SAD, SP, GAD, and major depressive disorder. In contrast to Verduin and Kendall's (2003) findings, children with SAD were least likely to have a comorbid anxiety disorder.

Etiology, Mechanisms, and Risk Factors

Attachment

Attachment theory suggests that the predisposition to anxiety can be exacerbated or alleviated by the type of attachment between mother and child (Manassis and Bradley 1994). Insecure mother-infant attachment has been shown to specifically predict separation anxiety in children. In a prospective, longitudinal study of 99 mother-child dyads (beginning when the child was 1 month old), attachment pattern, maternal sensitivity, and maternal separation anxiety were evaluated (Dallaire and Weinraub 2005). Insecurely attached children exhibited significantly more symptoms of SAD at age 6 years when compared to securely attached children. Regression analysis demonstrated that mother-child attachment pattern and maternal sensitivity each contributed uniquely to the prediction of children's separation anxiety at 6 years but that maternal separation anxiety did not.

Temperament

Behavioral inhibition is a genetically based temperamental trait that is defined as a child's reaction to novel or unfamiliar situations with reticence, distress, or avoidance (Kagan 1998). In prospective studies of toddlers with and without behavioral inhibition, children with behavioral inhibition were at an increased risk for SAD and other anxiety disorders at 3 years of age (Biederman et al. 1993).

Genetic and Environmental Factors

A recent study investigated genetic and environmental contributions to six childhood disorders, including SAD (Ehringer et al. 2006). The sample included 1,162 adolescent twin pairs and 426 adolescent siblings. This is one of the only studies that included nontwin siblings of twins in behavior genetic analyses of childhood psychiatric disorders. The study employed biometrical modeling to determine the relative contributions to the disorders of genes and shared and nonshared environmental influences. Lifetime SAD was more prevalent in monozygotic twins compared to dizygotic twins. The impact of shared environment on twins was similar to that for nontwin siblings. There was a moderate contribution of genetic factors, with most of the variance attributed to nonshared environmental factors. The study supported both genetic and nonshared environmental contributions to SAD.

Parental Anxiety

Offspring of parents with anxiety disorders are at risk for developing anxiety disorders. Biederman et al. (2001) reported that children of adults with major depression or panic disorder are more likely to develop SAD than children of controls. Merikangas et al. (1998) evaluated the diagnoses in children of parents with anxiety disorders and those with substance abuse. The offspring of adults with anxiety disorders were two times more likely to manifest an anxiety disorder compared with offspring of adults with substance abuse or control participants. The most common anxiety disorders in the children were SAD and GAD. In a sample of 57 pairs of anxious children and their mothers, maternal phobic anxiety was significantly associated with higher levels of separation anxiety in children (Bernstein et al. 2005a).

Parenting Style

Several factors in parenting style seem to be related to the emergence of anxiety in children: parental rejection, parental control, and parental intrusiveness (Rapee 1997; Wood 2006). Muris et al. (1998) reported that anxious parenting style and controlling behavior of parents were significantly correlated with SAD and overanxious disorder (OAD) symptoms in a general population of children. Forty anxious children (6–13 years) and their parents were administered the DSM-IV version of the Anxiety Disorders Interview Schedule (ADIS), anxiety symptom rating scales, and a new measure of parental intrusiveness developed by Wood (2006). Parental intrusiveness is defined as unnecessary assistance with children's self-help tasks, infantilizing behavior, and invasions of privacy (Wood 2006). A significant positive correlation was found between the score on the intrusiveness measure and the child's separation anxiety score on the ADIS. The intrusiveness measure was not significantly correlated with the GAD and SP scores on the ADIS.

Prevention

It is important to target both parents and youth in the prevention of childhood anxiety disorders, particularly SAD. Parent skills training programs can improve parent-child relationships, parenting style, family functioning, and anxiety management (Hirshfeld-Becker and Biederman 2002). In addition, school-based early intervention programs have been shown to be effective in treating children with mild to moderate anxiety disorders (e.g., Bernstein et al. 2005b; Dadds et al. 1997).

Course and Prognosis

The mean age at onset for SAD is usually between 7 and 9 years of age (Last et al. 1992). Some children develop SAD following a stressful life event (e.g., parental divorce, change in school, move to a new home), whereas other children progressively exhibit symptoms without a clear precipitating event. Some children with SAD recover and do not exhibit long-term effects; however, other children with SAD experience more chronic and persistent symptoms.

A longitudinal study sampled 3-year-old children (N=60) with clinical, subclinical, or nonclinical presentations of separation anxiety (Kearney et al. 2003). After approximately 3.5 years, many children who were initially diagnosed with SAD showed a decrease in symptoms and moved toward subclinical and nonclinical symptom presentations. Foley et al. (2004) further examined the course and outcomes of SAD in a community sample of twins (8–17 years). At 18-month follow-up, 20% of the children with SAD continued to meet diagnostic criteria. Predictors of persistent SAD included comorbid diagnosis of ODD, impairment due to ADHD symptoms, and reported maternal marital dissatisfaction. In addition, at the 18-month follow-up, children with persistent SAD were more likely to have a comorbid diagnosis of OAD and a new diagnosis of depressive disorder.

Childhood SAD may also be a risk factor for the development of anxiety disorders during adulthood (Manicavasagar et al. 1998). Data conflict as to whether SAD in children is directly related to the later development of panic disorder. Studies show that 50%–75% of youth diagnosed with panic disorder have a previous or comorbid diagnosis of SAD (Biederman et al. 1997; Masi et al. 2000). SAD in children may be related to a specific heritable form of early-onset panic disorder (Battaglia et al. 1995). In contrast, a 7-year longitudinal study (Aschenbrand et al. 2003) of youth who received treatment for an anxiety disorder during childhood showed that a diagnosis of SAD was predictive of a higher number of anxiety disorders at the 7-year follow-up compared to a diagnosis of GAD or SP during childhood, but not more predictive than other anxiety diagnoses of the development of panic disorder. Other research has suggested that SAD in children does not change into another anxiety disorder; rather, SAD persists with a different presentation that is more relevant to adult issues (e.g., fear of being alone) (Fagiolini et al. 1998; Manicavasagar et al. 2000). Shear et al. (2006) used data from the National Comorbidity Survey Replication to examine the persistence of SAD symptoms into adulthood. Results showed that 36% of those who were classified as having SAD during childhood continued to meet criteria for the disorder into adulthood. Similarly, Silove et al. (2002) found that adults with a history of childhood SAD endorsed significantly higher rates of SAD in adulthood (60%) compared to adults without a history of childhood SAD (8%).

Evaluation

A formal evaluation should be completed to distinguish the specific anxiety disorder, assess severity of symptoms, and determine functional impairment (American Academy of Child and Adolescent Psychiatry 2007). The American Academy of Child and Adolescent Psychiatry (AACAP) practice parameter also stresses the importance of assessing for diagnoses that may mimic anxiety disorders, such as physical conditions and/or other psychiatric disorders. The diagnosis of SAD can be made with a thorough diagnostic evaluation that includes an interview with the parent(s) and child. Oftentimes, children with SAD are not able to separate from parents to meet alone with the clinician, so the interview needs to be conducted with the parent and child together. A standardized interview may be used and is beneficial in differentiating among psychiatric disorders. The ADIS for DSM-IV is a semistructured interview for anxiety and other diagnoses that includes parent and child versions (Silverman and Albano 1996). It is also helpful to contact teachers, other school personnel, or daycare providers to gather additional information regarding the child's functioning in settings outside the home and away from parents.

Various rating scales have been developed to use in conjunction with a clinical interview. Broadband measures, such as the Behavior Assessment System for Children, Second Edition (BASC-2; Reynolds and Kamphaus 2004), offer multiple perspectives of the child's functioning (see Chapter 8, "Rating Scales"). The Multidimensional Anxiety Scale for Children (MASC; March et al. 1997) and the Screen for Child Anxiety Related Emotional Disorders Scale (SCARED; Birmaher et al. 1999) are self-report measures that include items directly related to separation anxiety, as well as other symptoms commonly associated with anxiety disorders (more detail in Chapter 8).

When distinguishing SAD from other anxiety disorders, it is important to understand what the child fears will happen when separated from a primary caregiver. Children with SAD fear that something bad will happen to them or their primary caretaker that will result in permanent separation. Children and adolescents diagnosed with other anxiety disorders (e.g., GAD, SP, panic disorder) may also worry about being separated from their primary caretaker; however, the reason for their fear is different. Children with SP may be concerned about being away from their parents due to the anxiety they experience in social and evaluative situations. Children with panic disorder may be resistant to being separated from their parents because they are fearful they may need their parents' help if a panic attack occurs. Children with GAD endorse multiple worries, which may include worry about the health and safety of themselves and family members, but these worries do not impair their ability to separate from their parents. Another distinguishing factor is that children with SAD exhibit minimal anxiety when with their primary caretaker, whereas children with other anxiety disorders often continue to worry even in the presence of their primary caretaker.

Treatment

The AACAP practice parameter for youth diagnosed with an anxiety disorder recommends that treatment planning consider a multimodal approach (American Academy of Child and Adolescent Psychiatry 2007). Effective treatment of children with SAD often includes child and parent psychoeducation, school consultation, cognitive-behavioral therapy (CBT), and selective serotonin reuptake inhibitors (SSRIs).

Pharmacological Treatments

Medication is considered as a part of the multimodal treatment plan when anxiety symptoms are moderate to severe and associated with substantial impairment. The age of the child is also considered. Older children are more likely to be prescribed medications compared to younger children. The first-choice medication for treating SAD is an SSRI.

Two randomized controlled trials support the use of SSRIs in the treatment of SAD. Both studies enrolled children with SAD, GAD, and/or SP. The Research Unit on Pediatric Psychopharmacology Anxiety Study Group (2001) study included 128 participants ages 6–17 years. After failing to improve after 3 weeks of psychosocial intervention, youth were randomized to 8 weeks of fluvoxamine or placebo. Dose ranges of fluvoxamine were 50–250 mg/day for children and 50–300 mg/day for adolescents. After 8 weeks, youth receiving fluvoxamine showed significantly greater improvement on a clinician-rated measure of anxiety compared to participants in the placebo group.

Birmaher et al. (2003) studied 74 children with SAD, GAD, and/or SP (7–17 years old) who were randomized to 12 weeks of fluoxetine (20 mg/day) or placebo. At posttreatment, 61% of children on fluoxetine as compared to 35% on placebo were rated as much or very much improved on a clinician rating scale. Interestingly, of the three anxiety disorders studied, SAD was least likely to respond to fluoxetine. However, this finding needs replication in a larger sample of children with anxiety disorders.

Alternative medications for SAD include tricyclic antidepressants (TCAs) and benzodiazepines (for review, see American Academy of Child and Adolescent Psychiatry 2007). TCAs generally have more side effects, especially cardiovascular effects, and are dangerous in overdose. Due to the possibility of tolerance and dependence, benzodiazepines are recommended only on a short-term basis in combination with an SSRI or TCA to target anxiety until the effect of the antidepressant begins.

Psychotherapeutic Treatments

Cognitive-behavioral therapy.

CBT is the best proven psychotherapeutic treatment for youth with SAD (Eisen and Schaefer 2005; Masi et al. 2001; see also Chapter 58, "Cognitive-Behavioral Treatment for Anxiety Disorders"). Six essential components of CBT have been identified for the treatment of anxiety disorders in youth: psychoeducation, somatic management, cognitive restructuring, problem solving, exposure, and relapse prevention (Velting et al. 2004). CBT is typically a time-limited intervention that focuses on the youth's current symptoms. Initial psychoeducation provides information to the parent and youth regarding behaviors that sustain SAD (e.g., avoidance of anxiety-provoking situations) and treatment approaches (e.g., thought identification, cognitive modification, behavioral exposures) that are effective in alleviating anxiety.

Children with SAD often report fearful thoughts related to anxiety-provoking situations (e.g., going to school, being away from the parent, attending sleepovers). Common anxious thoughts include "Mom will forget to pick me up from school"; "Mom will die when we are not together and I will never see her again"; and "I will get lost and never be able to see Mom again." Cognitive modification teaches youth to recognize their anxiety-provoking thoughts and to challenge these maladaptive thoughts with more realistic and rational thoughts.

As a result of anxious thoughts about separation, children change their behavior to prevent separation from their parents (e.g., school refusal, unwillingness to leave parents to go to a friend's house). Since youth with SAD believe that these dangerous and feared outcomes have a high likelihood of occurring, it is crucial to challenge these thoughts and predictions with behavioral exposure exercises. A hierarchy of exposures (e.g., from least to most anxiety provoking) is developed that is individualized to meet the child's needs. Exposures are planned with the child and parent and are a controlled method for the child to confront feared situations. Exposures are used to decrease the child's

anxiety by challenging the child's current inaccurate beliefs and helping the child develop new, more accurate beliefs about feared situations. As the child is exposed to the feared situations and the feared outcome does not occur, the child's anxiety gradually dissipates. Parents, who may also suffer from anxiety, may need support to withstand the child's distress and implement the exposure for long enough so that anxiety reduction occurs.

Parent-child interaction therapy.

Limited intervention research has been conducted with children under 7 years of age who are diagnosed with SAD. Parent-Child Interaction Therapy (PCIT) is empirically supported as a treatment for children with disruptive behavior disorders and has been adapted to be used in the treatment of young children with SAD (Pincus et al. 2005). PCIT helps parents learn to manage their child's behavioral difficulties and promotes a positive and accepting parent-child relationship, which often results in an improvement in attachment and warmth between the parent(s) and child. It is expected that this may ultimately help the child separate from the parent by strengthening the child's feeling of security. PCIT also incorporates parenting skills that are important in decreasing child anxiety (e.g., parental attention toward child, differential reinforcement, behavioral modification, clear commands).

Choate et al. (2005) completed a pilot study with three children (5–8 years old) with a primary diagnosis of SAD. Families monitored the child's separation anxiety behaviors prior to treatment and then participated in six to seven sessions of PCIT. None of the children met criteria for SAD immediately following treatment and at 3-months posttreatment. PCIT may be an effective treatment for children under 7 years of age with SAD, but further research is needed.

Multimodal Treatment

The Child-Adolescent Anxiety Multimodal Study compared the effectiveness of 12 weeks of sertraline, CBT, sertraline plus CBT, and placebo in the treatment of 488 children and adolescents with moderate to severe SAD, GAD, and/or SP (Walkup et al. 2008). At posttreatment, 55% who received sertraline, 60% who received CBT, 81% who received combination treatment, and 24% who received placebo were rated as very much or much improved on the Clinical Global Impressions-Improvement scale. Combination treatment was significantly superior to each of the monotherapies. Sertraline and CBT were equivalent. All active treatments were significantly more effective than placebo. This study demonstrates that an SSRI plus CBT results in the most positive outcome for youth with SAD, GAD, and/or SP. However, any of the three active treatments (SSRI, CBT, or combination) may be recommended, given the availability of specific interventions, cost, time constraints, and family preference (Walkup et al. 2008).

Other Treatment Modalities

Classroom-based accommodations may be part of the treatment plan for anxious children (American Academy of Child and Adolescent Psychiatry 2007). Children with SAD often have difficulty attending school due to their fear of separation from parents. Therefore, it is often beneficial to educate the teacher and school personnel regarding the impact of anxiety and effective strategies to help the child cope in the classroom. A 504 Plan or individualized education plan may also be a helpful way to provide specific accommodations and modifications for the child.

Research Directions

Research is needed to develop a better understanding of the pathway of SAD from childhood into adulthood. There continues to be controversy regarding the association between SAD in childhood and panic disorder in adulthood. In addition, there are questions concerning the possible presentation of SAD in adulthood. Researchers (e.g., Peleg et al. 2006) have started to consider the effect of maternal separation anxiety on the presentation of SAD in children.

School Refusal

Definition, Clinical Description, and Diagnosis

Unlike SAD, school refusal is not a DSM-IV diagnosis; it is a symptom associated with several diagnoses, including SAD, GAD, SP, major depression, and ODD. School refusal is often defined as difficulty attending school associated with emotional distress, especially anxiety and depression (King and Bernstein 2001). Terms such as *separation anxiety* and *school phobia* have been used synonymously with school refusal. However, the term *school refusal* is favored because it is descriptive and inclusive and does not imply etiology (King and Bernstein 2001). School refusal does not typ-

ically include youth who are not attending school due to truancy, antisocial features, or conduct disorder.

School refusal includes youth who are completely absent from school, initially attend school but leave during the school day, go to school after intense behavior problems (e.g., tantrums), or manifest extreme distress at school and plead with parents to let them stay home in the future (Kearney and Albano 2000). School refusers are a heterogeneous group of youth with various associated psychopathology (Suveg et al. 2005). Although the clinical picture can vary greatly, commonly seen features are pleas to parents to be allowed to stay home from school, distress when going to school, somatic complaints, and associated peer and family relationship difficulties (Last and Strauss 1990).

Kearney and Albano (2000) classify school refusal behavior as serving a function of negative reinforcement (i.e., to avoid unpleasant stimuli or social/evaluative situations at school) or positive reinforcement (i.e., to pursue pleasant situations outside of school). For example, children may refuse school to avoid one or more of the following: riding the school bus, going to gym class, encountering bullies, giving a speech, or interacting with teachers. In such cases, the school refusal behavior is a negative reinforcer. On the other hand, if the child is allowed to engage in pleasurable activities such as playing computer games or spending special time with a parent when refusing school, the school refusal serves as a positive reinforcer.

Epidemiology

Egger et al. (2003) examined the prevalence of school refusal as part of the longitudinal Great Smoky Mountains Study (GSMS; $n=1,422$) of psychiatric disorders in youth. The prevalence of three subtypes of school refusal in a community sample was presented: anxious school refusers who resisted going to school, did not go to school, or left school due to anxiety; truants who did not go to school or left school without permission and not due to anxiety; mixed school refusers who endorsed anxiety and truancy related to school attendance. The characteristics of these three types of school refusal are presented in Table 21–3.

Reviews have concluded that school refusal is present in approximately 1% of all youth and 5% of all clinic-referred youth (King et al. 1995). McShane et al. (2001) found that approximately 7% of youth evaluated over 5 years in a child and adolescent psychiatric facility with outpatient and inpatient services presented with school refusal. Similar to the community sample (Egger

TABLE 21–3. Characteristics of school refusal

Type of school refusal	Prevalence, %	Mean age at onset, years	Percentage of males
Anxious school refusers	1.6	10.9	47.9
Truants	5.8	13.1	65.1
Mixed school refusers	0.5	—	51.9

Source. Adapted from Egger et al. 2003.

et al. 2003), there was not a significant difference by gender (45% female, 55% male).

Ollendick and Mayer (1984) reported two peaks of onset of school refusal: 5–6 years and 10–11 years of age, which coincide with the beginning of kindergarten and the transition to middle school. In addition, McShane et al. (2001) found frequent onset of school refusal symptoms in the first or second year of high school in a clinical sample of 192 youth (10–17 years).

Comorbidity

School refusal often occurs in conjunction with psychiatric disorders, but the symptom presentation does not require the presence of a psychiatric disorder. In the GSMS community sample of school refusers (Egger et al. 2003), approximately 25% of youth with anxious school refusal (i.e., those who refuse school due to fear or anxiety) had at least one psychiatric disorder compared to only 6.8% of non–school refusal youth. Anxious school refusal was associated with depression (13.9%) and SAD (10.8%). The most common fears were regarding separation and a specific school situation.

In clinical samples of school refusers (Kearney and Albano 2004; McShane et al. 2001), more youth met criteria for a psychiatric diagnosis compared to the findings from the community sample. Greater than 50% of the participants from each of the samples had at least one psychiatric diagnosis. The primary categories of diagnoses were anxiety, mood, and disruptive behavior disorders. The two studies showed similar patterns of diagnoses among the participants with school refusal. The most prominent anxiety disorder among the school refusers was SAD (22%, Kearney and Albano 2004; 20%, McShane et al. 2001). Other common anxiety disorders included GAD, SP, specific phobia, and panic disorder. Major depressive disorder was the most prominent mood disorder (5%, Kearney and Albano 2004; 30%, McShane et al. 2001). The most prom-

inent disruptive behavior disorder was ODD (8.4%, Kearney and Albano 2004; 24%, McShane et al. 2001).

Etiology, Mechanisms, and Risk Factors

Egger et al. (2003) examined the psychosocial vulnerabilities of a community sample of youth with school refusal (anxious school refusers, truants, and mixed school refusers). Anxious school refusers were significantly more likely to live in a single-parent home, attend a dangerous school, and have a biological or nonbiological parent who had been treated for a psychiatric disorder. Truant youth experienced the following vulnerabilities: impoverished homes, single-parent homes, at least one adoptive parent, born to teenage parents, and minimal parental supervision. Mixed school refusers were more likely to have a parent who did not complete high school or was unemployed, have a parent who was treated for a psychiatric disorder, live in poverty, and move multiple times. Similar to the anxious school refusers, they were more likely to attend a dangerous school; similar to the truant youth, they were more likely to have minimal parental supervision.

Family Functioning

Family functioning is often viewed as a contributor to school refusal behavior. Parents of 64 school-refusing children completed the Family Environment Scale (FES) to assess various family subtypes (enmeshed, conflictive, isolated, detached, healthy) (Kearney and Silverman 1995). Parents of school-refusing children scored lower on the independence subscale and higher on the conflict subscale of the FES, which would indicate that the families were more enmeshed and had more conflict than normative families. The families also reported more isolative behavior than normative families. Approximately 39% of the families with school-refusing children endorsed healthy family profiles.

Family functioning was assessed by Bernstein et al. (1999) in 46 school-refusing adolescents (12–18 years) with comorbid anxiety and major depressive disorders. Adolescents, mothers, and fathers completed the Family Adaptability and Cohesion Evaluation Scale II. In general, the families appeared to be disengaged (on the cohesion subscale) and rigid (on the adaptability subscale).

Parental Psychopathology

Diagnostic interviews were used to assess the history and current presence of anxiety and depressive disorders in the parents of 51 anxious school-refusing youth (Martin et al. 1999). Eighty-one percent of parents had a history of a psychiatric disorder. In 41% of the school-refusing children, both parents had a history of a psychiatric disorder. Approximately 78% of mothers and 54% of fathers met criteria for a lifetime diagnosis of an anxiety disorder, and 51% of mothers and 22% of fathers met criteria for a lifetime diagnosis of a depressive disorder.

Stressful Life Events

Stressful life events are often triggers for the onset of school refusal behavior. McShane et al. (2001) reviewed medical records of youth with school refusal and identified the following events associated with the onset of symptoms: conflict at home (43%), conflict with peers (34%), academic difficulties (31%), move and/or change of school (25%), change in family composition (21%), and physical illness (20%).

Prevention

Promotion of healthy family relationships, encouragement of independent behavior in children, and support of children's involvement in school and extracurricular activities will serve to mitigate school refusal. Proactive problem solving about stressors in the school environment (e.g., bullies) will also be beneficial. At the earliest signs of school refusal, parents and school officials should promote a swift return to the classroom with support in place for the anxious child.

Course and Prognosis

In approximately 25% of cases, school refusal behavior remits spontaneously or resolves after minor interventions by parents (Kearney and Tillotson 1998). However, for cases that do not remit, short-term difficulties include academic failure and peer and family relationship problems. Negative outcomes at long-term fol-

low-up are lower likelihood of receiving advanced education, social isolation, job difficulties, and increased rates of psychopathology (Berg and Jackson 1985).

Flakierska-Praquin et al. (1997) evaluated 35 individuals 20–29 years after treatment for school refusal. Average age at follow-up was 34 years old. Initial diagnoses were based on retrospective chart reviews of 500 children (7–12 years old) who had received inpatient or outpatient psychiatric treatment. All 35 participants had an initial diagnosis of SAD. There were two comparison groups of 35 subjects each: a psychiatric group without a history of school refusal and a general population group. Adults with a history of school refusal had a significantly higher rate of outpatient psychiatric service use compared to the normal control group. Adults in the psychiatric control group were more likely to have criminal records than those in the other two groups. In addition, 14% of the school refusal group, 9% of the psychiatric control group, and 0% of the general population group continued to live with their parents. Adults with a history of school refusal had significantly fewer children than those in the comparison groups. These findings demonstrate long-term sequelae in adults with a history of school refusal.

Evaluation

There are no specific consensus guidelines for the assessment and treatment of school refusal. Since school refusal is often associated with anxiety, guidelines developed for childhood anxiety disorders (American Academy of Child and Adolescent Psychiatry 2007) are helpful. Youth with school refusal vary in their clinical presentation; therefore, it is most beneficial to use a multimodal assessment with multiple informants (e.g., youth, parents, school personnel) (King and Bernstein 2001; Ollendick and King 1998). Based on the vulnerabilities and symptoms associated with school refusal, a comprehensive evaluation may include several of the following components: clinical interview, semistructured diagnostic interview, examination of factors contributing to the school refusal, self-ratings and parent and teacher ratings of symptoms of anxiety and depression, evaluation of family functioning, and review of school attendance. It may also be helpful to complete a psychoeducational and language evaluation to rule out learning and language deficits that could be contributing to the school refusal behaviors.

The School Refusal Assessment Scale (SRAS; parent and child versions) was developed to assess the primary function of school refusal behavior (Kearney 2002; Kearney and Silverman 1993). The SRAS assesses the strength of four functional conditions that often maintain school refusal behavior: avoidance of school-related stimuli that trigger negative affect, escape from negative social and/or evaluative situations, getting attention from others, and/or receipt of tangible reinforcements when not in school. This assessment tool may be helpful in planning effective treatment for youth with school refusal.

Treatment

Similar to youth with anxiety disorders, youth with school refusal benefit most from a multimodal treatment approach. The function of the school refusal behavior should be considered in developing an effective individualized treatment protocol (Kearney and Albano 2000). Research on treatment efficacy in school refusal is primarily confined to pharmacotherapy and CBT.

Pharmacological Treatments

The first-choice medication for children and adolescents with school refusal is an SSRI. This is based on randomized controlled trials that demonstrate the efficacy of SSRIs for treating youth with anxiety disorders (Birmaher at al. 2003; Research Unit on Pediatric Psychopharmacology Anxiety Study Group 2001; Rynn et al. 2001; Wagner et al. 2004; Walkup et al. 2008). If school refusal is associated with depression, an SSRI may also be indicated (Emslie et al. 1997).

Several randomized controlled trials provide conflicting results regarding the efficacy of TCAs for anxiety-based school refusal (e.g., Klein et al. 1992). The lack of agreement is explained by small sample sizes, differing drug dosages, lack of control of adjunctive therapies, and different comorbidity patterns. In any case, the side-effect profile of TCAs places them out of the front line of treatment options.

In a study of multimodal treatment for 63 school-refusing adolescents with anxiety and major depressive disorders, adolescents were treated with 8 weeks of imipramine plus CBT versus 8 weeks of placebo plus CBT (Bernstein et al. 2000). Over the course of the study, school attendance significantly improved in the imipramine group, but not in the placebo group. Fifty-four percent of the imipramine group and 17% of the placebo group achieved remission (school attendance greater than 75%) at 8 weeks. The low remission rate in the placebo group reflected the severe symptoms of participants and supports the need for multimodal intervention in treating severe school refusal in teenagers. Naturalistic 1-year follow-up of these anxious-depressed adolescents found two-thirds met DSM-III-R (Ameri-

can Psychiatric Association 1987) criteria for an anxiety disorder and one-third met criteria for a depressive disorder (Bernstein et al. 2001). Furthermore, 77% had received outpatient psychotherapy, 20% received in-home therapy, 68% were prescribed psychotropic medications, 20% were hospitalized, and 15% had been placed outside the home. Ninety-seven percent attended school during the follow-up year.

Psychotherapeutic Treatments

Psychotherapeutic treatments aimed at school refusal are primarily cognitive-behavioral combined with a family systems approach that incorporates relaxation training, cognitive modification, social skills training, exposure-based activities, and contracting and contingency management (Kearney and Albano 2000). Relaxation training, cognitive modification, and social skills training are typically completed prior to engaging in exposure-based activities to prepare the youth for school reentry. Prior to school reentry, a plan must be developed with the youth that includes a hierarchy of steps toward full-day entry. Youth with mild or acute school refusal are more likely to start with immediate full-day return to school. School reentry is often a difficult process for youth with chronic school refusal; therefore, contingency contracts are helpful to motivate the youth to begin and continue the reentry process. Using homebound services or changing schools is generally not recommended.

In addition to using CBT techniques with the youth, it is crucial to work with parents and school personnel, who often play active roles in helping the youth return to school. Parents may need to learn behavioral management strategies. For instance, parents learn to set appropriate limits that do not reinforce the child's school refusal behaviors (e.g., escort child to school and limit access to attention and pleasurable activities when at home). School personnel are also key figures to ensure that the youth remains at school for the planned amount of time. Teachers can help integrate the child back into the classroom, and counselors can help manage anxiety if necessary. Youth, parents, and school personnel should work as a team to ensure successful school reentry.

CBT is an efficacious treatment for youth with school refusal; however, additional research needs to be conducted to gain "well established" empirical status. King et al. (1998) completed a 4-week treatment study of 34 school refusers (5–15 years). Participants were randomly assigned to CBT or waitlist control (WLC). At posttreatment, children who received CBT had a significantly better attendance record than children from the WLC. Furthermore, children from the CBT condition demonstrated significantly greater improvements on self-report measures of emotional distress and coping compared to children from the WLC. Sixteen of the children who received CBT completed a 3- to 5-year follow-up assessment (King et al. 2001). Thirteen of the 16 children had a normal school attendance at follow-up and did not endorse any new psychological problems.

Heyne et al. (2002) assigned 61 children (7–14 years) with school refusal (and at least one DSM-IV disorder) to one of three treatment conditions: child therapy (i.e., relaxation training, social skills training, cognitive therapy, and desensitization), parent-teacher training, and child therapy plus parent-teacher training. Overall, children from all treatment conditions demonstrated significant improvements in functioning at posttreatment. At follow-up, 69% of the participants no longer met criteria for an anxiety disorder, and 60% did not meet criteria for any disorder. Children in the combined treatment and parent-teacher training groups had a significantly better school attendance record than children in the child therapy group.

Research Directions

Further research is needed to define optimal treatments for school refusal and duration of acute and maintenance interventions. A focus on studying early intervention strategies will help to prevent difficult-to-treat chronic school refusal.

Summary Points

- Separation anxiety is normal for infants 6–30 months of age and typically intensifies between 13 and 18 months of age.
- The primary fear of children with SAD is that harm will come to themselves or their parents that will result in permanent separation.
- A multimodal treatment plan is beneficial for success in treating SAD and school refusal.
- An SSRI is the first-choice medication for treating SAD and school refusal.
- CBT is the psychosocial treatment of choice for treating SAD and school refusal.
- School refusal is not a DSM-IV diagnosis; it is a symptom that is commonly associated with anxiety or depressive disorders in youth.
- Youth with school refusal vary in their presentation; therefore, it is beneficial to conduct a multimodal assessment with multiple informants.
- School refusal behavior is often maintained through positive reinforcement (i.e., engagement in pleasant activities) and/or negative reinforcement (i.e., avoidance of unpleasant situations).

References

American Academy of Child and Adolescent Psychiatry: Practice parameter for the assessment and treatment of children and adolescents with anxiety disorders. J Am Acad Child Adolesc Psychiatry 46:267–283, 2007

American Psychiatric Association: Diagnostic and Statistical Manual of Mental Disorders, 3rd Edition, Revised. Washington, DC, American Psychiatric Association, 1987

American Psychiatric Association: Diagnostic and Statistical Manual of Mental Disorders, 4th Edition. Washington, DC, American Psychiatric Association, 1994

American Psychiatric Association: Diagnostic and Statistical Manual of Mental Disorders, 4th Edition, Text Revision. Washington, DC, American Psychiatric Association, 2000

Aschenbrand SG, Kendall PC, Webb A, et al: Is childhood separation anxiety disorder a predictor of adult panic disorder and agoraphobia? A seven-year longitudinal study. J Am Acad Child Adolesc Psychiatry 42:1478–1485, 2003

Battaglia M, Bertella S, Politi E, et al: Age at onset of panic disorder: influence of familial liability to the disease and of childhood separation anxiety disorder. Am J Psychiatry 152:1362–1364, 1995

Berg I, Jackson A: Teenage school refusers grow up: a follow-up study of 168 subjects, ten years on average after inpatient treatment. Br J Psychiatry 147:366–370, 1985

Bernstein GA, Warren SL, Massie ED, et al: Family dimensions in anxious-depressed school refusers. J Anxiety Disord 13:513–528, 1999

Bernstein GA, Borchardt CM, Perwien A, et al: Imipramine plus cognitive-behavioral therapy in the treatment of school refusal. J Am Acad Child Adolesc Psychiatry 39:276–283, 2000

Bernstein GA, Hektner JM, Borchardt CM, et al: Treatment of school refusal: one-year follow-up. J Am Acad Child Adolesc Psychiatry 40:206–213, 2001

Bernstein GA, Layne AE, Egan EA, et al: Maternal phobic anxiety and child anxiety. J Anxiety Disord 19:658–672, 2005a

Bernstein GA, Layne AE, Egan EA, et al: School-based interventions for anxious children. J Am Acad Child Adolesc Psychiatry 44:1118–1127, 2005b

Biederman J, Rosenbaum JF, Bolduc-Murphy EA, et al: A 3-year follow-up of children with and without behavioral inhibition. J Am Acad Child Adolesc Psychiatry 32:814–821, 1993

Biederman J, Faraone SV, Marrs A, et al: Panic disorder and agoraphobia in consecutively referred children and adolescents. J Am Acad Child Adolesc Psychiatry 36:214–223, 1997

Biederman J, Faraone SV, Hirshfeld-Becker DR, et al: Patterns of psychopathology and dysfunction in high-risk children of parents with panic disorder and major depression. Am J Psychiatry 158:49–57, 2001

Birmaher B, Brent DA, Chiappetta L, et al: Psychometric properties of the Screen for Child Anxiety Related Emotional Disorders Scale (SCARED): a replication study. J Am Acad Child Adolesc Psychiatry 38:1230–1236, 1999

Birmaher B, Axelson DA, Monk K, et al: Fluoxetine for the treatment of childhood anxiety disorders. J Am Acad Child Adolesc Psychiatry 42:415–423, 2003

Black B: Separation anxiety disorder and panic disorder, in Anxiety Disorders in Children and Adolescents. Edited by March JS. New York, Guilford, 1995, pp 212–234

Breton JJ, Bergeron L, Valla JP, et al: Quebec Child Mental Health Survey: prevalence of DSM-III-R mental health disorders. J Child Psychol Psychiatry 40:375–384, 1999

Choate M, Pincus D, Eyberg S, et al: Parent-child interaction therapy for treatment of separation anxiety disorder in young children: a pilot study. Cogn Behav Pract 12:126–135, 2005

Costello EJ, Angold A, Burns BJ, et al: The Great Smoky Mountains Study of Youth: goals, design, methods, and the prevalence of DSM-III-R disorders. Arch Gen Psychiatry 53:1129–1136, 1996

Dadds MR, Spence SH, Holland D, et al: Prevention and early intervention for anxiety disorders: a controlled trial. J Consult Clin Psychol 65:627–635, 1997

Dallaire DH, Weinraub M: Predicting children's separation anxiety at age 6: the contributions of infant-mother attachment security, maternal sensitivity, and maternal separation anxiety. Attach Hum Dev 7:393–408, 2005

Egger HL, Costello EJ, Angold A: School refusal and psychiatric disorders: a community study. J Am Acad Child Adolesc Psychiatry 42:797–807, 2003

Ehringer MA, Rhee SH, Young S, et al: Genetic and environmental contributions to common psychopathologies of childhood and adolescence: a study of twins and their siblings. J Abnorm Child Psychol 34:1–17, 2006

Eisen AR, Schaefer CE: Separation Anxiety in Children and Adolescents: An Individualized Approach to Assessment and Treatment. New York, Guilford, 2005

Emslie GJ, Rush J, Weinberg WA, et al: A double-blind randomized, placebo-controlled trial of fluoxetine in children and adolescents with depression. Arch Gen Psychiatry 54:1031–1037, 1997

Fagiolini A, Shear MK, Cassano GB, et al: Is lifetime separation anxiety a manifestation of a panic spectrum? CNS Spectr 3:63–72, 1998

Flakierska-Praquin N, Lindstrom M, Gillberg C: School phobia with separation anxiety disorder: a comparative 20- to 29-year follow-up study of 35 school refusers. Compr Psychiatry 38:17–22, 1997

Foley DL, Pickles A, Maes HM, et al: Course and short-term outcomes of separation anxiety disorder in a community sample of twins. J Am Acad Child Adolesc Psychiatry 43:1107–1114, 2004

Heyne D, King NJ, Tonge BJ, et al: Evaluation of child therapy and caregiver training in the treatment of school refusal. J Am Acad Child Adolesc Psychiatry 41:687–695, 2002

Hirshfeld-Becker DR, Biederman J: Rationale and principles for early interventions with young children at risk for anxiety disorders. Clin Child Fam Psychol Rev 5:161–172, 2002

Kagan J: Galen's Prophecy: Temperament in Human Nature. Boulder, CO, Westview Press, 1998

Kashani JH, Orvaschel H: A community study of anxiety in children and adolescents. Am J Psychiatry 147:313–318, 1990

Kearney CA: Identifying the function of school refusal behavior: a revision of the School Refusal Assessment Scale. J Psychopathol Behav Assess 24:235–245, 2002

Kearney CA, Albano AM: When Children Refuse School: A Cognitive-Behavioral Therapy Approach (Therapist Guide). San Antonio, TX, Psychological Corporation, 2000

Kearney CA, Albano AM: The functional profiles of school refusal behavior. Behav Modif 28:147–161, 2004

Kearney CA, Silverman WK: Measuring the function of school refusal behavior: the School Refusal Assessment Scale. J Clin Child Psychol 22:85–96, 1993

Kearney CA, Silverman WK: Family environment of youngsters with school refusal behavior: a synopsis with implications for assessment and treatment. Am J Fam Ther 23:59–72, 1995

Kearney CA, Tillotson CA: School attendance, in Handbook of Child Behavior Therapy. Edited by Watson TS, Gresham FM. New York, Plenum, 1998, pp 143–161

Kearney CA, Sims KE, Pursell CR, et al: Separation anxiety disorder in young children: a longitudinal and family analysis. J Clin Child Adolesc Psychol 32:593–598, 2003

King NJ, Bernstein GA: School refusal in children and adolescents: a review of the past 10 years. J Am Acad Child Adolesc Psychiatry 40:197–205, 2001

King NJ, Ollendick TH, Tonge BJ: School Refusal: Assessment and Treatment. Boston, MA, Allyn and Bacon, 1995

King NJ, Tonge BJ, Heyne D, et al: Cognitive-behavioral treatment of school-refusing children: a controlled evaluation. J Am Acad Child Adolesc Psychiatry 37:395–403, 1998

King NJ, Tonge BJ, Heyne D, et al: Cognitive-behavioral treatment of school-refusing children: maintenance of improvement at 3- to 5-year follow-up. Scand J Behav Ther 30:85–89, 2001

Klein RG, Koplewicz HS, Kanner A: Imipramine treatment of children with separation anxiety disorder. J Am Acad Child Adolesc Psychiatry 31:21–28, 1992

Last CG, Strauss CC: School refusal in anxiety-disordered children and adolescents. J Am Acad Child Adolesc Psychiatry 29:31–35, 1990

Last CG, Strauss CC, Francis G: Comorbidity among childhood anxiety disorders. J Nerv Ment Dis 175:726–730, 1987

Last CG, Perrin S, Hersen M, et al: DSM-III-R anxiety disorders in children: sociodemographic and clinical characteristics. J Am Acad Child Adolesc Psychiatry 31:1070–1076, 1992

Manassis K, Bradley S: The development of childhood anxiety disorders: toward an integrated model. J Appl Dev Psychol 15:345–366, 1994

Manicavasagar V, Silove D, Hadzi Pavlovic D: Subpopulations of early separation anxiety: relevance to risk of adult anxiety disorders. J Affect Disord 48:181–190, 1998

Manicavasagar V, Silove D, Curtis J, et al: Continuities of separation anxiety from early life into adulthood. J Anxiety Disord 14:1–18, 2000

March JS, Parker JDA, Sullivan K, et al: The Multidimensional Anxiety Scale for Children (MASC): factor structure, reliability, and validity. J Am Acad Child Adolesc Psychiatry 36:554–565, 1997

Martin C, Cabrol S, Bouvard MP, et al: Anxiety and depressive disorders in fathers and mothers of anxious school-refusing children. J Am Acad Child Adolesc Psychiatry 38:916–922, 1999

Masi G, Favilla L, Mucci M, et al: Depressive comorbidity in children and adolescents with generalized anxiety disorder. Child Psychiatry Hum Dev 30:205–215, 2000

Masi G, Mucci M, Millepiedi S: Separation anxiety disorder in children and adolescents: epidemiology, diagnosis, and management. CNS Drugs 15:93–104, 2001

McShane G, Walter G, Rey JM: Characteristics of adolescents with school refusal. Aust N Z J Psychiatry 35:822–826, 2001

Merikangas KR, Dierker LC, Szatmari P: Psychopathology among offspring of parents with substance abuse and/or anxiety disorders: a high-risk study. J Child Psychiatry 39:711–720, 1998

Muris P, Meesters C, Merckelbach H, et al: Worry in normal children. J Am Acad Child Adolesc Psychiatry 37:703–710, 1998

Ollendick TH, King NJ: Assessment practices and issues with school-refusing children. Behav Change 15:16–30, 1998

Ollendick TH, Mayer JA: School phobia, in Behavioral Theories and Treatment of Anxiety. Edited by Turner SM. New York, Plenum, 1984, pp 367–411

Peleg O, Halaby E, Whaby E: The relationship of maternal separation anxiety and differentiation of self to children's separation anxiety and adjustment to kindergarten: a study in Druze families. J Anxiety Disord 20:973–995, 2006

Pincus D, Eyberg S, Choate M: Adapting parent-child interaction therapy for young children with separation anxiety disorder. Education and Treatment of Children 28:163–181, 2005

Rapee RM: Potential role of childrearing practices in the development of anxiety and depression. Clin Psychol Rev 17:47–67, 1997

Research Unit on Pediatric Psychopharmacology Anxiety Study Group: Fluvoxamine for the treatment of anxiety disorders in children and adolescents. N Engl J Med 344:1279–1285, 2001

Reynolds CR, Kamphaus RW: Behavior Assessment System for Children, 2nd Edition. Circle Pines, MN, American Guidance Service, 2004

Rynn MA, Siqueland L, Rickels K: Placebo-controlled trial of sertraline in the treatment of children with generalized anxiety disorder. Am J Psychiatry 158:2008–2014, 2001

Shear K, Jin R, Ruscio AM, et al: Prevalence and correlates of estimated DSM-IV child and adult separation anxiety disorder in the National Comorbidity Survey Replication. Am J Psychiatry 163:1074–1083, 2006

Silove D, Manicavasagar V, Drobny J: Associations between juvenile and adult forms of separation anxiety disorder: a study of adult volunteers with histories of school refusal. J Nerv Ment Dis 190:413–415, 2002

Silverman WK, Albano AM: Anxiety Disorders Interview Schedule for DSM-IV: Child Version, Child and Parent Interview Schedules. San Antonio, TX, Psychological Corporation, 1996

Suveg C, Schenbrand SG, Kendall PC: Separation anxiety disorder, panic disorder, and school refusal. Child Adolesc Psychiatr Clin N Am 14:773–795, 2005

Velting ON, Setzer NJ, Albano AM: Update on and advances in assessment and cognitive-behavioral treatment of anxiety disorders in children and adolescents. Prof Psychol Res Pr 35:42–54, 2004

Verduin TL, Kendall PC: Differential occurrence of comorbidity within childhood anxiety disorders. J Clin Child Adolesc Psychol 32:290–295, 2003

Wagner KD, Berard R, Stein MB, et al: A multicenter, randomized, double-blind, placebo-controlled trial of paroxetine in children and adolescents with social anxiety disorder. Arch Gen Psychiatry 61:1153–1162, 2004

Walkup JT, Albano AM, Piacentini J, et al: Cognitive behavioral therapy, sertraline, or a combination in childhood anxiety. N Engl J Med 359:2753–2766, 2008

Wood JJ: Parental intrusiveness and children's separation anxiety in a clinical sample. Child Psychiatry Hum Dev 37:73–87, 2006

Chapter 22

Posttraumatic Stress Disorder

Judith A. Cohen, M.D.
Anthony P. Mannarino, Ph.D.

Posttraumatic stress disorder (PTSD) was first introduced into the *Diagnostic and Statistical Manual of Mental Disorders* (DSM) in 1980, making it one of the more recently accepted psychiatric disorders. PTSD is one of the few DSM diagnoses to have a recognizable etiologic agent, in that it must develop in direct response to a severe (sudden, terrifying, or shocking) life event (American Psychiatric Association 2000). Since the introduction of PTSD into DSM-III (American Psychiatric Association 1980), the disorder has been documented in children exposed to traumas such as domestic violence, natural disasters, medical trauma, war, terrorism, and community violence. Much has been learned about the developmental manifestations of PTSD and how challenging it is to evaluate this disorder in children. Progress has been made in identifying effective treatments for this disorder, but much remains unknown.

Definition, Clinical Description, and Diagnosis

In DSM-IV (American Psychiatric Association 1994) and its text revision, DSM-IV-TR (American Psychiatric Association 2000), PTSD is categorized as an anxiety disorder. It has several features in common with other anxiety disorders, particularly panic disorder and general anxiety disorder (GAD; see Table 22–1). PTSD is defined by the presence of the following: a) experiencing, hearing about, or witnessing a qualifying traumatic event (for example, child abuse; community, domestic, or school violence; natural or man-made disasters; war or terrorism; medical traumas; vehicular or other serious accidents; sudden or violent death of someone close to the child) in which the child's reaction involves intense fear, helpless-

TABLE 22–1. DSM-IV-TR Cluster B, C, and D PTSD symptoms in children and adolescents

Cluster B: Reexperiencing symptoms

Recurrent distressing thoughts about the trauma

Recurrent nightmares about the trauma

Repetitive play about the trauma

Trauma-specific reenactment

Illusions, flashbacks, feelings that trauma is recurring

Psychological distress at reminders

Physiological reactivity to reminders

Cluster C: Avoidant and numbing symptoms

Efforts to avoid thoughts, feelings, conversations

Efforts to avoid activities, places, people

Inability to recall important aspects of the trauma

Markedly decreased interest

Feelings of detachment/estrangement

Restricted range of affect

Sense of foreshortened future

Cluster D: Hyperarousal

Trouble falling or staying asleep

Increased irritability, anger, temper outbursts

Trouble concentrating

Hypervigilance

Exaggerated startle response

ness, or horror, or disorganized or agitated behavior; b) at least one persistent reexperiencing symptom; c) at least three persistent avoidant or numbing symptoms; d) at least two persistent hyperarousal symptoms; e) duration of these symptoms for more than 1 month; and f) clinically significant distress or impairment in at least one important area of functioning (American Psychiatric Association 2000, p. 467). Experts on early childhood trauma (Scheeringa et al. 2001, 2006; Zero to Three 2005) have developed alternative criteria for diagnosing PTSD in infants, toddlers, and preschoolers.

Scheeringa et al. (2006) have shown that decreasing the number of required Cluster C symptoms from three to two significantly improved diagnostic reliability of these criteria for prepubertal children. Another study showed that children with subthreshold PTSD symptoms have similar degrees of functional impairment to those meeting full diagnostic criteria (Carrion et al. 2002). Based on these studies, a reasonable approach is

for children with significant PTSD symptoms (i.e., a sufficient number or severity to cause clinical impairment) to receive evidence-informed treatment for PTSD, even in the absence of full diagnostic criteria.

Epidemiology and Risk Factors

PTSD is more common among girls than boys. Preliminary evidence suggests that youth with poorer performance on neurocognitive tests prior to trauma exposure are more vulnerable to developing PTSD (Parslow and Jorm 2007). A variety of risk factors have been identified for developing PTSD after disaster exposure and include increased media viewing of the disaster (Pfefferbaum et al. 1999), experiencing panic symptoms in the immediate aftermath of the disaster (Pfefferbaum et al. 2006; Thienkrua et al. 2006), having a delayed evacuation, having felt one's own or a family's member's life was in danger (Thienkrua et al. 2006), and presence of a predisaster anxiety disorder (LaGreca et al. 1998).

Comorbidity

Comorbidity appears to be the rule rather the exception in child cohorts with PTSD. These children commonly have depressive, other anxiety, and/or behavioral problems. Some child samples have shown comorbidity of up to 60% with depressive disorders; this is consistent with adult PTSD cohorts. Externalizing symptoms are common as well; comorbid conditions may include attention-deficit/hyperactivity disorder (ADHD) or oppositional or conduct disorders. Older children and adolescents may engage in substance use or abuse. These behaviors may represent attempts to avoid trauma reminders or may be signs of an independent substance use disorder. Dialogue is ongoing regarding whether youth develop "complex PTSD," and if so, how the clinical manifestations of this differ from the combination of PTSD and existing comorbid conditions (Briere and Spinazzola 2005).

Etiology

As noted above, in order to develop PTSD, children must have experienced or learned about a serious traumatic event. DSM-IV-TR defines this as "extreme"—that is, the type of event that has the potential to threaten the child's or a significant other's physical integrity, safety, or life. DSM-IV also states that the cause must be traumatic—i.e., shocking, terrifying, and/or unexpected. It is important to take into account developmental and cognitive factors when considering the nature of extreme stressors, however. For example, Lieberman et al. (2003) suggest that parental death from any cause is traumatic for children under 6 years old, because these children are so dependent on parents for their core sense of safety and security. As another example, even a death that was "expected" (such as one due to cancer) may be shocking and completely unanticipated by children who did not believe the person would die. Such children may develop PTSD or another condition, childhood traumatic grief (see Chapter 33, "Bereavement and Traumatic Grief"). In addition to the requirement of an extreme trauma, there is intriguing evidence of a genetic predisposition related to the development of PTSD (Seedat et al. 2001; M. Stein et al. 2002).

Prevention

Early identification of at-risk children may be possible through early screening of children exposed to trauma. This is particularly crucial after community-level traumas such as disasters, in which large numbers of children may be affected. School- or community-based screening and treatment may be the most efficient way to serve many of these children, who would not otherwise receive such interventions. Screening instruments such as the UCLA PTSD Reaction Index for DSM-IV or the Child PTSD Symptom Scale (CPSS; Foa et al. 2001) have been used successfully for school screening and treatment studies.

Widespread screening following a large-scale disaster may require triage by nonprofessional mental health workers. PsySTART is a 13-question instrument that can be used for rapid triage; it was used after the 2004 Asian tsunami to inquire about experiences rather than symptoms. The PsySTART tag successfully predicted risk factors for developing PTSD and depression 9 months posttsunami in 7- to 14-year-old children (Thienkrua et al. 2006).

Course and Prognosis

There is some evidence that "natural recovery" from PTSD occurs in children—i.e., that the overall percent-age of children qualifying for a PTSD diagnosis decreases over time (LaGreca et al. 1998), although other studies have not found a natural decrease over time (McFarlane 1987; Scheeringa et al. 2005). Researchers agree that for a core group of children, PTSD symptoms persist, and for these children, without effective intervention the prognosis is grim. Well-controlled longitudinal studies of adults who have experienced childhood traumas indicate that PTSD is a significant risk factor for increased suicide attempts, major depression, dissociation, and impaired global emotional functioning (Warshaw et al. 1993).

Clinical Evaluation

The following information pertains to clinical rather than forensic evaluations. PTSD is one of the most challenging disorders to accurately diagnose in children and adolescents. Clinicians face the paradox of needing children to describe experiences that the very essence of this disorder makes them avoid thinking and talking about. Many PTSD diagnostic criteria are not even comprehensible to young children, who are not developmentally capable of describing complex internal experiences or emotional states. Clinicians assessing these children should be familiar with the previously described diagnostic criteria for very young children and how to conduct a clinical interview with parents to elicit these children's PTSD symptoms (Zero to Three 2005).

Multiple Informants

As with any child psychiatric evaluation, assessing children for possible PTSD requires information from multiple sources. This should always include information from the child and parent or caretaker, although for very young children, information from the child will primarily consist of observational data. In assessing PTSD, the family may not want the school to know the child is receiving an evaluation due to privacy concerns and will need to be assured about confidentiality if this is appropriate. In some cases it may be necessary or possible to complete the evaluation without receiving teacher reports. In many instances, the evaluation of a child for PTSD will also include obtaining records and possibly additional information from a pediatrician, forensic evaluator, police investigator, or child protection worker, if there was alleged child abuse prior to coming to the evaluation. Agencies such as crime victims assistance programs, domestic violence shelters, child advocacy center, and/or other therapists or agencies or that provide services to the child and family might serve as useful supplemental sources of information.

Rating Scales and Standardized Interviews

Evaluators should consider using rating scales for assessing PTSD. Several validated self- and parent-report instruments are available for this purpose, including the UCLA PTSD Reaction Index for DSM-IV, the CPSS, and others. Some children are more comfortable acknowledging symptoms on a paper-and-pencil instrument than in a face-to-face interview, or vice versa. Providing both venues may optimize the evaluator's opportunity to learn about the child's symptoms. Semistructured interviews for PTSD (reviewed in American Academy of Child and Adolescent Psychiatry 1998) are also available, but are too time-consuming to be feasible for most clinical settings.

Differential Diagnosis

Other psychiatric conditions may manifest with symptoms similar to those seen in PTSD. Children with PTSD may appear to have ADHD due to poor attention, restlessness, hyperactivity, and disorganized and/or agitated play. Hyperarousal symptoms such as difficulty sleeping and poor concentration may also mimic ADHD. Unless clinicians obtain a careful history regarding the timing of onset or worsening of these symptoms in relation to trauma exposure, it may be impossible to distinguish these conditions. PTSD may also mimic oppositional defiant disorder due to hyperarousal symptoms presenting as angry outbursts or irritability. These symptoms may be particularly prominent if the child is exposed to modeling of anger as a successful strategy for controlling one's environment (for example, living with a perpetrator of domestic violence or in a context of ongoing bullying).

PTSD may present as panic disorder or social anxiety disorder if the child has striking anxiety and distress upon exposure to reminders of the trauma and avoidance of talking about the traumatic event. PTSD may be difficult to distinguish from other anxiety disorders if children develop phobias, fears, or avoidance of cues associated with their traumatic experiences. PTSD may also mimic major depressive disorder due to the presence of self-injury as a means of avoidant coping; sleep problems; social withdrawal; and/or affective numbing. PTSD may also be misdiagnosed as a primary substance use disorder since drugs and/or alcohol may be used to numb and avoid trauma reminders. Conversely, it is important to keep in mind that youth with a trauma history may have a primary substance use disorder with few trauma symptoms; such youth will likely benefit more from receiving interventions for substance use disorder rather than PTSD.

PTSD may be misdiagnosed as bipolar disorder. Some children with PTSD, particularly those who have been abused or exposed to ongoing domestic violence, may present with severe affective, behavioral, and/or cognitive dysregulation. These problems may be due to experiencing physiological changes as well as having been forced to tolerate ongoing abuse without protest. Such children may display extreme outbursts of anger, silliness, confusion, sexualized behavior, aggression, self-injury, and other symptoms suggestive of bipolar disorder. It is also possible for PTSD and bipolar disorder to coexist. Obtaining a history of trauma exposure and how this may be influencing symptoms is critically important in accurately diagnosing these children.

PTSD should also be distinguished from psychotic disorders, which PTSD may mimic due to the presence of flashbacks, hypervigilance, sleep disturbance, numbing, and/or social withdrawal. PTSD should also be differentiated from milder adjustment disorders. PTSD can mimic physical conditions including migraine, asthma, caffeinism, seizure disorder, hyperthyroidism and side effects from a variety of prescription medications and nonprescription drugs. PTSD is often associated with somatic symptoms such as headaches and abdominal pain. Children presenting with significant medical symptoms of unknown origin with a history of trauma should be considered for a mental health evaluation, which should include a complete assessment for PTSD symptoms.

Clinical Examination and Mental Status Findings

Evaluators may have particular difficulty distinguishing avoidance from oppositional behavior ("I don't want to talk about it") or appropriate resolution of a troubling experience ("I'm over it, and I'm tired of everyone asking me about that stuff"). One way to assess this is to ask the child to describe the experience "so I can reassure your parent who is concerned about you that everything is really okay." Another is to evaluate the child's adaptive functioning: if the child is doing well in most domains (school, friends, family, self-image, neurovegetative functioning) and has no apparent dysfunctional thoughts about the traumatic experience or PTSD or other psychiatric symptoms, the clinician may judge this avoidance to be adaptive. Avoidant symptoms may alternate with reexperiencing symptoms; at times children may have a predominance of one or the other. Finally, as always, the clinician should discuss these findings with the parent as the parent's reason for coming for the evaluation and other information may be pertinent in coming to any conclusion.

Treatment

Among the available treatments for childhood PTSD, there is more evidence for trauma-focused psychotherapy (i.e., therapies that specifically address and focus on children's traumatic experiences) than for pharmacotherapies. Therefore, in most cases, clinicians should provide children with evidence-based psychotherapy prior to starting medication unless there is a compelling reason to do otherwise. In some cases, there may be justification for starting medication immediately; for example, there may be a comorbid condition for which there is a proven pharmacological treatment, the child may be so dysregulated or dangerous that a medication is required for immediate safety, or the child is unable to function without the immediate addition of medication for another reason (e.g., sleep is severely impaired and the condition has not responded to reasonable psychosocial interventions). Since psychotherapeutic treatments are preferred as a first-line intervention in most cases, these are described first.

Psychotherapeutic Treatments

Several evidence-based treatment models are currently available for children with PTSD symptoms. These models have a number of common principles, concepts, and components that have guided their development and cut across their differences in orientation, style, format, and specific content. The National Child Traumatic Stress Network (www.NCTSN.org) is developing an in-depth information base and has a work group to identify core components of evidence-based practices for traumatized children (Chorpita et al. 2007). Underlying tenets of effective treatments for children with PTSD include the following:

1. Developmental sensitivity
2. Informed by the neurobiological impact of trauma on children
3. Include parents/caretakers/families (i.e., show an awareness of the centrality of the family constellation in children's lives)
4. Cultural sensitivity in the broadest sense of "culture"
5. Reestablish safety/trust
6. Address trauma reminders
7. Address significant areas of dysfunction (for example, cognitive distortions regarding the trauma; negative child-parent interactions; school problems) in order to regain optimal developmental trajectory and momentum

In matching evidence-based or evidence-informed treatments to specific children with PTSD or PTSD symptoms, clinicians should consider each child's developmental level; the setting in which it is either most efficient to provide services or most likely that the child/family will comply with receiving them; acceptability of different treatments in terms of duration, cost, privacy, and cultural match for a given family; comorbid conditions the child may have; type of trauma; and perhaps other individual factors. These factors are addressed in the following description of the well-established evidence-based models for childhood PTSD.

Trauma-Focused Cognitive-Behavioral Therapy

The core components of trauma-focused cognitive-behavioral therapy (TF-CBT) are summarized by the acronym PRACTICE: Psychoeducation, Parenting skills, Relaxation, Affective modulation, Cognitive processing, Trauma narrative, In vivo mastery of trauma memories, Conjoint child-parent sessions, and Enhancing safety (Cohen et al. 2005).

TF-CBT has the strongest evidence base for traumatized children with six published randomized controlled trials (RCTs) of more than 500 sexually abused and multiply traumatized children ages 3–17 years old. These trials demonstrated the superiority of TF-CBT over comparison treatments or a waitlist condition in improving PTSD as well as depressive, anxiety, behavioral, shame, and other symptoms in children (Cohen and Mannarino 1996, 1998; Cohen et al. 2004; Deblinger et al. 1996; King et al. 2000). Several of these studies also documented differential improvement in the personal symptoms and parenting skills for those parents who participated in TF-CBT treatment. TF-CBT has also been used for children exposed to traumatic grief (described in Chapter 33, "Bereavement and Traumatic Grief"), terrorism, natural disasters and domestic violence (e.g., Hoagwood and The CATS Consortium 2009).

Cognitive-Behavioral Interventions for Trauma in Schools

A parallel treatment model to TF-CBT, cognitive-behavioral intervention for trauma in schools (CBITS) provides similar PRACTICE components described in TF-CBT, with the exception that CBITS is provided in group therapy, which is conducted during the school day at the child's home school and therefore parental involvement typically does not occur. In the CBITS model, the trauma narrative occurs in individual "breakout" sessions with the group therapist. Advantages of school-based treatments such as CBITS include that they may greatly improve accessibility and acceptability of treatment for families who cannot or will not seek clinic-based services. Additionally, children may experience a decreased sense of stigmatization and improvement of other symptoms specifically through participating in group treatment. CBITS has been compared to a waitlist condition in one RCT and one quasi-RCT for children exposed to community violence, including primarily Latino immigrant children (Kataoka et al. 2003; B.D. Stein et al. 2003). It has also been used for children exposed to disasters.

Child-Parent Psychotherapy

For very young traumatized children, child-parent psychotherapy (CPP) is a relationship-based model delivered in joint child-parent treatment sessions focusing on improving interactions between the young child and his or her parent. Often the parent or caregiver has also experienced trauma as well, so this treatment allows both child and parent to learn improved ways of interacting, as well as correcting dysfunctional thoughts and developing a joint trauma narrative. In one RCT, young children (ages 3–7 years old) who participated in CPP with their domestic violence–exposed mothers experienced significantly greater improvement in PTSD and behavioral symptoms than those who received case management and individual psychotherapy (Lieberman et al. 2005). CPP has also been adapted for young children experiencing traumatic grief, as described in Chapter 33, "Bereavement and Traumatic Grief."

Cognitive-Based Cognitive-Behavioral Therapy

An individual trauma-focused CBT with a slightly different focus from TF-CBT has recently been tested for single-episode traumas in one RCT and found to be superior to a waitlist control for decreasing PTSD symptoms (Smith et al. 2007). In examining the impact of cognitive distortions, this study demonstrated that correcting cognitions partially mediated improvement in the CBT group only. This suggests that the underlying cognitive framework of the model is working as proposed.

Surviving Cancer Competently Intervention Program

A group and family-based CBT treatment for adolescent survivors of cancer, the Surviving Cancer Competently Intervention Program (SCCIP) is provided in a four-session, 1-day format to teens, siblings, and parents. SCCIP was compared to a waitlist control in one RCT and found to be superior in improving hyperarousal symptoms in teens (Kazak et al. 2004).

UCLA Trauma/Grief Program for Adolescents

The UCLA Trauma/Grief Program for Adolescents is a cognitive-behaviorally based group treatment model that includes five modules sequentially addressing trauma- and grief-related issues. It is typically provided in school settings. It has been used in quasi-randomized and open studies internationally and in the United States for youth exposed to disasters, terrorism, war, and community violence (Goenjian et al. 1997; Hoagwood and The CATS Consortium 2009; Layne et al. 2001; Saltzman et al. 2001). These studies have provided preliminary evidence that this model improves PTSD symptoms.

Trauma Systems Therapy

Trauma systems therapy (TST) combines an individual intervention such as TF-CBT with a more systematic approach for children with complex needs. For example, TST includes acute stabilization up to and including inpatient hospitalization; psychotropic medication management; intensive home-based behavioral or family-based interventions; and liaison with multiple other systems including medical, justice, child welfare, child protection, educational, and law enforcement. TST was associated with improvement in children's PTSD symptoms in one open trial (Saxe et al. 2005).

Other Psychosocial Treatments

Treatments are being developed and tested for traumatized children with "complex trauma" and a variety of comorbid conditions. One example is Seeking Safety, a treatment for adolescents with comorbid PTSD and substance use disorders. This treatment was originally developed and tested for adults. It has since been tested for adolescents in a small pilot study with positive outcomes for PTSD (Najavits et al. 2006). Treatments for youth with complex trauma, such as Structured Psychotherapy for Adolescents Recovering from Chronic Stress (SPARCS) and Life Skills/Life Story (www.NCTSN.org) are currently being tested in pilot studies with promising results.

In the wake of the September 11, 2001, terrorist attacks, interest has grown regarding optimal strategies for disseminating and implementing evidence-based treatments for traumatized children. One novel approach is using a Web-based curriculum to train large numbers of clinicians in the TF-CBT model. More than 35,000 learners from over 60 countries registered for this online course (www.musc.edu/tfcbt) during its first 36 months. Surveys showed that completers gained significant knowledge about TF-CBT and had high levels of satisfaction in using the course (B. Saunders, personal communication, May 2, 2007). The National Child Traumatic Stress Network (www.nctsn.org) is also using innovative dissemination strategies, including adaptation of the Institute for Healthcare Improvement's (www.ihi.org) learning collaborative model to spread innovative evidence-based treatments community-wide. TF-CBT, CPP, TST, and SPARCS learning collaboratives have been sponsored by the NCTSN, individual states, and other organizations within the United States and internationally. Preliminary data suggest that these are successfully spreading evidence-based treatments to participant agencies and communities.

Pharmacological Treatments

A number of neurotransmitter systems have been studied regarding the development and maintenance of PTSD symptoms. Many medications are prescribed for children with PTSD symptoms and include antiadrenergic agents, anticonvulsants, antidepressants, morphine, novel antipsychotics, and others, but little evidence exists regarding their efficacy. Only two double blind RCTs have been completed for childhood PTSD. The first study found that imipramine was superior to chloral hydrate when provided in a double blind fashion for 7 days for treating acute stress disorder symptoms among 25 hospitalized children ages 2–19 years with acute burns (Robert et al. 1999). Because of safety concerns related to cardiac conduction delays, imipramine would not be considered as a first-line treatment outside of hospital or other settings where electrocardiogram (ECG) monitoring is feasible. The second study found that TF-CBT+sertraline did not outperform TF-CBT+placebo in treating PTSD symptoms in 10–17-year-old children; both groups experienced significant improvement in PTSD as well as depressive and other symptoms (Cohen et al. 2007).

Small open trials have suggested the potential benefit of selective serotonin reuptake inhibitors (SSRIs) (e.g., Seedat et al. 2002), propranolol (Famularo et al. 1988), and clonidine (Harmon and Riggs 1996; Perry 1994) for treating childhood PTSD. Open trials have been conducted with two additional medications, neither of which would typically be routinely prescribed for traumatized children in outpatient settings. Saxe et al. (2001) conducted a naturalistic study examining morphine dosages for acutely burned children who required hospitalization. These researchers documented a linear association between mean morphine dosage (mg/kg/day) and 6-month reduction in PTSD symptoms, after controlling for subjective experience of pain. Morphine would likely be considered a first-line treatment for PTSD only among acutely injured or possibly other acutely traumatized children seen in hospital settings. An open trial using risperidone demonstrated remission from severe PTSD symptoms in 13 of 18 boys (Horrigan and Barnhill 1999). This cohort had high rates of serious comorbid conditions (e.g., bipolar disorder, ADHD, aggression); such factors would need to be weighed carefully when considering potential risks versus potential benefits of using atypical antipsychotic medications in children.

Due to the strong placebo effect in children, it is important not to assume that because a child's PTSD symptoms improve after taking a prescribed medication that this was due to the medication. Once the child seems to respond, the temptation is to leave the child on this medication, even if the symptoms then return. It is essential to carefully balance the potential risks and benefits in such situations, particularly since there is no empirical evidence to back up such prescribing practices. An alternative approach would be to decrease or to discontinue the medication, rather than increasing the dose, if symptoms recur, under an alternative assumption that the response was not due to medication in the first place but was rather a placebo response. This has the advantages of not continuing children on ineffective medications, avoiding unnecessary and possibly detrimental polypharmacy, and using a rational pharmacology approach to prescribing. Current recommendations are to provide children who have PTSD with trauma-focused psychotherapy as a first-line treatment, prior to starting medication, unless there is a clear indication that medication is warranted (American Academy of Child and Adolescent Psychiatry, in press).

Other Treatments

Eye movement desensitization and reprocessing (EMDR) is effective in decreasing PTSD symptoms in adults (Chemtob et al. 2000). It has been adapted for children and tested in one well-controlled trial, which showed that children receiving EMDR demonstrated more improvement in reexperiencing symptoms—but not in avoidance or hyperarousal symptoms—than a waitlist control group (Ahmad and Sundelin-Wahlstein 2008). Debate is ongoing regarding the mechanism of efficacy for EMDR; these authors noted that their adaptation was effective for children due to its similarity to cognitive therapy.

Unproven techniques, such as severely restricting movement through binding, restricting nutritional intake, or using "rebirthing" techniques, are sometimes used for traumatized children. These interventions have led to serious complications, including death. Professional organizations, including the American Academy of Child and Adolescent Psychiatry (www.aacap.org) and the American Professional Society on the Abuse of Children (www.apsac.org), recommend that these interventions not be used.

Research Directions

More research is needed regarding the interactions of genes, environmental risk, and protective factors and exposure to trauma. We also need to know more about whether psychosocial, pharmacological, and combined treatment have the potential to impact the adverse neurobiological effects of trauma. Important questions remain about how to treat children with PTSD who do not respond to the existing treatments, most notably those with serious comorbid psychiatric conditions such as substance use disorder, suicidality and other self-injurious behaviors, dissociation, and/or disruptive behavior problems. Only one RCT has been conducted using combined psychotherapy and pharmacotherapy, yet this is the treatment many children with PTSD with comorbid conditions receive in community settings and likely the types of treatments children with complex clinical presentations will need. More research of this type is needed; in light of the current FDA black box warnings and realistic safety concerns, it is unclear when or whether such research will occur.

Finally, it has become increasingly clear that developing and testing effective treatments for traumatized children are only the first of several necessary steps in improving outcomes for these children. In order to accomplish this goal, it will be essential to learn how to effectively disseminate and implement these treatments in the community settings where these children live and receive care. Even more critically important, we need to learn optimal strategies to identify and reach traumatized children who are not receiving any mental health services. Thus research efforts aimed at optimal training, dissemination, and implementation strategies for community therapists and identification and treatment strategies for traumatized children based in community settings such as schools, afterschool programs, daycare, or primary care settings will be crucial next steps for researchers.

Summary Points

- PTSD is one of the most difficult conditions to accurately diagnose in children. Clinicians need to anchor symptoms to a specific traumatic event; ask about symptoms in developmentally appropriate ways; obtain information from parents or other caretakers as well as from children; and realize that avoidance leads to underreporting in many cases.

- Although natural recovery can occur, many children do not spontaneously recover from PTSD. Children with subsyndromal PTSD symptoms often experience the same functional impairments as those meeting full diagnostic criteria. When the clinician is in doubt, children need treatment.

- Effective treatments are available for childhood PTSD throughout the developmental spectrum, from infants to adolescents.

- In general, treatment should start with psychotherapy, not pharmacotherapy, unless there is a clear reason to give medication (e.g., a comorbid diagnosis for which there is an effective pharmacotherapy, clear dangerousness requiring immediate medication, or symptoms so severe that psychotherapy is deemed unable to provide relief).

- Parents should be included in trauma-focused therapy whenever feasible; however, therapy should not be denied to children if parents are not available. School-based treatments can provide access to treatment for children who might not otherwise receive it.

- Resources for clinicians, parents, and teachers are available at: www.NCTSN.org.

References

Ahmad A, Sundelin-Wahlstein V: Applying EMDR on children with PTSD. Eur Child Adolesc Psychiatry 17:127–132, 2008

American Academy of Child and Adolescent Psychiatry: Practice parameters for the assessment and treatment of children and adolescents with posttraumatic stress disorder. J Am Acad Child Adolesc Psychiatry 37(suppl): 4S–28S, 1998

American Academy of Child and Adolescent Psychiatry: Revised practice parameters for the assessment and treatment of children and adolescents with posttraumatic stress disorder. J Am Acad Child Adolesc Psychiatry, in press

American Psychiatric Association: Diagnostic and Statistical Manual of Mental Disorders, 3rd Edition. Washington, DC, American Psychiatric Association, 1980

American Psychiatric Association: Diagnostic and Statistical Manual of Mental Disorders, 4th Edition. Washington, DC, American Psychiatric Association, 1994

American Psychiatric Association: Diagnostic and Statistical Manual of Mental Disorders, 4th Edition, Text Revision. Washington, DC, American Psychiatric Association, 2000

Briere J, Spinazzola J: Phenomenology and psychological assessment of complex posttraumatic states. J Trauma Stress 18:401–412, 2005

Carrion VG, Weems CF, Ray R, et al: Toward an empirical definition of pediatric PTSD: the phenomenology of PTSD symptoms in youth. J Am Acad Child Adolesc Psychiatry 41:166–173, 2002

Chemtob CM, Tolin DF, van der Kolk BA, et al: Eye movement desensitization and reprocessing, in Effective Treatments for PTSD. Edited by Foa EB, Keane TM, Friedman MJ. New York, Guilford, 2000, pp 139–154

Chorpita BF, Becker KD, Baleiden EL: Understanding the common elements of evidence-based practice: misconceptions and clinical examples. J Am Acad Child Adolesc Psychiatry 46:647–652, 2007

Cohen JA, Mannarino AP: A treatment outcome study for sexually abused preschool children: initial findings. J Am Acad Child Adolesc Psychiatry 35:42–50, 1996

Cohen JA, Mannarino AP: Interventions for sexually abused children: initial treatment outcome findings. Child Maltreatment 3:17–26, 1998

Cohen JA, Deblinger E, Mannarino AP, et al: A multisite, randomized controlled trial for children with sexual abuse-related PTSD symptoms. J Am Acad Child Adolesc Psychiatry 43:393–402, 2004

Cohen JA, Mannarino AP, Knudsen K: Treating sexually abused children: one year follow-up of a randomized controlled trial. Child Abuse Negl 29:135–145, 2005

Cohen JA, Mannarino AP, Perel JM, et al: A pilot randomized controlled trial of combined trauma-focused CBT and sertraline for childhood PTSD symptoms. J Am Acad Child Adolesc Psychiatry 46:811–819, 2007

Deblinger E, Lippmann J, Steer R: Sexually abused children suffering posttraumatic stress symptoms: initial treatment outcome findings. Child Maltreat 1:310–321, 1996

Famularo R, Kinscherff R, Fenton R: Propranolol treatment for childhood posttraumatic stress disorder, acute type: a pilot study. Am J Dis Child 142:1244–1247, 1988

Foa EB, Johnson K, Feeney NC, et al: The Child PTSD Symptom Scale (CSPP): a preliminary examination of its psychometric properties. J Clin Child Psychol 30:376–384, 2001

Goenjian AK, Karayan I, Pynoos RS, et al: Outcome of psychotherapy among early adolescents after trauma. Am J Psychiatry 154:536–542, 1997

Harmon RJ, Riggs PD: Clinical perspectives: clonidine for posttraumatic stress disorder in preschool children. J Am Acad Child Adolesc Psychiatry 35:1247–1249, 1996

Hoagwood KE, The CATS Consortium: Implementation of cognitive-behavioral therapy for children and adolescents affected by the World Trade Center disaster. Manuscript submitted for publication, 2009

Horrigan JP, Barnhill LJ: Risperidone and PTSD in boys. J Neuropsychiatry Clin Neurosci 11:126–127, 1999

Kataoka SH, Stein BD, Jaycox LH, et al: A school-based mental health program for traumatized Latino immigrant children. J Am Acad Child Adolesc Psychiatry 42:311–318, 2003

Kazak AE, Alderfer MA, Streisand R, et al: Treatment of posttraumatic stress symptoms in adolescent survivors of childhood cancer and their families: a randomized clinical trial. J Fam Psychol 18:493–504, 2004

King NJ, Tonge BJ, Mullen P, et al: Treating sexually abused children with posttraumatic stress symptoms: a randomized controlled trial. J Am Acad Child Adolesc Psychiatry 39:1347–1355, 2000

LaGreca AM, Silverman WK, Wasserstein SB: Children's predisaster functioning as a predictor of posttraumatic stress symptoms following Hurricane Andrew. J Consult Clin Psychol 66:883–892, 1998

Layne CM, Pynoos RS, Saltzman WR, et al: Trauma/grief-focused group psychotherapy: school-based postwar intervention with traumatized Bosnian adolescents. Group Dyn 5:277–290, 2001

Lieberman AF, Compton NC, Van Horn P, et al: Losing a Parent to Death in the Early Years: Guidelines for the Treatment of Traumatic Bereavement in Infancy and Early Childhood. Washington, DC, Zero to Three Press, 2003

Lieberman AF, Van Horn P, Ippen CG: Towards evidence-based treatment: child parent psychotherapy with preschoolers exposed to marital violence. J Am Acad Child Adolesc Psychiatry 44:1241–1248, 2005

McFarlane A: Posttraumatic phenomena in a longitudinal study of children following a natural disaster. J Am Acad Child Adolesc Psychiatry 26:764–769, 1987

Najavits LM, Gallow RJ, Weiss RD: Seeking Safety therapy for adolescent girls with PTSD and substance use disorders: a randomized clinical trial. J Behav Health Res 33:453–463, 2006

Parslow RA, Jorm AF: Pretrauma and posttrauma neurocognitive functioning and PTSD symptoms in a community sample of young adults. Am J Psychiatry 164:509–515, 2007

Perry BD: Neurobiological sequelae of childhood trauma: PTSD in children, in Catecholamine Function in Posttraumatic Stress Disorder: Emerging Concepts. Edited by Murburg MM. Washington, DC, American Psychiatric Press, 1994, pp 223–255

Pfefferbaum B, Nixon SJ, Krug RS, et al: Clinical needs assessment of middle and high school students following the 1995 Oklahoma City bombing. Am J Psychiatry 156:1069–1074, 1999

Pfefferbaum B, Stuber J, Galea S, et al: Panic reactions to terrorist attacks and probably PTSD in adolescents. J Trauma Stress 19:217–228, 2006

Robert R, Blakeney PE, Villarreal C, et al: Imipramine treatment in pediatric burn patients with symptoms of acute stress disorder: a pilot study. J Am Acad Child Adolesc Psychiatry 38:873–882, 1999

Saltzman WR, Pynoos RS, Layne CM, et al: Trauma- and grief-focused intervention for adolescents exposed to community violence: results of a school-based screening and group treatment protocol. Group Dyn 5:291–303, 2001

Saxe G, Stoddard F, Courtney D, et al: Relationship between acute morphine and the course of PTSD in children with burns. J Am Acad Child Adolesc Psychiatry 40:915–921, 2001

Saxe G, Ellis BH, Fogler J, et al: Comprehensive care for traumatized children: an open trial examines treatment using trauma systems therapy. Psychiatr Ann 35:443–448, 2005

Scheeringa MS, Peebles CD, Cook CA, et al: Toward establishing procedural, criterion and discriminant validity for PTSD in early childhood. J Am Acad Child Adolesc Psychiatry 40:52–60, 2001

Scheeringa M, Zeanah C, Myers L, et al: Predictive validity in a prospective follow-up of PTSD in preschool children. J Am Acad Child Adolesc Psychiatry 44:899–906, 2005

Scheeringa M, Wright MJ, Hunt JP, et al: Factors affecting the diagnosis and prediction of PTSD symptomatology in children and adolescents. Am J Psychiatry 163:644–651, 2006

Seedat S, Niehaus DJ, Stein DJ: The role of genes and family in trauma exposure and PTSD. Mol Psychiatry 6:360–362, 2001

Seedat S, Stein DJ, Ziervogel C, et al: Comparison of response to selective serotonin reuptake inhibitor in children, adolescents, and adults with PTSD. J Child Adolesc Psychopharmacol 12:37–46, 2002

Smith P, Yule W, Perrin S, et al: Cognitive behavioral therapy for PTSD in children and adolescents: a preliminary randomized controlled trial. J Am Acad Child Adolesc Psychiatry 46:1051–1061, 2007

Stein BD, Jaycox LH, Kataoka SH, et al: A mental health intervention for school children exposed to violence: a randomized controlled trial. JAMA 290:603–611, 2003

Stein M, Jang KL, Taylor S, et al: Genetic and environmental influences on trauma exposure and PTSD symptoms: a twin study. Am J Psychiatry 159:1675–1681, 2002

Thienkrua W, Cardozo BL, Chakkraband ML, et al: Symptoms of PTSD and depression among children in tsunami-affected areas in southern Thailand. JAMA 296:549–559, 2006

Warshaw MG, Fierman E, Pratt L, et al: Quality of life and dissociation in anxiety disordered patients with histories of trauma or PTSD. Am J Psychiatry 150:1512–1516, 1993

Zero to Three: DC:0–3: Diagnostic Classification of Mental Health and Developmental Disabilities of Infancy and Early Childhood, Revised Edition. Washington, DC, Zero To Three Press, 2005

Chapter 23

Obsessive-Compulsive Disorder

Daniel A. Geller, M.B.B.S., F.R.A.C.P.

Definition, Clinical Description, and Diagnosis

Obsessive-compulsive disorder (OCD) is characterized by the presence of *either* obsessions (*worries* is a more user-friendly term for children) *or* compulsions (*rituals* is a more user-friendly term for children). Although OCD is categorized among the anxiety disorders in DSM-IV (American Psychiatric Association 1994, 2000), especially in younger children, a variety of hidden or poorly articulated affects may drive the symptoms. There is active consideration of removing OCD from the DSM category of anxiety disorders and creating a new limited category for OCD "spectrum" disorders in DSM-V. Table 23–1 shows the current DSM-IV-TR criteria for OCD. The specifier "with poor insight" may be especially relevant to the diagnosis in youth since children's ability to explain their obsessions and the fears driving their compulsions may be quite limited.

Clinical Features

OCD in childhood is distinct in important ways from the disorder seen in adults. Pediatric OCD generally has a prepubertal age at onset, is male predominant, is characterized by a distinct pattern of obsessive-compulsive (OC) symptomatology and of psychiatric comorbidity, may be etiologically related to immune-mediated pathology (e.g., pediatric autoimmune neu-

---

This chapter is dedicated to the memory of Henrietta Leonard, M.D., esteemed clinician, researcher, teacher, mentor, and colleague.

TABLE 23–1. DSM-IV-TR diagnostic criteria for obsessive-compulsive disorder

A. Either obsessions or compulsions:

Obsessions as defined by (1), (2), (3), and (4):

  (1) recurrent and persistent thoughts, impulses, or images that are experienced, at some time during the disturbance, as intrusive and inappropriate and that cause marked anxiety or distress

  (2) the thoughts, impulses, or images are not simply excessive worries about real-life problems

  (3) the person attempts to ignore or suppress such thoughts, impulses, or images, or to neutralize them with some other thought or action

  (4) the person recognizes that the obsessional thoughts, impulses, or images are a product of his or her own mind (not imposed from without as in thought insertion)

Compulsions as defined by (1) and (2):

  (1) repetitive behaviors (e.g., hand washing, ordering, checking) or mental acts (e.g., praying, counting, repeating words silently) that the person feels driven to perform in response to an obsession, or according to rules that must be applied rigidly

  (2) the behaviors or mental acts are aimed at preventing or reducing distress or preventing some dreaded event or situation; however, these behaviors or mental acts either are not connected in a realistic way with what they are designed to neutralize or prevent or are clearly excessive

B. At some point during the course of the disorder, the person has recognized that the obsessions or compulsions are excessive or unreasonable.   **Note:** This does not apply to children.

C. The obsessions or compulsions cause marked distress, are time consuming (take more than 1 hour a day), or significantly interfere with the person's normal routine, occupational (or academic) functioning, or usual social activities or relationships.

D. If another Axis I disorder is present, the content of the obsessions or compulsions is not restricted to it (e.g., preoccupation with food in the presence of an eating disorder; hair pulling in the presence of trichotillomania; concern with appearance in the presence of body dysmorphic disorder; preoccupation with drugs in the presence of a substance use disorder; preoccupation with having a serious illness in the presence of hypochondriasis; preoccupation with sexual urges or fantasies in the presence of a paraphilia; or guilty ruminations in the presence of major depressive disorder).

E. The disturbance is not due to the direct physiological effects of a substance (e.g., a drug of abuse, a medication) or a general medical condition.

Specify if:

With Poor Insight: if, for most of the time during the current episode, the person does not recognize that the obsessions and compulsions are excessive or unreasonable

Source.   Reprinted from American Psychiatric Association: *Diagnostic and Statistical Manual of Mental Disorders*, 4th Edition, Text Revision. Washington, DC, American Psychiatric Association, 2000, pp. 462–463. Used with permission. Copyright © 2000 American Psychiatric Association.

ropsychiatric disorders associated with streptococcal infection [PANDAS]) in some cases, is more highly familial, and has a generally better prognosis than OCD beginning in adulthood. The secretive nature of OCD symptoms and the isolated and idiosyncratic functional deficits, which may be severe but domain specific and variable, contribute to the finding that OCD is underrecognized and underdiagnosed in youth.

Despite overlap between the phenotypic presentation in children and adults, issues such as limited insight and evolution of symptom profiles that follow developmental themes over time differentiate children and adults with OCD. In addition, children with OCD frequently display compulsions without well-defined obsessions and symptoms other than typical washing or checking rituals (e.g., blinking and breathing rituals) (Rettew et al. 1992). The majority of children exhibit both multiple obsessions and compulsions. Neither gender nor age at onset determine the type, number, or severity of OCD symptoms. Often, children's obsessions center upon fear of a catastrophic family event (e.g., death of a parent). Contamination, sexual or somatic obsessions, and scruples (overly moralistic thoughts) are the most commonly reported obsessions; and washing, repeating, checking, and ordering are the most commonly reported compulsions (Geller et al. 1998). While OCD symptoms tend to wax and wane, they persist in the majority of patients but change over time so that the presenting symptom constellation is not maintained (Rettew et al. 1992). Frequently, parents are noted to be intimately involved in their child's rituals, especially in reassurance seeking, a form of "verbal checking." Geller et al. (2001a) found that religious and sexual obsessions were overrepresented in adolescents compared with children and adults. Only hoarding was seen more often in children than in adolescents and adults. Factor analytic methods identify consistent symptom "dimensions" of OCD that may be more informative for understanding its causes. One four-factor solution explaining 60% of symptom variance is characterized by 1) symmetry/ordering/repeating/checking, 2) contamination/cleaning/aggressive behavior/somatic symptoms, 3) hoarding, and 4) sexual/religious symptoms (Stewart et al. 2007). This "dimensional" approach to phenotyping OCD may yield important biological signals in genetic, translational, and treatment studies where more traditional categorical approaches do not.

Pediatric OCD is characterized by male predominance (3:2 male to female). Boys may have an earlier age at onset than girls. Adult gender patterns (slight female preponderance) appear in late adolescence. The mean age at onset of OCD is 9–10 years and the majority of childhood onset is at ages 6–12.5 years. On average, age at assessment is 2 or more years after age at onset (Geller et al. 1998). Interest in the neuropsychological "endophenotype" of children with OCD grows out of clinical experience that many children have academic difficulties that are not wholly explained by their primary disorder. Given the potential involvement of frontal-striatal systems in OCD, several aspects of neuropsychological performance have been especially relevant to its study, especially measures of visuospatial integration, short-term memory, attention, and executive functions. Early studies of children with OCD yielded inconsistent results regarding significant neuropsychological deficits. More recently, Andres et al. (2007) examined neuropsychological performance in children and adolescents with OCD and found impairment in visual memory, visual organization, and velocity (processing speed). Deficits in visuospatial performance and processing speed are common, as is academic dysfunction.

Epidemiology

Prevalence rates of pediatric OCD are around 1%–2% in the United States and elsewhere (Apter et al. 1996;

Douglass et al. 1995; Flament et al. 1988). In the first epidemiological study of pediatric OCD, most subjects who were identified through screening who were later diagnosed with OCD had been previously undiagnosed. In the more recent British Child Mental Health Survey of more than 10,000 children and adolescents 5 to 15 years of age, the point prevalence was 0.25%, and almost 90% of cases identified had been undetected and untreated. In this study, lower socioeconomic status and lower intelligence quotients were associated with OCD in youth (Heyman et al. 2001). There are two peaks of incidence for OCD across the life span, one occurring in preadolescent children and a later peak in early adult life (mean age, 21 years) (Geller et al. 1998).

Comorbidity

OCD in youth is usually accompanied by other psychopathology. Community epidemiological studies find comorbid psychiatric diagnoses in over 50% of children with OCD (Douglass et al. 1995; Flament et al. 1988). This comorbid psychopathology often shows a distinct chronology, so that assessment and treatment approaches must evolve with time. Rates of comorbidity vary widely (Geller et al. 1998), but samples consistently find high rates of not only tic disorders but also mood, anxiety, ADHD, disruptive behavior, and specific developmental disorders and enuresis in youth with OCD (Figure 23–1).

Irrespective of age at ascertainment, an earlier age at onset predicts increased risk for ADHD and other anxiety disorders. In contrast, mood and psychotic disorders are associated with increasing chronological age and are more prevalent in adolescent subjects. Tourette's syndrome is associated with both age at onset (earlier onset is more likely to be associated with comorbid Tourette's syndrome) and chronological age (adolescents usually show remission of tics).

An important issue is whether comorbid disorders modify the expression of OCD. There is some evidence that this is so in the case of Tourette's syndrome, where specific symptoms (touching, tapping, repeating) appear more common than in patients without tic disorders (Leckman et al. 2003). By contrast, the OCD phenotype appears independent of the presence or absence of ADHD in symptoms, patterns of comorbid disorders, or OCD-specific functional impairment (Geller et al. 2003c). In any case, the presence (or absence) of comorbid psychopathology is important for clinicians to identify.

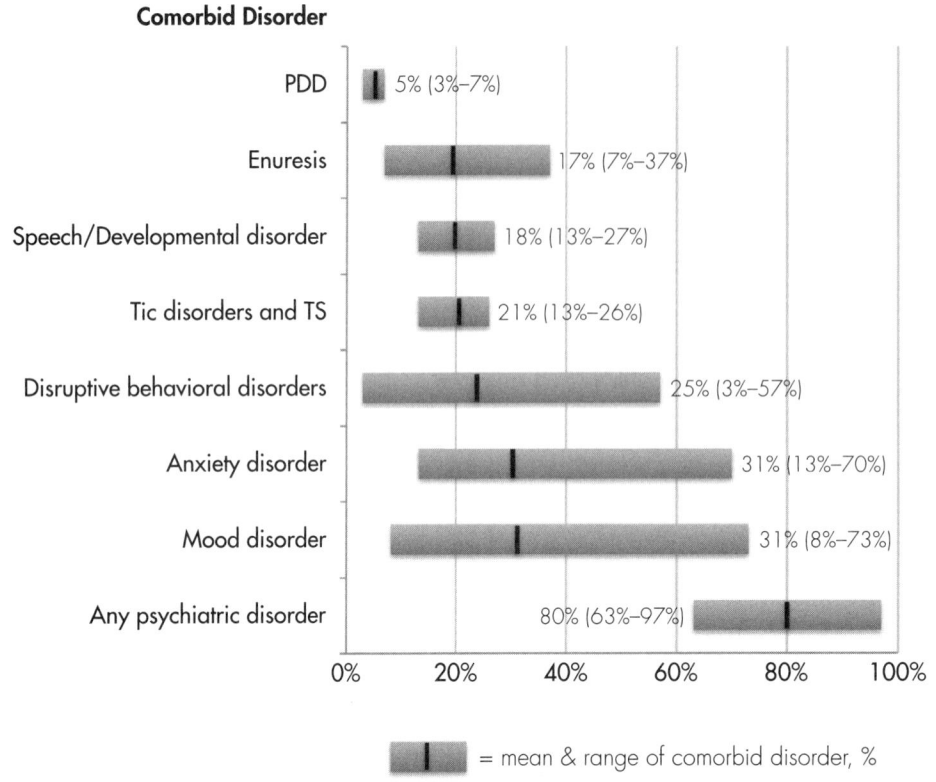

FIGURE 23–1.   Comorbid disorders in pediatric obsessive-compulsive disorder: review of clinical studies.

PDD=pervasive developmental disorder; TS=Tourette's syndrome.

Source.   Adapted from Geller et al. 1998.

Pathophysiology, Mechanisms, and Risk Factors

Several frontal cortico-striatal-thalamic circuits have been implicated in the pathophysiology of OCD, and several neurotransmitter systems modulate this feedback loop, including the excitatory amine glutamate, as well as dopamine- and serotonin-containing neurons (Rosenberg and Keshavan 1998). Pediatric imaging studies appear similar to those in adults, detecting structural abnormalities in the cingulate cortex, basal ganglia, and thalami of pediatric OCD patients (Rosenberg and Keshavan 1998). A handful of functional imaging studies conducted with children at rest and following treatment have yielded results compatible with those in adults. Fitzgerald et al. (2000) used multislice proton magnetic resonance spectroscopic imaging (^{1}H-MRS) in pediatric OCD patients and matched controls and found a significant reduction in N-acetylaspartate

(NAA)/choline and NAA/creatine/phosphocreatine levels bilaterally in the medial thalami of affected children compared with control subjects. Furthermore, reductions in left medial thalamic NAA levels were inversely correlated with OCD symptom severity. In a follow-up study of these youth, Rosenberg et al. (2001) observed that NAA and creatine normalized following treatment.

Using ^{1}H-MRS in 11 psychotropic drug–naive 8- to 17-year-olds with OCD before and after paroxetine treatment and 11 control children, Rosenberg et al. (2000) found significantly greater caudate glutamate concentrations in OCD children. Following paroxetine treatment, glutamate levels decreased in parallel with reduction in OCD symptoms and became similar to those of control subjects. In a single photon emission computed tomography (SPECT) study of 13 adults with early-onset (<10 years) versus later-onset OCD, and 22 healthy controls, early-onset cases showed decreased cerebral blood flow in the right thalamus, left anterior cingulate cortex, and bilateral inferior prefrontal cortex relative to late-onset subjects. In early-onset subjects only, severity of obsessive-compulsive symptoms cor-

TABLE 23–2. Diagnostic criteria for pediatric autoimmune neuropsychiatric disorders associated with streptococcal infection (PANDAS)

1. Obsessive-compulsive disorder and/or a tic disorder
2. Prepubertal onset between 3 and 12 years of age, or Tanner I or II
3. Episodic course (abrupt onset and/or exacerbations)
4. Symptom onset/exacerbations temporally related to *two* documented GABHS infections
5. Association with neurological abnormalities

Note. GABHS=group A beta-hemolytic streptococcus.
Source. Swedo et al. 1997.

related positively with left orbitofrontal regional cerebral blood flow suggesting that brain mechanisms in OCD may differ depending on the age at which symptoms are first expressed (Busatto et al. 2001).

Pediatric Autoimmune Neuropsychiatric Disorders Associated With Streptococcus

Perhaps no issue in OCD remains as controversial as the debate around PANDAS since its original description by Swedo et al. (1997). The central hypothesis of PANDAS derives from observations of neurobehavioral disturbance accompanying Sydenham's chorea, a sequel of rheumatic fever. An immune response to group A beta-hemolytic streptococcus (GABHS) infections leads to cross reactivity with and inflammation of basal ganglia with a distinct neurobehavioral syndrome that includes OCD and tics. Diagnostic criteria laid out by Swedo et al. (1997) (Table 23–2) have been used in a variety of studies of antibiotic prophylaxis (Garvey et al. 1999; Snider et al. 2005) and immune-modulating therapies (such as plasmapheresis), but detractors argue that GABHS is but one of many nonspecific physiological stressors that can trigger an increase in tics or OCD (Kurlan and Kaplan 2004). The weight of evidence at this time supports the belief that a subset of children with OCD and Tourette's syndrome have both onset and clinical exacerbations linked to GABHS (Kurlan et al. 2008).

Genetics

The contribution of genetic factors to the development of OCD has been explored in twin, family-genetic, and segregation analyses studies (Hanna et al. 2005; Nestadt et al. 2000; Pauls et al. 1995). The concordance rates for monozygotic twins are significantly higher than for dizygotic twins (van Grootheest et al. 2005). While family studies consistently demonstrate that OCD is familial (Lenane et al. 1990; Pauls et al. 1995), the risk of OCD in first-degree relatives appears to be greater for index cases with a childhood onset. For example, in their multisite family study of OCD, Nestadt et al. (2000) found a risk for OCD of around 12% in first-degree relatives, while relatives of pediatric OCD probands have shown age-corrected morbid risks of 24%–26% in more recent studies (do Rosario-Campos et al. 2005; Hanna et al. 2005). These findings suggest a greater genetic loading in pediatric-onset OCD. A further substantial proportion of relatives (5%–15%) are affected with subthreshold OC symptoms that may be genetic (Nestadt et al. 2000) but may also be relevant to family functioning. Segregation analyses suggest that familial patterns of OCD are consistent with genetic models that include genes of major effect (Alsobrook et al. 1999; Nestadt et al. 2000) with possible sex effects. It is highly likely that there are several genes that are important for the expression of this complex disorder. A genome-wide linkage scan for OCD showed evidence for susceptibility loci on chromosomes 3q, 7p, 1q, 15q, and 6q (Shugart et al. 2006).

Environmental Factors

While the above studies emphasize genetic factors, they also point clearly to major effects of *nongenetic* influences in the expression of OCD. For example, twin studies show that even among monozygotic twins, OCD is *not* fully concordant. In a cross-cultural sample of 4,246 twin pairs (Hudziak et al. 2004), genetic (45%–58%) and unique environmental (42%-55%) factors were about equally important. In a population sample of 527 female twin pairs (Jonnal et al. 2000), heritability for obsessions was 33% and for compulsions, 26%. Clearly, nonheritable etiological factors are as great or greater than genetic factors for risk of developing OCD. In fact, many if not most cases of OCD arise *with-*

out a positive family history of the disorder—so-called sporadic cases. Although sporadic occurrences do not rule out a genetic etiology (for example, due to spontaneous mutations), familial and sporadic "subtypes" of OCD have repeatedly been identified (Hanna et al. 2005; Nestadt et al. 2000; Pauls et al. 1995), leading to speculation about the differing impact of environmental and genetic factors on familial and nonfamilial forms of the disorder. Information regarding environmental triggers of the disorder may be especially relevant for the sporadic form, since the OCD cannot be explained by the presence of an affected relative.

Perinatal Factors in Pediatric OCD

Lensi et al. (1996) found a higher rate of *perinatal trauma* (defined by dystocic delivery, use of forceps, breech presentation, or prolonged hypoxia) in males with an earlier onset of OCD. Recently, Geller et al. (2008) found that children with OCD had mothers with significantly higher rates of illness during pregnancy requiring medical care and more birth difficulties (induced labor, forceps delivery, nuchal cord, or prolonged labor). Among the OCD-affected children, there were significant associations between adverse perinatal experiences and earlier age at onset, increased OCD severity, and increased risk for comorbid ADHD, chronic tic disorder, anxiety disorder, and major depressive disorder.

Role of the Family in Pediatric OCD

Parents are often intimately involved in their children's OC symptoms and may unwittingly reinforce compulsive behaviors by providing verbal reassurance or other "assistance" to their children (for example, handling objects that their children avoid, such as opening doors; laundering "contaminated" clothes and linens excessively; even wiping children on the toilet who will not do it themselves). Because OCD, and an anxiety diathesis in general, is highly familial, disentangling parental psychopathology from disturbed family functioning resulting from the child's OCD is critical, especially in younger patients. Increasingly, the central role of family members (both for maintenance of pathology as well as proxy therapy agents) for children affected with OCD has been recognized and is reflected both in a broader assessment

that evaluates family function and in newer models of treatment intervention.

Course and Prognosis

Precipitating psychosocial events are occasionally associated with the onset of OCD, sometimes dramatically. However, the majority of pediatric OCD cases have a gradual onset without a history of precipitating stressors. Sixteen samples reported in 22 studies with a total of 521 children with OCD and follow-up periods ranging from 1 to 15.6 years (mean 5.7 years) showed pooled mean persistence rates of 41% for *full* OCD and 60% for *full* or *subthreshold* OCD (Stewart et al. 2004). Earlier age at OCD onset, longer duration of OCD, and inpatient treatment predicted persistence. Comorbid psychiatric illness and poor initial treatment response were poor prognostic factors. Psychosocial function is frequently compromised, including being less likely to live with a partner, being unmarried, and still living with parents as adults and/or hiding symptoms from family. These studies report high levels of social/peer problems (55%–100%), isolation, and unemployment (45%). Educational level was not different from control subjects, with 30%–70% having attended college.

The long-term prognosis for pediatric OCD is better than originally thought (Stewart et al. 2004). Many children will remit partially or entirely. Adverse prognostic factors include very early age at onset, concurrent psychiatric diagnoses, poor initial treatment response, long duration of illness, and a positive first-degree family history of OCD.

Evaluation

Making the Diagnosis

The simplest probes derive from the DSM-IV-TR diagnostic criteria of the American Psychiatric Association (2000): "Do you ever have repetitive, intrusive or unwanted thoughts, ideas, images or urges that upset you or make you anxious and that you cannot suppress?" For younger children the question might be phrased, "Do you have worries that just won't go away?"

It is reasonable to offer some examples at this time such as "worries about things not being clean," or "worrying that something bad might happen to yourself or a loved one."

For compulsions a similar probe might be: "Do you ever have to do rituals or habits or other things over and over, even though you don't want to or you know they don't make sense, because you feel anxious or worried about something?" For younger children the question might be phrased, "Do you have rituals or habits that you can't stop?" Examples such as washing, checking, repeating, ordering, and counting can be offered.

Sometimes adults must infer obsessions from observing a child's behavior when the obsessions are not articulated or even acknowledged by the child. Examples include avoidance behaviors such as not entering a room or handling an object. If screening questions suggest that OC symptoms are present, clinicians should follow with more in-depth assessment using the DSM-IV-TR criteria of 1) time occupied by OC symptoms, 2) level of subjective distress, and 3) functional impairment, as well as a standardized inventory of symptoms and scalar assessment of severity, subjective distress, impairment, resistance, control, and insight, such as the Children's Yale-Brown Obsessive Compulsive Scale (CY-BOCS; Scahill et al. 1997).

The CY-BOCS is a 10-item anchored ordinal scale (0–4) that rates the clinical severity of the disorder by scoring the time occupied (0=no time, 4=more than 8 hours per day), degree of life interference (0=none, 4=extreme), subjective distress (0=none, 4=extreme), internal resistance (0=always, 4=none), and degree of control (0=excellent, 4=none) for both obsessions and compulsions. The CY-BOCS also includes a checklist of over 60 symptoms of obsessions and compulsions categorized by the predominant theme involved, such as contamination, hoarding, washing, checking, and so forth. Scores of 8–15 are considered to represent mild illness, 16–23 moderate illness, and ≥24 severe illness. Equally important are quantitative measures of avoidance, insight, indecisiveness, pathological responsibility and doubt, and slowness. The CY-BOCS is a clinician-administered instrument that is most informative when given to both children and their parents, and a "worst report" algorithm is likely to be most accurate.

While the CY-BOCS is the current standard assessment tool for pediatric OCD, there are several important limitations to this scale. The first is that the avoidance rating is not included in the quantitative score of the scale (though it is assigned an ordinal score from 0 to 4 later) and thus may underestimate severity when avoidance is a large part of the presenting behavior. Secondly, the scale is not linear. Marked reductions in time occupied by obsessions or compulsions are not reflected in a proportional drop in scale scores. It is for

this reason that a 25%–40% reduction in CY-BOCS scores is considered a clinically significant response.

Families may become deeply involved in their children's OCD. Parental efforts to relieve a child's anxiety may inadvertently lead to accommodation and reinforcement of OC behaviors. The very high intensity of affect and irritability displayed by some affected children may make it difficult for parents to react with the supportive yet detached responses needed for effective behavioral treatment. The familial nature of anxiety disorders and OCD are added factors in families' responses to a child with OCD. The role of individual family members in maintenance and management of OC symptoms is important to assess. Detailed and specific questions about activities of daily living may be needed to understand the cycle of OC behaviors at home.

Differential Diagnosis

Typical toddlers and preschoolers frequently engage in ritualistic behavior, such as mealtime or bedtime routines. As a rule, these routines do not cause impairment in family functioning and interruption of these rituals does not create severe distress in the child. For some children, however, excessive rituals early in life may be a marker for later onset of OCD (Leonard et al. 1990). Perhaps the most difficult differential diagnosis occurs in the context of a more pervasive developmental disorder (PDD) or autism spectrum disorder. Core symptoms of these disorders include stereotypic and repetitive behaviors and a restricted and narrow range of interests and activities that may easily be confused with OCD, especially in young children. A small number of children with OCD (5%–7%) may also meet criteria for Asperger's syndrome or PDD (Geller et al. 2001b). In OCD, symptoms are ego-dystonic and are associated with anxiety-driven obsessional fears. Children with PDD engage in repetitive stereotypic behaviors with apparent gratification and will become upset only when their preferred activities are interrupted. Left to their rituals, they do not display anxiety or discomfort. While younger children with OCD may not be able to articulate their concerns, evidence of anxiety is usually discernable. If symptoms are typical of OCD (such as washing, cleaning, or checking), one can infer obsessional concern.

Another diagnostic dilemma occurs in the context of poor insight into obsessional ideas that merges into overvalued ideation and even delusional thinking, suggesting psychosis. In children with OCD, insight is not static but varies with anxiety level and is best assessed when anxiety is at a minimum. While OC symptoms may herald a psychotic or schizophreniform disorder in youth, especially adolescents, other positive or negative symptoms of psychosis will usually be present or emerge to assist in differential diagnosis. The nature of obsessional ideation in these patients is often atypical (for example, a fear that he will turn into another person or that her parent has been replaced by an alien).

Clinical Examination

Best-estimate diagnostic formulations should include information from *all* available sources including the child, parents and other caregivers, teachers, and other clinicians involved. School and educational history provides an ecologically important and valid measure of function and of illness severity. OC symptoms that spill into the school setting imply more anxiety, stronger compulsions, less insight, and less resistance and control. Therefore educational impairment denoted by falling grades or the need for extra help or special class placement indicates more urgency for treatment and could justify more aggressive interventions, including medications. Consideration for neuropsychological assessment should be high in children with OCD who are struggling at school. Attention to GABHS infection as a potential precipitant for a PANDAS-associated OCD is indicated in acute and dramatic onsets or exacerbations in preadolescent patients, or when a child in remission suddenly relapses. Neurological signs such as chorea are evidence of rheumatic fever but may not occur for many months after infection. Softer neurological signs such as tremor, coordination difficulties, and soft motor abnormalities contribute to one criterion for the PANDAS diagnosis (Swedo et al. 1997). Since the immunology of streptococcus and its role in infection-triggered neuropsychiatric symptoms is poorly understood, recommendations regarding antibody assay are uncertain. When indicated, antistreptolysin O and anti-DNase B titers can be helpful. Intercurrent titers are also helpful in that subsequent exacerbations can be assayed to detect any sudden increase in antibody levels. Titers at intervals of less than 3 months are not likely to be helpful.

Treatment

Overview

Cognitive-behavioral therapy (CBT) is the first-line treatment for mild to moderate cases of OCD in children. Since the publication of a CBT treatment manual that operationalized and systematized this method (March and Mulle 1998), numerous studies have consistently shown its acceptability and efficacy (March et al. 2001; Piacentini et al. 2003). Severe OCD, concurrent psychopathology (e.g., comorbid anxiety or major depressive or disruptive behavior disorders), lack of family cohesion, poor insight, or lack of skilled CBT practitioners are factors to consider in deciding when to use medication. Scores of >23 on the CY-BOCS or Clinical Global Impressions—Severity scale (CGI-S) scores of "marked" to "severe" impairment provide a threshold for consideration of drug intervention. In addition, any situation that could impede the successful delivery of CBT should be cause for earlier consideration of medication treatment. Poor insight into the irrational nature of the obsessions and associated compulsions can lead to resistance to CBT. Chaotic or nonintact family situations will make close family involvement in implementation of CBT more difficult. Finally, there is a dire shortage of skilled CBT practitioners. Site-specific differences in CBT outcomes in the National Institute of Mental Health (NIMH)–funded Pediatric OCD Treatment Study (POTS; March et al. 2004) suggest that expert training will improve response rates to CBT. In the POTS study, CBT alone did not differ from sertraline alone and both were better than placebo.

Concurrent psychopathology may reduce the patient's acceptance of or compliance with CBT and may require medication itself. For example, a depressed adolescent with a mood-congruent anhedonic view of the future may see little point in making the effort to tolerate exposure and response prevention. While the response in children and adolescents treated with paroxetine was high (71%), the response rates in patients with comorbid ADHD, tic disorder, or ODD (56%, 53%, and 39%, respectively) were significantly less than in patients with OCD only (75%) (Geller et al. 2003a). Furthermore, comorbidity was associated with a greater rate of relapse (46% for ≥1 comorbid disorder [$P=0.04$] and 56% for ≥2 comorbid disorders [$P<0.05$] vs. 32% for no comorbidity). More recent analysis of data from the POTS (March et al. 2004) comparative treatment trial looked at symptom reduction on the CY-BOCS after 12 weeks of treatment. Those children with a comorbid tic disorder failed to respond to sertraline and did not separate statistically from placebo-treated patients, while response in youth with OCD without tics replicated previously published intent-to-treat outcomes. In children with tics, sertraline was helpful only when combined with CBT, while CBT alone was effective. The presence of disruptive behavior disorders may represent a thera-

TABLE 23–3. Dosage range for serotonin reuptake inhibitors in children with obsessive-compulsive disorder (OCD)

Drug	Starting dosage, mg		Typical dosage range, mg (mean dosage)[a]
	Preadolescent	Adolescent	
Clomipramine[b,c]	6.25–25	25	50–200
Fluoxetine[c,d]	2.5–10	10–20	10–80 (25)
Sertraline[c,d]	12.5–25	25–50	50–200 (178)
Fluvoxamine[b,c]	12.5–25	25–50	50–300 (165)
Paroxetine[e]	2.5–10	10	10–60 (32)
Citalopram[d]	2.5–10	10–20	10–60

[a]Mean daily doses used in controlled trials.
[b]Doses <25 mg/day may be administered by compounding 25 mg into 5 mL suspension.
[c]FDA approved for OCD in children and adolescents.
[d]Oral concentrate commercially available.
[e]Oral suspension commercially available.

peutic challenge for clinicians, especially cognitive-behavioral clinicians. Storch et al. (2008) found that those children with OCD and one or more comorbid diagnoses treated with CBT had lower response and remission rates relative to those without a comorbid diagnosis. The number of comorbid conditions was negatively related to outcome.

Pharmacological Treatments

The past decade has seen rapid advances in our knowledge of the pharmacotherapy of OCD. Clomipramine was the first agent approved for use in pediatric populations with OCD, in 1989. Subsequent multisite randomized controlled trials (RCTs), many of which were industry-sponsored, have demonstrated significant efficacy of the selective serotonin reuptake inhibitors (SSRIs) compared with placebo, including sertraline (March et al. 1998), fluvoxamine (Riddle et al. 2001), fluoxetine (Geller et al. 2001c), and paroxetine (Geller et al. 2002). No comparative treatment studies have yet been performed, and there is little to guide clinicians in the choice of therapeutic agents. Clomipramine and three SSRIs (fluoxetine, fluvoxamine, and sertraline) are approved by the U.S. Food and Drug Administration (FDA) for pediatric use, but paroxetine and citalopram are also used. Expert consensus guidelines for pediatric OCD (American Academy of Child and Adolescent Psychiatry 1998) suggest initiating at the lowest dose and titrating slowly (for example, 3 weekly increments), with close monitoring for response and adverse effects over the first 6 to 8 weeks (see Table 23–3). The FDA recommends weekly review

over the first 4 weeks, then every other week for 4 weeks, and at week 12 following initiation of SSRIs in children despite a lack of evidence that such a schedule alters outcome; visits at 2- to 3-week intervals are more typical in practice. Most important, clinicians should be available continuously for emergency communications during this period, and parents and youth should be encouraged to contact their physician with any concerns.

The cumulative data accrued from RCTs of pediatric OCD are now sufficient to examine the overall effect of medication treatment. One meta-analysis of all published RCTs (12) in children and adolescents with OCD (*N*=1,044) assessed evidence for differential efficacy based on type of drug, study design, and outcome measure (Geller et al. 2003b). There were four SSRIs (paroxetine, fluoxetine, fluvoxamine, and sertraline) and clomipramine, four study designs (parallel, withdrawal, substitution, and crossover), four dependent outcome measures (CY-BOCS, NIMH—Global Obsessive Compulsive Scale, CGI-S, and the Leyton Obsessional Inventory—Child Version), and two types of outcome scores (change and posttreatment). The effect size expressed as a pooled standardized mean difference for results of all studies was 0.46 (95% CI, 0.37–0.55) and showed a highly significant difference between drug and placebo treatment (z=9.87, P<0.001) (see Table 23–4).

Multivariate regression of drug effect controlled for other variables showed that clomipramine was significantly superior to each of the SSRIs but that the other SSRIs were comparably effective. Clinically speaking, overall effect sizes of medication treatment were mod-

TABLE 23–4. Effect size by drug in meta-analysis of pediatric obsessive-compulsive disorder trials

Drug	SMD	95% CI
Paroxetine	0.405	0.204–0.606
Fluoxetine	0.546	0.353–0.738
Fluvoxamine	0.375	0.167–0.584
Sertraline	0.327	0.160–0.493
Clomipramine	0.693	0.475–0.910

Note. CI=confidence interval; SMD=standardized mean difference.
Source. Adapted from Geller et al. 2003b.

est with improved CY-BOCS scores of about 6 points over placebo. Since then, the POTS (March et al. 2004) confirmed these findings with an effect size of 0.66 (95% CI, 0.12–1.2) for sertraline. A recent meta-analysis of 10 RCTs (Watson and Rees 2008) showed an overall drug effect size of 0.48 (95% CI, 0.36–0.61) and a clomipramine effect size of 0.85 (95% CI, 0.32–1.39). One limitation in interpreting published reports of medication trials is the numerous exclusion criteria used to select samples (Geller et al. 2003a). Because many comorbid conditions were excluded, the drug effect in clinical settings may be lower than meta-analyses suggest. Long-term studies suggest that there is a cumulative benefit over longer periods of drug exposure with gradually declining scalar scores and increasing remission rates for sertraline (Wagner et al. 2003) and paroxetine (Hollander et al. 2003) for up to 1 year.

Psychotherapeutic Treatments

Cognitive-Behavioral Therapy

The protocol used in the POTS (March et al. 2004) consists of 14 visits over 12 weeks spread across five phases: 1) psychoeducation, 2) cognitive training, 3) mapping OCD, 4) exposure and response prevention, and 5) relapse prevention and generalization training. Except for weeks 1 and 2, when patients come twice weekly, all visits are 1 hour per week. There is one between-visit, 10-minute telephone contact scheduled during each of weeks 3 through 12. Each session includes a statement of goals, review of the preceding week, provision of new information, therapist-assisted practice, homework for the coming week, and monitoring procedures.

The principle of *exposure and response prevention* (ERP) as illustrated in Figure 23–2 relies on the fact that anxiety usually attenuates after sufficient duration of contact with a feared stimulus. Repeated exposure is associated with decreased anxiety across exposure trials, with anxiety reduction largely specific to the domain of exposure, until the child no longer fears contact with specifically targeted phobic stimuli. Adequate exposure depends on blocking the negative reinforcement effect of rituals or avoidance behavior, a process termed *response prevention*. ERP is typically implemented gradually (sometimes termed *graded exposure*), with exposure targets under the patient's, or less desirably the therapist's, control (March et al. 2001).

In a recent meta-analysis of five RCTs of CBT in children (N=161) with OCD, Watson and Rees (2008) found a large mean pooled effect size of 1.45 (95% CI, 0.68–2.22). CBT studies have greater heterogeneity than pharmacotherapy trials. Although both treatments are significantly superior to control, CBT yields a larger treatment effect, consistent with treatment outcomes in adult OCD populations. These findings support the recommendations of the American Academy of Child and Adolescent Psychiatry (1998) practice parameters guidelines that CBT should comprise the first-line treatment for mild to moderate pediatric OCD, followed by pharmacotherapy.

Several variations in delivering CBT have been studied and reported, including those that use family-based approaches (Barrett et al. 2004; Storch et al. 2008), particularly with very young children where parents control most of the contingencies of their child's behavior. Another variation that may be helpful is CBT delivered in group settings, where positive elements of both group therapy and CBT are combined (Thienemann et al. 2001). Intensive CBT approaches work well for children who subscribe in advance to this approach (Franklin et al. 1998). Intensive approaches may be especially useful for treatment-resistant OCD or for patients who desire a very rapid response, and this can now be found in a few specialized intensive outpatient or residential treatment centers in the United States.

Combined Treatment

For greatest efficacy, the combination of CBT with medication is the treatment of choice. Recommendations from the POTS (March et al. 2004) were to start treatment with either CBT alone or CBT plus medication treatment. The combined treatment showed the greatest decrease in symptom scores and the greatest remission rate with an effect size that was more or less the arithmetic sum of the component treatments (effect size combined=1.4, CBT=0.97, and sertraline=0.67). Fifty-

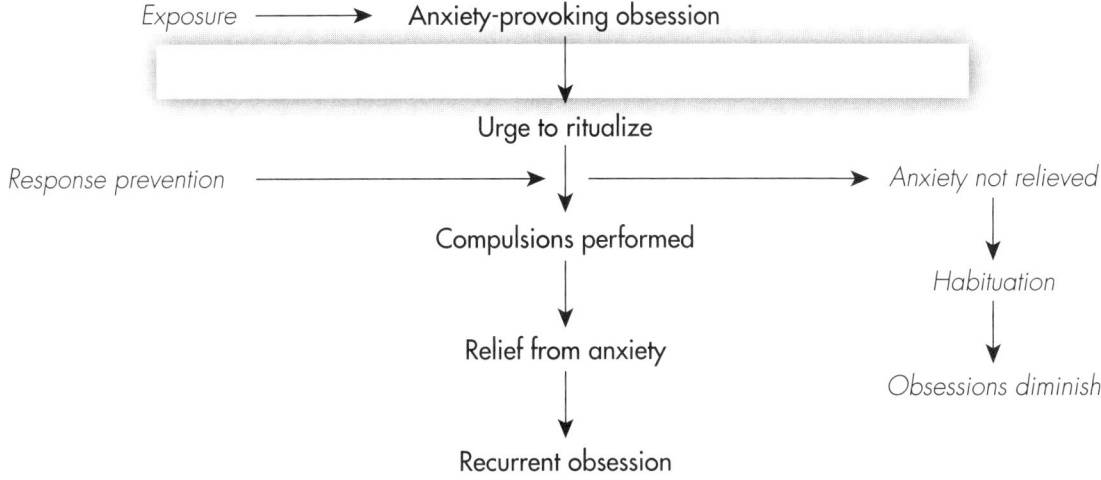

Exposure ⟶ Anxiety-provoking obsession

↓

Urge to ritualize

Response prevention ⟶ ⟶ Anxiety not relieved

↓ ↓

Compulsions performed Habituation

↓ ↓

Relief from anxiety Obsessions diminish

↓

Recurrent obsession

FIGURE 23–2. Theoretical basis of cognitive-behavioral treatment (exposure and response prevention).

four percent of children receiving combined treatment achieved a remission. It is possible that medication enhances the effect of CBT by decreasing anxiety and improving a child's ability to tolerate ERP. Although sertraline was the medication used in the POTS, other investigators have reported similar combination treatment approaches with different drugs including clomipramine (Foa et al. 2005) and fluvoxamine (Neziroglu et al. 2000), so that it is reasonable to extrapolate the POTS findings to other medications that have independently shown efficacy for OCD in children.

Augmentation Strategies

Medication augmentation strategies are reserved only for treatment-resistant cases. By expert consensus, the term "treatment resistant" applied to children with OCD indicates a child who has persistent and *substantial* OCD symptomatology in the face of *adequate* treatment known to be effective in childhood OCD. Persistent symptoms of at least moderate severity (e.g., CY-BOCS ≥16 or CGI-S of marked or severe impairment) are useful guidelines. At least two serotonin reuptake inhibitor trials are necessary to declare *adequate* medication therapy. Therefore, failure of *adequate* trials of at least two SSRIs or one SSRI and a clomipramine trial as well as a failure of *adequately* delivered CBT would constitute treatment resistance. Children should have a minimum of 10 weeks of each SSRI or clomipramine at maximum recommended (or tolerated) doses, with no change in dose for the preceding 3 weeks. In terms of *adequate* CBT dose, if a child has not shown *any* improvement after 8–10 total sessions (or 5–6 sessions of exposure), or has substantial residual OC psychopathology after completing standard CBT treatment, he

may be considered a CBT nonresponder. To summarize, failure of at least two monotherapies as well as combined treatment is required prior to considering the OCD as treatment resistant.

Adding clomipramine to an SSRI may be helpful. The rationale is to combine serotonergic effects of each while minimizing adverse events across differing drug classes. Even low-dose augmentation (25–75 mg/day) may be useful, but care must be taken when combining with CYP-450 2 D6 inhibitors such as fluoxetine or paroxetine due to potentially toxic increases in clomipramine levels, which must be monitored along with electrocardiogram indices. Clonazepam has also been used in combination with SSRIs in several small trials (Crockett et al. 2004). By far, the commonest drug augmentation strategies have employed atypical neuroleptics. High-quality RCTs employing atypicals have been done in adults with OCD (summarized by Bloch et al. 2006 in a comprehensive meta-analysis) but no controlled data exist in children, only case reports and open trials. However, expert consensus suggests that many children with treatment-resistant OCD will benefit from judicious augmentation with an atypical, particularly children with tic disorders, PDD symptoms, or mood instability.

Putative PANDAS cases of OCD have also attracted novel and experimental treatment interventions. Antibiotic prophylaxis with penicillin failed to prevent streptococcal infections in one study (Garvey et al. 1999) but was effective in a subsequent study with reduction in both infections and OCD symptoms in the year of prophylaxis compared to the previous baseline year (Snider et al. 2005). Data are not yet sufficient to meet minimal standards to recommend antibiotic prophylaxis for children with OCD, even when PANDAS is suspected as an etiology. Instead, standard treatments for both OCD and streptococcal infections are recommended. Plasmapharesis and other immune-modulating therapies remain experimental.

Other Treatment Modalities

Insight-oriented psychotherapy has proven disappointing in children and adolescents with OCD. Nevertheless, sequelae of OC symptoms should be considered for further treatment, especially when OCD has been longstanding. Children with OCD who have experienced the following may benefit from supportive individual or family psychotherapy: 1) decreased function in some important domain of life—for example, in school grades or ability to maintain friendships; and 2) loss of self-esteem or marked conflict at home that has disrupted primary relationships.

Concurrent psychopathology may also respond to non-CBT psychotherapeutic intervention. Particular attention to social function is recommended because of the long-term outcome data suggesting this is often compromised even in the context of successful educational outcomes. Collaborative engagement with other clinicians such as CBT therapists, educational psychologists, and school personnel—as well as immediate, and at times extended, family—is essential for best outcomes.

Research Directions

All levels of investigation—clinical, translational, and basic—are being pursued by the research community. Focus on the association at common polymorphisms in several serotonin transmitter system genes has shifted to include interest in glutamatergic mechanisms and the glutamate transporter gene *SLC1A1* (Arnold et al. 2006). Genetic research is hampered by low power to find genes in individual studies that could lead to incorrect acceptance of the null hypothesis. In response to this concern, the newly created International OCD Genetics Consortium seeks to use the power of genome-wide association methods and pooled data across sites promising hope that specific genes that increase risk for OCD will be identified.

Ever more powerful magnets provide a noninvasive and child-safe method for endophenotypic, translational, and pharmacogenomic brain imaging studies that should increase specificity of treatments to improve effect sizes and decrease adverse events. Novel therapeutic approaches employing glutamatergic, GABA-ergic and peptide neurotransmitter manipulation are likely and will be informed by genetic studies. Real challenges remain in identifying environmental triggers (such as intra-uterine, birth, and postnatal experiences and immune mediated pathophysiology) in genetically susceptible individuals, as only prospective "at-risk" longer-term studies can hope to understand the complex gene-environment interactions that underlie most cases of OCD.

Summary Points

- OCD affects 1%–2% of children and adolescents and is frequently underdiagnosed and undertreated due to the secretive nature of its symptoms.

- Families often become enmeshed in their children's rituals.

- Most often, OCD in children is accompanied by comorbid psychopathology that has a real impact on functioning and treatment outcome.

- Simple probes for the presence of anxiety, "worries," and rituals will identify most children with OCD.

- Gathering information from both parents and children is essential.

- Assessment should include a standardized quantitative or scalar measure of symptoms along with an inventory of "target" symptoms.

- CBT is the treatment of choice for mild to moderate childhood cases.

- Medications are reserved for cases of OCD that is more severe, has multiple comorbid conditions, is accompanied by poor insight, or is CBT resistant, or situations when adequate CBT resources cannot be found.

- SSRIs are the first recommended medicines for OCD at any age.

References

Alsobrook JP II, Leckman JF, Goodman WK, et al: Segregation analysis of obsessive-compulsive disorder using symptom-based factor scores. Am J Med Genet A 88:669–675, 1999

American Academy of Child and Adolescent Psychiatry: Practice parameters for the assessment and treatment of children and adolescents with obsessive-compulsive disorder. J Am Acad Child Adolesc Psychiatry 37(suppl):27S–45S, 1998

American Psychiatric Association: Diagnostic and Statistical Manual of Mental Disorders, 4th Edition. Washington, DC, American Psychiatric Association, 1994

American Psychiatric Association: Diagnostic and Statistical Manual of Mental Disorders, 4th Edition, Text Revision. Washington, DC, American Psychiatric Association, 2000

Andres S, Boget T, Lazaro L, et al: Neuropsychological performance in children and adolescents with obsessive-compulsive disorder and influence of clinical variables. Biol Psychiatry 61:946–951, 2007

Apter A, Fallon JT, King RA, et al: Obsessive-compulsive characteristics: from symptoms to syndrome. J Am Acad Child Adolesc Psychiatry 35:907–912, 1996

Arnold PD, Sicard T, Burroughs E, et al: Glutamate transporter gene SLC1A1 associated with obsessive-compulsive disorder. Arch Gen Psychiatry 63:717–720, 2006

Barrett P, Healy Farrell L, March JS: Cognitive-behavioral family treatment of childhood obsessive-compulsive disorder: a controlled clinical trial. J Am Acad Child Adolesc Psychiatry 43:46–62, 2004

Bloch MH, Peterson BS, Scahill L, et al: Adulthood outcome of tic and obsessive-compulsive symptom severity in children with Tourette Syndrome. Arch Pediatr Adolesc Med 160:65–69, 2006

Busatto GF, Buchpiguel CA, Zamignani DR, et al: Regional cerebral blood flow abnormalities in early-onset obsessive-compulsive disorder: an exploratory SPECT study. J Am Acad Child Adolesc Psychiatry 40:347–354, 2001

Crockett BA, Churchill E, Davidson JRT: A double-blind combination study of clonazepam with sertraline in obsessive-compulsive disorder. Ann Clin Psychiatry 16:127–132, 2004

do Rosario-Campos MC, Leckman JF, Curi M, et al: A family study of early-onset obsessive-compulsive disorder. Am J Med Genet B Neuropsychiatr Genet 136B:92–97, 2005

Douglass HM, Moffitt TE, Dar R, et al: Obsessive-compulsive disorder in a birth cohort of 18-year-olds: prevalence and predictors. J Am Acad Child Adolesc Psychiatry 34:1424–1431, 1995

Fitzgerald KD, Moore GJ, Paulson LA, et al: Proton spectroscopic imaging of the thalamus in treatment-naive pediatric obsessive-compulsive disorder. Biol Psychiatry 47:174–182, 2000

Flament M, Whitaker A, Rapoport JL, et al: Obsessive compulsive disorder in adolescence: an epidemiological study. J Am Acad Child Adolesc Psychiatry 27:764–771, 1988

Foa EB, Liebowitz MR, Kozak MJ, et al: Randomized, placebo-controlled trial of exposure and ritual prevention, clomipramine, and their combination in the treatment of obsessive-compulsive disorder. Am J Psychiatry 162:151–161, 2005

Franklin M, Kozak MJ, Cashman L, et al: Cognitive-behavioral treatment of pediatric obsessive-compulsive disorder: an open clinical trial. J Am Acad Child Adolesc Psychiatry 37:412–419, 1998

Garvey M, Perlmutter S, Allen A, et al: A pilot study of penicillin prophylaxis for neuropsychiatric exacerbations triggered by streptococcal infections. Biol Psychiatry 45:1564–1571, 1999

Geller D, Biederman J, Jones J, et al: Is juvenile obsessive compulsive disorder a developmental subtype of the disorder? A review of the pediatric literature. J Am Acad Child Adolesc Psychiatry 37:420–427, 1998

Geller D, Biederman J, Agranat A, et al: Developmental aspects of obsessive compulsive disorder: findings in children, adolescents and adults. J Nerv Ment Dis 189:471–477, 2001a

Geller D, Biederman J, Wagner KD, et al: Comorbid psychiatric illness and response to treatments, relapse rates, and behavioral adverse event incidents in pediatric OCD. Abstracts: Child and Adolescent Program of the 41st Annual National Institute of Mental Health (NIMH) New Clinical Drug Evaluation Unit (NCDEU) Meeting, Phoenix, Arizona, May 28–31, 2001. J Child Adolesc Psychopharmacol 11:320–340, 2001b

Geller D, Hoog SL, Heiligenstein JH, et al: Fluoxetine treatment for obsessive-compulsive disorder in children and adolescents: a placebo-controlled clinical trial. J Am Acad Child Adolesc Psychiatry 40:773–779, 2001c

Geller D, Wagner KD, Emslie GJ, et al: Efficacy of paroxetine in pediatric OCD: results of a multicenter study. Paper presented at the 155th annual meeting of the American Psychiatric Association Meeting, Philadelphia, PA, May 2002

Geller D, Biederman J, Stewart SE, et al: Impact of comorbidity on treatment response to paroxetine in pediatric obsessive compulsive disorder: is the use of exclusion criteria empirically supported in randomized clinical trials? J Child Adolesc Psychopharmacol 13(suppl):S19–S29, 2003a

Geller D, Biederman J, Stewart ES, et al: Which SSRI? A meta-analysis of pharmacotherapy trials in pediatric obsessive compulsive disorder. Am J Psychiatry 160:1919–1928, 2003b

Geller D, Coffey BJ, Faraone S, et al: Does comorbid attention-deficit/hyperactivity disorder impact the clinical expression of pediatric obsessive compulsive disorder. CNS Spectr 8:259–264, 2003c

Geller D, Wieland N, Carey K, et al: Perinatal factors affecting expression of obsessive compulsive disorder in children and adolescents. J Child Adolesc Psychopharmacol 18:373–379, 2008

Hanna G, Himle JA, Curtis GC, et al: A family study of obsessive-compulsive disorder with pediatric probands. Am J Med Genet A 134:13–19, 2005

Heyman I, Fombonne E, Simmons H, et al: Prevalence of obsessive-compulsive disorder in the British nationwide survey of child mental health. Br J Psychiatry 179:324–329, 2001

Hollander E, Allen A, Steiner M, et al: Acute and long-term treatment and prevention of relapse of obsessive-compulsive disorder with paroxetine. J Clin Psychiatry 64:1113–1121, 2003

Hudziak J, Van Beijsterveldt CE, Althoff RR, et al: Genetic and environmental contributions to the Child Behavior Checklist Obsessive-Compulsive Scale: a cross-cultural twin study. Arch Gen Psychiatry 61:608–616, 2004

Jonnal AH, Gardner CO, Prescott CA, et al: Obsessive and compulsive symptoms in a general population sample of female twins. Am J Med Genet A 96:791–796, 2000

Kurlan R, Kaplan EL: The pediatric autoimmune neuropsychiatric disorders associated with streptococcal infection (PANDAS) etiology for tics and obsessive-compulsive symptoms: hypothesis or entity? Practical considerations for the clinician. Pediatrics 113:883–886, 2004

Kurlan R, Johnson D, Kaplan EL, et al: Streptococcal infection and exacerbations of childhood tics and obsessive-compulsive symptoms: a prospective blinded cohort study. Pediatrics 121:1188–1197, 2008

Leckman JF, Pauls DL, Zhang H, et al: Obsessive-compulsive symptom dimensions in affected sibling pairs diagnosed with Gilles de la Tourette syndrome. Am J Med Genet A 116B:60–68, 2003

Lenane M, Swedo SE, Leonard HL, et al: Psychiatric disorders in first degree relatives of children and adolescents with obsessive compulsive disorder. J Am Acad Child Adolesc Psychiatry 29:407–412, 1990

Lensi P, Casssano GB, Correddu G, et al: Obsessive-compulsive disorder: familial-developmental history, symptomatology, comorbidity and course with special reference to gender-related differences. Br J Psychiatry 169:101–107, 1996

Leonard HL, Goldberger EL, Rapoport JL, et al: Childhood rituals: normal development or obsessive-compulsive symptoms. J Am Acad Child Adolesc Psychiatry 29:17–23, 1990

March JS, Mulle K: OCD in Children and Adolescents: A Cognitive-Behavioral Treatment Manual. New York, Guilford, 1998

March JS, Biederman J, Wolkow R, et al: Sertraline in children and adolescents with obsessive-compulsive disorder: a multicenter randomized control trial. JAMA 280:1752–1756, 1998

March JS, Franklin M, Nelson A, et al: Cognitive-behavioral psychotherapy for pediatric obsessive-compulsive disorder. J Clin Psychol 30:8–18, 2001

March JS, Foa EB, Gammon P, et al: Cognitive-behavior therapy, sertraline, and their combination for children and adolescents with obsessive-compulsive disorder: the Pediatric OCD Treatment Study (POTS) randomized controlled trial. JAMA 292:1969–1976, 2004

Nestadt G, Samuels J, Riddle M, et al: A family study of obsessive compulsive disorder. Arch Gen Psychiatry 57:358–363, 2000

Neziroglu F, Yaryura-Tobias JA, Walz J, et al: The effect of fluvoxamine and behavior therapy on children and adolescents with obsessive-compulsive disorder. J Child Adolesc Psychopharmacol 10:295–306, 2000

Pauls DL, Alsobrook JP II, Goodman WK, et al: A family study of obsessive-compulsive disorder. Am J Psychiatry 152:76–84, 1995

Piacentini J, Bergman RL, Keller M, et al: Functional impairment in children and adolescents with obsessive compulsive disorder. J Child Adolesc Psychopharmacol 13(suppl):61–69, 2003

Rettew DC, Swedo SE, Leonard HL, et al: Obsessions and compulsions across time in 79 children and adolescents with obsessive-compulsive disorder. J Am Acad Child Adolesc Psychiatry 31:1050–1056, 1992

Riddle MA, Reeve EA, Yaryura-Tobias JA, et al: Fluvoxamine for children and adolescents with obsessive-compulsive disorder: a randomized, controlled, multicenter trial. J Am Acad Child Adolesc Psychiatry 40:222–229, 2001

Rosenberg DR, Keshavan MS: Toward a neurodevelopmental model of obsessive-compulsive disorder. Biol Psychiatry 43:623–640, 1998

Rosenberg DR, MacMaster FP, Keshavan MS, et al: Decrease in caudate glutamatergic concentrations in pediatric obsessive-compulsive disorder patients taking paroxetine. J Am Acad Child Adolesc Psychiatry 39:1096–1103, 2000

Rosenberg DR, Amponsah A, Sullivan A, et al: Increased medial thalamic choline in pediatric obsessive-compulsive disorder as detected by quantitative in vivo spectroscopic imaging. J Child Neurol 16:636–641, 2001

Scahill L, Riddle MA, McSwiggin-Hardin M, et al: Children's Yale-Brown Obsessive Compulsive Scale: reliability and validity. J Am Acad Child Adolesc Psychiatry 36:844–852, 1997

Shugart YY, Samuels J, Willour VL, et al: Genomewide linkage scan for obsessive-compulsive disorder: evidence for susceptibility loci on chromosomes 3q, 7p, 1q, 15q, and 6q. Mol Psychiatry 11:763–770, 2006

Snider LA, Lougee L, Slattery M, et al: Antibiotic prophylaxis with azithromycin or penicillin for childhood-onset neuropsychiatric disorders. Biol Psychiatry 57:788–792, 2005

Stewart SE, Geller D, Jenike M, et al: Long-term outcome of pediatric obsessive compulsive disorder: a meta-analysis and qualitative review of the literature. Acta Psychiatr Scand 110:4–13, 2004

Stewart ES, Rosario MC, Brown TA, et al: Principal components analysis of obsessive-compulsive disorder symptoms in children and adolescents. Biol Psychiatry 61:285–291, 2007

Storch EA, Merlo LJ, Larson MJ, et al: Clinical features associated with treatment resistant pediatric obsessive-compulsive disorder. Compr Psychiatry 49:35–42, 2008

Swedo SE, Leonard HL, Mittleman B, et al: Identification of children with pediatric autoimmune neuropsychiatric disorders associated with streptococcal infections by a marker associated with rheumatic fever. Am J Psychiatry 154:110–112, 1997

Thienemann M, Martin J, Cregger B, et al: Manual-driven group cognitive-behavioral therapy for adolescents with obsessive-compulsive disorder: a pilot study. J Am Acad Child Adolesc Psychiatry 40:1254–1260, 2001

van Grootheest DS, Cath DC, Beekman AT, et al: Twin studies on obsessive-compulsive disorder: a review. Twin Res Hum Genet 8:450–458, 2005

Wagner KD, Cook EH, Chung H, et al: Remission status after long-term sertraline treatment of pediatric obsessive-compulsive disorder. J Child Adolesc Psychopharmacol 13(suppl):S53–S60, 2003

Watson HJ, Rees CS: Meta-analysis of randomized, controlled treatment trials for pediatric obsessive-compulsive disorder. J Child Psychol Psychiatry 49:489–498, 2008

PART VI

PSYCHOSES

Chapter 24

Early-Onset Schizophrenia

Jon S. Kuniyoshi, M.D., Ph.D.
Jon M. McClellan, M.D.

Schizophrenia is characterized by disturbances in perception, thought, emotion, affect, and social relatedness. Early-onset schizophrenia (EOS) is defined as onset prior to age 18 years, with childhood-onset schizophrenia (COS) referring to onset before age 13 years. EOS is considered to be continuous with adult-onset schizophrenia yet manifests with special developmental and social challenges. This chapter will provide information on history, etiology, neurobiological and genetic characteristics, clinical presentation, and an overview of psychosocial and pharmacological interventions to provide a basis for comprehensive care of children and adolescents with schizophrenia and related disorders.

History

Accounts of psychotic symptoms and madness date back to antiquity. In the early 1900s, Kraepelin described *dementia praecox* (i.e., dementia of the young) as a condition separate in character from disorders such as that caused by syphilis. Bleuler first coined the term *schizophrenia* to mean a splitting of the mind. Bleuler's four "A's," which he considered to be characteristics of schizophrenia, were ambivalence, autism, affective flattening, and loosening of associations.

Early descriptions of schizophrenia included rare cases of the syndrome in children. Later, Bender, Kanner, and others (Fish 1977) focused on the neurodevelopmental maturation of EOS and defined it by developmental deficits in language, perception, and movement, recognizable as early as infancy. This led to the clustering of conditions now considered autism and pervasive developmental disorders within the broader rubric of childhood schizophrenia.

In the 1970s, research differentiated the abnormal development of schizophrenia from that of autism (Kolvin 1971; Rutter 1972). Since that time, research has supported classifying the two conditions as distinct entities, with schizophrenia in youth defined using the same criteria as for adults. Early-onset forms appear to be continuous with the adult-onset illness in regard to symptoms, course of illness, outcome, and some shared neurobiological features.

Epidemiology

In the general population, the prevalence of schizophrenia is approximately 1% (American Psychiatric Association 2000). There are no community epidemiological studies examining EOS. Onset prior to age 13 years appears to be rare (American Academy of Child and Adolescent Psychiatry 2001). The rate of onset then increases sharply during adolescence, with the peak age at onset between ages 15 and 30 years (American Psychiatric Association 2000). In a study of all youth hospitalized for schizophrenia in Denmark over a 13-year period (*n*=312), only 4 youth were under age 13 years, and only 28 youth were younger than 15 years (Thomsen 1996). Although there are reported cases of schizophrenia in youth younger than 6 years of age, the diagnostic validity of the illness in preschoolers has not been established (American Academy of Child and Adolescent Psychiatry 2001).

EOS, especially COS, appears more often in males (American Academy of Child and Adolescent Psychiatry 2001). As age increases, this ratio tends to even out. Since the adult literature suggests that the average age at onset in males is approximately 5 years younger than that in females (Loranger 1984), the male predominance in EOS may be a cross-sectional effect.

Neurodevelopment and Etiology

Schizophrenia is viewed as a heterogeneous disorder with multiple etiologies. To date, no single set of causes of the disorder has been identified. The current evidence suggests that the development of schizophrenia is best explained by a multifactorial neurodevelopmental model, where multiple genetic and environmental exposures play a role.

Genetic Factors

Family, twin, and adoption studies all support a strong genetic component for schizophrenia. The lifetime risk of developing the illness is 5–20 times higher in first-degree relatives of affected probands compared to the general population. The rate of concordance among monozygotic twins is 40%–60%, whereas the rate of concordance in dizygotic twins and other siblings ranges from 5% to 15% (Cardno and Gottesman 2000).

Currently, most genetic research in psychiatry is based on the "common disease–common allele" model (Lohmueller et al. 2003), which theorizes that complex illnesses are caused by the collective impact of multiple alleles, each of which may only contribute a small effect. For schizophrenia, research based on this model has identified multiple candidate regions and candidate genes (Harrison and Weinberger 2005; Owen et al. 2004). However, causal relationships between the illness and candidate genes are difficult to establish, and associations are often not replicable. Genome-wide association studies have not replicated putative candidate genes or genomic regions previously thought to play a role in schizophrenia (Sanders et al. 2008; Sullivan et al. 2008).

For EOS, particularly COS, positive association studies have been found for candidate genes implicated in adults, including the dysbindin gene, neuregulin gene, *DAOA/G30*, *GAD1*, *Prodh2/DGCR6*, and *DISC1* (Harrison and Weinberger 2005; Owen et al. 2004). Youth with COS appear to have a higher rate of cytogenetic abnormalities than reported in adults with schizophrenia, including 22q11 deletion syndrome (Gothelf et al. 2007; Lewandowski et al. 2007; Maynard et al. 2003). Approximately 10%–30% of individuals with 22q11.2 deletion syndrome (also known as velocardiofacial or DiGeorge syndrome) develop schizophrenia-like psychotic disorders.

An alternative to the common disease–common allele model is the hypothesis that some mutations predisposing to schizophrenia are highly penetrant and individually rare, even specific to single cases or families (McClellan et al. 2006, 2007b). Recent research has demonstrated that individuals with schizophrenia harbor significantly more rare deletions and duplications that impact genes than healthy control subjects (Walsh et al. 2008; Xu et al. 2008). In particular, individuals with sporadic schizophrenia have an eight-fold risk of harboring a de novo structural mutation (Xu et al. 2008). Patients with onset of schizophrenia by age 18 years have a greater risk of having a rare genomic deletion or duplication mutation (Walsh et al. 2008). Genes disrupted in patients were more significantly likely to be involved with neural development (Walsh et al. 2008).

Environmental Factors

Genetic and environmental factors shape the neurodevelopment of an individual resulting in normative development or the expression of psychopathology (Grossman et al. 2003; Waddington et al. 1999). In the pathogenesis of schizophrenia, this may involve continuous interactive processes that impact both development and progression of the disorder (Waddington et al. 2001). Environmental exposures may mediate disease risk via a number of different mechanisms, including direct neurological damage, gene-environment interactions, epigenetic effects, and/or de novo mutations (McClellan et al. 2006). Numerous environmental exposures have been hypothesized to contribute to the development of schizophrenia. To date, the best replicated risk factors include paternal age and in utero exposure to maternal famine (St. Clair et al. 2005; Susser et al. 1996).

Neuroanatomical Abnormalities

Multiple regional brain volumetric reductions have been described in schizophrenia at first diagnosis, regardless of age (Rapoport et al. 2005; Thompson et al. 2001). Increased volumes of lateral ventricles and reductions in hippocampus, thalamus, and frontal lobe volumes have consistently been reported (Mehler and Warnke 2002; Rapoport et al. 1997). Using newer imaging technologies, in vivo cortical thickness differences in prefrontal temporal and parietal regions have been found in schizophrenia and related disorders (Narr et al. 2005a, 2005b).

The National Institute of Mental Health (NIMH) COS study has demonstrated significant gray matter volumetric reductions in their cohort. Longitudinal studies have shown a more rapid progressive loss of gray matter (3%–4% per year in COS vs. 1%–2% in controls), which occurs in a parietal-to-frontal pattern during adolescence (Thompson et al. 2001). Follow-up studies show that cortical thinning in COS may plateau in early adulthood, when it becomes similar to the schizophrenic adult regional pattern (Greenstein et al. 2006; Sporn et al. 2003). These changes appear specific to COS, as they occur in medication-naive patients (Narr et al. 2005a, 2005b) and are not found in those with transient psychosis (Gogtay et al. 2004b) nor in studies of adults (Greenstein et al. 2006; Sporn et al. 2003).

The volumetric reductions in gray matter found in COS are theorized to be due to the disruption of specific neurodevelopmental processes that occur during adolescence. One such hypothesized process is the pruning of overproduced synaptic projections. Pruning in the developing brain proceeds from subcortical to cortical regions, following a pattern in which more complex processes mature only after less complex maturation has been completed (Gogtay et al. 2004a; Toga et al. 2006). However, it is not clear whether cortical thinning associated with schizophrenia is the product of increased pruning or decreased myelination (Greenough et al. 1987; Grossman et al. 2003; Toga et al. 2006; Waddington et al. 2001).

The relationship between cortical volumetric reductions and clinical status is not well established. Volumetric reductions have been variably associated with either more (Cannon et al. 2002; Gur et al. 2000) or less severe (Gur et al. 1998; Vidal et al. 2006) symptoms. Impaired cognitive functioning has not been associated with increased rates of frontal cortical thinning (Gochman et al. 2005). Clinical and etiologic heterogeneity likely confounds the interpretation of findings.

Clinical Presentation

In DSM-IV-TR (American Psychiatric Association 2000), EOS is diagnosed using the same criteria as for adults (Table 24–1). Psychotic symptoms are the hallmark feature of schizophrenia and are generally divided into two broad clusters. Positive symptoms include hallucinations, delusions, and disorganized thought. Negative symptoms include affective flattening, alogia, avolition, and anhedonia. Among youth with a variety of psychotic illnesses, negative symptoms appear to be the most specifically associated with EOS (McClellan et al. 2002). Hallucinations, disordered thought, and affective flattening are common in EOS, whereas complex delusions and catatonia occur less frequently (Green et al. 1992; Werry et al. 1991). Thought disorder in EOS is generally characterized by loose associations and illogical thinking (Caplan et al. 1989).

In both youth and adults, schizophrenia is characterized by four phases: prodromal, acute, recovery, and residual. Patients cycle through the last three phases once the illness is established. Individuals often are first assessed during an active acute phase of disease, which is characterized by significant positive symptoms. During this phase, patients may be grossly disorganized, confused, and potentially dangerous to themselves or others.

TABLE 24–1. DSM-IV-TR diagnostic criteria for schizophrenia

A. *Characteristic symptoms:* Two (or more) of the following, each present for a significant portion of time during a 1-month period (or less if successfully treated):

    (1) delusions

    (2) hallucinations

    (3) disorganized speech (e.g., frequent derailment or incoherence)

    (4) grossly disorganized or catatonic behavior

    (5) negative symptoms, i.e., affective flattening, alogia, or avolition

    Note: Only one Criterion A symptom is required if delusions are bizarre or hallucinations consist of a voice keeping up a running commentary on the person's behavior or thoughts, or two or more voices conversing with each other.

B. *Social/occupational dysfunction:* For a significant portion of the time since the onset of the disturbance, one or more major areas of functioning such as work, interpersonal relations, or self-care are markedly below the level achieved prior to the onset (or when the onset is in childhood or adolescence, failure to achieve expected level of interpersonal, academic, or occupational achievement).

C. *Duration:* Continuous signs of the disturbance persist for at least 6 months. This 6-month period must include at least 1 month of symptoms (or less if successfully treated) that meet Criterion A (i.e., active-phase symptoms) and may include periods of prodromal or residual symptoms. During these prodromal or residual periods, the signs of the disturbance may be manifested by only negative symptoms or two or more symptoms listed in Criterion A present in an attenuated form (e.g., odd beliefs, unusual perceptual experiences).

D. *Schizoaffective and mood disorder exclusion:* Schizoaffective disorder and mood disorder with psychotic features have been ruled out because either (1) no major depressive, manic, or mixed episodes have occurred concurrently with the active-phase symptoms; or (2) if mood episodes have occurred during active-phase symptoms, their total duration has been brief relative to the duration of the active and residual periods.

E. *Substance/general medical condition exclusion:* The disturbance is not due to the direct physiological effects of a substance (e.g., a drug of abuse, a medication) or a general medical condition.

F. *Relationship to a pervasive developmental disorder:* If there is a history of autistic disorder or another pervasive developmental disorder, the additional diagnosis of schizophrenia is made only if prominent delusions or hallucinations are also present for at least a month (or less if successfully treated).

Classification of longitudinal course (can be applied only after at least 1 year has elapsed since the initial onset of active-phase symptoms):

    Episodic with interepisode residual symptoms (episodes are defined by the reemergence of prominent psychotic symptoms); *also specify if:* **With prominent negative symptoms**

    Episodic with no interepisode residual symptoms

    Continuous (prominent psychotic symptoms are present throughout the period of observation); *also specify if:* **With prominent negative symptoms**

    Single episode in partial remission; *also specify if:* **With prominent negative symptoms**

    Single episode in full remission

    Other or unspecified pattern

Source. Reprinted from American Psychiatric Association: *Diagnostic and Statistical Manual of Mental Disorders,* 4th Edition, Text Revision. Washington, DC, American Psychiatric Association, 2000, pp. 312–313. Used with permission. Copyright © 2000 American Psychiatric Association.

Recovery from the active phase marks a shift to a predominance of negative symptoms. The time to recovery generally takes 1–6 months or longer, depending on response to treatment. In youth, recovery is often incomplete. Longer duration of untreated psychosis and greater severity of negative symptoms at the time of diagnosis predict greater functional impairment over time (Brown and Pluck 2000; Clarke et al. 2006). Individuals who recover from an acute phase generally have persistent functional deficits, residual disordered thinking, and negative symptoms. Most youth with EOS demonstrate some degree of chronic impairment (Calderoni et al. 2001; Eggers et al. 2000; McClellan et al. 1993; Werry et al. 1991).

Prior to the onset of positive symptoms, individuals generally experience a decline in function that presages the illness. Abnormalities during the prodromal period include social isolation, academic difficulties, odd or idiosyncratic preoccupations, and mood symptoms. This phase can last from days to weeks or a more chronic course of years. COS tends to have a more chronic onset with signs in early childhood (Fish and Kendler 2005), while the presentation in adolescence can have either an acute or more insidious onset (Kolvin 1971; McClellan and McCurry 1998; McClellan et al. 1993; Werry et al. 1991).

In addition, the majority of youth with EOS have histories of premorbid problems, including cognitive delays, learning problems, behavioral difficulties and social withdrawal or oddities. Approximately 10%–20% of individuals with EOS have intellectual deficits, with borderline mental retardation or worse (Green et al. 1992; McClellan and McCurry 1998; McClellan et al. 1993; Werry et al. 1991). Commonly co-occurring and/or premorbid psychiatric disorders include attention-deficit/hyperactivity disorder, disruptive behavior disorders, and anxiety and mood disorders, and in adolescents, substance abuse (Bottas et al. 2005; Frazier et al. 2007; McClellan et al. 2003; Ross et al. 2006; Seedat et al. 2003; Westermeyer 2006). Although effective treatment for psychosis may lead to improvement in these domains, treatment planning needs to account for these conditions.

Differential Diagnosis: Other Psychotic Syndromes

The appropriate clinical management of schizophrenia relies upon the ability to accurately diagnose the condi-

tion. Therefore, it is important to recognize other syndromes and conditions that manifest with psychotic symptoms. Table 24–2 presents the differential diagnosis of EOS and lists both psychotic and nonpsychotic disorders that can manifest with reports of psychosis. Appropriate diagnostic evaluation (Table 24–3) requires strategies to evaluate for comorbid and confounding medical and psychiatric disorders and to assess detailed symptom phenomenology, prodromal symptoms, family history, and social stressors. The most important alternate diagnoses to consider when assessing a child for schizophrenia are reviewed below.

TABLE 24–2. Differential diagnosis of early-onset schizophrenia

Psychiatric

Psychotic disorder due to a general medical condition

Bipolar disorder

Major depressive episode with psychotic features

Schizoaffective disorder

Posttraumatic stress disorder

Obsessive-compulsive disorder

Pervasive developmental disorder

Conduct disorder

Psychosocial

Abuse

Traumatic stress

Chaotic family environment

Medical

Substance intoxication, both legal and illegal drugs

Delirium

Brain tumor

Head injury

Seizure disorder

Meningitis

Porphyria

Wilson's disease

Cerebrovascular accident

AIDS

Electrolyte imbalance

Blood glucose imbalance

Endocrine imbalance

TABLE 24–3. Components of a diagnostic evaluation for patients with psychotic symptoms

A comprehensive psychiatric history focusing on the longitudinal characterization of the patient's current and past symptoms. Information from multiple sources is helpful to improve accuracy.

A comprehensive psychosocial history including academic and interpersonal functioning and exposure to trauma or child maltreatment.

A comprehensive physical exam to rule out medical disease as a cause of psychotic symptoms.

Laboratory evaluations and neuroimaging as clinically indicated.

Rating scales and neuropsychological testing if warranted to assess for learning and developmental disability, which may contribute to or confound diagnosis.

Medical Conditions

Numerous medical conditions can result in symptoms of psychosis. Recognition and correction of these conditions can result not only in the remission of psychotic symptoms but also in the treatment of a potentially life-threatening illness. Psychosis caused by an underlying medical condition is often associated with delirium, a condition associated with significantly increased morbidity and mortality. This complex diagnosis with numerous potential etiologies (see Table 24–2) requires treatment that may include judicious psychopharmacological treatment with antipsychotic medication for symptom management until the underlying cause can be determined and eliminated (McClellan et al. 2007a). The potentially lethal nature of many of the underlying causes of delirium, psychosis, and other mental status changes requires a thorough medical and neurological examination at the time of first presentation of psychosis, especially in cases with acute onset or rapid progression of symptoms.

Intoxication

Both legal and illegal drugs can result in psychosis. In the case of prescribed medication, the treatment algorithm would include identification and elimination of the offending agent and possibly brief psychopharmacological treatment for symptom management. Prescription drugs associated with psychosis, especially when taken inappropriately, include corticosteroids, anesthetics, anticholinergics, antihistamines, amphetamines, and dextromethorphan.

While illicit drug use would ideally follow the same algorithm, elimination of the inciting substance can be problematic. Drugs of abuse that can result in psychosis include dextromethorphan, lysergic acid diethylamide (LSD), hallucinogenic mushrooms, psilocybin, peyote, cannabis, stimulants, salvia, and inhalants. Some drugs, such as methamphetamine, methylene-

dioxyamphetamine (MDA), and dextromethorphan, may result in more chronic impairment beyond the period of detoxification. Chronic psychotic states produced by these substances are similar in character to schizophrenia. There is continued debate as to whether these prolonged episodes represent independent drug effects or an environmental stimulus for the expression of schizophrenia in a vulnerable individual. Assessment of premorbid functioning may help with assessment and diagnosis.

Schizoaffective Disorder

Early-onset schizoaffective disorder has not been well defined. Youth with schizoaffective disorder have similar severe impairment to those with schizophrenia, in addition to experiencing concurrent mood disturbances (Frazier et al. 2007). Some follow-up studies have found that youth with schizoaffective disorder fare poorly (McClellan et al. 1999). Alternatively, Eggers (1989) found that 28% of his EOS sample at follow-up had schizoaffective psychoses, which predicted a better outcome. However, this was an ICD-9 diagnosis and may have included some subjects who would be diagnosed with bipolar disorder using DSM-IV-TR criteria.

Affective Psychosis

Psychotic mood disorders (especially bipolar disorder; see Chapter 19, "Bipolar Disorder") can manifest with a variety of affective and psychotic symptoms (McClellan et al. 1993; Werry et al. 1991). In children and adolescents with schizophrenia, negative symptoms may be mistaken for depression, especially since it is common for patients to experience dysphoria with their illness. Alternatively, mania in teenagers often manifests with florid psychosis, including hallucinations, delusions, and thought disorder (American

Academy of Child and Adolescent Psychiatry 2007). Psychotic depression may manifest with mood congruent or incongruent psychotic features, either hallucinations or delusions (American Academy of Child and Adolescent Psychiatry 1998).

This overlap in symptoms increases the likelihood of misdiagnosis at the time of onset (McClellan and McCurry 1999; McClellan et al. 1993). Longitudinal reassessment is needed to ensure accuracy of diagnosis. Family psychiatric history may also be a helpful differentiating factor, although a family history of depression is also common in youth with schizophrenia (American Academy of Child and Adolescent Psychiatry 2001).

Differentiating True Psychotic Symptoms From Other Phenomena

Many children report symptoms suggestive of hallucinations and delusions yet do not present with other evidence of psychosis, such as disorganization in thought and bizarre behavior. Most children reporting apparent psychotic symptoms do not have a true psychotic disorder (Garralda 1984). The assessment of psychosis in youth requires the gauging of potential symptom reports in the context of normal development. Overactive imaginations can be normal and characteristic of prepubertal children and developmentally disabled individuals. Atypical psychotic symptoms may be reported by youth with conduct disorder or other emotional disorders (McClellan and McCurry 1999; McClellan et al. 1993), including posttraumatic stress disorder (Hlastala and McClellan 2005). In these individuals, expression of psychotic symptoms can result in increased emotional support and therefore symptoms can result in reinforcement. Differentiation can be made by the presence or absence of disorganized thought and behavior, the qualitative nature of the symptom report, the context within which symptoms are reported, and the association of reports with onset of sleep or waking (e.g., hypnogogic and hypnopompic hallucinations) (Hlastala and McClellan 2005).

Autism and Other Pervasive Developmental Disorders

Autism and other pervasive developmental disorders (PDDs) are distinguished by the absence or transitory nature of psychotic symptoms and by the predominance of the characteristic abnormal language patterns, aberrant social relatedness, and ritualistic or repetitive repertoires of behavior (Green et al. 1984; Kolvin 1971; Volkmar and Cohen 1991). The earlier age at onset and the absence of a normal period of development are also indicative of PDD. The premorbid abnormalities in EOS tend to be less pervasive and severe than those with autism.

Children with Asperger syndrome lack the marked language disturbances associated with autism but present with deficits in social relatedness and contextual communication (especially with regard to social cues) and a restricted (and often unusual) range of interests. The lack of overt hallucinations and delusions distinguishes Asperger syndrome from schizophrenia (American Academy of Child and Adolescent Psychiatry 2001). However, it is not uncommon that youth with schizophrenia will have premorbid histories characterized by social oddities and aloofness, which may have been diagnosed as Asperger syndrome or PDD not otherwise specified. Once psychotic symptoms become apparent, the diagnosis of schizophrenia takes precedence.

Psychosocial Factors

Psychological or social factors, by themselves, do not appear to cause schizophrenia. However, psychosocial factors may interact with biological risk factors to mediate the timing of onset, course, and severity of the disorder. Family and parenting factors can certainly influence the disorder, both positively and negatively. Unfortunately, in the past, many families of youth with schizophrenia have been unfairly indicted as causing psychosis. Family support is essential for assistance in managing stressful situations and promoting appropriate social interaction, both of which are important for reducing symptoms.

Since family interactions influence the course and morbidity of illness, shaping family interactions should be a treatment focus in EOS. Criticism, emotional overinvolvement, and hostility in families (high in expressed emotion) have been associated with worse outcomes in adults with schizophrenia (Wearden et al. 2000). High expressed emotion is a strong predictor of future relapse of hospitalized patients (Butzlaff and Hooley 1998). However, high expressed emotion may be a response of caregivers to a family member more severely affected with mental illness, rather than a causal factor (Hooley and

Campbell 2002). In contrast, positive remarks from caregivers are associated with decreased negative symptoms and improved social functioning in adolescents and young adults (O'Brien et al. 2006). Higher scores on warmth scales in adults are associated with decreased relapse rate (Breitborde et al. 2007) and improved social functioning (Bertrando et al. 1992).

Interestingly, a study of Mexican American families found a curvilinear association between emotional overinvolvement and relapse (Breitborde et al. 2007). In this study, midlevel emotional overinvolvement and high-level warmth were associated with improved outcome, possibly reflective of the importance of family involvement tempered with a sense of independence. Thus it may be that a balance between independence and interdependence, combined with a greater environmental understanding of schizophrenic illness (Lopez et al. 2004), will be associated with decreased functional impairment. However, due to cultural variation these associations may not be present in all families with schizophrenia.

In African American families, high expressed emotion is not a predictor of relapse. High levels of critical and intrusive behavior are associated with improved outcome over a 2-year follow-up period in adults (Rosenfarb et al. 2006). As stated above, it is likely that cultural context influences how the patient perceives the family's behavior.

Peer Relationships

Experiential deprivation can develop in childhood as a result of decreased social interactions. Whether resulting from skill deficits or imposed restrictions, experiential deprivation and lack of empowerment are associated with functional deficits (Horan et al. 2005). During normal development, children transition from family-centered to peer-centered relationships. During adolescence, success in same-age relationships is a core developmental goal. Youth with schizophrenia are especially vulnerable to difficulties in interpersonal relationships. Even prior to the onset of the illness, most affected youth experience a prodromal period characterized by relationship difficulties and withdrawal (Cannon et al. 2001). Greater deficits in peer relations and social relatedness predict a poorer outcome. Therefore, intervention strategies are needed to address these issues.

Cultural and Diversity Issues

Cultural influences shape views and perspectives and need to be considered in interpretation of mental health symptoms and diagnosis. Societal beliefs should be considered in the context of interpreting psychotic symptoms or the impact of the diagnosis and treatment on family functioning. Religion often can have a large impact on an individual's belief system. Differentiating a psychotic thought process from culturally and religiously reinforced beliefs can be a challenge. Potential symptoms should be examined in the context of the individual's belief system. For example, a belief in God is often congruent with individual beliefs, but removing one's right hand because of a direct command from God violates most societal norms. By definition, delusions and hallucinations should be incongruent with the beliefs and values of the individual's environment and culture.

Schizophrenia prevalence rates from different cultures are similar (Draguns and Tanaka-Matsumi 2003). Interestingly, transitioning to a new culture may be associated with development of the illness. First- and second-generation immigrants have an increased risk of schizophrenia, with those coming from developing countries being at greater risk (Cantor-Graae and Selten 2005). Cultural influences may also occur within a region, such as the noted increased risk associated with urban environments (Spauwen et al. 2004). These findings suggest that increased stress, whether arising from illness or from family or societal roles, may result in an increased risk of schizophrenia and disease symptoms.

Treatment

Treatment of EOS requires a comprehensive, integrated approach combining medication therapies with psychosocial interventions. Developmentally appropriate interventions are needed that focus on cognitive, behavioral, and social functioning to reduce symptoms and improve quality of life. The management of EOS mirrors that of affected adults, with added special emphasis on developmental and family issues.

Controlled trials have established the short-term effectiveness of typical and atypical antipsychotics in treatment of adults with schizophrenia (Lehman et al. 2004), with improvements in overall functioning, reductions in psychotic symptoms, and decreased likelihood for relapse. Despite the widespread assumptions to the contrary, the newer atypical agents do not appear to be superior to the traditional neuroleptics in regard to long-term response or side-effect profiles (Jones et al. 2006; Kahn et al. 2008; Lieberman et al. 2005). Furthermore, many affected individuals are not able to be maintained on the same agent long-term (Jones et al. 2006; Kahn et al. 2008; Lieberman et al. 2005).

Medication treatment guidelines for EOS are based primarily on the adult literature. There are a few short-term controlled trials supporting the efficacy of traditional agents (e.g., haloperidol, loxapine, thioridazine, and thiothixene), as well as the second-generation antipsychotics olanzapine, risperidone, and aripiprazole (for review, see American Academy of Child and Adolescent Psychiatry 2001 and Kumra et al. 2008). Risperidone and aripiprazole have been approved by the U.S. Food and Drug Administration (FDA) for the treatment of adolescents with schizophrenia. Clozapine was found to be superior to both haloperidol (Kumra et al. 1996) and olanzapine (Shaw et al. 2006) in youth with treatment-resistant schizophrenia. However, clozapine's side-effect profile limits its use to patients who have failed other antipsychotic agents.

Procedures for the use of medication in EOS are available to help guide clinical practice (American Academy of Child and Adolescent Psychiatry 2001). In the acute phase, treatment is based on treatment history in the patient or his or her relatives, the side-effect profile of the medication, and, often, practical considerations of delivery options and insurance coverage. Immediate results are often due to sedation, and a trial of 4–6 weeks is needed to determine effectiveness. Rapid increases in dose can result in greater likelihood of side effects and increases the use of high doses that generally do not hasten recovery. If clinical utility has not been demonstrated after 6 weeks of treatment, another agent should be selected. The use of medication in the treatment of EOS will be covered in detail in Chapter 49, "Antipsychotic Medications."

Empirical evidence for psychosocial interventions in EOS is limited. However, clinical consensus suggests that children and adolescents will most likely benefit from comprehensive intervention strategies that focus on behavioral and family functioning and medication compliance.

For adults with schizophrenia, psychosocial interventions with some empirical support include psychoeducational strategies, family interventions, skills training, and relapse prevention. Cognitive-behavioral interventions focusing on identifying and challenging deficits in thought processes have shown lasting effects in symptom management, including medication compliance (Pilling et al. 2002). Assertive community intervention strategies show improvement in rates of hospitalization, housing stability, and relapse (Essock and Kontos 1995; Lehman 1998). Skills training has been as-

sociated with improved role functioning, self-efficacy, and patient satisfaction, though it has not been associated with symptom reduction or relapse prevention (Bellack et al. 2005).

Comprehensive strategies focusing on reintegration of patients into normative environments are essential to illness management. Providing interpersonal skills training to target social skills deficits can aid in stress reduction and skill acquisition. Interventions should be behaviorally focused and be tailored to the interpersonal skill and developmental level of the patient. These therapies can be used in children and adolescents but should be modified to account for developmental level.

For adults, family and environmentally based therapies have been demonstrated to improve compliance, decrease relapse, and lower hospital admissions (Huxley et al. 2000; Pilling et al. 2002). Behavioral, psychoeducational, and supportive family intervention strategies all appear to provide enduring positive effects (Glynn et al. 2006; Mueser et al. 1998; Tarrier et al. 1994). One small study of patients with EOS found that family psychoeducational therapy was associated with improvements in relapse rates and global functioning (Rund 1994). In this study, youth with greater premorbid functional deficits demonstrated more significant benefits. Although the literature is limited, it is reasonable to assume that family interventions are crucial elements of effective treatment for EOS. Key components include the provision of family education and support. Parental burden is high with this disorder, given the effects of the illness on family functioning, the grief at having an impaired child, the frustration inherent in dealing with a complex and often confusing mental health care system, and the financial burdens of caring for a chronically ill child. Efforts to provide support, decrease sense of isolation, validate frustrations, and empower families should improve outcomes and enhance quality of life.

Research Directions

Research is needed to advance knowledge of the etiologies, clinical presentation, and treatment of EOS. Over the next decade, there likely will be substantial gains regarding the identification of disease-risk genes, as well as the genetic mechanisms underlying both treatment response and adverse events. Characterization of genetic causes will ultimately further the understanding of the neuropathophysiology of the illness. In addition, processes mediated by these genes will become potential targets for new intervention and prevention strategies.

Summary Points

- Early-onset schizophrenia may represent a more severe variant of the adult-onset form.

- Childhood schizophrenia is a rare disorder (less than 1% prevalence). Most youth reporting psychotic-like symptoms do not truly have a psychotic illness. Caution is warranted for applying this diagnosis in young children.

- Premorbid signs and symptoms may occur early in childhood, yet at this point the presentations lack sufficient specificity to accurately predict the illness.

- Severity of negative symptoms and duration of untreated psychosis are associated with poor quality of life and long-term functioning.

- Genetic vulnerability and environmental exposures and experiences likely interact to influence the onset and progression of schizophrenia.

- A comprehensive treatment approach that combines psychopharmacology with psychotherapeutic and environmental interventions is needed for EOS.

- Comorbid illnesses are common and should be an additional focus of treatment.

References

American Academy of Child and Adolescent Psychiatry: Practice parameters for the assessment and treatment of children and adolescents with depressive disorders. J Am Acad Child Adolesc Psychiatry 37:63S–83S, 1998

American Academy of Child and Adolescent Psychiatry: Practice parameter for the assessment and treatment of children and adolescents with schizophrenia. J Am Acad Child Adolesc Psychiatry 40:4S–23S, 2001

American Academy of Child and Adolescent Psychiatry: Practice parameter for the assessment and treatment of children and adolescents with bipolar disorder. J Am Acad Child Adolesc Psychiatry 46:107–125, 2007

American Psychiatric Association: Diagnostic and Statistical Manual of Mental Disorders, 4th Edition, Text Revision. Washington, DC, American Psychiatric Association, 2000

Bellack AS, Dickinson D, Morris SE, et al: The development of a computer-assisted cognitive remediation program for patients with schizophrenia. Isr J Psychiatry Relat Sci 42:5–14, 2005

Bertrando P, Beltz J, Bressi C, et al: Expressed emotion and schizophrenia in Italy: a study of an urban population. Br J Psychiatry 161:223–229, 1992

Bottas A, Cooke RG, Richter MA: Comorbidity and pathophysiology of obsessive-compulsive disorder in schizophrenia: is there evidence for a schizo-obsessive subtype of schizophrenia? J Psychiatry Neurosci 30:187–193, 2005

Breitborde NJ, Lopez SR, Wickens TD, et al: Toward specifying the nature of the relationship between expressed emotion and schizophrenic relapse: the utility of curvilinear models. Int J Methods Psychiatr Res 16:1–10, 2007

Brown RG, Pluck G: Negative symptoms: the "pathology" of motivation and goal-directed behaviour. Trends Neurosci 23:412–417, 2000

Butzlaff RL, Hooley JM: Expressed emotion and psychiatric relapse: a meta-analysis. Arch Gen Psychiatry 55:547–552, 1998

Calderoni D, Wudarsky M, Bhangoo R, et al: Differentiating childhood-onset schizophrenia from psychotic mood disorders. J Am Acad Child Adolesc Psychiatry 40:1190–1196, 2001

Cannon M, Walsh E, Hollis C, et al: Predictors of later schizophrenia and affective psychosis among attendees at a child psychiatry department. Br J Psychiatry 178:420–426, 2001

Cannon TD, Thompson PM, van Erp TG, et al: Cortex mapping reveals regionally specific patterns of genetic and disease-specific gray-matter deficits in twins discordant for schizophrenia. Proc Natl Acad Sci USA 99:3228–3233, 2002

Cantor-Graae E, Selten JP: Schizophrenia and migration: a meta-analysis and review. Am J Psychiatry 162:12–24, 2005

Caplan R, Guthrie D, Fish B, et al: The Kiddie Formal Thought Disorder Rating Scale: clinical assessment, reliability, and validity. J Am Acad Child Adolesc Psychiatry 28:408–416, 1989

Cardno A, Gottesman II: Twin studies of schizophrenia: from bow-and-arrow concordances to star wars Mx and functional genomics. Am J Med Genet 97:12–17, 2000

Clarke M, Whitty P, Browne S, et al: Untreated illness and outcome of psychosis. Br J Psychiatry 189:235–240, 2006

Draguns JG, Tanaka-Matsumi J: Assessment of psychopathology across and within cultures: issues and findings. Behav Res Ther 41:755–776, 2003

Eggers C: Schizo-affective psychoses in childhood: a follow-up study. J Autism Dev Disord 19:327–342, 1989

Eggers C, Bunk D, Krause D: Schizophrenia with onset before the age of eleven: clinical characteristics of onset and course. J Autism Dev Disord 30:29–38, 2000

Essock SM, Kontos N: Implementing assertive community treatment teams. Psychiatr Serv 46:679–683, 1995

Fish B: Neurobiologic antecedents of schizophrenia in children: evidence for an inherited, congenital neurointegrative defect. Arch Gen Psychiatry 34:1297–1313, 1977

Fish B, Kendler KS: Abnormal infant neurodevelopment predicts schizophrenia spectrum disorders. J Child Adolesc Psychopharmacol 15:348–361, 2005

Frazier JA, McClellan J, Findling RL, et al: Treatment of Early-Onset Schizophrenia Spectrum Disorders (TEOSS): demographic and clinical characteristics. J Am Acad Child Adolesc Psychiatry 46:979–988, 2007

Garralda ME: Hallucinations in children with conduct and emotional disorders, II: the follow-up study. Psychol Med 14:597–604, 1984

Glynn SM, Cohen AN, Dixon LB, et al: The potential impact of the recovery movement on family interventions for schizophrenia: opportunities and obstacles. Schizophr Bull 32:451–463, 2006

Gochman PA, Greenstein D, Sporn A, et al: IQ stabilization in childhood-onset schizophrenia. Schizophr Res 77:271–277, 2005

Gogtay N, Giedd JN, Lusk L, et al: Dynamic mapping of human cortical development during childhood through early adulthood. Proc Natl Acad Sci USA 101:8174–8179, 2004a

Gogtay N, Sporn A, Clasen LS, et al: Comparison of progressive cortical gray matter loss in childhood-onset schizophrenia with that in childhood-onset atypical psychoses. Arch Gen Psychiatry 61:17–22, 2004b

Gothelf D, Feinstein C, Thompson T, et al: Risk factors for the emergence of psychotic disorders in adolescents with 22q11.2 deletion syndrome. Am J Psychiatry 164:663–669, 2007

Green WH, Campbell M, Hardesty AS, et al: A comparison of schizophrenic and autistic children. J Am Acad Child Psychiatry 23:399–409, 1984

Green WH, Padron-Gayol M, Hardesty AS, et al: Schizophrenia with childhood onset: a phenomenological study of 38 cases. J Am Acad Child Adolesc Psychiatry 31:968–976, 1992

Greenough WT, Black JE, Wallace CS: Experience and brain development. Child Dev 58:539–559, 1987

Greenstein D, Lerch J, Shaw P, et al: Childhood-onset schizophrenia: cortical brain abnormalities as young adults. J Child Psychol Psychiatry 47:1003–1012, 2006

Grossman AW, Churchill JD, McKinney BC, et al: Experience effects on brain development: possible contributions to psychopathology. J Child Psychol Psychiatry 44:33–63, 2003

Gur RE, Cowell P, Turetsky BI, et al: A follow-up magnetic resonance imaging study of schizophrenia: relationship of neuroanatomical changes to clinical and neurobehavioral measures. Arch Gen Psychiatry 55:145–152, 1998

Gur RE, Cowell PE, Latshaw A, et al: Reduced dorsal and orbital prefrontal gray matter volumes in schizophrenia. Arch Gen Psychiatry 57:761–768, 2000

Harrison PJ, Weinberger DR: Schizophrenia genes, gene expression, and neuropathology: on the matter of their convergence. Mol Psychiatry 10:40–68, 2005

Hlastala SA, McClellan J: Phenomenology and diagnostic stability of youths with atypical psychotic symptoms. J Child Adolesc Psychopharmacol 15:497–509, 2005

Hooley JM, Campbell C: Control and controllability: beliefs and behaviour in high and low expressed emotion relatives. Psychol Med 32:1091–1099, 2002

Horan WP, Ventura J, Nuechterlein KH, et al: Stressful life events in recent-onset schizophrenia: reduced frequencies and altered subjective appraisals. Schizophr Res 75:363–374, 2005

Huxley NA, Rendall M, Sederer L: Psychosocial treatments in schizophrenia: a review of the past 20 years. J Nerv Ment Dis 188:187–201, 2000

Jones PB, Barnes TR, Davies L, et al: Randomized controlled trial of the effect on quality of life of second- vs first-generation antipsychotic drugs in schizophrenia: Cost Utility of the Latest Antipsychotic Drugs in Schizophrenia Study (CUtLASS 1). Arch Gen Psychiatry 63:1079–1087, 2006

Kahn RS, Fleischhacker WW, Boter H, et al: Effectiveness of antipsychotic drugs in first-episode schizophrenia and schizophreniform disorder: an open randomised clinical trial. Lancet 371:1085–1097, 2008

Kolvin I: Studies in the childhood psychoses, I: diagnostic criteria and classification. Br J Psychiatry 118:381–384, 1971

Kumra S, Frazier JA, Jacobsen LK, et al: Childhood-onset schizophrenia: a double-blind clozapine-haloperidol comparison. Arch Gen Psychiatry 53:1090–1097, 1996

Kumra S, Oberstar JV, Sikich L, et al: Efficacy and tolerability of second-generation antipsychotics in children and adolescents with schizophrenia. Schizophr Bull 34:60–71, 2008

Lehman AF: Public health policy, community services, and outcomes for patients with schizophrenia. Psychiatr Clin North Am 21:221–231, 1998

Lehman AF, Lieberman JA, Dixon LB, et al: Practice guideline for the treatment of patients with schizophrenia, second edition. Am J Psychiatry 161:1–56, 2004

Lewandowski KE, Shashi V, Berry PM, et al: Schizophrenic-like neurocognitive deficits in children and adolescents with 22q11 deletion syndrome. Am J Med Genet B Neuropsychiatr Genet 144:27–36, 2007

Lieberman JA, Stroup TS, McEvoy JP, et al: Effectiveness of antipsychotic drugs in patients with chronic schizophrenia. N Engl J Med 353:1209–1223, 2005

Lohmueller KE, Pearce CL, Pike M, et al: Meta-analysis of genetic association studies supports a contribution of common variants to susceptibility to common disease. Nat Genet 33:177–182, 2003

Lopez SR, Nelson Hipke K, Polo AJ, et al: Ethnicity, expressed emotion, attributions, and course of schizophrenia: family warmth matters. J Abnorm Psychol 113:428–439, 2004

Loranger AW: Sex difference in age at onset of schizophrenia. Arch Gen Psychiatry 41:157–161, 1984

Maynard TM, Haskell GT, Peters AZ, et al: A comprehensive analysis of 22q11 gene expression in the developing and adult brain. Proc Natl Acad Sci USA 100:14433–14438, 2003

McClellan J, McCurry C: Neurodevelopmental Pathways in Schizophrenia. Semin Clin Neuropsychiatry 3:320–332, 1998

McClellan J, McCurry C: Early-onset psychotic disorders: diagnostic stability and clinical characteristics. Eur Child Adolesc Psychiatry 8(suppl):I13–19, 1999

McClellan J, Werry JS, Ham M: A follow-up study of early-onset psychosis: comparison between outcome diagnoses of schizophrenia, mood disorders, and personality disorders. J Autism Dev Disord 23:243–262, 1993

McClellan J, McCurry C, Snell J, et al: Early-onset psychotic disorders: course and outcome over a 2-year period. J Am Acad Child Adolesc Psychiatry 38:1380–1388, 1999

McClellan J, McCurry C, Speltz ML, et al: Symptom factors in early-onset psychotic disorders. J Am Acad Child Adolesc Psychiatry 41:791–798, 2002

McClellan J, Breiger D, McCurry C, et al: Premorbid functioning in early-onset psychotic disorders. J Am Acad Child Adolesc Psychiatry 42:666–672, 2003

McClellan J, Susser E, King MC: Maternal famine, de novo mutations, and schizophrenia. JAMA 296:582–584, 2006

McClellan J, Sikich L, Findling RL, et al: Treatment of Early-Onset Schizophrenia Spectrum Disorders (TEOSS): rationale, design, and methods. J Am Acad Child Adolesc Psychiatry 46:969–978, 2007a

McClellan J, Susser E, King MC: Schizophrenia: a common disease caused by multiple rare alleles. Br J Psychiatry 190:194–199, 2007b

Mehler C, Warnke A: Structural brain abnormalities specific to childhood-onset schizophrenia identified by neuroimaging techniques. J Neural Transm 109:219–234, 2002

Mueser KT, Bond GR, Drake RE, et al: Models of community care for severe mental illness: a review of research on case management. Schizophr Bull 24:37–74, 1998

Narr KL, Bilder RM, Toga AW, et al: Mapping cortical thickness and gray matter concentration in first episode schizophrenia. Cereb Cortex 15:708–719, 2005a

Narr KL, Toga AW, Szeszko P, et al: Cortical thinning in cingulate and occipital cortices in first episode schizophrenia. Biol Psychiatry 58:32–40, 2005b

O'Brien MP, Gordon JL, Bearden CE, et al: Positive family environment predicts improvement in symptoms and social functioning among adolescents at imminent risk for onset of psychosis. Schizophr Res 81:269–275, 2006

Owen MJ, Williams NM, O'Donovan MC: The molecular genetics of schizophrenia: new findings promise new insights. Mol Psychiatry 9:14–27, 2004

Pilling S, Bebbington P, Kuipers E, et al: Psychological treatments in schizophrenia, I: meta-analysis of family intervention and cognitive behaviour therapy. Psychol Med 32:763–782, 2002

Rapoport JL, Giedd J, Kumra S, et al: Childhood-onset schizophrenia: progressive ventricular change during adolescence. Arch Gen Psychiatry 54:897–903, 1997

Rapoport JL, Addington AM, Frangou S, et al: The neurodevelopmental model of schizophrenia: update 2005. Mol Psychiatry 10:434–449, 2005

Rosenfarb IS, Bellack AS, Aziz N: Family interactions and the course of schizophrenia in African American and White patients. J Abnorm Psychol 115:112–120, 2006

Ross RG, Heinlein S, Tregellas H: High rates of comorbidity are found in childhood-onset schizophrenia. Schizophr Res 88:90–95, 2006

Rund BR: Cognitive dysfunctions and psychosocial treatment of schizophrenics: research of the past and perspectives on the future. Acta Psychiatr Scand Suppl 384:9–16, 1994

Rutter M: Childhood schizophrenia reconsidered. J Autism Child Schizophr 2:315–337, 1972

Sanders AR, Duan J, Levinson DF, et al: No significant association of 14 candidate genes with schizophrenia in a large European ancestry sample: implications for psychiatric genetics. Am J Psychiatry 165:497–506, 2008

Seedat S, Stein MB, Oosthuizen PP, et al: Linking posttraumatic stress disorder and psychosis: a look at epidemiology, phenomenology, and treatment. J Nerv Ment Dis 191:675–681, 2003

Shaw P, Sporn A, Gogtay N, et al: Childhood-onset schizophrenia: a double-blind, randomized clozapine-olanzapine comparison. Arch Gen Psychiatry 63:721–730, 2006

Spauwen J, Krabbendam L, Lieb R, et al: Does urbanicity shift the population expression of psychosis? J Psychiatr Res 38:613–618, 2004

Sporn AL, Greenstein DK, Gogtay N, et al: Progressive brain volume loss during adolescence in childhood-onset schizophrenia. Am J Psychiatry 160:2181–2189, 2003

St. Clair D, Xu M, Wang P, et al: Rates of adult schizophrenia following prenatal exposure to the Chinese famine of 1959–1961. JAMA 294:557–562, 2005

Sullivan PF, Lin D, Tzeng JY, et al: Genomewide association for schizophrenia in the CATIE study: results of stage 1. Mol Psychiatry 13:570–584, 2008

Susser E, Neugebauer R, Hoek HW, et al: Schizophrenia after prenatal famine: further evidence. Arch Gen Psychiatry 53:25–31, 1996

Tarrier N, Barrowclough C, Porceddu K, et al: The Salford Family Intervention Project: relapse rates of schizophrenia at five and eight years. Br J Psychiatry 165:829–832, 1994

Thompson PM, Vidal C, Giedd JN, et al: Mapping adolescent brain change reveals dynamic wave of accelerated gray matter loss in very early-onset schizophrenia. Proc Natl Acad Sci USA 98:11650–11655, 2001

Thomsen PH: Schizophrenia with childhood and adolescent onset: a nationwide register-based study. Acta Psychiatr Scand 94:187–193, 1996

Toga AW, Thompson PM, Sowell ER: Mapping brain maturation. Trends Neurosci 29:148–159, 2006

Vidal CN, Rapoport JL, Hayashi KM, et al: Dynamically spreading frontal and cingulate deficits mapped in adolescents with schizophrenia. Arch Gen Psychiatry 63:25–34, 2006

Volkmar FR, Cohen DJ: Comorbid association of autism and schizophrenia. Am J Psychiatry 148:1705–1707, 1991

Waddington JL, Lane A, Larkin C, et al: The neurodevelopmental basis of schizophrenia: clinical clues from cerebro-craniofacial dysmorphogenesis, and the roots of a lifetime trajectory of disease. Biol Psychiatry 46:31–39, 1999

Waddington JL, Scully PJ, Quinn JF, et al: The origin and course of schizophrenia: implications for clinical practice. J Psychiatr Pract 7:247–252, 2001

Walsh T, McClellan JM, McCarthy SE, et al: Rare structural variants disrupt multiple genes in neurodevelopmental pathways in schizophrenia. Science 320:539–543, 2008

Wearden AJ, Tarrier N, Barrowclough C, et al: A review of expressed emotion research in health care. Clin Psychol Rev 20:633–666, 2000

Werry JS, McClellan JM, Chard L: Childhood and adolescent schizophrenic, bipolar, and schizoaffective disorders: a clinical and outcome study. J Am Acad Child Adolesc Psychiatry 30:457–465, 1991

Westermeyer J: Comorbid schizophrenia and substance abuse: a review of epidemiology and course. Am J Addict 15:345–355, 2006

Xu B, Roos JL, Levy S, et al: Strong association of de novo copy number mutations with sporadic schizophrenia. Nat Genet 40:880–885, 2008

PART VII

DISORDERS AFFECTING SOMATIC FUNCTION

Chapter 25

Obesity

Kelly Walker Lowry, Ph.D.

Definition, Clinical Description, and Diagnosis

Pediatric obesity has quickly become a national epidemic with significant medical and psychological consequences. Obesity results from an imbalance between food intake and energy output, leading to excessive levels of adipose tissue. Although once an adaptive survival mechanism, excessive adipose tissue now poses significant pathophysiological risk in the current environment of dietary abundance and limited physical activity (Daniels et al. 2005).

Direct measurement of adipose tissue can be difficult and costly. Assessment of obesity in most settings is done via calculation of body mass index (BMI), which has been well correlated with body fat, health risks, future adiposity, and future morbidity (Barlow and Expert Committee 2007). BMI is calculated by dividing weight in kilograms by the square of height in meters (kg/m^2). In youth, BMI percentiles for age and gender

are based on the Centers for Disease Control and Prevention (CDC) growth charts. A child with a BMI within the 85th–95th percentiles is considered overweight, a child with a BMI at or above the 95th percentile is considered obese, and a child with a BMI at or above the 99th percentile is considered to have severe childhood obesity (Barlow and Expert Committee 2007).

Epidemiology

Childhood obesity rates are increasing worldwide. Obesity appears to increase as countries adapt to Western or "American" lifestyles and cultural practices, which are characterized by high caloric intake and low levels of physical activity. The current environment has been labeled "obesogenic" to refer to an atmosphere that promotes obesity by providing frequent exposure and accessibility to high-calorie, high-fat foods and increasingly sedentary lifestyles.

TABLE 25–1. Common medical and psychological comorbidities

Medical

  Endocrinological

    Metabolic syndrome

    Type 2 diabetes mellitus

    Inflammation

    Polycystic ovary syndrome

    Hypothyroidism

  Cardiovascular

    Hypertension

    Lipid abnormalities

  Gastrointestinal

    Nonalcoholic fatty liver disease

    Gallstones

    Reflux

    Constipation

  Respiratory

    Obstructive sleep apnea

    Asthma

  Neurological

    Pseudotumor cerebri

  Orthopedic

    Blount disease

    Slipped capital femoral epiphysis

    Increased injury rates

Psychological

  Depression

  Eating-disordered behaviors

  Diminished self-esteem

  Body dissatisfaction

  Peer victimization

  Decreased quality of life

  Experiences of stigma

In 1963–1970, approximately 17.1% of children and adolescents in the United States were "at risk for overweight" or "overweight" (terms that have now been replaced with overweight and obese, respectively). By 2003–2006, approximately 32% of children and adolescents were overweight or obese (Ogden et al. 2008). Health care costs are rising due to childhood obesity. During 1979–1981, $35 million was spent annually on obesity-associated hospital costs. By 1997–1999, costs associated with youth obesity had more than tripled to $127 million annually (Wang and Dietz 2002).

Comorbidity

The presence of excessive adipose tissue places the individual at risk for significant medical and psychological comorbidities. It is beyond the scope of this chapter to review medical comorbidities in depth, but please refer to Table 25–1 for a brief overview of common medical and psychological comorbidities.

Youth who are overweight and obese are at increased risk for depression and depressive symptoms (Barlow and Expert Committee 2007; Daniels et al. 2005; Zametkin et al. 2004). Although most studies have used cross-sectional designs, one study prospectively examined the association between depressed mood and obesity in a sample of adolescents in grades 7–12 (Goodman and Whitaker 2002). Depressed mood at baseline predicted obesity at 1-year follow-up, even after controlling for race and socioeconomic status. Thus, depression in adolescence may be a risk factor for future obesity, perhaps via depressive symptoms such as increased appetite and decreased activity levels.

In a nonclinical sample of 15–17 year olds, the association between BMI and depressive symptoms was influenced by shame, parental employment, and parental separation (Sjoberg et al. 2005). A study of third graders found that the association between BMI and depressive symptoms was nonsignificant when controlling for concern regarding overweight (Erickson et al. 2000). Similar results were found in a study of students in grades 9–12. Adolescent BMI was associated with suicidal ideation, but the relationship was mediated by perceived weight, suggesting that adolescents' beliefs about body size may be a more important influence than actual weight on depressed mood and suicidal ideation (Eaton et al. 2005). Therefore, although obesity does appear to place youth at a greater risk for depression and depressive symptoms (and vice versa), careful consideration needs to be applied to other variables such as body dissatisfaction and family characteristics.

Overweight youth appear to have higher rates of eating disorders and eating-disordered behaviors than their nonoverweight peers (Britz et al. 2000). In a sample of 6- to 10-year-old overweight children, approximately 5% met criteria for binge-eating disorder (Morgan et al. 2002), and almost one-third of a sample of overweight adolescents reported engaging in binge eating (Berkowitz et al. 1993). The assessment and treatment of binge eating are of particular interest as treatment may also indirectly improve weight management.

Research suggests that some, but not all children who are overweight or obese may be at risk for lower self-esteem compared with children who are not overweight. Risk factors for lower self-esteem include early puberty, increased rates of peer victimization, greater body dissatisfaction, greater parental control over feeding practices, and internal attributions about weight status (i.e., feeling responsible for weight) (Lowry et al. 2007). Body satisfaction, also referred to as body image, may be lower in overweight and obese children and adolescents (Pesa et al. 2000; Thompson et al. 2007). Body satisfaction may be an important mediator in the association between weight status and psychological adjustment, as seen in one study where the relationship between self-esteem and body weight was no longer significant when controlling for body image (Pesa et al. 2000).

Children who are overweight or obese are at increased risk for peer victimization (Hayden-Wade et al. 2005; Storch et al. 2007; Thompson et al. 2007). Overweight children experience teasing that is more frequent, more severe, and more focused on appearance and body weight. Additionally, overweight or obese children appear to be more negatively influenced by peer victimization than nonoverweight youth (Hayden-Wade et al. 2005; Thompson et al. 2007).

Peer victimization and negative peer interactions may be a mechanism through which other symptoms of maladjustment arise. Peer victimization in overweight youth has been associated with poorer self-esteem, more depressive symptoms, increased anxiety, greater loneliness, higher parent report of internalizing and externalizing symptoms, higher incidence of bulimic behaviors, more weight concerns, lower confidence in physical appearance, and higher preference for isolative activities (Hayden-Wade et al. 2005; Storch et al. 2007). This research highlights the need to assess and address peer relationships and interactions in overweight youth and to consider that teasing may serve as a red flag for other psychological concerns.

Obese youth report lower health-related quality of life when compared to nonobese youth. In fact, one study examining quality of life in obese children ages 5–18 years old found that their scores were comparable to those of children newly diagnosed with cancer (Schwimmer et al. 2003). A study of adolescents found that overweight and obese adolescents self-reported significantly worse health-related quality of life than nonoverweight youth (Swallen et al. 2005).

Stigma regarding weight—i.e., *weight bias*—is pervasive and can have serious emotional and physical consequences. In addition to the social consequences associated with discrimination, stigma may perpetuate obesity. Stress can lead to increased cortisol levels and other metabolic abnormalities that may increase abdominal fat and contribute to obesity and other medical complications. Interestingly, stigmatizing beliefs are held not only by nonoverweight children. Overweight and obese youth are just as likely to endorse negative attitudes and stereotypes, which could have potentially disastrous effects on self-esteem (Puhl and Latner 2007).

Etiology, Mechanisms, and Risk Factors

Etiology

Medical and Genetic

Medical conditions or syndromes are thought to be responsible for less than 10% of all cases of childhood obesity. However, when present, these disorders can have substantial effects. Endogenous causes for obesity may include hormonal causes such as hypothyroidism, hypercortisolism, primary hyperinsulinism, pseudohypoparathyroidism, and acquired hypothalamic dysfunction. Familial lipodystrophy conditions including Beckwith-Wiedermann, Sotos, Weaver, and Ruvalcaba disorders may also be associated with pediatric obesity (Zametkin et al. 2004). Certain genetic syndromes have been linked with obesity, including Prader-Willi, Laurence-Moon/Bardet-Biedl, Alstrom, Borjeson-Forssman-Lehmann, Cohen, and Turner syndromes.

The influence of genetic factors on obesity is an exciting area of research. Twin studies have demonstrated that genetics may predict 20%–80% of the variance in child BMI (Zametkin et al. 2004). However, environmental factors likely play a much larger role in the development of childhood and adolescent obesity. The recent population level increase in obesity prevalence has occurred much too rapidly to be explained by genetic factors alone (Barlow and Expert Committee 2007).

Environmental

Environmental factors are strongly linked with pediatric obesity and overweight. Parental restriction of feeding has been consistently linked with child overeating and later development of overweight (Faith et al. 2004). However, some degree of feeding restriction is generally recommended in weight management programs to decrease consumption of less healthy food options. More research is needed to determine how much is too much restriction. More research is also needed to determine the direction of influence between child overeating and parental restriction. More successful parental feeding strategies appear to be the use of positive consequences and encouragement for what *to* eat (rather than what *not* to eat). Unfortunately, much less research has examined the effect of parenting behaviors on child physical activity habits and patterns.

Another significant environmental factor associated with childhood obesity is television viewing. The American Academy of Pediatrics (2001) recommends no more than 2 hours total of daily "screen time" (which includes television, video game, and computer exposure) for children over 2 years old and *no* screen time for children under 2 years old. Increased television viewing has repeatedly been associated with increased rates of obesity in children and adolescents. In addition to the passive and sedentary nature of television viewing, researchers have also highlighted the link between screen time and calorie consumption (Eisenmann et al. 2002).

Dietary practices also have a significant influence on pediatric obesity. In the last several decades, the average American diet has changed dramatically, with increased portion sizes and more frequent consumption of foods outside of the home. The quality of most American diets has deteriorated, with reduced consumption of fruits and vegetables, whole grains, and products rich in calcium. A recent report indicated that the most common vegetable consumed by 15- to 18-month-old children was french fries; 18%–33% of infants and toddlers consumed no servings of vegetables; and 23%–33% consumed no servings of fruit (Savage et al. 2007).

Changes in physical activity habits have also appeared to play a major role in the development of youth obesity. In addition to increased time spent in sedentary activities, children and teens spend considerably less time in moderate or vigorous physical activity. Schooltime physical activity hours and physical activity outside of school are declining. Causes for the decline include neighborhood safety concerns, limited supervised opportunities for activity, and limited options for activities in the built environment (such as parks and playgrounds). Furthermore, children who are already overweight or obese may be less likely to participate in physical activities or sports, due to feelings of shame or diminished athletic confidence.

Mechanisms

The mechanisms responsible for hunger, eating, and energy storage are complex and appear to be interconnected. Examination of appetite in human and animal studies has demonstrated the connection between efferent and afferent signals in the brain and periphery to influence eating. Leptin, ghrelin, adiponectin, plasma glucose, and insulin all have important roles in hunger, satiety, and fat distribution (Barlow and Expert Committee 2007; Zametkin et al. 2004). Research is currently being conducted regarding the neuroendocrinology and neuroscience of eating and will likely lead to breakthroughs in knowledge and treatment. However, it is unlikely that a single neurotransmitter or hormone will be identified as a solution to the obesity epidemic.

Risk Factors

Developmental

Multiple risk factors, or critical periods, across development have been associated with child and adolescent obesity. Prenatal factors including maternal diabetes or gestational diabetes have been linked with later development of child obesity. Infant birth weight greater than the 97th percentile has been shown to have a positive correlation with future BMI (Daniels et al. 2005; Whitaker and Dietz 1998). Results of research examining the effect of breast-feeding on weight status are mixed (Barlow and Expert Committee 2007). Early adiposity rebound, which refers to the point in early childhood when BMI begins to increase after reaching its nadir, has been suggested to be positively correlated with future overweight (Daniels et al. 2005). Finally, obesity in adolescence is a strong risk factor for adulthood obesity. Up to 80% of overweight teens become obese adults (Daniels et al. 2005), highlighting the need for early intervention.

Family and Social

An innovative study examining family and environmental factors associated with childhood obesity found that maternal psychological distress, family conflict, parental concerns about nutrition, and less positive family mealtime interactions were all more prevalent in families with overweight children compared to those of demographically matched nonoverweight

TABLE 25–2. Obesity-related assessment considerations when prescribing psychotropic medication to youth

Baseline assessment	Ongoing assessment
Height and weight (to calculate BMI)	Height and weight (to calculate BMI)
Blood pressure	Blood pressure
Resting heart rate	Resting heart rate
Family history of weight concerns and/or medical comorbidities	Inquire for changes such as:
Refer for baseline lab values if clinically indicated	More frequent urination
	Unintended weight loss
	Acanthosis

Note. BMI=body mass index.

peers (Zeller et al. 2007). These findings highlight the need for family-wide assessments and interventions.

Psychotropic Medication

The use of certain psychotropic medications is a strong risk factor for the development of obesity. Weight gain is not only a significant side effect, but has also been identified as a leading reason for adult nonadherence to psychotropic medication (Zametkin et al. 2004). Although such data are not available from child and adolescent samples, it is reasonable to assume that such behaviors may also be common in adolescent populations. Medications commonly associated with this effect include antipsychotics, mood stabilizers, and antidepressants (Devlin et al. 2000). For more information, see Chapter 47, "Antidepressants"; Chapter 48, "Mood Stabilizers"; and Chapter 49, "Antipsychotic Medications."

Patients and their parents should be informed of the potential risk for weight gain prior to medication initiation. Careful baseline evaluation and monitoring for weight gain and metabolic changes are required. (Please refer to Table 25–2 for specific assessment considerations.) A preventive weight maintenance or management program may be suggested at the onset of the medication trial. If problematic weight gain occurs, alternative medications may be considered and the prescribing physician should consider the benefits of psychotropic medication carefully along with the possible medical and psychological consequences of excessive weight gain (Devlin et al. 2000; Zametkin et al. 2004). Other treatment options may be available such as dose adjustment or switching to an alternative medication in the same class that is less associated with weight gain (Devlin et al. 2000).

Preliminary research has been conducted on the use of metformin to prevent excessive weight gain and/or metabolic changes associated with psychotropic medications. Youth ages 10–18 years (*N*=19) who

were prescribed olanzapine, risperidone, quetiapine, or valproate were then also prescribed 500 mg tid doses of metformin. At the end of 12 weeks, most of the patients experienced significant weight loss and reductions in BMI (Morrison et al. 2002). A randomized, double-blind, placebo-controlled trial was conducted with 39 youth ages 10–17. Participants had experienced weight gain more than 10% above baseline weight while being prescribed antipsychotic medication. Once metformin was prescribed, weight in the treatment group stabilized while youth in the placebo group continued to gain approximately 0.31 kg/week (Klein et al. 2006). More research on the safety and effectiveness of metformin in treating medication-induced obesity in youth is needed.

Prevention and Health Promotion

Prevention strategies have generally aimed at changing dietary and/or physical activity patterns or decreasing risk factors. A meta-analysis of 64 existing prevention programs with the primary outcome to prevent weight gain in children and adolescents found that 21% of the programs produced significant prevention effects pre- to postintervention (Stice et al. 2006). The largest effects were found for programs that targeted children and adolescents (vs. preadolescents), targeted girls, were briefer in nature, focused on weight (vs. also including additional health behaviors such as smoking), included pilot trials, and required participants to self-select into the intervention. Mandated dietary and physical activity improvements, delivery by trained interventionists, and parental involvement did not appear to be necessary for positive outcomes or larger treatment effects. More research is necessary to understand these findings, but perhaps the latter components are more important for the treatment of obesity rather than prevention.

The Expert Committee has recommended prevention behaviors for all youth, particularly those with risk factors for obesity such as parent obesity or maternal diabetes (Barlow and Expert Committee 2007). Strong evidence supports limiting consumption of sugar-sweetened beverages, increasing fruit and vegetable consumption, limiting screen time, eating breakfast daily, limiting restaurant meals, encouraging family meals, and limiting portion sizes. The committee also recommended consuming diets rich in calcium and fiber with balanced macronutrients, breastfeeding, moderate to vigorous physical activity 60 minutes daily, and limiting consumption of energy-dense foods. Prevention programs should be culturally sensitive when recommending dietary and physical activity changes.

Course and Prognosis

Overweight and obese children are at risk for becoming obese adults. One-third to one-half of obese 6-year-olds will become obese adults, and the risk rises with increasing child age. At least 80% of obese 10- to 14-year-old children with at least one obese parent may become obese adults. After age 10, the child's weight is a stronger predictor of adult weight than his or her parent's weight (Whitaker et al. 1997). Given the multiple medical, psychiatric, psychological, and social problems associated with pediatric overweight, the prognosis for untreated obesity can be dire. In one study, up to 30% of children treated across four treatment interventions had reached nonobese status at 10-year follow-up (Epstein et al. 2007); however, few interventions have reported such long-term effectiveness.

Evaluation

Medical Evaluation

Many obese children and adolescents will be monitored and identified by their primary care provider before reaching tertiary care centers or mental health specialists. The primary care provider should screen for the medical and psychiatric conditions discussed above and then refer to necessary specialists for additional treatment. The Expert Committee recommends that all children and adolescents be screened through calculation of BMI (Barlow and Expert Committee 2007). If indicated, it is then recommended that practitioners assess parental obesity, review family medical history, screen for obesity-related medical comorbidities, and review systems including sleep, respiratory, gastrointestinal, endocrine, nervous system, cardiovascular, psychiatric, orthopedic, skin, genetic, and lab testing. Behavioral assessment of parent and patient goals, dietary behaviors, and physical activity participation should also be conducted. Please refer to Barlow and Expert Committee (2007) for full Expert Committee recommendations regarding medical assessment.

Psychiatric Evaluation

Mental health professionals may work with obese youth where weight may or may not be the primary presenting problem or even a concern of parent or youth. It is important for the mental health professional to inquire if the child has recently completed a medical evaluation to screen for medical comorbidities and to refer if necessary, particularly if there are symptoms of metabolic or cardiovascular risk factors (such as acanthosis, nocturia, or elevated blood pressure).

The psychiatric evaluation of obese youth should screen for symptoms of depression and anxiety. Instruments such as the Children's Depression Inventory (CDI; Kovacs 1985) and the self-report Screen for Child Anxiety Related Emotional Disorders—Revised (SCARED-R; Muris et al. 1998) may be helpful. If clinically significant, the practitioner should follow up with a clinical interview to determine if the youth meets criteria for psychiatric diagnosis. If met, it is recommended that the youth undergo psychiatric treatment first or concurrently with participation in a weight management program, as untreated mental illness could adversely affect the youth's ability to effectively participate in a weight management program (Zametkin et al. 2004).

Assessments should also screen for eating-disordered behaviors (see Chapter 26, "Anorexia Nervosa and Bulimia Nervosa"). Clinicians should assess for binge eating, perhaps by inquiring about "loss of control" when eating. Other eating-disordered behaviors including use of diet pills, laxatives, diuretics, tobacco, purging, "crash dieting," and excessive exercise; these behaviors should also be assessed (Devlin et al. 2000; Zametkin et al. 2004). The Children's Eating Attitudes Test (ChEAT; Smolak and Levine 1994) is a measure that can be completed by children to assess for such disordered eating behaviors. Parental feeding strategies should also be evaluated. One well-standardized parent-report questionnaire to assess parental feeding strategies is the Children's Feeding Questionnaire (CFQ; Birch et al. 2001).

In addition to a brief overview of child or adolescent functioning, overweight and obese children and teens should be screened for the psychological comorbidities detailed earlier in this chapter. Poor self-esteem and body dissatisfaction, experiences of peer victimization and stigma, and decreased quality of life are all likely to affect child and family functioning and may impede success in weight management goals. When clinically indicated, assessment of the presence of substance use is also recommended (Zametkin et al. 2004). Psychiatric evaluation applies as described in Chapter 6, "The Process of Assessment and Diagnosis"; Chapter 7, "Diagnostic Interviews"; Chapter 8, "Rating Scales"; Chapter 9, "Pediatric Evaluation and Laboratory Testing"; Chapter 10, "Neurological Examination, Electroencephalography, and Neuroimaging"; and Chapter 11, "Psychological and Neuropsychological Testing." Please refer to Table 25–3 for a summary of key symptoms and sample questions.

Assessment of Readiness to Change

A final area of assessment is that of parent and youth readiness to change. Many parents misperceive their child's weight status and risk—and thus may fail to recognize their child as being overweight or obese (Eckstein et al. 2006). Parents and families who do not perceive risk or report concerns may not be ready to participate in interventions to change family dietary and physical activity habits. Instead, education regarding risk and motivational counseling (see Chapter 60, "Motivational Interviewing") may be a more appropriate intervention until the parent and/or youth is ready to commit to more rigorous treatment (Schwartz et al. 2007; Zametkin et al. 2004).

Treatment

According to the Expert Committee, "the primary goal of obesity treatment is improvement of long-term physical health through permanent healthy lifestyle habits" (Barlow and Expert Committee 2007, p. S181).

Notably, weight loss is not listed as a goal. For some children, due to ongoing growth, weight maintenance may be a more realistic goal, as stable weight with increasing height will result in lower BMI. Even small decreases in BMI may be accompanied by improvements in physical health, such as significant improvements in blood pressure, total cholesterol, low-density lipoprotein cholesterol, triglycerides, insulin, and aerobic fitness (Kirk et al. 2005).

Psychotherapeutic Treatments

Many treatment options exist, although some degree of psychotherapeutic intervention is a common component of almost all published efficacious interventions. Most interventions include a combination of the components discussed below: dietary changes, physical activity changes, and behavioral techniques.

Dietary

The most common dietary intervention used with children is the "Traffic Light Diet" (Epstein et al. 2007). This dietary approach classifies foods based on nutritional value into the three colors of a stoplight: green, yellow, and red. Green category foods include fruits and vegetables and should be eaten in abundance. Yellow category foods include lean meats and low-fat dairy items that should be the bulk of the diet and eaten in moderation. Red category foods include higher-calorie and higher-fat items such as cakes, candy, and french fries and should be limited. Many studies have demonstrated the effectiveness of this dietary approach, likely due to the ease of categorization of foods and understanding by children (Jelalian and Saelens 1999).

Dietary changes appear to be more successful when focusing on foods *to increase* rather than foods *to restrict.* One study compared increasing healthy foods to a group that focused on decreasing energy-dense foods to achieve weight control. Not only did the children in the *increasing* foods group demonstrate greater reductions in age- and gender-adjusted BMI scores, but parents also reported less concern at end of treatment and 24-month follow-up than for the *decreasing* foods group (Epstein et al. 2007).

Physical Activity

Physical activity interventions often target increasing physical activity and/or reducing sedentary behaviors, commonly by promotion of lifestyle exercise. Lifestyle exercise includes activities that can be incorporated

TABLE 25–3. Sample psychiatric evaluation for overweight or obese youth

Area of concern	Common symptoms	Sample questions (for child and/or parent) to assess for symptoms[a]
Depression	Anhedonia	Have you lost interest in activities that used to be enjoyable?
	Psychomotor retardation and/or fatigue	Do you feel tired more often or like you don't have much energy?
	Limited social interactions	How often do you spend time with friends or classmates?
	Recent rapid weight gain	Review medical history
	Decline in academic performance	What are your current grades? What were your grades last year?
Anxiety	Anxiety around eating	How do you feel when eating?
	Worries regarding weight and body size	How do you feel about your body shape and size?
	Use of food to cope with anxiety	When you feel worried, what helps you feel better?
Eating-disordered behaviors	Loss of control when eating	How do you feel when eating?
	Use of diet pills, laxatives, purging, excessive exercise, or tobacco to control weight	What methods have you used to change your weight?
	Binge eating	Do you ever eat more than other kids your age in one sitting?
	"Crash dieting"	What have you tried to lose weight?
	Eating in secret	How often do you eat when no one else is around, or how often do you try to hide eating?
	Skipping meals	How often do you miss or skip breakfast, lunch, or dinner in a given week?
Psychological adjustment	Poor self-esteem	How do you feel about yourself and your abilities?
	Body dissatisfaction	How do you feel about your body? Do you wish that parts of your body were different?
	Peer victimization (teasing and/or bullying behaviors)	Do you think that other students pick on you more frequently than they pick on other students?
	Limited peer relationships	Is it easy or more difficult for you to make friends?
	Feeling stigmatized due to weight	Do you think that others treat you differently because of your weight?
	Poor coping skills, particularly use of food-based coping	When you feel bad, what helps you feel better? Does food help you feel better if you are having a bad day?
Substance use	Unusual or erratic behavior change or change in friendships	Have you noticed any recent changes in your child's behavior or friendships?

TABLE 25–3. Sample psychiatric evaluation for overweight or obese youth *(continued)*

Area of concern	Common symptoms	Sample questions (for child and/or parent) to assess for symptoms[a]
Parenting behaviors	Level of concern for youth weight status	How concerned are you about your child's weight?
	Past attempts to manage child's weight	What have you tried in order to manage your child's weight?
	Feeding strategies	Who is in charge of meals and food in your home?
	Parent weight	Do you have concerns about your weight?
Family behaviors	Family dietary practices	Does your family eat together or "on the go"? How frequently do you eat out at restaurants or get fast food?
	Family physical activity practices	How does your family spend time together? Do family members exercise or participate in sports or recreational activities?
	Supports for adherence to an intervention program	Who will support you in your efforts to provide a healthier environment for your family? Do all family members agree with making changes?
	Cultural beliefs regarding weight, diet, and physical activity	Tell me about the meaning of food, activity, and weight in your family.
Environmental factors	Barriers to dietary or physical activity changes, such as access to healthy and affordable foods, neighborhood safety, and opportunities for safe and supervised physical activity	What things do you think may get in the way of making lifestyle changes to the family diet or physical activity?

[a]Questions may be directed to child and/or parent based on the child's developmental level and at the clinician's discretion.

into daily routines, such as using the stairs instead of the elevator or riding a bike instead of riding in a car. A meta-analysis of randomized controlled trials comparing lifestyle interventions to no-treatment or information-only/education-only controls indicated that lifestyle interventions are efficacious with moderate to large effect sizes at posttreatment and follow-up (Wilfley et al. 2007). There are mixed findings as to the effect of adding physical activity to dietary interventions when weight loss is the primary outcome. However, physical activity has been found to play a significant role in the long-term maintenance of weight loss in adults and may play a similar role in youth (Barlow and Expert Committee 2007).

Behavioral

Strong evidence exists for the short- and long-term efficacy of multicomponent behavioral treatment in children compared with placebo and education-only in-

terventions (Jelalian and Saelens 1999). Research on similar interventions in adolescents is less robust, but promising treatments in this population have been published. Successful interventions often include behavior modification, parent involvement, and exercise intervention components (Jelalian and Saelens 1999). However, determining the relative importance of intervention components remains challenging, since most programs use a combination of strategies.

Behavior modification strategies frequently include self-monitoring through the use of dietary logs, stimulus control through manipulation of the external environment, and contingency management through planning ahead for meals and activities. Setting goals for achieving dietary and physical activity behaviors is also common. Many interventions promote the use of reinforcement, both within the treatment program and at home to reinforce maintenance of behavior change (Jelalian and Saelens 1999). Problem solving and relaxation strategies have also been included in some interventions with mixed results (Duffy and Spence 1993; Epstein et al. 2007). Finally, promotion of coping strategies that are not food-based to deal with negative affect and negative peer interactions (such as teasing) has also been included in many programs.

Parenting behaviors are another primary focus of many behavioral interventions. The inclusion of separate yet simultaneous parent groups has been demonstrated as superior to child groups alone, particularly with school-age children (Epstein et al. 2007). Parenting strategies addressed in interventions frequently include giving praise, providing reinforcement, promoting family-wide change, altering the family food environment to promote healthy dietary choices and physical activity, and guiding parents in how to handle requests from children for less healthy foods. General parenting strategies for oppositional behavior are also commonly included (Barlow and Expert Committee 2007). Indeed, parental participation may be so valuable in intervening with children that researchers have begun to examine the effectiveness of conducting interventions with only parents. Parent-only groups compared to child-only and parent-plus-child groups have been shown to be as effective or superior in producing weight change outcomes and have the added benefit of being more cost-effective (Golan 2006).

Data on parent groups with adolescents are mixed, but a potential area of promise for adolescent interventions may be the use of peer groups and peer-based problem solving activities (Jelalian et al. 2006). The group setting can be a powerful mechanism to provide positive social experiences and teach adaptive social skills and coping. In these programs, "Outward Bound"–style group activities were used to promote self-confidence and group cohesiveness in adolescent participants through adventurous and developmentally appropriate activities.

Location

Psychotherapeutic interventions have been implemented in many locations including inpatient hospitals, outpatient medical centers, primary care offices, schools, community centers, camps, and via the Internet. Effective programs have been executed in all settings, but the dominant location noted in the empirical literature appears to be group treatment in outpatient medical centers. However, alternative locations, particularly in community centers and via the Internet, provide innovative venues for research and the possibility of reaching out to larger and more diverse groups of children and families.

Challenges

Encouraging findings for long-term effectiveness exist (Epstein et al. 2007), but are not consistently seen. A limitation of many programs is attrition, which may be as high as 55%. In one study, risk factors for attrition included being a recipient of Medicaid; black children; older youth; and participants presenting with greater report of depressive symptoms and lower self-concept (Zeller et al. 2004). These findings point to the need to better understand how to effectively reach participants who may be at risk for dropping out and the need to assess and target psychological risk factors early in treatment. More diversity in treatment samples is also needed.

Pharmacological Treatments

As is the case with most pharmacological development, weight loss medications have been much more extensively studied in adults than youth. However, two medications have now been approved by the U.S. Food and Drug Administration (FDA). Sibutramine was examined in a 54-week, randomized, double-blind trial of 498 adolescents ages 12–16 years. Participants received behavior therapy (diet and exercise) and either 10 mg of sibutramine or placebo. The treatment group experienced improved metabolic risk factors and approximately 3 kg more weight loss than the control group. Adverse effects included tachycardia, dry mouth, constipation, dizziness, insomnia, and hypertension (Berkowitz et al. 2006). Sibutramine has been approved by the FDA for use in patients age 16 years and older.

Orlistat was examined in a 54-week, randomized, double-blind study of 539 obese teens ages 12–16 years. Participants received a dose of orlistat or placebo 3 times daily plus a mildly hypocaloric diet, exercise, and behavioral therapy. Significant differences existed at 1 year posttreatment. The group that received orlistat decreased their average BMI by 0.55, but the placebo group increased their average BMI by 0.31. Adverse effects included mild to moderate gastrointestinal events (such as fatty/oily stool, oily spotting, or oily evacuation) in 9%–50% of the treatment group (Chanoine et al. 2005). Orlistat has been approved by the FDA for use in patients age 12 years and older.

Surgical Treatments

Bariatric surgery represents a new area of research and treatment for obese youth. The use of gastric bypass or gastric binding has led to substantial weight loss and improvement in comorbid medical conditions in youth (Inge et al. 2007). Inge et al. (2004) recommend the following selection criteria for youth and practitioners considering bariatric surgery: 1) at least 6 months or more of failed efforts to produce weight loss in a behavior-based weight management program, 2) physical maturity defined as 13 years or older for girls and 15 years or older for boys, 3) a BMI of 40 kg/m^2 or greater with a comorbid medical condition or a BMI of 50 kg/m^2 or greater without a comorbid medical condition, 4) commitment to medical and psychological evaluations prior to surgery, 5) agreement to avoid pregnancy for at least 1 year after surgery, 6) capability and willingness to adhere to nutritional guidelines, 7) informed assent to surgery, 8) decisional capacity, and 9) a supportive family environment.

Presurgical evaluation should include discussion of perioperative risks, postprocedural nutritional risks, and a lifelong commitment to altered dietary practices. Attendance at support group meetings prior to and following surgery has been recommended. Furthermore, surgical candidates should be provided with nutritional and psychological support after surgery (Barlow and Expert Committee 2007; Inge et al. 2004).

Ethical Considerations

Zametkin et al. (2004) highlighted ethical issues to consider when evaluating and treating overweight and obese youth. Weight bias and stigma represent a significant concern for many individuals. Clinicians should be careful to evaluate their own beliefs and possible countertransference toward overweight and obese individuals. Although parental influence in interventions will likely be an invaluable component of treatment, clinicians need to be cautious not to engage in "parent bashing" or blaming. Weight management and behavior changes are difficult for even the most resourceful and best intentioned individuals.

Finally, nonadherence is a significant concern in the treatment of most medical and psychiatric conditions. If parents or youth decline to participate in a weight management program, does this represent grounds for medical neglect? If so, at which weight category or level of medical comorbidity? If an adolescent with a condition necessitating treatment with antipsychotic medication expresses reluctance to take the medication out of concerns for weight gain, is it ethical to minimize weight gain risks to achieve adherence (Zametkin et al. 2004)? All of these issues need to be considered carefully. Collaboration with other professionals is recommended when faced with these issues.

Research Directions

Exciting research is being conducted in genetics and the neuroscience of eating, which will further our understanding of the mechanisms of adipose storage and risk for obesity development. Additional research on environmental influences on pediatric obesity development is needed, such as parental feeding strategies. Research on the effect of larger community and societal factors on childhood eating and activity levels is also needed and will likely inform future advocacy efforts in pediatric health promotion and even urban planning.

Information regarding the long-term effects of behavioral, pharmacological, and surgical interventions is needed, particularly regarding for which populations certain treatment protocols are most effective. Early research on the effects of bariatric surgery with adolescents appears promising, but little is known about the long-term medical and psychological effects of such treatments. Most obesity treatment research has focused on children and adolescents without comorbid psychiatric conditions. Given the potentially significant weight-related side effects of many psychotropic medications, effective interventions on how to best intervene with youth with psychiatric illness is vital. Finally, the need for culturally sensitive interventions is critical. Ethnic and racial discrepancies exist regarding prevalence rates of obesity, yet research is only beginning to address cultural differences in assessment and treatment.

Summary Points

- Rates of pediatric obesity have increased significantly in the last 30 years, and approximately 32% of U.S. children and adolescents are overweight or obese.

- Pediatric obesity is associated with significant medical and psychological comorbidities including depression, eating-disordered behaviors, poor self-esteem, peer victimization, poorer quality of life, and stigma.

- Many psychotropic medications have significant weight-gain side effects. Pediatric patients taking such medications should be carefully monitored for weight gain and obesity-related comorbidities.

- Pediatric obesity is a significant risk factor for adult obesity, and treatment becomes more difficult with increasing age.

- Psychiatric evaluation is important to assess for comorbidities and other conditions. Evaluation should assess for psychiatric symptoms as well as parent and family variables that may contribute to maladjustment and/or impede weight management treatment.

- Most treatments include some combination of dietary, physical activity, and behavioral components. Addressing parenting strategies may be beneficial, particularly in younger children. In adolescents, the use of peer groups may improve treatment results.

- Medication and surgical options are promising opportunities for treatment, but more research is needed to determine the long-term safety and efficacy of these interventions.

References

American Academy of Pediatrics: Children, adolescents, and television. Pediatrics 107:423–425, 2001

Barlow SE, Expert Committee: Expert committee recommendations regarding the prevention, assessment, and treatment of child and adolescent overweight and obesity: summary report. Pediatrics 120:S164–S192, 2007

Berkowitz RI, Stunkard AJ, Stallings VA: Binge-eating disorder in obese adolescent girls. Ann NY Acad Sci 699:200–206, 1993

Berkowitz RI, Fujioka K, Daniels SR, et al: Effects of sibutramine treatment in obese adolescents: a randomized trial. Ann Intern Med 145:81–90, 2006

Birch LL, Fisher JO, Grimm-Thomas K, et al: Confirmatory factor analysis of the Child feeding questionnaire: a measure of parental attitudes, beliefs and practices about child feeding and obesity. Appetite 36:201–210, 2001

Britz B, Siegfried W, Ziegler A, et al: Rates of psychiatric disorders in a clinical study group of adolescents with extreme obesity and in obese adolescents ascertained via a population-based study. Int J Obes Relat Metab Disord 24:1707–1714, 2000

Chanoine J, Hampl S, Jensen C, et al: Effect of orlistat on weight and body composition in obese adolescents: a randomized controlled trial. JAMA 293:2873–2883, 2005

Daniels SR, Arnett DK, Eckel RH, et al: Overweight in children and adolescents: pathophysiology, consequences, prevention, and treatment. Circulation 111:1999–2012, 2005

Devlin MJ, Yanovski SZ, Wilson GT: Obesity: what mental health professionals need to know. Am J Psychiatry 157:854–866, 2000

Duffy G, Spence SH: The effectiveness of cognitive self-management as an adjunct to a behavioral intervention for childhood obesity: a research note. J Child Psychol Psychiatry 34:1043–1050, 1993

Eaton DK, Lowry R, Brener ND, et al: Associations of body mass index and perceived weight with suicidal ideation and suicide attempts among US high school students. Arch Pediatr Adolesc Med 159:513–519, 2005

Eckstein KC, Mikhail LM, Ariza AJ, et al: Parents' perceptions of their child's weight and health. Pediatrics 117:681–690, 2006

Eisenmann JC, Bartee RT, Wang MQ: Physical activity, TV viewing, and weight in U.S. youth: 1999 youth risk behavior survey. Obesity 10:379–385, 2002

Epstein LH, Paluch RA, Roemmich JN, et al: Family-based obesity treatment, then and now: twenty-five years of pediatric obesity treatment. Health Psychol 26:381–391, 2007

Erickson SJ, Robinson TN, Haydel KF, et al: Are overweight children unhappy? Body mass index, depressive symptoms, and overweight concerns in elementary school children. Arch Pediatr Adolesc Med 154:931–935, 2000

Faith MS, Scanlon KS, Birch LL, et al: Parent-child feeding strategies and their relationship to child eating and weight status. Obes Res 12:1711–1722, 2004

Golan M: Parents as agents of change in childhood obesity: from research to practice. Int J Pediatr Obes 1:66–76, 2006

Goodman E, Whitaker RC: A prospective study of the role of depression in the development and persistence of adolescent obesity. Pediatrics 109:497–504, 2002

Hayden-Wade H, Stein R, Ghaderi A, et al: Prevalence, characteristics, and correlates of teasing experiences among overweight children vs nonoverweight peers. Obes Res 13:1381–1392, 2005

Inge TH, Krebs NF, Garcia VF, et al: Bariatric surgery for severely overweight adolescents: concerns and recommendations. Pediatrics 114:217–223, 2004

Inge TH, Xanthakos SA, Zeller MH: Bariatric surgery for pediatric extreme obesity: now or later? Int J Obes 31:1–14, 2007

Jelalian E, Saelens BE: Empirically supported treatments in pediatric psychology: pediatric obesity. J Pediatr Psychol 24:223–248, 1999

Jelalian E, Mehlenbeck R, Lloyd-Richardson E, et al: "Adventure therapy" combined with cognitive-behavioral treatment for overweight adolescents. Int J Obes 30:31–39, 2006

Kirk S, Zeller M, Claytor R, et al: The relationship of health outcomes to improvement in BMI in children and adolescents. Obes Res 13:876–882, 2005

Klein DJ, Cottingham EM, Sorter M, et al: A randomized, double-blind, placebo-controlled trial of metformin treatment of weight gain associated with initiation of atypical antipsychotic therapy in children and adolescents. Am J Psychiatry 163:2072–2079, 2006

Kovacs M: The Children's Depression Inventory (CDI). Psychopharmacol Bull 21:995–998, 1985

Lowry KW, Sallinen BJ, Janicke DM: The effects of weight management programs on self-esteem in pediatric overweight populations. J Pediatr Psychol 32:1179–1195, 2007

Morgan CM, Yanovski SA, Nguyen TT, et al: Loss of control over eating, adiposity, and psychopathology in overweight children. Int J Eat Disord 31:430–441, 2002

Morrison JA, Cottingham EM, Barton BA: Metformin for weight loss in pediatric patients taking psychotropic drugs. Am J Psychiatry 159:655–657, 2002

Muris P, Merckelbach H, Schmidt H, et al: The revised version of the Screen for Child Anxiety Related Emotional Disorders (SCARED-R): factor structure in normal children. Pers Individ Dif 26:99–112, 1998

Ogden CL, Carroll MD, Flegal KM: High body mass index for age among US children and adolescents, 2003–2006. JAMA 299:2401–2405, 2008

Pesa J, Syre T, Jones E: Psychosocial differences associated with body weight among female adolescents: the importance of body image. J Adolesc Health 26:330–337, 2000

Puhl RM, Latner JD: Stigma, obesity, and the health of the nation's children. Psychol Bull 133:557–580, 2007

Savage JS, Fisher JO, Birch LL: Parental influence on eating behavior: conception to adolescence. J Law Med Ethics 35:22–34, 2007

Schwartz RP, Hamre R, Dietz WH, et al: Office-based motivational interviewing to prevent childhood obesity: a feasibility study. Arch Pediatr Adolesc Med 161:495–501, 2007

Schwimmer JB, Burwinkle TM, Varni JW: Health-related quality of life of severely obese children and adolescents. JAMA 289:1813–1819, 2003

Sjoberg RL, Nilsson KW, Leppert J: Obesity, shame, and depression in school-aged children: a population-based study. Pediatrics 116:e389–e392, 2005

Smolak L, Levine MP: Psychometric properties of the children's eating attitudes test. Int J Eat Disord 16:275–282, 1994

Stice E, Shaw H, Marti N: A meta-analytic review of obesity prevention programs for children and adolescents: the skinny on interventions that work. Psychol Bull 132:667–691, 2006

Storch EA, Milsom VA, DeBraganza N, et al: Peer victimization, psychosocial adjustment, and physical activity in overweight and at-risk-for-overweight youth. J Pediatr Psychol 32:80–89, 2007

Swallen K, Reither E, Haas S, et al: Overweight, obesity, and health-related quality of life among adolescents: the National Longitudinal Study of Adolescent Health. Pediatrics 115:340–347, 2005

Thompson J, Shroff H, Herbozo S, et al: Relations among multiple peer influences, body dissatisfaction, eating disturbance, and self-esteem: a comparison of average weight, at risk of overweight, and overweight adolescent girls. J Pediatr Psychol 32:24–29, 2007

Wang G, Dietz WH: Economic burden of obesity in youths aged 6 to 17 years: 1979–1999. Pediatrics 109:E81-1, 2002

Whitaker RC, Dietz WH: Role of the prenatal environment in the development of obesity. J Pediatr 132:768–776, 1998

Whitaker RC, Wright JA, Pepe MS, et al: Predicting obesity in young adulthood from childhood and parental obesity. N Engl J Med 337:869–873, 1997

Wilfley DE, Tibbs TL, Van Buren DJ, et al: Lifestyle interventions in the treatment of childhood overweight: a meta-analytic review of randomized controlled trials. Health Psychol 26:521–523, 2007

Zametkin AJ, Zoon CK, Klein HW, et al: Psychiatric aspects of child and adolescent obesity: a review of the past 10 years. J Am Acad Child Adolesc Psychiatry 43:134–150, 2004

Zeller MH, Kirk S, Claytor R, et al: Predictors of attrition from a pediatric weight management program. J Pediatr 144:466–470, 2004

Zeller MH, Reiter-Purtill J, Modi AC, et al: Controlled study of critical parent and family factors in the obesigenic environment. Obesity 15:126–136, 2007

Chapter 26

Anorexia Nervosa and Bulimia Nervosa

Daniel Le Grange, Ph.D.
Kamryn T. Eddy, Ph.D.
David Herzog, M.D.

Eating disorders are relatively common psychiatric disorders most often observed in late adolescent and young adult females, with typical onset during adolescence (ages 12–18 years). Eating disorders may be chronic and relapsing conditions and are often associated with significant medical morbidity and psychiatric comorbidity. The etiology, maintaining factors, and treatment of eating disorders have been understudied, particularly in regard to children and adolescents. DSM-IV (American Psychiatric Association 1994) and its text revision, DSM-IV-TR (American Psychiatric Association 2000a), include three eating disorder diagnoses: 1) anorexia nervosa (AN) and 2) bulimia nervosa (BN), which each have specific criteria; and 3) eating disorder not otherwise specified (EDNOS), which is a more heterogeneous diagnosis capturing clinically significant eating disorder presentations that cannot be categorized as AN or BN.

In this chapter, we describe the diagnostic criteria for these eating disorders and consider their application to children and adolescents. We describe the epidemiology, comorbidity, and etiology of eating disorders, methods of prevention, developmental course and outcome, and assessment and treatment. While we include EDNOS where data are available, we focus on AN and BN because the most research has been done in these eating disorders.

Diagnosis

Anorexia Nervosa

DSM-IV-TR describes AN as a refusal to maintain weight (or lack of weight gain during a period of

TABLE 26–1. DSM-IV-TR diagnostic criteria for anorexia nervosa

A. Refusal to maintain body weight at or above a minimally normal weight for age and height (e.g., weight loss leading to maintenance of body weight less than 85% of that expected; or failure to make expected weight gain during period of growth, leading to body weight less than 85% of that expected).

B. Intense fear of gaining weight or becoming fat, even though underweight.

C. Disturbance in the way in which one's body weight or shape is experienced, undue influence of body weight or shape on self-evaluation, or denial of the seriousness of the current low body weight.

D. In postmenarcheal females, amenorrhea, i.e., the absence of at least three consecutive menstrual cycles. (A woman is considered to have amenorrhea if her periods occur only following hormone, e.g., estrogen, administration.)

Specify type:

Restricting type: during the current episode of anorexia nervosa, the person has not regularly engaged in binge-eating or purging behavior (i.e., self-induced vomiting or the misuse of laxatives, diuretics, or enemas)

Binge-eating/purging type: during the current episode of anorexia nervosa, the person has regularly engaged in binge-eating or purging behavior (i.e., self-induced vomiting or the misuse of laxatives, diuretics, or enemas)

Source.   Reprinted from American Psychiatric Association: *Diagnostic and Statistical Manual of Mental Disorders*, 4th Edition, Text Revision. Washington, DC, American Psychiatric Association, 2000, p. 589. Used with permission. Copyright © 2000 American Psychiatric Association.

TABLE 26–2. DSM-IV-TR diagnostic criteria for bulimia nervosa

A. Recurrent episodes of binge eating. An episode of binge eating is characterized by both of the following:

(1) eating, in a discrete period of time (e.g., within any 2-hour period), an amount of food that is definitely larger than most people would eat during a similar period of time and under similar circumstances

(2) a sense of lack of control over eating during the episode (e.g., a feeling that one cannot stop eating or control what or how much one is eating)

B. Recurrent inappropriate compensatory behavior in order to prevent weight gain, such as self-induced vomiting; misuse of laxatives, diuretics, enemas, or other medications; fasting; or excessive exercise.

C. The binge eating and inappropriate compensatory behaviors both occur, on average, at least twice a week for 3 months.

D. Self-evaluation is unduly influenced by body shape and weight.

E. The disturbance does not occur exclusively during episodes of anorexia nervosa.

Specify type:

Purging type: during the current episode of bulimia nervosa, the person has regularly engaged in self-induced vomiting or the misuse of laxatives, diuretics, or enemas

Nonpurging type: during the current episode of bulimia nervosa, the person has used other inappropriate compensatory behaviors, such as fasting or excessive exercise, but has not regularly engaged in self-induced vomiting or the misuse of laxatives, diuretics, or enemas

Source.   Reprinted from American Psychiatric Association: *Diagnostic and Statistical Manual of Mental Disorders*, 4th Edition, Text Revision. Washington, DC, American Psychiatric Association, 2000, p. 594. Used with permission. Copyright © 2000 American Psychiatric Association.

TABLE 26–3. DSM-IV-TR diagnostic criteria for eating disorder not otherwise specified

The eating disorder not otherwise specified category is for disorders of eating that do not meet the criteria for any specific eating disorder. Examples include

1. For females, all of the criteria for anorexia nervosa are met except that the individual has regular menses.

2. All of the criteria for anorexia nervosa are met except that, despite significant weight loss, the individual's current weight is in the normal range.

3. All of the criteria for bulimia nervosa are met except that the binge eating and inappropriate compensatory mechanisms occur at a frequency of less than twice a week or for a duration of less than 3 months.

4. The regular use of inappropriate compensatory behavior by an individual of normal body weight after eating small amounts of food (e.g., self-induced vomiting after the consumption of two cookies).

5. Repeatedly chewing and spitting out, but not swallowing, large amounts of food.

6. Binge-eating disorder: recurrent episodes of binge eating in the absence of the regular use of inappropriate compensatory behaviors characteristic of bulimia nervosa.

Source. Reprinted from American Psychiatric Association: *Diagnostic and Statistical Manual of Mental Disorders,* 4th Edition, Text Revision. Washington, DC, American Psychiatric Association, 2000, pp. 594–595. Used with permission. Copyright © 2000 American Psychiatric Association.

growth) of 85% of expected weight for height (ideal body weight). This occurs in the context of an overriding fear of weight gain and a lack of recognition of the physical changes that result from malnutrition (body image distortion or denial of the seriousness of the consequences of malnutrition) (American Psychiatric Association 2000a; Table 26–1).

Bulimia Nervosa

In DSM-IV-TR, BN is characterized by recurrent episodes of binge eating and inappropriate compensatory behaviors (e.g., self-induced vomiting; misuse of laxatives, diuretics, enemas; excessive exercising; or strict dieting or fasting). In addition to the behavioral component, individuals with BN are marked by beliefs and attitudes that overemphasize shape and weight as the sole or major way self-worth and self-esteem are maintained (American Psychiatric Association 2000a; Table 26–2).

Eating Disorder Not Otherwise Specified

EDNOS is a heterogeneous diagnosis comprising individuals with a range of clinically significant eating disorder symptom presentations (American Psychiatric Association 2000a). For EDNOS, DSM-IV-TR does not specify a criteria set but instead provides examples of symptom presentations that would fit within the EDNOS diagnosis (Table 26–3). In DSM-IV-TR, binge-

eating disorder (BED) is provided as one example of EDNOS but is also given a specific criteria set as a research diagnosis in need of further study (American Psychiatric Association 2000a; Table 26–4).

Application of DSM-IV-TR Criteria to Younger Populations

DSM-IV-TR does not make specific provisions for the diagnosis of eating disorders in children and adolescents and demonstrates little recognition that eating disorders in these younger patients may differ from those observed in adults. The multidisciplinary Workgroup for Classification of Eating Disorders in Children and Adolescents suggested that current DSM formulations are not sensitive to younger persons with eating disorders and recommended some adjustments to the current criteria (see Bravender et al. 2007). For the diagnosis of AN, the weight criterion (i.e., 85% ideal body weight or a BMI of 17.5 kg/m^2) is problematic for a population where growth is still expected. Instead, and as suggested by this workgroup, failure to grow as a result of malnutrition—an event particular to childhood—should serve as a substitute for meeting the usual weight criterion for AN. Similarly, menstrual criteria are difficult to apply in youth who are either premenarcheal (i.e., who may otherwise meet full criteria for AN) or who have not firmly established menstrual cycles (e.g., making it difficult to determine when three consecutive periods should have occurred). Additionally, there is no equivalence for amenorrhea

TABLE 26–4. DSM-IV-TR research criteria for binge-eating disorder

A. Recurrent episodes of binge eating. An episode of binge eating is characterized by both of the following:

   (1) eating, in a discrete period of time (e.g., within any 2-hour period), an amount of food that is definitely larger than most people would eat in a similar period of time under similar circumstances

   (2) a sense of lack of control over eating during the episode (e.g., a feeling that one cannot stop eating or control what or how much one is eating)

B. The binge-eating episodes are associated with three (or more) of the following:

   (1) eating much more rapidly than normal

   (2) eating until feeling uncomfortably full

   (3) eating large amounts of food when not feeling physically hungry

   (4) eating alone because of being embarrassed by how much one is eating

   (5) feeling disgusted with oneself, depressed, or very guilty after overeating

C. Marked distress regarding binge eating is present.

D. The binge eating occurs, on average, at least 2 days a week for 6 months.

   Note: The method of determining frequency differs from that used for bulimia nervosa; future research should address whether the preferred method of setting a frequency threshold is counting the number of days on which binges occur or counting the number of episodes of binge eating.

E. The binge eating is not associated with the regular use of inappropriate compensatory behaviors (e.g., purging, fasting, excessive exercise) and does not occur exclusively during the course of anorexia nervosa or bulimia nervosa.

in boys with AN. Further, the cognitive criteria may also be problematic as many young adolescent patients are not clear about what motivates their restrictive eating, and unlike older adolescent or adult patients, many report wishes to be healthy rather than a desire to lose weight. While youth often do not report body image distortion, they more clearly deny—through their actions and/or words—the seriousness of their current low weight.

DSM-IV-TR also makes few developmental concessions for adjusting the diagnosis of BN in children and adolescents. Most problematic, perhaps, are the frequency criteria for binge eating and purging (an average of twice a week for 3 months in duration). While these criteria more reasonably apply to older, more chronic patients, they pose significant diagnostic conundrums for adolescents with binge-eating and purging behaviors whose symptoms may be more intermittent or in flux with regard to intensity early in the course of the disorder.

Applying strict DSM-IV-TR definitions, a majority of adolescents with disturbed eating behaviors are categorized as EDNOS. In the only study examining relative rates of eating disorder diagnoses in an adolescent clinical sample, 57% in a cohort of 281 adolescents were categorized as EDNOS (Eddy et al. 2008). In this sample, individuals with EDNOS constituted a heterogeneous group with eating disorder presentations ranging from subthreshold AN to binge-eating disorder. This finding may indicate that EDNOS is an imprecise diagnosis that consequently does not shed much light on relevant treatment decisions. A broader view of the features that are common to all eating disorders (i.e., a "transdiagnostic" perspective) may lead to a more comprehensive understanding of eating difficulties (Fairburn et al. 2003). According to this perspective, certain clinically important commonalities exist across all types of eating disorders including abnormal eating patterns; sets of beliefs about food, weight, and/or shape; and emotional, social, and/or behavioral dysfunction secondary to disordered eating behaviors and attitudes. While this formulation of eating disorders remains controversial, it might be appealing to child and adolescent practitioners because of its emphasis on an overall developmental perspective.

It is also worth noting that in DSM-IV-TR, feeding disorders of infancy and early childhood are not categorized with the eating disorders. Some investigators have postulated a classification scheme to describe feeding patterns in children presenting to eating disorder clinics who have symptom presentations that bear little resemblance to AN or BN (Bryant-Waugh 2002).

This system would include youth exhibiting eating/feeding patterns such as selective or picky eating and food avoidance related to emotional issues (i.e., not secondary to shape/weight concerns). Indeed, drawing the line between an eating disorder and a feeding disorder in youth who have limited cognitive capacity to articulate weight/shape concerns may be problematic.

Epidemiology

Epidemiological research in eating disorders is limited and focused on adults. Research describing the prevalence, demographic characteristics, and clinical characteristics—particularly in the case of EDNOS—is needed.

Anorexia Nervosa

A recent national comorbidity survey including a representative sample of individuals ages 18 and older indicated that the lifetime prevalence of AN is 0.9% among females and 0.3% among males (Hudson et al. 2007). Notably, however, in most clinical samples, 90%–95% of those with AN are female. AN is most common among adolescent females (point prevalence in adults of 0.5%), with a typical onset during mid- to late-adolescence (American Psychiatric Association 2000b). Mid- to late-adolescent-onset AN is associated with a better prognosis compared with prepubertal or early adolescent onset; prepubertal AN may be associated with a more severe psychiatric profile. AN is most prevalent in industrialized societies. Although AN occurs across ethnicity and socioeconomic status, it tends to be less common among African American women than among white, Hispanic, and Asian American women.

Bulimia Nervosa

The national comorbidity survey indicated that the lifetime prevalence of BN is 1.5% among females and 0.5% among males (Hudson et al. 2007), although as with AN, females predominate in clinical samples of patients with BN. Rates of BN are likely to be increased among certain populations (e.g., college females). Interestingly, there is some suggestion that BN has decreased in prevalence within the last decade (Keel et al. 2006). Age at onset for BN tends to be later than that of AN, occurring more commonly in late adolescence

(Fairburn et al. 2000; Le Grange et al. 2004). Prepubertal onset of BN is relatively rare (Kent et al. 1992). Bulimic symptoms are widespread across ethnic and racial groups, although BN appears to be relatively less common among African American women compared with white and Hispanic women (Striegel-Moore et al. 2003).

Eating Disorder Not Otherwise Specified

The adult literature indicates that EDNOS predominates among those seeking treatment for eating disorder symptoms (Fairburn et al. 2007), and preliminary research suggests that this is also true among adolescents (Eddy et al. 2008). Yet, the only epidemiological research on EDNOS has been focused on BED among adults. Research on the epidemiology of BED is considered preliminary, but a recent national comorbidity survey indicated lifetime prevalence rates of 3.5% among women and 2.0% among men (Hudson et al. 2007). Rates of BED are as high as 20%–30% among specific populations, including overweight and obese individuals seeking weight loss treatment (Spitzer et al. 1992, 1993). Among overweight treatment-seeking youth, rates of BED are estimated to be up to 10% (Eddy et al. 2007), while less frequent binge eating and associated distress are more common (e.g., Eddy et al. 2007; Tanofsky-Kraff et al. 2004).

Comorbidity

Several studies of adults suggest that comorbid psychiatric illness is common for patients with eating disorders. Estimates of the lifetime prevalence of affective disorders range from 50% to 80%, and comorbid anxiety disorders are seen in 30%–65% of individuals with AN and BN (Herzog et al. 1996; Johnson et al. 2002). Alcohol and drug abuse are common in adults with eating disorders, particularly among individuals with bulimic symptoms (Herzog et al. 2006). Personality problems are also diagnosed frequently. AN has been associated with avoidant personality and BN with borderline personality disorder. Some researchers have described three personality subtypes among individuals with eating disorders (irrespective of diagnosis): 1) a high-functioning and perfectionistic type, 2) one that tends to be more constricted and overcontrolled, and 3) a group that tends to be more emotionally dysregulated and undercontrolled (Westen and Harnden-Fischer 2001).

While less is known about comorbidity among adolescents with eating disorders, preliminary research suggests that similar patterns apply. For example, a recent study of 80 adolescents with BN and subthreshold BN demonstrated that 62.5% of the sample had a comorbid diagnosis as determined by the Schedule for Affective Disorders and Schizophrenia for School-Age Children (Fischer and Le Grange 2007). The majority of these youth presented with a major mood disorder. In addition, 25% of the sample had previously attempted suicide or self-harm, 65.8% had consumed alcohol, and 30% had used illegal drugs. Further, in a recent study of adolescents with AN participating in a treatment trial, 36% were found to have a comorbid psychiatric disorder, with major depression and anxiety diagnoses being particularly common (Lock et al. 2006). Two large community samples of adolescent girls demonstrated a positive association between substance use/misuse and eating disorder symptoms (Granillo et al. 2005; Von Ranson et al. 2002). Inquiry into personality differences has suggested that different personality subtypes exist among adolescents with eating disorders (e.g., Thompson-Brenner et al. 2008). Adolescents with AN tend to be more avoidant, inhibited, and constricted with regard to personality style, while those with bulimic symptoms tend to be more affectively labile and undercontrolled (Thompson-Brenner et al. 2008).

Given the extent of co-occurring psychiatric conditions and high-risk behaviors in adult women with BN, as well as these preliminary adolescent data, comorbidity and high-risk health behaviors in adolescents with BN seem to mirror those of adults with BN. It would be important to keep in mind that it is possible that the current studies overestimate comorbidity in eating disorder patients, given that most of the limited inquiries are predominantly clinical samples and therefore may overrepresent more seriously compromised individuals.

Etiology and Risks for Adolescent Eating Disorders

While the precise pathogenesis of eating disorders remains unknown, it is likely multidimensional and influenced by biological, psychological, and sociocultural factors. A developmental psychopathological perspective of eating disorders postulates that certain biological vulnerabilities interact with the individual's exposure to a range of experiences (e.g., parenting that overemphasizes physical appearance; abuse; the media) that then influence beliefs and behaviors that support the development of eating disorders (Lock et al. 2001b; Steiner et al. 2003). A convergence of these biological, familial, and sociocultural influences reaches a critical threshold for those adolescents who develop an eating disorder. Most studies do not have a prospective developmental perspective, but they are nonetheless important in helping to conceptualize a possible etiological and developmental trajectory for eating disorders.

Vulnerability to the development of an eating disorder may be due to underlying biological factors. Heritable causation is being suggested because of increasing evidence for the familial clustering of eating disorders and eating attitudes (Kendler et al. 1995). Yet, there are no adequate longitudinal studies that control for shared and nonshared environments. Even so, it has been suggested that there is a 3%–10% increase in the prevalence of eating disorders in siblings, 27% in mothers, 16% in fathers, and 29% generally in first-degree relatives (Strober et al. 2000). Family history studies demonstrate that more than 50% of the risk for AN is attributable to genetic influences. There is also growing evidence that symptoms such as binge eating, self-induced vomiting, dietary restraint, body dissatisfaction, and weight preoccupation may be heritable (Bulik et al. 1997).

Neurobiological research has also demonstrated hormonal and neurohormonal systems differences in adult and late adolescent individuals with eating disorders (Pirke and Platte 1995). The degree to which these differences represent premorbid risk factors as opposed to secondary effects of disordered eating and starvation remains unclear, particularly as there is some suggestion that these systems differences normalize after refeeding. Further, it is unknown whether these findings can be generalized to adolescents. Neuroimaging studies suggest that there may be differences in serotonergic activity between individuals with AN and those with BN, although these findings are not definitive. For example, low levels of the neurotransmitter 5-hydroxytryptamine—serotonin—appear to be associated with binge-eating behaviors (Steiger et al. 2001). Dysregulated serotonin levels persist postrecovery in individuals with AN (Frank et al. 2004) and BN (Kaye et al. 1998). Further, the monoamine deficiencies in BN also persist postrecovery. Neurobiological findings that persist postrecovery suggest that these neurochemical alterations may contribute to the development of eating disorders.

Early experiences in one's family have been postulated to increase the developmental risk for eating disorders. Seminal work by Minuchin et al. (1978) hypothesized that families of patients with eating disorders are characterized by being overly enmeshed, conflict avoidant, and inflexible. More recently, Ward et al. (2001) suggested that insecure attachment (i.e., dismissive attachment styles) may contribute to risk for an eating disorder. Some research suggests that families of patients with AN are more controlling and organized compared with the families of patients with BN, which by comparison appear to be more chaotic, conflicted, and critical (Hoste and Le Grange 2008). However, comparisons to families with other psychopathology or nonclinical families have shown that these features are not uniquely associated with eating disorders (Casper and Troiani 2001). Thus, any potential role played by the family process in the etiology of eating disorders remains undetermined.

Interestingly, there appears to be no clear continuity between eating problems in early childhood, such as failure to thrive or picky eating, and the development of eating disorders during adolescence. Boys appear to be at greater risk for eating disorders in early childhood, while girls become more vulnerable during adolescence. In contrast, concern about weight and shape at a young age is considered to be a risk factor for later development of an eating disorder. Epidemiological research suggests that a significant minority of children express the desire to be thinner and try to lose weight. However less than 10% of these children score in the pathological range on a standard questionnaire of eating disorder pathology (Schur et al. 1999). Generally, girls endorse a desire to be thinner, while boys' weight/shape concerns are more focused on wishes to be bigger, or more muscular. These observations are consistent with gender-specific weight and shape concerns among adolescents, suggesting continuity between school-age children and adolescents in this respect.

A somewhat exaggerated focus on weight, shape, and dieting may be normative for many adolescents and could give rise to experimentation with various weight loss strategies, which may then increase risk for the development of eating disorders (Steiner et al. 2003). This increased focus on bodily appearance comes at a time when sexual attractiveness, social acceptance, and the ability to undertake actions related to these issues, independently of parents, are taking center stage and probably increase the likelihood of adolescents developing eating disorders. These adolescent challenges are negotiated in the context of the heightened influence of the fashion world (Ackard and Peterson 2000). As adolescent girls grow older, they appear to be less satisfied with their weight. This dissatisfaction is compounded by perceived media preference for lower weight (McCabe et al. 2001). It is therefore not surprising that dieting behaviors increase from middle school years (11–13 years of age) through adolescence, and it is estimated that dieting behavior may be as high as 60%–70% among high school girls. Adolescents may also experiment with other types of weight loss methods—including those that are extreme or harmful (e.g., fasting, purging).

In a test of the hypothesis that the development of eating problems is related to the onset of puberty, Attie and Brooks-Gunn (1989) prospectively followed 193 girls (7th–10th grade) for 2 years. They found that eating problems emerged in response to pubertal change, in particular the associated adipose accumulation, and that girls who were most dissatisfied with their bodies at puberty were at the highest risk for the development of eating difficulties. Other challenges typical of adolescence may also contribute to the development of an eating disorder (e.g., teasing by peers, discomfort in discussing problems with parents, and maternal preoccupation with dietary restriction). While some studies have indicated increased rates of sexual abuse history among women with eating disorders (Perez et al. 2002), the relationship between abuse and eating problems has not been systematically studied in younger patients.

Sociocultural risk factors such as the influence of the media, especially the thin ideal of the fashion industry, may be relevant to the development of eating disorders in adolescence (McCabe et al. 2001). It has been argued that comparison to these thin ideals gives rise to body dissatisfaction and disordered eating behaviors among young females (Ohring et al. 2001), while an increased emphasis on muscularity and lower body fat lead to increased shape and weight concerns and eating disorders in males (Leit et al. 2001). Migrating to a Western culture and the associated acculturation stress also pose some risk (Gunewardene et al. 2001; Le Grange et al. 2006). Eating-disordered behaviors serve to increase social acceptance and provide comfort in this new environment.

Prevention

Binford et al. (2004) provide a concise summary of the published controlled studies that have evaluated the mostly school-based, eating-disorder prevention programs. While research-based interventions have been able to bring about improved knowledge about eating disorders and positive changes in eating attitudes, findings have been disappointing, as the majority of these projects have not been able to show improvement in or prevention of eating disorder behaviors. While the authors attempt to understand these findings, they argue that efficacy in prevention programs might be demonstrated only if the programs target students in elementary school—i.e., before the onset of eating disorder symptoms.

Developmental Course and Outcomes

Differences in course and prognosis between AN and BN exist for adults and it is probable that these differences exist in adolescents as well. While both disorders may be chronic and relapsing and are associated with significant psychiatric and medical morbidity, AN is more strongly associated with poor outcome and mortality, while the outcomes for BN are more favorable. Across the eating disorders there is substantial diagnostic migration over time (Eddy et al. 2002; Tozzi et al. 2005).

Anorexia Nervosa

By definition, AN is associated with low weight, amenorrhea, and in turn, significant medical sequelae. A host of medical complications may set in as malnutrition worsens. Malnutrition is accompanied by evidence of physiological compromise (e.g., lowered body temperature, hypotension, changes in skin and hair texture and growth), along with changes in growth hormone, hypothalamic hypogonadism, bone marrow hypoplasia, structural brain abnormalities, cardiac dysfunction, and gastrointestinal difficulties. For children and adolescents, these changes are more pronounced due to their occurrence during significant stages of physical (and psychological) development. For adolescents with AN, the potential for significant growth retardation, pubertal delay or interruption, and peak bone mass reduction are significant. Osteopenia and osteoporosis are common—secondary to low weight in AN—and although bone mineral density improves somewhat with weight gain, osteopenia often persists (Misra and Klibanski 2006). Acutely, bradycar-

dia (very slow heart rate), hypothermia (very low body temperature), and dehydration may become life threatening (Fisher et al. 1995). Along with the physical effects of the illness come a range of psychological and social impairments, even if vocational and academic functioning are good.

Longitudinal research in adults with AN demonstrates mixed findings. Meta-analytic review of 119 studies including nearly 6,000 patients with AN indicated that over long-term follow-up, under one-half of surviving patients achieve full recovery, one-third improve but continue to experience eating disorder symptoms, and one-fifth remain chronically ill (Steinhausen 2002). Among those who achieve full recovery, one-third will relapse (Herzog et al. 1999). For adolescents, however, the course and outcome seem to be somewhat more favorable. In one longitudinal study of adolescents receiving inpatient treatment for AN, the vast majority (approximately 75%) achieved full recovery, with a median time to recovery of 5 years following participation in an intensive 6-month inpatient treatment (Strober et al. 1997). Further, follow-up studies of children and adolescents participating in family-based therapy for AN indicate substantial improvement and recovery with treatment (Le Grange and Lock 2005).

Diagnostic crossover between the AN subtypes and from AN to BN is common, occurring in approximately 50% of patients (Bulik et al. 1997; Eddy et al. 2002; Tozzi et al. 2005). Mortality in AN is estimated to be 0.56% per year, which is a 12-fold increase over that expected for young women in the general population (Herzog et al. 2000; Sullivan 1995). Suicide is particularly increased and accounts for at least half of the deaths in those with AN (Franko et al. 2004; Steinhausen 2002).

Bulimia Nervosa

BN is similarly associated with significant medical morbidity and may in addition lead to social impairment secondary to shame and the secrecy of the bulimic behaviors. While weight in BN may fluctuate, it generally remains in the healthy range. Instead, complications are secondary to binge/purge behaviors and include hypokalemia, esophageal tears, gastric disturbances, dehydration, and severe changes in blood pressure or heart rate when standing or sitting (orthostasis), which may require intermittent hospitalization (Fisher et al. 2001). Reported mortality rates are not increased in BN, although death may occur as a result of any of the above factors. In terms of the social impairment, with increased entrenchment of the disorder, a significant portion of the adolescent's day-to-day life is organized around the management of binge eating and the compensatory activities related to it. The adolescent may become more irritable, exhibit social withdrawal, demonstrate a decline in school performance, and report an increase in depressed mood. Further adding to the burden of BN are the frequently reported occurrence of other impulsive behaviors, such as alcohol use and shoplifting.

Longitudinal research indicates that the course of BN is unstable, with the vast majority of individuals with BN achieving some symptom relief over time and approximately 50% reaching full recovery (for review, see Keel and Mitchell 1997). Currently, long-term outcome studies are not available for adolescents with BN. Treatment studies show that with cognitive-behavioral guided self-care, less than 20% are binge and purge abstinent at the end of treatment (Schmidt et al. 2007), compared with an abstinence rate of 39% for participants in family-based treatment (Le Grange et al. 2007). At a 6-month follow-up, the percentage of abstinent patients improved to about 40% in the Schmidt study, while it decreased to 30% in the Le Grange study.

Diagnostic crossover from BN to AN is less common, occurring in up to one-quarter of patients (Tozzi et al. 2005).

Evaluation of Patients With Eating Disorders

Adolescents with eating disorders are often referred from a concerned pediatrician. Parents and pediatricians alike are reluctant to make a referral to psychiatric services. This reluctance may be due to a resistance to ascribe the eating behaviors to psychological factors that may incite feelings of shame or guilt in parents or due to a difficulty finding adequate or affordable mental health services. Youth with eating disorders often deny or minimize symptoms—either unconsciously, because of a distorted perception of their behavior and attitudes—or consciously, in an effort to keep clinicians and parents from recognizing the severity of their symptoms. Consequently, it is always necessary for the clinician to meet with the adolescent as well as his or her parents in order to obtain a more complete perspective on the referral.

Interview With the Adolescent

The assessment should start with a meeting with the adolescent. This meeting provides a developmentally appropriate "entry" into the family and demonstrates respect for the adolescent's developing identity. While many patients with an eating disorder might present a hostile, defensive, or challenging stance, the assessor should communicate support and warmth and ask open-ended questions to facilitate a better understanding of the individual patient and his or her family. The aims of this evaluation should include obtaining an understanding of some of the potential triggers that gave rise to the dieting behavior—for example, exposure to weight-related comments (e.g., teasing), onset of menses, experience with dating, family environment (e.g., quarrels or conflicts), experience with transitions (e.g., academic, friendship, or romantic relationship breakups, losses, traumas), or exposure to dieting (e.g., in social circle, in family). A comprehensive assessment should include information about history of weight loss efforts including calorie counting, restricting fat intake, restricting protein or meats, fasting or skipping meals, limiting fluid consumption, increased physical activity, avoidance of eating with others, eating in secret, hoarding food, binge eating, secretive eating, purging, and use of stimulants or diet pills. Additionally, intake evaluation should include inquiry about cognitions related to eating, weight, and shape (e.g., degree of body dissatisfaction).

Determining pretreatment levels of restriction, binge eating, compensatory behaviors, severity of weight and shape concerns, and preoccupation with eating is important as these become targets of intervention. AN is characterized by a cascade of restricting activities that typically starts with the exclusion of fats and sugars from the diet. Restricting proteins and meats follows this, and finally, restricting amounts. Although BN is also characterized by periods of dietary restriction, among individuals with BN these periods are less prolonged and are interrupted by lapses into binge eating and subsequently compensatory behaviors. For individuals with BN, patterns of failed dietary restriction, binge eating, and compensatory behaviors become cyclic. A binge may be "objective," (eating an amount in a finite period that is significantly more than for the average person) or "subjective" (eating a normal amount of food, but feeling out of control at the time of eating) (American Psychiatric Association 2000a). While AN and BN patients can present with both types of binge eating, AN patients are more likely than the typical BN patient to report exclusively "subjective" binge eating.

Interview With Parents

Once the meeting with the adolescent has concluded, the parents should be interviewed without the patient. In two-parent families, it is preferable for both to be present. The parents are able to provide more general information about the patient's development—e.g., complications during pregnancy, early feeding patterns, timing of developmental milestones, attachment style, transitions to preschool and elementary school, early temperament and personality, and family and peer relationships. The clinician should use the information obtained during the interview with the adolescent, compare it to the parents' version of events, and explore commonalties as well as differences. Together, both perspectives generate a comprehensive narrative of the events leading up to and sustaining the current clinical presentation.

Medical Examination

Because eating disorders can have profound medical complications, both medical and nutritional assessments are imperative. Clinicians conducting these assessments should be well versed in the medical aspects of malnutrition and binge-eating and purging behaviors to assess any medical problems that may be present. Patients with eating disorders often complain of dizziness, headaches, fainting spells, weakness, poor concentration, stomach and abdominal pain, and amenorrhea. Individuals who exhibit binge eating and purging commonly report throat pain, blood in emesis, small dotlike lesions in the sclera of the eyes, and swollen neck glands.

Standard medical assessment of an adolescent with an eating disorder would include 1) a complete physical to screen for signs of malnutrition (e.g., dehydration, tooth erosion, lanugo) and 2) laboratory tests to identify any abnormalities in blood, liver, and thyroid functioning. Medical assessment is helpful in determining the severity and chronicity of illness, and it is also needed to determine a differential diagnosis. Physical disorders such as diabetes mellitus, colitis, thyroid disease, Addison's disease, and brain tumors, among others, all may display clinical symptoms similar to those of AN. Similarly, neurological disorders that affect appetite regulation and eating patterns, gastrointestinal conditions, and hormonal disorders af-

fecting metabolism may manifest symptoms similar to those of BN. When conducting a physical assessment of individuals with eating disorders, these medical conditions should be evaluated and ruled out before proceeding with treatment targeting AN or BN.

A consultation between parents and a nutritionist with expertise in working with adolescents with eating disorders is helpful in clarifying the degree of weight loss in AN, as well as providing educational advice (to the parents) about the requirements of proper nutrition for restoring optimal health. A nutritionist can also help the clinician determine a reasonable weight range for recovery.

Psychometric Assessment

Specific structured interviews to evaluate eating disorder symptoms and confirm diagnosis are available. The most common screening instrument, the Eating Disorder Examination (EDE), is available for adults and older adolescents (Cooper and Fairburn 1987), as well as a version designed for use with children and young adolescents (Bryant-Waugh et al. 1996). Several self-report measures of eating disorder psychopathology are available: the Eating Disorder Inventory (EDI), which has normative data down to age 14 years (Shore and Porter 1990); the Eating Attitudes Test (EAT), which has a version applicable to school-age children (Maloney et al. 1988); and the Kids Eating Disorders Survey (KEDS), which is applicable to elementary and middle school–age children (Childress et al. 1993). Standardized interview and questionnaire assessments are clinically useful as they allow for the monitoring of progress over time, particularly with regard to specific symptoms.

Treatment for Adolescents With Eating Disorders

Adolescents with eating disorders require comprehensive psychiatric and medical care (Commission on Adolescent Eating Disorders 2005). Generally, a team approach is recommended to provide mental health care, medical treatment, and nutritional guidance. Level and intensity of treatment varies from outpatient to residential to inpatient. While decisions about level of care should be made on the basis of clinical severity, instead they are often driven by availability of resources and third-party coverage.

Currently, there are relatively few clinical treatment guidelines for eating disorders. It was therefore particularly timely when the National Institute for Health and Clinical Excellence (NICE) (National Collaborating Centre for Mental Health 2004) in the United Kingdom recently took a first step in summarizing guidelines for adult and adolescent eating disorders based on a comprehensive review of the literature. NICE recommends that treatment modalities be graded A to C. Grade A implies strong empirical support from several well-conducted randomized trials, while grade C implies expert consensus. By far the majority of the more than 100 recommendations that were made received only a grade C. There were two exceptions: cognitive-behavioral therapy (CBT) for adults with BN received an A, and family intervention for adolescent AN, with a focus on the eating disorder, received a B. No specific recommendation was made for adolescents with BN.

Methods of effective intervention differ somewhat according to the eating disorder diagnosis. For AN, inpatient treatment as well as one of two established outpatient approaches (psychodynamic individual therapy and family therapy) are generally implemented. In contrast, for BN, family therapy and cognitive-behavioral treatment are the only psychotherapeutic approaches that have been investigated. Pharmacotherapy for adolescent AN and BN has received little attention. Investigation into the effective treatment of eating disorders has accumulating substantial evidence for the efficacy of CBT for adult BN but has lagged behind in the study of treatments for AN.

Anorexia Nervosa

Inpatient Treatment

It is inevitable that the physical and/or psychological status of some patients will require inpatient treatment. The American Psychiatric Association (2000b) and the Society for Adolescent Medicine (2003; Golden et al. 2003) have articulated the criteria for admission to an inpatient setting. Admission to a pediatric ward would be warranted in the presence of severe and persistent medical complications that are life threatening. Indications of medical instability include, but are not limited to, weight ≤75% of ideal body weight, hypoglycemic syncope, fluid and electrolyte imbalance, cardiac arrhythmia, and severe dehydration. Medium (a few weeks) and longer-term (a month or more) admissions to a psychiatric facility that specializes in the treatment of eating disorders should be considered for severely underweight patients, particularly those who have been unresponsive to outpatient efforts at weight restoration, as well as those patients who present with serious comorbid psychiatric conditions that warrant more intensive supervision and treatment. For a more detailed description of inpatient treatment for eating disorders, see Golden et al. 2003.

Psychotherapy

Psychotherapeutic treatment of adolescents with AN has been dominated by two approaches: individual and family therapies, each with strong adherents and a theoretical position to support their views. Definitive evidence of the superiority of one of these approaches is lacking. However, inclusion of families in the treatment of adolescents with eating disorders seems to have a slight advantage.

Family-Based Treatment

The family therapy work by Minuchin et al. (1978) at the Child Guidance Clinic in Philadelphia exerted a considerable impact on ensuing treatment efforts in AN. The reasons for this impact were twofold: 1) the positive results from their first series of cases treated in family therapy and 2) the clear theoretical argument that underpins this approach. In their model of the *psychosomatic family*, they hypothesized that a specific family context is required for the eating disorder to develop. This family context is characterized by rigidity, enmeshment, overinvolvement and conflict avoidance, and usually evolves around the symptomatic behavior of the adolescent. This process was said to exist in tandem with a physiological vulnerability in the adolescent, which is due in part to her or his role as mediator in cross-generational alliances (Minuchin et al. 1978). While these authors emphasized that their model was not simply an account of a "family aetiology" for AN but instead highlighted the evolving, interactive nature of the process, they still considered the resulting psychosomatic family as a necessary condition for the development of AN. Consequently, the treatment proposed by the Philadelphia group was to *alter* family functioning.

Despite the optimism that Minuchin's findings created, serious methodological weaknesses underlie this research. In their uncontrolled case series, members of the treatment team conducted patient evaluations in the absence of comparison treatment groups and with follow-up that varied from 18 months to 7 years. Although this study did not purport to be a clinical trial, the theoretical principles and clinical application of

Minuchin's approach have served as the foundation for several subsequent family-based treatment studies.

A handful of randomized trials, mostly with modest sample sizes, have been conducted. The first controlled study to build on Minuchin's work, conducted at the Maudsley Hospital in London (Russell et al. 1987), compared outpatient family therapy with individual supportive therapy, following inpatient weight restoration. This family therapy included several components of Minuchin's approach, although it also differed in important ways. For instance, Russell and his colleagues encouraged the parents to persist in their efforts at weight restoration *until* treatment goals were achieved. For the most part, general adolescent and family issues were deferred until the eating disorder behavior was under control. In this study of 80 participants of all ages, all patients were initially admitted to the inpatient unit (average stay=10 weeks) for weight restoration before being randomly allocated to one of the two outpatient follow-up treatments. One of four subgroups (*n*=21) included young adolescents (age at onset ≤18, mean age at entry=16.6 years) with a short duration of illness (<3 years). After 1 year of outpatient treatment, this subgroup had a significantly better outcome with family therapy than their counterparts who were initially assigned to individual treatment. Ninety percent of patients who were originally assigned to family therapy had no further eating disorder symptoms compared with 36% of those who were in individual therapy (Russell et al. 1987). At 5-year follow-up, these benefits of family therapy were maintained (Eisler et al. 1997).

Since this seminal work, four studies have compared different forms of family intervention in adolescent AN (Eisler et al. 2000; Le Grange et al. 1992; Lock et al. 2005; Robin et al. 1999). In the first of these studies, the Maudsley group (Eisler et al. 2000; Le Grange et al. 1992) compared conjoint family therapy and separated family therapy (SFT). The therapeutic goals for both treatments were similar. However, in SFT the adolescent was seen independently from the parents, albeit by the same therapist. Both treatments were provided on an outpatient basis, and while none of the patients in the Le Grange et al. (1992) study required inpatient treatment during the course of study, 10% of Eisler et al.'s (2000) study patients were admitted to the inpatient unit during the course of treatment. Admission was usually initiated when the adolescent failed to gain weight despite the family's efforts and/or the study physician considered the patient to be at medical risk. Overall results for these two studies were similar, and regardless of the type of family treatment,

approximately 70% of patients had no further eating disorder symptoms at the end of treatment.

Similar to the long-term outcome of the original Maudsley study (Eisler et al. 1997), patients continued to improve after treatment ended in Eisler's study (Eisler et al. 2000). Results from a 5-year follow-up show that irrespective of the type of family treatment, 75% of patients had no further eating disorder symptoms, no deaths occurred in this cohort of 40 patients, and only 8% of those who achieved a healthy weight at the end of treatment reported any kind of relapse at follow-up (Eisler et al. 2007).

Following the Maudsley work, the first family therapy for AN study in the United States (Robin et al. 1999) compared two outpatient interventions in a controlled trial in a design that resembled the Maudsley investigations. These researchers compared behavioral systems family therapy (BSFT) with an ego-oriented individual therapy (EOIT) and reported significant improvement in AN symptoms at the end of treatment. More than two-thirds (67%) of patients reached target weight, and 80% regained menstruation. Patients continued to improve, and at 1-year follow-up, approximately 75% had reached their target weight and 85% had started or resumed menses. Meaningful differences were found between the two treatments. Patients in BSFT achieved significantly greater weight gain than those in EOIT, both at the end of treatment and at follow-up. Similarly, patients who received BSFT were significantly more likely to have returned to normal menstrual functioning at the end of treatment compared with those in EOIT. Both treatments were similar in terms of improvements in eating attitudes, depression, and self-reported eating-related family conflict. Neither group reported much family related conflict regarding eating, either before or after treatment. Robin and colleagues concluded that BSFT produced greater weight gain and higher rates of resumption of menstruation compared with EOIT. While both treatments produced comparable improvements in eating attitudes and depression, BSFT produced a more rapid treatment response.

The fourth controlled study following the original work of the Maudsley group was conducted by Lock et al. (2005). In this randomized dosage study, participants were allocated to either 10 sessions of manualized family-based treatment for AN (FBT-AN) delivered over 6 months or 20 sessions of FBT-AN over 12 months. For both treatment groups, these authors found significant weight gain and improvements in psychological symptoms of AN, as measured by the EDE. A 4-year follow-up confirmed that these initial

TABLE 26–5. Three phases of family-based treatment of anorexia nervosa

Phase 1: Restoring the adolescent's weight. Treatment is focused on the eating disorder symptoms and includes a family meal. Families are encouraged, with guidance from the therapist, to work out for themselves how best to restore weight for their anorexic child.

Phase 2: Handing control over eating back to the adolescent. The start of the second phase of treatment is usually signaled by the adolescent's acquiescence to the demands of the parents to increase her food intake and a positive change in the mood of the family. Symptoms remain central in the discussions, while weight gain with minimum tension is encouraged. All other issues that the family has had to postpone throughout the first phase of treatment can now be brought forward for review.

Phase 3: Discussion of adolescent development. The third phase is usually initiated when the adolescent has achieved and maintained a healthy weight and self-starvation has abated. Central to the discussion for this part of treatment is the establishment of a healthy relationship between the adolescent or young adult and his or her parents. That is, this relationship is no longer characterized by the illness constituting the basis of interaction. Adolescent developmental issues are also now brought to the fore.

weight gains and improvements in psychological symptoms were maintained, again showing no differences between the short- and long-term treatments (Lock et al. 2006).

An important advance that evolved in tandem with Lock's study was the manualization of the family therapy model that has been implemented in almost all of the Maudsley studies (Lock et al. 2001a), as well as a parent handbook to assist and guide parents through treatment (Lock and Le Grange 2005). This manual allows for FBT-AN to be tested more broadly in controlled *and* uncontrolled settings, while therapists now have a tool to add to their clinical armamentarium to address AN in their young patients. An outline of FBT-AN as it proceeds through three clearly defined phases is presented in Table 26–5.

Since Minuchin's seminal work, and in addition to the controlled trials, several case series of varying sample sizes have been published. These studies involved adolescents treated with family therapy, but they also included individual and inpatient treatments, albeit to a lesser extent. Most notable are three larger uncontrolled studies that have been published recently (Le Grange et al. 2005; Lock et al. 2006; Loeb et al. 2007), all of which used manualized FBT-AN. These studies add to the body of literature that supports the notion that parents are a resource and that it is feasible and useful to incorporate them into the treatment of their adolescent. Taken together, results are supportive of FBT-AN, although only provisional conclusions can be drawn from uncontrolled studies that describe a relatively small combined series of cases. However, in conjunction with Minuchin's work and the controlled studies, these preliminary investigations put forward a substantial literature in support of family-based treatment.

Pharmacotherapy

Psychopharmacological interventions for AN have been examined in adult samples, but the role of these agents in adolescents remains relatively unexplored. While the use of psychopharmacological agents is limited during times of acute medical compromise, low-dose atypical antipsychotics are sometimes used to address severe obsessional thinking, anxiety, and psychotic-like thinking. However, these agents pose problems with binge induction and little evidence of other benefits compared with controls. Several case reports and open-label trials describe the use of the newer antipsychotic agents (e.g., olanzapine) in the treatment of adolescent AN (Boachie et al. 2003; Dennis et al. 2006; Mehler et al. 2001). At doses of 5 mg per day and above, the patients reported decreased anxiety around eating, improved sleep, and decreased rumination about food and body concerns. Morning sedation was the most commonly reported adverse effect. Olanzapine appeared to be useful in addition to psychotherapy for these adolescents with AN.

Bulimia Nervosa

The NICE guidelines (National Collaborating Centre for Mental Health 2004) made no specific recommendation for the treatment of adolescents with BN, which reflects the fact that to date, systematic research in the treatment of BN has focused almost exclusively on adults. This is true despite the relatively common occurrence of binge-eating and purging behaviors during adolescence, and that many cases of BN onset in adolescence (Stice and Agras 1998). Significant progress has been made in understanding a range of efficacious treatments for adults with BN, such as

TABLE 26–6. Three phases of family-based treatment of bulimia nervosa

Phase 1: Reestablishing healthy eating. Treatment aims at empowering parents to disrupt binge eating, purging, restrictive dieting, and any other pathological weight-control behaviors. It also aims to externalize and separate the disordered behaviors from the affected adolescent to promote parental action and decrease adolescent resistance to their assistance.

Phase 2: Helping the adolescent eat independently. Once abstinence from disordered eating and related behaviors has been achieved, the second stage of treatment begins when parents transition control over eating and weight-related issues back to the adolescent under their supervision.

Phase 3: Adolescent developmental issues. The focus here is on ways the family can help address the effects of bulimia nervosa on adolescent developmental processes, both on the adolescent and the family as a whole.

CBT, interpersonal psychotherapy, and antidepressant medications. In these studies, the mean age of participants was 28.4 years, with a duration of illness of approximately 10 years, and usually a cutoff age for entry at 18 years (Agras et al. 2000). In contrast, case series data on CBT and two randomized controlled trials (RCTs) that have recently been completed (Le Grange et al. 2007; Schmidt et al. 2007) are the only treatment studies with an adolescent population that have been published.

Psychotherapies

Family-based treatment.

Dodge et al. (1995) first reported on the use of family therapy for BN in a small case series, demonstrating that family psychoeducation and parental coaching in disrupting binge/purge behaviors led to significant reductions in bulimic symptoms for adolescents. More recently, Le Grange and Lock (2007) described and manualized a family-based treatment for adolescents with BN (FBT-BN), derived from the approach that has demonstrated efficacy for adolescents with AN. Similar to FBT-AN, FBT-BN is agnostic about the causes of the disorder and assumes that adolescent development is negatively affected by characteristics of the eating disorder. These characteristics include secrecy, shame, and dysfunctional eating patterns, and in addition to impeding adolescent development, they are thought to have confused and disempowered parents and other family members. FBT-BN works in three stages (Table 26–6). However, there are several important differences between FBT-BN and FBT-AN. Notably, in FBT-BN, treatment is not focused on weight restoration, but rather on the regulation of eating patterns and the elimination of purging. An additional difference is that in BN, the treatment approach is more collaborative between parents and the affected adolescent. For adolescents with BN, the secretive na-

ture of the disorder, along with the shame and guilt associated with these symptoms, may lead to it being more easily overlooked by parents. Finally, adolescents with BN may be more likely to have psychiatric comorbidity than those with AN, which needs to be addressed in treatment.

To date, two RCTs for adolescents with BN and subthreshold BN have been published (Le Grange et al. 2007; Schmidt et al. 2007). Le Grange and colleagues compared manualized FBT-BN to individual supportive psychotherapy for adolescents (ages 12–19 years). Both directly following treatment and at 6-month follow-up, adolescents who had received FBT-BN were more likely to be binge/purge abstinent (39% vs. 18% following treatment and 29% vs. 10% at follow-up) compared with those who had received supportive psychotherapy. Schmidt et al. (2007) compared CBT guided self-care with family therapy in adolescent and young adult patients (ages 12–20 years). At 6-month follow-up, both treatments yielded significant improvements (family therapy=41% abstinent), without between-group differences. Notably, while the family treatments in both studies resembled one another, Schmidt et al. defined family as *any close other* rather than just parents. This broader definition may have been used in part due to the slightly older age of adolescents in this UK sample (17.6±0.3 years vs. 16.1±1.6 years) who may not have wanted their parents involved. Indeed, 25% of those eligible for the UK study declined participation because they did not want their parents involved in treatment (Perkins et al. 2004). While modifying "family" treatment to include other significant individuals in the patient's life may be sensible, this may not be the most effective way to approach FBT with younger adolescents where parental authority is key to the success of the treatment. These preliminary studies suggest that family-based therapy may be effective for the treatment of younger patients with BN.

Cognitive-behavioral therapy.

The cognitive-behavioral model of BN assumes that the maintenance of BN is based on dysfunctional attitudes toward body shape and weight. These beliefs lead to overvalued ideas about weight and increased body dissatisfaction, usually followed by attempts to control shape and weight by excessive dieting. Dieting can cause a sense of both psychological and physiological deprivation, leading to depressed mood. In addition, because of dietary restriction, hunger is increased, and this, in turn, leads to a greater probability of binge eating. Due to fears of weight gain associated with eating a large amount of usually calorie-dense food, inappropriate compensatory behaviors such as purging are seen as an attempt to allay these anxieties (Apple and Agras 1997). The clinical application of CBT has been tested in numerous controlled studies and has been found to be the most effective psychotherapeutic approach to the treatment of BN in adults. CBT is more effective than any other condition, including no treatment, nondirective therapy, pill placebo, manualized psychodynamic therapy (supportive-expressive), stress management, and antidepressant treatment (Agras et al. 2000).

There have been two published case series of adolescents with BN using CBT adapted for adolescents (Lock 2005; Schapman et al. 2006). The adolescent version of the treatment involves modifications to allow for increased parental involvement in treatment, use of concrete examples tailored for adolescents to illustrate points, and exploration of adolescent issues in the context of BN (e.g., separation/individuation). In addition to CBT for adolescents, CBT guided self-care has been compared with family therapy (Schmidt et al. 2007) in one of the two RCTs for this population. Results from this RCT suggest that CBT guided self-care was both an acceptable and feasible treatment for adolescents, with a treatment dropout rate of 29% and an abstinence rate of 36% (from both binge eating and purging) at the end of 12 months of treatment. These abstinence rates were similar to those found in more recent adult studies of CBT (Mitchell et al. 2006).

Pharmacotherapy

Randomized, controlled pharmacological clinical trials in adults with BN have largely indicated that antidepressants are superior to placebo in reduction of binge frequency (Walsh et al. 1997). Further, weight and shape concerns and mood disturbance also seem to demonstrate increased improvement with medication compared with placebo (Mitchell et al. 1993). However, controlled studies in adults directly evaluating the relative and combined effectiveness of CBT and antidepressant medication (Walsh et al. 1997) have suggested that when added to psychological treatments (e.g., CBT or interpersonal psychotherapy), medications did not generally improve treatment outcomes. Taken together, these data suggest that the use of antidepressants in adults with BN, offers only a marginal advantage over CBT alone.

To date, only one open-label medication trial has been published including adolescents (ages 12–18) with BN (Kotler et al. 2003). The findings from this study suggested that 8 weeks of fluoxetine (60 mg/day) was well tolerated in conjunction with supportive psychotherapy and yielded impressive improvement rates of approximately 70%. Controlled research with adolescents is needed, however, to determine the effectiveness of this medication in younger populations who may have different clinical profiles compared with adults with BN (Le Grange and Schmidt 2005).

Taken together, and notwithstanding the paucity of systematic data, there are strong clinical reasons to involve the parents in the treatment of adolescents with eating disorders. Family-based treatment provides an opportunity to reinforce pertinent behaviors and attitudes on the part of parents and other family members that can contribute to the recovery of the adolescent. At the same time, behaviors that reinforce symptomatic behavior can be minimized. This forum allows for the education about eating disorders to all family members, while also addressing the possible impact that the eating disorder may have on family relationships. Many adolescents with eating disorders may not welcome parental involvement in meal planning or assisting with efforts to decrease binge-eating and purging episodes. The clinician's task is to reassure everyone, not just the patient, that the parental involvement is supportive rather than critical (Le Grange and Lock 2007; Lock et al. 2001a). At the same time, family involvement helps the therapist to highlight for the parents the medical and psychological problems associated with the eating disorder and to elicit their support in helping their child. Such a perspective can help to shift parental attitudes toward the patient and the illness from exasperation and anger to a more productive and sympathetic position.

Research Directions

First, increased research into the similarities and differences in clinical, presentation, course, and outcome among youth with AN, BN and subthreshold variants compared with youth without these types of eating difficulties is needed. Second, conceptualization of eating disorders in a developmental context should lead to a clearer understanding of risk factors, treatment approaches, and prevention strategies. Third, we are sorely lacking in clinical trials for treatment of younger cohorts of patients. To date, there are only

seven published psychotherapy trials for adolescents with AN and BN, and one open-label pharmacotherapy study for adolescent BN. No doubt, advances in the treatment of AN and BN have been hampered by this lack of vigorous and systematic inquiry. Notwithstanding, findings suggest promising leads in terms of family-based treatment approaches.

Summary Points

- Eating disorders onset in the context of social, psychological, and physical development, making a developmental perspective on diagnosis and treatment essential.

- Inpatient treatment for adolescent eating disorders is useful for acute weight restoration but of limited use in reducing recidivism rates.

- The small number of outpatient treatment studies provides suggestive evidence that involving parents in treatment may be helpful (i.e., family-based treatment).

- There are no medications that appear to be routinely helpful with AN or BN, and pharmacological therapies remain largely unexplored.

- Taken together, the literature supports the importance of early identification of and intervention for eating disorders in order to improve outcomes.

References

Ackard D, Peterson D: Association between puberty and disordered, body image, and other psychological variables. Int J Eat Disord 29:187–194, 2000

Agras WS, Walsh BT, Fairburn CG, et al: A multicenter comparison of cognitive-behavioral therapy and interpersonal psychotherapy for bulimia nervosa. Arch Gen Psychiatry 57:459–466, 2000

American Psychiatric Association: Diagnostic and Statistical Manual of Mental Disorders, 4th Edition. Washington, DC, American Psychiatric Association, 1994

American Psychiatric Association: Diagnostic and Statistical Manual of Mental Disorders, 4th Edition, Text Revision. Washington, DC, American Psychiatric Association, 2000a

American Psychiatric Association: Practice guidelines for the treatment of patients with eating disorders (revision). Am J Psychiatry 157(suppl):1–39, 2000b

Apple RF, Agras WS: Overcoming Eating Disorders: A Cognitive-behavioral Treatment for Bulimia Nervosa and Binge Eating Disorder. Client Workbook. San Antonio, TX, Psychological Corporation, 1997

Attie I, Brooks-Gunn J: Development of eating problems in adolescent girls: a longitudinal study. Dev Psychol 25:70–79, 1989

Binford RB, Mussell MP, Rogers L, et al: Eating disorders: prevention and intervention strategies with children and adolescents, in Intervention With Children and Adolescents: An Interdisciplinary Perspective. Edited by Allen-Meares P, Fraser MW. Boston, MA, Pearson, 2004, pp 515–531

Boachie A, Goldfield GS, Spettigue W: Olanzapine use as an adjunctive treatment for hospitalized children with anorexia nervosa. Int J Eat Disord 33:98–103, 2003

Bravender T, Bryant-Waugh, R, Herzog D, et al: Classification of child and adolescent eating disturbances. Workgroup for Classification of Eating Disorders in Children and Adolescents (WCEDCA). Int J Eat Disord 40(suppl): S117–S122, 2007

Bryant-Waugh RJ: Overview of eating disorders, in Anorexia Nervosa and Related Eating Disorders in Children and Adolescence. Edited by Lask B, Bryant-Waugh R. East Sussex, UK, Psychology Press Ltd, 2002, pp 27–40

Bryant-Waugh RJ, Cooper PJ, Taylor CL, et al: The use of the Eating Disorder Examination with children: a pilot investigation. Int J Eat Disord 19:391–397, 1996

Bulik CM, Fear J, Pickering A: Predictors of the development of bulimia nervosa in women with anorexia nervosa. J Nerv Ment Dis 185:704–707, 1997

Casper R, Troiani M: Family functioning in anorexia by subtype. Int J Eat Disord 30:338–342, 2001

Childress A, Brewerton T, Hodges E, et al: The Kids Eating Disorder Survey (KEDS): a study of middle school students. J Am Acad Child Adolesc Psychiatry 32:843–850, 1993

Commission on Adolescent Eating Disorders: Treatment of eating disorders, in Treating and Preventing Adolescent Mental Health Disorders: What We Know and What We Don't Know. A Research Agenda for Improving the Mental Health of Our Youth. Edited by Evans DL, Foa EB, Gur RE, et al. Oxford, UK, Oxford University Press, 2005

Cooper Z, Fairburn CG: The Eating Disorder Examination: a semistructured interview for the assessment of the specific psychopathology of eating disorders. Int J Eat Disord 6:1–8, 1987

Dennis K, Le Grange D, Bremer J: Case report of olanzapine use in adolescent anorexia nervosa. Eat Weight Disord 11:e53–e56, 2006

Dodge E, Hodes M, Eisler I, et al: Family therapy for bulimia nervosa in adolescents: an exploratory study. J Fam Ther 17:59–77, 1995

Eddy K, Keel P, Dorer D, et al: Longitudinal comparison of anorexia nervosa subtypes. Int J Eat Disord 31:191–202, 2002

Eddy K, Tanofsky-Kraff M, Thompson-Brenner H, et al: Eating disorder pathology among overweight treatment-seeking youth: clinical correlates and cross-sectional risk modeling. Behav Res Ther 45:2360–2371, 2007

Eddy K, Celio Doyle A, Hoste R, et al: Eating disorder not otherwise specified (EDNOS): an examination of EDNOS presentations in adolescents. J Am Acad Child Adolesc Psychiatry 47:156–164, 2008

Eisler I, Dare C, Russell GFM, et al: Family and individual therapy in anorexia nervosa: a five-year follow-up. Arch Gen Psychiatry 54:1025–1030, 1997

Eisler I, Dare C, Hodes M, et al: Family therapy for adolescent anorexia nervosa: the results of a controlled comparison of two family interventions. J Child Psychol Psychiatry 41:727–736, 2000

Eisler I, Simic M, Russell GFM, et al: A randomised controlled treatment trial of two forms of family therapy in adolescent anorexia nervosa: a five-year follow-up. J Child Psychol Psychiatry 48:552–560, 2007

Fairburn CG, Cooper Z, Doll H, et al: The natural course of bulimia nervosa and binge eating disorder in young women. Arch Gen Psychiatry 57:659–665, 2000

Fairburn CG, Cooper Z, Shafran R: Cognitive-behavioral therapy for eating disorders: a "transdiagnostic" theory and treatment. Behav Res Ther 41:509–528, 2003

Fairburn CG, Cooper Z, Bohn K, et al: The severity and status of eating disorder NOS: implications for DSM-V. Behav Res Ther 45:1705–1715, 2007

Fischer S, Le Grange D: Comorbidity and high-risk behaviors in treatment seeking adolescents with bulimia nervosa. Int J Eat Disord 40:751–753, 2007

Fisher M, Golden N, Katzman D, et al: Eating disorders in adolescents: a background paper. J Adolesc Health 16:420–437, 1995

Fisher M, Schneider M, Burns J, et al: Differences between adolescents and young adults at presentation to an eating disorder program. J Adolesc Health 28:222–227, 2001

Frank GK, Bailer UF, Henry S, et al: Neuroimaging studies in eating disorders. CNS Spectr 9:539–548, 2004

Franko DL, Keel PK, Dorer DJ, et al: What predicts suicide attempts in women with eating disorders? Psychol Med 34:843–853, 2004

Golden NH, Katzman DK, Kreipe RE, et al: Eating disorders in adolescents: position paper of the Society for Adolescent Medicine. J Adolesc Health 33:496–503, 2003

Granillo T, Jones-Rodriguez G, Carvajal SC: Prevalence of eating disorders in Latina adolescents: associations with substance use and other correlates. J Adolesc Health 36:214–220, 2005

Gunewardene A, Huon G, Zheng R: Exposure to westernization and dieting: a cross-cultural study. Int J Eat Disord 29:289–293, 2001

Herzog DB, Nussbaum KM, Marmor AK: Comorbidity and outcome in eating disorders. Psychiatr Clin North Am 19:843–859, 1996

Herzog DB, Dorer DJ, Keel PK, et al: Recovery and relapse in anorexia and bulimia nervosa: a 7.5-year follow-up study. J Am Acad Child Adolesc Psychiatry 38:829–837, 1999

Herzog DB, Greenwood DN, Dorer DJ, et al: Mortality in eating disorders: a descriptive study. Int J Eat Disord 28:20–26, 2000

Herzog DB, Franko DL, Dorer DJ, et al: Drug abuse in patients with eating disorders. Int J Eat Disord 39:434–442, 2006

Hoste R, Le Grange D: Expressed emotion among white and ethnic minority families of adolescents with bulimia nervosa. Eur Eat Disord Rev 16:395–400, 2008

Hudson JI, Hiripi E, Pope HG, et al: The prevalence and correlates of eating disorders in the National Comorbidity Survey Replication. Biol Psychiatry 61:348–358, 2007

Johnson JG, Cohen P, Kotler L, et al: Psychiatric disorders associated with risk for the development of eating disorders during adolescence and early adulthood. J Consult Clin Psychol 70:1119–1128, 2002

Kaye WH, Grendall K, Strober M: Serotonin neuronal function and selective serotonin reuptake inhibitor treatment in anorexia nervosa. Biol Psychiatry 44:825–838, 1998

Keel PK, Mitchell JE: Outcome in bulimia nervosa. Am J Psychiatry 154:313–321, 1997

Keel PK, Heatherton TF, Dorer DJ, et al: Point prevalence of bulimia nervosa in 1982, 1992, and 2002. Psychol Med 36:119–127, 2006

Kendler KS, Walters EE, Neale MC, et al: The structure of genetic and environmental risk factors for six major psychiatric disorders in women. Arch Gen Psychiatry, 52:374–383, 1995

Kent A, Lacey H, McClusky SE: Premenarchal bulimia nervosa. J Psychosom Res 36:205–210, 1992

Kotler L, Devlin B, Davies M, et al: An open trial of fluoxetine in adolescents with bulimia nervosa. J Child Adolesc Psychopharmacol 13:329–325, 2003

Le Grange D, Lock J: The dearth of psychological treatment studies for anorexia nervosa. Int J Eat Disord 37:79–91, 2005

Le Grange D, Lock J: Treating Bulimia in Adolescents: A Family-Based Approach. New York, Guilford, 2007

Le Grange D, Schmidt U: The treatment of adolescents with bulimia nervosa. J Ment Health 14:587–597, 2005

Le Grange D, Eisler I, Dare C, et al: Evaluation of family treatments in adolescent anorexia nervosa: a pilot study. Int J Eat Disord 12:347–357, 1992

Le Grange D, Loeb KL, Orman S, et al: Bulimia nervosa: a disorder in evolution? Arch Pediatr Adolesc Med 158: 478–482, 2004

Le Grange D, Binford R, Loeb KL: Manualized family-based treatment for anorexia nervosa: a case series. J Am Acad Child Adolesc Psychiatry 44:41–46, 2005

Le Grange D, Binford R, Peterson C, et al: DSM-IV threshold versus subthreshold bulimia nervosa. Int J Eat Disord 39:462–467, 2006

Le Grange D, Crosby RD, Rathouz PJ, et al: A randomized controlled comparison of family-based treatment and supportive psychotherapy for adolescent bulimia nervosa. Arch Gen Psychiatry 64:1049–1056, 2007

Leit R, Pope HG, Gray J: Cultural expectations of muscularity in men: the evolution of playgirl centerfolds. Int J Eat Disord 29:90–93, 2001

Lock J: Adjusting cognitive behavior therapy for adolescents with bulimia nervosa: results of case series. Am J Psychotherapy 59:267–281, 2005

Lock J, Le Grange D: Help Your Teenager Beat an Eating Disorder. New York, Guilford, 2005

Lock J, Le Grange D, Agras WS, et al: Treatment Manual for Anorexia Nervosa: A Family-Based Approach. New York, Guilford, 2001a

Lock J, Reisel B, Steiner H: Associated health risks of adolescents with disordered eating: how different are they from their peers? Results from a high school survey. Child Psychiatry Hum Dev 31:249–265, 2001b

Lock J, Agras WS, Bryson S, et al: A comparison of short- and long-term family therapy for adolescent anorexia nervosa. J Am Acad Child Adolesc Psychiatry 44:632–639, 2005

Lock J, Couturier J, Agras WS: Comparison of long-term outcomes in adolescents with anorexia nervosa treated with family therapy. J Am Acad Child Adolesc Psychiatry 45:666–672, 2006

Loeb KL, Walsh BT, Lock J, et al: Open trial of family-based treatment for adolescent anorexia nervosa: evidence of successful dissemination. J Am Acad Child Adolesc Psychiatry 46:792–800, 2007

Maloney MJ, McGuire JB, Daniels SR: Reliability testing of a children's version of the Eating Attitude Test. J Am Acad Child Adolesc Psychiatry 27:541–543, 1988

McCabe M, Ricciardelli L, Finemore J: The role of puberty, media and popularity with peers on strategies to increase weight, decrease weight and increase muscle tone among adolescent boys and girls. J Psychosom Res 52:145–153, 2001

Mehler C, Wewetzer C, Schulze U, et al: Olanzapine in children and adolescents with chronic anorexia nervosa. Eur Child Adol Psychiatry 10:151–157, 2001

Minuchin S, Rosman B, Baker I: Psychosomatic Families: Anorexia Nervosa in Context. Cambridge, MA, Harvard University Press, 1978

Misra M, Klibanski A: Anorexia nervosa and osteoporosis. Rev Endocr Metab Disord 7:91–99, 2006

Mitchell JE, Raymond N, Specker S: A review of the controlled trials of pharmacotherapy and psychotherapy in the treatment of bulimia nervosa. Int J Eat Disord 14:229–247, 1993

Mitchell J, Agras WS, Wonderlich S: Treatment of bulimia nervosa: where are we and where are we going? Int J Eat Disord 39:95–101, 2006

National Collaborating Centre for Mental Health: Eating Disorders: Core Interventions in the Treatment and Management of Anorexia Nervosa, Bulimia Nervosa and Related Eating Disorders. London, UK, British Psychological Society and Gaskell, 2004

Ohring R, Graber J, Brooks-Gunn J: Girls' recurrent and concurrent body dissatisfaction: correlates and consequences over 8 years. Int J Eat Disord 31:404–415, 2001

Perez M, Voelz Z, Pettit J, et al: The role of acculturative stress and body dissatisfaction in predicting bulimic symptomatology across ethnic groups. Int J Eat Disord 31:442–454, 2002

Perkins S, Winn S, Murray J, et al: A qualitative study of the experience of caring for a person with bulimia nervosa, part 1: the emotional impact of caring. Int J Eat Disord 36:256–268, 2004

Pirke M, Platte P: Neurobiology of eating disorders in adolescents in Eating Disorders in Adolescence: Anorexia and Bulimia Nervosa. Edited by Steinhausen H. New York, DeGruyter, 1995, pp 171–179

Robin AL, Siegel PT, Moye AW, et al: A controlled comparison of family versus individual therapy for adolescents with anorexia nervosa. J Am Acad Child Adolesc Psychiatry 38:1482–1489, 1999

Russell GFM, Szmukler GI, Dare C, et al: An evaluation of family therapy in anorexia nervosa and bulimia nervosa. Arch Gen Psychiatry 44:1047–1056, 1987

Schapman A, Lock J, Couturier J: Cognitive-behavioral therapy for adolescents with binge eating syndromes: a case series. Int J Eat Disord 39:252–255, 2006

Schmidt U, Lee S, Beecham J, et al: A randomized controlled trial of family therapy and cognitive behavioral guided self-help for adolescents with bulimia nervosa and related conditions. Am J Psychiatry 164:591–598, 2007

Schur E, Sanders M, Steiner H: Body dissatisfaction and eating attitudes in young children. Int J Eat Disord 27:74–82, 1999

Shore R, Porter J: Normative and reliability data for 11–18 year olds on the Eating Disorder Inventory. Int J Eat Disord 9:201–207, 1990

Society for Adolescent Medicine: Eating disorders in adolescents: position paper for the Society for Adolescent Medicine. J Adolesc Health 33:496–503, 2003

Spitzer RL, Devlin MJ, Walsh BT, et al: Binge eating disorder: a multisite field trial for the diagnostic criteria. Int J Eat Disord 11: 191–203, 1992

Spitzer RL, Yanovski S, Wadden T, et al: Binge eating disorder: its further validation in a multisite trial. Int J Eat Disord 13:137–153, 1993

Steiger H, Gauvin L, Israel M, et al: Association of serotonin and cortisol indices with childhood abuse in bulimia nervosa. Arch Gen Psychiatry 58:837–843, 2001

Steiner H, Kwan W, Walker S, et al: Risk and protective factors for juvenile eating disorders. Eur Child Adolesc Psychiatry 12(suppl):38–46, 2003

Steinhausen HC: The outcome of anorexia nervosa in the 20th century. Am J Psychiatry 159:1284–1293, 2002

Stice E, Agras WS: Predicting onset and cessation of bulimic behaviors during adolescence. Behav Ther 29:257–276, 1998

Striegel-Moore RH, Dohm FA, Kraemer HC, et al: Eating disorders in white and black women. Am J Psychiatry 160:1326–1331, 2003

Strober M, Freeman R, Morrell W: The long-term course of severe anorexia nervosa in adolescents: survival analysis of recovery, relapse, and outcome predictors over 10–15 years in a prospective study. Int J Eat Disord 22:339–360, 1997

Strober M, Freeman A, Lampert C, et al: Controlled family study of anorexia nervosa and bulimia nervosa: evidence of shared liability and transmission of partial syndromes. Am J Psychiatry 157:393–401, 2000

Sullivan PF: Mortality in anorexia nervosa. Am J Psychiatry 152:1073–1074, 1995

Tanofsky-Kraff M, Yanovski SZ, Wilfley DE, et al: Eating-disordered behaviors, body fat, and psychopathology in overweight and normal-weight children. J Consult Clin Psychol 72:53–61, 2004

Thompson-Brenner H, Eddy KT, Satir D, et al: Personality subtypes in adolescent eating disorders: validation of a classification approach. J Child Psychol Psychiatry 49:170–180, 2008

Tozzi F, Thornton LM, Klump KL, et al: Symptom fluctuation in eating disorders: correlate of diagnostic crossover. Am J Psychiatry 162:732–740, 2005

Von Ranson KM, Iacono WG, McGue M: Disordered eating and substance use in an epidemiological sample, I: associations within individuals. Int J Eat Disord 31:389–403, 2002

Walsh BT, Wilson GT, Loeb KL, et al: Medication and psychotherapy in the treatment of bulimia nervosa. Am J Psychiatry 154:523–531, 1997

Ward A, Ramsey R, Turnbull SJ, et al: Attachment in anorexia nervosa: a transgenerational perspective. Br J Med Psychol 74:497–505, 2001

Westen D, Harnden-Fischer J: Personality profiles in eating disorders: rethinking the distinction between axis I and axis II. Am J Psychiatry 158:547–562, 2001

Chapter 27

Tic Disorders

Kenneth E. Towbin, M.D.

Tics are sudden, quick, repetitive, stereotyped, "relatively involuntary" muscle contractions that can occur in any part of the body. Tic disorders are highly prevalent in children and adolescents but cause severe impairment in only a small minority. However, tic disorders also are model neuropsychiatric conditions that provide a unique window into the interplay of genetic risk, psychology, experience, and environment. Exploring tic disorders has led to a deeper understanding of neural pathways and circuits in the brain that subserve sensory and motor function, linking the frontal lobes, the striatum, and thalamus. The study of tic disorders has increased our knowledge of the relationship between cognition and motor activity and illuminated the role of striatum in motor planning and execution. Treatments now include interventions that draw directly on this preclinical and clinical work.

The term *tic disorders* comprises four diagnostic entities: transient tics, chronic motor tics, chronic phonic tics, and Tourette's disorder. Tourette's disorder (also called Tourette's syndrome, both hereafter called

"Tourette's") takes its name from Georges Gilles de la Tourette (1982) who, while a student under Charcot, first described the condition.

Symptoms and Comorbidity

Tics are repetitive, brief, sudden, stereotyped movements that can occur in any voluntary muscle. Tics affect the same muscles over days and hours but also migrate to different parts of the body and spread to include more regions over months and years. Specific tics appear and disappear or reappear after a long hiatus. Generally, tics appear in the face first (e.g., eye blinks, grimaces) and then progress to more caudal muscles in the neck, shoulders, arms, trunk, back, and legs.

Tics are best understood as "relatively involuntary." They may be suppressed successfully for minutes to hours, but they cannot be constrained indefinitely. The capacity to postpone tics varies throughout the day and across situations. One measure of tic severity is how much effort a person must exert in order to suppress a tic and how successfully he can inhibit them. Tics may be unwittingly influenced by suggestion. It is common for someone with tics to experience more symptoms while describing them. Tics also can mimic others' movements (echopraxia), words (echolalia), or sounds in the environment. It is common for a new tic to begin with a stimulus, such as a temporary physical irritation or a forceful emotional experience, and to continue long after that stimulus has ended.

Tics characteristically show variable frequency and intensity throughout the day, across months, and through years. This waxing and waning is not random. Tics occur in clusters and bundles of clusters that have been described as "bouts" and "bouts of bouts" (Peterson and Leckman 1998). Tics may also occur during sleep, unlike other movement disorders (Kostanecka-Endress et al. 2003).

Tics often increase in association with emotionally stimulating events, whether exciting and pleasing or stressful or distressing events. Some individuals find that their symptoms cease during effortful acts such as performing in public (Sacks 1985), executing skilled procedures (Sacks 1995), or during competitive athletics, but are worse just before or afterward.

Tics are often categorized as either simple or complex. *Simple tics* are those confined exclusively to one or a few muscle groups and are very brief, such as a grimace, shoulder shrug, a cough, or a sniff sound. *Complex tics* involve multiple muscle groups and integrated actions, such as thrusting one arm forward while slapping the contralateral thigh with the corresponding hand or repeatedly uttering the first line of a jingle. Complex tics may entail many serial movements and/or sounds, such as stopping midstride and in succession touching a hand to the floor, hopping once, barking, and completing a pirouette. These distinctions do not carry diagnostic or prognostic implications, although a display of complex repetitive behavior without simple tics should lead one to question the presence of a tic disorder.

Individuals with tics commonly report two types of mental events—*premonitory urges* (Leckman et al. 1993) and *obsessions and/or compulsions* (OCs; see Chapter 23, "Obsessive-Compulsive Disorder"). OCs are reported in 50%–90% of persons with Tourette's (Gaze et al. 2006) and may arise with or precede tics (Leckman et al. 2006a). OCs involving obsessions with symmetry and compulsions of counting, arranging, ordering, and repeating until "just right" appear to be more prevalent in persons with tic disorders plus obsessive-compul-

sive disorder (OCD) than those with only OCD (Hasler et al. 2005; Leckman et al. 2001, 2003; Mataix-Cols et al. 1999; Nestadt et al. 2003). In comparison to people with only OCD, persons with Tourette's more commonly may have aggressive, sexual, and religious obsessions (Leckman et al. 1994, 2003; Zohar et al. 1997) and less commonly have obsessions about contamination, germs, neatness and cleanliness, and compulsions of hoarding, cleaning, and washing (Robertson 2000).

Premonitory urges, reported by 75%–80% of persons with chronic tic disorders (CTDs) and Tourette's (Banaschewski et al. 2003; Kwak et al. 2003; Leckman et al. 1993), precede tics and may have a physical quality, such as localized tingling, itch-like sensations, or tensions in muscles, or an ideational feature such as thoughts or urges related to making sounds, movements, or gestures. Acknowledging these mental events has resulted in a blurring of a distinction between compulsions and complex tics. It is now recognized that many people with complex tics report thoughts, mental events, or unpleasant sensations prior to tics, and these thoughts, urges, or tensions are analogous to the thoughts and urges experienced by people with compulsions (Banaschewski et al. 2003; Kwak et al. 2003).

Attention-deficit/hyperactivity disorder (ADHD) is seen in 20%–90% of persons with Tourette's and CTDs (Robertson 2006). School-age children with Tourette's report rates of 25% (Kadesjo and Gillberg 2000).

Other impairments common in clinically referred children with Tourette's and CTD are aggressive behaviors and temper outbursts, oppositional behavior, behavioral inflexibility, and problems in social understanding and reciprocity. Despite their common association, these are not considered "core" features of Tourette's. However, Tourette's and tics are more common among individuals with autism spectrum disorders (Baron-Cohen et al. 1999; Canitano and Vivanti 2007), and conversely, autism spectrum disorders are more common among those with Tourette's (Berthier et al. 1993). Reports of elevated rates of behavioral problems are likely a result of ascertainment bias than Tourette's itself and more closely related to comorbid ADHD symptoms (Budman et al. 2000).

The typical onset of tic disorders is childhood and early adolescence. The peak incidence is ages 4–7 (Khalifa and von Knorring 2005; Leckman et al. 1998), and symptoms often are at their worst during late childhood and early adolescence (Coffey et al. 2004; Khalifa and von Knorring 2005). For 85% of individuals, late adolescence and early adulthood bring relief

TABLE 27–1. DSM-IV-TR criteria for Tourette's disorder

A. Both multiple motor and one or more vocal tics have been present at some time during the illness, although not necessarily concurrently. (A *tic* is a sudden, rapid, recurrent, nonrhythmic, stereotyped motor movement or vocalization.)

B. The tics occur many times a day (usually in bouts) nearly every day or intermittently throughout a period of more than 1 year, and during this period there was never a tic-free period of more than 3 consecutive months.

C. The onset is before age 18 years.

D. The disturbance is not due to the direct physiological effects of a substance (e.g., stimulants) or a general medical condition (e.g., Huntington's disease or postviral encephalitis).

Source. Reprinted from American Psychiatric Association: *Diagnostic and Statistical Manual of Mental Disorders*, 4th Edition, Text Revision. Washington, DC, American Psychiatric Association, 2000, p. 114. Used with permission. Copyright © 2000 American Psychiatric Association.

TABLE 27–2. DSM-IV-TR criteria for chronic motor or vocal tic disorder

A. Single or multiple motor or vocal tics (i.e., sudden, rapid, recurrent, nonrhythmic, stereotyped motor movements or vocalizations), but not both, have been present at some time during the illness.

B. The tics occur many times a day nearly every day or intermittently throughout a period of more than 1 year, and during this period there was never a tic-free period of more than 3 consecutive months.

C. The onset is before age 18 years.

D. The disturbance is not due to the direct physiological effects of a substance (e.g., stimulants) or a general medical condition (e.g., Huntington's disease or postviral encephalitis).

E. Criteria have never been met for Tourette's disorder.

Source. Reprinted from American Psychiatric Association: *Diagnostic and Statistical Manual of Mental Disorders*, 4th Edition, Text Revision. Washington, DC, American Psychiatric Association, 2000, p. 115. Used with permission. Copyright © 2000 American Psychiatric Association.

as tics become quieter (Bloch et al. 2006b; Coffey et al. 2004). Adults who continue to have tics generally have no more than mild symptoms.

Differential Diagnosis

The DSM-IV-TR (American Psychiatric Association 2000) criteria for Tourette's disorder, chronic motor or vocal tic disorder, and transient tic disorder are shown in Tables 27–1 through 27–3. If tics are present for a year, then the diagnosis is CTD (motor or phonic) or Tourette's disorder. Differentiating Tourette's disorder from CTD is straightforward. If during the course of the disorder there have been phonic and motor tics, even if they are not present at the same time, then the diagnosis is Tourette's disorder. If exclusively motor or exclusively

phonic tics occur during the individual's lifetime, this a chronic motor or phonic tic disorder, respectively. Tics occurring for less than a year are transient tics. In DSM-IV (American Psychiatric Association 1994, 2000), an individual is not required to have impairment from tics in order to receive the diagnosis.

The differential diagnosis of tic disorders is summarized in Table 27–4.

Clearly, some patients experience sudden onset or exacerbation of symptoms in association with streptococcal or other infections, though uneven evidence leaves doubt about whether a separate condition called PANDAS (postinfectious autoimmune neurological disorders associated with streptococcal infection) is valid (Kurlan and Kaplan 2004; Loiselle et al. 2004; Singer et al. 2005; Swedo and Grant 2005). If valid, PANDAS might explain roughly 10%–12% of children with OCD or Tourette's (Singer et al. 2000).

TABLE 27–3. DSM-IV-TR criteria for transient tic disorder

A. Single or multiple motor and/or vocal tics (i.e., sudden, rapid, recurrent, nonrhythmic, stereotyped motor movements or vocalizations).

B. The tics occur many times a day, nearly every day for at least 4 weeks, but for no longer than 12 consecutive months.

C. The onset is before age 18 years.

D. The disturbance is not due to the direct physiological effects of a substance (e.g., stimulants) or a general medical condition (e.g., Huntington's disease or postviral encephalitis).

E. Criteria have never been met for Tourette's disorder or chronic motor or vocal tic disorder.

Specify if:

Single episode or **recurrent**

Source. Reprinted from American Psychiatric Association: *Diagnostic and Statistical Manual of Mental Disorders,* 4th Edition, Text Revision. Washington, DC, American Psychiatric Association, 2000, p. 116. Used with permission. Copyright © 2000 American Psychiatric Association.

Epidemiology

The lifetime prevalence rate for Tourette's is 0.4%–1.8% (Apter et al. 1993; Costello et al. 1996; Hornsey et al. 2001; Jin et al. 2005; Kadesjo et al. 2000; Khalifa and von Knorring 2003; Peterson et al. 2001a; Robertson 2003). Many studies are flawed by failures to ascertain a representative community population, apply clear definitions, and make diagnoses from direct interviews and observations (Hirtz et al. 2007). The rates for CTD are 2–4 times that for Tourette's (Apter et al. 1992; Costello et al. 1996), and estimates for transient tics range from 5% to 18% (Costello et al. 1996; Lapouse and Monk 1964; Peterson et al. 2001a). There is a 1.5- to 10-fold greater prevalence among males (Freeman et al. 2000; Hornsey et al. 2001; Jin et al. 2005; Khalifa and von Knorring 2003). Tourette's has been observed in all races, but rates and symptoms may differ among ethnic groups (Jin et al. 2005; Mathews et al. 2007).

Comorbid diagnoses are common with Tourette's. In nonclinic populations with Tourette's, ADHD has been observed in 40%–60% (Kadesjo et al. 2000; Kurlan et al. 2002; Sheppard et al. 1999), and 10%–80% have OCD (Apter et al. 1993; Kurlan et al. 2002). Among those with Tourette's seeking clinical care, 30% have comorbid anxiety disorders (Coffey et al. 2000) and 10%–75% have major depression (Robertson et al. 2006).

Genetics

Twin and family studies provide sturdy evidence that Tourette's and CTD are fundamentally genetic conditions. The twin concordance rates for Tourette's is 53%–56% for monozygotic pairs and 8% in dizygotic sibs (Hyde et al. 1992; Price et al. 1985). When criteria are broadened to allow for a cotwin having Tourette's or CTD, the concordance rates climb to 77%–94% for monozygotic and 23% for dizygotic pairs, strongly pointing to a genetic etiology. However, one cannot presume that genetic factors are the exclusive cause when the concordance rate for monozygotic twins is less than 100%.

Further support from many family studies (Eapen et al. 1993; Hebebrand et al. 1997; Kano et al. 2001; Pauls et al. 1991; Walkup et al. 1996) in different sites, countries, and ethnic groups all confirm high recurrence rates among family members. In families of European origin and ascertained by the presence of a Tourette's proband, the prevalence of Tourette's or CTD in first-degree relatives ranges from 15% to 53%. When these rates are compared to the general population prevalence of Tourette's or CTD of 1%–1.8%, the 10- to 50-fold difference strongly suggests a genetic contribution. Such studies also find rates of OCD and OC symptoms among relatives of Tourette's probands that are 10–20 times the general population prevalence (Bloch et al. 2006b; Pauls et al. 1991; Walkup et al. 1996).

Although, Tourette's and ADHD co-occur commonly, family studies suggest a complex genetic relationship between them. A proband having only Tourette's does not predict having only ADHD in relatives, and ADHD-only does not predict Tourette's-only in relatives. However, a proband having Tourette's-only or ADHD-only does predict ADHD+Tourette's in relatives (Stewart et al. 2006). Thus, in Tourette's+ADHD, unlike ADHD-only, ADHD may be a symptom of the same etiology as their tics.

TABLE 27–4. Differential diagnosis of Tourette's and tics

Disorder	Movement type	Migrate	Suppressible	Wax and wane	Stimulus response	Comment
Tics	Sudden simple or complex clonic	Yes	Yes	Yes	Yes/No	Increase with attention
Dystonias	Sudden, simple clonic	No	No	No	No	Increase with effort
Myoclonus	Simple clonic					Increase with effort
Dyskinesia	Complex slow choreiform	Yes	No	No	No	Increase with distraction
Restless legs	Complex slow	No	No	No	No	Movement relieves tension
Chorea	Slow, continuous	No	No	Yes/No	No	Increase with effort
Akathisia	Complex	No	Briefly	Yes	No	Relieved by movement
Stereotypy	Slow complex	Yes	Yes	Yes	Yes/No	Often pleasurable
Hyperekplexia	Sudden complex	No	No	No	Yes	Related to startle
Parkinson's disease	Tremor					Gait disturbance, hyperreflexia, family history
Huntington's disease	Chorea					Prominent behavioral and mental changes acquired

Whole genome scans have identified candidate genes that await further specification and replication. There is evidence for genetic susceptibility for chromosomes 2 (Simonic et al. 2001; Tourette Syndrome Association International Consortium 2007), 3 (Tourette Syndrome Association International Consortium 2007), 4 (Tourette Syndrome Association International Consortium 1999), 5 (Tourette Syndrome Association International Consortium 2007; Yoon et al. 2007), 6, 8 (Simonic et al. 2001; Tourette Syndrome Association International Consortium 1999), 13 (Abelson et al. 2005), 14 (Tourette Syndrome Association International Consortium 2007), and 21 (Abelson et al. 2005; Keen-Kim et al. 2006).

Neuroanatomy and Neurophysiology

Tics are associated with abnormal functioning in cortico-striatal-thalamo-cortical (CSTC) loop circuits (Parent and Hazrati 1995). Cortical fibers end in somatotopically arranged segments of the striatum (caudate nucleus and putamen) and subthalamic nucleus. The striatum and subthalamic nucleus send efferents to the globus pallidus (interna and externa), which in turn sends fibers to the globus pallidus interna (GPi). From the GPi, the pathway courses to the thalamus, which completes the loop with separate, parallel efferents to the cortex. Circuits originating in the motor and dorsolateral cortex are considered to be the most important for tic disorders.

At the cellular level in the striatum, medium-size spiney neurons and dopamine play a key role in producing tics. Medium-size spiney neurons receive afferents using glutamate (excitatory), γ-aminobutyric acid (GABA; inhibitory), dopamine (D1 excitatory, D2 inhibitory), and serotonin (Mink 2006) and send inhibitory GABA efferents to the GPi. Thus, impairment of these neurotransmitter systems would affect spiney neuron function, produce movements, and explain the influence of dopamine and serotonin synapses on tic expression. At the synaptic level, tics are associated with an excessive response in presynaptic "phasic" (or burst) dopamine release (Grace et al. 2007; Harris and Singer 2006).

The association of tics and dysregulation of CSTC circuits is supported by data from magnetic resonance imaging (MRI) (Bohlhalter et al. 2006; Marsh et al. 2007; Peterson et al. 1998, 2001b), positron emission tomography (PET) (Albin et al. 2003; Jeffries et al. 2002), and deep brain stimulation (Visser-Vandewalle et al. 2003). Although the ventral striatum appears to be a critical region, it is premature to conclude tic disorders are caused by problems there (Albin and Mink 2006); a strong association between tics and CTSC dysregulation could arise from, or be a partial compensation for, flawed signaling in the other regions such as the cerebellum, operculum, insula, or thalamus (Butler et al. 2006; Lerner et al. 2007). A current theory (Leckman et al. 2006b) suggests that the normal relationship between striatum and thalamus is disrupted by malfunctioning "pacemaker" firings of matrisomes in the striatum. Disorganizing thalamic discharges (Leckman et al. 2006b) subsequently lead to excessive activation in the frontal cortex (Leckman et al. 2006b) or excessive disorganized intercommunication between motor and orbitofrontal CTSC loops (Jeffries et al. 2002) leading to motor, premonitory, and emotional symptoms (Leckman et al. 2006b).

Assessment

Since tic symptoms wax and wane, assessment and re-evaluation are a routine part of treatment. The initial evaluation requires time to understand the patient in order to learn what he knows about his symptoms, his impairment, and his adaptation. Tics may influence physical, mental, familial, cultural, academic/occupational, and community realms. Focusing on each of these domains is crucial in thinking about the severity of symptoms and the kinds of interventions that are likely to be helpful. People with tic disorders often find conversations about their symptoms to be uncomfortable and may take strides to camouflage, minimize, and suppress tics. For some, focusing on tics may immediately increase symptoms, while others may be only vaguely aware of them.

Severity is deduced from the frequency, intensity, and impairment of each tic. This requires clinical judgment, however, because there is an imperfect correlation of impairment with frequency or intensity. For example, a frequent tic, such as eye blinks, may be hardly noticeable and cause no interference, while audible coprolalia, even if very rare, may be quite impairing. A patient may have pain from repeated movements that are hardly visible to anyone. A complex movement that demands removing both hands from the steering wheel during highway driving, even if infrequent, can be life-threatening. Thus, cataloging the entire array of tics—motor and phonic—is vital. Valid and reliable rating scales, such as the Yale Global Tourette Severity Scale (Leckman et al. 1989), Hopkins Motor and Vocal Tic Scale (Walkup et al. 1992), or the combined Tic Rating Scale (Goetz and Kompoliti 2001; Kompoliti and Goetz 1997) may be helpful. These scales include a global measure that allows a clinician to summarize the observations into a single quantity.

A comprehensive assessment should include asking about inner phenomena like premonitory urges and obsessive-compulsive symptoms, which can be distracting and intrusive. The details of obsessions and the recognized senselessness of their elaborate, rule-governed behaviors often are embarrassing and a burden to discuss. Patients often regard their sexual, aggressive, or religious (often contra-religious) thoughts to be disgraceful. Checklists and standard self-report measures such as the Yale-Brown Obsessive Compulsive Scale—Child version (Scahill et al. 1997; Storch et al. 2004), the Leyton Obsessional Inventory (Berg et al. 1986; Cooper 1970), and a modified form of the Child Behavior Checklist (Hudziak et al. 2006; Nelson et al. 2001) can promote gathering this information, but they should facilitate, not supplant, conversation. It may take multiple meetings before children or adolescents will feel enough trust and reassurance to reveal their symptoms.

It is important to assess for co-occurring problems related to learning problems, mood disorders, and anxiety disorders. Patients with Tourette's often have executive function problems that interfere with learning and work. Impairment from symptoms can lead to depression and secondary anxiety, including profound fears about competence (generalized anxiety) and social acceptance/embarrassment (social anxiety).

A patient's symptoms may cause as much stress for the family as for the individual. Tic disorders are familial in three ways: they are biologically genetic, they affect the dynamics among the immediate family members, and they can influence how the family relates to the community and extended family members. A child with Tourette's is highly likely to have a parent who is wrestling with the same or similar disorder; 15%–60% of first-degree family members of children with Tourette's have tic disorders or OCD (Robertson and Cavanna 2007). The family may be directly affected by the child's symptoms. Frequent, loud vocalizations or noisy, forceful motor tics such as stomping or banging can disturb everyone at home. They can interfere with family activities. Siblings who experience this may be angry and distance themselves from the patient. The demands on parents to support the patient by giving time and energy to assure optimal academic and therapeutic care for one child can mean less attention and patience for others at home. Parents can develop anxiety disorders or depression as they encounter barriers to care or support that might help the patient. With increasing stress there may be more friction between spouses, between parents and children, and between siblings. There may be effects on the family's relationship with the wider community and extended relatives who do not understand the symptoms of Tourette's and wrongly view the child with Tourette's as rude or unruly. The family may be criticized for their responses, resulting in increasing isolation and loss of social and emotional support.

For children who have both learning problems and ADHD symptoms, neuropsychological assessments can assist in recommending school accommodations. Obstacles to assistance for youth with Tourette's can force parents and school staff into adversarial exchanges and mar the child's relationships with classmates and teachers. When symptoms are covert, it may be difficult for teachers and peers to understand why the patient needs accommodations or does not act like other students and that disruptive symptoms are biological, brain-based, difficult to control, and create a burden for the patient.

Treatment

General Comments

The cornerstone of treatment is observation. Clinicians, patients, parents, and teachers benefit from knowing what symptoms are present and how they change over time and with different circumstances (Himle et al. 2006), how much a child struggles with his or her symptoms, and what strategies he or she uses to reduce them. Observing can be as simple as a log or diary of the most prominent tics, when they change, and what efforts the child has made to contain them. A more rigorous behavioral approach, called Self-Monitoring, relies on detailed observations at specific periods (Azrin and Peterson 1988). Observation alone can have a potent effect on reducing symptoms by raising awareness and increasing helpful coping responses. However, in unusual circumstances, observation can "backfire"—i.e., increase tics—by reminding the patient about symptoms or by expanding parental anxiety, increasing scrutiny, and leading the patient to feel greater pressure to contain and monitor his symptoms.

The initial focus should be on providing accurate information to patients and parents and assuring they comprehend the problem. This includes hearing the patient's and family's conceptions about the etiology and nature of symptoms, revising them as necessary, and teaching about the course and outcome of tic disorders. Education aims to reduce fears about the future, decrease blame, and promote cohesion in the family's efforts to resolve problems that arise from the patient's symptoms.

Specific Interventions

Behavioral Interventions

There is growing evidence that recently developed behavioral interventions can reduce the severity and frequency of tics. In addition, there is greater recognition that medication is not effective for everyone, and for other patients undesirable side effects can offset an otherwise good result.

In adults, randomized, controlled studies suggest that habit reversal training can be more successful than waitlist conditions (Peterson and Azrin 1992) or active treatment, such as supportive therapy (Deckersbach et al. 2006; Wilhelm et al. 2003). Habit reversal relies on a *competing response procedure*—an action that when carried out, makes it impossible to produce the tic, can be sustained for several minutes, and would not be readily visible to someone who was casually observing the patient. A premier example would be isometric tensing of muscles in opposition to a tic, or breathing in a certain way to subvert a vocal tic (Azrin et al. 1988). Tics with premonitory urges are perfect candidates for this kind of behavioral maneuver, although the number of children treated with these methods remains small.

Another technique known as relaxation training, in which muscles are systematically tensed and then relaxed, is a component of many behavioral treatments, although a study employing this treatment alone reported no difference from a control condition (Bergin et al. 1998).

Behavioral treatments require time, practice, determination, and dedication. A course of treatment typically takes several months or 12–14 sessions. Behavioral treatments generally work best for those who can form a strong relationship with the behavioral therapist.

Pharmacological Treatment

The approach to treating tic disorders with medication requires the clinician to think about more than

whether tics are present and what medication should be used to reduce them. First, tic severity should be considered broadly. The burden of tics is not exclusively related to frequency or severity. The impact tics are having on the individual, the family, and the patient's social environment all must be weighed. Two patients with the same level of tic severity can have radically different treatment plans. The foremost objective is to maintain a strong working relationship with each patient because treatment of tics is usually a long-term endeavor. Reducing tics at the expense of a patient's sense of control over her treatment, her comfort, and self-image is too costly. A child who feels "worked on" rather than working in collaboration with her doctor will not continue the relationship or the medication.

The objective of treatment is to reduce, not eliminate, tics. Determining when a sufficient reduction of tics has been reached is a subjective judgment that balances the patient's needs and quality of life against side effects and the risks of each medication. Weighing the risk-to-benefit ratio should always include the patient. For example, a lean patient may prefer the least sedating medication possible even if it might cause slight weight gain. The opposite may be true for a patient who is watching in horror as his weight rises. Waxing and waning of tics creates uncertainty about whether changes in symptoms are results of medication or natural variation. When patients have mild tics, the decision is among drug treatment with alpha-adrenergic agonists, no medication, and perhaps behavioral treatments. Starting with symptom monitoring is the best first intervention. Decisions about medication can then be tailored to the patient's antecedent pattern of symptoms. When tics are moderate to severe, a patient might prefer and do better with low doses of risperidone or pimozide than a higher dose of alpha-adrenergic agonists. Clearly, no one drug or dose fits everyone. When raising doses, the clinician must proceed gradually and use small increments.

The side-effect profile and the timing of starting or increasing medication are critically important. An art of caring for patients with tics is to learn the triggers and pattern of tic severity and work prospectively, when possible, to manage medication doses. For example, if the patient starts medication during final exams or at the start of summer camp, the passing of the initial stress may lead to a natural reduction in symptoms that could be falsely attributed to the drug. Moreover, increased sedation during exams may be costly for the patient. When patients are uncomfortable, clinicians can be pressed to increase doses quickly, but doing so can produce side effects that neutralize whatever relief was sought by reducing tics.

Another principle of treatment is constant reevaluation. If symptoms are well controlled for a sufficient period, perhaps 6–9 months, it is important to consider reducing medication. This is particularly helpful starting in mid- to late adolescence since tics may naturally wane during this time. It is also important when there are medication side effects that are difficult to tolerate. As with dose increases, decrements should be taken in small steps and with an eye toward timing and consequences. Since the majority of patients with tics will have only minor residual symptoms by late adolescence or early adulthood, it is incumbent on clinicians to attempt reducing medications in patients of this age who are doing well. Rebound symptoms may be observed when doses are reduced, so educating patients and families about this and allowing sufficient time to elapse to reestablish equilibrium before the next decrement are important.

Dopamine antagonists.

Medications that block dopamine are the mainstay of treatment for moderate to severe tics. These medications are the most studied for tic disorders and provide the most consistent, robust, and positive results. Chapter 49 ("Antipsychotic Medications") has a detailed discussion of the use and side effects of these drugs. Pimozide is a dopamine-blocking agent that carries the risks and side effects of other agents in this class. Pimozide, like ziprasidone, can produce changes in cardiac conduction leading to QTc prolongation. In clinical trials using dopamine-blocking agents for tic disorders, intolerance of side effects led to discontinuation in 10%–40% of participants.

Alpha-2 adrenergic agonists.

These agents are discussed in Chapter 50, "Alpha-Adrenergics, Beta-Blockers, Benzodiazepines, Buspirone, and Desmopressin." In low doses, clonidine down-regulates norepinephrine and leads to decreased serotonin production in the median raphe (Bunney and DeRiemer 1982). The downstream effect of decreased serotonin is to decrease dopamine release in the substantia nigra (Bunney and DeRiemer 1982). Using this knowledge, investigators reported modest positive results with clonidine in two randomized controlled trials (Gaffney et al. 2002; Leckman et al. 1991). Gaffney et al. (2002) reported a similar reduction of tics with clonidine or risperidone. Two other studies (Goetz et al. 1987; Singer et al. 1995) showed no improvement in tics. The more benign side-effect profile of clonidine has led some authorities to consider it

the first-line pharmacological agent for treatment of mild to moderate tics (Gilbert 2006; Gilbert and Singer 2001; Swain et al. 2007). However, problems with sedation, cognitive dulling, multiple dosing throughout the day, more modest reductions in symptoms, and depression can be dissuasive. Nevertheless, clonidine does not produce extrapyramidal side effects, weight gain, or tardive dyskinesia.

The other major alpha-2 adrenergic agonist, guanfacine, has been investigated in two studies that generated opposite results. At this point, the evidence in support of guanfacine for tics is meager. Scahill et al. (2001) measured a modest 31% reduction in tic severity during their investigation of guanfacine for ADHD symptoms in children with tics.

Table 27–5 summarizes randomized controlled clinical drug trials. Several review papers are available (Sandor 2003; Scahill et al. 2006; Swain et al. 2007). All these agents possess risks and side effects that require close monitoring and include cardiac and neurological assessments. Dopamine antagonists also require attention to metabolic disorders.

Treatment of associated symptoms.

The treatment of ADHD symptoms and OCD are discussed in Chapter 15 ("Attention-Deficit/Hyperactivity Disorder") and Chapter 23 ("Obsessive-Compulsive Disorder"), respectively. In OCD, there is good evidence that obsessions and compulsions in persons with a personal or family history of tic disorders may not respond as well to behavioral or pharmacological treatment as those without such a history. First-line intervention using cognitive-behavioral therapy (CBT) or a combination of serotonin reuptake inhibitors (SRIs) with CBT is recommended. There is evidence that those who do not respond to SRIs may benefit from augmentation with low doses of dopamine antagonists (e.g., risperidone, haloperidol, or pimozide) (Bloch et al. 2006a; Goodman et al. 2006; McDougle 1997; Skapinakis et al. 2007). Particular care should be taken when combining pimozide with sertraline, as drug-drug interactions may increase the risk of QTc prolongation (Alderman 2005).

The treatment of ADHD symptoms in the context of Tourette's or chronic tics has been revised in the last decade. Tics may be observed in patients receiving standard stimulant medications such as methylphenidate (MPH) or dextroamphetamine (d-AMP), and they may increase in patients with preexisting tics. Case reports (Erenberg 2005; Robertson 2006) have led some experts to recommend against using stimulants in patients with ADHD and Tourette's, and that the U.S. Food and Drug Administration (FDA) assert that

TABLE 27–5. Pharmacological treatment of tic disorders: agents that have randomized, placebo-controlled trials

Drug	Relevant studies	Typical dosage range, mg/day	Significant side effects	Efficacy	Comments
Dopamine antagonists			**All in this group carry risks of sedation, cognitive dulling, elevation in serum prolactin, extrapyramidal side effects, and tardive dyskinesia (TD).**		
Haloperidol	Ross et al. 1978; Sallee et al. 1997; Shapiro et al. 1989	0.25–8		25%–30% reduction in symptoms.	
Metoclopramide	Nicolson et al. 2005	20–40	Sedation. May have lower risk for adverse cognitive effects.	39% reduction in symptoms.	Small study
Pimozide	Bruggeman et al. 2001; Gilbert et al. 2004; Ross et al. 1978; Sallee et al. 1997; Shapiro et al. 1989	0.5–8	Higher risk of QTc prolongation; less severe sedation and extrapyramidal effects compared to haloperidol. Less weight gain than risperidone (Gilbert et al. 2004).	22%–53% reduction in symptoms.	
Risperidone	Bruggeman et al. 2001; Gaffney et al. 2002; Gilbert et al. 2004; Scahill et al. 2003	0.25–4	Risk of weight gain, 0.75–1 lb/wk; prolactin elevation; possibly lower risk of TD compared to pimozide, haloperidol.	26%–56% reduction in symptoms.	
Ziprasidone	Sallee et al. 2000	10–100	Particularly increased risk of QTc prolongation.	40% reduction in tics compared to 16% on placebo.	

TABLE 27–5. Pharmacological treatment of tic disorders: agents that have randomized, placebo-controlled trials *(continued)*

Drug	Relevant studies	Typical dosage range, mg/day	Significant side effects	Efficacy	Comments
α₂-Adrenergic agonists			**All display sedation and risk of hypotension.**		
Clonidine	Gaffney et al. 2002; Goetz et al. 1987; Leckman et al. 1991	0.15–0.25		Mixed. 20%–30% reduction in tics reported. Gaffney et al. 2002 compared with risperidone and found no difference in efficacy. Goetz et al. 1987 found no difference from placebo.	Requires 0.05–0.1 mg doses given 3–5 times/day
Guanfacine	Cummings et al. 2002; Scahill et al. 2001	0.5–4		Contradictory studies: Scahill et al. 2001 report 31% reduction; Cummings et al. 2002 reported no effect on tics.	Twice a day divided dosing needed

stimulants are contraindicated in children with tics and Tourette's. Experts have recommended alpha-adrenergic agonists such as clonidine or guanfacine as the first-line agents for ADHD symptoms in patients with Tourette's (Robertson 2006; Swain et al. 2007). However, longitudinal studies report that tics did not increase with MPH or d-AMP treatment, that increases are clinically trivial (Erenberg 2005; Kurlan 2003; Roessner et al. 2006; Tourette's Syndrome Study Group 2002), and that tics may even decrease with stimulants (Tourette's Syndrome Study Group 2002). Thus, current guidelines are equivocal on the first-line agents for ADHD in Tourette's (Gilbert 2006). Alpha-adrenergic agonists may be effective but carry greater risk of sedation. MPH and d-AMP appear to be more effective for ADHD symptoms than clonidine or guanfacine (Scahill et al. 2001; Tourette's Syndrome Study Group 2002). Exacerbation of tics is seen in about 25% of Tourette's patients whether they are given stimulants, clonidine, the combination, or placebo (Tourette's Syndrome Study Group 2002). Tics that arise after starting stimulants may decline over 3 months (Castellanos et al. 1997). There are data that atomoxetine may be useful in patients with tic disorders, too (Allen et al. 2005; Gilbert 2006).

Advocacy

The Tourette Syndrome Association (TSA) has been providing solid information, legislative activity, family support, research, and education on behalf of patients and families since 1972. It can be useful for families to learn about the TSA by visiting its Web site (www.tsa-usa.org) and for healthcare providers and teachers to be aware of TSA-sponsored professional programs (www.tsa-tsa.org).

Research Directions

The primary foci of future work will be in genetics, pathophysiology, and treatment interventions. A growing body of work points to candidate genes, and there are good reasons to believe that larger samples and ever more refined strategies will elucidate the primary genetic contributions to Tourette's. Identifying these genes will also allow a more refined understanding of the environmental contributions to Tourette's.

Pathophysiology studies have provided keen insights on the function of the CSTC circuit, but important questions remain about the function and impairment of striatal medium-size spiney neurons and pathways from the motor and dorsolateral cortex that figure prominently in tic disorders.

More effective, safer treatments are needed. Recent investigations using surgically implanted electrodes into the globus pallidus, internal capsule, nucleus accumbens, or thalamus for control of intractable tics (Neimat et al. 2006; Servello et al. 2008; Visser-Vandewalle 2007) have been promising. Which sites are optimal for relief are not yet clear (Neimat et al. 2006; Servello et al. 2008; Visser-Vandewalle 2007), and the role for deep brain stimulation in the care of severe Tourette's and tic disorders has yet to be spelled out. Guidelines are being set out for this potentially helpful but high-risk intervention (Mink et al. 2006; Riley et al. 2007). On the pharmacological front, there may be a role for serotonin antagonists and for exploration of safer antidopaminergic agents.

Summary Points

- Tics are repetitive, brief, sudden, stereotyped movements that can occur in any voluntary muscle. Tics characteristically wax and wane, often migrate through the body, and can range in severity from very mild to quite severe.
- Tics can be transient or chronic. *Chronic tics* that include both phonic and motor elements, even if they occur at different times, are called Tourette's disorder.
- Tic disorders often co-occur with ADHD and with OCD. Impairment caused by these disorders can be greater than from the tics themselves.
- Some tics may be preceded by mental or sensory events called premonitory urges.
- Tics are associated with abnormal functioning in CSTC loop circuits.
- Tics and Tourette's are genetic disorders and probably result from multiple genes acting together.

- Tics affect physical, mental, familial, and academic/occupational domains.
- Currently, the most effective treatment for tics is dopamine-blocking agents, although these drugs also can have serious side effects.

References

Abelson JF, Kwan KY, O'Roak BJ, et al: Sequence variants in SLITRK1 are associated with Tourette's syndrome. Science 310:317–320, 2005

Albin RL, Mink JW: Recent advances in Tourette syndrome research. Trends Neurosci 29:175–182, 2006

Albin RL, Koeppe RA, Bohnen NI, et al: Increased ventral striatal monoaminergic innervation in Tourette syndrome. Neurology 61:310–315, 2003

Alderman J: Coadministration of sertraline with cisapride or pimozide: an open-label, nonrandomized examination of pharmacokinetics and corrected QT intervals in healthy adult volunteers. Clin Ther 27:1050–1063, 2005

Allen AJ, Kurlan RM, Gilbert DL, et al: Atomoxetine treatment in children and adolescents with ADHD and comorbid tic disorders. Neurology 65:1941–1949, 2005

American Psychiatric Association: Diagnostic and Statistical Manual of Mental Disorders, 4th Edition. Washington, DC, American Psychiatric Association, 1994

American Psychiatric Association: Diagnostic and Statistical Manual of Mental Disorders, 4th Edition, Text Revision. Washington, DC, American Psychiatric Association, 2000

Apter A, Pauls DL, Bleich A, et al: A population-based epidemiological study of Tourette syndrome among adolescents in Israel. Adv Neurol 58:61–65, 1992

Apter A, Pauls DL, Bleich A, et al: An epidemiologic study of Gilles de la Tourette's syndrome in Israel. Arch Gen Psychiatry 50:734–738, 1993

Azrin NH, Peterson AL: Habit reversal for the treatment of Tourette syndrome. Behav Res Ther 26:347–351, 1988

Banaschewski T, Woerner W, Rothenberger A: Premonitory sensory phenomena and suppressibility of tics in Tourette syndrome: developmental aspects in children and adolescents. Dev Med Child Neurol 45:700–703, 2003

Baron-Cohen S, Scahill VL, Izaguirre J, et al: The prevalence of Gilles de la Tourette syndrome in children and adolescents with autism: a large scale study. Psychol Med 29:1151–1159, 1999

Berg CJ, Rapoport JL, Flament M: The Leyton Obsessional Inventory-Child Version. J Am Acad Child Adolesc Psychiatry 25:84–91, 1986

Bergin A, Waranch HR, Brown J, et al: Relaxation therapy in Tourette syndrome: a pilot study. Pediatr Neurol 18:136–142, 1998

Berthier ML, Bayes A, Tolosa ES: Magnetic resonance imaging in patients with concurrent Tourette's disorder and Asperger's syndrome. J Am Acad Child Adolesc Psychiatry 32:633–639, 1993

Bloch MH, Landeros-Weisenberger A, Kelmendi B, et al: A systematic review: antipsychotic augmentation with treatment refractory obsessive-compulsive disorder. Mol Psychiatry 11:622–632, 2006a

Bloch MH, Peterson BS, Scahill L, et al: Adulthood outcome of tic and obsessive-compulsive symptom severity in children with Tourette syndrome. Arch Pediatr Adolesc Med 160:65–69, 2006b

Bohlhalter S, Goldfine A, Matteson S, et al: Neural correlates of tic generation in Tourette syndrome: an event-related functional MRI study. Brain 129:2029–2037, 2006

Bruggeman R, van der Linden C, Buitelaar JK, et al: Risperidone versus pimozide in Tourette's disorder: a comparative double-blind parallel-group study. J Clin Psychiatry 62:50–56, 2001

Budman CL, Bruun RD, Park KS, et al: Explosive outbursts in children with Tourette's disorder. J Am Acad Child Adolesc Psychiatry 39:1270–1276, 2000

Bunney BS, DeRiemer S: Effect of clonidine on dopaminergic neuron activity in the substantia nigra: possible indirect mediation by noradrenergic regulation of the serotonergic raphe system. Adv Neurol 35:99–104, 1982

Butler T, Stern E, Silbersweig D: Functional neuroimaging of Tourette syndrome: advances and future directions. Adv Neurol 99:115–129, 2006

Canitano R, Vivanti G: Tics and Tourette syndrome in autism spectrum disorders. Autism 11:19–28, 2007

Castellanos FX, Giedd JN, Elia J, et al: Controlled stimulant treatment of ADHD and comorbid Tourette's syndrome: effects of stimulant and dose. J Am Acad Child Adolesc Psychiatry 36:589–596, 1997

Coffey BJ, Biederman J, Smoller JW, et al: Anxiety disorders and tic severity in juveniles with Tourette's disorder. J Am Acad Child Adolesc Psychiatry 39:562–568, 2000

Coffey BJ, Biederman J, Geller D, et al: Reexamining tic persistence and tic-associated impairment in Tourette's disorder: findings from a naturalistic follow-up study. J Nerv Ment Dis 192:776–780, 2004

Cooper J: The Leyton Obsessional Inventory. Psychol Med 1:48–64, 1970

Costello EJ, Angold A, Burns BJ, et al: The Great Smoky Mountains Study of Youth: functional impairment and serious emotional disturbance. Arch Gen Psychiatry 53:1137–1143, 1996

Cummings DD, Singer HS, Krieger M, et al: Neuropsychiatric effects of guanfacine in children with mild Tourette syndrome: a pilot study. Clin Neuropharmacol 25:325–332, 2002

Deckersbach T, Rauch S, Buhlmann U, et al: Habit reversal versus supportive psychotherapy in Tourette's disorder: a randomized controlled trial and predictors of treatment response. Behav Res Ther 44:1079–1090, 2006

Eapen V, Pauls DL, Robertson MM: Evidence for autosomal dominant transmission in Tourette's syndrome. United Kingdom cohort study. Br J Psychiatry 162:593–596, 1993

Erenberg G: The relationship between Tourette syndrome, attention deficit hyperactivity disorder, and stimulant medication: a critical review. Semin Pediatr Neurol 12:217–221, 2005

Freeman RD, Fast DK, Burd L, et al: An international perspective on Tourette syndrome: selected findings from 3,500 individuals in 22 countries. Dev Med Child Neurol. 42:436–447, 2000

Gaffney GR, Perry PJ, Lund BC, et al: Risperidone versus clonidine in the treatment of children and adolescents with Tourette's syndrome. J Am Acad Child Adolesc Psychiatry 41:330–336, 2002

Gaze C, Kepley HO, Walkup JT: Co-occurring psychiatric disorders in children and adolescents with Tourette syndrome. J Child Neurol 21:657–664, 2006

Gilbert D: Treatment of children and adolescents with tics and Tourette syndrome. J Child Neurol 21:690–700, 2006

Gilbert D, Singer HS: Risperidone was as effective as pimozide for Tourette's disorder. Evid Based Ment Health 4:75, 2001. Available at: http://ebmh.bmj.com/cgi/content/extract/4/3/75. Accessed June 10, 2009.

Gilbert DL, Batterson JR, Sethuraman G, et al: Tic reduction with risperidone versus pimozide in a randomized, double-blind, crossover trial. J Am Acad Child Adolesc Psychiatry 43:206–214. 2004

Gilles de la Tourette G: Étude sur une affection nerveuse caractérisée par l'incoordination motrice, accompagnée d'écholalie et de coprolalia, in Gilles de la Tourette Syndrome. Edited by Friedhoff AJ, Chase TN. New York, Raven, 1982, pp 1–16

Goetz CG, Kompoliti K: Rating scales and quantitative assessment of tics. Adv Neurol 85:31–42, 2001

Goetz CG, Tanner CM, Wilson RS, et al: Clonidine and Gilles de la Tourette's syndrome: double-blind study using objective rating methods. Ann Neurol 21:307–310, 1987

Goodman WK, Storch EA, Geffken GR, et al: Obsessive-compulsive disorder in Tourette syndrome. J Child Neurol 21:704–714, 2006

Grace AA, Floresco SB, Goto Y, et al: Regulation of firing of dopaminergic neurons and control of goal-directed behaviors. Trends Neurosci 30:220–227, 2007

Harris K, Singer HS: Tic disorders: neural circuits, neurochemistry, and neuroimmunology. J Child Neurol 21:678–689, 2006

Hasler G, LaSalle-Ricci VH, Ronquillo JG, et al: Obsessive-compulsive disorder symptom dimensions show specific relationships to psychiatric comorbidity. Psychiatry Res 135:121–132, 2005

Hebebrand J, Klug B, Fimmers R, et al: Rates for tic disorders and obsessive compulsive symptomatology in families of children and adolescents with Gilles de la Tourette syndrome. J Psychiatr Res 31:519–530, 1997

Himle MB, Chang S, Woods DW, et al: Establishing the feasibility of direct observation in the assessment of tics in children with chronic tic disorders. J Appl Behav Anal 39:429–440, 2006

Hirtz D, Thurman DJ, Gwinn-Hardy K, et al: How common are the "common" neurologic disorders? Neurology 68:326–337, 2007

Hornsey H, Banerjee S, Zeitlin H, et al: The prevalence of Tourette syndrome in 13–14-year-olds in mainstream schools. J Child Psychol Psychiatry 42:1035–1039, 2001

Hudziak JJ, Althoff RR, Stanger C, et al: The Obsessive Compulsive Scale of the Child Behavior Checklist predicts obsessive-compulsive disorder: a receiver operating characteristic curve analysis. J Child Psychol Psychiatry 47:160–166, 2006

Hyde TM, Aaronson BA, Randolph C, et al: Relationship of birth weight to the phenotypic expression of Gilles de la Tourette's syndrome in monozygotic twins. Neurology 42:652–658, 1992

Jeffries KJ, Schooler C, Schoenbach C, et al: The functional neuroanatomy of Tourette's syndrome: an FDG PET study III: functional coupling of regional cerebral metabolic rates. Neuropsychopharmacology 27:92–104, 2002

Jin R, Zheng RY, Huang WW, et al: Epidemiological survey of Tourette syndrome in children and adolescents in Wenzhou of P.R. China. Eur J Epidemiol 20:925–927, 2005

Kadesjo B, Gillberg C: Tourette's disorder: epidemiology and comorbidity in primary school children. J Am Acad Child Adolesc Psychiatry 39:548–555, 2000

Kano Y, Ohta M, Nagai Y, et al: A family study of Tourette syndrome in Japan. Am J Med Genet 105:414–421, 2001

Keen-Kim D, Mathews CA, Reus VI, et al: Overrepresentation of rare variants in a specific ethnic group may confuse interpretation of association analyses. Hum Mol Genet 15:3324–3328, 2006

Khalifa N, von Knorring AL: Prevalence of tic disorders and Tourette syndrome in a Swedish school population. Dev Med Child Neurol 45:315–319, 2003

Khalifa N, von Knorring AL: Tourette syndrome and other tic disorders in a total population of children: clinical assessment and background. Acta Paediatr 94:1608–1614, 2005

Kompoliti K, Goetz CG: Tourette syndrome: clinical rating and quantitative assessment of tics. Neurol Clin 15:239–254, 1997

Kostanecka-Endress T, Banaschewski T, Kinkelbur J, et al: Disturbed sleep in children with Tourette syndrome: a polysomnographic study. J Psychosom Res 55:23–29, 2003

Kurlan R: Tourette's syndrome: are stimulants safe? Curr Neurol Neurosci Rep 3:285–288, 2003

Kurlan R, Kaplan EL: The pediatric autoimmune neuropsychiatric disorders associated with streptococcal infection (PANDAS) etiology for tics and obsessive-compulsive symptoms: hypothesis or entity? Practical considerations for the clinician. Pediatrics 113:883–886, 2004

Kurlan R, Como PG, Miller B, et al: The behavioral spectrum of tic disorders: a community-based study. Neurology 59:414–420, 2002

Kwak C, Dat VK, Jankovic J: Premonitory sensory phenomenon in Tourette's syndrome. Mov Disord 18:1530–1533, 2003

Lapouse R, Monk MA: Behavior deviations in a representative sample of children: variation by sex, age, race, social class, and family size. Am J Orthopsychiatry 34:436–446, 1964

Leckman JF, Riddle MA, Hardin MT, et al: The Yale Global Tic Severity Scale: initial testing of a clinician-rated scale of tic severity. J Am Acad Child Adolesc Psychiatry 28:566–573, 1989

Leckman JF, Hardin MT, Riddle MA, et al: Clonidine treatment of Gilles de la Tourette's syndrome. Arch Gen Psychiatry 48:324–328, 1991

Leckman JF, Walker DE, Cohen DJ: Premonitory urges in Tourette's syndrome. Am J Psychiatry 150:98–102, 1993

Leckman JF, Grice DE, Barr LC, et al: Tic-related vs non-tic-related obsessive compulsive disorder. Anxiety 1:208–215, 1994

Leckman JF, Zhang H, Vitale A, et al: Course of tic severity in Tourette syndrome: the first two decades. Pediatrics 102:14–19, 1998

Leckman JF, Zhang H, Alsobrook JP, et al: Symptom dimensions in obsessive-compulsive disorder: toward quantitative phenotypes. Am J Med Genet 105:28–30, 2001

Leckman JF, Pauls DL, Zhang H, et al: Obsessive-compulsive symptom dimensions in affected sibling pairs diagnosed with Gilles de la Tourette syndrome. Am J Med Genet B Neuropsychiatr Genet 116:60–68, 2003

Leckman JF, Bloch MH, Scahill L, et al: Tourette syndrome: the self under siege. J Child Neurol 21:642–649, 2006a

Leckman JF, Vaccarino FM, Kalanithi PS, et al: Annotation: Tourette syndrome: a relentless drumbeat—driven by misguided brain oscillations. J Child Psychol Psychiatry 47:537–550, 2006b

Lerner A, Bagic A, Boudreau EA, et al: Neuroimaging of neuronal circuits involved in tic generation in patients with Tourette syndrome. Neurology 68:1979–1987, 2007

Loiselle CR, Lee O, Moran TH, et al: Striatal microinfusion of Tourette syndrome and PANDAS sera: failure to induce behavioral changes. Mov Disord 19:390–396, 2004

Marsh R, Zhu H, Wang Z, et al: A developmental fMRI study of self-regulatory control in Tourette's syndrome. Am J Psychiatry 164:955–966, 2007

Mataix-Cols D, Rauch SL, Manzo PA, et al: Use of factor-analyzed symptom dimensions to predict outcome with serotonin reuptake inhibitors and placebo in the treatment of obsessive-compulsive disorder. Am J Psychiatry 156:1409–1416, 1999

Mathews CA, Jang KL, Herrera LD, et al: Tic symptom profiles in subjects with Tourette syndrome from two genetically isolated populations. Biol Psychiatry 61:292–300, 2007

McDougle CJ: Update on pharmacologic management of OCD: agents and augmentation. J Clin Psychiatry 58(suppl):11–17, 1997

Mink JW: Neurobiology of basal ganglia and Tourette syndrome: basal ganglia circuits and thalamocortical outputs. Adv Neurol 99:89–98, 2006

Mink JW, Walkup J, Frey KA, et al: Patient selection and assessment recommendations for deep brain stimulation in Tourette syndrome. Mov Disord 21:1831–1838, 2006

Neimat JS, Patil PG, Lozano AM: Novel surgical therapies for Tourette syndrome. J Child Neurol 21:715–718, 2006

Nelson EC, Hanna GL, Hudziak JJ, et al: Obsessive-compulsive scale of the child behavior checklist: specificity, sensitivity, and predictive power. Pediatrics 108:E14, 2001

Nestadt G, Addington A, Samuels J, et al: The identification of OCD-related subgroups based on comorbidity. Biol Psychiatry 53:914–920, 2003

Nicolson R, Craven-Thuss B, Smith J, et al: A randomized, double-blind, placebo-controlled trial of metoclopramide for the treatment of Tourette's disorder. J Am Acad Child Adolesc Psychiatry 44:640–646, 2005

Parent A, Hazrati LN: Functional anatomy of the basal ganglia, I: the cortico-basal ganglia-thalamo-cortical loop. Brain Res Brain Res Rev 20:91–127, 1995

Pauls DL, Raymond CL, Stevenson JM, et al: A family study of Gilles de la Tourette syndrome. Am J Hum Genet 48:154–163, 1991

Peterson AL, Azrin NH: An evaluation of behavioral treatments for Tourette syndrome. Behav Res Ther 30:167–174, 1992

Peterson BS, Leckman JF: The temporal dynamics of tics in Gilles de la Tourette syndrome. Biol Psychiatry 44:1337–1348, 1998

Peterson BS, Skudlarski P, Anderson AW, et al: A functional magnetic resonance imaging study of tic suppression in Tourette syndrome. Arch Gen Psychiatry 55:326–333, 1998

Peterson BS, Pine DS, Cohen P, et al: Prospective, longitudinal study of tic, obsessive-compulsive, and attention-deficit/hyperactivity disorders in an epidemiological sample. J Am Acad Child Adolesc Psychiatry 40:685–695, 2001a

Peterson BS, Staib L, Scahill L, et al: Regional brain and ventricular volumes in Tourette syndrome. Arch Gen Psychiatry 58:427–440, 2001b

Price RA, Kidd KK, Cohen DJ, et al: A twin study of Tourette syndrome. Arch Gen Psychiatry 42:815–820, 1985

Riley DE, Whitney CM, Maddux BN, et al: Patient selection and assessment recommendations for deep brain stimulation in Tourette syndrome. Mov Disord 22:1366; author reply 1367–1368, 2007

Robertson MM: Tourette syndrome, associated conditions and the complexities of treatment. Brain 123:425–462, 2000

Robertson MM: Diagnosing Tourette syndrome: is it a common disorder? J Psychosom Res 55:3–6, 2003

Robertson MM: Attention deficit hyperactivity disorder, tics and Tourette's syndrome: the relationship and treatment implications: a commentary. Eur Child Adolesc Psychiatry 15:1–11, 2006

Robertson MM, Cavanna AE: The Gilles de la Tourette syndrome: a principal component factor analytic study of a large pedigree. Psychiatr Genet 17:143–152, 2007

Robertson MM, Williamson F, Eapen V: Depressive symptomatology in young people with Gilles de la Tourette Syndrome: a comparison of self-report scales. J Affect Disord 91:265–268, 2006

Roessner V, Robatzek M, Knapp G, et al: First-onset tics in patients with attention-deficit-hyperactivity disorder: impact of stimulants. Dev Med Child Neurol 48:616–621, 2006

Ross MS, Moldofsky H: A comparison of pimozide and haloperidol in the treatment of Gilles de la Tourette's syndrome. Am J Psychiatry 135:585–587, 1978

Sacks OW: Ricky ticcy ray, in The Man Who Mistook His Wife for a Hat and Other Clinical Tales. New York, Summit Books, 1985, pp 92–101

Sacks OW: A surgeon's life, in An Anthropologist on Mars: Seven Paradoxical Tales. New York, Knopf, 1995, pp 77–107

Sallee FR, Nesbitt L, Jackson C, et al: Relative efficacy of haloperidol and pimozide in children and adolescents with Tourette's disorder. Am J Psychiatry 154:1057–1062, 1997

Sallee FR, Kurlan R, Goetz CG, et al: Ziprasidone treatment of children and adolescents with Tourette's syndrome: a pilot study. J Am Acad Child Adolesc Psychiatry. 39:292–299, 2000

Sandor P: Pharmacological management of tics in patients with TS. J Psychosom Res 55:41–48, 2003

Scahill L, Riddle MA, McSwiggin-Hardin M, et al: Children's Yale-Brown Obsessive Compulsive Scale: reliability and validity. J Am Acad Child Adolesc Psychiatry 36:844–852, 1997

Scahill L, Chappell PB, Kim YS, et al: A placebo-controlled study of guanfacine in the treatment of children with tic disorders and attention deficit hyperactivity disorder. Am J Psychiatry 158:1067–1074, 2001

Scahill L, Leckman JF, Schultz RT, et al: A placebo-controlled trial of risperidone in Tourette syndrome. Neurology 60:1130–1135, 2003

Scahill L, Erenberg G, Berlin CM Jr, et al: Contemporary assessment and pharmacotherapy of Tourette syndrome. NeuroRx 3:192–206, 2006

Servello D, Porta M, Sassi M, et al: Deep brain stimulation in 18 patients with severe Gilles de la Tourette syndrome refractory to treatment: the surgery and stimulation. J Neurol Neurosurg Psychiatry 79:136–142, 2008

Shapiro E, Shapiro AK, Fulop G, et al: Controlled study of haloperidol, pimozide and placebo for the treatment of Gilles de la Tourette's syndrome. Arch Gen Psychiatry 46:722–730, 1989

Sheppard DM, Bradshaw JL, Purcell R, et al: Tourette's and comorbid syndromes: obsessive compulsive and attention deficit hyperactivity disorder: a common etiology? Clin Psychol Rev 19:531–552, 1999

Simonic I, Nyholt DR, Gericke GS, et al: Further evidence for linkage of Gilles de la Tourette syndrome (GTS) susceptibility loci on chromosomes 2p11, 8q22 and 11q23–24 in South African Afrikaners. Am J Med Genet 105:163–167, 2001

Singer HS, Brown J, Quaskey S, et al: The treatment of attention-deficit hyperactivity disorder in Tourette's syndrome: a double-blind placebo-controlled study with clonidine and desipramine. Pediatrics 95:74–81, 1995

Singer HS, Giuliano JD, Zimmerman AM, et al: Infection: a stimulus for tic disorders. Pediatr Neurol 22:380–383, 2000

Singer HS, Hong JJ, Yoon DY, et al: Serum autoantibodies do not differentiate PANDAS and Tourette syndrome from controls. Neurology 65:1701–1707, 2005

Skapinakis P, Papatheodorou T, Mavreas V: Antipsychotic augmentation of serotonergic antidepressants in treatment-resistant obsessive-compulsive disorder: a meta-analysis of the randomized controlled trials. Eur Neuropsychopharmacol 17:79–93, 2007

Stewart SE, Illmann C, Geller DA, et al: A controlled family study of attention-deficit/hyperactivity disorder and Tourette's disorder. J Am Acad Child Adolesc Psychiatry 45:1354–1362, 2006

Storch EA, Murphy TK, Geffken GR, et al: Psychometric evaluation of the Children's Yale-Brown Obsessive-Compulsive Scale. Psychiatry Res 129:91–98, 2004

Swain JE, Scahill L, Lombroso PJ, et al: Tourette syndrome and tic disorders: a decade of progress. J Am Acad Child Adolesc Psychiatry 46:947–968, 2007

Swedo SE, Grant PJ: Annotation: PANDAS: a model for human autoimmune disease. J Child Psychol Psychiatry 46:227–234, 2005

Tourette Syndrome Association International Consortium: A complete genome screen in sib pairs affected by Gilles de la Tourette syndrome: the Tourette Syndrome Association International Consortium for Genetics. Am J Hum Genet 65:1428–1436, 1999

Tourette Syndrome Association International Consortium: Genome scan for Tourette disorder in affected-sibling-pair and multigenerational families. Am J Hum Genet 80:265–272, 2007

Tourette's Syndrome Study Group: Treatment of ADHD in children with tics: a randomized controlled trial. Neurology 58:527–536, 2002

Visser-Vandewalle V: DBS in Tourette syndrome: rationale, current status and future prospects. Acta Neurochir Suppl 97:215–222, 2007

Visser-Vandewalle V, Temel Y, Boon P, et al: Chronic bilateral thalamic stimulation: a new therapeutic approach in intractable Tourette syndrome. Report of three cases. J Neurosurg 99:1094–1100, 2003

Walkup JT, Rosenberg LA, Brown J, et al: The validity of instruments measuring tic severity in Tourette's syndrome. J Am Acad Child Adolesc Psychiatry 31:472–477, 1992

Walkup JT, LaBuda MC, Singer HS, et al: Family study and segregation analysis of Tourette syndrome: evidence for a mixed model of inheritance. Am J Hum Genet 59:684–693, 1996

Wilhelm S, Deckersbach T, Coffey BJ, et al: Habit reversal versus supportive psychotherapy for Tourette's disorder: a randomized controlled trial. Am J Psychiatry 160:1175–1177, 2003

Yoon DY, Rippel CA, Kobets AJ, et al: Dopaminergic polymorphisms in Tourette syndrome: association with the DAT gene (SLC6A3). Am J Med Genet B Neuropsychiatr Genet 144:605–610, 2007

Zohar AH, Pauls DL, Ratzoni G, et al: Obsessive-compulsive disorder with and without tics in an epidemiological sample of adolescents. Am J Psychiatry 154:274–276, 1997

Chapter 28

Elimination Disorders

Edwin J. Mikkelsen, M.D.

Enuresis

Enuresis has been described throughout recorded time. A comprehensive summary by Glicklich (1951) found descriptions going back to the Papyrus Ebers of 1550 B.C. The history of enuresis is also rich with regard to the various treatment modalities that have been used over the years. Unfortunately, many of these would now appear to be sadistic in nature, given our current base of knowledge.

Definition and Clinical Description

The word *enuresis* is derived from the Greek word *enourein,* meaning "to void urine." A pathological connection is not inherent in the derivation but has been acquired over time. The word has come to denote nocturnal events, but that also is not inherent in the original derivation.

The phenomenology of enuresis is simply the voiding of urine, which usually occurs during sleep. However, it can also occur during the day while the individual is awake. The word *diurnal* is used to describe events that occur during the day. Individuals who have episodes both during the day and night are referred to as having diurnal and nocturnal enuresis. The volume of urine that is voided is not specified and technically could vary considerably while still being considered an *enuretic event.* The concrete nature of the enuretic event makes data collection relatively simple. It also makes it possible to quantify the magnitude of treatment effects by comparing the pre- and posttreatment weekly averages.

The author wishes to thank Ms. Patsy Kuropatkin for her invaluable assistance with preparation of this manuscript.

TABLE 28–1. DSM-IV-TR diagnostic criteria for enuresis

A. Repeated voiding of urine into bed or clothes (whether involuntary or intentional).

B. The behavior is clinically significant as manifested by either a frequency of twice a week for at least 3 consecutive months or the presence of clinically significant distress or impairment in social, academic (occupational), or other important areas of functioning.

C. Chronological age is at least 5 years (or equivalent developmental level).

D. The behavior is not due exclusively to the direct physiological effect of a substance (e.g., a diuretic) or a general medical condition (e.g., diabetes, spina bifida, a seizure disorder).

Specify type:

Nocturnal only

Diurnal only

Nocturnal and diurnal

Source. Reprinted from American Psychiatric Association: *Diagnostic and Statistical Manual of Mental Disorders,* 4th Edition, Text Revision. Washington, DC, American Psychiatric Association, 2000, p. 121. Used with permission. Copyright © 2000 American Psychiatric Association.

Diagnosis

The DSM-IV-TR (American Psychiatric Association 2000) criteria for enuresis are reproduced in Table 28–1.

There are two subtypes of enuresis, based on the natural history of the disorder. The term *primary enuresis* is used to describe those individuals who have never achieved continence, whereas *secondary enuresis* refers to those who were able to achieve continence but then subsequently resumed wetting. A time period of 6 months to 1 year is usually accepted as the length of time continence must have been maintained, although the DSM-IV-TR criteria do not specify the required duration of continence. The vast majority of children with enuresis wet involuntarily. The DSM-IV-TR notation that the wetting may be "involuntary or intentional" is unfortunate, as those whose events are intentional clearly differ in many ways.

Epidemiology

The epidemiology of enuresis has proven to be relatively consistent in large, cross-sectional national studies. Although these studies vary with regard to the frequency of the enuretic events and the ages of the cross-sectional samples, they are similar enough to be compared. The first comprehensive epidemiological investigations were Rutter's Isle of Wight Study (Rutter 1989). Those findings clearly indicated that the prevalence of enuresis diminished with advancing age, as only 1.1% of 14-year-old males were wetting once a week. The corresponding frequency for 14-year-old females was 0.5%. Subsequent large epidemiological

studies have been generally consistent with these initial findings (Bower et al. 1996; Soderstrom et al. 2004). In general, the prevalence for 5-year-olds is in the 5%–10% range and drops to 3%–5% by age 10 (American Psychiatric Association 2000). All of the studies document the disproportionate occurrence in males.

Medical Comorbidity

The primary concern with regard to medical comorbidity is the presence of a urinary tract infection. This is even more relevant in females. The presence of structural urinary tract abnormalities has been extensively investigated. Although some studies report a small percentage of children for whom this may be a factor, the consensus is that there is not enough evidence to warrant routinely subjecting children to these invasive studies (Kawauchi et al. 1996).

Enuresis has also been reported as a side effect of treatment with selective serotonin reuptake inhibitors (SSRIs) (Hergüner et al. 2007).

A recent study (Sans Capdevila et al. 2008) reports an association between habitual snoring and obstructive sleep apnea with nocturnal enuretic events. The potential medical causes of enuresis are outlined in Table 28–2.

Psychological Comorbidity

Children with secondary enuresis are more apt to present with comorbid psychiatric disorders than children with primary enuresis (von Gontard et al. 1999). The other major area of investigation has been with

TABLE 28–2. Medical causes of enuresis

Urinary tract infection

Diabetes insipidus

Diabetes mellitus

Urethritis

Seizure disorder

Sickle cell trait

Sleep apnea

Neurogenic bladder

Sleep disorders

Genitourinary malformation or obstruction

Side effect of or idiosyncratic reaction to a
medication[a]

[a]Per case reports regarding selective serotonin reuptake
inhibitors; be vigilant for chronological correlations.
Source.   Adapted from Dulcan et al. 2003.

comorbid attention-deficit/hyperactivity disorder
(ADHD) (Baeyens et al. 2004; Biederman et al. 1995).
These studies support the hypothesis that the enuresis
is comorbid with the ADHD and is not secondarily related to the ADHD. Other than the association of enuresis with ADHD, the primary finding has been that
behavioral disorders in children with enuresis are
nonspecific (Mikkelsen et al. 1980). This finding is consistent with a number of studies that link enuresis with
a generalized developmental delay in maturation
(Touchette et al. 2005).

Etiology, Mechanism, and Risk Factors

There have been discrete historical periods of research
concerning the etiology and pathophysiology of enuresis. Early psychodynamic theories, which conceived of enuresis as a willful expression of anger or
resentment, have been largely abandoned. The development of all-night polysomnographic studies led to
research that focused on enuresis as a sleep disorder
that was characterized as a "disorder of arousal," with
the enuretic events occurring in "deep sleep." However, subsequent studies with larger sample sizes indicated that enuretic events occurred during phases of
the sleep cycle in direct proportion to the amount of
time spent in that phase (Mikkelsen 2001).

The success of various pharmacological treatments
(which will be discussed in more detail below) has also
led to speculation regarding etiology. The first widely

demonstrated effective pharmacological treatment
was imipramine. Initially, it was thought that the efficacy of imipramine could be related to its anticholinergic effects on the urinary sphincter, as urinary
retention can be a side effect. However, a large, double-blind study that compared imipramine with meth-
scopolamine (an anticholinergic agent that does not
cross the blood-brain barrier) found imipramine to be
significantly more effective, suggesting a central effect, although a precise mechanism could not be elucidated (Mikkelsen and Rapoport 1980; Mikkelsen et al.
1980). In a more recent study, Hunsballe et al. (1997)
suggested that imipramine produced a decrease in os-
molar clearance and urinary output, which might contribute to its well-documented efficacy in enuresis.

The most recent era in pharmacological treatment
with desmopressin acetate (DDAVP) has generated a
number of hypotheses concerning the child's levels of
plasma atrial natriuretic peptide (ANP) and the ability
to concentrate urine during the night (Miller et al.
1992). Rittig et al. (1991) compared 15 children with
nocturnal enuresis and 11 matched control subjects
with regard to the circadian variation of ANP, creatinine clearance, and the excretion of sodium and potassium. Although the two groups did not differ in ANP
levels, the children with enuresis demonstrated increased natriuresis, kaliuresis, and polyuria during the
initial hours of sleep. As the abnormalities did not correlate with differing levels of ANP, the authors specu-
lated that the difference might be related to an abnormal tubular factor. Subsequent research has supported
this hypothesis (Natochin and Kuznetsova 1999).

Another line of investigation has focused on the
circadian production of plasma arginine vasopressin
(AVP), as abnormalities with the production of this
peptide could explain both the response to DDAVP
and the pathophysiology of enuresis. A study by
Medel et al. (1998) investigated morning levels of AVP
in control subjects and in children with enuresis and
found significant differences. Also of interest was the
observation that these levels correlated with response
or lack of response to DDAVP. However, the recognition that AVP is secreted in a pulsatile manner (Wood
et al. 1994) suggested that frequent sampling of
plasma samples would be needed to draw any firm
conclusions regarding the significance of AVP levels.
Subsequent studies, which have used more frequent
sampling of AVP, have not produced consistent results (Lackgren et al. 1997; Wood et al. 1994). The most
detailed series of investigations (Aikawa et al. 1998,
1999) with regard to AVP secretion used hourly measurements for 24 hours. The first group of studies

found that children with enuresis had significantly lower AVP levels than control subjects in the 11:00 P.M. to 4:00 A.M. time period. The authors then identified two subgroups of children with enuresis based on urinary osmotic pressure and volume of nocturnal urine production. One subgroup of children had low urinary osmotic pressure coupled with large nocturnal urine production, while the other had normal osmotic pressure and relatively small nocturnal urine production. The authors report that the first group had significantly lower mean nocturnal AVP levels. The AVP levels were also measured after treatment with DDAVP, and a significant increase in AVP levels was found. However, this was a group effect and was not found in every child. A recent study with a somewhat different design also implicated lower nocturnal AVP as a significant factor in a subset of individuals (Rittig et al. 2008).

The child's inherent bladder capacity is an obvious potential contributor to enuresis. In an early study, Shaffer et al. (1984) investigated the relationship between bladder capacity and behavioral disturbance as they related to the development of enuresis. The results were suggestive of a general underlying developmental delay, in that the children who were identified as having a behavioral disturbance also had more developmental delays and smaller functional bladder capacity.

A subsequent study found no difference in functional bladder capacity when comparing control subjects, children with enuresis, and those whose enuresis had remitted (Wille 1994). Studies involving ultrasound to determine both the bladder capacity and the thickness of the bladder wall did suggest that these factors were significantly related to response to DDAVP (Sreedhar et al. 2008). However, a recent study that investigated a number of factors that might be predictive of response, including functional bladder capacity, indicated a correlation with daytime fluid intake, suggesting no simple explanation for DDAVP responders and nonresponders (Dehoorne et al. 2007).

It has long been known that enuresis tends to run in families. The advent of the modern era of genetic linkage studies has led to several large pedigree studies. All of the linkage studies involve families with a history of multiple affected generations with high rates of enuresis. Loeys et al. (2002) reported heterogeneous results in a genetic linkage study of 32 families with pedigrees that were positive for multiple individuals with primary nocturnal enuresis. The results indicated linkage to chromosome 12q (four families); 13q 13–14 (six families); and 22q 11 (nine families).

Other studies have also implicated multiple chromosomes. Thus, although this line of research is promising, it appears that there will not be a simple parsimonious genetic explanation for the well-documented, multigenerational transmission of enuresis.

A family history of enuresis continues to be the most significant risk factor for primary enuresis. A Scandinavian epidemiological study found that the risk of enuresis for a child was 7.1 times greater if the father had enuretic events beyond the age of 4 (Jarvelin et al. 1988).

Course and Prognosis

Typically, there is a relatively high rate of spontaneous remission between ages 5–7 years and after age 12 years. DSM-IV-TR refers to a spontaneous remission rate of approximately 5%–10% per year. However, yearly remission rates as high as 14%–16% have been reported (American Academy of Child and Adolescent Psychiatry 2004). Thus, enuresis is a self-limited disorder, and the vast majority of children who are affected will eventually experience a spontaneous remission. The persistence of enuresis into late adolescence is rare.

Evaluation

The evaluation of the child with enuresis should include a thorough history obtained both from the parents and the child. This will include historical data with regard to the major developmental milestones, as well as prior attempts at toilet training. The toilet training history should also include a description of the techniques used, the duration of the trials, and the results. This interview will also provide an opportunity to explore for possible environmental and emotional contributions to the enuresis. For example, is the child afraid of the dark, and does he or she wet the bed due to fear of getting up to go to the bathroom? Another example would be the child with attentional problems and daytime wetting because he or she puts off going to the bathroom until it's too late.

The objective nature of the enuretic event simplifies the evaluation process. It is useful to approach the problem in a nonjudgmental manner that emphasizes that the enuretic events are not voluntary. A simple calendar-tracking method can be used to record the frequency of enuretic events. This will both establish the diagnosis and provide a baseline for measuring treatment effects. Both the parents and child should be instructed to collect frequency data. It will also be useful to note the time of day in addition to the date for those children with daytime wetting. This information can then be incorporated into a "Voiding Diary" (Reiner 2008). A urinalysis should be obtained to rule out a urinary tract infection. Invasive diagnostic studies are usually not warranted unless there is some reason to suspect an anatomical abnormality.

Behavioral disturbances that accompany enuresis may represent either an emotional reaction to having enuresis or a comorbid psychiatric disorder. The primary psychological effect related to enuresis is a decrease in self-esteem, which will often improve with effective treatment.

Treatment

The primary consideration with regard to treatment is that enuresis is a self-limited disorder with a substantial rate of spontaneous remission with each successive year. The frequency of the enuretic events should also be a consideration. A child who experiences enuretic episodes virtually every night is in a different category than the child who barely meets the threshold for diagnosis.

Pharmacological Treatments

The first era of pharmacological treatment followed MacLean's observation that imipramine was an effective treatment. His initial report in 1960 (MacLean 1960) was subsequently supported by multiple double-blind studies (Mikkelsen and Rapoport 1980). The treatment was generally found to be safe, although there were some tragic reports of fatal overdoses in children who thought that if taking a few pills would make the enuresis go away for a night, then taking the whole bottle would completely cure them. Treatment with imipramine does require cardiac monitoring and periodic blood levels to guard against toxicity. The usual protocol for imipramine treatment is to obtain a baseline electrocardiogram and to begin at 25 mg, with a slow titration of 25 mg increments at weekly intervals until continence is achieved. If dosages in the 75–125 mg range have not produced a positive response, it becomes less likely that the child will respond to imipramine. A dosage of 5 mg/kg/day is considered to be the upper limit. As the rate of spontaneous remission is significant, it makes sense to withdraw the medication every 3 months to determine if the enuresis has remitted (Mikkelsen et al. 1980). Multiple large studies have reported that the efficacy of imipramine correlated with the steady-state concentration of imipramine combined with its active metabolite, de-

sipramine (de Gatta et al. 1990; Rapoport et al. 1980). The variation in serum levels of children receiving the same dosage of imipramine has been reported to be as great as sevenfold (Fritz et al. 1994). Imipramine is still used for children who are refractory to other methods of treatment, either as an adjunctive or stand-alone treatment.

The advent of treatment with DDAVP largely supplanted the use of imipramine. Initially, DDAVP was administered by nasal inhalation, although an oral formulation was later developed. Moffatt et al. (1993) published a review article that identified 18 randomized, controlled studies including 689 subjects. Many of these subjects had not responded to prior treatment. The range of efficacy, as measured by the decrease in frequency of enuretic events, was 10%–91%. In most subjects, wetting resumed after DDAVP was discontinued; only 5.7% were reported to maintain continence after discontinuation of DDAVP.

The most common side effects were abdominal pain, headaches, epistaxis, and nasal stuffiness. In general, children whose enuretic events were less frequent and those who were older than 9 years of age had better outcomes.

The most significant side effect that has been identified with intranasal use of DDAVP is hyponatremia and related seizures. Excess fluid intake has been identified as a contributing factor, leading to a recommendation that children not ingest more than 8 ounces of fluid on nights when DDAVP is used (Robson et al. 1996). The risk appears to be greater during the initial stage of treatment, and younger children appear to be at a greater risk. It is thought that greater bioavailability related to prolonged half-life may contribute to the development of side effects (Dehoorne et al. 2006b). It also appears that the oral preparation may present less risk of hyponatremia. Robson et al. (2007) have reported that postmarketing data revealed 151 cases of DDAVP-related hyponatremia; 145 of these were related to the nasal preparation, as compared to 6 who were receiving the oral form. In recognition of the risk of hyponatremic seizures, some of which were fatal, the U.S. Food and Drug Administration Agency (FDA) recently issued a warning that the intranasal preparation of DDAVP should no longer be used for the treatment of primary nocturnal enuresis. The alert also indicated that treatment with the oral formulation should be interrupted during acute illness that could produce a fluid or electrolyte imbalance.

The observation that wetting will usually resume after DDAVP is discontinued has led to long-term follow-up studies of chronic use. A large, multicenter Swedish study involving 399 children ages 6–12 with primary nocturnal enuresis used a 4-week baseline observational period, followed by a 6-week dose titration period, and then 1 year of long-term treatment that included a week without treatment every 3 months to identify those who had a spontaneous remission. Doses used ranged from 20 μg to 40 μg. The average weekly frequency of wet nights during the last 3-month treatment period was 0.8, as compared to 5.3 nights during the baseline phase of the study. As in other studies, older age correlated significantly with positive response (Hjalmas et al. 1998).

The introduction of the oral form of DDAVP has made it much easier to administer. Also, as noted above, the FDA no longer approves of the use of the nasal formulation due to an increased risk of hyponatremia and seizures. A large, multicenter study that compared 20 μg of the nasal spray to 200 μg and 400 μg doses of oral DDAVP found no significant differences in treatment response, although the 400 μg oral preparation appeared to be superior to the 200 μg dose (Janknegt et al. 1997).

A randomized, placebo-controlled study using 200 μg, 400 μg, and 600 μg doses of oral DDAVP suggested a linear dose response with increasing dose correlated with the decrease in frequency of enuretic events (Skoog et al. 1997). The long-term use of oral DDAVP was found to be safe in a large Canadian study (Wolfish et al. 2003).

A recent innovation in treatment with DDAVP has been the development of a sublingual oral lyophilisate formulation referred to as "MELT," which is well tolerated and preferred by many children (Lottmann et al. 2007). A relatively small dose in the range of 120 μg to 240 μg has been found to be effective (Vande Walle et al. 2006). This formulation of DDAVP is not available in the United States at this time but is presently in Phase III clinical studies.

A number of studies have attempted to determine the pretreatment factors that are associated with a positive response to DDAVP. Those that have been repeatedly identified include lower frequency of baseline enuretic events, older age, and greater bladder capacity (Kruse et al. 2001). An extensive investigation by Dehoorne et al. (2006a), involving children who were nonresponsive to DDAVP, suggested that this was due to increased urinary osmolality and nocturnal polyuria, which could be related to their dietary habits and fluid intake.

Psychotherapeutic Treatment

There is no evidence that a traditional psychotherapeutic approach will produce any benefit for primary enuresis, although it may be helpful in ameliorating the child's embarrassment and diminished self-esteem (Collier et al. 2002). A therapeutic-educational approach is also useful in helping the family to initiate treatment in a nonjudgmental, supportive manner.

Children who have secondary enuresis are more apt to have psychological stressors contributing to the loss of continence and may be more likely to benefit from psychotherapy (American Academy of Child and Adolescent Psychiatry 2004). A psychotherapeutic approach may also be useful for comorbid psychiatric disorders.

Other Treatment Modalities

Behavioral treatment with the bell and pad method of conditioning was first described in 1904 and has been an accepted treatment strategy for several decades (Rappaport 1997).

In this method of treatment, the child sleeps on a pad that has wires attached to an alarm. When the enuretic event occurs, the urine completes the electrical circuit and the alarm sounds. The most recent review of the literature (Glazener et al. 2005) found an initial response rate of approximately two-thirds, and the rate of sustained remission was close to 50%. It has long been known that there are two distinct subgroups of children who experience remission with the bell and pad: those who learn to wake up to urinate and those who sleep through the night without wetting. Butler et al. (2007) undertook a pre- and postalarm treatment study to investigate possible physiological explanations for success. Seventy-five percent of their subjects met success criteria, and of these, 89% predominately slept through the night on dry nights. Those who experienced success manifested an increase in posttreatment ability to concentrate urine. In approximately half of these subjects, this appeared to be due to an increase in vasopressin.

The most recent innovation in this behavioral methodology uses an externally attached ultrasonic monitor that sounds an alarm at a specific threshold of bladder capacity (Pretlow 1999).

A number of other behavioral strategies have been reported, including retention-control training, evening fluid restriction, reward systems, and nighttime awakening to urinate. A thorough review of the published literature regarding these interventions (Glazener and Evans 2004) indicated that the methodology and small sample size of these reports precluded a rigorous meta-analysis.

In his recent book for parents, children, and professionals, Bennett (2005) describes a protocol that begins with simple behavioral interventions and progresses to treatment with the bell and pad. The author reports that 85% of the children he has treated with this protocol achieved continence with a relapse rate of only 15%. The book contains a useful section that provides an overview of the commercially available forms of the bell and pad.

Combined Treatment Methods

The concomitant use of the bell and pad method of treatment with DDAVP has produced variable results. A study by Leebeek-Groenewegan et al. (2001) indicated that the combination produced a more rapid response but did not improve the overall success rate. However, a study that paired imipramine with the alarm or DDAVP with the alarm found that neither was superior to the alarm alone (Naitoh et al. 2005). Another approach has been to add DDAVP after 6 weeks of bell and pad treatment that was not completely effective or after 2 weeks for children with no response at that point and multiple nocturnal events (Kamperis et al. 2008). The authors note that those children who required the addition of DDAVP had greater nocturnal urine production.

Comparison of Treatments

In a large, longitudinal study, Monda and Husmann (1995) compared the results of observation only with treatment with imipramine, DDAVP, or the bell and pad method. The length of follow-up was 12 months. However, treatment was weaned after 6 months, so that the response at 6 months represents the effects of active treatment and the 12-month data represent the frequency with which continence was maintained after cessation of active treatment. These results clearly indicate the superiority of the bell and pad method of treatment with regard to the degree of relapse after the cessation of active treatment. A subsequent systematic review of the literature involving the alarm, imipramine, and DDAVP confirmed this finding (Glazener and Evans 2002).

Research Directions

Despite advances in genetic research, it does not appear that a single genetic mechanism will be identified that explains all cases. Although there has been substantial progress with regard to the underlying pathophysiology, there is still no conclusive explanation. It seems reasonable to hypothesize that combining genetic and pathophysiological investigations may make it possible to identify clinically distinct subtypes.

Encopresis

The history of encopresis is less well documented than that of enuresis. There are also far fewer research studies investigating the cause of encopresis, as compared to the interest in enuresis.

Definition and Clinical Description

Encopresis is defined as the passage of feces into inappropriate places by a child who has reached a chronological age or developmental level at which he or she could be reasonably expected to be able to control the expulsion of feces. A distinction is made between retentive encopresis, which usually involves constipation with overflow incontinence, and nonretentive encopresis. An important distinction can also be made between involuntary and voluntary encopresis.

Diagnosis

DSM-IV-TR criteria for encopresis are reproduced in Table 28–3. A distinction is not made in DSM-IV-TR whether the encopresis is involuntary or voluntary. As with enuresis, a distinction is made between primary and secondary encopresis, with the latter term referring to those who have developed fecal continence and then relapse. The categorization of encopresis into two subtypes is clinically quite significant. The category "with constipation and overflow incontinence" represents *retentive encopresis,* whereas the category "without constipation and overflow incontinence" corresponds to *nonretentive encopresis.* The frequency required to establish the diagnosis is at least one event per month, for 3 months. The age required is a chronological age of 4 years, or equivalent developmental level.

Epidemiology

Encopresis is less prevalent than enuresis. Unfortunately, the sampling strategy and frequency of encopretic episodes vary considerably in large, cross-sectional studies. However, there is enough consistency to warrant comparison. The first large study (Bellman 1966) found a prevalence of 1.5% among a cohort of 8,863 children ages 7–8 years. The male-to-female ratio was 3:1. Subsequent epidemiological studies have been generally consistent with these

TABLE 28–3. DSM-IV-TR diagnostic criteria for encopresis

A. Repeated passage of feces into inappropriate places (e.g., clothing or floor) whether involuntary or intentional.

B. At least one such event a month for at least 3 months.

C. Chronological age is at least 4 years (or equivalent developmental level).

D. The behavior is not due exclusively to the direct physiological effects of a substance (e.g., laxatives) or a general medical condition except through a mechanism involving constipation.

Code as follows:

787.6 With constipation and overflow incontinence

307.7 Without constipation and overflow incontinence

Source. Reprinted from American Psychiatric Association: *Diagnostic and Statistical Manual of Mental Disorders,* 4th Edition, Text Revision. Washington, DC, American Psychiatric Association, 2000, p. 118. Used with permission. Copyright © 2000 American Psychiatric Association.

initial findings (Heron et al. 2008; van der Wal et al. 2005). As with enuresis, the prevalence of encopresis decreases as the child ages.

Medical and Psychological Comorbidity

There are occasionally children who present with both enuresis and encopresis (Rutter et al. 1981). Chronic constipation is usually present in those who have retentive encopresis, as this is part of the underlying pathophysiology of this disorder. Children with encopresis have more behavioral difficulties than control subjects, although there is no specific pattern (Joinson et al. 2006; Mellon et al. 2006). Obviously, those children who voluntarily defecate in inappropriate places will likely have a comorbid psychiatric disorder. Voluntary encopresis and hoarding of feces may be seen as a sequela of sexual abuse, but this symptom is not diagnostic of sexual abuse (Mellon et al. 2006). Potential medical causes of encopresis appear in Table 28–4.

Etiology, Mechanism, and Risk Factors

Retentive Encopresis

Chronic constipation is, by definition, the major factor in the evolution of retentive encopresis. The fecal incontinence that is observed is overflow incontinence from the retained fecal mass. Loening-Baucke (2004) has extensively investigated the physiological correlates of retentive encopresis with regard to the child's ability to defecate a rectal balloon. In general, these studies support the hypothesis that children with this

TABLE 28–4. Medical causes of encopresis

Constipation
Hirschsprung's disease
Medical conditions producing diarrhea
Side effect or idiosyncratic reaction to a medication (maintain vigilance for chronological correlation)
Painful lesion
Hemorrhoids (contributing to constipation)
Thyroid disease
Hypercalcemia
Lactase deficiency
Pseudo-obstruction
Spina bifida
Cerebral palsy with hypotonia
Rectal stenosis
Anal fissure
Anorectal trauma, including sexual abuse

Source. Adapted from Dulcan et al. 2003.

type of encopresis may have an inherent physiological predisposition to develop constipation. For example, in one of these studies, 56% of the subjects were unable to defecate the rectal balloon (Loening-Baucke 2004). The follow-up component of this study indicated that 64% of those who could defecate the rectal balloon were improved at 1 year of follow-up, as opposed to only 14% of those who could not defecate the balloon. Related studies have also revealed abnormalities with regard to the functioning of the anal sphincter (Loening-Baucke and Cruikshank 1986). However, it is also possible that the physiological difficulties with expulsion are the result of chronic constipation.

Nonretentive Encopresis

The pathophysiology of nonretentive encopresis is less clear and has not received the research attention that has been devoted to retentive encopresis. Presumably, the mechanism would be related either to the child not sensing the need to defecate until it is too late, and/or abnormalities of anal sphincter physiological function.

Course and Prognosis

The natural history of encopresis indicates that for the majority of individuals the disorder will eventually resolve, and reports of encopresis continuing into adolescence are rare. However, the rate of spontaneous remission is not well documented.

The concrete nature of the encopretic event makes the diagnosis relatively straightforward. The major distinction will be between retentive and nonretentive encopresis. This can usually be determined by clinical history, including a description of the encopretic events. A simple flat plate of the abdominal X ray will also reveal the presence of extensive constipation. The physiological studies discussed above, which investigated the bowel and anal sphincter physiology, were research studies and are not used on a routine clinical basis. Etiologies such as Hirschsprung's disease are rare but should be considered. In those situations where the defecation appears to be voluntary, more extensive psychological investigation is required. Even though the encopretic event is usually a clearly defined event, a thorough history is required to ensure that a more benign explanation (such as poor cleaning after defecation) accounts for the apparent soiling. Other emotional environmental factors could include the child's reluctance to use the toilets at school or attentional problems that may predispose him or her to wait until it is too late to get to the bathroom. As with enuresis, a calendar that tracks the frequency and time of day and date will be useful.

Treatment

Pharmacological Treatment

Case reports anecdotally describe the efficacy of tricyclic antidepressants, such as imipramine and amitriptyline, for nonretentive encopresis (Mikkelsen 2001). Presumably, this is due to anticholinergic effects on the anal sphincter, as the therapeutic effect is usually described as occurring before the antidepressant effect would be expected to occur.

Cisapride (Propulside) has been described as effective for retentive encopresis, as it stimulates bowel activity (Nurko et al. 2000). However, this agent is no longer available in the United States, due to deaths that were likely caused by the individual's genetic inability to metabolize the drug.

Psychotherapeutic Treatments

Psychotherapy may be indicated for those children who voluntarily defecate feces in inappropriate places and/or hoard the feces, depending on the dynamics and psychiatric comorbidity.

Behaviorally Based Treatment

Levine and Bakow (1976) described a treatment approach that involves educational, psychological, behavioral, and physiological components. The educational and psychological components are designed to inform the family about the functioning of the bowel and to address any interpersonal issues related to the encopresis. The physiological component involves bowel catharsis, followed by daily administration of laxatives. Daily, timed intervals on the toilet, coupled with rewards for success, represent the behavioral aspects of the treatment plan. The success rate for this overall treatment strategy was reported to be 78%. A comparison study that investigated variations of this approach found little additional benefit from augmenting the basic strategy with biofeedback or enhanced toilet training (Borowitz et al. 2002). This approach continues to be a primary treatment modality (Reiner 2008).

Loening-Baucke (1990) developed a treatment approach utilizing biofeedback that was derived from his physiological studies discussed earlier (see subsection "Retentive Encopresis"). The purpose of the biofeedback was to improve defecation dynamics, and the results indicated that the biofeedback was superior to traditional approaches. A subsequent, long-term follow-up study involved 129 children with constipation, encopresis, and abnormal defecation dynamics, who were treated with conventional treatment—and 63 children who received conventional treatment plus biofeedback training. The length of follow-up was 4.1±1.5 years. The success rates were remarkably similar for both groups, with 86% of the conventionally treated children showing improvement, as compared with 87% of those who also received biofeedback. Follow-up found a recovery rate of 62% for the conventionally treated group, 50% of whom had initially responded positively to the conventional and biofeedback group, and 23% of those from that group who had no initial improvement. Perhaps the most significant finding was that complete remission was significantly correlated with length of time at follow-up. The author concluded that biofeedback treatment was not significantly more effective than conventional treatment and that the natural course of the disorder was to resolve over time (Loening-Baucke 1995). Subsequent reviews of biofeedback treatment have reached similar conclusions (Brazzelli and Griffiths 2001). However, positive results with biofeedback, coupled with laxative use, have more recently been reported (Croffie et al. 2005).

Research Directions

Encopresis has not been as extensively investigated as enuresis (Mikkelsen 2001). The natural history and evolution of the disorder is also not as well characterized as that of enuresis. It is also not clear if the physiological deficits in bowel and sphincter physiology that have been identified in some studies represent an inherent physiological vulnerability or the results of chronic constipation.

Summary Points

Enuresis

- Enuresis is ultimately a self-limited disorder with relatively high rates of spontaneous remission of 12%–14%.

- Pharmacological treatment with imipramine or DDAVP is equally effective, although DDAVP has fewer side effects and is the most widely used intervention.

- A recent FDA alert drew attention to the risk of hyponatremia, seizures, and, in some cases, death related to DDAVP. The notification stated that the nasal preparation should no longer be used for enuresis and that the use of the oral preparation should be interrupted during illnesses that would disrupt fluid balance.

- Behavioral treatment with the bell and pad method of conditioning is as effective as pharmacological treatment, and relapse is significantly less apt to occur after the cessation of active treatment.

- Children with secondary enuresis are more apt to have a psychological or stressful underlying condition.

- Treatment decisions for primary nocturnal enuresis should be predicated on the severity of the enuresis, the response of the child and family to the enuretic events, the possibility of spontaneous remission, the reported efficacy of the intervention, the rate of relapse after active treatment is stopped, and the side-effect risk related to the intervention. This equation will usually indicate that the bell and pad method of treatment is the most appropriate first choice for treatment.

Encopresis

- There are two primary subtypes of encopresis: retentive, which involves constipation and related overflow incontinence, and nonretentive encopresis. A third category would be those youth who voluntarily defecate in inappropriate places, although DSM-IV-TR does not formally recognize this group.

- A distinction is made between primary and secondary encopresis, with the latter term referring to those who achieve continence and then relapse.

- Retentive encopresis has been more extensively studied with regard to physiology and treatment. The most accepted form of treatment is a protocol that contains educational, psychological, behavioral, and physiological components.

- Those children whose encopresis is of a voluntary nature clearly require full psychological evaluation and may respond to psychotherapeutic interventions or treatment of the underlying and/or comorbid psychopathology.

- The natural history of encopresis is to move toward continence. However, the natural history and rate of spontaneous remission are not as well understood as those of enuresis.

References

Aikawa T, Kashara T, Uchiyama M: The arginine-vasopressin secretion profile of children with primary nocturnal enuresis. Eur Urol 33(suppl):41–44, 1998

Aikawa T, Kashara T, Uchiyama M: Circadian variation of plasma arginine vasopressin concentration, or arginine vasopressin in enuresis. Scand J Urol Nephrol 202:47–49, 1999

American Academy of Child and Adolescent Psychiatry: Practice parameter for the assessment and treatment of children and adolescents with enuresis. J Am Acad Child Adolesc Psychiatry 43:1540–1550, 2004

American Psychiatric Association: Diagnostic and Statistical Manual of Mental Disorders, 4th Edition, Text Revision. Washington, DC, American Psychiatric Association, 2000

Baeyens D, Roeyers H, Hoebeke P, et al: Attention deficit/hyperactivity disorder in children with nocturnal enuresis. J Urol 171:2576–2579, 2004

Bellman M: Studies on encopresis. Acta Paediatr Scand 56 (Suppl 170):S1–S151, 1966

Bennett HJ: Waking Up Dry: A Guide to Help Children Overcome Bedwetting. Elk Grove Village, IL, American Academy of Pediatrics, 2005

Biederman J, Santangelo SL, Faraone SV: Clinical correlates of enuresis in ADHD and non-ADHD children. J Child Psychol Psychiatry 36:865–877, 1995

Borowitz SM, Cox DJ, Sutphen JL, Kovatchev B: Treatment of childhood encopresis: a randomized trial comparing three treatment protocols. J Pediatr Gastroenterol Nutr 34:378–384, 2002

Bower WF, Moore KH, Shepherd RB, et al: The epidemiology of childhood enuresis in Australia. Br J Urol 78:602–606, 1996

Brazzelli M, Griffiths P: Behavioural and cognitive interventions with or without other treatments for defaecation disorders in children. Cochrane Database Syst Rev 4:CD002240, 2001

Butler RJ, Holland P, Gasson S, et al: Exploring potential mechanisms in alarm treatment for primary nocturnal enuresis. Scand J Urol Nephrol 41(suppl):407–413, 2007

Collier J, Butler RJ, Redsell SA, et al: An investigation of the impact of nocturnal enuresis on children's self-concept. Scand J Urol Nephrol 36(suppl):204–208, 2002

Croffie JM, Ammar MS, Pfefferkorn MD, et al: Assessment of the effectiveness of biofeedback in children with dyssynergic defecation and recalcitrant constipation/encopresis: does home biofeedback improve long-term outcomes. Clin Pediatr 44(suppl):63–71, 2005

de Gatta MF, Galindo P, Rey F, et al: The influence of clinical and pharmacological factors on enuresis treatment with imipramine. Br J Clin Pharmacol 30:693–698, 1990

Dehoorne JL, Raes AM, van Laecke E, et al: Desmopressin resistant nocturnal polyuria secondary to increased nocturnal osmotic excretion. J Urol 716(suppl):749–753, 2006a

Dehoorne JL, Raes AM, van Laecke, et al: Desmopressin toxicity due to prolonged half-life in 18 patients with nocturnal enuresis. J Urol 176(suppl):754–757, 2006b

Dehoorne JL, Walle CV, Vansintjan P, et al: Characteristics of a tertiary center enuresis population, with special emphasis on the relation among nocturnal diuresis, functional bladder capacity and desmopressin response. J Urol 177(suppl):1130–1137, 2007

Dulcan MK, Martini DR, Lake MB: Concise Guide to Child and Adolescent Psychiatry, 3rd Edition. Washington, DC, American Psychiatric Association, 2003

Fritz GK, Rockney RM, Yeung AS: Plasma levels and efficacy of imipramine treatment for enuresis. J Am Acad Adolesc Psychiatry 33:60–64, 1994

Glazener CM, Evans JH: Desmopressin for nocturnal enuresis in children. Cochrane Database Syst Rev 3:CD002112, 2002

Glazener CM, Evans JH: Simple behavioural and physical interventions for nocturnal enuresis in children. Cochrane Database Syst Rev 2:CD003637, 2004

Glazener CM, Evans JH, Peto RE: Alarm interventions for nocturnal enuresis in children. Cochrane Database Syst Rev 2:CD002911, 2003. Update in Cochrane Database Syst Rev 2:CD002911, 2005

Glicklich LB: An historical account of enuresis. Pediatrics 8:859–876, 1951

Hergüner S, Kilingaslan A, Görker I, et al: Serotonin-selective reuptake inhibitor-induced enuresis in three pediatric cases. J Child Adolesc Psychopharmacol 17(suppl):367–370, 2007

Heron J, Joinson C, Croudace T, et al: Trajectories of daytime wetting and soiling in a United Kingdom 4- to 9-year-old population birth cohort study. J Urol 179(suppl):1970–1975, 2008

Hjalmas K, Hanson E, Hellstrom AL, et al: Long-term treatment with desmopressin in children with primary monosymptomatic nocturnal enuresis: an open multicentre study. Swedish Enuresis Trial (SWEET) Group. Br J Urol 82:704–709, 1998

Hunsballe JM, Rittig S, Pedersen EB, et al: Single dose imipramine reduces nocturnal urine output in patients with nocturnal enuresis and nocturnal polyuria. J Urol 158:830–836, 1997

Janknegt RA, Zweers HM, Delaere KP, et al: Oral desmopressin as a new treatment modality for primary nocturnal enuresis in adolescents and adults: a double-blind, randomized, multicenter study. Dutch Enuresis Study Group. J Urol 157:513–517, 1997

Jarvelin MR, Vikevainen-Tervonen L, Moilanen I, et al: Enuresis in seven-year-old children. Acta Paediatr Scand 77:148–153, 1988

Joinson C, Heron J, Butler U, et al: Psychological differences between children with and without soiling problems. Pediatrics 117(suppl):1575–1584, 2006

Kamperis K, Hagstroem S, Rittig S, et al: Combination of the enuresis alarm and desmopressin: second-line treatment for nocturnal enuresis. J Urol 179(suppl):817–818, 2008

Kawauchi A, Kitamori T, Imada N, et al: Urological abnormalities in 1,328 patients with nocturnal enuresis. Eur Urol 29:231–234, 1996

Kruse S, Hellstrom AL, Hanson E, et al: Treatment of primary monosymptomatic nocturnal enuresis with desmopressin: predictive factors. BJU Int 88(suppl):572–576, 2001

Lackgren G, Neveus T, Stenberg A: Diurnal plasma vasopressin and urinary output in adolescents with monosymptomatic nocturnal enuresis. Acta Paediatr 86:385–390, 1997

Leebeek-Groenewegan A, Blom J, Sukhai R, et al: Efficacy of desmopressin combined with alarm therapy for monosymptomatic nocturnal enuresis. J Urol 166(suppl):2456–2458, 2001

Levine MD, Bakow H: Children with encopresis: a study of treatment outcome. Pediatrics 58:845–852, 1976

Loening-Baucke V: Modulation of abnormal defecation dynamics by biofeedback treatment in chronically constipated children with encopresis. J Pediatr 116:214–222, 1990

Loening-Baucke V: Biofeedback treatment for chronic constipation and encopresis in childhood: long-term outcome. Pediatrics 96:105–110, 1995

Loening-Baucke V: Functional fecal retention with encopresis in childhood. J Pediatr Gastroenterol Nutr 38(suppl):79–84, 2004

Loening-Baucke VA, Cruikshank BM: Abnormal defecation dynamics in chronically constipated children with encopresis. J Pediatr 108:562–566, 1986

Loeys B, Hoebeke P, Raes A, et al: Does monosymptomatic enuresis exist? A molecular genetic exploration of 32 families with enuresis/incontinence. BJU Int 90(suppl):76–83, 2002

Lottmann H, Froeling F, Alloussi S, et al: A randomised comparison of oral desmopressin lyophilisate (MELT) and tablet formulations in children and adolescents with primary nocturnal enuresis. Int J Clin Pract 61(suppl):1454–1460, 2007

MacLean REG: Imipramine hydrochloride (Tofranil) and enuresis. Am J Psychiatry 117:511, 1960

Medel R, Dieguez S, Brindo M, et al: Monosymptomatic primary enuresis: differences between patients responding or not responding to oral desmopressin. Br J Urol 3:46–49, 1998

Mellon MW, Whiteside SP, Friedrich WN: The relevance of fecal soiling as an indicator of child sexual abuse: a preliminary analysis. J Dev Behav Pediatr 27(suppl):25–32, 2006

Mikkelsen EJ: Enuresis and encopresis: ten years of progress. J Am Acad Child Adolesc Psychiatry 40:1146–1158, 2001

Mikkelsen EJ, Rapoport JL: Enuresis: psychopathology, sleep stage, and drug response. Urol Clin North Am 7:361–377, 1980

Mikkelsen EJ, Rapoport JL, Nee L, et al: Childhood enuresis, I: sleep patterns and psychopathology. Arch Gen Psychiatry 37:1139–1144, 1980

Miller K, Atkin B, Moody ML: Drug therapy for nocturnal enuresis: current treatment recommendations. Drugs 44:47–56, 1992

Moffatt ME, Harlos S, Kirshen AJ, et al: Desmopressin acetate and nocturnal enuresis: how much do we know? Pediatrics 92:420–425, 1993

Monda JM, Husmann DA: Primary nocturnal enuresis: a comparison among observation, imipramine, desmopressin acetate and bed-wetting alarm systems. J Urol 154:745–748, 1995

Naitoh Y, Kawauchi A, Yamao Y, et al: Combination therapy with alarm and drugs for monosymptomatic nocturnal enuresis not superior to alarm monotherapy. Urology 66(suppl):632–635, 2005

Natochin YV, Kuznetsova AA: Defect of osmoregulatory renal function in nocturnal enuresis. Scand J Urol Nephrol 202:40–43, 1999

Nurko S, Garcia-Aranda JA, Worona LB, et al: Cisapride for the treatment of constipation in children: a double-blind study. J Pediatr 136:135–140, 2000

Pretlow RA: Treatment of nocturnal enuresis with an ultrasound bladder volume controlled alarm device. J Urol 162:1224–1228, 1999

Rapoport JL, Mikkelsen EJ, Zavadil A, et al: Childhood enuresis, II: psychopathology, tricyclic concentration in plasma, and antienuretic effect. Arch Gen Psychiatry 37:1146–1152, 1980

Rappaport L: Prognostic factors for alarm treatment. Scand J Urol Nephrol 183:55–57, 1997

Reiner WG: Pharmacotherapy in the management of voiding and storage disorders, including enuresis and encopresis. J Am Acad Child Adolesc Psychiatry 47(suppl):491–498, 2008

Rittig S, Knudsen UB, Norgaard JP, et al: Diurnal variation of plasma atrial natriuretic peptide in normals and patients with enuresis nocturna. Scand J Clin Lab Invest 51:209–217, 1991

Rittig S, Schaumburg HL, Siggaard C, et al: The circadian defect in plasma vasopressin and urine output is related to desmopressin response and enuresis status in children with nocturnal enuresis. J Urol 179(suppl):2389–2395, 2008

Robson WL, Norgaard JP, Leung AK: Hyponatremia in patients with nocturnal enuresis treated with DDAVP. Eur J Pediatr 155:959–962, 1996

Robson WL, Leung AK, Norgaard JP: The comparative safety of oral versus intranasal desmopressin for the treatment of children with nocturnal enuresis. J Urol 178(suppl):24–30, 2007

Rutter M: Isle of Wight revisited: Twenty-five years of child psychiatric epidemiology. J Am Acad Child Adolesc Psychiatry 28:633–653, 1989

Rutter M, Tizard J, Whitmore K (eds): Education, Health and Behavior. New York, Krieger, Huntington, 1981

Sans Capdevila O, Crabtree VM, Kheirandish-Gozal L, et al: Increased morning brain natriuretic peptide levels in children with nocturnal enuresis and sleep-disordered breathing: a community-based study. Pediatrics 121(suppl):e1208–e1214, 2008

Shaffer D, Gardner A, Hedge B: Behavior and bladder disturbance of enuretic children: a rational classification of a common disorder. Dev Med Child Neurol 26:781–792, 1984

Skoog SJ, Stokes A, Turner KL: Oral desmopressin: a randomized double-blind placebo controlled study of effectiveness in children with primary nocturnal enuresis. J Urol 158:1035–1040, 1997

Soderstrom U, Hoelcke M, Alenius L, et al: Urinary and faecal incontinence: a population-based study. Acta Paediatr 93(suppl):386–389, 2004

Sreedhar B, Yeung CK, Leung VY, et al: Ultrasound bladder measurements in children with severe primary nocturnal enuresis: pretreatment and posttreatment evaluation and its correlation with treatment outcome. J Urol 179(suppl):1568–1572, 2008

Touchette E, Petit D, Paquet J, et al: Bed-wetting and its association with developmental milestones in early childhood. Arch Pediatr Adolesc Med 159(suppl):1129–1134, 2005

van der Wal MF, Benninga MA, Hirasing RA: The prevalence of encopresis in a multicultural population. J Pediatr Gastroenterol Nutr 40(suppl):345–348, 2005

Vande Walle JG, Bogaert GA, Mattsson S, et al: A new fast-melting oral formulation of desmopressin: a pharmacodynamic study in children with primary nocturnal enuresis. BJU Int 97(suppl):603–609, 2006

von Gontard A, Mauer-Mucke K, Pluck J, et al: Clinical behavioral problems in day- and night-wetting children. Pediatr Nephrol 13:662–667, 1999

Wille S: Functional bladder capacity and calcium-creatinine quota in enuretic patients, former enuretic and non enuretic controls. Scand J Urol Nephrol 28:353–357, 1994

Wolfish NM, Barkin J, Gorodzinsky F, et al: The Canadian enuresis study and evaluation: short- and long-term safety and efficacy of an oral desmopressin preparation. Scand J Urol Nephrol 37(suppl):22–27, 2003

Wood CM, Butler RJ, Penny MD, et al: Pulsatile release of arginine vasopressin (AVP) and its effect on response to desmopressin in enuresis. Scand J Urol Nephrol 163:93–101, 1994

Chapter 29

Sleep Disorders

Anna Ivanenko, M.D., Ph.D.
Kyle P. Johnson, M.D.

Child and adolescent mental health clinicians serve on the front line of recognizing sleep disorders in children and adolescents since so many children we assess have sleep complaints. These sleep problems may represent either 1) primary sleep disorders, such as obstructive sleep apnea (OSA), restless legs syndrome (RLS), or narcolepsy; or 2) insomnia comorbid with psychiatric conditions, such as depression or anxiety. Mental health professionals must keep sleep disorders in mind when assessing children with neurocognitive, emotional, behavioral, and motivational problems, because chronic sleep disruption can cause these difficulties.

Sleep Requirements

Sleep and circadian rhythms develop from infancy into adult expression as a reflection of central nervous system (CNS) maturation. The most dramatic changes in sleep architecture and sleep requirements occur during the first year of life. Newborns enter sleep through the rapid eye movement (REM) sleep state and demonstrate a greater proportion of REM sleep in respect to total sleep amount than adults, with almost 50% of total sleep time being occupied by REM sleep. REM sleep reduces to an average 20% of total sleep time within the first 12 months of child development and remains at about that percentage through the life span. In infants, REM and non-REM (NREM) sleep alternate during the night with a periodicity of approximately 50 minutes (the ultradian cycle). The ultradian cycle gradually increases in length to an average of 90 minutes in adults.

According to a recent study of 944 infants and toddlers ages 2 weeks to 2 years, the average 24-hour sleep duration across these 2 years was 12.5 hours (Montgomery-Downs and Gozal 2006). A significant decline in daytime sleep (scheduled naps) occurs within the first 5 years of life. Infants are reported to sleep an average of 9 hours per night and nap for 4 hours during the day. Toddlers sleep approximately 11.7 hours in a 24-hour period, including one nap. The majority of children give up their daytime naps by age 5 years, although there are some who require napping at an older age (National Sleep Foundation 2006).

From the infant's birth to age 6 months, the circadian system undergoes robust development. Entrainment to day and night begins in utero under the influence of maternal melatonin. The circadian rhythm of body temperature begins to manifest in the first week after birth. The wake circadian rhythm attains significance by day 45, with increased melatonin secretion at sunset, followed by the circadian rhythm of sleep by day 56 after birth. By 6 months of age, the infant is usually entrained to the light-dark cycle and social rhythm of the household.

Another developmental shift in regulation of sleep homeostasis and the circadian system occurs with the beginning of puberty. Research has shown that the average sleep requirement during adolescence increases to approximately 9.5 hours, with a tendency toward delayed sleep and awakening, thus creating a timing conflict between the school-social schedule and the sleep schedule.

Epidemiology

Sleep disorders are highly prevalent across the life span. Numerous epidemiological studies have been conducted using parental and self-reports. Fewer studies have used objective sleep measurements like actigraphy or polysomnography. Most of the surveys refer to symptoms of disrupted sleep—such as problems initiating and maintaining sleep, frequent nocturnal awakenings, delayed sleep onset, and restless sleep; behaviors associated with sleep, such as sleepwalking, sleeptalking, snoring, and witnessed apneas with gasping for air; and excessive daytime sleepiness.

Approximately 25% of children will experience sleep-related problems at some point of their development. A number of surveys completed by the parents of a community sample of children found sleep problems in 20% of 5-year-old children and 6% of 11-year-olds (Rona et al. 1998) and a 37%–50% prevalence of sleep problems in school-age children (Blader et al. 1997; Owens et al. 2000b). A high rate of problems in sleep initiation, sleep maintenance, and excessive daytime sleepiness due to chronic sleep loss has been reported by adolescents. A survey of 1,014 adolescents revealed a 10.7% lifetime prevalence of insomnia with a median age at onset of 11 years (Johnson et al. 2006). Of interest, 52.8% of the adolescents with insomnia had a comorbid psychiatric disorder.

Children with chronic medical, neurodevelopmental, and psychiatric disorders present with a much higher rate of sleep disorders. Between 30% and 80% of children with mental retardation and from 50% to 70% of children with autism spectrum disorders have been reported to have sleep problems (Johnson 1996; Stores and Wiggs 1998).

Classification of Sleep Disorders

There are two major classification systems for sleep disorders: *International Classification of Sleep Disorders, Second Edition* (ICSD-2; American Academy of Sleep Medicine 2005), and the *Diagnostic and Statistical Manual of Mental Disorders, Fourth Edition* (DSM-IV; American Psychiatric Association 1994; 2000). Sleep behavior disorder and regulatory disorder with sleep problem are also included in the *Diagnostic Classification, Zero to Three* (DC: 0–3R; Zero to Three 2005).

According to DSM-IV, sleep disorders are divided into four major classes: dyssomnias, parasomnias, sleep disorders related to another mental disorder, and other sleep disorders, which include sleep disorders due to a medical condition and substance-induced sleep disorder (Table 29–1).

ICSD-2 is a more comprehensive classification of sleep disorders that includes a wide variety of sleep-related conditions, including a revised definition of primary insomnia that emphasizes a behavioral insomnia of childhood subdivided into two types: sleep-onset association type and limit-setting type.

Evaluation

Sleep History

Taking a sleep history is the first and most important step in assessing children and adolescents for sleep disorders. Due to a high rate of sleep comorbidities with other psychiatric disorders, it is essential to obtain a sleep history in pediatric patients as they present to the clinician's office with behavioral and emotional problems.

BEARS is an easy-to-remember mnemonic introduced to help clinicians to gather sleep symptoms. It stands for Bedtime, Excessive daytime sleepiness, Awakenings, Regularity, and Snoring (Mindell and

TABLE 29–1. DSM-IV-TR classification of sleep disorders

Primary sleep disorders
  Dyssomnias
    Primary insomnia
    Narcolepsy and primary hypersomnia
    Breathing-related sleep disorder
  Dyssomnia not otherwise specified
  Circadian rhythm sleep disorders
    Delayed sleep phase syndrome
    Jet lag
    Shift work
    Unspecified
  Parasomnias
    Nightmare disorder
    Sleep terror disorder
    Sleepwalking disorder
    Parasomnia not otherwise specified

Sleep disorders related to another mental disorder

Other sleep disorders

Sleep disorders due to a general medical condition

Substance-induced sleep disorders

Owens 2003). It is important to understand a child's customary sleep habits and patterns, both during the weekdays and weekends; night-to-night variability in sleep duration; number of nocturnal awakenings; and sleep-related behaviors.

Medical history, physical examination, and neurodevelopmental and psychiatric history are the required parts of a comprehensive sleep evaluation.

Questionnaires

Several questionnaires have been developed and validated to assess for the most common sleep problems in children and adolescents. The Pediatric Sleep Questionnaire (PSQ) has been validated for the assessment of sleep-disordered breathing, daytime sleepiness, snoring, and behavioral problems like hyperactivity, impulsivity, and inattention in children ages 2–18 years (Chervin et al. 2000). The Children's Sleep Habits Questionnaire (CSHQ) yields eight subscales that reflect the major domains of behavioral and medical sleep disorders and a total score indicating the extent and severity of sleep-related problems (Owens et al. 2000a). The

Sleep Disorders Inventory for Students (SDIS) is a validated parent- and self-report questionnaire for children ages 2–10 years (SDIS-C) and adolescents ages 11–18 years (SDIS-A) that can be used for screening of sleep disorders in a variety of clinical and school settings (available at Child Uplift, Inc., P.O. Box 146, Fairview, WY 83119; www.sleepdisorderhelp.com).

The Epworth Sleepiness Scale is a clinical tool recently modified for use in children and adolescents (Drake et al. 2003) that is very helpful for screening the subjective propensity to fall asleep in certain situations and for measuring treatment outcome.

A sleep log/sleep diary (Figure 29–1) is a valuable tool that provides nightly information on the child's bedtime, sleep-onset time, rise time, and number of nocturnal awakenings and is usually recommended to be completed for a period of 2 weeks. Sleep logs are usually filled out by parents or caregivers of younger children and by adolescents themselves. Sleep logs are based on observations and/or self-perception and lack objective assessment of sleep.

Actigraphy uses a small, portable motion sensor that counts and stores movements per minute using a specially designed algorithm. The device is typically worn on the nondominant wrist and collects continuous objective sleep-wake data including total amount of sleep, sleep efficiency, and number and duration of awakenings. It is a very valuable tool to assess night-to-night variability of sleep and can detect subtle circadian sleep disturbances.

Nocturnal polysomnography (PSG) is currently the gold standard procedure to study sleep-disordered breathing and other types of intrinsic sleep disorders in children. It includes recordings of electroencephalogram, electro-oculogram, electromyogram, airflow, respiratory and abdominal efforts, oxygen saturation, end-tidal carbon dioxide, and limb muscle activity. PSG requires the child and one of the parents or caregivers to spend a night in a sleep laboratory. PSG is indicated for the diagnosis of OSA, central apnea, alveolar hypoventilation, snoring, and upper airway resistance syndrome in children. PSG is also used to establish the diagnosis of periodic limb movement disorder (PLMD) and to evaluate for nocturnal seizures and parasomnias, such as REM behavior sleep disorder.

The Multiple Sleep Latency Test (MSLT) is used to assess daytime sleepiness and includes a series of four to five naps conducted at 2-hour intervals, with the first nap beginning 2 hours after the final morning awakening. The MSLT is routinely preceded the night before by a PSG. The MSLT is a routine part of the sleep laboratory assessment of narcolepsy and idio-

Name:

DOB: / /

Date Started: / /

Date Ended: / /

List Medications:

Day	6p	7	8	9	10	11	Midnight 12	1	2	3	4	5	6	7	8	9	10	11	Noon 12	1	2	3	4	5	Comments

Day	6p	7	8	9	10	11	Midnight 12	1	2	3	4	5	6	7	8	9	10	11	Noon 12	1	2	3	4	5	Comments
Ex																									

Key: ↑ = out of bed; ↓ = in bed; ■ = sleep.

FIGURE 29–1. Sleep log/sleep diary.

pathic hypersomnia and helps to objectively measure the degree of somnolence due to sleep apnea or as a result of chronic sleep loss.

The Maintenance of Wakefulness Test is similar to the MSLT procedure, but the patient is asked to remain awake while sleep latency is measured. The test is used in adolescents with disorders of excessive daytime sleepiness to assess their ability to maintain adequate levels of alertness, especially when beginning to drive.

Dyssomnias

Primary Insomnia

The DSM-IV-TR criteria for primary insomnia are presented in Table 29–2.

Prevalence

Sleep initiation and maintenance insomnia—including bedtime resistance, disruptive nocturnal awakenings, and other behavioral sleep problems—are most commonly observed in young children, with a prevalence of 25%–50% in preschool-age children.

Clinical Characteristics

The revised edition of ICSD-2 introduced unique diagnostic entities of behavioral insomnia of childhood: limit-setting type and sleep-onset association type. Limit-setting type of behavioral insomnia refers to parental difficulties establishing behavioral limits and enforcing bedtimes and is commonly associated with stalling and refusing to go to bed. Sleep-onset associa-

tion type is characterized by maladaptive sleep-onset associations such as rocking, feeding, watching TV, or parental presence. Behavioral sleep problems result in delayed sleep onset, fragmented nocturnal sleep, insufficient sleep time, and daytime sleepiness. They also contribute to nighttime awakenings, because once the child wakes up at night, he or she is unable to reinitiate sleep without recreating the same sleep association.

Treatment

Nonpharmacological interventions are the first choice of treatment. Behavioral interventions include parental education, "sleep hygiene," extinction, graduated extinction, scheduled awakenings, and positive bedtime routines and cognitive-behavioral therapy (Kuhn and Elliott 2003; Mindell 1999). Intervention for insomnia in children should start with establishing appropriate and realistic parent and child expectations and treatment goals. Age-appropriate sleep duration and bedtime should be discussed with the parents. School schedule and extracurricular activities should be taken into consideration when establishing the treatment protocol. It is very important to set and reinforce regular bed and rise times. Introducing a positive relaxing bedtime routine is an important step in preparing a child to fall asleep. Morning rise time is especially important as a powerful environmental cue for entrainment of the sleep-wake cycle. The sleeping environment should be controlled to exclude television, video games, computer, and the like. Children should be encouraged to sleep in their own bed on a consistent basis. Establishment of appropriate nap time is very important since it will affect nocturnal sleep onset and sleep duration time.

TABLE 29–2. **DSM-IV-TR diagnostic criteria for primary insomnia**

A. The predominant complaint is difficulty initiating or maintaining sleep, or nonrestorative sleep, for at least 1 month.

B. The sleep disturbance (or associated daytime fatigue) causes clinically significant distress or impairment in social, occupational, or other important areas of functioning.

C. The sleep disturbance does not occur exclusively during the course of narcolepsy, breathing-related sleep disorder, circadian rhythm sleep disorder, or a parasomnia.

D. The disturbance does not occur exclusively during the course of another mental disorder (e.g., major depressive disorder, generalized anxiety disorder, a delirium).

E. The disturbance is not due to the direct physiological effects of a substance (e.g., a drug of abuse, a medication) or a general medical condition.

Source. Reprinted from American Psychiatric Association: *Diagnostic and Statistical Manual of Mental Disorders,* 4th Edition, Text Revision. Washington, DC, American Psychiatric Association, 2000, p. 604. Used with permission. Copyright © 2000 American Psychiatric Association.

Numerous behavioral techniques have been described for childhood sleep disorders, including standard extinction in which parents ignore the child's undesired behavior, except for safety purposes. Extinction is difficult for many parents to implement; therefore, graduated extinction has been more frequently used in clinical practice. This approach allows parents to check the child at time intervals of increasing duration until the desired behavior is achieved. Cognitive therapy has been successfully implemented to treat insomnia in older children and adolescents. Cognitive strategies include restructuring of thoughts and attitudes, systemic desensitization, positive reinforcement, and relaxation techniques.

There are no well-designed controlled studies of sedative-hypnotics in children, and there are no FDA-approved pharmacological agents for use in pediatric insomnia. For the current status of knowledge on pharmacological treatment of pediatric insomnia, please review Consensus Statement by Mindell et al. (2006) and Chapter 51, "Medications Used for Sleep."

Narcolepsy and Primary Hypersomnia

The DSM-IV-TR criteria for narcolepsy are presented in Table 29–3.

Prevalence

The prevalence of narcolepsy in the adult population is approximately 2–5 per 10,000 with the rate in children presumably half of that.

Clinical Characteristics

Narcolepsy is a rare neurological disorder characterized by daytime sleepiness, cataplexy (sudden loss of muscle tone triggered by emotional arousal such as laughter), hypnagogic hallucinations, and sleep paralysis. The classic tetrad of narcolepsy including all of the above symptoms is rare in children. Most pediatric patients present with excessive daytime sleepiness and sleep attacks often masked by behavioral and emotional symptoms such as irritability, hyperactivity, inattention, and increased sleep needs at younger age. A newly discovered neuropeptide, hypocretin (also known as orexin), has been linked to the pathophysiology of narcolepsy. The diagnosis of narcolepsy requires sleep laboratory evaluation to include PSG and MSLT with evidence of pathological sleepiness and at least two sleep-onset REM periods.

Idiopathic hypersomnia is a diagnosis of exclusion and is characterized by sleepiness with long-lasting, nonrefreshing sleep that is not associated with frequent periods of sleep onset with REM.

Treatment

Treatment options for narcolepsy and idiopathic hypersomnia are similar and include pharmacotherapy and behavioral intervention. Good sleep habits with a regular sleep-wake schedule and adequate amount of nocturnal sleep are essential parts of management of excessive daytime sleepiness. Scheduled daytime naps of 25–30 minutes each are beneficial in increasing daytime alertness. Patients should avoid alcohol and recreational substances, and adolescents need to be cautioned about the risks of driving or operating machinery when sleepy. Education and support for these conditions are available through The Narcolepsy Network (www.narcolepsynetwork.org), a nonprofit organization for patients, families, and professionals.

Long-term administration of pharmacological agents is often required to reduce sleepiness and improve daytime alertness. A long-acting alerting medication, modafinil, can provide all-day benefits following morning administration. Psychostimulants such as methylphenidate or dextroamphetamine have been used alone or in combination with modafinil in treating excessive sleepiness in children and are generally well-tolerated. In a small sample of children with narcolepsy and idiopathic hypersomnia, modafinil at dosages of 200–600 mg/day was shown to reduce daytime sleepiness without significant side effects (Ivanenko et al. 2003). A recent study indicated that sodium oxybate (Xyrem) was effective for the treatment of excessive daytime sleepiness associated with narcolepsy in children and adolescents (Murali and Kotagal 2006) and was not associated with any significant side effects. Tricyclic antidepressants (clomipramine, imipramine, protriptyline); mixed action antidepressants, like venlafaxine; and serotonin reuptake inhibitors may be used to treat cataplexy and other symptoms of narcolepsy, such as sleep paralysis and hypnagogic hallucinations.

Kleine-Levin Syndrome

Prevalence

Kleine-Levin syndrome (KLS) is a rare disorder with typical onset during adolescence. The exact prevalence of KLS is unknown, especially in the pediatric population.

TABLE 29–3. DSM-IV-TR diagnostic criteria for narcolepsy

A. Irresistible attacks of refreshing sleep that occur daily over at least 3 months.

B. The presence of one or both of the following:

(1) cataplexy (i.e., brief episodes of sudden bilateral loss of muscle tone, most often in association with intense emotion)

(2) recurrent intrusions of elements of rapid eye movement (REM) sleep into the transition between sleep and wakefulness, as manifested by either hypnopompic or hypnagogic hallucinations or sleep paralysis at the beginning or end of sleep episodes

C. The disturbance is not due to the direct physiological effects of a substance (e.g., a drug of abuse, a medication) or another general medical condition.

Source. Reprinted from American Psychiatric Association: *Diagnostic and Statistical Manual of Mental Disorders,* 4th Edition, Text Revision. Washington, DC, American Psychiatric Association, 2000, p. 615. Used with permission. Copyright © 2000 American Psychiatric Association.

Clinical Characteristics

Recurrent episodes of hypersomnia are the main feature of KLS. Sleepiness is profound and episodes of continuous sleep may last up to 20 hours. A flu-like prodrome may precede an episode of hypersomnia, and associated symptoms may or may not be present and are not required for the diagnosis. Episodes of hypersomnia vary in duration from less than 1 week and up to 30 days. Sexually acting-out behavior is more commonly present in males. The etiology of KLS is unknown, but a prominent theory suggests dysfunction of the hypothalamus and midbrain limbic system. While establishing the diagnosis of KLS, the clinician should rule out organic causes of periodic hypersomnia, as well as psychiatric causes such as bipolar disorder.

Treatment

Treatment of KLS is symptomatic, focused on the relief of hypersomnia and associated symptoms. Modafinil and psychostimulants have been used in the management of excessive sleepiness. There have been reports of successful use of lithium carbonate in the treatment of KLS.

Restless Legs Syndrome and Periodic Limb Movement Disorder

Prevalence

RLS is a common sensorimotor disorder, occurring in 5%–10% of adults with an estimated prevalence in the pediatric population of 2% (Picchietti et al. 2007).

Clinical Characteristics

RLS is defined as an urge to move the legs, usually accompanied by uncomfortable and unpleasant sensations in the legs. Periodic limb movements of sleep are characterized by episodes of repetitive stereotypical limb movements. The presence of insomnia or excessive daytime sleepiness is required to establish the diagnosis of PLMD. Children frequently report symptoms of RLS differently from adults, which makes the diagnosis of RLS in children more challenging. New diagnostic criteria have been established for children and adolescents (Allen et al. 2003). As RLS and PLMD have been more extensively studied, the association between these disorders and attention-deficit/hyperactivity disorder (ADHD) in children has become evident (Cortese et al. 2005). Many children with ADHD have been found to have RLS or PLMD and vice versa.

Treatment

Behavioral interventions for RLS and PLMD are mainly focused on preserving a stable sleep-wake schedule, avoiding sleep deprivation, reducing caffeine intake, eliminating tobacco and alcohol, and avoiding stimulating activities close to bedtime. Pharmacological interventions include iron supplementation that is usually recommended if the child's serum ferritin level is below 35 µg/L. Serum ferritin level should be monitored every 3–4 months and iron therapy discontinued when serum ferritin rises above 35–50 µg/L (Simakajornboon et al. 2003).

Clinical evidence suggests that dopaminergic medications such as pramipexole and ropinirole are effective in pediatric cases of RLS (Walters et al. 2000). Ropinirole and pramipexole are U.S. Food and Drug

Administration (FDA)–approved for RLS treatment in adults, but not in children. Gabapentin is another medication known to reduce symptoms of RLS in children. Other classes of medication, such as benzodiazepines (clonazepam) and alpha-agonists (clonidine), and carbamazepine have been successfully used to relieve RLS symptoms in children.

Breathing-Related Sleep Disorder

The DSM-IV-TR criteria for breathing-related sleep disorder are presented in Table 29–4.

Obstructive Sleep Apnea

Prevalence.
Although habitual snoring has been reported in as many as 12% of children, the general prevalence of pediatric OSA is approximately 1%–3% (Marcus 2001). The prevalence rates are much higher among children with neuromuscular and craniofacial abnormalities with rates approaching 85% in some children with genetic syndromes (Brooks 2002).

Clinical characteristics.
Symptoms of OSA include persistent snoring, witnessed apneas with gasping for air, restless sleep, and nocturnal diaphoresis. OSA is often the result of adenotonsillar hypertrophy, obesity, sinus problems, or craniofacial abnormalities (Redline et al. 1999). Sleep-disordered breathing has been associated with subjectively reported daytime somnolence and even more commonly with neurocognitive symptoms, including inattention and hyperactivity in children (O'Brien and Gozal 2004). OSA is defined as episodes of complete or partial cessations of airflow for the duration of two respiratory cycles in children and associated with oxygen desaturations or arousals. Polysomnography is recommended to establish a diagnosis of OSA, assess the severity and nature of the sleep-disordered breathing, and (performed before and after treatment) to assess treatment efficacy (American Academy of Pediatrics 2002). Due to serious neurocognitive and physical consequences of OSA, it is very important to recognize and treat it early in life to prevent a negative effect on child development.

Treatment.
The treatment of choice for pediatric OSA is surgery, typically adenotonsillectomy (American Academy of Pediatrics 2002). Postsurgery polysomnography dem-onstrates that adenotonsillectomy is curative in approximately 80% of cases (Lipton and Gozal 2003). Children with allergic rhinitis and/or sinusitis may benefit from inhaled nasal steroids (Brouillette et al. 2001), antihistamines, and decongestants.

Continuous positive airway pressure (CPAP) is recommended for children who have either failed surgical intervention or are not surgical candidates (American Academy of Pediatrics 2002; Marcus et al. 1995). The use of CPAP was recently approved by the FDA for children who are 7 years and older and weigh more than 40 pounds. An attended laboratory titration of CPAP should be performed to determine the effective pressure setting. Supplemental oxygen is not recommended for routine use in children with OSA, due to the risks of developing hypoventilation.

Parasomnias

Prevalence

Parasomnias are much more frequently seen in children than adults and usually represent normal neurophysiology of sleep development. They usually appear at around the second year of life and continue into the preschool or school-age years. Parasomnias are much more prevalent in children with psychiatric and neurological disorders and can be also exacerbated or induced by psychopharmacological agents. Most parasomnias resolve by adolescence.

Clinical Characteristics

Parasomnias represent partial CNS arousals characterized by autonomic and motor activity. Parasomnias like sleepwalking, sleeptalking, night terrors, confusional arousals, and nocturnal enuresis occur during slow-wave sleep. Children usually have no recollection of the nocturnal events on the next day. Nightmares and REM behavior sleep disorder occur in REM sleep and are usually associated with vivid dream recall. Sleepwalking and especially REM behavior sleep disorder are potentially dangerous conditions occasionally associated with injuries to self or others. Parasomnias are highly heritable and usually present in many family members. Although they usually represent a benign developmental condition, parasomnias can be associated with severe sleep disruption and may cause significant family distress and daytime sleepiness.

TABLE 29–4. DSM-IV-TR diagnostic criteria for breathing-related sleep disorder

A. Sleep disruption, leading to excessive sleepiness or insomnia, that is judged to be due to a sleep-related breathing condition (e.g., obstructive or central sleep apnea syndrome or central alveolar hypoventilation syndrome).

B. The disturbance is not better accounted for by another mental disorder and is not due to the direct physiological effects of a substance (e.g., a drug of abuse, a medication) or another general medical condition (other than a breathing-related disorder).

Coding note: Also code sleep-related breathing disorder on Axis III.

Source. Reprinted from American Psychiatric Association: *Diagnostic and Statistical Manual of Mental Disorders,* 4th Edition, Text Revision. Washington, DC, American Psychiatric Association, 2000, p. 622. Used with permission. Copyright © 2000 American Psychiatric Association.

Treatment

The behavioral abnormalities in all of these disorders can be triggered by factors that disrupt sleep. Therefore, strict adherence to sleep hygiene principles is necessary. Children should avoid sleep deprivation, stressful situations, and caffeine close to bedtime. Treatment of other sleep, emotional, and behavioral disorders is known to reduce the frequency and intensity of parasomnias.

In cases of likely self-injury and high parental distress, parental education and reassurance should be provided with the emphasis on preventing injury and helping the child to return to bed. In all cases, removing potentially dangerous objects close to the bedside, such as bedside tables and sharp objects; keeping knives and firearms out of the reach of a child; locking house entrance doors and windows; and installing bedroom alarm devices are examples of safety precautions that parents can take.

In severe cases of parasomnias, medications such as clonazepam (0.01 mg/kg, usual starting dose 0.25 mg qhs), diazepam (0.04–0.25 mg/kg), or lorazepam (0.05 mg/kg) can be considered (Sheldon 2004).

Circadian Rhythm Sleep Disorder

The DSM-IV-TR criteria for circadian rhythm sleep disorder are presented in Table 29–5.

Prevalence

It is estimated that circadian rhythm sleep disorders affect over 10% of children. Delayed sleep-phase syndrome (DSPS) occurs in 5%–10% of adolescents but may begin at a much younger age. Advanced sleep-phase syndrome is more common in preschoolers.

Clinical Characteristics

Circadian rhythm sleep disorders are the disruption of the internal body rhythms that regulate sleep-wake-fulness and are characterized by normal sleep that occurs at the "wrong" time relative to social demands.

DSPS is normally associated with changes seen during puberty in the regulation of sleep homeostasis and the circadian clock. These changes result in the delay of sleep phase in relation to the dark and light cycle. Early rise times on school days create significant sleep deficiency. Adolescents with DSPS present with excessive daytime sleepiness, especially in the morning hours, that results in academic impairment, mood problems, attentional deficits, and family conflict. A recently conducted national survey of sleep patterns and habits among adolescents revealed chronic insufficient sleep during the school week, with a high correlation between sleep loss and depressive symptoms (National Sleep Foundation 2006).

Treatment

Sleep hygiene, family and child education, and the gradual advancement of sleep phase are essential parts of treatment for DSPS. Bright light therapy (5,000–10,000 lux) with morning exposure usually produces phase advancement in several days. Melatonin administered approximately an hour before bedtime helps to facilitate sleep phase advancement. Chronotherapy, another behavioral technique that may be applied to adolescents with severe DSPS, is a gradual delay in bedtime by 3-hour increments until the desired bedtime is reached.

TABLE 29–5. DSM-IV-TR diagnostic criteria for circadian rhythm sleep disorder

A. A persistent or recurrent pattern of sleep disruption leading to excessive sleepiness or insomnia that is due to a mismatch between the sleep-wake schedule required by a person's environment and his or her circadian sleep-wake pattern.

B. The sleep disturbance causes clinically significant distress or impairment in social, occupational, or other important areas of functioning.

C. The disturbance does not occur exclusively during the course of another sleep disorder or other mental disorder.

D. The disturbance is not due to the direct physiological effects of a substance (e.g., a drug of abuse, a medication) or a general medical condition.

Specify type:

.31 **Delayed sleep phase type:** a persistent pattern of late sleep onset and late awakening times, with an inability to fall asleep and awaken at a desired earlier time

.35 **Jet lag type:** sleepiness and alertness that occur at an inappropriate time of day relative to local time, occurring after repeated travel across more than one time zone

.36 **Shift work type:** insomnia during the major sleep period or excessive sleepiness during the major awake period associated with night shift work or frequently changing shift work

.30 **Unspecified type**

Source. Reprinted from American Psychiatric Association: *Diagnostic and Statistical Manual of Mental Disorders,* 4th Edition, Text Revision. Washington, DC, American Psychiatric Association, 2000, p. 629. Used with permission. Copyright © 2000 American Psychiatric Association.

Sleep Problems in Children With Psychiatric Disorders

Attention-Deficit/Hyperactivity Disorder

There is a large body of literature indicating high prevalence of sleep disorders in children with ADHD, based on subjective parental and self-reports and objective instrumental assessments of sleep. Difficulty settling down to sleep, delayed sleep onset with frequent nocturnal awakenings, restless sleep, and reduced total amount of sleep have been reported in children with ADHD. Both behavioral and intrinsic sleep disorders have been associated with symptoms of ADHD. Snoring and OSA have been implicated in the possible pathophysiology of ADHD symptoms in some children. A strong association among RLS, PLMD, and ADHD was shown in a number of studies, with 26%–64% of children with ADHD meeting criteria for PLMD on polysomnography (Picchietti et al. 1998, 1999) and over 44% of children with PLMD having a clinical diagnosis of ADHD (Crabtree et al. 2003).

This high prevalence of sleep disorders in children with ADHD makes sleep assessment an important part of evaluation and treatment of ADHD.

Mood Disorders

Problems with sleep initiation, sleep maintenance, and hypersomnia are some of the most prevalent symptoms among children and adolescents with depressive disorders. Early studies of children with major depression indicated that up to two-thirds of depressed youth reported sleep-onset and sleep-maintenance insomnia, with over half of these children having early morning awakenings with inability to return to sleep (Ivanenko et al. 2005). A longitudinal study of 1,710 adolescents showed that 88% of those with major depressive disorder reported sleep disturbances (Roberts et al. 1995). A more recent study of 553 depressed children assessed with the Interview Schedule for Children and Adolescents—Diagnostic Version revealed that 72.7% had sleep disturbance, 53.5% had insomnia alone, 9% had hypersomnia, and 10.1% had both insomnia and hypersomnia. The degree of sleep dysfunction correlated with the severity of depression, with more sleep-disturbed children having more depressive symptoms and anxiety disorders (Liu et al. 2007). Sleep laboratory studies examining polysomnographic characteristics in children and adolescents with major depressive disorder have found more sleep abnormalities such as longer sleep latency and shorter REM latency in adolescents than in prepubertal children, indicating that maturational factors play a significant role in the pathophysiology of sleep dysfunction associated with major depression.

Autism Spectrum Disorders

Sleep difficulties are estimated to occur in 44%–86% of children with autism or autism spectrum disorders (ASD; Richdale 1999; Stores and Wiggs 1998). The most frequently reported sleep problems in ASD are difficulties falling asleep; frequent nocturnal and early morning awakenings; irregular sleep-wake cycle; restless sleep; and parasomnias such as sleepwalking, night terrors, confusional arousals, and REM behavior sleep disorder. Several hypotheses have been proposed to explain these sleep difficulties including disrupted and poorly entrained circadian rhythms due to failure to recognize social and environmental cues, neurostructural and neurochemical abnormalities involving systems regulating sleep, and altered melatonin production.

Effective behavioral treatments of sleep disorders in children with ASD include sleep hygiene, stimulus control, scheduled nocturnal awakenings, positive bedtime routine, daytime nap restriction, and graduated extinction. Chronotherapy with light therapy and melatonin were studied in children with ASD with demonstrated effectiveness in regulating sleep-wake cycle, improving sleep continuity, and reducing sleep-onset latency (Lord 1998; Malow 2004).

Substance Abuse

Sleep complaints are highly prevalent among adolescents using illicit drugs, alcohol, and cigarettes. The most common sleep-related symptoms in adolescents abusing substances are excessive daytime sleepiness, insomnia, and DSPS. Johnson and Breslau (2001) conducted a survey of 13,831 adolescents ages 12–17 years, which revealed that almost 6% of study participants reported sleep problems, with a dose-dependent relationship between alcohol and illicit drug use and severity and frequency of sleep disturbances. Other psy-

chiatric disorders are frequently comorbid with sleep disorders and substance abuse, making this relationship more complicated, especially when it comes to treatment options. However, the same study indicated that those adolescents with illicit drug abuse history experienced more persistent sleep problems, regardless of other psychiatric comorbidities. A six-session group therapy was formulated and tried in adolescents with substance use disorders and sleep problems that included stimulus control instructions, bright light exposure, sleep hygiene, cognitive therapy, and mindfulness-based stress reduction (Bootzin and Stevens 2005). The results of this study suggested effectiveness of this complex approach for the treatment of sleep problems and drug abuse in adolescents.

Anxiety Disorders

Anxiety and sleep problems are closely tied together, especially during childhood. A longitudinal study of sleep and behavioral and emotional problems revealed that the presence of sleep problems at age 4 is significantly correlated with the development of depression and anxiety by age 15 (Gregory and O'Connor 2002). Children with secure affective attachments to their primary caregivers are significantly less likely to develop sleep problems and will have fewer nighttime awakenings, fewer problems at bedtime, and less excessive daytime sleepiness. It has been shown that higher functioning families with fewer psychiatric difficulties tend to have children who are more cooperative at bedtime and obtain longer sleep throughout the night (Seifer et al. 1996). While most children experience some fears at bedtime, children with anxiety disorders experience far more fear and anxiety at bedtime. Nightmares occur in 75% of 4- to 12-year-old children. However, children who have been exposed to major stressors, including trauma and abuse, have more persistent nightmares, frequently representing flashbacks of their traumatic experiences, with increased levels of autonomic arousal causing awakenings. In addition, children who were abused have significantly poorer sleep efficiency, less quiet sleep, and more nocturnal activity on sleep studies than nonabused children, even when controlling for psychiatric disorders. Systemic desensitization to fears, imagery rehearsal therapy with positive bedtime routines, and cognitive-behavioral therapy have demonstrated efficacy in the treatment of sleep symptoms associated with anxiety disorders.

Summary Points

- Sleep disorders are highly prevalent in children of all ages.

- Children and adolescents with psychiatric conditions have a higher prevalence of sleep disorders.

- Primary sleep disorders may manifest with symptoms of inattention, academic difficulties, poor impulse control, mood changes, excessive daytime sleepiness, and fatigue—resembling symptoms of ADHD, depressive disorders, and learning disabilities.

- Early identification and treatment of sleep disorders are important in improving negative developmental outcomes.

- Referral to the sleep laboratory is indicated for children with suspected sleep-disordered breathing, excessive daytime sleepiness, and parasomnias.

- The first-choice treatment for children with nocturnal anxiety, behavioral insomnia of childhood, and nightmares includes behavioral interventions.

- Pharmacological interventions for children with sleep disturbances should be considered only in the context of behavioral interventions and should preferably be short-term.

References

Allen RA, Picchietti D, Hening WA, et al: Restless legs syndrome: diagnostic criteria, special considerations, and epidemiology: a report from the restless legs syndrome diagnosis and epidemiology workshop at the National Institutes of Health. Sleep Med 4:101–119, 2003

American Academy of Pediatrics, Section of Pediatric Pulmonology, Subcommittee on Obstructive Sleep Apnea Syndrome: Clinical practice guideline: diagnosis and management of childhood obstructive sleep apnea syndrome. Pediatrics 109:704–712, 2002

American Academy of Sleep Medicine: International Classification of Sleep Disorders, 2nd Edition. Westchester, IL, American Academy of Sleep Medicine, 2005

American Psychiatric Association: Diagnostic and Statistical Manual of Mental Disorders, 4th Edition. Washington, DC, American Psychiatric Association, 1994

American Psychiatric Association: Diagnostic and Statistical Manual of Mental Disorders, 4th Edition, Text Revision. Washington, DC, American Psychiatric Association, 2000

Blader JC, Koplewicz HS, Abikoff H, et al: Sleep problems in elementary school children: a community study. Arch Pediatr Adolesc Med 151:473–480, 1997

Bootzin RR, Stevens SJ: Adolescents, substance abuse, and the treatment of insomnia and daytime sleepiness. Clin Psychol Rev 25:629–644, 2005

Brooks LJ: Genetic syndromes affecting breathing during sleep in children, in Sleep Medicine. Edited by Lee-Chiong TL, Sateia MJ, Carskadon MA. Philadelphia, PA, Hanley and Belfus, 2002, pp 305–314

Brouillette RT, Manoukian JJ, Ducharme FM, et al: Efficacy of fluticasone nasal spray for pediatric obstructive sleep apnea. J Pediatr 138:838–844, 2001

Chervin R, Hedger K, Dillon JE, et al: Pediatric Sleep Questionnaire (PSQ): validity and reliability of scales for sleep-disordered breathing, snoring, sleepiness, and behavioral problems. Sleep Med 1:21–32, 2000

Cortese S, Konofal E, Lecendreux M, et al: Restless legs syndrome and attention-deficit/hyperactivity disorder: a review of the literature. Sleep 28:1007–1013, 2005

Crabtree VM, Ivanenko A, O'Brien LM, et al: Periodic limb movement disorder of sleep in children. J Sleep Res 12:73–81, 2003

Drake C, Nickel C, Burduvali E, et al: The Pediatric Daytime Sleepiness Scale (PDSS): sleep habits and school outcomes in middle-school children. Sleep 26:455–458, 2003

Gregory AM, O'Connor TG: Sleep problems in childhood: a longitudinal study of developmental change and association with behavioral problems. J Am Acad Child Adolesc Psychiatry 41:964–971, 2002

Johnson CR: Sleep problems in children with mental retardation and autism. Child Adolesc Psychiatr Clin N Am 5:673–681, 1996

Johnson EO, Breslau N: Sleep problems and substance use in adolescents. Drug Alcohol Depend 64:1–7, 2001

Johnson EO, Roth T, Schultz L, et al: Epidemiology of DSM-IV insomnia in adolescents: lifetime prevalence, chronicity, and an emergent gender difference. Pediatrics 117:247–256, 2006

Ivanenko A, Tauman R, Gozal D: Modafinil in the treatment of excessive daytime sleepiness in children. Sleep Med 4:579–582, 2003

Ivanenko A, Crabtree VM, Gozal D: Sleep and depression in children and adolescents. Sleep Med Rev 9:115–129, 2005

Kuhn BR, Elliott AJ: Treatment efficacy in behavioral pediatric sleep medicine. J Psychosom Res 54:587–597, 2003

Lipton AJ, Gozal D: Treatment of obstructive sleep apnea in children: do we really know how? Sleep Med Rev 7:61–80, 2003

Liu X, Buysse DJ, Gentzler AL, et al: Insomnia and hypersomnia associated with depressive phenomenology and comorbidity in childhood depression. Sleep 30:83–90, 2007

Lord C: What is melatonin? Is it useful treatment for sleep problems in autism? J Autism Dev Disord 28:345–346, 1998

Malow BA: Sleep disorders, epilepsy, and autism. Ment Retard Dev Disabil Res Rev 10:122–125, 2004

Marcus CL: Sleep-disordered breathing in children. Am J Respir Crit Care Med 164:16–30, 2001

Marcus CL, Ward SL, Mallory GB, et al: Use of nasal continuous positive airway pressure as treatment of childhood obstructive sleep apnea. J Pediatr 127:88–94, 1995

Mindell JA: Empirically supported treatments in pediatric psychology: bedtime refusal and night wakings in young children. J Pediatr Psychol 24:465–481, 1999

Mindell JA, Owens JA: Sleep problems in pediatric practice: clinical issues for pediatric nurse practitioner. J Pediatr Health Care 17:324–331, 2003

Mindell JA, Emslie G, Blumer J, et al: Pharmacological management of insomnia in children and adolescents: consensus statement. Pediatrics 117:1223–1232, 2006

Montgomery-Downs HE, Gozal D: Sleep habits and risk factors for sleep-disordered breathing in infants and young toddlers in Louisville, Kentucky. Sleep Med 7:211–219, 2006

Murali H, Kotagal S: Off-label treatment of severe childhood narcolepsy-cataplexy with sodium oxybate. Sleep 29:1025–1029, 2006

National Sleep Foundation: Sleep in America poll, 2006. Washington, DC, National Sleep Foundation, 2006. Available at: http://www.sleepfoundation.org/atf/cf/{F6BF2668-A1B4-4FE8-8D1A-A5D39340D9CB}/2006_summary_of_findings.pdf. Accessed April 26, 2009.

O'Brien LM, Gozal D: Neurocognitive dysfunction and sleep in children: from human to rodent. Pediatr Clin North Am 51:187–202, 2004

Owens J, Spirito A, McGuinn M: The Children's Sleep Habits Questionnaire (CSHQ): psychometric properties of a survey instrument for school-aged children. Sleep 23:1043–1051, 2000a

Owens J, Spirito A, McGuinn M, et al: Sleep habits and sleep disturbance in school-aged children. J Dev Behav Pediatr 21:27–36, 2000b

Picchietti D, England SJ, Walters AS, et al: Periodic limb movement disorder and restless legs syndrome in children with attention-deficit hyperactivity disorder. J Child Neurol 13:588–594, 1998

Picchietti D, Underwood DJ, Farris WA, et al: Further studies on periodic limb movement disorder and restless legs syndrome in children with attention-deficit hyperactivity disorder. Mov Disord 14:1000–1007, 1999

Picchietti D, Allen RP, Walters AS, et al: Restless legs syndrome: prevalence and impact in children and adolescents: the Peds REST study. Pediatrics 120:253–266, 2007

Redline S, Tishler PV, Schluchter M, et al: Risk factors for sleep-disordered breathing in children: association with obesity, race, and respiratory problems. Am J Respir Crit Care Med 159:1527–1532, 1999

Richdale AL: Sleep problems in autism: prevalence, cause and intervention. Dev Med Child Neurol 41:60–66, 1999

Roberts RE, Lewinsohn PM, Seeley JR: Symptoms of DSM-III-R major depression in adolescence: evidence from an epidemiological survey. J Am Acad Child Adolesc Psychiatry 34:1608–1617, 1995

Rona RJ, Li L, Gulliford MC, et al: Disturbed sleep: effects of sociocultural factors and illness. Arch Dis Child 78:20–25, 1998

Seifer R, Sameroff AJ, Dickstein S, et al: Parental psychopathology and sleep variation in children. Child Adolesc Psychiatr Clin N Am 5:715–727, 1996

Sheldon SH: Parasomnias in childhood. Pediatr Clin North Am 51:69–88, 2004

Simakajornboon N, Gozal D, Vlasic V, et al: Periodic limb movements in sleep and iron status in children. Sleep 26:735–738, 2003

Stores G, Wiggs L: Abnormal sleep patterns associated with autism. Autism 2:157–169, 1998

Walters AS, Mandelbaum DE, Lewin DS, et al: Dopaminergic therapy in children with restless legs/periodic limb movements in sleep and ADHD: dopaminergic therapy study group. Pediatr Neurol 22:182–186, 2000

Zero to Three: Diagnostic Classification, 0–3R: Diagnostic Classification of Mental Health and Developmental Disorders of Infancy and Early Childhood, Revised Edition. Arlington, VA, Zero To Three, 2005

PART VIII

SPECIAL TOPICS

Chapter 30

Evidence-Based Practices

John Hamilton, M.D., M.Sc.
Eric Daleiden, Ph.D.

> *The limits of my language are the limits of my mind. All I know is what I have words for.*

> —Ludwig Wittgenstein

Definitions

In the context of child and adolescent psychiatry, evidence-based approaches involve the application of empirical data to the improvement of care and patient outcomes. Evidence-based approaches are based on the notion that not all treatments are equally effective. Various reviews of child and adolescent treatments have found evidence for differential effects of psychopharmacological and psychosocial interventions (e.g., Pappadopulos et al. 2004; Weisz et al. 2004). Two examples of evidence-based approaches are the evidence-based medicine model and the evidence-based practice (EBP) model. EBP is an umbrella term that includes evidence-based medicine but covers a diversity of approaches and professions including psychosocial approaches like empirically supported treatments (Hamilton 2006).

Not surprisingly, various ways to evaluate or "grade" treatments have emerged. Each strategy places differential emphasis on the nature of evidence, study quality, independent replication, cost-effectiveness, potential for harm or benefit, and effectiveness across populations and settings. The main point here is that a simple "yes or no" dichotomy—i.e., "evidence based" or "not evidence-based"—loses much information. This chapter, therefore, does not attempt to set the bar for the adjectival phrase "evidence-based" as applied to a treatment but rather tries to show ideas and examples of how to align daily real-world practice with the evidence base in a feasible way using EBPs.

This chapter also discusses implementation of EBPs in multidisciplinary organizations so that effective psychosocial and psychopharmacological interventions are available for patients with common disorders. Implementation refers to a purposeful set of specific activities for putting defined programs or professional behaviors into practice such that "independent observers can detect its presence and strength" (Fixsen et al. 2005). EBP targets good use of evidence, including patient and family preference, for both psychosocial and psychopharmacological interventions.

Interestingly, most implementation of EBPs has not directly attempted to include so-called nonspecific influences in client-clinician interaction. Although termed "nonspecific" factors because they transcend individual treatments and clinicians, they nevertheless explain a significant proportion of the variance in psychosocial interventions (Shirk and Karver 2003). Such nonspecific influences as the youth's relationship with the provider, warmth and empathy of the provider toward the youth, and the provider's relationship with the parents are important predictors of some aspects of outcome, such as premature termination (Garcia and Weisz 2002). Fortunately, clinicians and organizations can attend to both nonspecific and specific factors affecting outcome (Kendall et al. 1998).

Effective implementation and efficacious treatments must come together in practice to achieve desired youth and family outcomes. EBP is *finding and using feasible treatments proven in the most valid studies to deliver the most rapid, complete, and long-lasting improvement in functioning and symptoms with the least harm.* EBP welcomes the use of clinical expertise in formulating the context of symptoms (Jellinek and McDermott 2004) but sees formulation by itself, separate from active efforts to integrate the literature and local evidence into clinical care, as inadequate.

Historical Notes

In the 1980s, David Sackett and Gordon Guyatt were leaders in publishing a series of iconoclastic articles in the *Canadian Medical Association Journal*. Sackett and Guyatt were especially interested in an empirical approach to the clinical history and examination, an approach that challenged many established practices. Eventually, a series of 25 articles was published in the *Journal of the American Medical Association* from 1993 to 2000 as the "Users' Guides to the Medical Literature," and later published in expanded form (Guyatt and Rennie 2002). This focus on empirical results, an interest in statistics, populations, and the results of randomized trials, began in 1981 but took off when mixed with computers and the Internet in the 1980s and 1990s, becoming known as evidence-based medicine.

In the 1980s and 1990s, child and adolescent psychology and psychiatry were themselves changing markedly. Rapid growth occurred in both medications and empirically supported psychosocial treatments for psychiatric disorders in youth. Advances in diagnostic criteria allowed the study of specific treatment procedures applied to defined symptom clusters. Clearly defined protocols detailed specific treatment procedures. In addition, consumer groups, governments, and other purchasing agents increasingly demanded treatments that "worked," were cost-effective, and minimized harm. Randomized clinical trials and meta-analyses emerged as gold-standard methodologies for resolving scientific disputes.

EBP in child psychiatry confronts the task of bringing these diverse interests, evidence bases, and treatment procedures together and applying the results to improve care for youth.

Finding Evidence

Strategic Search of the Literature

Skills to access and summarize the literature efficiently are essential to implementing EBP. This section suggests how to craft search strategies using available resources: a workable combination of thoroughness and efficiency. Exhaustive thoroughness is worthless if it is not feasible, while inadequate searches may yield misinformation. Resources to perform a search vary enormously, from a team of scholars dedicated to the issue for a year to a single practitioner logging on to public databases with a few minutes before dinner.

The first step in searching the evidence is to identify sources of information. Public, commercial, and hybrid delivery services are available to the practitioner. For example, PubMed is a public service of the U.S. National Library of Medicine, whereas Ovid Technology and EBSCOhost are commercial vendors that sell access to a variety of databases (including full-text access to selected journals). The EBP practitioner must become familiar with multiple databases and arrange to have at least some readily available in the practice setting. Although information sources are constantly evolving, four are especially useful in child and adolescent psychiatry.

MEDLINE

PubMed supplies over 17 million citations from MEDLINE and other life science journals; it includes links to some full-text articles. PubMed is the public site where the database MEDLINE can be accessed, but commercial vendors also support access through their standard interface. MEDLINE uses Medical Index Subject Headings (MeSH) to categorize journal articles. Most importantly, MEDLINE accessed at the PubMed site has a sophisticated Clinical Queries site that is extremely useful in searching for information from only randomized controlled trials (RCTs). If a question primarily concerns the efficacy or potential harm of a therapy or medication, begin at this Clinical Queries site. Here software enables the user to create a highly specific search that will retrieve only RCTs. Use MeSH terms, found on the MeSH Database at the PubMed site. The PubMed "Help" section shows how to "explode" or restrict MeSH subheadings, as well as how to use search tools such as Boolean operators and wild cards. Each database has a tutorial function that explains its wildcards and its thesaurus; these are database specific.

If the subject is one with many RCTs returned in Clinical Queries, look for a meta-analysis around the issue in question. In addition, create branching chains of references from the most useful. Once you find an especially relevant article, enter the author's name in the search box and find other pieces by the same author. Read through the bibliographies of the most relevant articles to find other articles. Also note the MeSH subject term for a reference you find very helpful and use it for an MeSH search. These approaches quickly create an expanding web of relevant references.

PsycINFO

PsycINFO is a database of the American Psychological Association. Over 2,000 journals, 98% peer-reviewed, make up 78% of the database. Books and book chapters and selected dissertations from Dissertation Abstracts International each make up 11%. This database includes abstracts for articles published after 1994. Rather than using MeSH, each abstract is indexed using the thesaurus of Psychological Index Terms, available online, with over 7,900 controlled terms. Each abstract can be indexed with up to 15 terms. In PsycINFO it is possible to search constructs like "identity," "bullying," or "self-esteem" as official Thesaurus terms, which is an advantage over MEDLINE. Full-text access to the American Psychological Association journals in PsycINFO is available for a fee through the PsycARTICLES database.

Journal of the American Academy of Child and Adolescent Psychiatry

The *Journal of the American Academy of Child and Adolescent Psychiatry* (JAACAP) site has some unique advan-

tages. Articles tend to be highly relevant, and the search engine allows both full-text searching and full-text retrieval for American Academy of Child and Adolescent Psychiatry (AACAP) members. Its disadvantages are no dropdown "limits" boxes in the search engine and no controlled vocabulary, and results obtained are limited to a single journal.

Nevertheless, the easy availability of full-text articles and its often high relevance make this Web site useful. For example, a clinician wondering about how much to encourage an adolescent to receive psychotherapy in addition to fluoxetine for generalized anxiety disorder (GAD) recalled that JAACAP had published an RCT on fluoxetine in youth with anxiety disorders. Entering "fluoxetine and anxiety" in JAACAP's search engine, the clinician immediately found the full text of the RCT as the third reference listed and noted the modest effect size on clinical global improvement of 0.26 and no effect on functional outcome (Birmaher et al. 2003). She used these data to remind herself that she should not rely on this medication as the sole treatment.

Cochrane Library and CENTRAL

Cochrane Library's two most relevant databases are Clinical Trials (also called CENTRAL), which is composed of individual controlled trials, and Systematic Reviews. Cochrane Library's Clinical Trials site strives to be complete, with over 350,000 registered controlled trials; importantly, it includes *only* controlled trials and only published trials. Its advantage over a search for RCTs at the PubMed site is that Clinical Trials is more complete. For example, in Cochrane's Clinical Trials, "citalopram" yields 505 references. In MEDLINE via PubMed, "citalopram" searched as an MeSH term plus limits "randomized controlled trial" yields 287. The additional references from CENTRAL reflect its inclusion of databases in addition to MEDLINE.

Search Strategies

1. *Define what you want to know and what resources and time are available.* Start with knowing what databases are available and whether they include full-text articles. Tailor the search to the question. For example, an estimate of how much weight an adolescent on a given dose of olanzapine for a year is likely to gain may be gleaned from a single full-text article in a few minutes. On the other hand, a team of clinicians reviewing the literature on psychotherapies for oppositional defiant disorder (ODD) and seeking to choose the most effective

treatment feasible at their site may need to review multiple databases and many articles to come to a conclusion over the course of months.

2. *Start broad and then go narrow.* Cast a wide net initially—a broad, "sensitive" search retrieving far more references than could be actually read—then tighten the search using explicit "limits" that eliminate some references and retain others. In MED-LINE, consider using the subheadings under MeSH terms to tighten the search. For example, adding "Major" (abbreviated [MAJR]) after the term restricts the search to only those articles where the subject is a major topic heading in that journal article. Using the "Limits" feature in databases also narrows the number of references. Consider specifying only meta-analyses or only RCTs, only a specific age group such as adolescents, or only references from the last 10 years.

3. *Use transparent methods.* A search is transparent if the reader can use the description to achieve the same results at each step. Transparency is highly desirable since it increases credibility and makes redoing searches easy. To create transparency, describe the results for each search term, and then combine sets of references using Boolean operators. Software at search sites can save how many hits (i.e., retrieved references) resulted at each stage and the effects of combining sets and of adding each limit. Avoid adding multiple limits simultaneously since the effect of each limit is then less transparent. "Hand searching" as the final step means visually scanning each reference for relevance and quality. Finally, if a list of authors is searched by name as being especially expert on the subject, then define the explicit inclusion criteria used to make up the list.

4. *Follow leads.* Follow up on any leads and use them to create an expanding chain of relevant references. Often getting a start in the "right" niche in the literature quickly leads to other useful references. For example, after hearing a presentation on trauma-focused cognitive-behavioral therapy (TF-CBT) for adolescents, a clinician wanted to learn more and searched "trauma-focused CBT" in PsycINFO as keywords; of 7 references, 4 concerned youth and 3 were by the same author, Judith A. Cohen. Searching "Cohen, Judith A" as author in PsycINFO's search engine returned 74 articles.

5. *"Browse" if you have time.* Searching MEDLINE regarding the rash due to lamotrigine in bipolar adolescents, a clinician was hand searching individual abstracts (because the number of hits was low) when he found a striking reference (Varghese et al. 2006), a report of cases of rashes so severe they needed hospitalization in a burn unit. This reference would not have appeared in searching only RCTs, yet it suggests extreme caution in using lamotrigine.

6. *Consider using Cochrane Library's guidelines.* If the search is a major effort defining evidence for a program, for example, and the answerable question involves the effects of an intervention, consider applying the methodology suggested in *Cochrane Handbook for Systematic Reviews of Interventions* (Cochrane Library 2008). This handbook contains the methodology used by authors of Cochrane's systematic reviews to search for evidence. This transparent, well-defined, consensus-driven methodology is useful for more definitive searches if time and resources permit.

Literature Summaries: Preappraised Evidence

Practitioners can choose to either evaluate individual studies themselves or rely on other appraisals. In many practice settings, preappraised evidence is most feasible. *Preappraised* means that someone familiar with how to critique a study for bias has already appraised each study for potential flaws:

1. *Cochrane Library's Systematic Reviews.* If the topic is well studied, such as the use of stimulants in attention-deficit/hyperactivity disorder (ADHD), consider starting with Systematic Reviews. All Cochrane Library Systematic Reviews (CLSR) use explicit methodology regarding which studies are included and how results are summarized (Guyatt et al. 2002). Theoretically, this is ideal because someone else has done the hard work of sifting relevant data. In practice, systematic reviews on topics in child psychiatry are often nonexistent or under development and therefore listed as "Protocol."

The CLSR database uses rigorous methods. The purpose of a systematic review is to minimize biases that are common in narrative reviews while conducting research synthesis in a manner that is clear and open to critical assessment. The CLSR therefore sets a high standard for the review of a topic. The standard methodology takes into account the most common flaws in RCTs as well as such issues as the "file drawer" problem (not including unpublished studies). In addition, CLSR publishes its results online with an opportunity for rebuttals. Unfortunately, as yet CLSR has little to offer on common disorders in child psychiatry. The Campbell Collaboration (www.campbellcollaboration.org) and its Register of Interventions and Policy Evaluations (C2-RIPE) database are younger siblings of Cochrane specifically oriented to education, criminal justice, and social welfare rather than health care. They may mature into useful tools for clinicians but currently provide limited content relevant here.

2. *Organizational consensus statements.* Many professional organizations publish practice guidelines. AACAP, the American Psychiatric Association, and the National Institute for Health and Clinical Excellence (NICE) in the United Kingdom all publish guidelines on the Internet. The NICE guidelines (www.nice.org.uk), for example, use the exemplary methodology associated with systematic reviews, but their child psychiatry topics are limited to only the most prevalent disorders, such as ADHD and depression. By definition, a systematic review uses transparent methodology designed to minimize multiple sources of bias. An expert consensus statement differs from a systematic review in that it often includes expert opinion rather than drawing conclusions almost exclusively from published data. Treatment algorithms represent a particularly convenient form of practice guideline that integrate consensus and evidence into prescriptive decision trees or process flow charts (Chorpita et al. 2005b; Kashner et al. 2003).

3. *Evidence-Based Mental Health.* The Internet site for the journal *Evidence-Based Mental Health* contains commentary, including critical appraisal, on many significant studies in adult and child psychiatry. There is a fee to have access to all full-text reviews, but many are available at no charge. Hospitals and universities may subscribe and have access to full-text reviews.

Critical Appraisal

Actually slogging through the time-consuming effort of verifying the methodology of an RCT is often beyond the threshold of most clinicians' ambitions, skills, and available time. However, some groups, such as those in teaching environments in universities, actually do perform these tasks (March et al. 2005). Re-

cent publicly available software makes this task easier (Martin and Srihari 2006). Current guidelines to appraise the quality of an RCT prior to publication have been widely accepted by journal editors and may make critical appraisal by readers of the future less likely to find methodological flaws (Altman et al. 2001). Still, even at top journals, authors have the freedom to draw conclusions and generalize beyond specific study data.

Embedded Information Delivery

A key factor in the use of information is the extent to which it is available at the time a decision is being made. Therefore, information technology has increasingly focused on delivering information when and where it is being used. Evidence-based guidelines and notification systems are becoming increasingly integrated into electronic health record systems, where they appear as prompts on the practitioner's screen. Practitioners are advised to review the information technology they use, so as to identify whether context-sensitive flags, keywords, "smart phrases," or other "tickler" strategies are built into the system. If so, practitioners should understand the source and limitations of such information to promote proper application to each specific patient.

Finding and evaluating evidence is an important step in EBP, but mere exposure to relevant evidence is unlikely to systematically change care practices or improve youth and family outcomes. Implementation of EBPs requires attention to the context of care and use of specific strategies to promote professional development and effective practice.

Implementation

This section focuses on several key issues from the literature on implementing change within organizations.

Practitioners and Organizational Life

Organizations effective at implementing innovations tend to have cultures that include knowledge sharing,

TABLE 30–1. Proven implementation strategies used to implement evidence-based practices (EBPs): examples

Implementation element	Example
Knowledge sharing	Easy-to-use manual (Chorpita 2007) based on exposure is bought for each interested staff member.
Strong visionary leadership	Physician and team leader are committed to EBPs, and coinvestigators are committed to research of EBPs.
Open to experimentation	EBP project is presented as part of an ongoing and necessary "reengineering" process occurring organization-wide.
Available resources	Continuing education money is available to bring in trainers.
Staff training and coaching	External therapist models how to educate anxious youth and parents about exposure in a group setting with therapists observing; PMT trainers offer a 1-day basic course for therapists.
Monitoring and feedback	Team tracks RADS scores in depressed youth and SWAN results in children with attention-deficit/hyperactivity disorder.
Demonstration of positive results	Anxiety-group parents return to individual therapists very pleased, creating enthusiasm in therapists for project.
Alignment of interests with principles of organizational leaders	EBPs are framed as part of reengineering and "matching performance of the best" initiatives of organizational leaders.

Note.   PMT=parent management training; RADS=Reynolds Adolescent Depression Scale; SWAN=SWAN Scale ADHD Rating Form (Swanson 2004).

strong leadership with a clear strategic vision, visionary staff in key positions, openness to experimentation and risk taking, available "extra" resources, available staff training and coaching, and effective monitoring and feedback systems (Fixsen et al. 2005; Greenhalgh et al. 2004). Practitioners create their own context by giving meanings to what they perceive within their work setting and by choosing what to initiate and how to respond to expectations within their organizational culture (Dopson and Fitzgerald 2005). Like others working in organizations, clinicians find their mental life alternates between moments when they experience the often chaotic flux of a complex organization and moments when they assign meaning to the events unfolding. The meanings players assign to events (in this case, efforts to implement EBPs) are crucial.

Table 30–1 illustrates a practitioner-driven effort to increase use of EBPs at a clinic in a large prepaid health plan. The table adds two additional elements: framing the project as consistent with current initiatives from high-level management and demonstrating positive results to therapists early on in the project. If well-defined evidence-based programs do not already exist within a clinician's organization or practice, individual professionals can nevertheless strive to align their knowledge, skills, and behaviors with state-of-the-art practices as well as work to change an organization to be more aligned with the evidence.

Defining the Overall Context With Who, What, and How

Three elements define the context of initiatives to implement evidence-based processes:

- First, who's involved? Each level of an organization may rely on different sources of evidence and value different outcomes. For example, administrators may monitor access and satisfaction surveys, whereas practitioners in the same system may attend to how quickly patients report feeling better.
- Second, what is considered evidence? What constitutes evidence and who gets to define evidence are at the heart of many debates about the value and relevance of EBP (Westen et al. 2004), and a variety of systems to rate evidence are available. These rating systems use such factors as proper randomization and use of an active control (not a waiting list), number of replications, effectiveness across populations, settings, time, cost-effectiveness, beneficial versus harmful effects, and certainty about the size of these effects.

- A third critical element of evidence-based initiatives is how treatments are defined at the level of treatment families, specific protocols, or practices within protocols (Figure 30–1). A *treatment family* is a set of protocols that share common features or mechanisms of action, similar to a class of medications. *Specific protocols* describe the treatment activities (e.g., procedures, sequence, and dosage) that were actually tested in research studies: this is the familiar "manualized" approach to a specific disorder. A common practices approach analyzes specific protocols into more elementary components of practice and then aggregates these components across studies to identify common elements. Figure 30–1 illustrates these three strategies for specifying the "how" of EBP for anxiety and avoidant problems (Chorpita and Daleiden 2007).

The common practices approach is called the *core component method* or *distillation and matching* because the common core components effective in many different manualized treatments for the same class of problems have been "distilled" to choose only those elements proven to be present in many of the manuals with demonstrated efficacy for that class of problems. They can then be matched to individual clients. Grouping core components of efficacious treatments using these ideas has important implications for the aggregation of findings across studies and the application of evidence to guide adaptation of treatment procedures to the local context (Chorpita et al. 2005a).

Specific Leverage Points Within an Organization

The *context* of organizational life is critically important in planning and carrying out implementation. Figure 30–2 further "unpacks" this overburdened concept. Although contexts may be described by many parameters and care processes differ dramatically by context, the model in Figure 30–2 provides a convenient heuristic for further discussion beyond "who and how." At the broadest levels, context includes the regulatory, funding, and working environment where the professional is functioning. Consider now the contextual factors of Figure 30–2 individually, beginning with pretreatment and interventions and then working toward broader and less immediate aspects of context.

Pretreatment Points of Contact

Often parents or youth have contact with a system prior to seeing a clinician. Some clinics, for example,

offer an orientation session for parents before their child sees a clinician. The orientation explains eligibility rules and educates, informs, and motivates parents, and often adolescents as well, about what to expect and the kinds of treatment available for common disorders. Integrating evidence-based content into such frontline presentations where potential clients and care systems initially make contact can create demand for EBPs and promote a match between client characteristics and effective treatment. Youth and families may then help maintain EBPs by asking for and expecting services supported by evidence when they do arrive at clinicians' offices.

What to Treat and How

Assessment instruments are readily available to improve the assessment of general functioning, as well as symptoms of various dimensions of psychopathology. Thus, one obvious application of the evidence base to the assessment process is the selection of well-validated instruments, since assessment is essential for developing a client-specific evidence base and evaluating care. The assessment process itself is a great opportunity to introduce EBP recommendations into the care process and to define intervention targets for monitoring.

The assessment, diagnosis, and case formulation processes guide decisions about what to treat and how to treat. In fact, the formalization and wide-scale adoption of structured diagnostic systems have promoted a literature and funding structure often organized around diagnostic categories. In addition, many meta-analyses and systematic reviews use these categories in aggregating studies.

Although diagnosis is often a good place to start in matching treatments to a particular client's circumstances, careful consideration of the match between what clients say is important to them and outcomes documented in studies is essential to serve the best interests of youth and families. Fortunately, the evaluation of multiple outcomes is becoming more common in clinical trials. For example, the Multimodal Treatment Study of Children With ADHD (MTA) measured 19 outcomes ranging from ADHD symptoms to parent-child relations to academic achievement (MTA Cooperative Group 1999). In choosing an appropriate treatment, it is important to know what the youth and family want to achieve (e.g., better grades) and choose treatments that achieve that outcome. The distinction between the target population (e.g., all adolescents with major depressive disorder) and the outcome domain (e.g., improved school functioning) is critical in

1. Treatment Families
    Cognitive-Behavioral Therapy (27 Protocols)
    Education (3 Protocols)
    Exposure (29 Protocols)
    Modeling (9 Protocols)

2. Specific Protocols (4 examples from the 72 study groups with practices summarized below)
    Kendall, P. C., Hedtke, K. A. (2006). Cognitive-behavioral therapy for anxious children: Therapist manual (3rd Ed.). Ardmore, PA: Workbook Publishing.

    Klingman, A., Melamed, B. G., Cuthbert, M. I., Hermecz, D. A. (1984). Effects of participant modeling on information acquisition and skill utilization. Journal of Consulting and Clinical Psychology 52, 414–422.

    March, J. S., Mulle, K. (1998). OCD in children and adolescents: A cognitive behavioral treatment manual. New York, NY: Guilford.

    Wilson, N. H., Rotter, J. C. (1986). Anxiety management training and study skills counseling for students on self-esteem and test anxiety and performance. School Counselor, 34, 18–31.

3. Common Practices

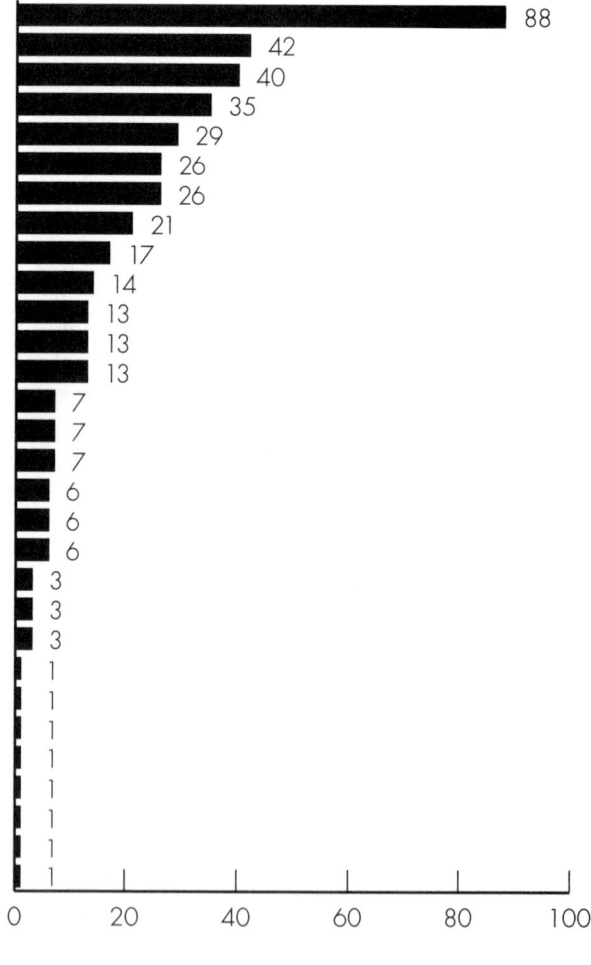

Percentage of study groups using the practice (N = 72)

FIGURE 30–1.   Three ways to describe those practices receiving Level I (Best Support) for anxiety and avoidant problems of youth (Chorpita and Daleiden 2007).

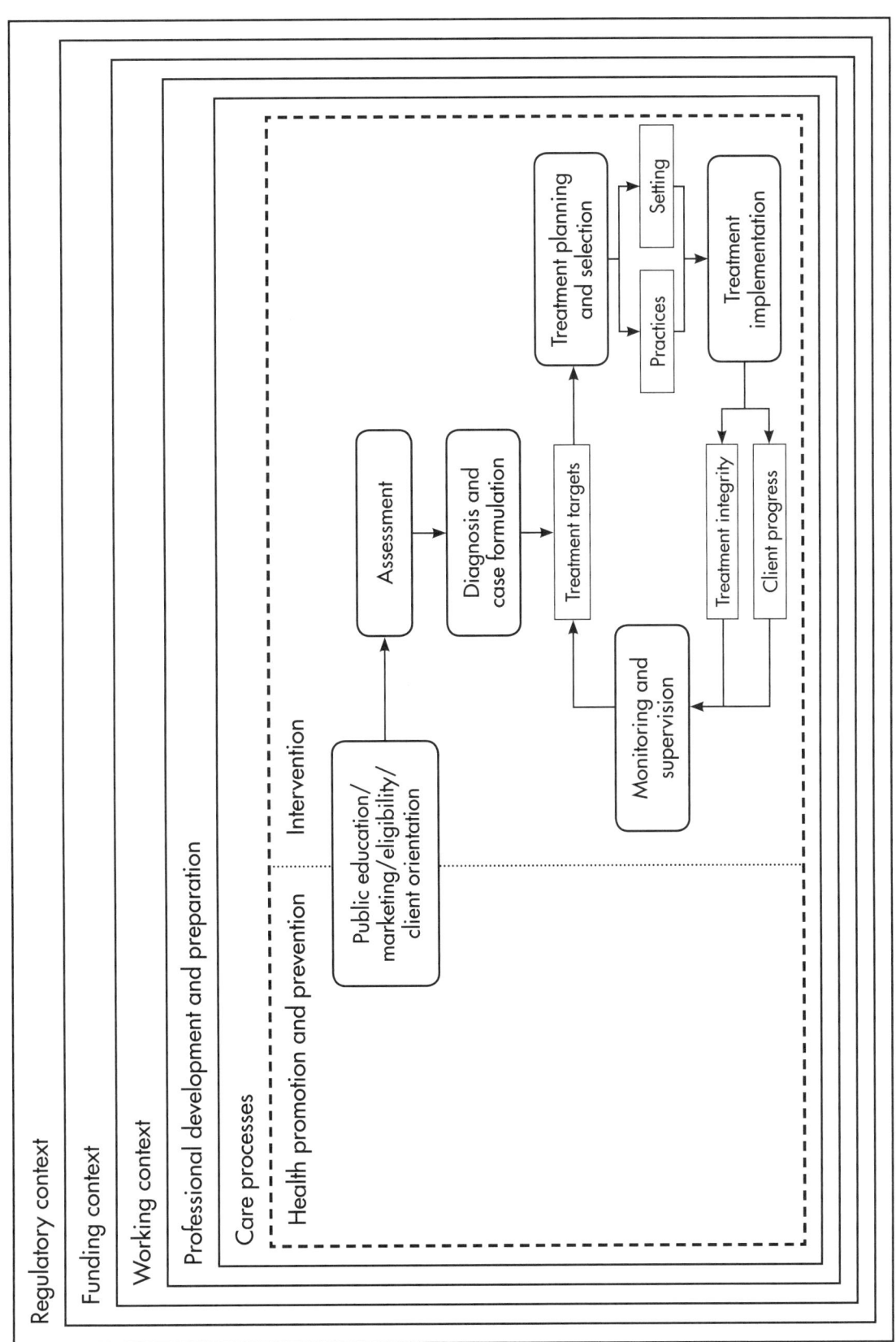

FIGURE 30–2. Multiple organizational contexts impact implementation of evidence-based practices.

TABLE 30–2. Level of evidence supporting varied interventions for anxious/avoidant behaviors

Problem area	Level 1/ Best support	Level 2/ Good support	Level 3/ Moderate support	Level 4/ Minimal support	Level 5/ No support
Anxious or avoidant behaviors	Cognitive-behavioral therapy (CBT); education, exposure, modeling	Assertiveness training, CBT and medication; CBT with parents; hypnosis; relaxation	None	Biofeedback; play therapy, psychodynamic therapy; rational emotive therapy	Client-centered therapy; eye movement desensitization and reprocessing; relationship counseling; teacher psychoeducation

Source. Adapted from the Child and Adolescent Mental Health Division 2007.

finding and applying the intervention literature. In addition to specifying treatment targets, case formulation should involve specifying the working etiological model of the client's symptoms. Fortunately, well-supported EBPs are often associated with specific causal models of change.

Not Simply Picking a "Good Manualized Treatment" and Doing It

The traditional evidence-based treatment approach has been closely aligned to the treatment selection decision: if a clinician has a convenient list of interventions supported by evidence and listed by problem area, then the clinician can easily review treatment options. Such a list of empirically supported treatments has been a primary product of the evidence-based treatment literature reviews (e.g., Chambless et al. 1996). Because interventions in such reviews are usually defined as specific, manualized treatment protocols, selection of a specific manual or protocol often determines other common clinical decisions, such as the sequencing of interventions, and how to monitor progress and measure adherence to treatment.

Hawaii's Child and Adolescent Mental Health Division (2007) posts on the Internet its "blue menu," a one-page summary of interventions at the treatment-family level for common disorders based on the quality of evidence supporting each. The "blue menu" is useful in uniting multiple stakeholders—parents, youth, providers, and others—around the evidence. For example, the portion of the table referring to youth with anxiety disorders is shown in Table 30–2.

Note that the focus in Table 30–2 is a "problem area" rather than a diagnosis. The levels of support are modifications of the American Psychological Association's ranking system. Note also in Table 30–2 that cells contain treatment procedures classified by type (e.g., CBT, biofeedback) rather than a specific, branded therapy with a specific manual. As noted earlier (see Figure 30–1), analyzing therapeutic elements that consistently show up as the common elements across multiple manuals of effective treatments (e.g., exposure for anxiety used in 88% of study groups across treatment families) *allows the distillation of multiple manuals into a single set of therapeutic activities* (Chorpita et al. 2005a). Common elements have also been called core components because they result from an analysis of known effective treatments for specific problem areas. Organizational efforts to implement EBPs may be aided by incorporating core components rather than exclusively focusing on entire manuals; this may help bypass some practitioners' resistance to manuals (Kendall et al. 1998).

Delivering Care

Selecting a good treatment is not the same as doing a good treatment. The litmus test for treatment implementation is whether an independent observer reviewing a session could detect the occurrence of the evidence-based activities (Fixsen et al. 2005). Thus, a treatment protocol or practice needs to translate into specific practitioner behaviors. Practitioners must have the capacity to perform the behaviors (e.g., knowledge, materials, and tools) and the discipline to execute the behaviors in each session. How does a single person or group of individuals motivated to use EBPs move toward that goal?

Establishing a readily accessible library of treatment materials is a key piece of EBP infrastructure. For example, having a readily available selection of manuals on doing CBT in anxious youth is useful for practitioners trying to implement EBPs for anxious youth. In addition to material access, practitioners must become knowledgeable about the content of treatment protocols and recall that knowledge during the treatment session. Knowledge may be developed by reading materials and searching the Internet, attending training, and role-playing treatment practices. For example, a Web site applicable to youth exposed to trauma includes specific, step-by-step instructions for each component of therapy, printable sample scripts for introducing concepts and techniques to clients, and streaming video demonstrations of the therapy procedures, as well as continuing education credits (Medical University of South Carolina 2007). Finally, recalling knowledge and applying skills within treatment sessions may be facilitated through the use of prepared materials, memory tickler systems, and on-the-job coaching.

Treatment developers have also worked to redesign treatment protocols to increase their accessibility and adaptability within treatment sessions. For example, a well-studied manualized treatment for depression, the Adolescent Coping With Depression course, provides a curriculum and detailed specification for each treatment session and is also available on the Internet (Lewinsohn et al. 1990). The core components approach was also developed in part to increase practitioner knowledge about the content of treatment protocols and to support EBP implementation by promoting learning of reusable practices. Using modular design techniques (Chorpita et al. 2005b), a modern manual for problems with anxiety offers an approach to bringing the core components of empirically supported treatments into busy clinics in a feasible way, including handouts, records, and worksheets that can be reproduced (Chorpita 2007). Thanks to the generosity of many treatment developers, these new resources make many more EBPs feasible in most settings. These include Internet-based continuing education unit teaching with streaming videos, Internet-based sophisticated workbooks for depressed adolescents at no cost, and the new focus on core components rather than intact, full-scale manuals.

Patients' gains reinforce initial efforts to learn EBPs. The acceptance of TF-CBT increased over time as clinicians and supervisors both gained experience and saw clients improve (Hoagwood et al. 2007). Parent management training (PMT) trainers report similar results: once clinicians try showing parents of youth with ODD how to praise their children effectively for the "positive opposite" (i.e., desired behavior) and children begin to change, therapists become enthusiastic about PMT.

Monitoring and Supervision

Monitoring refers to the measurement and review of such aspects of treatment as patient progress, treatment practices, and fidelity to supported practices. Practitioners can use the resulting data to reflect whether their patients are improving, what practice habits are forming, and how often their treatments are faithful to proven treatment elements. Studies repeatedly support the value of monitoring and feedback (Fixsen et al. 2005). Preliminary evidence also suggests that large-scale implementation of EBPs within a system of care based in part on ongoing monitoring for individual cases may significantly improve youth and family outcomes (Daleiden et al. 2006). Monitoring outcome also contributes to the effectiveness of using a medication algorithm for depressed youth in improving outcomes compared to a historical control (Emslie et al. 2004). Monitoring can also include treatment integrity: the type and quality of the practices implemented and adherence of actual care practices to the planned treatment using self-report, chart review, observation, or taping. A focus on monitoring adherence to evidence-based treatments, for example, can add to a peer supervision group of practitioners.

Many research studies are conducted with ongoing client monitoring and supervision of practitioners. Fixsen et al. (2005) review striking evidence that on-the-job coaching is a critical component for generalizing behavior from training and role-play sessions to actual intervention sessions. For example, direct supervision by an expert in the specific treatments being administered is ideal, but peer consultation, periodic self-review of session audiotapes or videotapes, targeted searching and reading in the context of specific clinical decisions, targeted input from lecturers at regional and national meetings, training videos, and instructional Web sites are also useful.

Funding Context

Funding mechanisms and availability also differ markedly across contexts. Many funding sources do not reimburse EBPs differently than usual care, and some funding sources provide only temporary funding to encourage initiating EBPs. In one context, large closed-staff health maintenance organizations (HMOs) rely primarily on prepayments from a defined population rather than income from billing procedures. Clinicians at such HMOs therefore operate in a context more like the National Health Service in the United Kingdom or other locales with a nationalized system of health care: reimbursement in the usual sense has a minimal role, allowing some flexibility in developing programs without concern about unit-cost reimbursement. In this prepaid context, delivering high service volumes and timely access to services that promote consumer satisfaction is critical to ensuring economic viability and administrative support for evidence-based programs.

Professional Development and Preparation

Client-practitioner interactions remain at the heart of behavioral health care practices. Supportive contexts, program policies, and integrated information delivery are organizational tools for increasing the use of evidence. These tools capitalize on the unique expertise that both clients (experts in their goals and histories) and practitioners (experts in assessment, psychopathology, and treatment) bring to this interaction. Continuing education and active communication with networks of professional peers help practitioners maintain their expertise and bring it to patient encounters (Davis 1998; Rogers 2003).

Research Directions

Several research areas related to using EBPs are especially promising in their potential to influence the public health of youth:

1. Electronic medical records now allow researchers easier access to data of all kinds relevant to EBP, including patterns of medication use by practitioner and by diagnosis. Research in how to use these data to enhance practice in systems will be important.
2. Common protocols that address multiple youth problems are needed to address the feasibility challenge of having a different treatment program for each youth problem. One approach is the development of "multiple problem" treatment manuals. An ongoing study, for example, by the Network on Youth Mental Health, sponsored by the John D. and Catherine T. MacArthur Foundation, is testing three conventional, evidence-based treatment manuals versus a multiproblem modular manual that allows individualization guided by an algorithm.
3. Recent reviews (e.g., Fixsen et al. 2005; Greenhalgh et al. 2004) have highlighted the importance of treatment implementation and identified key factors for promoting changes in care. Continued study of practice development activities, supervision activities, organizational structure, and funding mechanisms is needed.
4. Promising research is examining professional networks to promote EBP and research, such as the CAPTN (Child and Adolescent Psychiatry Trials Network).
5. Further research into combining medication and psychosocial intervention into a common treatment platform in real-world settings is needed, especially for youth with multiple comorbid disorders (when so much evidence is based on focal disorders).

Summary Points

- EBP is not an end in itself but rather a tool to achieve better outcomes more often and more quickly.
- In practitioners' offices, both effective implementation and efficacious treatments are needed to achieve desired outcomes.
- Think about implementation as a "play within a play": practitioners' behavior that is faithful to treatments known to "work" is the play you watch within the larger play of a service delivery system making efforts to improve care through proven implementation drivers like practice-based coaching, facilitative administrators, and reminders.
- Agreeing where to set the bar to qualify as "evidence-based" can be a useful discussion in defining a hierarchy of evidence acceptable to all stakeholders.
- Anticipate disputes about what evidence is.

- Overly rigid definitions of EBP—such as expecting exhaustive worldwide searches in everyday clinical work—alienate practitioners and generate a reputation for infeasibility.

- Use the Clinical Queries section of PubMed to retrieve results from RCTs and find results efficiently.

- Implementation is primarily a social process. You're convincing a social network as well as individual practitioners.

- Periodically ask a colleague to review your treatment notes or a taped session. Ask him or her to comment on how much of the time you are using EBPs during sessions.

References

Altman D, Schulz KF, Moher D, et al: The revised CONSORT statement for reporting randomized trials: explanation and elaboration. Ann Intern Med 134:663–694, 2001

Birmaher B, Axelson DA, Monk K, et al: Fluoxetine for the treatment of childhood anxiety disorders. J Am Acad Child Adolesc Psychiatry 42:415–423, 2003

Chambless DL, Baker MJ, Baucom DH, et al: An update on empirically validated therapies. Clin Psychol 49:5–18, 1996

Child and Adolescent Mental Health Division: "Blue menu"—evidence-based child and adolescent psychosocial interventions. Honolulu, HI, Child and Adolescent Mental Health Division, Hawaii State Department of Health, 2007. Available at: http://www.hawaii.gov/health/mental-health/camhd/library/pdf/ebs/ebs022.pdf. Accessed January 2, 2008.

Chorpita BF: Modular Cognitive-Behavioral Therapy: Guides to Individualized Evidence-Based Treatment. New York, Guilford, 2007

Chorpita BF, Daleiden EL: Biennial Report: Effective Psychosocial Interventions for Youth With Behavioral and Emotional Needs. Honolulu, HI, Child and Adolescent Mental Health Division, Hawaii Department of Health, 2007. Available at: http://www.hawaii.gov/health/mental-health/camhd/library/pdf/ebs/ebs012.pdf. Accessed January 2, 2008.

Chorpita BF, Daleiden EL, Weisz JR: Identifying and selecting the common elements of evidence-based interventions: a distillation and matching model. Ment Health Serv Res 7:5–20, 2005a

Chorpita BF, Daleiden EL, Weisz JR: Modularity in the design and application of therapeutic interventions. Appl Prev Psychol 21:1–16, 2005b

Cochrane Handbook for Systematic Reviews of Interventions Version 5.0.0 [updated February 2008]. The Cochrane Collaboration, 2008. Available at: http://www.cochrane.org/resources/handbook. Accessed January 6, 2008.

Daleiden EL, Chorpita BF, Donkervoet C, et al: Getting better at getting them better: health outcomes and evidence-based practice within a system of care. J Am Acad Child Adolesc Psychiatry 45:749–756, 2006

Davis D: Does CME work? An analysis of the effect of educational activities on physician performance or health care outcomes. Int J Psychiatr Med 29:21–39, 1998

Dopson S, Fitzgerald L: The active role of context, in Knowledge to Action? Evidence-Based Health Care in Context. Edited by Dopson S, Fitzgerald L. Oxford, UK, Oxford University Press, 2005, pp 79–103

Emslie GJ, Hughes CW, Crismon ML, et al: A feasibility study of the childhood depression medication algorithm: the Texas Children's Medication Algorithm Project (CMAP). J Am Acad Child Adolesc Psychiatry 43:519–527, 2004

Fixsen D, Naoom SF, Blase KA, et al: Implementation Research: A Synthesis of the Literature (FMHI Publication #231). Tampa, FL, University of South Florida, Louis de la Parte Florida Mental Health Institute, The National Implementation Research Network, 2005

Garcia JA, Weisz JR: When youth mental health care stops: therapeutic relationship problems and other reasons for ending youth outpatient treatment. J Consult Clin Psychol 70:439–443, 2002

Greenhalgh T, Robert G, Bate P, et al: How to spread good ideas: a systematic review of the literature on diffusion, dissemination, and sustainability of innovations in health service delivery and organisation, 2004. Available at: http://www.sdo.nihr.ac.uk/files/project/38-final-report.pdf. Accessed April 21, 2009.

Guyatt GH, Rennie D (eds): Users' Guides to the Medical Literature: A Manual for Evidence-Based Clinical Practice. Chicago, IL, American Medical Association Press, 2002

Guyatt GH, Hayward R, Richardson WS, et al: Moving from evidence to action, in Users' Guide to the Medical Literature: A Manual for Evidence-Based Clinical Practice. Edited by Guyatt GH, Rennie D. Chicago, IL, American Medical Association Press, 2002, pp 175–199

Hamilton J: Evidence-based practice for outpatient clinical teams. J Am Acad Child Adolesc Psychiatry 45:364–370, 2006

Hoagwood K, Vogel JM, Levitt JM, et al: Implementing an evidence-based trauma treatment in a state system after September 11: the CATS project. J Am Acad Child Adolesc Psychiatry 46:773–779, 2007

Jellinek M, McDermott J: Formulation: putting the diagnosis into a therapeutic context and treatment plan. J Am Acad Child Adolesc Psychiatry 43:913–916, 2004

Kashner TM, Carmody TJ, Suppes T, et al: Catching up on health outcomes: The Texas Medication Algorithm Project. Health Serv Res 38:311–331, 2003

Kendall PC, Hedtke KA: Cognitive-Behavioral Therapy for Anxious Children: Therapist Manual. Ardmore, PA, Workbook Publishing, 2006

Kendall PC, Chu B, Gifford A, et al: Breathing life into a manual: flexibility and creativity with manual-based treatments. Cogn Behav Pract 5:177–198, 1998

Klingman A, Melamed BG, Cuthbert MI, et al: Effects of participant modeling on information acquisition and skill utilization. J Consult Clin Psychol 52:414–422, 1984

Lewinsohn P, Clarke GN, Hops H, et al: Cognitive-behavioral group treatment of depression in adolescents. Behav Ther 21:385–401, 1990

March JS, Chrisman A, Breland-Noble A, et al: Using and teaching evidence-based medicine: the Duke University Child and Adolescent Psychiatry Model. Child Adolesc Psychiatr Clin N Am 14:273–296, 2005

Martin A, Srihari V: Geometrically evident: framing studies using the Graphic Appraisal Tool for Epidemiology (GATE). J Am Acad Child Adolesc Psychiatry 45:1521–1526, 2006

Medical University of South Carolina: TF-CBT Web: A Web-Based Learning Course for Trauma-Focused Cognitive-Behavioral Therapy. Charleston, Medical University of South Carolina, 2007. Available at: http//tfcbt.musc.edu. Accessed January 6, 2008.

MTA Cooperative Group: A 14-month randomized clinical trial of treatment strategies for attention-deficit/hyperactivity disorder. Arch Gen Psychiatry 56:1073–1086, 1999

Pappadopulos EA, Tate Guelzow B, Wong C, et al: A review of the growing evidence base for pediatric psychopharmacology. Child Adolesc Psychiatric Clin N Am 23:817–855, 2004

Rogers EM: Diffusion of Innovations, 5th Edition. New York, Free Press, 2003

Shirk SR, Karver M: Prediction of treatment outcome from relationship variables in child and adolescent therapy: a meta-analytic review. J Clin Consult Psychol 71:452–464, 2003

Swanson J: SWAN Rating Scale. University of California, Irvine, 2004. Available at: http://www.adhd.net. Accessed January 6, 2008.

Varghese W, Haith LR, Patton ML, et al: Lamotrigine-induced toxic epidermal necrolysis in three patients treated for bipolar disorder. Pharmacotherapy 26:699–704, 2006

Weisz JR, Hawley KM, Doss AJ: Empirically tested psychotherapies for youth internalizing and externalizing problems and disorders. Child Adolesc Psychiatr Clin N Am 13:729–815, 2004

Westen D, Novotny CM, Thompson-Brenner H: The empirical state of empirically supported psychotherapies: assumptions, findings, and reporting in controlled clinical trials. Psychol Bull 130:631–663, 2004

Chapter 31

Child Abuse and Neglect

Paramjit T. Joshi, M.D.
Peter T. Daniolos, M.D.
Jay A. Salpekar, M.D.

Child abuse continues to be a serious pediatric and social problem all over the world. Although earlier studies attempted to separate the impact of physical from sexual abuse, contemporary research is focusing on the impact of polyvictimization, as it is the rare child who experiences only one type of abuse. It has become clear that the worst outcomes are seen in children who experience a multitude of adversities and that such youth are most likely to experience poor mental and physical health. Prevention efforts, timely intervention, and fostering resiliency of abused children can help mitigate some of the long-term effects of abuse.

Definitions

In the Child Abuse Prevention, Adoption, and Family Services Act of 1988, *physical abuse* was defined as "the physical injury of a child under 18 years of age by a person who is responsible for the child's welfare, under circumstances which indicate that the child's health or welfare is harmed or threatened" (Kaplan et al. 1998). For the National Incidence Study, physical abuse was defined as being present when a child younger than age 18 experiences nonaccidental injury (harm standard) or risk of injury (endangerment standard) as a result of having been hit with a hand or other object or having been kicked, shaken, thrown, burned, stabbed, or choked by a parent or parent substitute (Sedlak and Broadhurst 1996). *Child neglect* is differentiated from child abuse and refers to the failure of the responsible caretaking adults to provide adequate physical care and supervision.

Sexual abuse most commonly refers to any activity within a spectrum ranging from inappropriate physical touching to sexual intercourse or rape. For decades, child sexual abuse has eluded specific definition, despite the efforts of researchers, therapists, and child advocates (Haugaard 2000). Important considerations include the wide range of normal sexual behavior and development among children and adolescents (Ryan 2000). Children may exhibit a wide range of sexual behaviors, even in circumstances where abuse may not be present (Friedrich et al. 1998). Eroticized behavior, increased sexual interest, and sexual play may result from numerous influences beyond potential abuse, including inadvertent observation of adults engaged in sexual activity, oedipal fantasies, manic or hypomanic states, or exposure to pornographic materials and television (Yates 1997). *Sexual play* generally involves mutually interested children at similar ages and developmental stages and does not involve coercion (American Academy of Pediatrics Committee on Child Abuse and Neglect 1999). *Incest* refers to the sexual abuse of children within the context of the nuclear family, generally involving sexual activity between a parent and child or among siblings.

Legal definitions of sexual abuse generally involve sexual contact between an adult and a minor child (Green 1997). If both the perpetrator and the victim are minors, abuse can be understood to have occurred if there is a significant discrepancy in age or there is coercion. Some have defined age discrepancies of 4–5 years as being more definitive for an abuse scenario, but there is not a commonly accepted age difference defining abuse of a minor by another minor.

Epidemiology

The work of Kempe et al. (1962), who first described the battered child syndrome, led to the recognition of child abuse as a major pediatric, psychiatric, and social problem. By 1965, child protective services were established throughout the United States, and laws were passed that required medical reporting and legal investigation of child abuse and neglect. However, sexual abuse still appears to be significantly underreported. A report issued by the National Child Abuse and Neglect Data System of the U.S. Department of Health and Human Services in 2001 noted that the overall number of children victimized by child abuse and neglect has continued to decrease since 1993. Reasons for this decline are not well understood. Parents continue to be the main perpetrators. Almost 60% of all victims experienced neglect, whereas 21.3% experienced physical abuse and 11.3% were sexually abused (U.S. Department of Health and Human Services 2001a, 2001b).

The number of child fatalities caused by maltreatment remains unchanged, with younger children at greatest risk, especially those under age 3 years (Kaplan et al. 1999) and boys. Other risk factors include having been born to a mother under 21 years of age, non-European American ethnicity, or products of multiple births. Homicides occurring during the first week of life are almost exclusively perpetrated by mothers. Mothers and fathers were equally likely to fatally injure their children ages 1 week to 13 years. However, fathers committed 63% of parent-perpetrated homicides among 13- to 15-year-olds and were responsible for 80% of those occurring in 16- to 19-year-olds (Kuntz and Bahr 1996).

Some studies report that 10%–25% of girls are sexually victimized in some manner before age 18 (Fergusson et al. 1996). The most common age of initial sexual abuse is 8–11 years. Male parents or male parent figures continue to be the most common perpetrators of sexual abuse. Women are reported as abusers in a distinct minority of cases, and adolescents are reported to be the perpetrators in 20% of cases (American Academy of Pediatrics Committee on Child Abuse and Neglect 1999).

Sexual abuse of boys has been less well studied and may be more significantly underreported and untreated. Boys seem less likely to disclose sexual abuse, generally for fear of disbelief, retribution, or social stigma and reluctance to admit vulnerability (Holmes and Slap 1998). Perpetrators of sexual abuse against boys are most likely to be male and unrelated to the victim. Studies have also shown that sexually abused boys are more likely to ultimately express a homosexual identity compared with boys without such a history. However, if the perpetrator is female, boys may be even more disinclined to report abuse and less likely to be supported by caregivers when abuse is reported (Holmes and Slap 1998).

Etiology

Most experts believe that physical and sexual abuse results from a combination of factors within both parents and children, in conjunction with their specific environment, with youth from single-parent and step-families having higher rates of victimization. Single-parent household risk was linked to lower socioeconomic status and violent neighborhoods and schools (Turner et al. 2007). Child abuse tends to occur in multiproblem families with significant instability and characterological or personality disorder in the parents. Other risk factors include parental mental illness, substance abuse, lack of social support, poverty, minority ethnicity, lack of acculturation, presence of four or more children in a family, young parental age, stressful events, and exposure to family violence. While sexual abuse is prevalent in all socioeconomic classes, physical abuse and neglect may be more common in lower socioeconomic classes. However, abusers have racial, religious, and ethnic distributions similar to those of the general population (Fergusson et al. 1996; Ryan 2000). Risk factors in the child include prematurity, mental retardation, and physical handicaps (Cicchetti and Toth 1995). Children with cognitive deficits may have impaired judgment and decreased ability to verbally communicate feelings.

Perpetrators have a wide variety of character and personality pathology. However, a common theme among abusers is that they regard their victims not as independent beings but instead as narcissistic extensions of themselves, existing only for the purposes of their own gratification (Glasser et al. 2001). Abusers select children based on age, gender, and physical characteristics that match their own appearance or age when they were first abused. Abusers have been described as passive and inadequate in most aspects of their lives; contact with children gives them feelings of power and control. Sexual perpetrators may associate themselves with events or circumstances where they have access to children. Examples include youth group activities, schools, recreational facilities, or locations near playgrounds or other areas that youth may frequently be found. Abusers may seek to "groom" victims, offering them gifts or money in order to gain their trust prior to engaging in any abusive behavior. Perpetrators are usually gender specific regarding their victims; those who select both male and female victims may have more severe psychopathology (Hilton and Mezey 1996). Victimization by known perpetrators is generally more common than sexual abuse from an unknown or extrafamilial source.

Approximately 30%–50% of the instances of sexual abuse and 15% of those arrested for forcible rape are perpetrated by those under age 18, most initially engaging in abusive acts before age 15 (American Academy of Child and Adolescent Psychiatry 1999). In a study by Ryan (2000), nearly 40% of abusive youth reported having been sexually abused themselves. More than 60% were known to school systems as having problems with truancy, behavioral difficulties, or learning problems. The majority of female adolescents who abuse have also been abused themselves. These

adolescents were generally abused at younger ages and were three times as likely to have been abused by a female. Further, sexually abusive youth most frequently have comorbid conduct disorder, mood disorders, and anxiety disorders. The number of psychiatric diagnoses is higher with a lower age of first offense (American Academy of Child and Adolescent Psychiatry 1999).

Studies of women who "broke the cycle of abuse" suggests that continuity is not the rule; many abused children grow up to be competent, nonabusive parents. Maltreated mothers who were able to break this cycle of abuse reported receiving emotional support from a foster parent or relative when they were children, which in turn enhanced their self-worth and ability to be effective parents (Egeland et al. 1993). It is widely believed that abuse during childhood can lead to victims abusing their own offspring. However, methodological issues in many studies have limited confirmation of this phenomenon (Ertem et al. 2000).

Polyvictimization is more the rule than the exception; in addition to sexual and physical abuse, it includes bullying, property damage, witnessing peer or sibling victimization, and witnessing others (such as parents) being victimized. Leventhal (2007) finds that polyvictims are more likely to score in the clinical range on mental illness measures. Whether a child has been sexually abused versus physically abused, for example, matters less in the long term as compared to the overall level of adversity and the number of victimizations experienced by the child (Finkelhor et al. 2007; Leventhal 2007). Poor outcomes are more likely in individuals who have experienced greater adversity. It is not adequate to simply ask about physical or sexual abuse. Instead one needs to explore the depth of adversity that a child has experienced in order to gauge the risk of subsequent psychopathology and to identify and guide needed treatment interventions.

Clinical Presentation

Children who are victims of abuse exhibit a variety of emotional and behavioral symptoms. Photographic documentation of all injuries is crucial. One must consider the possibility of physical abuse in every child who presents with an injury. The clinician should obtain a careful and thorough history and complete a comprehensive physical examination, including radiological and laboratory studies, in every injured child. Indicators suggesting possible abuse include lack of a reasonable

TABLE 31–1. Behavioral observations

The clinician needs to be sensitive to and aware of certain frequently observed behaviors that have been associated with abuse in children:

- Unusually fearful and docile, distrustful, and/or guarded
- Wary of physical contact
- On the alert for danger
- Attempts to meet parents' needs by role reversal
- Afraid to go home
- Angry reactions and delinquent behaviors
- Hypersexual behavior, self-exposing
- Artwork or play with themes of sexual activity or aggression
- Substance abuse
- Suicidality
- Fire-setting behavior
- Sleep difficulties, nightmares

explanation for the injury; contradictory, changing, or vague history of the injury; observation of an inappropriate history for the injury; excessive or inadequate level of concern; and delay in seeking medical attention (Cheung 1999). In addition, a parent blaming an injury on a sibling or claiming that it was self-inflicted, or a parent having unrealistic and premature expectations of the child, could also be suggestive of abuse. The behavioral observations and findings on clinical examination are described in Tables 31–1, 31–2, and 31–3.

Special attention needs to be paid when examining an infant or toddler for physical abuse. In 1972, pediatric radiologist John Caffey coined the term *whiplash shaken baby syndrome* to describe a constellation of clinical findings in infants and toddlers, including retinal hemorrhages, subdural or subarachnoid hemorrhages, and little or no evidence of external cranial trauma. It was postulated that whiplash forces caused subdural hematomas by tearing cortical bridging veins. Serious injuries in infants are rarely accidental unless there is a clear explanation. Head injuries are the leading cause of traumatic childhood death and of child abuse fatalities.

Radiological documentation of skeletal injuries may be the best early evidence of alleged abuse. A skeletal survey to identify recent and old fractures is indicated in a child less than age 2 years with suspicious bruising or fractures. Such surveys are not as helpful in children over age 5 years (American Academy of Pediatrics Committee on Child Abuse and Ne-

glect 2001). Bone scans should be performed to identify subtle fractures in children less than age 5 years. A magnetic resonance imaging (MRI) study can better identify epiphyseal separations if they are suspected from the plain films. Ultrasound may also be indicated to identify epiphyseal injury. However, thoraco-abdominal trauma is best evaluated initially by computed tomographic (CT) scanning (Toomey and Bernstein 2001). Both MRI and CT scans can assist in determining when the injuries occurred and can also substantiate repeated injuries by documenting changes in the chemical states of hemoglobin in affected areas. In the event of suspected brain or head injury, a CT scan is the first-line imaging investigation, with its sensitivity to intraparenchymal, subarachnoid, subdural, and epidural hemorrhage and also to mass effect. Due to its relative insensitivity to subarachnoid blood and fractures, an MRI study is considered complementary to a CT scan and should ideally be obtained 2–3 days later if possible. Because MRI may fail to detect acute bleeding, its use should be delayed for 5–7 days in acutely ill children (American Academy of Pediatrics Section on Radiology 2000; Cheung 1999).

Specific findings such as a dilated hymen or anus, bruising, scarring, or perianal tearing are important findings to discern and to document appropriately (American Academy of Child and Adolescent Psychiatry 1999). The presence of sexually transmitted diseases may or may not confirm the occurrence of sexual activity or abuse. Generally, gonorrhea, genital herpes, or syphilis definitively diagnosed in a child outside of the perinatal period usually confirms the occurrence of sexual activity and possible sexual abuse. The presence of human immunodeficiency virus (HIV), chlamydia, or anogenital condylomata acuminata should raise suspicion for sexual abuse but still may not represent diagnostic certainty. Definitive findings confirming sexual activity include pregnancy or the presence of semen. Pregnancy in an adolescent should always lead to an inquiry as to the possibility of sexual abuse.

Emergency room physicians are commonly called on to perform acute evaluations that include crisis management and evidence collection. Physical examination should be done promptly. However, if the abuse has occurred in the previous 72 hours, physical examinations should be performed immediately with the goal of obtaining reliable physical evidence. It is recommended that a physician trained in conducting sexual abuse evaluations perform the examination. The examination should be done a minimum number of times by the smallest possible number of clinicians. The assessment should be done as part of a comprehensive physical ex-

TABLE 31–2. Medical findings after physical abuse

The physician should closely examine an injured child for suspicious physical findings suggesting abuse (Cheung 1999):

Cutaneous injuries, such as bruises or lacerations in the shape of an object or multiple bruises in areas that are difficult to injure in play (e.g., upper arms, medial thighs).

Stocking-glove distribution burns, suggesting immersion, burns on the perineum, burns in recognizable shapes (e.g., an iron), cigarette burns, and especially multiple burns in various stages of healing.

Head injuries, including complex skull fractures with intracranial hemorrhage, retinal hemorrhage, bilateral ocular injury, dental injury, or traumatic hair loss with scalp hematomas.

Ear injuries, including twisting injuries of the lobe and ruptured tympanic membranes.

Skeletal injuries, including posterior rib fractures (especially when there are multiple fractures), multiple fractures in different stages of healing, metaphyseal fractures in long bones of infants, spiral fractures, and femur fractures in a nonambulatory child; also, radiological signs of subperiosteal hemorrhage, epiphyseal separation, periosteal shearing, and periosteal calcification.

Abdominal injuries, including hepatic hematoma, laceration, or hemorrhage and duodenal hematoma or perforation.

Chest injuries, such as pulmonary contusion, pneumothorax, and pleural effusion.

TABLE 31–3. Medical findings of sexual abuse

Vague somatic complaints such as abdominal pain and headaches

Secondary enuresis and/or encopresis

Redness or irritation of the vulva; anogenital injuries such as lacerations, scarring, or bruising of genitalia; and anal dilatation or scarring

Repeated urinary tract infections and/or hematuria

Anal fissures or blood in the stool

amination to deemphasize the genital findings. Sexually abused children frequently do not have corroborating physical findings. Obtaining evidence from a physical examination is exquisitely important; if physical evidence is present, perpetrators are 2.5 times more likely to receive legal consequences (American Academy of Child and Adolescent Psychiatry 1997).

The American Academy of Pediatrics Committee on Child Abuse and Neglect (1999) has outlined comprehensive guidelines for the necessary physical examination after sexual abuse; among them are the following:

- The examination should not cause additional emotional trauma. Appropriate time must be allowed to account for the child's anxiety.
- Careful explanation of every step should precede the examination.
- Particular attention needs to be given to examination of the mouth, genitals, perineal region, anus, buttocks, and thighs.

- A supportive adult known to the child as well as a nursing chaperone should be present.
- The examination should be thorough, including developmental, growth, mental, and emotional factors as well as physical findings.
- History taking should be thorough and ideally should be obtained before the physical examination. Care should be taken not to suggest answers to questions.
- If collection of forensic samples is imperative and the child is unable to cooperate, use of sedation should be considered.
- Appropriate agency reporting and thorough documentation of findings, including the child's statements and behavior, are essential.
- The physician should offer reassurance about healing and recovery.

Diagnostic Considerations and Comorbidity

Increasing evidence suggests that children who are victims of abuse have varying symptoms and sequelae, stemming from the variability in timing, duration, frequency, and specific characteristics of the abuse as well as an individual child's resilience and vulnerability to mental illness. In reviewing the psychological effects of abuse, Cicchetti and Toth (1995) noted a wide range of effects, including affective dysregulation, disruptive and aggressive behaviors, insecure and atypical attachment patterns, impaired peer relationships with either increased aggression or social withdrawal, and academic underachievement. High rates of other comorbid psychiatric disorders have been reported and include major depression, conduct disorder, oppositional defiant disorder (ODD), agoraphobia, overanxious disorder, ADHD, and substance abuse (Kaplan et al. 1998).

Four factors have been suggested to describe the extent to which a child is traumatized by sexual abuse. These include 1) traumatic sexualization, 2) powerlessness, 3) stigmatization, and 4) betrayal, each leading to feelings of fear, anxiety, and helplessness in the child. Schetky and Green (1988) cite other factors that influence the sexually abused child's symptomatology and outcome. These are the age and developmental level of the child; the onset, duration, and frequency of the abuse; the degree of coercion and physical trauma; the relationship between the child and the perpetrator; the child's preexisting personality; and the interaction between acute and long-term variables.

Early sexual abuse is linked to sexual high-risk behaviors as well. Childhood sexual and emotional abuse were found to be independently associated with subsequent engagement in sex work after controlling for sociodemographic variables in the At Risk Youth Study, a prospective cohort study of street-involved youth in Vancouver, Canada (Stoltz et al. 2007). In this study, children who were sexually abused remained vulnerable to sexual predation and were more likely to engage in higher risk-taking behavior. The authors highlight the need to focus on not only sexual abuse but also emotional abuse as leading to an increased likelihood for involvement in sex work.

McCrae et al. (2006) evaluated data on children investigated for sexual abuse from the National Survey of Child and Adolescent Well-being, looking at not only abuse rates but characteristics of abuse (such as penetration) and co-occurring family problems. They found that among 3- to 7-year-olds, behavioral symptoms were associated with caregiver domestic violence and mental illness. Among 8- to 11-year-olds, depressive symptoms were associated with severe abuse and multiple family problems, and posttraumatic stress was associated with chronic unresolved abuse. Characteristics of sexual abuse related to poor outcomes include duration, use of force, penetration, and a perpetrator who is close to or related to the child. The highest rates of symptoms other than depression were observed in children with severe sexual abuse, such as intercourse or oral sex. More girls than boys suffered from depression. African American children ages 8–11

showed elevated behavioral symptoms regardless of socioeconomic class. This suggests that cultural views of sexual abuse may heighten shame in victims and that lower health care utilization and disparities or help-seeking differences may lead to greater psychological problems.

Senn et al. (2006) found that those whose sexual abuse involved penetration and/or force reported more adult sexual high-risk behavior, including numerous sexual partners and previous sexually transmitted disease diagnoses, than those who were not sexually abused or were abused without force or penetration. For men, sexual abuse with force and penetration was associated with the greatest involvement in the sex trade. For women, those abused with penetration, regardless of whether force was used, had the most sex trade activity. The authors suggest that more severe abuse leads to maladaptive coping responses and the emergence of traumatic sexualization. The traumagenic model postulates that sexually abused youth emerge as adults who believe that sex is necessary in order to obtain affection from others. Such youth may also develop a sense of powerlessness linked to sexuality, and as adults they take more sexual risks and are less likely to refuse intercourse.

Neurodevelopmental Impact of Abuse

Traumatic events are overwhelming and lead to disrupted brain homeostasis and a maladaptive compensatory response (Perry and Pollard 1998). Sustained stress leads to overstimulation of the hypothalamic-pituitary-adrenal (HPA) axis and subsequently to elevated cortisol levels (Bremner et al. 2003). Theoretically, all parts of the brain—cortex, limbic system, midbrain, and brainstem—may be affected, and powerful traumatic memories may be created. Altered cortical homeostasis impacts cognitive or narrative memory, altered limbic homeostasis impacts emotional memory, altered midbrain homeostasis impacts motor memory, and altered brainstem homeostasis may impact physiological-state memories (Perry and Pollard 1998).

Altered brain homeostasis overall impacts natural stress responses of hyperarousal and dissociation. Hyperarousal, or a fight-or-flight state, naturally involves activation of the sympathetic nervous system via norepinephrine-specific neurons stemming from the locus coeruleus of the midbrain. Interaction between the locus coeruleus and the HPA axis results in increased release of adrenocorticotropin and cortisol to prepare the body for defense (Perry and Pollard 1998). Arousal, startle responses, vigilance, irritability, and sleep are all affected by this activation. Abused youth exhibit impaired sleep efficiency, and prolonged sleep latency. Chronic activation of the HPA axis and resulting cortisol system alteration may damage the hippocampus. Adults with posttraumatic stress disorder (PTSD) due to severe sexual or physical abuse have decreased hippocampal size as detected with MRI and positron emission tomographic scans (Bremner et al. 2003). Such findings may explain the memory impairment often present in victims of abuse. Studies of abused children have revealed hippocampal and limbic abnormalities, which may predispose these children to memory deficits and emotional dysregulation. Following the acute fear response, the brain may create a set of memories that can be rapidly triggered by reminders of the trauma. Affected children thus remain in a persistent state of fear, with hypersensitivity and emotional overreactivity. In many cases, the most adaptive response to the pain of the abuse may be to activate dissociative mechanisms involving disengagement from the external world by using primitive psychological defenses such as depersonalization, derealization, numbing, and—in extreme cases—catatonia. Dissociation may then be protective, allowing the child to psychologically survive the abuse. Over time, the defense often becomes maladaptive, emerging at inappropriate times (Perry and Pollard 1998).

Cognitive, academic, and language delays have been consistently documented in maltreated youth. Studies of preschool children report significantly decreased intelligence as compared with control subjects (Vondra et al. 1990). Wodarski et al. (1990) studied a group of physically abused youth and found that 60% of the neglected youths and 55% of the abused youth had repeated at least one grade as compared with 24% of the comparison group. A 3-year follow-up study of this population found that the language and mathematics scores dropped in the abused group. In severely abused children, frontotemporal and anterior brain electroencephalographic abnormalities have been noted as well.

Attachment Dysregulation

A child's internal representation of his or her attachment figure depends on the availability and responsiveness of the caregiver. Research has shown that the way a child thinks about his or her relationship with primary caregivers is related to the child's self-esteem, social competence, peer relationships, arousal, distress, and psychopathology. Over time, the infant develops a set of expectations about future interactions based on previous experiences and interactions with the primary caregiver (Bowlby 1982). An infant securely attaches to a mother who is sensitive to the infant's needs. Insensitive or unresponsive parenting leads to insecure attachments that have been subcategorized as anxious/avoidant, anxious/ambivalent, and disorganized attachment. Abusive parenting is associated with insecure attachments, often of the disorganized type, which in turn often leads to later psychopathology in the infant. In a review of the impact of child maltreatment on subsequent attachment patterns (Morton and Browne 1998), 11 of 13 controlled studies found that significantly more maltreated infants displayed insecure attachments. Children exposed to abusive parenting are excessively sensitized in their arousal level, emotional regulation, and behavioral reactivity and are at risk for later developing neuropsychiatric problems (Perry and Pollard 1998). Conversely, Gunnar (1998) suggests that the security of attachment between an infant and caregiver buffers stress by downregulating the HPA axis. Compared with insecurely attached infants, 18-month-old children with secure attachments to their mothers were found to have decreased cortisol levels when frightened by a clown (Nachmias et al. 1996). Numerous studies have identified the key role of a responsive, predictable, and nurturing caregiver in the development of a healthy neurobiological stress response (Perry and Pollard 1998). During the first 2 years of life, there is a genetically programmed overproduction of axons, dendrites, and synapses in the brain, with subsequent pruning of those not used. The environment thus impacts which synaptic connections are maintained and survive (Glaser 2000), possibly explaining the power of physical abuse in derailing secure attachments and healthy outcomes over the long term. The work of Lyons-Ruth et al. (1990) and Beardslee et al. (1997) has shown that healthy infant-parent attachment promotes optimal development and protects against adverse outcomes.

Aggression

The most frequent outcome of abuse is aggression. Abused preschool children engage in aggressive behavior more frequently than their peers, and they more often attribute hostile intent to their peers. Abused children have also been reported to be at risk for violent criminal behavior in adolescence (Herrenkohl et al. 1997) and in adulthood (Widom 1989). Adolescents with a history of abuse are also reported to engage in more aggression with their peers and within their dating relationships. Pathological defense mechanisms may also play a role, including identification with the aggressor. Lewis (1996) writes that abusive experiences provide a model for violence, teach aggression through reinforcement, inflict pain, and cause central nervous system injuries associated with impulsivity, emotional lability, and impaired judgment. Furthermore, this experience creates a sense of being endangered and thus increases paranoid feelings and diminishes the child's capacity to recognize feelings and put them into words, not actions.

Substance Abuse and Self-Injurious Behavior

Children may resort to behaviors that facilitate opioid-mediated dissociation, such as rocking, head banging, and self-mutilation, with these painful stimuli activating the brain's endogenous opiates. Abused children are also more likely to develop substance abuse, likely in a self-medicating fashion. Alcohol serves to reduce anxiety, opiates trigger soothing dissociation, and stimulants activate mesolimbic dopaminergic reward areas in children deprived of true rewards in their lives (Perry and Pollard 1998).

Glassman et al. (2007) noted that emotional and sexual abuse had the strongest link to nonsuicidal self-injury (NSSI). The authors theorized that NSSI is mediated by self-criticism after emotional abuse, with "individuals who are excessively criticized and verbally or emotionally abused...engag(ing) in excessive self-criticism and us(ing) NSSI as a form of direct 'self-abuse'" (p. 2484). Their study is consistent with prior research supporting the association between NSSI and histories of physical or sexual abuse. The study is unique, however, in showing a strong link between childhood emotional abuse and NSSI. In exploring the etiology, the authors suggest that emotional abuse may lead to a self-critical cognitive style, which in turn leads to NSSI as a form of self-punishment. Underlying depression may intensify NSSI behaviors.

Attention-Deficit/Hyperactivity Disorder

Several studies have documented a higher prevalence of ADHD in abused children and adolescents. It is possible that children who have ADHD are more likely to provoke abusive behaviors in adults. Impulsive par-

ents could directly transmit ADHD genetically to their children. However, it is also proposed that the trauma of abuse itself plays a causal role in the development of ADHD symptoms (Weinstein et al. 2000).

Depression and Suicide

Abused infants are prone to affective withdrawal and diminished capacity for pleasure and have a tendency to exhibit negative affect such as sadness and distress (Green 1997). Major depression or dysthymia was reported in 27% of children of latency age who had been abused (Green 1997). One study reports that approximately 8% of children and adolescents with documented abuse have a current diagnosis of major depressive disorder, 40% have lifetime major depressive disorder diagnoses, and at least 30% have lifetime disruptive disorder diagnoses (ODD or conduct disorder). These prevalence rates are several times higher than those found in community samples of children and adolescents (Kaplan et al. 1999). Depression may be a consequence of abuse or may result in a child being more vulnerable to abuse. Studies also report an association between abuse in childhood and subsequent suicidal behavior and risk taking (Kaplan et al. 1999). Furthermore, Green (1997) reported increased self-mutilation and suicidal ideation or attempts in children subjected to parental beatings or threatened by abandonment from their adult caretakers. Depression and suicidal behavior are overrepresented among adolescent inpatients with a history of sexual abuse. Further, sexually abused girls may be particularly at risk for suicide attempts, independent of other psychopathology (Bergen et al. 2003).

Danielson et al. (2005) studied differences in adolescent depression severity and symptoms based on the type of abuse (e.g., sexual abuse, physical abuse, both combined) and gender. Results showed differences in depression severity and symptoms based on the type of abuse and gender. Adolescents who experienced both sexual and physical abuse were more likely to be depressed, have suicidal ideation, or have PTSD than those who experienced physical abuse only or those who did not experience any abuse at all. Longer duration of abuse was related to greater depression severity, sleep disturbances, and greater anxiety. Consistent with prior research, greater guilt was experienced by those who were abused by a relative. Such youth also endorsed more problems with appetite and thoughts of death, which may be related to underlying hopelessness and anger in children abused by a relative. Finally, female adolescents were more depressed than males. The authors urge clinicians to explore for underlying abuse histories in patients with mood disorders, given the clear link between trauma and the later development of depression. Such an assessment is imperative, as it may lead to the identification of a child currently in an abusive environment.

A prospective study of depression in abused and neglected children grown up found that abuse and neglect were associated with increased risk for major depressive disorder in adulthood (Widom et al. 2007). Children who were physically abused or experienced multiple types of abuse were at increased risk of lifetime major depression, whereas neglect increased risk for current major depression. Surprisingly, childhood sexual abuse was not associated with increased risk of major depression. Significantly more of the abused and neglected children who met criteria for major depression in adulthood also met the criteria for at least one other lifetime diagnosis, including PTSD, drug use/dependence, antisocial personality disorder, and dysthymia.

Dissociative Disorders

Dissociative disorders may result from abuse. Children who dissociate may experience brief psychotic symptoms such as hearing command auditory hallucinations. Severely abused children commonly hear voices commanding them to harm themselves or others. As a result, they may be misdiagnosed with a psychotic disorder such as schizophrenia. A dissociating child may also be misdiagnosed with an externalizing disorder—ADHD, ODD, or impulse control disorder. A study of a group of severely abused youngsters in residential treatment facilities found that 23% of the boys met DSM-IV criteria for dissociative identity disorder (American Psychiatric Association 1994; Yeager and Lewis 2000). Dissociative disorders are difficult to discern in younger children, especially prior to age 7 when faculties of concrete reasoning are less well developed. Dissociation may be present in victims of sexual abuse more often than in victims of physical abuse. Some children may have dissociative experiences as defense mechanisms or as a manner of reexperiencing or gaining understanding and mastery over the abusive experience.

Anxiety Disorders and Posttraumatic Stress Disorder

Anxiety disorders may take many forms, including phobias, social anxiety, generalized anxiety disorder, and PTSD. Symptoms of PTSD include fear reactions, reexperiencing phenomena, flashbacks, sleep disruption, exaggerated startle response, and hyperacuity, as well as general anxiety and deterioration of functioning. The chronicity and severity of abuse increase the likelihood of a PTSD diagnosis. Children often display disorganized or agitated behavior rather than the fear, helplessness, and horror described in adults. Repetitive play involving themes of the trauma is common rather than the classic flashbacks or recurrent and intrusive recollections of the trauma.

In her review of trauma leading to PTSD, Terr (1996) wrote that traumatic events, including physical abuse, cause psychic trauma when the child understands that something terrible is happening and that he or she is in danger, senses his or her own helplessness, and registers and stores an implicit or explicit traumatic memory. Soon after a traumatic event, play can be "grim, monotonous, and at times, dangerous." The child often does not make a connection between the play and the trauma. Terr cites protective factors, including intelligence, humor, and relatedness. Only later does the clinician see more clearly intrusive thoughts, fears, and repeated dreams. A foreshortened sense of the future is common in abused children and can lead to reckless risk taking. Unconscious reenactment of the trauma can lead to retraumatization of the child. In some cases, this reenactment can be dangerous to the child or to others. Pelcovitz et al. (1994) studied the prevalence of PTSD in physically abused adolescents and found that these youth may be more at risk for behavioral, emotional, and social difficulties than for clear PTSD. This is in contrast to the previous work of Green (1997), who found that physically abused adolescents were at risk for developing PTSD. Pelcovitz et al. (1994) suggest that physically abused adolescents may "enact" their victimization rather than express their reactions to the abuse via symptoms of PTSD. The authors point out the differences between physical and sexual assaults, with sexual abuse often accompanied by a higher level of secrecy and shame, which may reinforce emergent PTSD symptoms. External signs of physical abuse, such as bruises and fractures, may lead to more support, facilitating integration of the trauma. Pelcovitz et al. add that an alternative possibility is that the physically abused youth in their study did not manifest PTSD symptoms because they remained in an abusive environment. There may be a delay in the onset of PTSD symptoms until after the trauma has ended.

Multiple Somatic Health Problems

An association has been found between childhood abuse and adult health problems, including poor self-rated health, pain, physical disabilities, and frequent emergency room and health professional visits (Chartier et al. 2007; Springer et al. 2007). Sexual risk taking leads to increased teenage pregnancy and exposure to HIV and sexually transmitted diseases (Kaplan et al. 1999).

Prevention

The cornerstone of treatment of children who are victims of abuse is first to make certain that the child is protected from further injury and to ensure the safety of the child from further abuse and from potential sequelae of the abuse. Making a report to child protective services needs to occur as soon as possible, preferably in the context of the initial evaluation or first disclosure. Kaplan et al. (1998) reviews three types of child abuse primary prevention strategies: 1) competency enhancement with parent education programs; 2) media campaigns, hotlines, and parent socialization programs; and 3) targeting of high-risk groups, such as single parents and teenage parents, those of low socioeconomic status, and those with neurocognitively compromised children. Research has shown that maltreated children with healthier ego resiliency, ego overcontrol, and higher self-esteem fared better in their overall adjustment (Glaser 2000). A focus of treatment should therefore be helping abused youth gain better control over their urges and actions and better self-awareness, ultimately creating a coherent narrative of their life story. This is a complex undertaking, due in part to the likelihood that ego control and ego resilience are in part temperamentally determined and that self-esteem is influenced by nurturance (Glaser 2000). Because brain development is related to environmental forces, intense and early intervention offers the greatest hope for healthier outcomes.

Leventhal (2001) described two home-based models for preventing child abuse and neglect. Both models focus on high-risk families. The Healthy Families model uses the Kempe Family Stress Inventory to identify high-risk families, covering areas such as parental history of abuse, violence, substance abuse, mental illness, or criminal acts. In the Olds model, first-time mothers are eligible if they have two of the following characteristics: 1) have less than 12 years of education, 2) are unmarried, or 3) are of low socioeconomic status. Research on the effectiveness of these two models has shown that there is a resulting stronger alliance with the parents and that the effects are

sustained over many years. However, when high levels of domestic violence are present, it is difficult for parents to improve their parenting by the use of home visits.

The Centers for Disease Control and Prevention developed important summary recommendations to raise awareness and improve efforts for primary prevention (McMahon and Puett 1999). Primary prevention includes educating children about "bad touch" and empowering them to resist abusers. School-based primary prevention programs have been shown to be effective in raising awareness, particularly when used over the long-term and with older as well as younger children (Hebert et al. 2001). Efforts have also included providing outreach to adults who are abusers or victims themselves.

Leventhal (2001) writes that fathers need specific attention, because as much as two-thirds of serious physical abuse is caused by males in the family. Typically these men have little experience caring for young children, have difficulties with their own impulse control, and tend to be violent toward their partners. One strategy is to empower women to leave their partners and to make better future decisions in selecting partners. Another strategy is to help men be more nurturing and effective as parents. Prevention strategies based on attachment theory focus on improving the caregiver–child relationship, which in turn buffers the child against life stressors. A number of studies have attempted to change insecure attachment relationships to secure ones (Morton and Browne 1998). Interventions focusing on enhancing parental sensitivity were more successful in changing attachment status than were more in-depth interventions that focused on the intrapsychic representational model.

Lyons-Ruth et al. (1990) examined attachment patterns among infants at social risk, measuring development, mother–infant interaction, and maternal depression and social contacts while also evaluating the efficacy of home visits in improving the security of a child's attachment to the caregiver. The home-visiting service had four goals:

1. Providing an accepting relationship
2. Increasing the family's competence in accessing resources
3. Modeling and reinforcing more interactive, positive, and developmentally appropriate exchanges between mother and infant, emphasizing the mother's dual role as teacher and source of emotional security for her infant

4. Decreasing social isolation with a weekly parenting group or a monthly social hour using psychodynamic and behavioral interventions

At 18 months of age, infants of depressed mothers who received home-visiting services compared to unserved infants of depressed mothers outperformed by a mean of 10 points on the Bayley Mental Development Index. They were also twice as likely to be classified as securely attached in their relationships with their mothers. Because a secure attachment has been associated with lower risk of abuse, this could be a powerful intervention to decrease the risk of physical maltreatment.

McCrae et al. (2006) suggest that rather than a one-size-fits-all intervention based on caregiver's assumptions, treatment should be tailored based on the overall level of adversity experienced by the child, avoiding assumptions that all children with a certain type of abuse need a certain type of treatment. Services need to be anchored in a deep understanding of the individual child's life experience, his or her current needs, and an understanding of the impact of the trauma on the child.

Child and Parent Treatment

The major goals of treatment are first to protect the child and strengthen the family and then to address the impact of past abuse in treatment of the child and the family. The ecological model calls for a focus on the multidimensional aspects of child abuse rather than just on the abusive parent (as has been done in traditional child abuse programs). Attachment theory has emphasized the interactive aspects of maltreatment and the importance of intervening in changing the parent–child relationship, with the hope of facilitating a more secure attachment between child and parent. Therapeutic techniques vary depending on the developmental level of the child. Treatment of ensuing psychiatric disorders such as major depression and PTSD should be done promptly and should involve consultation with a child and adolescent psychiatrist. In any abuse-specific therapy, it is important to consider the notion of retraumatization. Therapists must be exceedingly sensitive to issues of resistance and the pace necessary for successful treatment. Many victims may not directly confront the realities of their abuse but instead may benefit sufficiently from a problem-oriented approach or supportive approach. Despite

this fact, it is prudent for the therapist early on to make clear the reason for the initiation of the therapy and to point out behavior patterns that may be maladaptive as a result.

Family-based therapy needs to improve the parent's devalued self-image, reverse distortions of his or her child that can lead to scapegoating, interpret any links between the current abuse and the parent's own abuse history, and provide the parent with a positive model of raising children. Green (1997) suggests using therapeutic nurseries to treat infants and pathological parent–child interactions with dyadic parent–child therapy serving as the foundation of treatment. Psychotherapy of the child should include creating a therapeutic environment, in either individual or group settings, which allows the child to master the trauma, in part through controlled repetitions of the event using symbolic reenactments with dolls, puppets, drawings, and so forth.

> The retrieval and integration of traumatic memories will gradually enable the child to verbalize memories and feelings associated with the abuse rather than acting them out in a repetitive manner. Impulse control is strengthened by imposing limits on the direct expression of aggression, such as hitting or destroying play materials, and encouraging the verbalization of anger. Self-esteem gradually improves during the child's exposure to the climate of acceptance generated by the therapist that gradually neutralizes the child's mistrust and hypervigilance. (Green 1997, p. 694)

The child must be told that the abuse is not his or her fault and that he or she is not to be blamed. Terr (1996) reminds clinicians of the need to explore issues of betrayal, overexcitement, and personal responsibility, especially in children who have been abused within their own families. Play therapy may be useful in the treatment of a traumatized young child (Terr 1996). Play and drawing allow for safe displacement of the complex thoughts and feelings stemming from the abuse and help the child to use nonverbal and symbolic expressions of events that are too painful to be expressed in words. A goal of therapy should be helping the child use healthier coping responses.

Clinicians should be sensitive to the consequences that may ensue following the results of such disclosure and should not make impossible promises regarding reporting events to the appropriate authorities. Adolescent girls may be more resistant to discussing certain topics of abuse with a male counselor. Individual cases merit specific consideration in terms of the mode, duration, and frequency of therapy; flexibility on the part of the therapist is essential. The overall goals of treatment have to be clearly focused on behavioral and functional issues that need improvement.

Group therapy may benefit older adolescents who have relatively positive self-esteem. It is crucial that a safe space is created before group or individual therapy begins. This population can be easily retraumatized by overzealous therapists who neglect first building a trusting and safe alliance with the patient. Ideal candidates for group therapy have emotional and cognitive capacities both to benefit from the experience and to not impair the treatment of others. Specific activities, including role-playing and games to improve communication skills, can be effective in group settings (Celano et al. 1996). Before recommending group treatment, the clinician should consider any pending legal proceedings involving the patient. It may be inadvisable to involve a victim in group treatment before the individual is to give legal testimony because the information may be rejected or perceived as having been contaminated by suggestion from others.

Family therapy or individual therapy for parents is often necessary to assist caregivers in coming to terms with their own responses to the child's victimization. Nonoffending parents often have issues of guilt or depression regarding the fact that they were unable to prevent the child's victimization. Treatment that includes individual therapy for nonoffending parents can improve the psychosocial functioning of the abused child (Celano et al. 1996). Furthermore, a parent's own issues of childhood sexual abuse may emerge and may ultimately be disclosed coincidentally with the child's treatment. Family therapy can help to establish appropriate boundaries and roles for family members and can help avoid scapegoating the victim (Hilton and Mezey 1996).

Cognitive-behavioral therapy has also been shown to be superior to supportive counseling in a 12-month follow-up study (Cohen et al. 2004). Randomized controlled trials show that trauma-focused cognitive-behavioral therapy improves not only PTSD symptoms but also the attributions of abuse, shame, depression, and other behavior problems. Trauma-focused cognitive-behavioral therapy (TF-CBT) has also been found to be superior to comparison and control conditions in improving comorbid depression, anxiety, and externalizing symptoms (Cohen et al. 2004).

Although a full review of psychopharmacological interventions is beyond the scope of this chapter, medications may improve the outcome of abused children, especially if they are manifesting symptoms of PTSD. A recent study on the treatment of childhood PTSD by Cohen et al. (2007) found no clear benefit to adding sertraline to TF-CBT. TF-CBT+sertraline was not superior to TF-CBT+placebo except with regard to Children's Global Assessment Scale outcomes. Thus, it appears that for most children with PTSD, including those with major depressive disorder, a trial of initial TF-CBT or other trauma–focused psychotherapy alone is warranted before adding medication. According to anecdotal reports (Kaplan et al. 1999; Terr 1991), propranolol decreased hyperarousal and hypervigilance in abused children. Clonidine has also helped to reduce symptoms of hyperarousal, aggression, and insomnia in abused preschool children with PTSD (Harmon and Riggs 1996). Guanfacine was found to help alleviate sleep disturbances in boys with PTSD (Leonard 1999).

Positive outcomes can be enhanced with rapid, early, and effective psychotherapeutic interventions. Positive outcomes are possible despite egregious abuse scenarios. Prognosis after abuse depends on many factors, including familial, demographic, and treatment characteristics. A degree of stability within the family plays an important role. In general, parent support and involvement in treatment along with the affected child yield a significantly better outcome.

Resilience

Heller et al. (1999) reviewed the literature on resilience to the effects of child maltreatment. Dispositional or temperamental attributes of the child include above-average intelligence, high self-esteem, internal locus of control, external attribution of blame, presence of spirituality, ego resilience, and high ego control. Familial cohesion, including competent foster care, has been related to developing resilience in children. Extrafamilial support such as a positive school experience promotes resilience, which in turn likely increases individual self-worth and a sense of control over one's destiny. Rutter (1990) has argued that the field must move beyond focusing on single resilience factors to considering the developmental processes that promote adaptive functioning. Rutter has also suggested that resilience is probably not a fixed state but is rather a malleable and organic trait, which can be enhanced with a nurturing environment; resilience may buffer the impact of abuse and promote a positive sense of one's worth.

The ecological model of recovery involves integrating affects and cognitions related to the trauma within a coherent and continuous sense of self, a particularly key task for adolescent identity formation. After a sense of safety and security is established, the next crucial step is to develop an improved self-esteem and a safe attachment with an adult. It is postulated that this then lends itself to the integration of trauma-related memories, affects, and cognitions within a coherent sense of self. This then leads to the active establishment of healthy interpersonal relationships where abusive experiences can be renegotiated. Daigneault et al. (2007) suggest that this path likely leads to resilience in certain adolescents.

Daigneault et al. (2007) studied four factors that could predict resilience: interpersonal trust, maternal conflicts, family violence, and out-of-home placements. Interpersonal trust emerged as the most predictive of resilience. The investigators reported that empowerment was also a key factor, noting, "Adolescents exhibiting resilient trajectories…reported feeling more empowered; using more appropriate coping strategies to deal with sexual abuse and its consequences; and using fewer avoidant coping strategies; using fewer types of drugs; being more trustful of others; and engaging in less conflict with their mothers" (p. 424).

Thus, those treating such youth need to develop a trusting relationship and promote a sense of empowerment and self-efficacy. Providing a degree of control and power over treatment is important based on this research, after a safe space has been created in the therapy, in order to promote underlying resiliency. Traumatized individuals often reexperience feelings of powerlessness within their psychotherapy.

Legal Considerations

Legal considerations are important in the initial stages of evaluation. Physicians and mental health clinicians are mandated by all 50 states to report suspected cases of child sexual abuse. The specific requirements in terms of timing, level of suspicion, and other details vary according to state guidelines. Most important is prompt referral to a child protective services organization to ensure appropriate collection and validation of forensic information.

The forensic evaluation should be performed by a clinician who is trained in forensic assessment; this individual usually should not be the physician or therapist who is involved in ongoing treatment (Yuille et al. 1993). Confidentiality issues must be clarified before a forensic evaluation. The fact that an evaluation is be-

ing done for purposes of court proceedings needs to be made clear to the parents and child from the outset. Treating clinicians should document direct statements of disclosure in the medical record, preferably as quotations. Depending on specific legal circumstances, such information may obviate the need for direct testimony from the child victim. Guidelines for forensic evaluation of children have been published by the American Academy of Child and Adolescent Psychiatry (1999) and by the American Professional Society on the Abuse of Children (1990).

Research Directions

Future research will need to expand the current understanding of the etiology of maltreatment. As Ertem et al. (2000) noted, widespread assumptions about abuse—such as the adage "once abused, an abuser you will become"—need to be challenged, and when they are found to be fictitious, they should be discarded. The role of genetic factors has been shown to moderate the outcome of maltreated children. Functional polymorphisms in the promoter region of the serotonin transporter (5-HTTLPR) gene have been reported to moderate the influence of early maltreatment and stressful life events on the development of depression (Caspi et al. 2003). Future studies could 1) examine the relevant genetic, environmental, and protective factors to identify children early on who would be most vulnerable to adverse outcomes; and 2) delineate environmental and neural mechanisms to help promote resilience. Resilience, a major protective factor, needs to be better studied and understood so that it can be fostered and supported to minimize the impact of an adverse environment. A better understanding is also needed of the complex interactions between risk and protective factors and the protective role of the caregiving relationship in mediating both extrinsic and intrinsic risk factors (Glaser 2000).

Neurodevelopmental research must continue to explore the impact of abuse and neglect on the developing brain and the subsequent emotional and behavioral dysregulation and derailment of social development. This understanding can support the development of more effective psychotherapeutic interventions. The role of dissociation in the symptoms displayed by the abused child also needs to be better understood. Stress has been shown to have a suppressive effect on hippocampal neurogenesis, which may negatively affect the consolidation of memory and may play a role in the development of dissociation. There is great variability in the various measures of juvenile victimization that have been developed. Juvenile victimization would greatly benefit from assessment instruments that are comprehensive, methodologically sound, and

relevant to settings such as health and mental health clinics, criminal justice institutions, and child protection agencies (Hamby and Finkelhor 2000). It is critically important that future efforts focus on the development of well-defined, reliable measurement tools.

Summary Points

- Child abuse and neglect continue to be a serious problem worldwide, with some estimates of prevalence ranging up to 30% or higher.

- Family structure, child mental or physical illness, caregiver psychopathology, and disadvantaged environments are key risk factors for abuse.

- Multiple instances of abuse or polyvictimization are more common than previously thought and may be more associated with subsequent impaired function.

- Perpetrators often select victims based on age, gender, or other characteristics that serve to meet their own dysfunctional emotional needs.

- Evaluation of abused children must include thorough physical examination, appropriate documentation, and exclusion of other potential causes of injury.

- Child sexual abuse is linked to future high-risk sexual behaviors.

- The most frequent behavioral outcome of child abuse is dysregulated aggression.

- Childhood abuse is linked to adult health problems, including frequent emergency room and health professional visits.

- Treatment focus should include protecting the child, strengthening the family, and understanding the impact of the trauma on the child.

- Treatment approaches that can improve interpersonal trust are the most predictive of resilience and improved outcome following abuse.

References

American Academy of Child and Adolescent Psychiatry: Practice parameters for the forensic evaluation of children and adolescents who may have been physically or sexually abused. J Am Acad Child Adolesc Psychiatry 36:423–442, 1997

American Academy of Child and Adolescent Psychiatry: Practice parameters for the assessment and treatment of children and adolescents who are sexually abusive of others. J Am Acad Child Adolesc Psychiatry 38(suppl): 55S–76S, 1999

American Academy of Pediatrics Committee on Child Abuse and Neglect: Guidelines for the evaluation of sexual abuse of children: subject review. Pediatrics 103:186–191, 1999

American Academy of Pediatrics Committee on Child Abuse and Neglect: Shaken baby syndrome: rotational cranial injuries—technical report. Pediatrics 108:206–210, 2001

American Academy of Pediatrics Section on Radiology: Diagnostic imaging of child abuse. Pediatrics 105:1345–1348, 2000

American Professional Society on the Abuse of Children: Guidelines for Psychosocial Evaluation of Suspected Sexual Abuse in Young Children. Chicago, IL, American Professional Society on the Abuse of Children, 1990

American Psychiatric Association: Diagnostic and Statistical Manual of Mental Disorders, 4th Edition. Washington, DC, American Psychiatric Association, 1994

Beardslee WR, Salt P, Versage EM, et al: Sustaining change in parents receiving preventive interventions for families with depression. Am J Psychiatry 154:510–515, 1997

Bergen HA, Martin G, Richardson AS, et al: Sexual abuse and suicidal behavior: a model constructed from a large community sample of adolescents. J Am Acad Child Adolesc Psychiatry 42:1301–1309, 2003

Bowlby J: Attachment and Loss, Vol I: Attachment, 2nd Edition. London, Hogarth Press, 1982

Bremner JD, Vythilingam M, Vermetten E, et al: MRI and PET study of deficits in hippocampal structure and function in women with childhood sexual abuse and posttraumatic stress disorder. Am J Psychiatry 160:924–932, 2003

Caspi A, Sugden K, Moffitt TE, et al: Influence of life stress on depression: moderation by a polymorphism in the 5-HTT gene. Science 301:386–389, 2003

Celano M, Hazzard A, Webb C, et al: Treatment of trauma-genic beliefs among sexually abused girls and their mothers: an evaluation study. J Abnorm Child Psychol 24:1–17, 1996

Chartier MJ, Walker JR, Naimark B: Childhood abuse, adult health, and health care utilization: results from a representative community sample. Am J Epidemiol 165:1031–1038, 2007

Cheung KK: Identifying and documenting findings of physical child abuse and neglect. J Pediatr Health Care May/June:142–143, 1999

Cicchetti D, Toth SL: A developmental psychopathology perspective on child abuse and neglect. J Am Acad Child Adolesc Psychiatry 34:541–565, 1995

Cohen JA, Deblinger E, Mannarino AP, et al: A multisite, randomized controlled trial for children with sexual abuse-related PTSD symptoms. J Am Acad Child Adolesc Psychiatry 43:393–402, 2004

Cohen JA, Mannarino AP, Perel JM, et al: A pilot randomized controlled trial of combined trauma-focused CBT and sertraline for childhood PTSD symptoms. J Am Acad Child Adolesc Psychiatry 46:811–819, 2007

Daigneault I, Hebert M, Tourigny M: Personal and Interpersonal characteristics related to resilient developmental pathways of sexually abused adolescents. Child Adolesc Psychiatr Clin N Am 16:415–434, 2007

Danielson CK, deArellano MA, Kilpatrick DG, et al: Child maltreatment in depressed adolescents: differences in symptomatology based on history of abuse. Child Maltreat 10:37–48, 2005

Egeland B, Carlson E, Sroufe LA: Resilience as process. Dev Psychopathol 5:517–528, 1993

Ertem IO, Leventhal JM, Dobbs S: Intergenerational continuity of child physical abuse: how good is the evidence? Lancet 356:814–819, 2000

Fergusson DM, Horwood LJ, Lynskey MT: Childhood sexual abuse and psychiatric disorder in young adulthood, II: psychiatric outcomes of childhood sexual abuse. J Am Acad Child Adolesc Psychiatry 34:1365–1374, 1996

Finkelhor D, Ormrod RK, Turner HA: Poly-victimization: a neglected component in child victimization. Child Abuse Negl 31:7–26, 2007

Friedrich WN, Fisher J, Broughton D, et al: Normative sexual behavior in children: a contemporary sample. Pediatrics 101:E9, 1998

Glaser D: Child abuse and neglect and the brain: a review. J Child Psychol Psychiatry 41:97–116, 2000

Glasser M, Kolvin I, Campbell D, et al: Cycle of child sexual abuse: links between being a victim and becoming a perpetrator. Br J Psychiatry 179:482–494, 2001

Glassman LH, Weierich MR, Hooley JM, et al: Child maltreatment, nonsuicidal self-injury, and the mediating role of self-criticism. Behav Res Ther 45:2483–2490, 2007

Green AH: Physical abuse of children, in Textbook of Child and Adolescent Psychiatry, 2nd Edition. Edited by Weiner JM. Washington, DC, American Psychiatric Press, 1997, pp 687–697

Gunnar M: Quality of early care and buffering of neuroendocrine stress reactions: potential effects on the developing human brain. Prev Med 27:208–211, 1998

Hamby SL, Finkelhor D: The victimization of children: recommendations for assessment and instrument development. J Am Acad Child Adolesc Psychiatry 39:829–840, 2000

Harmon RJ, Riggs PD: Clonidine for posttraumatic stress disorder in preschool children. J Am Acad Child Adolesc Psychiatry 35:1247–1249, 1996

Haugaard JJ: The challenge of defining child sexual abuse. Am Psychol 55:1036–1039, 2000

Hebert M, Lavoie F, Piche C, et al: Proximate effects of a child sexual abuse prevention program in elementary school children. Child Abuse Negl 25:505–522, 2001

Heller SS, Larrieu JA, D'Imperio R, et al: Research on resilience to child maltreatment: empirical considerations. Child Abuse Negl 23:321–338, 1999

Herrenkohl RC, Egolf BP, Herrenkohl EC: Preschool antecedents of adolescent assaultive behavior: a longitudinal study. Am J Orthopsychiatry 67:422–432, 1997

Hilton MR, Mezey GC: Victims and perpetrators of child sexual abuse. Br J Psychiatry 169:408–421, 1996

Holmes WC, Slap GB: Sexual abuse of boys: definition, prevalence, correlates, sequelae, and management. JAMA 280:1855–1862, 1998

Kaplan SJ, Pelcovitz D, Salzinger S, et al: Adolescent physical abuse: risk for adolescent psychiatric disorders. Am J Psychiatry 155:954–959, 1998

Kaplan SJ, Pelcovitz D, Labruna V: Child and adolescent abuse and neglect research: a review of the past 10 years, part I: physical and emotional abuse and neglect. J Am Acad Child Adolesc Psychiatry 38:1214–1222, 1999

Kempe CH, Silverman FN, Steele BF, et al: The battered child syndrome. JAMA 181:17–24, 1962

Kuntz J, Bahr SJ: A profile of parental homicide against children. J Fam Violence 11:347–362, 1996

Leonard H: Guanfacine alleviates sleep disorders in boys with PTSD. The Brown University Child and Adolescent Psychopharmacology Update, p 1, October 1999

Leventhal JM: The prevention of child abuse and neglect: successfully out of the blocks. Child Abuse Negl 25:431–439, 2001

Leventhal JM: Children's experiences of violence: some have much more than others. Child Abuse Negl 31:3–6, 2007

Lewis DO: Development of the symptom of violence, in Child and Adolescent Psychiatry: A Comprehensive Textbook, 2nd Edition. Edited by Lewis M. Baltimore, MD, Williams & Wilkins, 1996, pp 334–344

Lyons-Ruth K, Connell DB, Grunebaum H: Infants at social risk: maternal depression and family support services as mediators of infant development and security of attachment. Child Dev 61:85–98, 1990

McCrae JS, Chapman MV, Christ SL: Profile of children investigated for sexual abuse: association with psychopathology symptoms and services. Am J Orthopsychiatry 76:468–481, 2006

McMahon PM, Puett RC: Child sexual abuse as a public health issue: recommendations of an expert panel. Sex Abuse 11:257–266, 1999

Morton N, Browne KD: Theory and observation of attachment and its relation to child maltreatment: a review. Child Abuse Negl 22:1093–1104, 1998

Nachmias M, Gunnar M, Mangelsdorf S, et al: Behavioral inhibition and stress reactivity: the moderating role of attachment security. Child Dev 67:508–522, 1996

Pelcovitz D, Kaplan S, Goldenberg B, et al: Posttraumatic stress disorder in physically abused adolescents. J Am Acad Child Adolesc Psychiatry 33:305–312, 1994

Perry BD, Pollard R: Homeostasis, stress, trauma and adaptation: a neurodevelopmental view of childhood trauma. Child Adolesc Psychiatr Clin N Am 7:33–51, 1998

Rutter M: Psychosocial resilience and protective mechanisms, in Risk and Protective Factors in the Development of Psychopathology. Edited by Rolf J, Masten AS, Cicchetti K, et al. New York, Cambridge University Press, 1990, pp 181–214

Ryan G: Childhood sexuality: a decade of study, part I—research and curriculum development. Child Abuse Negl 24:33–48, 2000

Schetky D, Green A: Child Sexual Abuse: A Handbook for Health Care and Legal Professionals. New York, Brunner/Mazel, 1988

Sedlak AJ, Broadhurst DD: The Third National Incidence Study of Child Abuse and Neglect. Washington, DC, U.S. Department of Health and Human Services, 1996

Senn TE, Carey MP, Vanable PA, et al: Characteristics of sexual abuse in childhood and adolescence influence sexual risk behavior in adulthood. Arch Sex Behav 36:637–645, 2006

Springer KW, Sheridan J, Kuo D, et al: Long-term physical and mental health consequences of childhood physical abuse: results from a large population-based sample of men and women. Child Abuse Negl 31:517–530, 2007

Stoltz JA, Shannon K, Kerr T, et al: Associations between childhood maltreatment and sex work in a cohort of drug-using youth. Soc Sci Med 65:1214–1221, 2007

Terr LC: Childhood traumas: an outline and overview. Am J Psychiatry 148:10–20, 1991

Terr LC: Acute responses to external events and posttraumatic stress disorder, in Child and Adolescent Psychiatry: A Comprehensive Textbook, 2nd Edition. Edited by Lewis M. Baltimore, MD, Williams & Wilkins, 1996

Toomey S, Bernstein H: Child abuse and neglect: prevention and intervention. Curr Opin Pediatr 13:211–215, 2001

Turner HA, Finkelhor D, Ormrod R: Family structure variations and predictors of child victimization. Am J Orthopsychiatry 77:282–295, 2007

U.S. Department of Health and Human Services: HHS reports new child abuse and neglect statistics. HHS News, April 2, 2001a

U.S. Department of Health and Human Services: Trends in the Well-Being of America's Children and Youth 2001. Washington, DC, Office of the Assistant Secretary for Planning and Evaluation, 2001b, pp 142–143

Vondra JI, Barnett DE, Cicchetti D: Self-concept, motivation, and competence among preschoolers from maltreating and comparison families. Child Abuse Negl 14:525, 1990

Weinstein D, Staffelbach D, Biaggio M: Attention-deficit hyperactivity disorder and posttraumatic stress disorder: differential diagnosis in childhood sexual abuse. Clin Psychol Rev 20:359–378, 2000

Widom CS: Child abuse, neglect, and adult behavior. Criminology 27:251–271, 1989

Widom CS, DuMont K, Czaja SJ: A prospective investigation of major depressive disorder and comorbidity in abused and neglected children grown up. Arch Gen Psychiatry 64:49–56, 2007

Wodarski JS, Kurtz PD, Gaudin JM Jr, et al: Maltreatment and the school age child: major academic, socioemotional, and adaptive outcomes. Social Work 35:506–513, 1990

Yates A: Sexual abuse of children, in Textbook of Child and Adolescent Psychiatry, 2nd Edition. Edited by Wiener JM. Washington, DC, American Psychiatric Press, 1997, pp 699–709

Yeager CA, Lewis DO: Mental illness, neuropsychologic deficits, child abuse, and violence. Child Adolesc Psychiatr Clin N Am 9:793–813, 2000

Yuille JC, Hunter R, Joffe R, et al: Interviewing children in sexual abuse cases, in Child Witnesses: Understanding and Improving Testimony. Edited by Goodman GS, Bottoms BL. New York, Guilford, 1993, pp 95–115

Chapter 32

HIV and AIDS

Larry K. Brown, M.D.
Laura B. Whiteley, M.D.
April A. Peters, M.Div.

Human immunodeficiency virus may be the proto-typical biopsychosocial disease with issues at every level, from the cellular to the social, that are important to consider in psychiatric management. As will be discussed in this chapter, issues that are important in the treatment of infected patients include adherence to medical care, stigma, disclosure of infection, bereavement, and the emergence of cognitive impairment.

Epidemiology

In the United States, nearly 1.2 million people are estimated to be infected with HIV/AIDS, but fortunately, pediatric AIDS is now rare (Centers for Disease Control and Prevention 2008). Maternal transmission of HIV decreased by three-quarters between 1994 and 2004 in the United States, resulting in fewer than 200 new cases of maternal transmission in 2003. This reduction can largely be attributed to more widespread HIV testing and anti-retroviral therapy for pregnant women. In contrast, HIV infection among adolescents, especially those in minority communities, is increasing. Black or African American youth constitute nearly 70% of the infections for adolescents. There has been a 40% increase in adolescents and young adults living with HIV/AIDS in the United States since 2000. Females account for nearly 40% of the infections in adolescents ages 13–19 and most were infected through heterosexual contact, whereas male-to-male sexual contact accounts for three-quarters of the infections among adolescent males (Centers for Disease Control and Prevention 2007a). Teens are at risk for HIV due to emergent risk behavior as indicated by data from the Youth Risk Behavior Surveillance (Centers for Disease Control and Prevention 2006b). By the twelfth grade,

63% of teens have had sexual intercourse, and 14.3% have had sex with four or more partners. Among sexually active teens, 23.3% used alcohol or drugs at the time of their last intercourse and nearly 40% report not using a condom at last intercourse. Of the estimated 19 million new sexually transmitted diseases (STDs) that occur each year, roughly half occur in young people ages 15–24 years (Centers for Disease Control and Prevention 2006a; Weinstock et al. 2004). For chlamydia, the most commonly reported STD in the United States, the rate for female adolescents (ages 15–19) was 2,796/100,000, the highest among all age groups (Centers for Disease Control and Prevention 2006a; Weinstock et al. 2004). Clearly, many adolescents are at risk for acquiring HIV.

Etiology

HIV and Its Transmission

HIV is a retrovirus containing RNA and a reverse transcriptase to translate its RNA into DNA within the human host. Once HIV infects its host, it is a virus capable of causing profound immunodeficiency. AIDS is a collection of symptoms and infections that occur because of the significant damage to the immune system caused by HIV. Treatments exist to slow the progression of HIV and AIDS; however, there remains no known cure.

Transmission of HIV typically occurs through sexual behaviors, perinatal transmission, and injection substance abuse. Other routes of infection include exposure to HIV during medical procedures or blood transfusions. Among adolescents and young adults in the United States, sexual intercourse is the leading cause of new, nonperinatal HIV infection (Grant et al. 2006). Unprotected receptive sexual acts convey more risk for infection with HIV than unprotected insertive sexual acts. During vaginal receptive sex, women are especially susceptible to infection due to vaginal microbial ecology and physiology, as well as to a higher prevalence of STDs. Other STDs increase transmission of HIV due to disruption of the epithelial barrier by ulceration and accumulation of susceptible cells (macrophages and lymphocytes) in semen and vaginal secretions (Fleming and Wasserheit 1999). Anal intercourse for both men and women is an even greater risk due to the fragility of rectal mucosa and the resulting exposure to blood. Transmission of HIV from oral sex was thought unlikely in the early years of the epidemic. However, more recent studies suggest that oral intercourse, especially receptive oral intercourse, can lead to transmission of HIV (Rothenberg et al. 1998).

Pediatric HIV and AIDS are predominantly a result of perinatal transmission during pregnancy, labor, delivery, or breast-feeding (Centers for Disease Control and Prevention 2007b). Although one-quarter of infants born to untreated HIV-infected mothers are infected, transmission can be decreased to 2% by suppression of viral load below 1,000 HIV RNA using prenatal antiretroviral therapy and delivery by cesarean section (International Perinatal HIV Group 1999). It remains difficult to clearly determine the rate of HIV transmission due to breast-feeding. Current recommendations for HIV-infected women are to avoid breast-feeding if formula is available for the infant. The risk of breast-feeding should be weighed against the risk of dehydration, malnutrition, and other infections from water or formula (World Health Organization 2004). Although intravenous drug use is infrequent among children and adolescents, it is a route of maternal acquisition of HIV. In the mid-1990s, 42% of children with AIDS had mothers who used intravenous drugs.

Pediatric and adolescent exposure to HIV infection during medical procedures or blood transfusions has been reduced enormously in developed countries due to the enforcement of universal precautions and improved blood donor selection and HIV screening techniques.

Course of the Disease

The Centers for Disease Control and Prevention (CDC) has developed a classification system to describe the spectrum of HIV disease for children and infants separate from that of adolescents and adults (www.cdc.gov/hiv), in which the course and stage of the disease are defined by the appearances of a variety of mucocutaneous and opportunistic infections. Comorbid conditions that are associated with progressive immunosuppression are shown in Table 32–1.

The course of maternally transmitted or childhood HIV/AIDS differs from HIV/AIDS acquired during adolescence (Kline 2008). HIV adversely affects the developing central nervous system (CNS) and linear growth and weight gain. Overall, children and adolescents with AIDS appear to have slightly better survival rates than adults with AIDS. Children, adolescents, and young adults in whom AIDS was diagnosed during 1996–2004 lived longer than persons with AIDS in any other age group. Nine years after receiving a diagnosis of AIDS, 81% of those younger than 13 and 76% of those ages 13–24 were alive (Centers for Disease Control and Prevention 2007b; Mofenson et al. 2004).

TABLE 32–1. Conditions that emerge with advancing immunosuppression in HIV/AIDS

CD4 cell count (cells/mm^3)	Condition
200–500	Bacterial sinusitis/pneumonia Herpes simplex Herpes zoster Kaposi's sarcoma Thrush Tuberculosis reactivation
100–200	*Pneumocystis carinii* pneumonia
50–100	Cerebral toxoplasmosis Cervical carcinoma Cryptosporidiosis Peripheral neuropathy Progressive multifocal leukoencephalopathy Primary tuberculosis Systemic fungal infections
0–50	Central nervous system lymphoma Cytomegalovirus disease Disseminated *Mycobacterium avium-intracellulare* complex HIV-associated dementia Non-Hodgkin's lymphoma

Source. Adapted from American Psychiatric Association 2000b, p. 19.

Comorbidities

Neurological Manifestations

Neurological complications of HIV/AIDS are common and not limited to opportunistic infections (see Table 32–1). All levels of the neuraxis can be involved and include the brain, meninges, nerves, and spinal cord. HIV infects macrophages and monocytes but not other nervous system cells. The brain is a repository for HIV even when peripheral HIV viral levels are low. HIV may penetrate into brain tissue as early as 2 weeks after infection. The majority of patients with advanced HIV/AIDS will live with clinically evident neurological dysfunction sometime during the course of their illness (Koppel et al. 1985). In the United States and Europe, where antiretroviral therapy is relatively available, peripheral neuropathy and HIV-associated

cognitive dysfunction are the most common neurological sequelae from HIV/AIDS (McGuire 2003).

The mechanism of HIV-associated cognitive impairment is not completely understood. Mechanisms of neurotoxicity implicated include direct neuronal injury by virus proteins (Tat, gp120), products of macrophage activation (proinflammatory cytokines and chemokines interleukin 1, interleukin 6, tumor necrosis factor alpha, interferon gamma, monocyte chemoattractant protein 1, macrophage inflammatory proteins 1alpha and 1beta), neuroreceptor blockade, autoimmunity, and antibody-mediated cellular toxicity (Goodkin 2006; Shapshak et al. 1999, 2004). The term *dementia* is not commonly used to describe HIV-associated cognitive deficits or the impact of HIV on the developing nervous system in children. Cognitive decline is referred to as either HIV encephalopathy or HIV-associated progressive encephalopathy. However, "dementia due to HIV disease" in children is specifically mentioned in DSM-IV-TR (American Psychiatric Association 2000a).

HIV-associated encephalopathy in children is characterized by a triad of symptoms: impaired brain growth, progressive motor dysfunction, and loss or plateau of developmental milestones. It has an estimated prevalence of 13%–23% among infected children and is associated with lack of immune response and ongoing viremia (Goodkin 2006). The course is influenced by the timing of infection in the neurological development of the child, the strain of HIV, and genetic vulnerabilities. Three patterns of abnormal neurocognitive development have been described: 1) rapid progressive encephalopathy with loss of attained milestones, 2) subacute progression of encephalopathy with relatively stable periods, and 3) static encephalopathy with a failure to achieve new milestones (Pumariega et al. 2006). Findings from autopsy studies of children with progressive encephalopathy include inflammatory changes, calcifications of basal ganglia vessels, white matter degeneration, astrocytosis, and overall decreased brain weight. Vascular lesions ranging from aneurysm to infarctions are observed frequently (Patsalides et al. 2002).

Studies assessing cognitive status in HIV-infected children show that expressive language is significantly more impaired than receptive language. Visuomotor skills and spatial learning and memory are also frequently impaired (Frank et al. 1997; Keller et al. 2004). Wechsler Intelligence Scale for Children (WISC) scores and academic achievement scores of older HIV-infected children have also been shown to be below average. Screening for HIV cognitive impairment is in-

TABLE 32–2. Etiologies of delirium in patients with HIV/AIDS

Intracranial	Extracranial
Seizure disorders	Substance withdrawal
Central nervous system neoplasms/lymphoma	Renal failure
Toxoplasmosis	Liver failure or hepatitis
Cryptococcal meningitis	Infection/sepsis
Encephalitis due to HIV, herpes, cytomegalovirus	Endocrine dysfunction
Progressive multifocal leukoencephalopathy	Metabolic abnormalities
Pneumocystis jiroveci pneumonia	Hypoxia
	Anemia, leukopenia, thrombocytopenia
	Hypoalbuminemia
	Hypoglycemia
	Side effects of HIV medications (zidovudine, efavirenz)

Source.   Adapted from American Psychiatric Association 2000b, p. 23.

fluenced by the fact that impairment is more subcortical than cortical, and therefore clinical symptoms tend to involve motor functions, memory, mood (with flattening of emotional range), apathy, and coarsening of personality. For adolescents and adults, the HIV Dementia Scale is more sensitive to subcortical deficits than the Folstein Mini-Mental State Examination, which is directed mostly at cortical deficits and may not detect impairment until very late in the course of HIV cognitive decline. Other tests directed at assessing psychomotor speed and subcortical processing, such as the Grooved Pegboard or Trail Making Test Part B, may be clinically useful for adolescents. For children, the WISC and the Children's Memory Scale can be used to monitor cognitive status. It is important to consider the effect of environmental variables such as poverty, poor prenatal and postnatal care, and malnutrition on test results when evaluating the cognitive functioning of infected children.

Various etiologies of delirium in HIV-infected individuals are shown in Table 32–2. Little is known regarding the rate, etiology, and management of delirium in HIV-infected children and adolescents (Scharko et al. 2006). Decline in mental status in any HIV-infected patient warrants full physical examination, appropriate laboratory evaluation, and neurological evaluation, including diagnostic imaging of the brain and lumbar puncture if indicated. It is also essential to review prescribed and nonprescribed medications as well as recreational drug and alcohol use.

Psychiatric Comorbidities

Youth with HIV can present with a wide spectrum of psychiatric illnesses. Studies of HIV-infected adoles-

cents in medical care (sample sizes between 200 and 300) have found that most adolescents report significant psychosocial stresses, nearly half report high levels of depression on screening measures, and nearly half continue to have unprotected sex (Murphy et al. 2000, 2001). In one study using structured diagnostic interviews with a small number of HIV-infected adolescents, 44% presented with current major depression, 85% had at least one DSM diagnosis, and 53% had a history of psychiatric disorders prior to HIV infection (Pao et al. 2000). In addition to symptoms of anxiety and depression, parents of HIV-infected school-age children also report more conduct and hyperactivity problems in their children (Bose et al. 1994). A longitudinal study of 1,800 maternal-infected youth less than 15 years old found an increased incidence of psychiatric hospitalization compared to a sample of noninfected youth and the general pediatric population (Gaughan et al. 2004).

Substance use disorders may be more prevalent in adolescents with HIV. Among 323 HIV-infected adolescents, the frequency of alcohol and/or marijuana use was greater than use in national samples (Murphy et al. 2001). Other studies have shown that 56% of HIV-infected youth reported using marijuana in the previous month, emphasizing the importance of diligent screening (Hosek et al. 2005).

Often primary psychiatric symptoms such as depression, anxiety, mania, and psychosis are difficult to differentiate from secondary symptoms (due to general medical conditions). The timing of symptom onset in relation to infection, as well as family psychiatric history, should be considered along with the necessary medical investigation for treatable and reversible causes of psychiatric symptoms. Mood or mental status change in children or adolescents with HIV should alert the clinician to the possibility of illnesses such as opportunistic infections, neoplasms affecting the CNS, metabolic dysfunction, and drug interactions.

Pain from a variety of etiologies commonly complicates HIV disease and psychiatric presentation. Individuals with HIV often experience physical pain that increases distress, negatively affects quality of life, and influences sleep patterns. As in other chronic illnesses, pain needs to be understood within a developmental context so that preventive and therapeutic intervention strategies can be developed (Bose et al. 1994).

Treatment Overview

As HIV has become more a chronic illness, an ideal treatment model for youth living with HIV/AIDS involves the cooperation of pediatricians and psychiatrists, as well as other mental health, social services, and medical providers. With a multidisciplinary approach, the medical and psychosocial issues influencing symptoms and treatment can be determined and addressed. Ideally, care should be coordinated by a team with access to community resources as well as knowledge of the disease and the newest therapies. Very little data are available regarding the use of psychotropic medications in adolescents and children with HIV/AIDS. It is likely that many of the same psychiatric treatments and approaches can be used for infected as for noninfected patients. Thus, this section will draw on clinical principles relevant to noninfected youth and research with HIV-infected adults. Evaluation and support for psychological and psychosocial needs of affected families are crucial to the optimal management of the infected youth. Poverty, a lack of resources, social isolation, and parental history of substance abuse all influence the adjustment of children with HIV. Family-centered approaches that provide developmentally appropriate supports for the infected youth and his or her siblings and parents may reduce isolation and improve family functioning (Mellins and Ehrhardt 1994; Wight et al. 2003). Issues of adaptation to a chronic illness are confronted by youth with HIV and their families and include adherence to medical care, disclosure of infection to others, and change in the meaning of the illness due to a new developmental level or new family circumstances.

Antiretroviral Medications

Adherence to Care

Treatment of HIV illness with antiretroviral medications is aimed at suppressing viral replication and preventing deterioration of the immune system. The emergence of drug-resistant HIV during therapy remains a major challenge to treatment. HIV has a high spontaneous mutation rate, and emergence of drug resistance during treatment is frequent. The achievement of viral suppression necessitates a combination of antiretroviral agents, each with different mechanisms of action. There are four main categories of antiretroviral medications, each with numerous side effects, including behavioral and cognitive side effects (Table 32–3).

TABLE 32–3. Antiretroviral medication classes and neuropsychiatric side effects

Drug class	Antiretroviral medications	Neuropsychiatric side effects
Nucleoside and nucleotide reverse transcriptase inhibitors	abacavir, didanosine, emtricitabine, lamivudine, stavudine, tenofovir, zalcitabine, zidovudine	Agitation, mood changes, sleep disturbances, impaired concentration, confusion, seizures, peripheral neuropathy, mania, headache, somnolence, auditory hallucinations
Nonnucleoside reverse transcriptase inhibitors	delavirdine, efavirenz, nevirapine	Agitation, mood changes, sleep disturbances, depersonalization, suicidality, psychosis, catatonia, delirium
Protease inhibitors	atazanavir, fosamprenavir, indinavir, lopinavir, nelfinavir, ritonavir, saquinavir	Agitation, mood changes, sleep disturbances
Fusion inhibitors	enfuvirtide	Mood changes

Near-perfect adherence to an antiretroviral regimen is important, and data show that medication adherence is a predictor of therapeutic effect and related to lower viral load (Feingold et al. 2000; Flynn et al. 2004). Unfortunately, adherence to medications for HIV by youth is suboptimal (Reddington et al. 2000). Family disruption; poor provider-patient relationship; fear of social stigma; anxiety; depression; and substance abuse all negatively influence adherence to medication regimens and other aspects of care (Simoni et al. 2007). Accessibility to treatment, education, good patient-provider relationships, and successful treatment of anxiety and depression increase adherence (Simoni et al. 2007). Assessment of the barriers to compliance at each visit with a health care provider can increase commitment to medication regimens if done in a supportive, nonjudgmental way. Behavioral strategies such as visual reminders (calendars and daily schedules) and incentives for desirable behavior, as well as psychopharmacological treatment of underlying behavioral difficulties, can be implemented. Cognitive-behavioral therapies for improved adherence to care are being studied and are promising (Lemanek et al. 2001).

Neurocognitive Functioning

The use of antiretroviral medications can improve cognitive deficits or symptoms of progressive encephalopathy and adaptive functioning in children for a period of time. Treatment with antiretroviral medications has been associated with improvements in communication and socialization, as well as improved performance on age-appropriate assessments, such as the WISC, McCarthy Scales of Children's Abilities, and the Bayley Scales of Infant Development. Unfortunately, antiretroviral treatment has not been shown to prevent neurocognitive decline permanently. Often neuropathological and neuropsychological deficits are enduring due to the development of resistance to antiretroviral medications (Civitello 2003).

Psychopharmacological Treatment

The optimal psychopharmacological treatment of HIV-infected children and adolescents is a subject of debate and in need of further research. A balance of the risks and benefits associated with the use of psychotropic medication should be determined in each individual. It is likely that many of the same approaches and psychiatric treatments can be used for infected as

noninfected youth. The general principles when prescribing a psychotropic medication to patients with HIV or AIDS are to start with lower doses and titrate the medication slowly, to be aware of potential drug-drug interactions between psychotropic and antiretroviral medications, to be cognizant of possible side effects of drugs being prescribed, and to use the simplest drug regimen possible. Nonnucleoside reverse transcriptase inhibitors and protease inhibitors are metabolized by and inhibit various cytochrome P450 (CYP450) isoenzymes including 3A4, 2B6, 1A2, 2D6, 2C9, and 2C19. Theoretically, psychotropic medications that are also metabolized by and/or inhibit these isoenzymes can cause toxicity. Ritonavir, a protease inhibitor, is most likely to cause drug-drug interactions as it is a potent inhibitor of 3A4 and a paninhibitor of other isoenzymes. Although the risk of negative drug-drug interactions exists between psychotropic and antiretroviral medications, untreated psychiatric disorders can lead to a decrease in the patient's quality of life, an increase in suicidal behavior, and an increased need for health care.

Antidepressants

The selective serotonin reuptake inhibitors (SSRIs) are the most commonly prescribed class of medications for anxiety and depression in HIV-infected adults (Ruiz et al. 2000). In children and adolescents with HIV, SSRIs have been used and well tolerated; however, the efficacy of SSRIs in children and adolescents with HIV is unknown. The SSRIs are metabolized by several CYP450 enzymes, making it likely that other CYP450 enzymes will take over if one is inhibited. It is believed that most SSRIs can be given safely with many antiretroviral regimens. There is evidence in adults that coadministration of escitalopram with ritonavir does not result in a clinically significant interaction, but there have been case reports of serotonin syndrome in adults while taking ritonavir and fluoxetine (DeSilva et al. 2001; Gutierrez et al. 2003).

Venlafaxine, duloxetine, and mirtazapine are considered to be relatively safe in adults taking antiretroviral regimens. Venlafaxine and duloxetine are metabolized mostly by CYP2D6, which is inhibited by ritonavir—although it is unclear if this interaction is clinically significant. Mirtazapine is metabolized by CYP1A2, 2D6, and 3A4, making it likely that if one enzyme is inhibited, other enzymes could take over the metabolism of the drug. Bupropion, which is metabolized primarily by CYP2B6 and inhibits 2D6 moderately, should be used cautiously with ritonavir, efavirenz, and nelfinavir, since inhibition may increase its plasma levels. Due to the adverse effects of nausea, hypotension, syncope, priapism, respiratory distress associated with trazodone, and the rare but fatal hepatotoxicity associated with nefazodone, the use of these drugs with antiretroviral medications such as ritonavir, which inhibit their metabolism, is discouraged (Bialer et al. 2006).

Mood Stabilizers

Although the efficacy of mood stabilizers in HIV-infected children and adolescents has not been established, they are in clinical use. With lithium, care must be given to concurrent administration of antibiotics, cardiovascular/antihypertensive drugs, and nonsteroidal anti-inflammatory agents that are known to contribute to lithium toxicity. Lithium has the potential to aggravate HIV-associated nephropathy, but data are limited. Valproate and lamotrigine are also used, since they may be efficacious in controlling secondary mania that develops in the context of HIV disease. Ritonavir and nelfinavir may cause a decrease in levels of the mood stabilizers by induction of glucuronyl transferase, but data in adults are unclear regarding the clinical significance of these potential interactions. In all cases, close monitoring of available serum levels is prudent (Bialer et al. 2006; Ruiz et al. 2000).

Antipsychotics

The general regimen is the use of high-potency antipsychotics starting at a low dose and with lower target doses in patients with advanced HIV disease. Typical neuroleptics, with the exception of pimozide, inhibit and are metabolized by CYP2D6. Therefore, coadministration with ritonavir could theoretically lead to increased levels and potential toxicity. In contrast, the atypical antipsychotics are metabolized by multiple CYP450 enzymes and may be better tolerated. It is recommended to avoid the coadministration of clozapine with the protease inhibitor ritonavir (American Psychiatric Association 2000b; Bialer et al. 2006; Ruiz et al. 2000).

Anxiolytics

The mainstays of psychotropic treatment for anxiety disorders in adults are antidepressants and benzodiazepines. In patients with HIV on antiretroviral therapy, lorazepam, temazepam, and oxazepam are preferable due to their lack of active metabolites. They have no known drug interactions with antiretrovirals. These benzodiazepines are also preferred in patients with compromised liver function due to concomitant

illnesses such as hepatitis C. Benzodiazepines are not considered first-line treatments for anxiety in children and adolescents with or without HIV, and SSRIs are more commonly used.

Stimulants

Hyperactivity associated with HIV encephalopathy and primary attention-deficit/hyperactivity disorder in children with HIV has been treated with methylphenidate and clonidine, with safety and good results (Pumariega et al. 2006). In adults, stimulants have been used with success to treat depression, cognitive decline, and fatigue (Bialer et al. 2006), although there are no such data for their use for these symptoms in youth.

Psychotherapeutic Treatment

Suicidality

Although there has been a decline in stigma associated with HIV, as well as promising medical advancements, children and adolescents with HIV continue to experience psychological distress (Brown et al. 2000a). It is unknown how advances in antiretroviral therapy and decreasing stigma have affected suicidality. It is also unknown if stresses at specific stages of illness (e.g., diagnosis, disclosure to family) are associated with greater suicidality. The general prevalence of suicidality in adolescents and our lack of information about its timing underscore the importance of screening for suicidality throughout the course of treatment for HIV.

Sexual Abuse

Sexual abuse is prevalent among youth with HIV. Such abuse is associated with a variety of negative outcomes including suicide attempts, alcohol and/or drug use, and use of crack cocaine. Among infected youth, it is also associated with more conduct problems, incarceration, and greater sexual risk behavior (Anaya et al. 2005). The identification of abuse can lead to appropriate legal and family notification and treatment, as it would for noninfected youth.

High-Risk Sexual Behavior

Most infected youth experience turmoil concerning HIV infection that influences their perception of sexuality and intimate relationships. Psychoeducational and therapeutic approaches have been proven to be effective in improving safer sexual behaviors and reinforcing safer peer norms. For example, a motivation and skills intervention with HIV-infected adolescents with hemophilia, comprised of individual and peer group activities, increased safer sex and the perception of peer approval for safer sexual behaviors (Brown et al. 2000b). Other research has demonstrated that group programs result in less distress, more social support, and safer sexual behavior (Rotheram-Borus et al. 2001a, 2001b). During psychotherapy, issues such as denial of infection and its negative effect on safe sex practices can be addressed. Overall, effective psychoeducational approaches are likely to enhance motivation for responsible behavior by acknowledging anger concerning infection, improving skills in group settings, and reinforcing safer peer norms.

Bereavement

Children and adolescents with HIV not only have to cope with their own mortality but often have to cope with the illness and loss of a family member. Bereavement is complicated by social stigma. If secrecy surrounds the death of a family member or parent with AIDS, this may lead children and adolescents to believe that their illness is shameful. Therapy with HIV-infected youth who are experiencing the loss of a family member can allow open expression of the patient's fears and fantasies in order to prevent pathological grief reactions. Interventions can also support extended family members, including siblings, when appropriate. For example, a lengthy cognitive-behavioral multifamily group intervention dealing with adaptation to HIV/AIDS has been described and tested by Rotheram-Borus et al. (1998).

Disclosure and Stigma

The cultural, social, and economic contexts are important when considering issues of stigma in HIV-infected youth. In the United States, despite increasing social acceptance of HIV infection, stigma remains a profound issue and affects issues such as disclosure of one's infection. Caregivers of young children may anticipate stigma and postpone disclosure of an HIV diagnosis to their children. Caregivers may realistically worry that stigma and shame will lead to further ostracism, impairing a child's sense of emotional well-being and competence. However, case reports suggest that less secrecy about HIV helps children feel decreased shame and can lead to more positive family relationships. Because studies suggest that disclosure is associated with higher self-esteem for children and less depression for parents, the American Academy of Pediatrics recommends that disclosure of the diagno-

sis to an HIV-infected child should be individualized to include the child's cognitive ability, developmental stage, clinical status, and social circumstances (American Academy of Pediatrics 1999). Symptomatic children, particularly those requiring hospitalization, should be informed of their HIV status, as the likelihood of children inadvertently learning about their status in the hospital setting is high. Disclosure should optimally be conducted in a controlled situation with parents and knowledgeable professionals. Adolescents should know their HIV status and be fully informed of the illness to maximize their health behavior, including sexual behavior. Adolescents may be reluctant to disclose their infection to partners and may worry that suggesting condom use with a committed partner will lead to suspicion or disclosure of their infection. Similarly, worries about inadvertent disclosure of infection to friends may inhibit adolescents from attending medical appointments regularly or being adherent with medication regimens. For all youth, being knowledgeable about their medical status and its implications and having the skills to reveal their infection to important people in their lives are reasonable goals that are likely to result in less distress, greater medical adherence, and safer behavior. Achieving these goals should be viewed as a process that takes into account the resources and barriers of each patient and family.

Prevention

Prevention Programs

HIV prevention is important in child and adolescent mental health settings because adolescents with psychiatric disorders are at increased risk of infection due to involvement in sexual risk activities and substance use. In addition, factors such as previous trauma, chaotic family situations, poverty, limited educational and employment opportunities, and lack of access to appropriate medical care can further increase risk. Although few programs have been designed specifically for adolescents with psychiatric disorders, effective prevention programs have been developed for adolescents in the community.

Successful HIV programs, based on social learning theory, have aimed to enhance motivation for safer sex and to consolidate communication and condom use skills. Such programs have been shown to delay the onset of sexual initiation and/or reduce sexual risk be-

TABLE 32–4. Assessing sexual risk in the clinical interview

Use understandable, nontechnical language geared to the patient's cognitive level and culture. Younger patients are especially likely to have misunderstandings or misconceptions about HIV and sex.

Use specific, rather than general, language. "Have you had vaginal sex?" is preferable to the nonspecific "Are you sexually active?"

Avoid gender-specific language. Do not presume the gender of sexual partners.

Inquire directly about substance use/abuse, especially use during sex.

Ask about plans for beginning or continuing sex and its effects on the patient's life and relationships.

The number of sexual partners and condom use at last intercourse are two of the most reliable indicators of sexual risk.

Find out about the nature of the partner relationship (e.g., screen for dating violence) and whether this is a "main" partner (less likely to use a condom).

Determine whether the teen has the skills for condom use and negotiation with partners.

havior (Johnson et al. 2006; Pedlow and Carey 2004). Motivation for safe behavior is increased by acquiring recognition of personal vulnerability to HIV and other STDs. Relevant skills, such as condom use and appropriate assertive and sexual communication with partners, can be practiced in small-group settings. These groups are opportunities to promote positive peer norms for safer sex and abstinence and to help adolescents learn to cope with peer pressure.

While interventions with these components are found to be helpful in most community settings, meta-analyses and reviews have found that they work less well in clinical and detention settings (Brown et al. 1997; Johnson et al. 2003, 2006; Pedlow and Carey 2004). Adolescents with psychiatric disorders fail to benefit from these interventions as the material is not geared to their impairments and the constellation of complex problems that they face. Issues of impulsivity, sensitivity to rejection, family dysfunction, and substance use may not be sufficiently addressed. Also, skills for managing anxiety associated with the context of sexual activity may be especially problematic for adolescents in mental health treatment due to their general distress, difficulty with affect management, or previous traumas such as sexual abuse (Lescano et al. 2004).

Clinical Intervention

Mental health professionals are well positioned to reduce HIV risk in teens in psychiatric care (Donenberg and Pao 2005). Clinicians can approach safe sexual behavior directly with patients by asking about sexual behavior, condom use, and the place of sex in the adolescent's life. Questions about sexual behavior and risk should be part of a standard clinical interview, and critical elements can be found in Table 32–4.

A comprehensive assessment of sexual behavior and risk is quite significant in its own right and conveys the importance of sexual behavior to therapy and treatment. It also conveys concern about the patient's well-being and indicates that the adolescent has control over his or her sexual behavior. As teens talk more about their behavior, their awareness of and motivation to change their behavior can increase (Brown and Lourie 2001). Motivational interviewing (Miller and Rollnick 2002) using open-ended questioning elicits the patient's own thoughts about risk and change. For example, informing a patient that three-quarters of teens his age did not smoke marijuana in the last month or that 85% of teens have not had four or more sexual partners can help the teen contextualize his own behavior (Centers for Disease Control and Prevention 2006b). Also, dramatic relief ("What would your life be like if you were infected with HIV?") may elicit an emotional response that can be used as the basis for change. As well, teens can be encouraged to engage in self-reevaluation ("You said your boyfriend might use condoms, but you choose not to ask him to") and rethink previous decisions.

Beyond adolescents' own attitudes and risk behaviors, it is also crucial to understand their perceptions of the norms of their peer group and the influence of sexual partners. Adolescents often overestimate the extent and prevalence of sexual risk among their friends. For those who are dependent on risk-taking peers, the challenges of negotiating safe behavior within peer group pressure can be highlighted. Understanding the nature of the relationship with an adolescent's sex partner is also crucial. Teens tend not to have the same partner for long. Instead, many practice brief serial monogamy with a partner they love or feel a commitment toward. Despite the emotional connection, the risk is great, given the possibility of infection of their partner by previous partners.

In addition, recent research suggests that about one-third of adolescents have a "casual" partner and that sexual behavior differs by partner type (Lescano et al. 2006). Teens are more likely to use condoms with casual partners, but still not consistently, so a substantial risk remains. Adolescents tend to overestimate the safety of using condoms "most of the time" with casual partners and underestimate the risk of not using condoms with partners with whom they feel a commitment.

Role of the Family

Parents and families play an important role in teenagers' sexual attitudes and behavior (Donenberg et al. 2001, 2002; Fisher and Feldman 1998). Many family factors are associated with teenagers' sexual risk taking: limited parental monitoring, availability, and support; coercive family exchanges; frequent parental criticism and hostility; poor family communication; and parent-adolescent conflict are implicated in the etiology and maintenance of risky sexual behavior (Bettinger et al. 2004; McBride et al. 2003; Voisin 2002). Fortunately, more comfortable and direct family communication can have a substantial impact, increasing condom use (Holtzman and Rubinson 1995; Lehr et al. 2000; Leland and Barth 1993; Romer et al. 1999; Whitaker and Miller 2000; Whitaker et al. 1999), decreasing number of sexual partners (Holtzman and Rubinson 1995; Leland and Barth 1993), increasing condom self-efficacy (Dittus et al. 1999; Hutchinson and Cooney 1998), and increasing communication with sexual partners (Hutchinson and Cooney 1998; Whitaker et al. 1999). Talking prior to sexual debut appears to be especially important (Miller et al. 1998). Clinicians can help families initiate and/or consistently monitor the teen's behavior. In conjunction with vigilant monitoring, parents need to acknowledge that adolescents have a developmental need for some privacy and autonomy. These issues are made difficult by parents' anxiety at considering their children to be emerging sexual beings. Another task is to help the teen see the family as a potential source of support, not just a source of conflict. The clinician can help to begin a joint conversation between the teen and parents about sexual behavior, and the clinician can model and direct respectful interaction between the parties.

Summary Points

HIV Infection

- HIV infection continues to rise in adolescents, especially in minority and disadvantaged communities.
- HIV/AIDS is now a chronic, not acute, condition in developed countries.
- Adherence to medical care is critical to prevent antiretroviral resistance and is influenced by developmental, motivational, and family factors.
- A change in mood or mental state may be due to advancing HIV disease, opportunistic infections, medication side effects, or new social stress.
- Psychological issues to address are stigma, disclosure of infection, and bereavement and trauma.
- Cognitive impairment is possible and usually subcortical in nature.
- Most psychotropic medications can be used, but be aware of possible antiretroviral interactions via the CYP system.

HIV Prevention

- Youth with psychiatric disorders are at greater risk due to impairments, substance use, previous trauma, and poor family functioning.
- A careful evaluation of sexual behavior is therapeutic.
- Address personal relevance of HIV/STDs and motivation and skills for safer sexual behavior.
- Condom use may be sporadic, less frequent with a "committed" partner, and impaired due to anxiety.
- Family communication and parental monitoring are helpful.

References

American Academy of Pediatrics: Disclosure of illness status to children and adolescents with HIV infection. Pediatrics 103:164–166, 1999

American Psychiatric Association: Diagnostic and Statistical Manual of Mental Disorders, 4th Edition, Text Revision. Washington, DC, American Psychiatric Association, 2000a

American Psychiatric Association: Practice guideline for the treatment of patients with HIV/AIDS. Am J Psychiatry 157(suppl):1–62, 2000b

Anaya HD, Swedeman D, Rotherman-Borus MJ: Differences among sexually abused and nonabused youth living with HIV. J Interpers Violence 20:1547–1559, 2005

Bettinger JA, Celentano DD, Curriero FC, et al: Does parental involvement predict new sexually transmitted diseases in female adolescents? Arch Pediatr Adolesc Med 158:666–670, 2004

Bialer PA, Kato K, Latoussakis V: Psychotropic drug interactions with antiretroviral medications, in Psychiatric Aspects of HIV/AIDS. Edited by Kato K, Latoussakis V. Baltimore, MD, Lippincott Williams & Wilkins, 2006, pp 149–160

Bose S, Moss HA, Brouwers P, et al: Psychologic adjustment of human immunodeficiency virus-infected school age children. J Dev Behav Pediatr 15:526–533, 1994

Brown LK, Lourie KJ: Motivational interviewing and the prevention of HIV among adolescents, in Adolescents, Alcohol, and Substance Abuse: Reaching Teens Through Brief Interventions. Edited by Monti PM, Colby SM, O'Leary TA. New York, Guilford, 2001, pp 244–274

Brown LK, Danovsky MB, Lourie KJ, et al: Adolescents with psychiatric disorders and the risk of HIV. J Am Acad Child Adolesc Psychiatry 36:1609–1617, 1997

Brown LK, Lourie KJ, Pao M: Children and adolescents living with HIV and AIDS: a review. J Child Psychol Psychiatry 41:81–96, 2000a

Brown LK, Schultz JR, Parsons JT, et al: Sexual behavior change among HIV-infected adolescents with hemophilia. Pediatrics 106:1–6, 2000b

Centers for Disease Control and Prevention: Trends in Reportable Sexually Transmitted Diseases in the United States, 2005. Atlanta, GA, Centers for Disease Control and Prevention, 2006a. Available at: http://www.cdc.gov/std/stats05/trends2005.htm. Accessed July 13, 2007.

Centers for Disease Control and Prevention: Youth risk behavior surveillance—United States 2005. MMWR Surveill Summ 55:1–83, 2006b

Centers for Disease Control and Prevention: HIV/AIDS Surveillance in Adolescents and Young Adults (Through 2005). Atlanta, GA, Centers for Disease Control and Prevention, 2007a. Available at: http://www.cdc.gov/hiv/topics/surveillance/resources/slides/adolescents/. Accessed July 16, 2007.

Centers for Disease Control and Prevention: HIV/AIDS Surveillance Report 2005, Vol 17, Revised Edition. Atlanta, GA, Centers for Disease Control and Prevention, 2007b

Centers for Disease Control and Prevention: HIV prevalence estimates—United States, 2006. MMWR Morb Mortal Wkly Rep 57:1073–1076, 2008

Civitello L: Neurologic aspects of HIV infection in infants and children: therapeutic approaches and outcome. Curr Neurol Neurosci Rep 3:120–128, 2003

DeSilva K, Le Flore DB, Marston BJ, et al: Serotonin syndrome in HIV-infected individuals receiving antiretroviral therapy and fluoxetine. AIDS 15:1281–1285, 2001

Dittus PJ, Jaccard J, Gordon VV: Direct and nondirect communication of maternal beliefs to adolescents: adolescent motivations for premarital sexual activity. J Appl Soc Psychol 29:1927–1963, 1999

Donenberg GR, Pao M: Youth and HIV/AIDS: psychiatry's role in a changing epidemic. J Am Acad Child Adolesc Psychiatry 44:728–747, 2005

Donenberg GR, Emerson E, Bryant FB, et al: Understanding AIDS-risk behavior in clinically disturbed adolescents: links to psychopathology and peer relationships. J Am Acad Child Adolesc Psychiatry 40:642–653, 2001

Donenberg GR, Wilson HW, Emerson E, et al: Holding the line with a watchful eye: the impact of perceived parental monitoring on risky sexual behavior among adolescents in psychiatric care. AIDS Educ Prev 14:138–157, 2002

Feingold AR, Rutstein RM, Meislich D, et al: Protease inhibitor therapy in HIV-infected children. AIDS Patient Care STDS 14:589–593, 2000

Fisher L, Feldman SS: Familial antecedents of young adult health risk behavior: a longitudinal study. J Fam Psychol 12:66–80, 1998

Fleming D, Wasserheit J: From epidemiological synergy to public health policy and practice: the contribution of other sexually transmitted diseases to sexual transmission of HIV infection. Sex Transm Infect 75:3–17, 1999

Flynn PM, Rudy BJ, Douglas SD, et al: Virologic and immunologic outcomes after 24 weeks in HIV-positive adolescents receiving highly active antiretroviral therapy. J Infect Dis 190:271–279, 2004

Frank EG, Foley GM, Kuchuk A: Cognitive functioning in school-age children with HIV. Percept Mot Skills 85:267–272, 1997

Gaughan DM, Hughes MD, Oleske J, et al: Psychiatric hospitalizations among children and youths with human immunodeficiency virus infection. Pediatrics 113:544–551, 2004

Goodkin K: Virology, immunology, transmission, and disease stage, in Psychiatric Aspects of HIV/AIDS. Edited by Fernandez F, Ruiz P. Philadelphia, PA, Lippincott Williams & Wilkins, 2006, pp 11–22

Grant AM, Jamieson DJ, Elam-Evans LD, et al: Reasons for testing and clinical and demographic profile of adolescents with nonperinatally acquired HIV infection. Pediatrics 117:468–475, 2006

Gutierrez MM, Rosenberg J, Abramowitz W: An evaluation of the potential for pharmacokinetic interaction between escitalopram and the cytochrome P450 3A4 inhibitor ritonavir. Clin Ther 25:1200–1210, 2003

Holtzman D, Rubinson R: Parent and peer communication effects on AIDS-related behavior among U.S. high school students. Fam Plann Perspect 27:235–240, 268, 1995

Hosek SG, Harper GW, Domanico R: Predictors of medication adherence among HIV-infected youth. Psychol Health Med 10:166–179, 2005

Hutchinson MK, Cooney TM: Patterns of parent-teen sexual risk communication implications for intervention. Fam Relat 47:185–194, 1998

International Perinatal HIV Group: The mode of delivery and the risk of vertical transmission of human immunodeficiency virus type 1: a meta-analysis of 15 prospective cohort studies. N Engl J Med 340:977–987, 1999

Johnson BT, Carey MP, Marsh KL, et al: Interventions to reduce sexual risk for the human immunodeficiency virus in adolescents, 1985–2000. Arch Pediatr Adolesc Med 157:381–388, 2003

Johnson BT, Carey MP, Chaudoir SR, et al: Sexual risk reduction for persons living with HIV. J Acquir Immune Defic Syndr 41:642–650, 2006

Keller MA, Venkatraman TN, Thomas A, et al: Altered neurometabolite development in HIV-infected children: correlation with neuropsychological tests. Neurology 62:1810–1817, 2004

Kline MW: Pediatric HIV Infection. Houston, TX, Baylor International Pediatric AIDS Initiative, 2008. Available at: http://bayloraids.org/resources/pedaids. Accessed February 29, 2008.

Koppel BS, Wormser G, Tuchman AJ, et al: Central nervous system involvement in patients with acquired immune deficiency syndrome (AIDS). Acta Neurol Scand 71:337–353, 1985

Lehr ST, DiIorio C, Dudley WN, et al: The relationships between parent-adolescent communication and safer sex behaviors in college students. J Fam Nurs 6:180–196, 2000

Leland NL, Barth RP: Characteristics of adolescents who have attempted to avoid HIV and who have communicated with parents about sex. J Adolesc Res 8:58–76, 1993

Lemanek KL, Kamps J, Chung NB: Empirically supported treatments in pediatric psychology: regimen adherence. J Pediatr Psychol 26:253–275, 2001

Lescano CM, Brown LK, Puster K, et al: Sexual abuse and adolescent HIV risk: a group intervention framework. J HIV AIDS Prev Child Youth 6:43–57, 2004

Lescano CM, Vazquez EA, Brown LK, et al: Condom use with "casual" and "main" partners: what's in a name? J Adolesc Health 39:443, 2006

McBride CK, Paikoff RL, Holmbeck GN: Individual and familial influences on the onset of sexual intercourse among urban African American adolescents. J Consult Clin Psychol 71:159–167, 2003

McGuire D: Neurologic manifestations of HIV, in HIV InSite Web site. San Francisco, University of California–San Francisco, 2003. Available at: http://hivinsite.ucsf.edu/InSite?page=kb-04-01-02. Accessed July 7, 2007.

Mellins CA, Ehrhardt AA: Families affected by pediatric AIDS: sources of stress and coping. J Dev Behav Pediatr 15:S54–S60, 1994

Miller KS, Levin ML, Whitaker DJ, et al: Patterns of condom use among adolescents: the impact of mother-adolescent communication. Am J Public Health 88:1542–1544, 1998

Miller WR, Rollnick S: Motivational Interviewing: Preparing People for Change, 2nd Edition. New York, Guilford, 2002

Mofenson LM, Oleske J, Serchuck L, et al: Treating opportunistic infections among HIV-exposed and infected children: recommendations from CDC, the National Institutes of Health, and the Infectious Diseases Society of America. MMWR Recomm Rep 53:1–92, 2004

Murphy DA, Moscicki AB, Vermund SH, et al: Psychological distress among HIV-positive adolescents in the REACH study: Effects of life stress, social support and coping. J Adolesc Health 27:391–398, 2000

Murphy DA, Durako SJ, Moscicki A, et al: No change in health risk behaviors over time among HIV-infected adolescents in care: role of psychological distress. J Adolesc Health 29:57–63, 2001

Pao M, Lyon M, D'Angelo LJ, et al: Psychiatric diagnoses in HIV seropositive adolescents. Arch Pediatr Adolesc Med 154:240–244, 2000

Patsalides AD, Wood LV, Atac GK, et al: Cerebrovascular disease in HIV-infected pediatric patients: neuroimaging findings. Am J Roentgenol 179:999–1003, 2002

Pedlow CT, Carey MP: Developmentally appropriate sexual risk reduction interventions for adolescents: rationale, review of interventions, and recommendations for research and practice. Ann Behav Med 27:172–184, 2004

Pumariega AJ, Shugart M, Pumariega JB: HIV/AIDS among children and adolescents in Psychiatric Aspects of HIV/AIDS. Edited by Fernandez F, Ruiz P. Baltimore, MD, Lippincott Williams & Wilkins, 2006, pp 149–160

Reddington C, Cohen J, Baldillo A, et al: Adherence to medication regimens among children with human immunodeficiency virus infection. Pediatr Infect Dis J 19:1148–1153, 2000

Romer D, Stanton B, Galbraith J, et al: Parental influence on adolescent sexual behavior in high-poverty settings. Arch Pediatr Adolesc Med 153:1055–1062, 1999

Rothenberg R, Scarlett M, del Rio C, et al: Oral transmission of HIV. AIDS 12:2095–2105, 1998

Rotheram-Borus MJ, Murphy DA, Miller S, et al: An intervention for adolescents whose parents are living with AIDS. Clin Child Psychol Psychiatry 2:201–219, 1998

Rotheram-Borus MJ, Lee M, Murphy DA, et al: Efficacy of a preventive intervention for youths living with HIV. Am J Public Health 91:400–405, 2001a

Rotheram-Borus MJ, Murphy DA, Wight RG, et al: Improving the quality of life among young people living with HIV. Eval Program Plann 24:227–237, 2001b

Ruiz P, Guynn RW, Matorin AA: Psychiatric considerations in the diagnosis, treatment and prevention of HIV/AIDS. J Psychiatr Pract 6:129–139, 2000

Scharko AM, Baker EH, Kothari HM, et al: Case study: delirium in an adolescent girl with human immunodeficiency virus-associated dementia. J Am Acad Child Adolesc Psychiatry 45:104–108, 2006

Shapshak P, Segal DM, Crandall KA, et al: Independent evolution of HIV type 1 in different brain regions. AIDS Res Hum Retroviruses 15:811–820, 1999

Shapshak P, Duncan R, Minagar A, et al: Elevated expression of INF-gamma in the HIV-1 infected brain. Front Biosci 1:1073–1081, 2004

Simoni JM, Montgomery A, Martin E, et al: Adherence to antiretroviral therapy for pediatric HIV infection: a qualitative systematic review with recommendations for research and clinical management. Pediatrics 119:e1371–e1381, 2007

Voisin DR: Family ecology and HIV sexual risk behaviors among African American and Puerto Rican adolescent males. Am J Orthopsychiatry 72:294–302, 2002

Weinstock H, Berman S, Cates W: Sexually transmitted diseases among American youth: incidence and prevalence estimates 2000. Perspect Sex Reprod Health 36:6–10, 2004

Whitaker D, Miller KS: Parent-adolescent discussions about sex and condoms: impact on peer influences of sexual risk behavior. J Adolesc Research 15:251–273, 2000

Whitaker D, Miller KS, May DC, et al: Teenage partners' communication about sexual risk and condom use: the importance of parent-teenager discussions. Fam Plann Perspect 31:117–121, 1999

Wight R, Aneshensel C, Le Blanc A: Stress buffering effects of family support in AIDS care giving. AIDS Care 15:595–613, 2003

World Health Organization: HIV Transmission Through Breastfeeding: A Review of Available Evidence. Geneva, Switzerland, World Health Organization, 2004, pp 1–25

Chapter 33

Bereavement and Traumatic Grief

Judith A. Cohen, M.D.
Anthony P. Mannarino, Ph.D.

Nearly all children lose to death someone close to them. One in 20 children will experience the death of a parent before reaching adulthood; one in seven will experience the death of an immediate family member (sibling, parent, or grandparent) by the age of 18 (Social Security Administration 2000). Thus in one way or another, many children have some experience with bereavement.

Uncomplicated Bereavement

The terms bereavement, grief and mourning are often used interchangeably, but they have different meanings.

Bereavement is the condition of having had someone close die. *Grief* is the intense emotion that one feels upon having someone close die. *Mourning* encompasses the religious, ethnic, community, and/or cultural practices associated with bereavement. *Uncomplicated bereavement* in children resembles depression in many ways, sharing great sadness or grief, crying, withdrawing from others, not wanting to eat, being unable to sleep or pay attention in school, losing interest in normal activities, and perhaps (especially in younger children) searching or asking for the deceased person. Like adults, children experience "pangs" of grief: sudden, seemingly unprovoked, intense waves of painful feelings. In contrast to adults, children often show these symptoms intermittently and may seem perfectly normal at other times, being able to play or laugh even during very solemn times, such as when they are at memorial services or when the rest of the family is crying. This may lead adults to wonder whether children are inured or callous to the more constant grief that adults tend to experience. The intermittent nature of children's expressions of grief is characteristic of children's general affective states, which are often more changeable and reactive than those of adults.

Although Kübler-Ross described grief reactions as occurring in stages, we now understand uncomplicated childhood grief as consisting of typical tasks, which may be accomplished over varying periods of time. These tasks do not necessarily occur in sequential order; children may return to a previous task while working through a later one. Worden (1996) and Wolfelt (1996) described the following tasks of uncomplicated child bereavement:

1. Accepting the reality of the death
2. Fully experiencing the pain of the death
3. Adjusting to an environment and self-identity without the deceased
4. Converting the relationship with the deceased from one of interaction to one of memory
5. Finding meaning in the deceased's death
6. Experiencing a continued supportive relationship with adults in the future

Task 1

Children may have a particularly difficult time accepting the reality of death, since they have had less experience with death than adults, and younger children may have less ability to cognitively comprehend the permanence of death. This is why very young children may ask, "When is mommy coming home?" despite having had repeated explanations that mommy is "dead" and "can never come home again." In some cases seeing the dead body, attending funerals, seeing adults weeping, and being present at other mourning rituals may help them to accept the reality of death by confronting it more directly. In these situations, it is important for an adult to be available to the child, to answer questions and provide emotional support. If all of the available adults are emotionally distraught, it may be preferable for the child to skip these activities rather than to attend without a supportive adult.

Task 2

As bereaved adults know, grief is one of the most painful emotions that humans can experience, and children experience this overwhelming pain no less than adults. With uncomplicated grief, children eventually regain their previous level of functioning but still feel sadness at predictable times, such as "anniversary" dates (e.g., the deceased's birthday, the anniversary of the deceased's death, Mother's Day if the deceased was the child's mother).

Task 3

As children recover from acute grief, they also have to adjust to their environment without their significant other. At first, everything around them may remind them of the deceased, especially if the deceased person lived with them. The first time children do each thing without the significant other, it is a reminder that "he isn't here with me anymore." This may be an impetus for renewed pangs of grief. Typically a gradual adjustment process occurs whereby it becomes easier for children to tolerate the deceased's absence. Children also have to develop new identities in which some important qualities or characteristics of the deceased person are typically adopted as the traits of children's own internalized self. For example, adopting an important belief or credo of the deceased is one way for the child to incorporate part of the deceased into his or her own self-identity. Thus, although the deceased is no longer alive, a treasured aspect of that person continues as a "living presence" in the children's lives.

Task 4

In this task children must come to accept that they can no longer see, speak to, go places with, or regularly interact with the deceased person. The deceased is no longer a living, breathing person. All that is left of the deceased is memories and the love and other good things that the person gave them while they were alive. Children must make the difficult and painful step in accepting that the deceased is no longer and will never again be available on a day-to-day basis. The person is gone and can be accessed only in the child's memory.

Task 5

Like adults, children struggle to understand how someone who meant so much could be taken away. Some children may question their religious faith, whereas others, to find comfort, may lean more heavily on their belief in a deity. Regardless of developmental level, children seek answers for why the death happened. Children may wonder whether someone was "to blame," perhaps the doctor (if the deceased died of an illness) or even the child himself or herself (if there is no one else obvious to blame). This is why it is important for adults to provide accurate information to children about the cause of death, even if by violent means. Children often surprise adults in their ability to make profound meaning of death and to move forward in their lives.

Task 6

After the death of a significant other, some children hesitate to get close to adults, fearing that since they are older than children, they are likely to die soon, too. However, at this time children especially need the ongoing support of adults, whether their parents or, in the tragic event that one or both of their parents died, other loving and caring adults. Providing reassurance about the adult in question and having an open discussion about the child's concerns about another death are often sufficient in these situations; if not, children may need additional interventions, including a mental health assessment if this is indicated.

Each of the above tasks requires the child to tolerate thoughts and memories about the deceased person, however painful these may be. For some children this is too painful, and these children may avoid memories of the deceased. Such children may develop childhood traumatic grief, which is described later in this chapter.

Intervention: Peer Support Groups

Because the timing of children negotiating each of these tasks has not been well studied, there is little empirical information available to parents or professionals regarding normal versus pathological responses for bereaved children and when parents should seek help for these children. Most bereaved children in the United States receive no mental health interventions; for those children who do receive services, the most commonly provided appear to be bereavement peer support groups such as those developed by the Dougy Center (www.dougy.org). The Dougy model consists of peer support groups facilitated by adult volunteers. Providers of children's support groups do not conceptualize these groups as "therapy," nor do they regard child attendees as having pathological responses. Rather, they view almost all responses to grief as being normal; for this reason, many do not believe in the existence of traumatic grief in children (Schurmann 2006). Children in bereavement peer support groups engage in a variety of activities to remember and memorialize their special deceased person in the company of other children who are also grieving. An example might be to draw a memory of a happy time that the child shared with the deceased person to put in a group quilt or in a memory box. Other examples might be to have a group discussion about what children believe happens when someone they love dies or that there are many different "normal" ways to grieve—that children grieve in their own time and at their own pace. Creative activities in many media (e.g., making memory candles, writing a memorial song, creating a memorial dance) are also often part of bereavement support group activities.

Peer support group activities would *not* include therapeutic interventions such as cognitive processing or exposure components described below. Little is known about empirical outcomes for children in peer support groups, as these have not been systematically studied. However, for children with uncomplicated bereavement, peer support is well accepted by families and children who access these services.

Childhood Traumatic Grief

Childhood traumatic grief (CTG) is a newly recognized condition. Discussion is ongoing about the defining features of CTG, even to the extent of whether it should be called CTG or *childhood complicated grief,* reflecting differences in conceptualizations regarding the degree of overlap among CTG, adult complicated grief, and posttraumatic stress disorder (PTSD). While one research group (Melham et al. 2007) has conceptualized CTG as being closer to complicated grief and more distinct from PTSD (i.e., not necessarily related to the traumatic nature of the death), others have viewed CTG and PTSD as more closely related. However, all of the research findings agree on two key points: 1) highly significant correlations between children's CTG scores and PTSD scores and 2) CTG (or childhood complicated grief) and PTSD are distinct conditions (Layne et al. 2001; Melham et al. 2004, 2007).

In the absence of more definitive empirical answers, this chapter will apply the definition from the child trauma and child development literature. CTG includes the following features (Brown et al. 2004; Cohen and Mannarino 2004; Layne et al. 2001):

1. The child's significant other died under traumatic circumstances (i.e., life-threatening, shocking, and/or terrifying).
2. The child has symptoms of PTSD.
3. The child's PTSD symptoms are impinging on the child's ability to resolve the typical tasks of grieving.
4. The child has some degree of functional impairment.

CTG is different from uncomplicated bereavement in several ways. First, the nature of the death is often (but not always) qualitatively different in cases of CTG, with these deaths typically being from sudden, unexpected, gory, and/or violent causes such as suicide, homicide, accidents, war, terrorism, and disasters. When CTG-related deaths are from medical causes, they are often sudden conditions such as heart attacks or strokes rather than from anticipated causes such as cancer. However, CTG can also result from chronic medical conditions, because children may not understand or believe that death is anticipated, and thus for them, the death was unexpected and sudden. In a similar fashion, deaths from anticipated causes can be frightening or shocking to children if they witness severe cyanosis, gasping for air, attempts at resuscitation, excessive bleeding, or similar events. Thus, any cause of death can lead to CTG if the child subjectively experiences the death as traumatic.

Some PTSD symptoms, including sleep difficulties, loss of interest in usual activities, and trouble concentrating are expected in bereaved children (DSM-IV-TR; American Psychiatric Association 2000). However, core PTSD symptoms, such as intrusive reexperiencing of the deceased's death and persistent avoidance of death reminders, are less typical of uncomplicated bereavement. A complete discussion of how to evaluate children for PTSD symptoms is included in Chapter 22, "Posttraumatic Stress Disorder."

A diagnosis of CTG requires not only that there are PTSD symptoms but also that these symptoms are impinging on the child's ability to resolve bereavement tasks. Children with this condition develop avoidance of trauma reminders—in this case, reminders of the deceased's death. These children are unable to tolerate thoughts or memories of the deceased, even happy memories, without these thoughts segueing into thoughts about how the person died. Since these thoughts are by definition terrifying, shocking, and upsetting, they reinforce avoidance of reminiscing about the deceased. Children with CTG are thus "stuck" on the traumatic aspects of the death, such that they are unable to move through the tasks of bereavement that require them to tolerate sustained memories of the dead

person. Children with CTG have some degree of functional impairment, whether in school, with friends, with family, or in their ability to accomplish their tasks of daily living such as playing and doing homework.

There are currently few validated assessment instruments to evaluate CTG. The UCLA/BYU Expanded Grief Inventory (EGI) is the only published instrument that assesses CTG and has been validated by two independent groups (Brown et al. 2004; Layne et al. 2001). The EGI includes a 24-item CTG scale in which children respond to items on a 5-point Likert scale. The EGI is appropriate for children ages 7–17 years of age and can be obtained from the National Child Traumatic Stress Network (NCTSN; www.nctsn.org). Another option is to use the child-modified version of the Inventory of Complicated Grief (ICG-R; Melham et al. 2007). No instrument is available to assess CTG in younger children.

Treatment

Attempts to develop appropriate interventions for CTG have begun. Treatments for children exposed to suicide (e.g., Pfeffer et al. 2002) or war (e.g., Gordon et al. 2004) may be applicable. Since these models do not specifically focus on the traumatic aspects of the death (for example, neither model includes development of a trauma narrative or a trauma reminder component) and neither study included assessment of CTG, they are not described in detail here. However, both studies will provide valuable information to clinicians treating CTG.

Traumatic Grief–Cognitive Behavioral Therapy

Traumatic grief–cognitive behavioral therapy (TG-CBT) is derived from trauma-focused cognitive-behavioral therapy (TF-CBT), an evidence-based treatment for PTSD that is described in detail in Chapter 22, "Posttraumatic Stress Disorder." Like TF-CBT, TG-CBT is typically provided in parallel sessions to the child and the parent or primary caretaking adult, with some joint child-parent sessions included in the latter parts of the trauma- and grief-focused modules of treatment. TG-CBT also provides children and parents with the "PRACTICE" trauma-focused components used in TF-CBT and then adds the following grief-focused components (Cohen et al. 2006a):

- *Receiving grief psychoeducation*—Age-appropriate information about grief, bereavement, and mourning rituals is provided. Grief-focused books and games are used to assist children in talking about death and help them ask about difficult or confusing aspects of death. Parents are asked about their mourning rituals. If these vary from those of their extended family or culture, therapists explore with parents how to reconcile these differences for themselves and their children.

- *Grieving the loss and resolving ambivalent feelings about the deceased*—Children identify what they have lost ("what I miss") and address potential ambivalent or unresolved issues with the deceased person ("what I don't miss"). Parents address similar issues in their parallel sessions. Various techniques are used—for example, making a name anagram to identify things the child misses and writing a letter to the deceased to resolve ambivalent feelings or unresolved issues.
- *Preserving positive memories*—Therapists assist children in creating lasting memories of the deceased—for example, through picture albums, videotapes, poems, collages, or a memory box containing mementos of the deceased. For children who lost all of the deceased's belongings (e.g., in a disaster or war), the use of drawings or family and friends' pictures or memories of the deceased may be helpful.
- *Redefining the relationship*—Therapists assist children in converting the relationship with the deceased person to one of memory—for example, through a balloon exercise. In this exercise, children first list everything they can still hold on to that they had in the relationship in a picture of a balloon tied to a figure on the ground. In a second balloon drawn floating toward the sky, children list all of the things that are gone forever from the relationship. Children then think about who can do some of these things in the deceased person's absence.
- *Discussing treatment closure issues*—Helping children and parents prepare for future reminders of the traumatic death (e.g., birthdays, anniversaries of the death) can be accomplished through the use of a circular calendar, in which the months of the year are written in a circle like the numbers on a clock. Since the circular calendar does not end but keeps circling around to these same dates, it illustrates that the child may experience recurrences of reminders of the traumatic death when these dates occur in future years. Therapists assist children and parents in making concrete plans for how to cope with these future reminders and address treatment termination issues.

Empirical support.

TG-CBT has been tested in two open trials and a small randomized controlled trial (RCT). The two open trials (Cohen et al. 2004, 2006b) included children with CTG secondary to various causes of death. Children receiving TG-CBT experienced significant improvement in CTG, PTSD, and other symptoms. In the RCT for children whose uniformed parents died on September 11, 2001, mothers in the TG-CBT group experienced significantly greater improvement in PTSD and general psychopathology than those in the child-centered therapy group (Brown et al. 2004). Children did not have elevated CTG or PTSD scores at pretreatment, and there were no significant group differences in child outcomes.

UCLA Trauma/Grief Program for Adolescents

This treatment model (Layne et al. 2001) is provided in groups for adolescents and has been adapted for youth as young as 11 years of age. It consists of the following five modules:

1. *Traumatic experiences*—The initial module focuses on assessment, psychoeducation, normalizing, and validating of the posttraumatic stress reaction; the module also includes exposure through the construction of a group joint trauma narrative. Cognitive restructuring techniques are used to a) clarify distortions and misattributions that lead to distress and b) facilitate the development of a realistic and positive perspective.
2. *Trauma and loss reminders*—The next module focuses on efforts to normalize and promote effective coping with trauma and loss reminders. This includes identifying the nature and frequency of reminders, linking these reminders with distress symptoms, and identifying maladaptive coping responses. It also involves using reminders to understand the personal meaning of traumatic events for each group member, using cognitive reprocessing techniques to improve affective modulation, and improving group members' ability to seek social support.
3. *Posttraumatic stress and adversities*—The third module includes identifying and decreasing the negative effects of traumatic events. These may include school problems; peer and family relationships; health problems; problems with the community, neighborhood, or living conditions; and financial difficulties. Through training in effective problem solving, communication skills, and other skills, this module also helps youth adapt to and accept changes in life circumstances that may have resulted from the trauma or loss that led to the death.

If appropriate, family, community, and/or other interventions are included in this module to reduce secondary adversities.

4. *Bereavement and the interplay of trauma and grief*—This module assists youth in identifying grief reactions and understanding that grief follows an individual course, thus increasing tolerance for loss reminders. The group may reconstitute nontraumatic mental images of the deceased to facilitate positive reminiscing, process conflict-laden feelings about the deceased, and focus on social skills in order to improve participants' ability to talk about their losses.

5. *Resumption of developmental progression*—The final module seeks to help older adolescents establish appropriate independence from parents; develop the capacity for intimate relationships; and enhance moral development, ambition, and motivation for educational and occupational achievement and citizenship. This module also includes assisting participants in replacing maladaptive core beliefs with more adaptive ways of viewing themselves and society.

Empirical support.

This model has been tested in two open studies: 1) in Bosnian adolescents postwar and 2) in adolescents exposed to community violence in Los Angeles (Layne et al. 2001; Saltzman et al. 2001). Both studies demonstrated that participants experienced significant improvement in CTG and PTSD symptoms as well as improved adaptive functioning (e.g., in academic achievement).

Grief and Trauma Intervention for Elementary-Age Children

Salloum et al. (2001) described a pilot group model for adolescent survivors of homicide victims. Salloum (2004) subsequently adapted this model for adolescents exposed to other traumatic experiences. The goals of this model include reducing traumatic reactions associated with the traumatic death, providing education about trauma and grief, and offering a safe environment for children to share thoughts and feelings (Salloum 2004). It also addresses bereavement tasks of self-protection, acceptance/reworking, and identity/development. It includes an ecological perspective and Rynearson's (2001) restorative retelling approach, which begins with bolstering resilience, then participating in a healing narrative experience, and ending with reconnecting. This 10-session treatment model includes the following stages:

- *Orientation (session 1)*—This stage includes an introduction and orientation to the treatment model and helps participants to identify supports, share the nature of the relationship to the deceased, and briefly describe the nature of the violence or trauma witnessed.

- *Inclusion (sessions 2–4)*—This stage includes administering the pretreatment assessment instruments, providing education about reactions to violence or trauma, initially sharing how the deceased died through selection of one of three worksheets (loss-focused, trauma-focused, or other), exploring the relationship of the deceased person to the child, formalizing goals of the group, providing grief and trauma psychoeducation, recognizing types of losses, identifying past coping techniques, listing different ways of coping, and helping children find creative healthy ways of coping. Relaxation training begins in this stage and continues in the following stage.

- *Mutuality/goal achievement (sessions 5–8)*—Safety issues are discussed, and traumatic reactions are identified; techniques for decreasing traumatic reactions are explored, and training in relaxation techniques is continued. Feeling identification; making connections among feelings, thoughts, and trauma reminders; identification of special dates and anniversaries; exploration of feelings of anger and revenge; anger management training; and education about special issues are provided during this stage. Sessions 6–7 also include pull-out individual sessions focusing on trauma/loss exposure during which children create restorative narratives or retelling of the death experiences.

- *Separation/termination (sessions 9–10)*—Activities in this stage include identifying supports, compiling a list of coping techniques, addressing spirituality/religion, examining family reactions and interactions, exploring children's sense of meaning in life, recognizing progress toward goals and how to achieve future goals, administering posttreatment assessment, and terminating the sessions.

Empirical support.

This treatment model has been tested in two open studies and is currently being tested in an RCT for elementary school–age children whose family members or other significant others died after Hurricane Katrina. The pilot studies included youth exposed to homicide or other violence (Salloum et al. 2001; A. Salloum, "Group Therapy for Children Experiencing Grief and Trauma Due to Homicide and Violence: A

Pilot Study," unpublished manuscript, 2006) and both studies demonstrated significant improvement in PTSD symptoms.

Child-Parent Psychotherapy for Traumatic Grief in Early Childhood

Child-parent psychotherapy (CPP) is a relationship-based treatment for infants and preschoolers exposed to domestic violence. CPP involves joint sessions with parents and their young children that focus on resolving maladaptive behaviors, supporting developmentally appropriate interactions, and guiding the child and parent in creating a joint narrative of the traumatic events while working toward their resolution (Lieberman et al. 2005). After the terrorist attacks of September 11, 2001, and the formation of the NCTSN, Lieberman and her colleagues adapted CPP for very young children whose parents died under traumatic circumstances. This adaptation has been published, widely disseminated, and used internationally (Lieberman et al. 2003).

Since CPP is a relationship-based model, the CTG adaptation does not include specific treatment components but initially consists of creating a safe environment for the treatment, such as identifying a surrogate primary caregiver for children whose only parent died; preserving reassuring, nonfrightening reminders of the deceased parent; deciding whether or not to take a young child to the parent's wake or funeral; and helping new caregivers to establish and maintain predictable routines. After this has been achieved, this model consists of specific treatment themes, such as what and how to tell the child about the parent's death, explaining the idea of death to a young child, giving meaning to the parent's death, alleviating the child's fears, addressing intrusive memories and traumatic reminders, consolidating positive and negative feelings about the lost parent, maintaining the child's connection with the memory of the deceased parent, managing anniversaries, and modeling manageable separation through the therapist's vacations and, ultimately, through treatment termination.

Empirical support.

CPP has been supported in an RCT for young children experiencing domestic violence, including some children whose primary caretaker died as a result of this violence (Lieberman and Van Horn 2005). To date, the CTG adaptation of the CPP model has not been empirically evaluated as a separate model.

Summary Points

- Many children will experience bereavement before reaching adulthood, and the majority of these children will not require any mental health interventions.

- Peer bereavement support groups are the most common intervention provided to bereaved children in the United States; little information is available regarding their efficacy in assisting children to resolve typical tasks of grieving or in recognizing children in need of more intensive mental health services.

- Some children who lose important people under traumatic circumstances develop CTG, which is an evolving condition in terms of definition, assessment, and risk factors. The current conceptualization of CTG consists of a subjectively traumatic death followed by trauma symptoms that impinge on a child's ability to work through typical bereavement tasks.

- Treatment models are being developed to address the particular needs of children with CTG; most of these are group models, but some are individual child and parent or conjoint child-parent models.

- Preliminary evidence suggests that integrating trauma- and grief-focused components is effective in reducing CTG, PTSD, and related difficulties for children and adolescents with CTG.

- More research is needed to fully understand the construct and treatment of CTG. Unfortunately, domestic and community violence, accidents, suicide, drug abuse, medical traumas, disasters, and war will likely result in many more children developing traumatic grief in the future.

References

American Psychiatric Association: Diagnostic and Statistical Manual of Mental Disorders, 4th Edition, Text Revision. Washington, DC, American Psychiatric Association, 2000

Brown EJ, Goodman RF, Cohen JA, et al: Treatment of childhood traumatic grief: a randomized controlled trial. Paper presented at "Childhood Traumatic Grief" symposium at Strengthening Our Future: Developing Healthy Children and Youth, Strong Families and Safe Communities, Kansas City, MO, April 2004

Cohen JA, Mannarino AP: Treatment of childhood traumatic grief. J Clin Child Adolesc Psychol 33:819–831, 2004

Cohen JA, Mannarino AP, Knudsen K: Treating childhood traumatic grief: a pilot study. J Am Acad Child Adolesc Psychiatry 43:1225–1233, 2004a

Cohen JA, Mannarino AP, Deblinger E: Treating Trauma and Traumatic Grief in Children and Adolescents. New York, Guilford, 2006a

Cohen JA, Mannarino AP, Staron V: Modified cognitive behavioral therapy for childhood traumatic grief (CBT-CTG): a pilot study. J Am Acad Child Adolesc Psychiatry 45:1465–1473, 2006b

Gordon JS, Staples JK, Blyta A, et al: Treatment of posttraumatic stress disorder in postwar Kosovo high school students using mind-body skills groups: a pilot study. J Trauma Stress 17:143–147, 2004

Layne CM, Pynoos RS, Saltzman WS, et al: Trauma/grief-focused group psychotherapy: school-based postwar intervention with traumatized Bosnian adolescents. Group Dyn 5:277–290, 2001

Lieberman AF, Van Horn P: Don't Hit My Mommy! A Manual for Child-Parent Psychotherapy With Young Witnesses of Family Violence. Washington, DC, Zero to Three Press, 2005

Lieberman AF, Compton NC, Van Horn P, et al: Losing a Parent to Death in the Early Years: Guidelines for the Treatment of Traumatic Bereavement in Infancy and Early Childhood. Washington, DC, Zero to Three Press, 2003

Lieberman AF, Van Horn P, Ippen CG: Toward evidence-based treatment: child-parent psychotherapy with preschoolers exposed to marital violence. J Am Acad Child Adolesc Psychiatry 44:1241–1248, 2005

Melham NM, Day N, Shear MK, et al: Traumatic grief among adolescents exposed to a peer's suicide. Am J Psychiatry 161:1411–1416, 2004

Melham NM, Moritz G, Walker M, et al: Phenomenology and correlates of complicated grief in children and adolescents. J Am Acad Child Adolesc Psychiatry 46:493–499, 2007

Pfeffer CCR, Jiang H, Kakuma T, et al: Group intervention for children bereaved by suicide of a relative. J Am Acad Child Adolesc Psychiatry 41:505–513, 2002

Rynearson EK: Retelling Violent Death. Philadelphia, PA, Brunner Routledge, 2001

Salloum A: Group Work With Adolescents After Violent Death: A Manual for Practitioners. Philadelphia, PA, Brunner Routledge, 2004

Salloum A, Avery L, McClain RP: Group psychotherapy for adolescent survivors of homicide victims: a pilot study. J Am Acad Child Adolesc Psychiatry 40:1261–1267, 2001

Saltzman WR, Pynoos RS, Layne CM, et al: Trauma- and grief-focused intervention for adolescents exposed to community violence: results of a school-based screening and group treatment protocol. Group Dyn 5:291–303, 2001

Schurmann D: Childhood traumatic grief, in Plenary. Edited by Lurier A, Cohen J, Goodman R, et al. Presented at the 10th National Symposium on Children's Grief Support, Chicago, IL, June 2006

Social Security Administration: Intermediate assumptions of the 2000 Trustees Report. Washington, DC, Office of the Chief Actuary of the Social Security Administration, 2000

Wolfelt AD: Healing the Bereaved Child: Grief Gardening, Growth Through Grief and Other Touchstones for Caregivers. Fort Collins, CO, Companion Press, 1996

Worden JW: Children and Grief: When a Parent Dies. New York, Guilford, 1996

Chapter 34

Ethnic, Cultural, and Religious Issues

Mary Lynn Dell, M.D., M.T.S., Th.M.

Over the past 30 years, North America has experienced unparalleled changes in the ethnicities and nationalities that residents claim as their primary identity or background. Racial groups officially recognized by the 2000 U.S. Census included white, black or African American, Native American or Alaska Native, Asian, Native Hawaiian and other Pacific Islander, and other. Of these, African Americans comprised the largest group of persons of color, followed by Hispanics/Latinos. The total U.S. population increased by 13.2% between 1990 and 2000, with several nonwhite groups making significant gains in absolute numbers and percentages (U.S. Bureau of the Census 2001). A substantial and ever-growing percentage of children and families, whether permanent residents or transients, are immersed in a "home" of family-of-origin culture while surrounded by a variety of U.S. local and national environments. The explosion of cultural, eth-nic, and religious diversity of society and its implications for patient care require our intentional study and consideration.

History of Cultural Psychiatry and Key Definitions

The roots of cultural psychiatry go back to eighteenth-century observations that immigrant groups from Europe presented different types of emotional problems than those born and living in the continental United States. By the late nineteenth and early twentieth centuries, clinical case reports detailed unusual symptom patterns in numerous minority, indigenous, and tribal groups from around the world. Emil Kraepelin, father of comparative psychiatry, described differences he observed in non-Western societies in the late 1800s. Beginning with Sigmund Freud and continuing with Jung, Adler, and Horney, psychoanalysts highlighted the importance of cultural factors in neuroses and psychotherapy. By the mid-twentieth century, anthropologists, social workers, psychologists, and even theologians shared an overlapping interest in culture and mental health. Over the past 50 years, academic psychiatry departments on both coasts and in Hawaii led the way in research, writing, and training. The American Psychiatric Association established the Transcultural Psychiatry Committee, which has authored statements since the 1960s. The inclusion of Appendix I, "Outline for Cultural Formulation and Glossary of Culture-Bound Syndromes," in DSM-IV (American Psychiatric Association 1994) attests to the relevance of this discipline to psychiatric practice. The outline for cultural formulation is especially helpful clinically, guiding clinicians through a systematic consideration of a patient's cultural identity, cultural explanations of a patient's illness, cultural factors related to psychosocial environment and levels of functioning, and cultural elements of the relationship between the patient and the clinician (Caraballo et al. 2006; Ton and Lim 2006; Tseng 2001).

Several terms are used interchangeably, although with somewhat different meanings in this multidisciplinary mental health specialty, and thus require definition. The Committee on Cultural Psychiatry for the Group for the Advancement of Psychiatry (2002) defines *culture* as "a set of meaning, behavioral norms, and values used by members of a particular society as they construct their unique view of the world. These… include social relationships, language, nonverbal expression of thoughts and emotions, religious beliefs, moral thought, technology, and financial philosophy" (pp. 6–7). Culture is dynamic, shapes and is shaped by individuals, and evolves over time as it is passed on to succeeding generations. It shapes meanings and expressions of disease, illness, pain, and suffering, which in turn influence a people's receptivity to medical and psychiatric care. *Ethnicity* encompasses one's identity with a group of people sharing common origins, history, customs, and beliefs. Ethnicity may include geographical, national, and religious identities, such as Irish Catholic, Vietnamese American, or Greek Orthodox. *Race* refers to physical, biological, and genetic qualities of humans, particularly as these features lead to categorization of visible similarities or differences.

Race as a concept is not scientifically valid and does not lend itself well to objective, reliable description; yet it proves itself a powerful factor not only in human politics but also in psychiatric diagnosis, access to care, and therapeutic relationships. *Cultural psychiatry*, then, is the discipline concerned with matters of culture, ethnicity, and race as they affect description, assessment, diagnosis, biopsychosocial formulation, treatment planning, and training in all aspects of psychiatric practice (Group for the Advancement of Psychiatry 2002; Ton and Lim 2006).

Cultural Aspects of Typical Child Development and Family Life

In virtually all cultures, marriage and family are the foundational units in which children are conceived, grow, and develop. Marriage is the socially sanctioned unit, usually intended to be long-lasting, if not permanent, from which a family is created and nurtured. Families, in turn, function as groups through which individuals grow physically, emotionally, and socially; learn to relate to the outside world; and transmit cultural beliefs, histories, and behaviors to the next generation.

While the biological functioning of males and females is essential to procreation, marriage and family life are patterns that vary across cultures and time. These cultural variations include functions of the marital union, way in which spouses are chosen, location of the marital unit and its subsequent family, lines of authority and power, inheritance, and household and family structure. These different patterns of family organization and functioning have been described by anthropologists, providing a common language for scholars and clinicians alike who deal professionally with matters of culture (Tseng 2001, 2003).

Family life cycles emerge from biology and childbearing yet are influenced significantly by cultural patterns and religious beliefs and rituals. Many cultures worldwide now follow the stages of a Western family life cycle, including marriage, childbearing, childrearing, empty nest, and widowing. However, the time spent in each stage is affected by gender roles, education, acceptable ages for marriage and parenthood, number and autonomy of offspring, remarriage, and occupational and work lives. In addition, particular cultures and religious traditions celebrate and react to family and individual life cycle events differently.

For instance, Judaism's emphasis on a child's transition into adulthood at age 13 is shared by many cultures, while American funerals can be either very solemn or celebratory occasions depending on the history and ethnicity of the family and cultural group (Kaslow et al. 1995; Tseng 2001).

Theory and practical study of individual child and adolescent development have been dominated by Western schemas, especially Freud's psychosexual, Piaget's cognitive, and Erikson's psychosocial frameworks. Methodologically sound studies of development outside of Western Europe and North America are few, though scholarship on cross-cultural child development generally spans a continuum. On one end is the position that because children are biologically humans and thus very similar, cultural influences are minimal, if any. The other extreme is that culture is such a huge factor in the family, social, and psychological makeup of children that few, if any, generalizations can be made across cultures (Koss-Chioino and Vargas 1992; Tseng 2001). Cross-cultural studies have consistently documented that certain qualities of temperament and mother-child interactions are found more often in certain cultures than in others. Later in development, different cultures mark adulthood at varying times, some with unique rites or rituals of passage often tied temporally to puberty. Young people tend to take on adult roles and responsibilities after such a public acknowledgment of their maturation, especially in non-Western cultures (Tseng 2001).

Culture and Psychopathology

Culture-Bound Syndromes

In the seventeenth and eighteenth centuries, Western Europeans and Americans exploring Asia, Africa, South America, Arctic regions, the Pacific Islands, and other unfamiliar parts of the world noted unusual but distinct medical and/or psychiatric syndromes indigenous to countries or circumscribed geographical regions. Mental illnesses as manifested in particular cultural groups have fascinated psychiatrists, anthropologists, and scholars and have been the subject of considerable research. The term *culture-bound syndromes* was introduced in 1967 to describe disorders that are 1) discrete and well-defined, 2) accepted as a specific disorder in the country of origin, 3) a response

to specific precipitants in that culture, and 4) found to occur much more in the "home" culture than in other cultures (Guarnaccia and Rogler 1999; Levine and Gaw 1995). A glossary of 25 culture-bound syndromes was included in DSM-IV in 1994, signaling that these were no longer rare entities of academic interest only (American Psychiatric Association 1994). The increasing cultural diversity of American society, including immigrants from other countries retaining their homeland's beliefs and practices of mental health, as well as the authority attributed to DSM worldwide, compels clinicians to be familiar with these syndromes. (Guarnaccia and Rogler 1999; Tseng 2001). While important to adult cultural psychiatry, little evidence exists that the symptoms and behaviors of specific culture-bound syndromes are common in childhood or adolescence. However, clinicians should remember that children and adolescents from some diverse cultures may have been exposed to adults suffering from culture-bound syndromes and thus should be observed or evaluated for anxiety, depression, acute stress, or posttraumatic stress disorders arising from those experiences.

Cultural Aspects of DSM-IV-TR Diagnostic Entities

Exact psychiatric diagnosis in culturally diverse children living in the United States is difficult, primarily due to factors beyond the simple counting of symptoms on a checklist. Poverty, suboptimal living conditions, language and communication issues with children and their caregivers, value differences across generational lines, poor health care, and excessive stresses of daily living blur lines between usual and understandable emotional reactions, adjustment problems, coping mechanisms, expectable cultural variation, and genuine psychiatric illness. Many cultural minorities are suspicious of majority health care providers, and even when desirous of evaluation and treatment, they may face considerable challenges with transportation, child care, missed work for appointments, and navigation of referral processes and increasingly complex and technical paperwork for payment. Frequently, children have more than one diagnosis. At other times, they may not meet strict criteria for any DSM diagnosis, but symptoms and the overall clinical picture beg nonetheless for therapeutic intervention. While all children and their families have unique qualities, some generalizations may be helpful in the assessment and diagnosis of DSM entities.

Anxiety may be understandable if a child feels unsafe or worries about family members. For immigrant and minority culture families who live in inner cities in suboptimal housing with violence close by and who struggle with having enough to eat and adequate clothing, anxiety and apprehension are integral parts of daily life. These acute and chronic psychosocial and environmental stresses complicate the differential diagnosis of adjustment disorder with anxious mood, panic disorder, and generalized anxiety disorder. Overt expression of anxiety varies culturally as well—people from Asian cultures may be less expressive or withdraw when stressed or anxious, while Latino and Eastern European groups may be much more verbal and expressive in response to identical situations. What may look like social phobia in a majority culture white adolescent may be typical behavior in a recently relocated African girl. Many children immigrating from other countries have witnessed and suffered through war, persecution, refugee camps, natural disasters, and grave illnesses, putting them at greater risk for acute and posttraumatic stress disorders and their emotional and physiological sequelae (American Psychiatric Association 2000; Canino and Spurlock 2000; Tseng 2001).

The past experiences, ongoing stresses, and exposure to violence that foster anxiety, in addition to a high likelihood of losses, also predispose culturally diverse children and adolescents to depressive disorders. African American, Native American, and Latino youth may be prone to low self-esteem and status in school and peer groups, thereby increasing risk for depressive symptoms. Cultural minority children may live with a pervasive sense of hopelessness for the future, reinforcing any tendencies toward mood disorders. Higher rates of suicide in some minorities, particularly Native Americans, are well documented (American Psychiatric Association 2000; Canino and Spurlock 2000; Fleming 2006; Tseng 2003).

Clinicians should be alert to dissociation, as a single symptom or disorder, in culturally diverse children. Exposure to trauma, as either witnesses or victims, may result in children distancing themselves from real or perceived experiences as a defense mechanism. The clinician should always inquire about and be alert to indications of rape, torture, or abuse. On the other hand, some world religious traditions foster dissociation in rituals and practices, or dissociation may be a part of isolated culture-bound syndromes (American Psychiatric Association 2000; Tseng 2003).

Attention-deficit/hyperactivity disorder is diagnosed more frequently in the United States and industrialized nations, perhaps reflecting diagnostic bias and greater school attendance compared to less developed countries. Cultural factors must be considered when assessing attentional symptoms and externalizing behaviors in minority youth. Families from some cultures, including the Chinese and Japanese, express and tolerate impulsivity and oppositionality less than typical U.S. majority families. For culturally diverse youth living in unsafe urban areas, verbal bravado and physical aggression may be employed adaptively for the protection and safety of self, siblings, and property. Clinicians need to assess level of functioning and adaptive behaviors across the multiple domains of home, school, work, and social networks as they determine the presence and severity of attentional, conduct, and other disruptive behavior disorders (American Psychiatric Association 2000; Canino and Spurlock 2000; Tseng 2001).

DSM-IV-TR notes that "there are wide cultural variations in attitudes toward substance consumption, patterns of substance abuse, accessibility of substances, physiological reactions to substances, and prevalence of substance-related disorders" (American Psychiatric Association 2000, p. 205). In addition, individual cultures and religious traditions differ on acceptable practices for children and adolescents, especially regarding alcohol. In some Western European cultures, children are served small amounts of wine with daily meals by their parents. Other cultures may be guided by faith traditions that forbid all alcohol consumption or restrict it only to specific religious observances. In the majority Euro-American culture of the United States, one finds the full spectrum from abstinence to slight to moderate alcohol consumption, to abuse and dependence in adolescents and young adults. Alcohol abuse and dependence may exist in >50% of adults in some local communities of Native American and Native Alaskans, with substantial rates of use by adolescents in these groups (Fleming 2006). While alcohol consumption is normative in many Japanese, Korean, and other Asian communities, American Asians are very reluctant to discuss substance use and resultant problems (Du 2006). For disadvantaged cultural minority groups, assessment and treatment of substance use disorders are complicated by issues of socioeconomics, living conditions, poor school attendance, unemployment, lack of treatment facilities, and often the reluctance to use services that do exist (Canino and Spurlock 2000; Du 2006; Fleming 2006; Primm 2006; Tseng 2001).

Physicians must remember to consider medical problems with neuropsychiatric manifestations as they work with culturally diverse children. Children born in other countries and adopted by families in the

United States may have been exposed to infectious agents or toxins, in utero or early infancy, with central nervous system sequelae. The poverty and trying living conditions of some cultural minorities increase the possibility of limited or no prenatal care or regular pediatric care in infancy and childhood, insufficient nutrition to foster optimal brain development, or toxic effects of lead-based paint on pottery or of herbal remedies. Routine inquiry should be made about exposure to alcohol, tobacco, and illicit substances during pregnancy. Even if these injuries cannot be reversed, early identification may slow the rate of adverse effects and facilitate appropriate medical care, educational placements, and interventions with other family members.

Culture, Ethnicity, and Psychopharmacology

Cultural psychopharmacology is truly one of the most multidisciplinary fields in medicine today, encompassing psychiatry, pharmacology, genetics, pediatrics, neurology, toxicology, epidemiology, and molecular physiology. This discussion will provide a brief summary of key points. Interested readers are referred to more extensive reviews (Gaw 2001; Munoz et al. 2007; Smith 2006; Tseng 2003).

For decades psychiatrists have detected variability among ethnic groups regarding *pharmacokinetics*, the biological processes of drug absorption, distribution, metabolism, and excretion; and *pharmacodynamics*, the physiological and biochemical effects of medications at sites in the human body. Differences in therapeutic drug doses, efficacy, half-lives, drug-drug interactions, tolerability, and short- and long-term side effects have been well documented among different races and ethnic groups. Interest in this topic has soared with the growth of *pharmacogenetics*, the study of genetic influences on drug responses. Especially relevant to ethnopsychopharmacology is the discovery of genetic polymorphisms of the cytochrome P450 (CYP) liver enzymes responsible for oxidative metabolism of many psychotropic medications (Gaw 2001).

The four most significant CYP enzymes at this time appear to be CYP2D6, CYP2C19, CYP3A4, and CYP1A2. The majority of antidepressants, antipsychotics, benzodiazepines, mood stabilizers, and several other neuropsychiatrically active substances serve as substrates for these four CYP enzymes. Genetic polymorphisms of these enzymes help explain drug

metabolism differences among ethnic groups, as well as genetic differences among individuals in the same ethnic group. These genetic variations also factor into the pharmacokinetic considerations regarding induction and inhibition of drug metabolism by other active substances, including other psychotropic medications. Table 34–1 summarizes key points about the four important CYP enzymes, their psychotropic medication substrates, and relevance to observed ethnic psychopharmacological variations (Gaw 2001; Munoz et al. 2007; Smith 2006; Tseng 2003).

Some generalizations about certain ethnic groups and their responses to psychotropic drug classes are possible. For instance, Hispanics respond to lower doses of tricyclic antidepressants and antipsychotics, both typical and atypical, especially risperidone. They have a higher rate of side effects to tricyclics. African Americans respond to lower doses of selective serotonin reuptake inhibitors (SSRIs) and have higher risk for tardive dyskinesia with typical neuroleptics. Asians have good responses to lower doses of tricyclics, typical and atypical antipsychotics, benzodiazepines, and lithium. Asians also have a higher prolactin response to atypical antipsychotics than other ethnic groups (Munoz et al. 2007).

Clinicians should consider genetic and biological variables other than CYP that affect the way certain ethnicities respond to medications. African Americans and those from Mediterranean cultures may have a deficiency of glucose-6-phosphate dehydrogenase. Asian populations may have deficiencies of alcohol dehydrogenase and aldehyde dehydrogenase, leading to a toxic build-up of metabolites after alcohol consumption. Genetic variations in serum drug-binding proteins, such as alpha glycoprotein, affect the amount of unbound free drug concentrations in the blood. Diet, tobacco and cannabis abuse, and the use of herbal and folk medicines may factor into psychopharmacological considerations of some individuals and ethnic groups more than others (Gaw 2001; Munoz et al. 2007).

The following suggestions have been offered for prescribing for ethnic minorities, most of which are core principles for pediatric psychopharmacology:

1. Start at a low dose and increase slowly.
2. Inquire about diet, smoking, and herbal and folk remedies.
3. Check plasma levels when possible.
4. With the patient's permission, include key family members.
5. Before giving up on any medication, consider trying a different formulation (such as a liquid form,

TABLE 34–1.　Four important cytochrome P450 (CYP) enzymes in cultural psychopharmacology

CYP2D6

Antidepressant substrates: fluoxetine, paroxetine, duloxetine, venlafaxine, desipramine, nortriptyline

Antipsychotic substrates: haloperidol, clozapine, risperidone, olanzapine, phenothiazines

Important other substrates: codeine, hydrocodone, caffeine

>30 mutations, many ethnically specific, that inactivate, impair, or accelerate function

Seven CYP2D6 mutations responsible for 99% genetic variations

Africans and Asians are slower metabolizers (one-third of Asians have gene mutations that decrease activity)

Arabs and Ethiopians may be ultra-rapid metabolizers

CYP2C19

Antidepressant substrates: citalopram, escitalopram, sertraline, venlafaxine, clomipramine, amitriptyline

Benzodiazepine substrates: diazepam, temazepam

Inhibited by fluoxetine, sertraline, fluvoxamine

20% of East Asians (Chinese, Japanese, Koreans) are poor metabolizers

Only 3%–5% of whites are slow metabolizers

CYP3A4

Antidepressant substrates: sertraline, mirtazapine, reboxetine

Antipsychotic substrates: aripiprazole, clozapine, quetiapine, ziprasidone

Benzodiazepine substrates: alprazolam, clonazepam, diazepam, midazolam

Anticonvulsant/mood stabilizer substrates: carbamazepine, gabapentin, lamotrigine

Asian Indians, East Asians, and Mexicans have lower activity

Africans and African Americans have higher activity

CYP1A2

Antidepressant substrates: fluvoxamine, clomipramine, imipramine, amitriptyline

Antipsychotic substrates: haloperidol, olanzapine, clozapine, phenothiazines

Other common substrates: caffeine, acetaminophen

Induced by tobacco, high protein diets, cruciferous vegetable

Higher rates of smoking in Asians, Latinos, and Japanese affect drug levels

Source.　Gaw 2001; Munoz et al. 2007; Smith 2006; Tseng 2003.

if available, instead of tablet or capsule form), especially in children and adolescents (Smith 2006).

Finally, clinicians must remember the role of cultural attitudes and the psychodynamics involved in the prescription process, especially for cultural minorities. Individuals from other cultures may distrust physicians and Western medicine in general or clinicians from a perceived powerful majority in particular. Some groups may be more stoic than others, waiting to seek help until either greater intervention is needed or little can be done. Spoken-language barriers affect seeking care, and misunderstandings of gestures and body language may contribute to patients' uneasiness in medical settings. Religious beliefs, particularly pertaining to the cause of affliction, influence the seeking of treatment and the expectations of

whether or not medical care will be successful. This is likely to be even more true for psychiatric disorders. One must inquire about patients' basic medical knowledge in a respectful way that neither under- nor overestimates their understanding of germ theory and biological psychiatric illness, as well as what medications should do and how they should be taken. In some cultures, people, and especially elderly persons, attribute great knowledge to physicians and want to please them at all costs, even giving them the answers they believe the doctor wants to hear instead of factual reports. Even the method of drug administration—intramuscular versus oral—and the size, color, and packaging of the medication may have significant meaning. Psychiatrists are well advised not to jump to conclusions that the patient is being intentionally noncompliant or nonadherent to recommended psychopharmacotherapy. Extra time spent in consideration of cultural factors in the treatment process may yield helpful insights into ongoing assessment and care (Ahmed 2001; Dell et al. 2008; Smith 2006).

Religion, Spirituality, and Culture

Basic Definitions and Relevance to Care

For centuries, patients, faith communities, and a majority of clinicians have recognized the importance of religion and spirituality in health, illness, and medical and psychiatric care. There is recent renewed interest in the relationships among religion, spirituality, culture, and psychiatry and medicine. In a sense, religion and spirituality can be considered as a subset or category of culture. On the other hand, unlike other cultural elements, this topic transcends diverse societies and deals with individual and collective values, norms, core beliefs, and relationships with the divine—matters of "ultimate importance" to members of a culture. This unique role of religion and spirituality in virtually all cultures and their pervasive influences on mental health and illness merit special consideration.

Religion is an organized system of beliefs, principles, rituals, practices, and related symbols that brings individuals and groups to sacred or ultimate reality and truth. It includes relationships with others, whether inside a community of individuals with shared beliefs or external to a like-minded community. *Spirituality* includes religion and faith communities but is not restricted to organized religion and group membership. It may encompass an individual's understandings of and quest for ultimate meaning in life's deepest, most perplexing questions and mysteries (Koenig et al. 2001). One can be religious only, spiritual only, both religious and spiritual, or neither and can pass between these descriptions on multiple occasions in a lifetime.

Two terms important to understanding religion and spirituality in North America, especially regarding Protestantism, are *evangelicalism* and *fundamentalism.* Evangelicals are Protestants with a conservative approach to the Bible, believing that one must have a close, personal relationship with Jesus Christ in order to be a Christian. Typically, though not always, evangelical Christians believe all aspects of life should be guided by biblical teachings, including family life, major life decisions, politics, and entertainment, to name but a few. Fundamentalists are a subset of evangelicals, noted for literal interpretation of scripture or a belief in the absolute authority of the Bible. Modernism, especially science, may be suspect unless compatible with strict biblical precepts. Fundamentalists, compared to more liberal evangelicals, are often less likely to participate in secular society without wanting, or even insisting, that society change to conform to their values. In the United States, the term fundamentalism primarily is applied to very conservative Protestantism. However, the concept of *fundamentalism,* including strict interpretation of sacred writings, traditional lifestyle practices guided by religious teachings, and suspicion of or resistance to modernity, may be found worldwide in Judaism, Islam, Hinduism, and other major world faith traditions (Ammerman 1991; Hood et al. 2005; Wentz 2003).

Ironically, Sigmund Freud, often caricatured as unfriendly to religion and spirituality, coined a term that is helpful in understanding this potentially sensitive subject matter and its importance in psychiatry and culture. *Weltanschauung,* or *worldview,* refers to a philosophy of life or belief system that addresses life's most common, basic questions. These include the meaning and purpose of life, life direction and goals, what is good and desirable in life, happiness, relationships with others, suffering, and death. A worldview may or may not include or share aspects with an organized religious tradition (Freud 1933/1962).

Many, if not most, practical elements in the lives of children and families are influenced to varying degrees by religious convictions, practices, or values stemming from spiritual beliefs. Examples include childrearing practices and attitudes toward medical and psychiatric care, substance use, sexuality, dating, and money. Seemingly mundane matters, such as choice of what clothing is appropriate for school and what children are permitted to view on television and the Internet, are rooted in core values formed by religious beliefs or lack thereof. Even children, adolescents, and families who claim no religious or spiritual belief are immersed in a secular culture that reflects majority values shaped or influenced by religious principles. As these issues are often identified as concerns by children and families presenting to child and adolescent psychiatrists and influence diagnosis and treatment planning, clinicians are well advised to attune themselves to both the overt and subtle religious and spiritual themes in the lives of their patient populations (Josephson and Dell 2004).

Religious and Spiritual Diversity in North American Culture

The fact that a discussion of religious and cultural diversity is included in a psychiatric textbook is partly a consequence of the way the United States chose to address the relationship between religion and government at the time of its founding. Separation of church and state and the First Amendment, guaranteeing freedom of religion, fostered a social climate conducive to division of existing major faith traditions when differences of belief or practice arose and the establishment of totally new religious groups or denominations, in addition to welcoming the variety of traditions brought from other countries by subsequent generations of immigrants (Atwood 2005). Those of us living in a culture where religious difference is not suppressed or persecuted must remember that even the most objective mention of religion to someone from a land or cultural heritage in which religious conformity was paramount for civil order and personal safety may elicit a hesitant response requiring sensitivity and understanding on the part of the clinician.

In American colonial times, religious diversity meant that Congregationalists settled in New England, Quakers in Pennsylvania, Anglicans in Virginia, and Roman Catholics in Maryland. To these over the next century and a half were added waves of German, Irish, Eastern European, Scandinavian, and other immigrants, bringing more diversity to American Protestantism, Catholicism, and Judaism. Perhaps only in the last 20 years has North America truly embodied its melting pot reputation, seeing an influx of nearly all religious traditions from all parts of the world. Psychiatrists are treating increasingly diverse patients from many cultural and religious backgrounds. While mental health clinicians do not need to be experts in comparative religion, more psychiatrists are desiring familiarity with basic beliefs and daily rituals of faith traditions found in geographical areas where they practice. Table 34–2 summarizes basic facts regarding seven major traditions commonly encountered today.

Diversity also describes beliefs and practices within major world faith traditions, as well as between them. The concept of *continuum of belief and practice* is helpful clinically and refers to the following observations:

1. Most major world faith traditions have subgroups, branches, or denominations that identify themselves as a distinct subgroup of the larger tradition. These subgroups may be distinguished by the nature and extent of their religious practices and observances. For example, the three largest groups within Judaism—Orthodox, Conservative, and Reform—generally fall on a continuum from orthodox belief and strict observance of religious law and custom to less defined and ritualized belief and practice.

2. Most major faith traditions consist of followers or members who, as both individuals and local faith communities, fall on a continuum from observant to nonobservant, politically conservative to liberal, and rigid and excluding of others to open and welcoming of those who have differing viewpoints. For example, in any single Protestant denomination are members who believe that homosexuality is sinful and others who believe that sexual orientation is biologically determined and same-sex relationships are acceptable—with both groups self-identifying as faithful members of the same denomination.

As already noted, the relationships among religion, spirituality, and culture are complex, always influencing and shaping each other. For instance, what does it mean when a patient claims a Baptist religious preference on her clinic registration form? The twelfth edition of the authoritative *Handbook of Denominations in the United States* (Mead et al. 2005) lists 31 distinct Baptist denominations, 11 more than recognized 4 years previously in the eleventh edition (Mead et al. 2001). Is her family Southern Baptist, upper middle class, Euro-American, and suburban with conservative political leanings? Or is the patient African American and active in a smaller, historically black, poorer denomination whose theology and beliefs are rooted in the Deep South long before the Civil War? The geographical area of the country, the characters of the civil communities in which we live, and extended-family histories, myths, and legends can tell practitioners as much or more about priorities, values, and clinically relevant lifestyle issues as one's religious affiliation. In the context of the increasing multiculturalism and ethnic diversity of the early twenty-first century, the intertwining of religion, ethnicity, and immigration/acculturation must be appreciated. For instance, three different families may mark themselves as Catholic on hospital registration forms—a family from the Bronx whose two sets of grandparents moved from Puerto Rico as teenagers but whose present-day grandchildren know little to no Spanish; a second-generation Italian Catholic family from south Philadelphia whose children attend parochial schools and whose non-English-speaking grandmother attends daily morning Mass and provides most of the after-school child care;

TABLE 34–2. Major faith traditions: important facts

Christianity

Three major groups—Catholic (Roman and others), Orthodox (Greek, Russian, and others), Protestant

80% of U.S. adults (51% Protestant, 24% Catholic, 0.6% Orthodox, ~3% other)

Abrahamic, monotheistic, early members from Jewish and non-Jewish backgrounds

Based on life and teachings of Jesus, son of God

Sacred text is the Bible, including Old (Hebrew Scriptures) and New Testaments

Judaism

12 million worldwide

6 million in the United States, 1.7% of U.S. adults

Originated in ancient Mesopotamia, traces heritage to patriarch Abraham

Can refer to both a religion and ethnicity

Defined primarily by practices and ethics found in sacred texts instead of doctrines

Three major groups in the United States: Orthodox (10%), Conservative (35%), Reform (40%)

Islam (Muslim)

Second largest world religion, 20% of world's population (Indonesia, Middle East, Bangladesh, Pakistan, Nigeria)

0.6% of U.S. adults, >6 million people, and third largest religion in the United States

Abrahamic—shares historical and theological elements with Judaism and Christianity

Muhammad viewed as last messenger of God (*Allah*)

Qur'an is sacred text

Important practices *(five pillars)*: profession of belief, prayer, fasting, charity, pilgrimage to Mecca

Three major branches: *Sunnis, Shi'as, Sufis*

Buddhism

Fourth largest religious tradition in the world—Tibet, Sri Lanka, Thailand, China, Korea, Japan

0.7% of U.S. adults

Originated in 5th century B.C.E. India with teachings of Siddhartha Gautama, "the Buddha"

Three branches: East Asian, Tibetan, Theravada

Elements include nonextremism *(Middle Way)*, teachings of Buddha *(Dharma)*, view of suffering *(Four Noble Truths)*, and state of complete selflessness and dissolution of self's boundaries *(Nirvana)*

Emphasizes right living, compassion, morality, self-discipline

Hinduism

83% of population in India, not widespread in rest of world

0.4% of U.S. adults, primarily of Asian Indian lineage

No clear historical beginning, but roots identifiable as early as 3000 B.C.E.

Complex system of beliefs, ideals, practices; God and Truth are one; many gods and goddesses represent Truth and Divinity

Key concepts: cycle of birth, death, rebirth in another body *(reincarnation)*; current experiences are fruits of past actions *(karma)*; ethical teachings *(dharma)*; social class system *(castes)*

Important duties: personal cleanliness; food preparation and eating habits; marriage and family relationships; quiet meditation

African American religious traditions

More African Americans claim formal religious affiliation than all other ethnic groups

Predominantly Christian, with both predominantly black denominations and black churches in predominantly white denominations

Two-thirds of historically black Protestant churches in the United States are Baptist

TABLE 34–2. Major faith traditions: important facts *(continued)*

African American religious traditions *(continued)*

Centers of community life—education, social justice, social work, culture

Churches and clergy were leaders in civil rights movement

Nation of Islam—organized African American Muslim group founded in 1930

Native American religion and spirituality

<0.3% U.S. adults

Nearly as many forms as nations, tribes, cultures

Spirituality is a personal relationship connecting individual's spirit to creation, present world, sense of place, other people, and animals

Many rituals involving nature, human development, and rites of passage

Modern expressions may be admixed with traditional aspects of Christianity

Opposition to majority consumerism, materialism, politics, economics, and environmental abuse and neglect is also attractive to many non–Native Americans

Source. Cutting 2006; Eckel 2003; Esposito 2003; Gill 2003; Johnson 2006; Larson 2003; Neusner 2003; Pew Research Center 2008; Raman 2006; Scarlett 2006.

and a bilingual Mexican American family in El Paso, Texas, whose adult members go back and forth to Mexico based on work status and affordability of necessary medical care. Catholicism may be important to all but is lived out differently in their radically different life circumstances.

In 2007, the Pew Research Center interviewed 35,000 Americans ages 18 and older in an effort to explore the contemporary U.S. religious landscape (Pew Research Center 2008). Their findings support the importance of religion and spirituality in the United States. Approximately 84% of the sample claimed a religious affiliation, with an additional 6% stating they were religious but not affiliated. While the study documented increasing religious diversity both in major traditions claimed (i.e., Buddhism, Hinduism, Islam) and in denominational or subgroup differences within the larger religion, Protestantism just barely remained the majority tradition at 51.3%. Of importance for medical and psychiatric history taking are the findings that 1) 28% of Americans have left the tradition in which they were raised for a different religion or none at all, 2) 25% of Americans under the age of 30 claimed no affiliation at all, and 3) over half of adults who were unaffiliated as a child have chosen a faith tradition to claim as an adult. In addition, ongoing Latino immigration is increasing the absolute number of Catholics in the United States (Pew Research Center 2008).

Religion, Spirituality, and Culture in Assessment and Treatment Planning

Obviously, if time permits, a wealth of helpful clinical information can be obtained in individual work with the child and in family sessions regarding religion and spirituality and their roles in both pathology and possible treatment (Moncher and Josephson 2004; Sexson 2004). However, in many situations involving multicultural patients and families, repeat visits are limited; therefore, simple, straightforward assessment tools can be helpful.

The screening mnemonic FICA, described in Table 34–3, is simple and easy to use and remember, and is a good tool for obtaining basic information. Primarily developed for and used in adult populations, it can be used with parents and older children, provided that developmentally appropriate language is used by the interviewer. These questions serve as a starting point to discuss past religious and spiritual experiences, current practices, satisfaction with religious and spiritual elements of life, and supportive resources (Caraballo et al. 2006; Puchalski and Romer 2000).

The mnemonic BELIEF, described in Table 34–4, was developed for evaluating families in the medical setting and is helpful in mental health settings as well. The examiner inquires about issues prompted by each letter of the word. This device is especially helpful in establishing trust and rapport for the future when matters of religious or spiritual significance might arise (McEvoy 2003).

TABLE 34–3. FICA religion/spirituality screening tool

F—Is religious **faith** part of your day-to-day life?

I—How has faith **influenced** your life, past and present?

C—Are you currently part of a religious or spiritual **community?**

A—What are the spiritual needs you would like to have **addressed?**

Source. Reprinted with permission from Puchalski C, Romer AL: "Taking a Spiritual History Allows Clinicians to Understand Patients More Fully." *Journal of Palliative Medicine* 3:129–137, 2000. The publisher for this copyrighted material is Mary Ann Liebert, Inc., publishers.

TABLE 34–4. BELIEF religion/spirituality screening tool

B—the family's **belief** system

E—the family's **ethics,** or value system

L—how the family practices their religion or spirituality, or **lifestyle**

I—the family's **involvement** in a religious or spiritual community

E—participation of child and/or family in religious **education**

F—**future** issues in health care that might have religious or spiritual meaning or implications (e.g., contraception, circumcision, immunizations)

Source. Reprinted with permission from McEvoy M: "Culture and Spirituality as an Integrated Concept in Pediatric Care." *MCN: The American Journal of Maternal Child Nursing* 28:39–43, 2003. Used with permission.

Finally, clinicians and the families they treat often overlook treatment resources available through local religious institutions and faith-based organizations. These resources include food pantries, clothes closets, emergency cash assistance, shelters, health clinics, transportation to medical appointments, English as a Second Language (ESL) classes, daycare for children and elders, recreational activities, and practical training in areas such as job interviewing and computer skills. These services are becoming increasingly valuable as other government and health care funds diminish in amount and availability (Dell 2004).

Research Directions

Three areas of cultural psychiatry provide fertile soil for research, especially as ethnic and racial minorities increase in both absolute numbers and percentages of the total population, intermarry, have children, and become acculturated into mainstream North Ameri-

can life. Biologically, pharmacogenetics and neuropsychopharmacology will continue to pursue better understandings of the ethnic differences in drug metabolism and interactions. These efforts will be ongoing in light of the rapid rate of new drug development and the infinite number of new genetic combinations created by marriage and conception, especially those of bicultural and multicultural heritages. Similarly, psychological, sociological, and anthropological studies will enhance understanding of the psychodynamics and group dynamics of multiculturalism, and how a diverse society influences and is influenced by not only biology, but also cultural variables. Finally, the area of religion, spirituality, and health will continue to look for connections between the beliefs and practices of world faith traditions, spirituality, and pathways to improved mental and physical health.

Summary Points

- Child, adolescent, and family development is influenced by both genetics and the psychological and experiential aspects of culture.

- Susceptible individuals in some cultures display unusual psychiatric and behavioral syndromes, often stress and anxiety induced, that are specific to particular societies. These culture-bound syndromes have been included in DSM, attesting to acceptance of these entities by the psychiatric profession.

- Different cultural groups and ethnicities demonstrate variable enzymatic activity of the cytochrome P450 system that is genetically influenced, if not determined.

- Religion and spirituality form a subset of culture that affects and is affected by all other elements of culture. These relationships are becoming increasingly complex and important as the United States increases in ethnic and religious pluralism.

- Familiarity with general facts about major world faith traditions is helpful in clinical practice. However, there is considerable variation in individual belief and practice, so clinicians are well advised to inquire about the belief systems and customs of specific patients and families.

References

Ahmed I: Psychological aspects of giving and receiving medications, in Culture and Psychotherapy: A Guide to Clinical Practice. Edited by Tseng W-S, Streltzer J. Washington, DC, American Psychiatric Press, 2001, pp 123–134

American Psychiatric Association: Diagnostic and Statistical Manual of Mental Disorders, 4th Edition. Washington, DC, American Psychiatric Association, 1994

American Psychiatric Association: Diagnostic and Statistical Manual of Mental Disorders, 4th Edition, Text Revision. Washington, DC, American Psychiatric Association, 2000

Ammerman NT: North American Protestant fundamentalism, in Fundamentalisms Observed. Edited by Marty ME, Appleby RS. Chicago, IL, University of Chicago Press, 1991, pp 1–65

Atwood CD: Religion in America, in Handbook of Denominations in the United States, 12th Edition. Edited by Mead FS, Hill SS, Atwood CD. Nashville, TN, Abingdon Press, 2005, pp 15–23

Canino IA, Spurlock J: Culturally Diverse Children and Adolescents: Assessment, Diagnosis, and Treatment, 2nd Edition. New York, Guilford, 2000

Caraballo A, Hamid H, Lee JR, et al: A resident's guide to the cultural formulation, in Clinical Manual of Cultural Psychiatry. Edited by Lim RF. Washington, DC, American Psychiatric Publishing, 2006, pp 243–269

Cutting C: Islam, in Encyclopedia of Religious and Spiritual Development. Edited by Dowling EM, Scarlett WG. Thousand Oaks, CA, Sage Publications, 2006, pp 212–217

Dell ML: Religious professionals and institutions: untapped resources for clinical care. Child Adolesc Psychiatric Clin N Am 13:85–110, 2004

Dell ML, Vaughan BS, Kratochvil CJ: Ethics and the prescription pad. Child Adolesc Psychiatr Clin N Am 17:93–111, 2008

Du N: Asian American patients, in Clinical Manual of Cultural Psychiatry. Edited by Lim RF. Washington, DC, American Psychiatric Publishing, 2006, pp 69–117

Eckel MD: Buddhism in the world and in America, in World Religions in America, 3rd Edition. Edited by Neusner J. Louisville, KY, Westminster John Knox Press, 2003, pp 142–153

Esposito JL: Islam in the world and in America, in World Religions in America, 3rd Edition. Edited by Neusner J. Louisville, KY, Westminster John Knox Press, 2003, pp 172–185

Fleming CM: American Indian and Alaska native patients, in Clinical Manual of Cultural Psychiatry. Edited by Lim RF. Washington, DC, American Psychiatric Publishing, 2006, pp 175–203

Freud S: The question of a weltanschauung (1933), in The Standard Edition of the Complete Psychological Works of Sigmund Freud, Vol 22. Translated and edited by Strachey J. London, Hogarth Press, 1962, pp 158–167

Gaw AC: Concise Guide to Cross-Cultural Psychiatry. Washington, DC, American Psychiatric Publishing, 2001

Gill S: Native Americans and their religions, in World Religions in America, 3rd Edition. Edited by Neusner J. Louisville, KY, Westminster John Knox Press, 2003, pp 9–23

Group for the Advancement of Psychiatry, Committee on Cultural Psychiatry: Cultural Assessment in Clinical Psychiatry. Washington DC, American Psychiatric Publishing, 2002

Guarnaccia PJ, Rogler LH: Research on culture-bound syndromes: new directions. Am J Psychiatry 156:1322–1327, 1999

Hood RW Jr, Hill PC, Williamson WP: The Psychology of Religious Fundamentalism. New York, Guilford, 2005

Johnson T: Native American Indian spirituality, in Encyclopedia of Religious and Spiritual Development. Edited by Dowling EM, Scarlett WG. Thousand Oaks, CA, Sage Publications, 2006, pp 313–315

Josephson AM, Dell ML: Religion and spirituality in child and adolescent psychiatry: a new frontier. Child Adolesc Psychiatric Clin N Am 13:1–15, 2004

Kaslow NJ, Celano M, Dreelin ED: A cultural perspective on family theory and therapy. Psychiatr Clin North Am 18:621–633, 1995

Koenig HG, McCullough ME, Larson DB: Handbook of Religion and Health. New York, Oxford University Press, 2001

Koss-Chioino JD, Vargas LA: Through the cultural looking glass: a model for understanding culturally responsive psychotherapies, in Working with Culture. Edited by Vargas LA, Koss-Chioino JD. San Francisco, CA, Jossey-Bass, 1992, pp 1–22

Larson GJ: Hinduism in India and in America, in World Religions in America, 3rd Edition. Edited by Neusner J. Louisville, KY, Westminster John Knox Press, 2003, pp 124–141

Levine RE, Gaw AC: Culture-bound syndromes. Psychiatr Clin North Am 18:523–536, 1995

McEvoy M: Culture and spirituality as an integrated concept in pediatric care. MCN Am J Matern Child Nurs 28:39–43, 2003

Mead FS, Hill SS, Atwood CD: Handbook of Denominations in the United States, 11th Edition. Nashville, TN, Abingdon Press, 2001

Mead FS, Hill SS, Atwood CD: Handbook of Denominations in the United States, 12th Edition. Nashville, TN, Abingdon Press, 2005

Moncher FJ, Josephson AM: Religious and spiritual aspects of family assessment. Child Adolesc Psychiatric Clin N Am 13:49–70, 2004

Munoz R, Primm A, Ananth J, et al: Life in Color: Culture in American Psychiatry. Chicago, IL, Hilton, 2007, pp 105–125

Neusner J: Judaism in the world and in America, in World Religions in America, 3rd Edition. Edited by Neusner J. Louisville, KY, Westminster John Knox Press, 2003, pp 106–123

Pew Research Center: The U.S. religious landscape survey reveals a fluid and diverse pattern of faith, in Pew Forum on Religion and Public Life. Washington, DC, Pew Research Center, 2008. Available at: http://pewresearch.org/pubs/743/united-states-religion. Accessed March 8, 2008.

Primm AB: African American patients, in Clinical Manual of Cultural Psychiatry. Edited by Lim RF. Washington, DC, American Psychiatric Publishing, 2006, pp 35–68

Puchalski C, Romer AL: Taking a spiritual history allows clinicians to understand patients more fully. J Palliat Med 3:129–137, 2000

Raman VV: Hinduism, in Encyclopedia of Religious and Spiritual Development. Edited by Dowling EM, Scarlett WG. Thousand Oaks, CA, Sage Publications, 2006, pp 199–203

Scarlett WG: Buddhism, in Encyclopedia of Religious and Spiritual Development. Edited by Dowling EM, Scarlett WG. Thousand Oaks, CA, Sage Publications, 2006, pp 59–60

Sexson SB: Religious and spiritual assessment of the child and adolescent. Child Adolesc Psychiatric Clin N Am 13:35–47, 2004

Smith MW: Ethnopsychopharmacology, in Clinical Manual of Cultural Psychiatry. Edited by Lim RF. Washington, DC, American Psychiatric Publishing, 2006, pp 207–235

Ton H, Lim RF: The assessment of culturally diverse individuals, in Clinical Manual of Cultural Psychiatry. Edited by Lim RF. Washington, DC, American Psychiatric Publishing, 2006, pp 3–31

Tseng W-S: Handbook of Cultural Psychiatry. San Diego, CA, Academic Press, 2001

Tseng W-S: Clinician's Guide to Cultural Psychiatry. San Diego, CA, Academic Press, 2003

U.S. Bureau of the Census: U.S. Census 2000 Population Change and Distribution: Census 2000 Brief. Washington, DC, U.S. Bureau of the Census, 2001

Wentz RE: American Religious Traditions: The Shaping of Religion in the United States. Minneapolis, MN, Fortress Press, 2003

Chapter 35

Youth Suicide

Tina R. Goldstein, Ph.D.
David A. Brent, M.D.

Definitions

In order to correct a history of inconsistent and unclear terminology regarding suicide-related behavior, O'Carroll et al. (1996) developed a defined set of terms. These guidelines will be utilized throughout the chapter and are summarized in Table 35–1.

Epidemiology

Suicidal ideation can be thought of along a continuum from passive, nonspecific ideation (e.g., "I wish I had never been born") to active, specific ideation with intent and/or plan. At any point in time, 15%–25% of adolescents endorse some degree of suicidal ideation. Ideation that is specific and active is much less com-

mon, however, with estimates between 2% and 6% (Lewinsohn et al. 1996).

Estimates of the lifetime prevalence of suicide attempts in adolescents range from 1% to 10% (Lewinsohn et al. 1996). In a recent survey, 8% of high school students reported attempting suicide within the prior year, 2% of whose attempts were medically serious (Eaton et al. 2006).

In the United States in 2005, suicide was the third leading cause of death among youth and young adults and accounted for 13% of the mortality in this age group (Centers for Disease Control and Prevention 2007). The suicide rate in this age group increased by 8% from 2003 to 2004 (the largest single-year increase since 1990; for further discussion, see the subsection "Selective Serotonin Reuptake Inhibitors" in the "Treatment" section later in this chapter), although overall, the last decade has witnessed a decline.

TABLE 35–1. Suicide terminology

Term	Definition
Suicide	Fatal, self-inflicted, destructive act with explicit or implicit intent to die
Suicide attempt	Nonfatal, self-inflicted, destructive act (not necessarily resulting in injury) with explicit or implicit intent to die
Suicidal ideation	Thoughts of harming or killing oneself
Suicidality	All suicide-related behaviors and thoughts
Nonsuicidal self-injurious behavior	Any self-inflicted destructive act performed without intent to die but with full intent of inflicting physical harm to oneself (viewed as distinct from suicidal behavior)

Note. The term "suicide gesture" is not recommended by the National Institute of Mental Health task force, nor is it included among the operational definitions because it confounds lethality with intent.
Source. O'Carroll et al. 1996.

Characteristics

Age

The rates of attempted and completed suicide increase dramatically with age throughout childhood into adolescence. Various explanations may account for this relationship, including elevated risk for psychopathology incurred during adolescence, increased capacity to prepare and execute a suicide plan with cognitive maturity, and decreased supervision with age. Although prepubertal children do endorse suicidal ideation, their cognitive immaturity appears to limit their ability to plan and execute lethal suicide attempts. Suicidal behavior is rare in preschool-age children; when present in this age group, physical and/or sexual abuse is common (Rosenberg et al. 1987).

Gender

The rate of completed suicide among youth is significantly higher for males than females, with a ratio of nearly 6 to 1 in 2001 (Anderson and Smith 2003). However, females endorse much higher rates of specific suicidal ideation (6% vs. 2%) and have higher suicide attempt rates than males (10% vs. 4%) (Lewinsohn et al. 1996). The higher rate of completed suicide among male youth may be attributable to higher rates of associated risk factors, including substance use and antisocial behaviors, and the tendency for males to employ more violent and lethal means of attempting suicide.

Race and Socioeconomic Status

In general, the suicide rate in the United States is higher among white than nonwhite youth. However, Ameri-

can Indian youth in the United States exhibit a particularly elevated suicide rate. Furthermore, the rate of completed suicide among young African American males has been growing disproportionately in more recent years (Joe and Kaplan 2002). Hispanic youth, while not at increased risk for completed suicide as compared with other ethnic groups, do have significantly higher rates of suicidal ideation and attempt (Grunbaum et al. 2004). Little is known about suicidality among Asian American youth, who have a low likelihood of disclosure of suicidal ideation and a tendency to underutilize mental health services (Leong et al. 2007).

With regard to socioeconomic status, in the United States increased suicide risk is conveyed by lower socioeconomic status—with the exception of young African American males, for whom completed suicide is associated with higher socioeconomic status (Gould et al. 1996).

Risk Factors

Suicidal Ideation

Youth with frequent and severe suicidal ideation (i.e., high levels of intent and/or planning) have about a 60% chance of making a suicide attempt within 1 year of ideation onset (Kessler et al. 1999).

Previous Suicidal Behavior

The strongest predictor of future suicide is a history of suicide attempt (Brent et al. 1999). Follow-up studies of adolescent suicide attempters report a reattempt rate ranging from 6% to 15% per year, with the greatest risk occurring within 3 months of the initial attempt (Goldston et al. 1999). The period immediately following discharge from an inpatient psychiatric unit appears to be associated with particularly high risk (Kjelsberg et al. 1994). Youth with a history of attempting suicide using methods high in medical lethality, such as hanging, shooting, or jumping, are at especially high risk for eventual completed suicide (Beautrais 2004). However, it is not necessarily the case that an attempt of low lethality reflects low suicidal intent, particularly among younger children who may overestimate the lethality of means.

Availability of Lethal Means

Evidence from case-control studies indicates that firearms are much more common in the homes of suicide completers than in those of attempters and control subjects. If a loaded gun is in the home, it is highly likely to be selected as a means of suicide. In one study, a loaded gun in the home was associated with a 30-fold increased risk for completed suicide, even among youth with no apparent psychopathology (Brent and Bridge 2003).

Psychiatric Disorders

The overwhelming majority—nearly 90%—of youth who die by suicide have evidence of serious psychopathology (Brent et al. 1988). Youth who attempt suicide also demonstrate high rates of psychopathology, in the range of 60% (Gould et al. 1998). Mood disorders convey the most potent risk, with over 80% of attempters and 60% of completers meeting criteria for at least one major mood disorder (Brent 1993; Gould et al. 1998). Unipolar depression and bipolar disorder are most closely linked to suicidal behavior in youth (Brent et al. 1988). Depressed youth with a chronic course of illness lasting 2 years or more are at particularly elevated risk for both attempted and completed suicide.

Other psychiatric conditions frequently associated with youth suicide and suicide attempt include disruptive, anxiety, and substance use disorders. Comorbidity is the rule rather than the exception among youth who attempt and complete suicide, with up to 70% of suicidal youth meeting criteria for multiple psychiatric conditions (Lewinsohn et al. 1996). As the number of comorbid conditions increases, so does the risk for suicide attempt (Brent et al. 1999).

Comorbid substance abuse increases the risk of attempted and completed suicide, through both the negative impact of substance use on mood disorder and

the increased risk of lethal suicidal behavior while under the influence. This is particularly true among older adolescent males when coupled with conduct disorder. Although conduct disorder and related disruptive disorders are more likely to eventuate in suicide and suicidal behavior when comorbid with substance use, disruptive disorders also independently contribute to suicide risk (Fergusson et al. 1995).

Psychological Factors

Psychological factors linked to suicide risk include impulsive aggression in response to frustration or provocation (Brent et al. 2002). Hopelessness also correlates strongly with suicidal intent and predicts risk for reattempt and completed suicide beyond its association with depression (Goldston et al. 2001).

In terms of personality traits, *neuroticism*—the tendency to experience prolonged and severe negative affect in response to stress—has repeatedly been associated with suicide attempts in youth, above and beyond its association with other risk factors (Roy 2002). Although perfectionism is another personality trait associated with suicide attempts in youth, studies have failed to find a link between perfectionism and completed suicide (Shaffer et al. 1996).

There is accumulating evidence from population-based studies that same-sex attraction and sexual behavior, particularly among males, is associated with increased risk for attempted suicide (Remafedi 1999). The relationship between homosexuality and suicidality may be mediated by 1) gender nonconformity and subsequent parental and peer rejection and bullying and/or 2) the increased risk for depression and substance abuse found among adolescents who identify as homosexual.

Medical Disorders

Specific chronic medical conditions, including diabetes and epilepsy, have been associated with suicidality in pediatric populations, even after controlling for other risk factors (Goldston et al. 1997). Research also supports a prospective association between suicide attempts and functionally impairing physical illness or injury (Lewinsohn et al. 1996).

Family Factors

The parents of youth who attempt suicide or complete suicide have higher-than-expected rates of mood disor-

TABLE 35–2. Summary of studies examining biological factors associated with suicidality

Study	Finding
Greenhill et al. 1995	Altered serotonergic function among depressed adolescent suicide attempters
Pandey 2004; Pandey et al. 1997, 2002	Increased receptor binding ($5\text{-}HT_{2A}$) of the serotonin metabolite 5-hydroxyindoleacetic acid, decreased protein kinase A and C activity, downregulation of cAMP-response element binding protein (CREB), and increased activity of brain-derived neurotropic factor in the prefrontal cortex and hippocampus in postmortem studies comparing adolescent suicide completers with nonpsychiatric deceased controls
Dahl et al. 1991; Matthew et al. 2003	Altered adrenocortical function in suicidal depressed adolescents, as evidenced by elevated cortisol levels in the late evening hours
Dahl et al. 1992; Ryan et al. 1988	Blunting of sleep-stimulated growth hormone secretion

der, substance abuse, and antisocial behavior (Brent et al. 1996, 1999). Research suggests both environmental and genetic mechanisms for the familial transmission of suicidal behavior, and evidence suggests that suicidal behavior is transmitted in families distinct from its association with familial psychiatric illness. The first-degree relatives of adolescent suicide attempters and completers exhibit a suicide attempt rate two to six times higher than that found in the general population, even after controlling for higher rates of psychopathology (Fergusson et al. 2003). Likewise, the offspring of mood-disordered adults with a history of suicide attempt are at four to six times greater risk for suicide attempt as compared with offspring of mood disordered adults with no history of suicide attempt (Melhem et al. 2007). Greater familial loading has been found to be specifically associated with earlier age at onset of suicidal behavior in offspring, suggesting that early-onset suicidality may be a particularly familial form that is mediated by impulsive aggression.

The family environments of suicide attempters are characterized by high levels of discord and violence and are perceived as less supportive and more conflictual than those of nonattempters (Brent et al. 1994; Gould et al. 1996). Both physical and sexual abuse also have a potent association with attempted and completed suicide in youth, as does parental loss or absence (Brent et al. 1994; Gould et al. 1996).

Biological Factors

Table 35–2 presents findings from studies examining the neurobiology associated with youth suicide.

Protective Factors

A positive parent-child connection as evidenced by active parental supervision, leisure and meal times spent together, and clear behavioral and academic expectations has been shown to be associated with lower levels of suicidal behavior (Borowsky et al. 2001). Similarly, adolescents who report a positive connection with school, academic success, a prosocial peer group, and religious affiliation show lower rates of suicidal behavior (Fergusson et al. 2003).

Based on the literature of risk and protective factors for youth suicidal behavior to date, Bridge et al. (2006) propose a developmental-transactional model of youth suicidal behavior whereby suicidal behavior is conceptualized as resulting from sociocultural, developmental, psychiatric, psychological, and family environmental factors.

Assessment

Suicidal ideation should be assessed according to both severity (intent) and pervasiveness (frequency and intensity). Suicidal ideation characterized by a high degree of severity and pervasiveness is associated with greater likelihood of suicide attempt in adolescents (Lewinsohn et al. 1996). In addition, prior suicidal behavior should be carefully reviewed.

Suicidal Intent

Suicidal intent is the extent to which the individual wishes to die. Given findings that adolescents may disclose suicidal ideation on self-report ratings but deny this information during interviews, assessment of suicidal risk should incorporate both means of assessment. The individual's behavior should also be carefully assessed.

With regard to suicidal intent, four components should be explored (Kingsbury 1993): 1) belief about intent (i.e., the extent to which the individual is wishing to die); 2) preparatory behavior (e.g., giving away prized possessions; writing a suicide note); 3) prevention of discovery (i.e., planning the attempt so that rescue is unlikely); and 4) communication of suicidal intent. High intent—as evidenced by expressing a wish to die, planning the attempt ahead of time, timing the attempt to avoid detection, and confiding suicide plans prior to the attempt—is associated with recurrent suicide attempts and with suicide completion.

Suicide Plan and Access to Means

Assessment should include inquiry regarding specific plans for inflicting self-harm, as well as access to means considered (see the subsection "Means Restriction" in the "Treatment" section later in this chapter).

Medical Lethality

Suicide attempts of high medical lethality (e.g., hanging, shooting) are frequently characterized by high suicidal intent, and individuals who use more medically lethal means are at higher risk to complete suicide. However, evidence also indicates that an impulsive attempter with relatively low intent but ready access to lethal means may also engage in a medically serious and even fatal attempt (Brent et al. 1999).

It is important to differentiate nonsuicidal self-injurious behavior from suicide attempt (see terminology in Table 35–1). Examples include scratching, cutting, or burning oneself as a means of relieving or expressing emotional pain. Given that the risk factors for nonsuicidal self-harm and suicidal behavior overlap, many youth engage in both behaviors, and therefore the presence of one should alert the clinician to inquire about the other.

Precipitants

The most common precipitant for adolescent suicidal behavior is interpersonal conflict or loss, most often involving a parent or a romantic relationship. Legal and disciplinary problems also frequently precipitate suicidal behavior, particularly among youth with conduct disorder and substance abuse. Precipitants that are chronic and ongoing, especially recurrent physical or sexual abuse, are associated with poorer outcomes, including recurrence of suicidal behavior and even subsequent completion (Brent et al. 1999).

Motivation

Motivation is the reason the individual cites for his or her suicidality. Individuals with high suicidal intent indicate their primary motivation is either to die or to permanently escape an emotionally painful situation, and these youth are at elevated risk for reattempt (Cohen-Sandler et al. 1982). Many youth who attempt suicide report they are motivated by the desire to influence others or to communicate a feeling. Understanding the motivation for the suicide attempt has important implications for treatment, as intervention may focus on helping youth identify their needs more explicitly and find less dangerous ways to get their needs met.

Consequences

The consequences of suicidality refer to any environmental contingencies that occur in response to suicidality. Particularly salient is whether there are naturally occurring contingencies in the environment that reinforce suicidal threats or attempts (e.g., increased attention and support, decreased demands and responsibilities). However, positive reinforcement from the environment does not necessarily indicate that the individual acted purposefully to gain the reinforcement.

Treatment

Few clinical trials have examined the treatment of adolescent suicidal behavior. In fact, most treatment studies of depressed adolescents exclude suicidal youth and do not report outcomes related to suicidality. Data from psychosocial and pharmacological studies suggest that the treatment of depression may not be sufficient to reduce suicidal risk; rather, specific treatments targeting suicidality may be required (Emslie et al. 2006).

Approaches to the treatment of youth suicidality that show promise include clinical interventions like safety planning and hospitalization, as well as psychosocial treatment packages that involve cognitive, emotion regulation, and interpersonal approaches. Although no pharmacological treatment has demonstrated efficacy in treating suicidality per se in youth, medications that target aggression and emotional dysregulation such as lithium and atypical neuroleptics may hold promise.

Clinical Management

Safety Plans

A safety plan is a hierarchically arranged list of strategies that the patient agrees to employ in the event of a suicidal crisis. The development of a safety plan is considered one of the most critical parts of the assessment and treatment of suicidal youth and involves collaboration among the clinician, patient, and family. On an outpatient basis, the safety plan is implemented once it is determined that the patient is safe to maintain as an outpatient; in fact, the safety plan may be used to help determine appropriate level of care (i.e., the inability to collaborate on a safety plan may be indicative of need for a higher level of care). However, care should be taken to avoid the use of coercion when negotiating the safety plan so as not to mask the adolescent's suicidal risk.

The first strategy is to eliminate the availability of lethal means in the patient's environment, including firearms, ammunition, and pills. Next, a no-harm agreement is negotiated among the adolescent, parents, and clinician that in the event the adolescent has suicidal urges, he or she will implement coping skills, inform a responsible adult, and/or call the clinician or emergency room. The clinician then works with the patient to develop a plan for coping with suicidal urges. The patient is asked to identify the warning signs of a suicidal crisis; these may include specific thoughts (e.g., "I hate my life"), emotions (e.g., despair), and/or behaviors (e.g., social isolation). Risk factors for that individual may also be identified (e.g., not getting enough sleep). The safety plan involves a stepwise increase in level of intervention from internal coping strategies to external strategies. Primarily, patients are encouraged to consider internal strategies or coping skills they can employ without the assistance of other people (e.g., distracting by playing a computer

game). In the event that internal strategies are insufficient, patients should identify key figures who can be enlisted to help, including responsible adults. Their contact information should be made readily available to the patient.

Family cooperation in the development of a safety plan is extremely important. An important family component to the safety plan is the negotiation of a truce around "hot topics" or possible precipitants to future suicidality. This truce gives permission for the patient and parents to table issues that trigger conflict until they have learned how to disagree without leading to suicidality.

Few studies have examined the effectiveness of safety plans. One quasi-experimental study showed a reduction in suicide attempts among youth at high risk for suicide in a runaway shelter after implementing a one-session intervention that included a written safety plan with no-harm contract (Rotheram-Borus and Bradley 1991). A recent review found that no-harm contracts alone are not a sufficient method for suicide prevention (Lewis 2007).

Means Restriction

Few studies have been conducted to evaluate the effectiveness of restriction of access to lethal means. Studies in psychiatric and pediatric outpatient settings have not found a significant effect of parental psychoeducation on securing access to lethal means (Brent et al. 2000). However, removal of guns from the homes of at-risk youth is strongly recommended. Specific elements of psychoeducation regarding access to lethal means may be critical in decreasing risk—insisting on removal of the gun (rather than merely securing it), speaking directly to the gun owner, and ascertaining the perceived risks of removing the gun. Some parents will be unwilling to remove guns but would be willing to secure them (Brent et al. 2000). Therefore, risk reduction may be achieved by exploring alternatives to removal, including storing guns locked, unloaded, and/or disassembled.

Inpatient Hospitalization

Although psychiatric hospital admission is believed to provide a safe environment for suicidal patients to resolve acute suicidal crises, there is no research to support the efficacy of inpatient hospitalization in reducing suicidality. Among individuals hospitalized for a suicide attempt, the highest risk period for suicide and reattempt occurs after discharge from the hospital (Kjelsberg et al. 1994), making the transition particularly important.

Several studies have attempted to target this risk period. Carter et al.'s (2005) "Postcards From the Edge" study demonstrated that adolescents and adults who were randomly assigned to receive written contact via postcard during the year following self-poisoning exhibited fewer suicide reattempts and fewer days hospitalized as compared with those who did not receive written contact. For adolescent suicide attempters, adherence with posthospitalization treatment may be maximized by having hospital staff schedule the initial outpatient appointment.

Psychotherapy Approaches

Cognitive-Behavioral Therapy

Brent et al.'s (1997) study of depressed adolescents included suicidal teens; findings indicate that cognitive-behavioral therapy (CBT) was superior to both family and supportive therapies in the treatment of depressive symptoms, but all three treatments were associated with similar reductions in suicidality. In the multisite Treatment for Adolescents With Depression Study (TADS) in which fluoxetine, CBT, and the combination were compared with each other and with placebo, both fluoxetine and the combination produced substantial improvements in depression relative to placebo and CBT alone, but only the combination was associated with decreased suicidal ideation as compared to placebo (March et al. 2004).

Rotheram-Borus et al. (2000) compared brief family CBT alone to an "enhanced" CBT condition in which an additional family psychoeducation session was delivered in the emergency room for female adolescent suicide attempters. The "enhanced" CBT group showed increased adherence to CBT treatment and lower suicidal ideation at posttreatment. At 18-month follow-up, the rates of attempts and suicidal ideation were not different between the two groups.

Dialectical Behavior Therapy

Dialectical behavior therapy (DBT)—a treatment that focuses on the development of mindfulness, emotional regulation, distress tolerance, and interpersonal skills—has been shown to reduce recurrent suicidal and self-harm behavior in personality disordered adults. Miller et al. (2006) modified DBT for use with suicidal adolescents by decreasing the length of treatment and incorporating family members into treatment. Katz et al. (2004) compared inpatient treatment with and without DBT for adolescents hospitalized for suicidal ideation or attempt. Both groups showed similar reduction in self-reported depression, suicidal ideation, and hopelessness; there were no differences in reattempts, rehospitalization, or adherence to outpatient treatment.

Home-Based Family Therapy

Harrington et al. (1998) compared a five-session home-based family therapy plus routine care with routine care alone for adolescent suicide attempters. Overall, the home-based family therapy intervention was no better than routine care for reducing ideation or reattempt. However, among the subgroup of suicide attempters in the sample who were not depressed, the home-based treatment reduced suicidal ideation more so than routine care.

Multisystemic Therapy

Huey et al. (2004) compared multisystemic therapy (MST)—an intensive family-based treatment delivered in the patient's natural environment that involves case management and both individual and family treatment—with psychiatric hospitalization and usual care for youth presenting to the emergency room with suicidal ideation, suicide attempt, homicidal ideation, or psychosis. Rates of reattempt were significantly lower in the MST group than in the usual-care group at 1-year follow-up. However, high rates of hospitalization in the MST group render these findings difficult to interpret. Additionally, there were no group differences for suicidal ideation, depression, or hopelessness.

Youth-Nominated Support Teams

Youth-nominated support teams (YST-1) aim to augment the connection between suicidal adolescents and individuals in their social network by providing psychoeducation to those individuals nominated by suicidal adolescents as supportive (most commonly parents, nonparental relatives, nonadult relatives, peers, or teachers) and facilitating weekly contact between the nominated individuals and the suicidal adolescents (King et al. 2006). A randomized study comparing YST-1 plus usual care to usual care alone for adolescents hospitalized for suicidal ideation or attempt found no between-group differences in the rate of suicide attempt. Suicidal ideation declined in both groups, but among girls, the YST-1 group showed a greater decline in suicidal ideation. However, the low (35%) acceptance rate into randomization, as well as the high attrition rate in the experimental condition because of adolescents' unwillingness or inability to involve at least two supportive individuals, may limit the utility of this approach.

Developmental Group Therapy

Wood et al. (2001) compared a six-session skills-based group therapy plus usual care to usual care alone for adolescents who had engaged in at least two episodes of self-harm within the past year. The developmental group therapy approach focused on family conflict, problem solving, interpersonal relationships, anger management, school problems, depression, and hopelessness. As compared with usual care, the experimental treatment group showed an overall reduction in conduct and school problems as well as repeated self-harm episodes.

Skills-Based Therapy

Donaldson et al. (2005) conducted a randomized trial comparing a brief skills-based therapy (SBT, including problem-solving and emotion regulation skills) with supportive relationship therapy (SRT) for adolescent suicide attempters. Both groups showed similar improvements in depression and suicidal ideation. A trend emerged for subjects receiving SBT to have a higher rate of reattempts than those in SRT at 3 and 6 months and a higher dropout rate. This study suggests SRT might be at least as efficacious as the experimental treatment.

School-Based Prevention

Eggert et al. (1995) developed a semester-long personal growth class focused on enhancing protective factors against suicide (e.g., school attendance, self-esteem, personal control, and prosocial peer group). They compared the class plus screening for suicidality with a more intensive version of the class (two semesters) and suicidality screening alone. All three groups received school-based case management. Surprisingly, the brief screening intervention was as efficacious as both class interventions in reduction of suicidal ideation and associated risk factors, with one exception—the personal growth class resulted in greater improvements in self-rated personal control. Brief screening and contact with a case manager may be an effective and sufficient intervention to reduce suicidal risk, although this approach awaits replication.

Pharmacological Approaches

Selective Serotonin Reuptake Inhibitors

No studies have expressly examined the effect of fluoxetine or any other selective serotonin reuptake inhibitors (SSRIs) on impulsive aggression in youth. Findings from the TADS indicate that fluoxetine is superior to placebo for the treatment of depression in youth but is not associated with greater decreases in suicidal ideation. It is important to note, however, that all groups exhibited a significant decrease in suicidal ideation (March et al. 2004). Recent findings from the Treatment of Resistant Depression in Adolescents (TORDIA) study of teens who did not respond to an adequate initial SSRI trial indicate that switch to a different SSRI was just as efficacious as switch to venlafaxine; there were no differences in rates of suicidality between groups (Brent et al. 2008).

There is concern regarding a possible association between SSRI treatment and emergent suicidality in children and adolescents. Indeed, the TADS documented a twofold increase in suicide-related adverse events among youth receiving active medication as compared with those taking placebo. Similarly, the U.S. Food and Drug Administration's meta-analysis of short-term placebo-controlled trials of SSRIs and other antidepressants in youth also indicated an increased risk of suicidal ideation or attempt in patients taking antidepressants. Most commonly, suicidality occurred early in treatment and consisted of increased or new-onset suicidal ideation, with very few suicide attempts and no suicide completions. The mechanism by which SSRIs might increase risk for suicidal behavior is not known; possible explanations include increased irritability and agitation, disinhibition, and potentiation of a mixed state in those with a preexisting bipolar diathesis.

It is imperative to consider the public health implications of these data from a broader perspective. Although causation has not been demonstrated, there is a significant correlation in time between an increase in SSRI prescriptions and sales and a decline in both the overall suicide rate and the suicide rate among adolescents (Ludwig and Marcotte 2005). Additionally, the decrease in SSRI prescriptions following the public health warning of a possible association between SSRIs and suicide in youth was associated with a marked increase in youth suicide in the United States (Gibbons et al. 2007). Furthermore, a recent meta-analysis supports the assertion that many more youth will show a good clinical response to SSRIs than will become suicidal (Bridge et al. 2007).

Lithium

Among children and adolescents, data support the use of lithium for the treatment of aggression (Malone et al. 2000). Examination of the use of lithium for the treatment of suicidality in youth appears warranted.

Divalproex

Divalproex has demonstrated efficacy in the treatment of impulsive aggression, mood lability, and behavioral symptoms in studies of children, adolescents, and adults (Hollander et al. 2003).

Neuroleptics

The use of neuroleptics for the treatment of youth suicidality has not been evaluated. However, atypical neuroleptics have been shown to be efficacious in the treatment of aggressive behavior in children and adolescents (Findling et al. 2000).

Research Directions

The public health implications of youth suicide in this country are serious. Although progress has been made in improving our understanding of risk and protective factors for suicidality in youth, a great deal remains to be known about the effective prevention and treatment of suicidality in this population. Recommended directions for future research include increased inclusion of suicidal youth in studies of mood disorders, treatment studies aimed at prevention for those at highest risk, and studies examining the neurobiology associated with suicidality in youth. Pending data from a five-site pilot project funded by the National Institute of Mental Health (Treatment of Adolescent Suicide Attempters; TASA) may be helpful in further informing future directions for treatment.

Summary Points

- The strongest predictor of future suicide is a history of suicide attempt.
- The majority of youth who die by suicide have evidence of serious psychopathology, with mood disorders conveying the most potent risk for attempt and completion.
- Psychological factors associated with suicidality include hopelessness and a tendency to impulsive aggression.
- Assessment of suicidal ideation should include attention to both severity (intent) and pervasiveness (frequency and intensity).
- Assessment with suicidal individuals should include explicit questions regarding plans for self-harm, as well as determination of access to lethal means.
- Clinical management of suicidal youth includes safety planning with the adolescent and family members, means restriction, and inpatient hospitalization when warranted.
- Despite recent concerns regarding increased suicide risk among children and adolescents taking SSRIs, research indicates that more youth will show a good clinical response to SSRIs than will become suicidal.
- Data from psychosocial and pharmacological studies suggest that treatment of depression may not be sufficient to reduce suicidal risk in youth; rather, specific treatments targeting suicidality may be required and may include pharmacological and psychosocial interventions.

References

Anderson RN, Smith BL: Deaths: leading causes for 2001. Natl Vital Stat Rep 52:1–85, 2003

Beautrais AL: Further suicidal behavior among medically serious suicide attempters. Suicide Life Threat Behav 34:1–11, 2004

Borowsky IW, Ireland MA, Resnick MD: Adolescent suicide attempts: risks and protectors. Pediatrics 107:485–493, 2001

Brent DA: Depression and suicide in children and adolescents. Pediatr Rev 14:380–388, 1993

Brent DA, Bridge J: Firearms availability and suicide: Evidence, interventions, and future directions. Am Behav Sci 46:1192–1210, 2003

Brent DA, Perper JA, Goldstein CE, et al: Risk factors for adolescent suicide: a comparison of adolescent suicide victims with suicidal inpatients. Arch Gen Psychiatry 45:581–588, 1988

Brent DA, Perper JA, Moritz G, et al: Familial risk factors for adolescent suicide: a case-control study. Acta Psychiatr Scand 89:52–58, 1994

Brent DA, Bridge J, Johnson BA, et al: Suicidal behavior runs in families: a controlled family study of adolescent suicide victims. Arch Gen Psychiatry 53:1145–1152, 1996

Brent DA, Holder D, Kolko D, et al: A clinical psychotherapy trial for adolescent depression comparing cognitive, family, and supportive therapy. Arch Gen Psychiatry 54:877–885, 1997

Brent DA, Baugher M, Bridge J, et al: Age and sex-related risk factors for adolescent suicide. J Am Acad Child Psychiatry 38:1497–1505, 1999

Brent DA, Baugher M, Birmaher B, et al: Compliance with recommendations to remove firearms by families participating in a clinical trial for adolescent depression. J Am Acad Child Psychiatry 39:1220–1226, 2000

Brent DA, Oquendo M, Birmaher B, et al: Familial pathways to early onset suicide attempt: risk for suicidal behavior in offspring of mood-disordered suicide attempters. Arch Gen Psychiatry 59:801–807, 2002

Brent DA, Emslie GJ, Clarke GN, et al: Switching to venlafaxine or another SSRI with or without cognitive behavioral therapy for adolescents with SSRI-resistant depression: the TORDIA randomized control trial. JAMA 299:901–913, 2008

Bridge J, Goldstein TR, Brent DA: Adolescent suicide and suicidal behavior. J Child Psychol Psychiatry 47:372–394, 2006

Bridge J, Iyengar S, Salary CB, et al: Clinical response and risk for reported suicidal ideation and suicide attempts in pediatric antidepressant treatment: a meta-analysis of randomized controlled trials. JAMA 297:1683–1696, 2007

Carter GL, Clover K, Whyte IM, et al: Postcards from the EDge project: randomised controlled trial of an intervention using postcards to reduce repetition of hospital treated deliberate self-poisoning. Br Med J 331:805 (epub), 2005.

Centers for Disease Control and Prevention: Compressed mortality file: underlying cause-of-death, in CDC Wonder. Atlanta, GA, Centers for Disease Control and Prevention, 2007. Available at: http://wonder.cdc.gov/mortSQL.html. Accessed May 10, 2007.

Cohen-Sandler R, Berman AL, King RA: Life stress and symptomatology: determinants of suicidal behavior in children. J Am Acad Child Psychiatry 21:178–186, 1982

Dahl RE, Ryan ND, Puig-Antic J, et al: 24-Hour cortisol measures in adolescents with major depression: a controlled study. Biol Psychiatry 30:25–36, 1991

Dahl RE, Ryan ND, Williamson DE, et al: Regulation of sleep and growth hormone in adolescent depression. J Am Acad Child Psychiatry 31:615–621, 1992

Donaldson D, Spirito A, Esposito-Smythers C: Treatment for adolescents following a suicide attempt: results of a pilot trial. J Am Acad Child Adolesc Psychiatry 44:113–120, 2005

Eaton D, Kann L, Kinchen SA, et al: Youth risk behavior surveillance: United States, 2005. MMWR Surveill Summ 55:1–108, 2006

Eggert LL, Thompson EA, Herting JR, et al: Reducing suicide potential among high-risk youth: tests of a school-based prevention program. Suicide Life Threat Behav 25:276–296, 1995

Emslie G, Kratochvil C, Vitiello B, et al: Treatment for Adolescents with Depression Study (TADS): safety results. J Am Acad Child Psychiatry 45:1440–1455, 2006

Fergusson DM, Horwood LJ, Lynskey MT: The stability of disruptive childhood behaviors. J Abnorm Child Psychol 23:379–396, 1995

Fergusson DM, Beautrais AL, Horwood LJ: Vulnerability and resiliency to suicidal behaviours in young people. Psychol Med 33:61–73, 2003

Findling RL, McNamara NK, Branicky LA, et al: A double-blind pilot study of risperidone in the treatment of conduct disorder. J Am Acad Child Psychiatry 4:509–516, 2000

Gibbons RD, Brown CH, Hur K, et al: Early evidence on the effects of regulators' suicidality warnings on SSRI prescriptions and suicide in children and adolescents. Am J Psychiatry 164:1356–1363, 2007

Goldston DB, Kelley AE, Reboussin DM, et al: Suicidal ideation and behavior and noncompliance with the medical regimen among diabetic adolescents. J Am Acad Child Psychiatry 36:1528–1536, 1997

Goldston DB, Daniel SS, Reboussin DM, et al: Suicide attempts among formerly hospitalized adolescents: a prospective naturalistic study of risk during the first 5 years after discharge. J Am Acad Child Psychiatry 38:660–671, 1999

Goldston DB, Daniel SS, Reboussin DM, et al: Cognitive risk factors and suicide attempts among formerly hospitalized adolescents: a prospective naturalistic study. J Am Acad Child Psychiatry 40:91–99, 2001

Gould MS, Fisher P, Parides M, et al: Psychosocial risk factors of child and adolescent completed suicide. Arch Gen Psychiatry 53:1155–1162, 1996

Gould MS, King R, Greenwald S, et al: Psychopathology associated with suicidal ideation and attempts among children and adolescents. J Am Acad Child Psychiatry 37:915–923, 1998

Greenhill L, Waslick B, Parides M, et al: Biological studies in suicidal adolescent inpatients. Scientific Proceedings of the Annual Meeting of the American Academy of Child and Adolescent Psychiatry 11:124, 1995

Grunbaum JA, Kann L, Kinchen SA, et al: Youth risk behavior surveillance: United States, 2003. MMWR Surveill Summ 53:1–96, 2004

Harrington R, Kerfoot M, Dyer E, et al: Randomized trial of a home-based family intervention for children who have deliberately poisoned themselves. J Am Acad Child Psychiatry 37:512–518, 1998

Hollander E, Tracy KA, Swann AC, et al: Divalproex in the treatment of impulsive aggression: efficacy in Cluster B personality disorders. Neuropsychopharmacology 28:1186–1197, 2003

Huey SJ, Henggeler SW, Rowland MD, et al: Multisystemic therapy effects on attempted suicide by youths presenting psychiatric emergencies. J Am Acad Child Psychiatry 43:183–190, 2004

Joe S, Kaplan MS: Firearm-related suicide among young African-American males. Psychiatr Serv 53:332–334, 2002

Katz LY, Cox BJ, Gunasekara S, et al: Feasibility of dialectical behavior therapy for suicidal adolescent inpatients. J Am Acad Child Psychiatry 43:276–282, 2004

Kessler RC, Borges G, Walters EE: Prevalence of and risk factors for lifetime suicide attempts in the national comorbidity survey. Arch Gen Psychiatry 56:617–626, 1999

King CA, Kramer A, Preuss L, et al: Youth-nominated support team for suicidal adolescents: a randomized controlled trial. J Consult Clin Psychol 74:199–206, 2006

Kingsbury SJ: Clinical components of suicidal intent in adolescent overdose. J Am Acad Child Psychiatry 32:518–520, 1993

Kjelsberg E, Neegaard E, Dahl AA: Suicide in adolescent psychiatric inpatients: incidence and predictive factors. Acta Psychiatr Scand 89:235–241, 1994

Leong F, Leach M, Yeh C, et al: Suicide among Asian Americans: What do we know? What do we need to know? Death Stud 31:417–434, 2007

Lewinsohn PM, Rohde P, Seeley JR: Adolescent suicidal ideation and attempts: prevalence, risk factors, and clinical implications. Clin Psychol Sci Pract 3:25–46, 1996

Lewis LM: No-harm contracts: a review of what we know. Suicide Life Threat Behav 37:50–57, 2007

Ludwig J, Marcotte DE: Antidepressants, suicide, and drug regulation. J Policy Anal Manage 24:249–272, 2005

Malone R, Delaney MA, Luebbert JF, et al: A double-blind placebo-controlled study of lithium in hospitalized aggressive children and adolescents with conduct disorder. Arch Gen Psychiatry 57:649–654, 2000

March JS, Silva S, Petrycki S, et al: Fluoxetine, cognitive-behavioral therapy, and their combination for adolescents with depression: Treatment for Adolescent Depression Study (TADS) randomized controlled trial. JAMA 292:807–820, 2004

Matthew SJ, Coplan JD, Goetz RR, et al: Differentiating depressed adolescent 24 hour cortisol secretion in light of their adult clinical outcome. Neuropsychopharmacology 28:1336–1343, 2003

Melhem NM, Brent DA, Ziegler M, et al: Familial pathways to early-onset suicidal behavior: familial and individual antecedents of suicidal behavior. Am J Psychiatry 164:1364–1370, 2007

Miller AL, Rathus JH, Linehan MM: Dialectical Behavior Therapy With Suicidal Adolescents. New York, Guilford, 2006

O'Carroll PW, Berman AL, Maris RW, et al: Beyond the Tower of Babel: a nomenclature for suicidology. Suicide Life Threat Behav 26:237–252, 1996

Pandey GN: Decreased catalytic activity and expression of protein kinase C isozymes in teenage suicide victims: a postmortem brain study. Arch Gen Psychiatry 61:685–693, 2004

Pandey GN, Dwivedi Y, Pandey SC, et al: Protein kinase C in the postmortem brain of teenage suicide victims. Neurosci Lett 228:111–114, 1997

Pandey GN, Dwivedi Y, Rizavi HS, et al: Higher expression of serotonin 5-HT2A receptors in the postmortem brains of teenage suicide victims. Am J Psychiatry 159:419–429, 2002

Remafedi G: Suicide and sexual orientation: nearing the end of the controversy? Arch Gen Psychiatry 56:885–886, 1999

Rosenberg ML, Smith JC, Davidson LE, et al: The emergence of youth suicide: an epidemiologic analysis and public health perspective. Ann Rev Public Health 8:417–440, 1987

Rotheram-Borus MJ, Bradley J: Triage model for suicidal runaways. Am J Orthopsychiatry 61:122–127, 1991

Rotheram-Borus MJ, Piacentini J, Cantwell C, et al: The 18-month impact of an emergency room intervention for adolescent female suicide attempters. J Consult Clin Psychol 68:1081–1093, 2000

Roy A: Family history of suicide and neuroticism: a preliminary study. Psychiatry Res 110:87–90, 2002

Ryan ND, Puig-Antich J, Rabinovich H, et al: Growth hormone response to desmethylimipramine in depressed and suicidal adolescents. J Affect Disord 15:323–337, 1988

Shaffer D, Gould MS, Fisher P, et al: Psychiatric diagnosis in child and adolescent suicide. Arch Gen Psychiatry 53:339–348, 1996

Wood A, Trainor G, Rothwell J, et al: Randomized trial of group therapy for repeated deliberate self-harm in adolescents. J Am Acad Child Adolesc Psychiatry 40:1246–1253, 2001

Chapter 36

Gender Identity and Sexual Orientation

Kenneth J. Zucker, Ph.D.

Gender Identity Disorder

Definition, Clinical Description, and Diagnosis

Gender identity refers to a person's basic sense of self as a male, a female, or some other "third" type of gendered subjectivity. By the age of 3, most children demonstrate the rudimentary capacity to self-label their gender identity. Thus, most preschoolers can answer "correctly" the basic question "Are you a boy or a girl?" However, most preschoolers do not appreciate that gender is an invariant aspect of the self. Thus, 3-year-olds may not understand that they will grow up to be a man or a woman, or they may believe that if they engage in cross-gender surface behaviors this will alter their gender. It is not until a few years later that children appear to master the concept of gender constancy (Zucker et al. 1999). Children also attach affective meaning to being a boy or a girl. There is, for example, a tendency among young children to "overvalue" their own gender and "devalue" the other gender, a phenomenon that developmental and social psychologists have studied under the rubric of "in-group" and "out-group" biases (Susskind and Hodges 2007).

Children and youth are referred for clinical evaluation when their gender identity (and corresponding gender role behaviors) does not "match" their biological sex. In children, this disjunction is easily observed in a variety of surface behaviors that index cross-gender identification: sex-of-playmate preference, roles in fantasy play, cross-dressing, and toy and activity interests. These youngsters either will also express an intense desire to become a member of the opposite sex or will actually "mislabel" their own gender (in relation to their birth sex). There is also a marked rejection of activities and behaviors associated with their own sex, and sometimes there are verbal and behavioral manifestations of an intense dislike of sex-related anatomic features. In adolescents, behavioral signs of cross-gender identification are also apparent, but more importantly, one can observe an intensification of the discomfort with somatic features that are associated with their biological sex. From a developmental perspective, in adolescents the clinical phenomenology of *gender dysphoria*—the subjective discomfort with one's gender identity (in relation to one's birth sex)— matches more closely to that observed in adults who are struggling with their gender identity. Because of this developmental variation in clinical presentation, DSM-IV (American Psychiatric Association 1994, 2000) has distinct criteria sets for gender identity disorder (GID) in children and in adolescents and adults.

Epidemiology

Epidemiological studies have not examined GID in youth (for an overview, see Zucker and Lawrence 2009). There is consensus that GID is relatively uncommon. For example, based on the number of adults requesting sex reassignment surgery (SRS) in the Netherlands, Bakker et al. (1993) suggested a prevalence of 1 in 11,000 men and 1 in 30,400 women. On the original version of the Child Behavior Checklist (Achenbach and Edelbrock 1983), there are two "gender" items: "behaves like opposite sex" and "wishes to be of opposite sex." For both referred and nonreferred children, depending on the age and sex of the child, the percentage of mothers who endorsed the item "wishes to be of opposite sex" with a rating of very true or often true ranged from 0% to 2%.

There are sex differences in referral rates for children and youth with GID. In my own clinic, the male-female ratio for children ages 2–12 years from 1975 to 2007 was 4.6:1 (N=502), but for adolescents, the male-female ratio was only 1.4:1 (N=158). It is possible that the natural history of GID is such that the true prevalence drops between childhood and adolescence (a point that is discussed more fully in the section "Course and Prognosis"). There is considerable evidence that parents, teachers, and peers are less tolerant of cross-gender behavior in boys than in girls; however, in adolescence, social pressures may be equally salient for boys and girls with pervasive cross-gender behavior. In our clinic, the number of child referrals per year has remained quite stable over the past 20 years; in contrast, the number of adolescent referrals per year tripled between the years 2004–2007 (Zucker et al. 2008).

This increase in adolescent referrals likely has a multifactorial explanation. One possible factor is the increase in media attention given to transgendered youth. Along with the increasing use of the Internet for social purposes, it is likely that youth are more able to "come out" and discuss more openly their gender identity concerns and that this facilitates clinical referral.

Comorbidity

Children and youth with GID should be evaluated systematically for the presence of other behavior problems and/or psychiatric disorders. On average, both children and youth with GID show as many general behavior problems as do referred youth in general (Cohen-Kettenis et al. 2003; Wallien et al. 2007; Zucker et al. 2002). In boys with GID, internalizing disorders predominate, whereas in girls with GID there is a mixture of internalizing and externalizing disorders. There are probably three broad reasons for the co-occurrence of these other behavior problems. First, children with GID experience social ostracism (particularly from same-sex peers) for their cross-gender behavior (Cohen-Kettenis et al. 2003). Second, family psychopathology, including both maternal and paternal psychiatric disorder, probably functions as a general risk factor. Third, even when there is reasonable support for a child's or youth's cross-gender behavior or identity, the subjective experience of growing up with an atypical gender identity can prove extremely stressful. This becomes even more salient during the adolescent years when the discordance between one's subjective gender identity and somatic sex (in terms of pubertal changes) is magnified.

Causal Mechanisms

Identification of causal mechanisms regarding GID requires a consideration of what is known about normative gender development, including both biological and psychosocial factors (for review, see Ruble et al. 2006). Detailed reviews of etiological hypotheses for GID can be found elsewhere (Cohen-Kettenis and Pfäfflin 2003), and only a summary will be provided here.

Regarding biological factors, the vast majority of children with GID do not have a disorder of sex development (DSD; formerly known as physical intersex conditions). A variable minority of children with DSDs, including genetic females with congenital adrenal hyperplasia and genetic males with various androgen resistance syndromes who are raised as females, do, however, show indicators of cross-gender behavior and identification, and some will go through a gender change (Meyer-Bahlburg 2005). One interpretation of these data is that prenatal hormonal factors play a role in cross-gender behavior and subsequent gender dysphoria. For most children with GID, however, there is no direct evidence of a sex-atypical prenatal hormonal milieu. Accordingly, researchers have attempted to identify other biological factors that might implicate prenatal hormonal factors or biological markers that affect sex-dimorphic neural structures but not sex-dimorphic genital differentiation.

There is some evidence that within-sex variation in sex-dimorphic behavior has a heritable component, but studies of identical twins discordant for GID suggest that genetic factors do not tell the whole story (Segal 2006). Activity level (AL) is a sex-dimorphic dimension of temperament; in children with GID, AL appears to be sex-inverted (Zucker and Bradley 1995), which may be related to genetic factors, subtle prenatal hormonal factors, or temperament. Boys with GID have an elevated rate of left-handedness (Zucker et al. 2001), which may be a sign of prenatal developmental perturbations. They are also later in birth order relative to their brothers (Blanchard et al. 1995), which may be a marker of a progressive maternal immune response to male-specific antigens that results in a demasculinization of the male fetal brain (Blanchard and Klassen 1997). One null finding shows the complexity in studying biological influences on GID. Wallien et al. (2008) examined the digit ratios of the second and fourth fingers (2D:4D) in both boys and girls with GID. 2D:4D shows a well-established normative sex difference, with a smaller ratio in males than in females, which has been attributed to between-sex variation in prenatal androgen exposure. Wallien et al. found a significant 2D:4D sex difference in a control group of boys and girls but no evidence for an altered digit ratio in GID children.

Psychosocial hypotheses have considered various factors, including parental prenatal gender preferences, parent-child relationship factors, and the role of social reinforcement of cross-gender behavior. There is no evidence that parents of children with GID disproportionately wished for a child of the opposite sex during the pregnancy. There is evidence that parental response during the early phase of GID differentiation has been one of tolerance or encouragement of cross-gender behavior, although it is not clear if this can be best interpreted as a predisposing factor or a perpetuating factor. Many parents report that when their child first engaged in cross-gender behavior, it was interpreted as either "cute" or "only a phase" and so their response was to go along with the child's interests. Such parents become concerned only when the behavior persists or when the child begins to experience social ostracism by peers. There is a variety of evidence that children with GID feel closer to the opposite-sex parent, which may promote cross-gender identification, although the child's interests may be a cause, not a result.

Course and Prognosis

Follow-up studies of both boys and girls with GID have provided data on at least three types of psychosexual outcomes: 1) persistence of GID with a co-occurring homosexual or bisexual sexual orientation; 2) desistence of GID with a co-occurring homosexual or bisexual sexual orientation; and 3) desistence of GID with a co-occurring heterosexual sexual orientation.

Follow-Up Studies of Boys

Green's (1987) study constitutes the most comprehensive long-term follow-up of GID boys. Forty-four feminine boys and 30 control boys were evaluated at a mean age of 18.9 years (range, 14–24). Sexual orientation in fantasy and behavior (using Kinsey ratings) was assessed by means of a semistructured interview. Of the previously feminine boys, 75%–80% were either bisexual or homosexual at follow-up versus 0%–4% of the control boys. Only 1 youth, at age 18 years, was gender-dysphoric to the extent of considering SRS.

Data from six other follow-up reports on 55 boys with GID were summarized by Zucker and Bradley (1995). At follow-up (range, 13–26 years), if 13 uncertain cases are excluded, 27 (64.2%) of the remaining 42 cases had "atypical" (i.e., homosexual, transsexual, or transvestitic) outcomes. In these studies, the percentage of boys who showed persistent GID was higher than that reported by Green (1987) (11.9% vs. 2.2%, respectively), but the percentage of those who were homosexual (62.1%) was somewhat lower.

Zucker and Bradley (1995) reported follow-up data on 40 boys at a mean age of 16.7 years (range, 13–23). Of these, 8 (20%) were classified as gender-dysphoric at follow-up. The remaining 80% had a "normal" or male-typical gender identity. Regarding sexual orientation in fantasy, 20 (50%) were classified as heterosexual, 17 (42.5%) were classified as bisexual/homosexual, and 3 (7.5%) were classified as "asexual" (i.e., they did not report any sexual fantasies). Regarding sexual orientation in behavior, 9 (22.5%) were classified as heterosexual, 11 (27.5%) were classified as bisexual/homosexual, and 20 (50.0%) were classified as "asexual" (i.e., they did not report any interpersonal sexual experiences).

Wallien and Cohen-Kettenis (2008) provided follow-up data on 40 boys (range, 16–28 years) seen for GID at the sole clinic for children and youth in the Netherlands. They reported a GID persistence rate of 20%. Depending on the metric, the percentage of probands with either a bisexual or homosexual sexual orientation ranged from 68% to 81% and the percentage of probands with a heterosexual sexual orientation ranged from 19% to 32%.

Follow-Up Studies of Girls

Drummond et al. (2008) evaluated 25 girls with GID at a follow-up mean age of 23.2 years (range, 15–36). Of these 25 girls, 3 (12%) had persistent GID, two of whom had a homosexual sexual orientation and the third was asexual. The remaining 22 (88%) girls had a "normal" gender identity.

Regarding sexual orientation in fantasy (Kinsey ratings) for the 12 months preceding the follow-up assessment, 15 (60%) girls were classified as exclusively heterosexual, 8 (32%) were classified as bisexual/homosexual, and 2 (8%) were classified as "asexual" (i.e., they did not report any sexual fantasies). Regarding sexual orientation in behavior, 11 (44%) girls were classified as exclusively heterosexual, 6 (24%) were classified as bisexual/homosexual, and 8 (32%) were classified as "asexual" (i.e., they did not report any interpersonal sexual experiences).

Wallien and Cohen-Kettenis (2008) provided follow-up data on 18 girls, with a GID persistence rate of 50%. All of the persisters had a homosexual sexual orientation and all of the desisters had a heterosexual sexual orientation.

Persistence and Desistance in a Comparative-Developmental Perspective

From these follow-up studies, only a minority of children followed prospectively had a persistence of GID into adolescence and young adulthood. It is possible that gender identity shows relative malleability during childhood, with a gradual narrowing of plasticity as the gendered sense of self consolidates as adolescence approaches.

Follow-up studies of adolescents with GID show a much higher rate of GID persistence than do children.

Cohen-Kettenis and van Goozen (1997), for example, reported that 22 (66.6%) of 33 adolescents went on to receive sex reassignment surgery (SRS). At initial assessment, the mean age of the 22 adolescents who received SRS was 17.5 years (range, 15–20). Of the 11 who did not receive SRS, 8 were not recommended for it because they were not diagnosed with transsexualism (corresponding to the DSM-IV diagnosis of GID); the 3 remaining patients were given a diagnosis of transsexualism but the "real-life test" (i.e., living for a time as the opposite sex prior to the institution of contrasex hormonal treatment and surgery) was postponed because of severe concurrent psychopathology and/or adverse social circumstances. These data, therefore, suggest a very high rate of GID persistence, which is eventually treated by SRS.

Evaluation

The assessment and diagnosis of GID should, of course, rely on a clinical interview that involves the principal caregivers. For most parents, this can be carried out in the presence of the child, although in some cases, parents are more comfortable when they are interviewed separately. Most adolescents are comfortable discussing their gender dysphoria and other concerns in the presence of parents or other caregivers, but some prefer to be seen separately. Discussion of an adolescent's sexual orientation is usually best carried out in an individual interview.

Zucker (2005b) reviewed a variety of standardized assessment measures for children and youth who may have GID that can complement a standard clinical interview. Given that dimensional assessment of psychiatric disorders will likely be introduced in DSM-V, these measures will become increasingly relevant. Three examples will be provided, all of which are easy to use by the clinician in a mental health setting or private practice and do not involve more complicated and cumbersome stimuli (e.g., various toys and dress-up apparel used in free-play assessments):

1. The Gender Identity Interview for Children contains 12 items. Each item is coded on a 3-point response scale. Using factor analysis, Zucker et al. (1993) identified two factors, which were labeled *affective gender confusion* (7 items) and *cognitive gender confusion* (4 items), that accounted for 38.2% and 9.8% of the variance, respectively. Both mean factor scores significantly differentiated gender-referred probands ($n=85$) from controls ($n=98$). Cutoff scores of either three or four deviant responses

yielded high specificity rates (88.8% and 93.9%, respectively) but lower sensitivity rates (54.1% and 65.8%, respectively). Table 36–1 shows responses to the Gender Identity Interview for Children from a 6-year-old girl (IQ=107) who was referred for gender identity concerns.

2. The Gender Identity Questionnaire for Children (GIQC) is a parent-report questionnaire (Johnson et al. 2004). The GIQC consists of 16 items pertaining to various aspects of sex-typed behavior that are reflected in the GID diagnostic criteria, each rated on a 5-point response scale. A factor analysis based on 325 gender-referred children and 504 controls (siblings, clinic-referred, and nonreferred), with a mean age of 7.6 years, identified a one-factor solution containing 14 items, accounting for 43.7% of the variance. The gender-referred children had a significantly larger total deviant score than did the control subjects, with a large effect size of 3.70, using Cohen's *d*. With a specificity rate set at 95% for the controls, the sensitivity rate for the probands was 86.8%.

3. The Gender Identity/Gender Dysphoria Questionnaire for Adolescents and Adults (GIDYQ-AA) is a self-report questionnaire (Deogracias et al. 2007). The GIDYQ-AA consists of 27 items pertaining to various aspects of gender dysphoria, each rated on a 5-point response scale using the past 12 months as a time frame. In the female version, for example, items include "In the past 12 months, have you felt more like a man than like a woman?" and "In the past 12 months, have you wished to have an operation to change your body into a man's (e.g., to have your breasts removed or to have a penis made)?" A factor analysis based on 389 university students (heterosexual and nonheterosexual in their sexual orientation) and 73 clinic-referred patients with GID identified a one-factor solution containing all 27 items, accounting for 61.3% of the variance. The GIDYQ-AA strongly discriminated the GID patients from both the heterosexual and nonheterosexual controls. Using a cutpoint of 3.00, sensitivity was 90.4% for the gender identity patients and specificity was 99.7% for the controls.

Therapeutics

In adolescents, like adults, the gender dysphoria may wax and wane, but there is little in the way of empirical evidence, or even clinical experience, that psychotherapeutic techniques or interventions are particularly effective. Hormonal and surgical interventions may be the most effective way to resolve gender dysphoria in carefully selected adolescent patients (Cohen-Kettenis and van Goozen 1997; Smith et al. 2001, 2005).

In contrast, for children, there is clinical evidence that psychological treatments for GID can contribute to its remission. Although there is a literature on a variety of therapeutic approaches (behavior therapy, psychotherapy and psychoanalysis, parent counseling, group therapy, and so forth), there is not one randomized, controlled treatment trial for children with GID. Although there have been some treatment effectiveness studies, much is lacking in these investigations. As a result, the clinician must rely largely on the "wisdom" that has accumulated in the case report literature and the conceptual underpinnings that inform the various approaches to intervention.

In the absence of best-practice therapeutic guidelines, the case formulation (i.e., the clinician's underlying conceptual model) is what will organize the approach to treatment (see Zucker 2008). There are three contemporary positions on therapeutics (for a detailed review, see Zucker 2007).

The most common therapeutic approach has been to help the child feel more comfortable with a gender identity that matches the biological sex. Multimethod approaches are typically used, including individual therapy with the child, parent counseling, and parent-guided interventions in the naturalistic environment, including limit setting on cross-gender behaviors, encouragement of alternative activities, and promotion of same-sex peer relationships (see Meyer-Bahlburg 2002).

In contrast, some contemporary therapists (and parents) have adopted a very different therapeutic position. They view the child's early manifestation of a cross-gender identification as a fixed and "essential" aspect of the child's identity. The diagnosis of GID is rejected (except perhaps for insurance purposes), and the child is labeled as "transgendered." The child's cross-gender identification is accepted and encouraged, including at least an informal change in the child's social gender (e.g., enrolling a biological male at school as a girl). An intermediate position also rejects the diagnosis of GID but does not necessarily view cross-gender identification as immutable. In place of the GID diagnosis, such children are characterized as "gender variant," and one goal is to help the child negotiate the social complexities that result from his or her cross-gender identification (Ehrensaft 2007; Menvielle et al. 2005).

TABLE 36–1. Interview transcript of the Gender Identity Interview for Children

---

Interviewer (I): Are you a boy or a girl?

Child (C): Boy.

I: Are you a girl?

C: Boy.

I: When you grow up, will you be a mommy or a daddy?

C: Daddy.

I: Could you ever be a mom?

C: No.

I: Are there any good things about being a girl?

C: No.

I: Are there any things that you don't like about being a girl?

C: Yes.

I: Tell me some of the things you don't like about being a girl.

C: Wearing dresses, wearing ponytails. I think I don't remember all the rest.

I: Do you think it is better to be a boy or a girl?

C: Boy.

I: Why?

C: Because boys like cars. 'Cuz they can have spiky hair. That's all.

I: In your mind, do you ever think you would like to be a boy?

C: Yes.

I: Can you tell me why?

C: Because I just like being a boy. Because they don't wear dresses.

I: In your mind, do you ever get mixed up and you're not really sure if you are a boy or a girl?

C: No.

I: Do you ever feel more like a boy than like a girl?

C: Yes.

I: Tell me more about that.

C: I feel like that a lot of times. Every day. That's pretty much all of it.

I: You know what dreams are, right? Well, when you dream at night, are you ever in the dream?

C: Yes.

I: In your dreams, are you a girl, a boy, or sometimes a girl and sometimes a boy?

C: A boy.

I: Tell me about the dreams…

C: I was spying with the Jonas Brothers, Zach and Cody, Drake and Josh and me…and they call me Nick… when I was in the dream when my daddy was a ghost… [Note: The patient's father died suddenly 14 months prior to the evaluation.]

I: Do you ever think that you really are a boy?

C: Yes.

I: Tell me more about that.

C: All the time.

Note.   See Zucker et al. 1993 for a description of this measure.

Sexual Orientation

In 1973, the American Psychiatric Association delisted homosexuality from DSM as a mental disorder. There are, however, reasons why mental health professionals need to remain current about what is known about people with a minority sexual orientation. First, it represents a form of cultural competence in delivering clinical care. Second, it requires sensitivity in training clinicians (Townsend et al. 1997). Third, there may be unique (or heightened) mental health challenges associated with a minority sexual orientation. Fourth, there remain many youth who struggle with their emerging minority sexual orientation, and the practitioner needs to know how best to help them in the consolidation of their sexual identity.

Definition and Assessment

The most salient dimension of sexual orientation is the sex of the person to whom one is attracted sexually. In clinical practice and in many areas of research, structured interview assessments or self-report questionnaires are used to ask about a person's sexual orientation. Such approaches tend to evaluate distinct domains (e.g., sexual orientation in fantasy vs. sexual orientation in behavior). Another domain pertains to a person's self-labeling of sexual identity (e.g., using common terms such as gay, lesbian, queer, homosexual, bisexual). Most adolescents are familiar with these terms.

In recent years, there has been a considerable body of research demonstrating, especially in people with a minority sexual orientation, that the various components (fantasy, attraction, behavior, self-labeling) do not always "hang together" (e.g., Savin-Williams 2006). Thus, by one metric, a person might be "classified" as homosexual, but not by another. In clinical practice, a typical example might be of a youth who has an exclusively homoerotic sexual orientation in fantasy, but, for various reasons, is reluctant to self-label as gay, lesbian, or homosexual.

Is Sexual Orientation a Stable or Fluid Trait?

A common question encountered in clinical practice is whether a person's sexual orientation is a stable or a fluid trait. For example, a youth struggling with his or her sexual orientation may want to know if sexual orientation change is possible (e.g., that the current experience is "only a phase") or if sexual orientation is fixed. A good clinical assessment can ascertain a youth's sexual orientation along the parameters described earlier (i.e., in fantasy, in attraction, in behavior, and in self-labeling). Some individuals who experience a disjunction among these four parameters may experience distress and one issue is how best to help them cope. For example, a youth with an exclusively homoerotic sexual orientation in fantasy but who does not identify as gay may have this disjunction for a variety of reasons (e.g., religious imperatives that condemn homosexuality, familial attitudes). Thus, one therapeutic approach might be to help the youth understand the origins of his or her "internalized" homophobia. Some youth who desire a heterosexual intimate life may be able to engage in overt heterosexual behavior despite their homoerotic sexual orientation in fantasy.

Several decades of treatment studies, largely of men, designed to change a person's sexual orientation from homosexual to heterosexual suggest that for most people, sexual orientation is a stable trait (i.e., the underlying sexual orientation in fantasy does not change) (for review, see Drescher and Zucker 2006). For women, however, the picture is more mixed. In women, data suggest considerable stability of a minority sexual orientation but with a fair degree of fluidity within the subcategories of lesbian, bisexual, and unlabeled (Diamond 2005).

Models of Sexual Identity Formation

Since the 1970s, many researchers have considered "stage" models with regard to sexual identity formation (for review, see Savin-Williams and Cohen 2004). In their original form, there was the assumption that there was an almost universal temporal sequence in sexual identity development milestones (e.g., nascent awareness of same-sex sexual attraction, a period of sexual identity confusion, then a period of self-identification as gay or lesbian, and, finally, a commitment to that identity and a "coming-out" to others). Although early research found support for these temporal stages, more recent research has identified different temporal trajectories, including sex, ethnic, and cohort effects (see Diamond 2008). Thus, for the practicing clinician, there should be an awareness that there is no one pattern in sexual identity formation and consolidation.

Mental Health Issues

A variety of well-conducted epidemiological studies have shown that gay, lesbian, and bisexual adults have higher rates of various mental disorders and substance abuse than do heterosexual adults (Cochran 2001; Meyer 2003). Studies of youth with a minority sexual orientation have also identified elevations in an array of mental health and substance abuse problems, familial and peer maltreatment or victimization, and relational violence. In addition, "internalized homophobia" (i.e., the struggle a youth has in accepting his or her minority sexual orientation) has been deemed a mental health risk factor (Lock and Kleis 1998). Moreover, sexual minority male youth are at increased risk for HIV/AIDS (Goodenow et al. 2002).

One controversial mental health issue pertaining to sexual minority youth concerns suicidality (ideation, attempts) and suicide completion. In clinical practice, it is common to learn that a youth's depression or suicidality is related to dealing with his or her sexual orientation; however, for many youth, they do not immediately acknowledge the connection. Moreover, it is not uncommon to learn that the clinician did not ask about the youth's sexual orientation, so the underlying issue is not actually addressed. Although it is unlikely that the proportion of suicide completions is grossly overrepresented among gay youth, there is consensus that suicidality (ideation and/or attempts) is elevated and should not be overlooked (Silenzio et al. 2007; Wichstrøm and Hegna 2003). As noted by Savin-Williams and Ream (2004), however, it is not clear whether sexual orientation per se is the risk factor or, rather, there is a variety of factors that lead to psychiatric vulnerability in sexual minority youth (i.e., minority stress parameters).

Research Directions

Regarding GID in children and youth, there are several important clinical questions to be addressed over the next 5 years. Perhaps the most important issue concerns the diagnosis itself. Critics want to see the diagnosis eliminated from DSM-V on the grounds that the diagnosis unnecessarily pathologizes within-sex variation in gender-related behaviors (Hill et al. 2007) or that the diagnosis was introduced to DSM-III in 1980 (American Psychiatric Association 1980) as a backdoor maneuver to prevent later homosexuality (see Zucker and Spitzer 2005). Others have argued that the diagnostic criteria require tightening in order to better differentiate children and youth with bona fide gender dysphoria from those who simply show extreme cross-gender behavior (see Bockting 2009; Zucker 2005a). In addition, therapeutic approaches to GID have been sorely understudied empirically. There is also still much to be learned about the natural history of GID.

Regarding sexual orientation in youth, perhaps the issue of greatest relevance to the clinician is to better understand the factors that differentiate youth with a minority sexual orientation who have various mental health problems from those who do not. After all, it is the former who are likely to come to the attention of the clinician, not the latter. With the emergence of more representative samples of sexual minority youth, it should be possible to identify these differences epidemiologically, which will avoid the pitfalls of reliance on nonrepresentative, clinically referred samples.

Summary Points

- Gender identity self-labeling appears early in development, but cognitive limitations preclude a full appreciation of its constancy until middle childhood.
- Children with GID often show comorbid behavioral and emotional problems, which require clinical evaluation and treatment in their own right.
- Causal mechanisms for GID remain poorly understood.
- Most prospective studies of children with GID show high rates of remission, which is in contrast to prospective studies of youth and adults.
- There are well-established dimensional assessment techniques that complement a clinical diagnostic interview.
- Well-controlled therapeutic studies of children with GID remain to be done.
- Sexual orientation is a multidimensional construct, and there are disjunctions among these parameters, especially for sexual minority youth.

- Sexual orientation may be a more stable trait in males than in females.
- Sexual orientation in youth is associated with a number of mental health problems, and it is imperative to identify the risk factors associated with these problems.

References

Achenbach TM, Edelbrock C: Manual for the Child Behavior Checklist and Revised Child Behavior Profile. Burlington, University of Vermont, Department of Psychiatry, 1983

American Psychiatric Association: Diagnostic and Statistical Manual of Mental Disorders, 3rd Edition. Washington, DC, American Psychiatric Association, 1980

American Psychiatric Association: Diagnostic and Statistical Manual of Mental Disorders, 4th Edition. Washington, DC, American Psychiatric Association, 1994

American Psychiatric Association: Diagnostic and Statistical Manual of Mental Disorders, 4th Edition, Text Revision. Washington, DC, American Psychiatric Association, 2000

Bakker A, van Kesteren PJM, Gooren LJG, et al: The prevalence of transsexualism in the Netherlands. Acta Psychiatr Scand 87:237–238, 1993

Blanchard R, Klassen P: H-Y antigen and homosexuality in men. J Theor Biol 185:373–378, 1997

Blanchard R, Zucker KJ, Bradley SJ, et al: Birth order and sibling sex ratio in homosexual male adolescents and probably prehomosexual feminine boys. Dev Psychol 31:22–30, 1995

Bockting W: Are gender identity disorders mental disorders? Recommendations for revision of the World Professional Association for Transgender Health's Standards of Care. International Journal of Transgenderism 11:53–62, 2009

Cochran SD: Emerging issues in research on lesbians' and gay men's mental health: does sexual orientation really matter? Am Psychol 56:931–947, 2001

Cohen-Kettenis PT, Pfäfflin F: Transgenderism and Intersexuality in Childhood and Adolescence: Making Choices. Thousand Oaks, CA, Sage Publications, 2003

Cohen-Kettenis PT, van Goozen SHM: Sex reassignment of adolescent transsexuals: a follow-up study. J Am Acad Child Adolesc Psychiatry 36:263–271, 1997

Cohen-Kettenis PT, Owen A, Kaijser VG, et al: Demographic characteristics, social competence, and behavior problems in children with gender identity disorder: a cross-national, cross-clinic comparative analysis. J Abnorm Child Psychol 31:41–53, 2003

Deogracias JJ, Johnson LL, Meyer-Bahlburg HFL, et al: The gender identity/gender dysphoria questionnaire for adolescents and adults. J Sex Res 44:370–379, 2007

Diamond LM: A new view of lesbian subtypes: stable versus fluid identity trajectories over an 8-year period. Psychol Women Q 29:119–128, 2005

Diamond LM: Sexual Fluidity: Understanding Women's Love and Desire. Cambridge, MA, Harvard University Press, 2008

Drescher J, Zucker KJ (eds): Ex-Gay Research: Analyzing the Spitzer Study and Its Relation to Science, Religion, Politics, and Culture. New York, Harrington Park Press, 2006

Drummond KD, Bradley SJ, Badali-Peterson M, et al: A follow-up study of girls with gender identity disorder. Dev Psychol 44:34–45, 2008

Ehrensaft D: Raising girlyboys: a parent's perspective. Studies in Gender and Sexuality 8:269–302, 2007

Goodenow C, Netherland J, Szalacha L: AIDS-related risk among adolescent males who have sex with males, females, or both: evidence from a statewide survey. Am J Public Health 92:203–210, 2002

Green R: The "Sissy Boy Syndrome" and the Development of Homosexuality. New Haven, CT, Yale University Press, 1987

Hill DB, Rozanski C, Carfagnini J, et al: Gender identity disorders in childhood and adolescence: a critical inquiry. International Journal of Sexual Health 19:57–75, 2007

Johnson LL, Bradley SJ, Birkenfeld-Adams AS, et al: A parent-report Gender Identity Questionnaire for Children. Arch Sex Behav 33:105–116, 2004

Lock J, Kleis BN: A primer on homophobia for the child and adolescent psychiatrist. J Am Acad Child Adolesc Psychiatry 37:671–673, 1998

Menvielle EJ, Tuerk C, Perrin EC: To the beat of a different drummer: the gender-variant child. Contemp Pediatr 22:38–39, 41, 43, 45–46, 2005

Meyer IH: Prejudice, social stress, and mental health issues in lesbian, gay, and bisexual populations: conceptual issues and research evidence. Psychol Bull 129:674–697, 2003

Meyer-Bahlburg HFL: Gender identity disorder in young boys: a parent- and peer-based treatment protocol. Clin Child Psychol Psychiatry 7:360–377, 2002

Meyer-Bahlburg HFL: Introduction: gender dysphoria and gender change in persons with intersexuality. Arch Sex Behav 34:371–373, 2005

Ruble DN, Martin CL, Berenbaum SA: Gender development, in Handbook of Child Psychology, 6th Edition, Vol 3: Social, Emotional, and Personality Development. Edited by Damon W, Lerner RM (series eds), Eisenberg N (vol ed). New York, Wiley, 2006, pp 858–932

Savin-Williams RC: Who's gay? Does it matter? Curr Dir Psychol Sci 15:40–44, 2006

Savin-Williams RC, Cohen KM: Homoerotic development during childhood and adolescence. Child Adolesc Psychiatr Clin N Am 13:529–549, 2004

Savin-Williams RC, Ream GL: Suicide attempts among sexual-minority male youth. J Clin Child Adolesc Psychol 32:509–522, 2004

Segal NL: Two monozygotic twin pairs discordant for female-to-male transsexualism. Arch Sex Behav 35:347–358, 2006

Silenzio VMB, Pena JB, Duberstein PR, et al: Sexual orientation and risk factors for suicidal ideation and suicide attempts among adolescents and young adults. Am J Public Health 97:2017–2019, 2007

Smith YLS, van Goozen SHM, Cohen-Kettenis PT: Adolescents with gender identity disorder who were accepted or rejected for sex reassignment surgery: a prospective follow-up study. J Am Acad Child Adolesc Psychiatry 40:472–481, 2001

Smith YLS, van Goozen SHM, Kuiper AJ, et al: Sex reassignment: outcomes and predictors of treatment for adolescent and adult transsexuals. Psychol Med 35:89–99, 2005

Susskind J, Hodges C: Decoupling children's gender-based in-group positivity from out-group negativity. Sex Roles 56:707–716, 2007

Townsend MH, Wallick MM, Pleak RR, et al: Gay and lesbian issues in child and adolescent psychiatry training as reported by training directors. J Am Acad Child Adolesc Psychiatry 36:764–768, 1997

Wallien MS, Cohen-Kettenis PT: Psychosexual outcome of gender-dysphoric children. J Am Acad Child Adolesc Psychiatry 47:1413–1423, 2008

Wallien MS, Swaab H, Cohen-Kettenis PT: Psychiatric comorbidity among children with gender identity disorder. J Am Acad Child Adolesc Psychiatry 46:1307–1314, 2007

Wallien MS, Zucker KJ, Steensma TD, et al: 2D:4D finger-length ratios in children and adults with gender identity disorder. Horm Behav 54:450–454, 2008

Wichstrøm L, Hegna K: Sexual orientation and suicide attempt: a longitudinal study of the general Norwegian adolescent population. J Abnorm Psychol 112:144–151, 2003

Zucker KJ: Gender identity disorder in children and adolescents. Annu Rev Clin Psychol 1:467–492, 2005a

Zucker KJ: Measurement of psychosexual differentiation. Arch Sex Behav 34:375–388, 2005b

Zucker KJ: Gender identity disorder in children, adolescents, and adults, in Gabbard's Treatments of Psychiatric Disorders, 4th Edition. Edited by Gabbard GO. Washington, DC, American Psychiatric Publishing, 2007, pp 683–701

Zucker KJ: Children with gender identity disorder: is there a best practice? [Enfants avec troubles de l'identité sexuée: y-a-t-il une pratique la meilleure?] Neuropsychiatr Enfance Adolesc 56:358–364, 2008

Zucker KJ, Bradley SJ: Gender Identity Disorder and Psychosexual Problems in Children and Adolescents. New York, Guilford, 1995

Zucker KJ, Lawrence AA: Epidemiology of gender identity disorder: recommendations for the Standards of Care of the World Professional Association for Transgender Health. International Journal of Transgenderism 11:8–18, 2009

Zucker KJ, Spitzer RL: Was the gender identity disorder of childhood diagnosis introduced into DSM-III as a backdoor maneuver to replace homosexuality? An historical note. J Sex Marital Ther 31:31–42, 2005

Zucker KJ, Bradley SJ, Lowry Sullivan CB, et al: A Gender Identity Interview for Children. J Pers Assess 61:443–456, 1993

Zucker KJ, Bradley SJ, Kuksis M, et al: Gender constancy judgments in children with gender identity disorder: evidence for a developmental lag. Arch Sex Behav 28:475–502, 1999

Zucker KJ, Beaulieu N, Bradley SJ, et al: Handedness in boys with gender identity disorder. J Child Psychol Psychiatry 42:767–776, 2001

Zucker KJ, Owen A, Bradley SJ, et al: Gender-dysphoric children and adolescents: a comparative analysis of demographic characteristics and behavioral problems. Clin Child Psychol Psychiatry 7:398–411, 2002

Zucker KJ, Bradley SJ, Owen-Anderson A, et al: Is gender identity disorder in adolescents coming out of the closet? (Letter to the editor). J Sex Marital Ther 34:287–290, 2008

Chapter 37

Aggression and Violence

Jeffrey H. Newcorn, M.D.
Iliyan Ivanov, M.D.
Anil Chacko, Ph.D.
Jeffrey M. Halperin, Ph.D.

Aggression is one of the most frequent indications for child and adolescent psychiatric referral, often in association with severe and emergent symptomatology—yet aggression is a normal behavior, present in all people to some extent. The nature, meaning, and prevalence of aggression in children differ as a function of developmental level and context, and it is important to distinguish "pathological," "maladaptive," or "antisocial" manifestations of aggression from "prosocial" or adaptive behaviors (e.g., self-defense). Aggression is generally considered to be a highly stable behavioral trait. Nevertheless, only half of school-age children who are aggressive continue to manifest this behavior in adolescence. When aggression persists, it is highly impairing and often carries severe consequences for academic achievement and occupational attainment,

family and peer relationships, and psychological development, as well as risk for dire outcomes—including antisocial personality disorder, substance abuse, and criminality.

Definition and Clinical Description

Pathological or maladaptive aggression occurs outside an expectable social context and occurs either in the absence of antecedent social cues and/or with an intensity, frequency, duration, and/or severity that is disproportionate to its causes. It generally does not terminate in an appropriate time frame and/or in response to feedback. Pathological aggression can occur in the context of specific psychiatric disorders, or it can be a nonspecific manifestation of anger or frustration. Numerous subtypes of aggression have been described, but most classification schemes dichotomize aggression with respect to the ability to modulate and control the behavior and/or the intended goal. Examples include the following:

- *Proactive* (i.e., goal-directed, usually associated with leadership skills and positive peer perceptions) versus *reactive* (i.e., responding to a threat, retaliating)
- *Predatory* (i.e., deliberate and controlled) versus *affective* (i.e., impetuous and poorly controlled)
- *Instrumental* (implies goal-directed behavior that offers some benefit to the aggressor) versus *hostile* (attempting to cause pain to the victim with no independent gain) subtypes

However, in actuality, most children exhibit a combination of these behaviors (Dodge and Coie 1987).

Epidemiology

Aggression and violence among youth represent a major public health concern. A 1997 U.S. Office of Juvenile Justice and Delinquency Prevention survey found that 9% of high school students carried a weapon to school within the last 30 days; 44% of guns used in crimes were owned by persons younger than age 25, with 11% belonging to juveniles younger than 17; and an estimated 1,400 homicides involved a juvenile offender (Centers for Disease Control and Prevention, National Center for Chronic Disease Prevention and Health Promotion 2000).

Most research on youth violence has focused on boys, since males commit violent acts more frequently than females. The most widely accepted developmental taxonomy of aggression distinguishes life-course-persistent from adolescent-limited antisocial behavior. Life-course-persistent aggression, which refers to the childhood onset of severe conduct problems (i.e., before age 10), emerges from early neurodevelopmental and family adversity risk factors, persists longitudinally, and almost always predicts poor adult adjustment. Fortunately, life-course-persistent aggression represents only a subgroup of the larger pool of aggressive youth—yet it is precisely these few individuals and families (10%) who commit more than 50% of crimes in the United States (Donnellan et al. 2005).

Aggression is more prominent in girls than was previously believed, with prevalence estimates ranging from 4% to 9%. An Office of Juvenile Prevention survey found that in the 1990s, there was a 23% increase in the number of violent crime arrests in adolescent females (vs. 11% in males) and an increase in the severity of adolescent female crime (Centers for Disease Control and Prevention, National Center for Chronic Disease Prevention and Health Promotion 2000). The underidentification of aggression in girls may be related to its later age at onset (Monuteaux et al. 2007) and its "relational" nature—perhaps reflecting the vulnerability of girls to family dysfunction and/or traumatic experiences. One study of incarcerated adolescents found that females reported posttraumatic stress disorder (PTSD) symptoms 50% more often than their male counterparts (Teplin et al. 1996). Aggressive girls exhibit more covert aggression and less intense behavioral disturbance than boys—yet despite these apparently less intense characteristics, aggression in girls predicts substantial subsequent impairment.

Aggression frequently occurs in the context of specific psychiatric diagnoses, although it is a defining characteristic for only some of these (e.g., conduct disorder [CD]). In addition, it may be an associated feature in youth with attention-deficit/hyperactivity disorder (ADHD), oppositional defiant disorder (ODD), substance abuse disorders, depression, bipolar disorders, anxiety disorders (including PTSD), psychotic disorders (including but not limited to schizophrenia), pervasive developmental disorders, Tourette's disorder, and organic mental disorders (see chapters on these disorders). Nevertheless, a large subgroup of aggressive youth does not meet criteria for any specific psychiatric diagnosis.

Several medical conditions carry risk for transient or more permanent aggressive behavior—due to inhibitory dyscontrol, impaired insight and judgment, and/or disorientation—including delirious states secondary to infections (e.g., meningitis, encephalitis) or endocrine abnormalities and seizure disorders (occurring during either ictal or postictal periods). These conditions may manifest with acute onset of aggression, even if there is no preexisting pattern of antisocial acts; however, if treated properly the aggression is generally time limited. In contrast, individuals who develop aggressive behavior following traumatic brain injury often have a more chronic course.

Etiology, Mechanisms, and Risk Factors

The different types of aggression appear to be associated with distinct neurobiological mechanisms. Prosocial aggression (e.g., male dominance) appears to be heavily influenced by testosterone, while impulsive aggression is more consistently related to serotonin (5-HT). Inhibition of 5-HT synthesis, depletion of 5-HT stores, or destruction of 5-HT neurons can produce aggressive behavior. Cerebrospinal fluid levels of the 5-HT metabolite 5-hydroxyindoleacetic acid (5-HIAA) have been inversely correlated with measures of aggressive behavior in both male and female primates. In addition, low 5-HT function early in life predicts excessive aggression, risk taking, and premature death in nonhuman male primates. Numerous studies have examined the relationship between arousal and aggression using physiological measures. Heart rate is generally decreased and less variable at baseline and in response to stimuli; findings from skin conductance studies have been less consistent.

Findings from neuroimaging studies implicate the orbital prefrontal cortex (which inhibits limbic and other subcortical regions), anterior cingulate cortex (which manages incoming affective stimuli), and ventromedial prefrontal cortex (which regulates emotion processing). Studies of traumatic brain injury patients indicate that prefrontal cortex insults are associated with increased aggression, whereas medial-temporal lobe insults decrease aggression. Youth with CD were shown to have reduced volume of the right temporal lobe and possibly prefrontal cortex (Kruesi et al. 2004). Reduced activation in both anterior cingulate cortex and amygdala (Stadler et al. 2007) may reflect impairments in the recognition and cognitive control of emotional stimuli, which presumably increases risk for aggression.

Neurochemistry

Convergent data from studies in animals and human adults have found an inverse relationship between central 5-HT function and impulsive aggression—but this has not been established in children. Given that aggression in children is fairly heterogeneous and only approximately 50% of aggressive children become aggressive adults, it might be that low 5-HT function is only present in a subgroup of aggressive youth. In support of this hypothesis, blunted prolactin response to fenfluramine at ages 7–11 (indicative of low 5-HT activity) predicted aggressive outcome in adolescence, above and beyond the effect of early childhood aggression (Halperin et al. 2006). Continued follow-up indicated that the children who initially had lower prolactin response to fenfluramine were at increased risk for antisocial personality disorder (ASPD) and borderline personality disorder in adulthood (Flory et al. 2007). Low 5-HT responsivity in childhood was necessary but not sufficient for aggressive outcome at follow-up; concomitant psychosocial risk was also required. However, psychosocial risk was not associated with aggression at follow-up in youth with higher 5-HT responsivity in childhood—suggesting that this may be a protective factor (Marks et al. 2007). These findings underscore the importance of examining interaction of environmental and biological risks.

Hormones

Aggression is associated with hormonal changes that occur in response to stress. Aggression has been linked with both elevated peripheral cortisol, which is characteristic of acute stress or anxiety states, and reduced cortisol, which may accompany posttraumatic stress. Reduced cortisol has been specifically related to the early onset and persistence of aggression (Murakami et al. 2006). It is not clear whether the observed associations reflect direct or indirect effects, and whether aggression and cortisol levels appear to be related through associations with one or more other factors, but not each other.

Prominent gender differences in the nature and level of aggression (i.e., male > female) have stimulated research examining the potential role of male sex steroids. In animals, testosterone levels generally reflect prosocial dominance behavior, not antisocial or pathological aggression. Testosterone concentration and aggressive behavior are correlated in boys only after puberty—suggesting the importance of developmental mechanisms. Moreover, testosterone is primarily associated with aggression following provocation—very likely through interactions with a variety of neurotransmitters.

Genetic Factors
Familiality/Heritability

Considerable data indicate that aggression runs in families. Twin studies consistently report higher concordance rates for aggression among monozygotic compared with dizygotic twins (Button et al. 2004), with heritability estimates ranging from 0.28 to 0.72. However, the variability in heritability across studies indicates that genes account for only a portion of the variance. A host of adverse environmental factors—including poverty, low socioeconomic status, marital discord, harsh parenting, poor supervision, parental psychopathology, and crowded living conditions—have been linked to aggressive behavior in youth. It has been hypothesized that families with limited resources (e.g., psychological, cognitive, educational, social, financial) are likely to have less structured households, resulting in less parental supervision and heightened risk for aggression. However, this seemingly face valid explanation offers little insight into the interplay of biological and environmental risk factors for aggression. Both adoption and molecular genetic studies indicate that there is greater susceptibility to adverse environmental factors in genetically vulnerable individuals. For instance, among adopted-away children whose biological parents were diagnosed with ASPD, children who had both biological vulnerability (i.e., family history of ASPD) and environmental risk (i.e., adverse adoptive environment) were found to have higher levels of aggression than children with biological vulnerability who were raised in more stable environments as well as those with environmental but not biological risk (Cadoret et al. 1995).

Candidate Genes

The candidate genes most consistently linked to aggression are the monoamine oxidase A (MAOA) and 5-HT transporter (5-HTT) genes. MAOA is an enzyme that metabolizes monoamine neurotransmitters, including 5-HT. MAOA knockout mice display elevated levels of 5-HT (and the other monoamines), and males exhibit high levels of aggression. Restricted expression of MAOA in these mice lowers monoamine levels and reverses aggressive behavior. In humans, a rare mutation in the MAOA gene was found to be associated with impulsively violent behavior over multiple generations. Findings in both males and females suggest that the risk for physical aggression during adulthood may be increased by the interaction of low MAOA activity and exposure to early trauma (Caspi et al. 2002). Similarly, youth homozygous for the long (LL) variant of the 5-HTT gene and parental antisocial behavior were shown to have high levels of antisocial behavior. Youth with one or more 5-HTT short variants also had high levels of externalizing behavior but in conjunction with genetic risk for alcoholism (Miczek et al. 2007). Males with the short vari-

ant were more likely to have symptoms of CD, aggression, and ADHD; females had lower levels of these behaviors. Other studies have focused on the role of genes related to 5-HT synthesis, reuptake, metabolism, and receptor functions. Two polymorphisms of the tryptophan hydroxylase gene have been associated with increased scores on the total and irritability/assaultiveness scales of the Buss-Durkee Hostility Inventory and with impulsive-aggressive suicidal behavior.

Social-Environmental Factors
Psychosocial Stress and Trauma

Childhood trauma is a risk factor for subsequent violent behavior. Studies of victimized women find that physical and sexual abuse in childhood increase risk for violence against domestic partners and spouses. Individuals with documented neglect and abuse are four times more likely to develop personality disorders than the general population. Physical and sexual abuse both increase risk for ASPD and borderline personality disorder, conditions for which aggression is a core symptom. The bases for this association have been elucidated using animal models. Rodents exposed to early environmental stress (i.e., decreased frequency of maternal licking, grooming, and arched back nursing) have altered neurophysiological and neuroendocrine parameters mediated by neural circuits linking the amygdala, hippocampus, and prefrontal cortex, affecting domains such as processing of emotional information and stress responsivity (Zhang et al. 2004). These findings are consistent with data indicating that victims of childhood abuse and neglect often have difficulty processing and modulating emotional reactions to life events and that the inability to properly regulate physiological arousal in the context of affect-laden experiences can easily escalate to aggressive behavior (Caspi et al. 2002).

Family Structure and Function

A variety of family-based risk factors contribute to the etiology or maintenance of aggression in youth, including large sibships, parental separation, single-parent households, child neglect, parental conflict, poverty, harsh discipline practices, poor supervision, and parental criminality (see Chapter 16, "Oppositional Defiant Disorder and Conduct Disorder").

Peer Interactions

Delinquent peer membership, repeated victimization by peers, and residence in a neighborhood with high rates of crime, poverty, and/or unemployment all increase risk for youth violence. Early peer rejection is also an important (and often underappreciated) predictor of aggression. Several studies have found that peer rejection is associated with impulsive and emotionally reactive behaviors. Essentially, the effect is that of a social stressor, which augments adverse behavior in predisposed youth (who also are at increased risk for peer rejection). The impact of peer rejection is particularly evident when it occurs early in childhood—with significant effects found to be present even after controlling for ADHD and aggression (Miller-Johnson et al. 2002). However, interactions among multiple risk factors are the rule, and the direction of the effects is uncertain. For example, is peer rejection associated with increased risk for aggression, or is peer acceptance protective, perhaps by minimizing the impact of other risk factors (Dodge et al. 2003)?

Community and Social Factors

The occurrence of high-visibility incidents of youth violence in schools (e.g., Columbine and Heritage High School shootings) highlights the link between community factors and aggression. Aggressive, antisocial acts occur more frequently in crowded, high-poverty, high-crime areas, and a variety of community-based factors influence their development and maintenance (Caspi et al. 2000). An important component of peer-related transmission of risk is the reciprocal, positive reinforcement of antisocial acts that occurs between deviant group members (i.e., deviancy training). The grouping of aggressive, antisocial youth in residential treatment or special education settings has therefore been questioned. Although deviancy training appears to be less significant in treatment settings (Weiss et al. 2005), it is clearly operative in adolescent gangs and, possibly, classroom placements in schools with high numbers of aggressive youth. However, family and parent-related factors mediate these relationships (Capaldi and Patterson 1994), suggesting that intervention at multiple levels is possible.

Academic Factors

A substantial literature indicates that aggressive children have cognitive deficits, primarily in the verbal domain. It may be that childhood cognitive and learning problems are etiologically related to aggression, but inadequate education and resultant underachievement could also be consequences of aggression. Patterson et al. (1989) hypothesized that cognitive problems and academic failure may result in subsequent rejection by normally achieving peers and a clustering of children at higher risk for delinquency. However, it remains unknown whether there is a specific relationship between learning (particularly reading) problems and aggression and whether this apparent association is attributable to the frequent co-occurrence of low intelligence and attention problems.

Environmental Toxins

Prenatal or postnatal exposure to a variety of toxins, substances of abuse, or infectious agents is associated with increased risk for aggression. Maternal use of alcohol, nicotine, and/or other drugs during pregnancy substantially increases risk for both ADHD and conduct problems in offspring, due to toxic effects on neurodevelopment of catecholamine systems and/or alterations in gene expression. However, interpretation is complicated by the elevated rates of ADHD, substance abuse, and conduct and antisocial disorders in mothers who use alcohol, nicotine, or other drugs during pregnancy, suggesting that gene-environment interactions are likely involved.

Prevention
Early Intervention

A number of programs have been developed to aid in the prevention of aggression and conduct problems in at-risk children and families (e.g., Fast Track Conduct Problems Prevention Research Group, First Step, Incredible Years Teacher Training, Linking the Interests of Family and Teacher, Montreal Program, Seattle Social Development Project). Typically, prevention programs are implemented during preschool or early elementary school, continuously over 2–5 years, with the goals of increasing social competence, social problem solving, and resilience. Results point to long-term benefits in reducing antisocial behavior and aggression for many programs (e.g., Chicago Child Parent Center, High Scope Perry Preschool Project, Houston Parent Child Developmental Center, Syracuse University Family Development Project, Yale Child Welfare Research Program). Characteristics of successful programs include: 1) multimodal intervention for children and parents, parent support, teacher involvement, and early childhood education; 2) delivery of interventions consistently on a daily to weekly basis; 3) duration of 2 years or longer; 4) specific interventions to remediate coercive family processes and harsh and inconsistent parenting techniques through skill building and development of problem-solving and coping skills; 5) interventions that begin in early childhood; 6) application of individual management techniques; and 7) collaboration among community, school, family, and mental health professionals.

School-Based Violence Prevention Programs

School-based violence prevention programs for adolescents have been developed and disseminated (see Chapter 63, "School-Based Interventions"), particularly following highly visible violent events in schools, such as the shootings at Columbine High School. A meta-analysis of 44 school-based violence prevention programs found at least moderate success, with effect sizes ranging from 0.36 to 0.59 (Mytton et al. 2002).

Preventive Parent Training

Several preventive parent training programs emphasize the development of social skills, problem-solving techniques, and anger management strategies in reducing child aggression and conduct problems (e.g., Earlscourt Social Skills Program, Incredible Years Dinosaur Program, DARE to Be You community-based program). Multiple-family group approaches have also been used in the prevention of childhood aggression (Costello et al. 2001). These approaches target both child behavioral symptoms and overall functioning but are primarily intended to improve parental skills and family interactions critical to enhancing youth mental health over time (McKay et al. 2002).

Course and Prognosis

Aggression is considered to be a relatively stable trait, and aggression in childhood often predicts continuation or even escalation of behavior problems over time, leading to ASPD, domestic abuse, and/or incarceration. Nevertheless, many aggressive children do not become aggressive adults. Antecedent problems present during the preschool years, including poor peer relationships and inadequate problem-solving patterns, predict the development of impulsive aggression; physical abuse is also present in 20%–25% of these youth. Planned aggression starts about 2 years later and is fueled by aggressive role models and a positive valence of aggression rather than physical abuse (Dodge et al. 1990).

Several models have attempted to describe the escalation from childhood ADHD to aggression and criminal behavior and the predictors of escalation and/or persistence. While no single theory can predict individual course, several points are generally accepted:

1. Antisocial behavior emerges in an orderly fashion that begins with oppositionality and seemingly trivial nondelinquent antisocial acts (e.g., aggressiveness, arguing, fighting with siblings, talking back to adults, yelling, lying, noncompliance, temper tantrums) that presage more serious delinquent acts (e.g., physical fighting, stealing, fire setting).
2. Predictors of continuity include early onset, increased variety, and high frequency of problem behaviors; increases in one area (e.g., frequency) are often associated with increases in other areas (e.g., variety).
3. Children who practice both overt and covert antisocial acts (i.e., versatile offenders) differ from those who partake in only covert antisocial activities (e.g., theft only or substance abuse only). Versatile child offending is associated with increased family adversity and greater police contact.
4. Physical aggression in childhood is one of the most important predictors of later diversified offending (McKay and Halperin 2001), although family history of aggression and/or affective lability in childhood also increases risk for persistence and escalation.

Evaluation

Clinical Assessment

Treatment planning with aggressive youth is based on a comprehensive understanding of psychological, behavioral, cognitive, and differential diagnostic considerations related to the nature, context, and severity of aggression and to the risk and protective factors that characterize the individual patient and family. There are several important components of this examination:

1. Interview the patient and relevant others to understand how and why the aggressive behavior developed whether it is situation specific, what the consequences have been, and whether there is any current ideation/plan. Imminent risk to any individual carries a legal obligation to warn the potential target (i.e., *Tarasoff* decision).
2. Determine whether there are specific stresses and/or contextual factors related to the aggressive behavior—as these may be amenable to manipulation either directly or indirectly (e.g., via psychosocial intervention).
3. Determine whether there is substance abuse, and if so, the nature and extent of the abuse (because substances of abuse may be disinhibiting or lead to instrumental aggression).
4. Obtain information regarding individual, family, and peer risk factors—including family history of aggression, criminality, substance abuse, personality disorders, family relationships (including parenting styles, disciplinary practices and family violence), academic function (including ADHD, learning disabilities, and academic achievement), and current and past peer interactions—noting changes in affectively charged relationships, such as a break-up with a close friend or boyfriend or girlfriend.
5. Obtain detailed information regarding ADHD and disruptive and aggressive behavior to aid in understanding the developmental trajectory of the aggressive behavior.

Mental Status Examination

The primary focus of the mental status examination should be differential diagnosis, because aggression often accompanies other psychiatric diagnoses. It is also important to assess cognitive capacity, and specifically verbal skills (which relate to the capacity for insight, judgment, and problem-solving skills), as well as personality characteristics such as adaptability, affect regulation, and cognitive flexibility (which are necessary for shifting focus away from affectively charged topics or events before they escalate to aggressive behavior). It is important to evaluate the capacity for empathy, the degree of connection to others, and the extent to which there is hostile attribution bias (i.e., ascribing hostile intent even when there is none) or more frank distortions of factual content, the most severe example being paranoid thinking. These fac-

tors inform not only the assessment of risk but also the patient's capacity to engage in treatment.

Psychometric Instruments

A variety of psychometric instruments can be used for assessing youth and monitoring treatment. Aggression rating scales and structured interviews can augment the unstructured clinical assessment. Broad-band rating scales (e.g., Achenbach and Conners scales) can be used to get an overview of the child's or adolescent's mental health functioning and screen for aggressive behavior. However, the behavior disorder and aggression items on broad-based scales often evaluate oppositional behavior and covert aggressive behaviors rather than overt physical aggression. The latter is more easily evaluated using one of many narrow-band rating scales. Table 37–1 provides a description of frequently used aggression rating scales (Barkley 2006; Buss and Perry 1992; Halperin et al. 2002, 2003; Miller et al. 1995; Miller-Johnson et al. 2002; Sorgi et al. 1991; Yudofsky et al. 1986).

Psychological Testing

Neuropsychological testing may aid in the assessment of cognitive functions that may confer relative or specific risk for aggression—such as intellectual capacity, learning disorders, language skills, verbal reasoning, attention, vigilance, inhibitory control, and academic achievement. Projective tests may provide information relative to how the patient is likely to think in unstructured or stressful situations.

Differential Diagnosis

Aggressive behavior can be either a specific core symptom or an associated feature of a psychiatric disorder. Conditions to carefully consider include ADHD and disruptive behavior disorders (i.e., ODD and CD); mood disorders (including major depression, dysthymic disorder, and bipolar disorder); anxiety disorders (including PTSD and obsessive-compulsive disorder); substance abuse disorders; tic disorders (including Tourette's disorder); specific (e.g., learning) and/or pervasive developmental disorders; psychotic disorders; somatization disorder; and a variety of medical conditions, including seizure disorders (ictal or interictal) and acute metabolic syndromes producing delirium and/or confusional states. The latter are generally associated with physical symptoms (e.g., tachycardia, fever, blood pressure fluctuations, dyspnea, muscle ri-

TABLE 37–1. Frequently used rating scales for aggression in children and adolescents

Scale	Description/features/comments	References
Buss-Durkee Hostility Inventory Buss-Perry Hostility Inventory	Originally developed for college students; a modified version for youth with updated items, eliminated items not relevant to youth, and improved readability for youth with lower vocabulary skills.	Buss and Durkee 1957 Buss and Perry 1992
Children's Aggression Scale (parent and teacher versions)	Contains five factors: verbal aggression, aggression against objects and animals, provoked physical aggression, unprovoked physical aggression, and use of weapons. Distinguishes aggression 1) inside vs. outside the home and 2) against children vs. adults.	Halperin et al. 2002, 2003
Home and School Situations Questionnaires	Focus on the environmental context in which behavior problems occur (e.g., household or classroom situations) in youth ages 4–11 years old.	Barkley and Edelbrock 1987
New York Teacher Rating Scale	Teacher report that includes DSM items for both oppositional defiant disorder and conduct disorder, as well as a number of other items of disruptive and/or aggressive behavior.	Miller et al. 1995
Overt Aggression Scale (OAS)	Observer-rated instrument originally designed for inpatient settings. Rates severity of verbal aggression, physical aggression, physical aggression against self, and physical aggression against others.	Yudofsky et al. 1986
OAS—Modified	Self/other modification of OAS suitable for outpatient settings; rates behavior over a 1-week interval. The same four domains of aggression are included, but a 5-point response format allows assessment of both severity and frequency.	Sorgi et al. 1991

gidity) and altered mental status. The rationale for careful differential diagnosis is that treatment of underlying or associated conditions may lead to improvement or resolution of the aggressive behavior. This is most often seen when the underlying medical or psychiatric condition is acute but is less likely to occur when there is more chronic physical or psychiatric illness.

Pediatric Evaluation and Laboratory Tests

Medical and neurological evaluations are required to rule out conditions (e.g., toxins, seizures, infections,

head trauma, substance use) associated with reversible changes of mental state. See Chapter 9, "Pediatric Evaluation and Laboratory Testing," and Chapter 10, "Neurological Examination, Electroencephalography, and Neuroimaging," for further discussion.

Treatment

Several psychosocial and pharmacological interventions have demonstrated efficacy and feasibility for the treatment of aggression. Psychosocial intervention can be utilized for either impulsive or planned aggression; medication is generally only effective in the treatment of impulsive aggression. Improvement is often relative, and multimodal intervention is the norm.

Psychotherapeutic Treatments

Empirically supported psychosocial interventions target one or more of the behaviors that characterize or serve to maintain the aggressive behavior (e.g., affect regulation, verbal aggression, property destruction, physical aggression). Behavioral parent training (BPT; see Chapter 55, "Behavioral Parent Training") is the best-studied and best-validated treatment for youth aggression (Brestan and Eyberg 1998). BPT attempts to break the negative reinforcement cycle between parents and their children, which contributes to the development and proximal maintenance of aggressive behaviors. BPT teaches parents how to manipulate antecedents (e.g., rules, commands) and consequences (e.g., rewards, time out) related to the aggressive behavior; the anticipated result is a shift away from an aversive parent-child relationship to one that is mutually reinforcing. Components of BPT include didactic instruction, videotaped vignettes to elicit discussion, and modeling and role-playing of the use of specific strategies. Treatment may be conducted in either individual or group formats.

Cognitive-behavioral treatment (CBT) has also been utilized successfully. Aggressive youth often have hostile attribution biases, make errors in interpreting social cues, and have positive expectations related to their aggressive behavior. CBT primarily targets these social-cognitive deficits by teaching youth to effectively recognize and interpret social cues; generate multiple interpretations for others' behavior; and implement nonaggressive, prosocial problem-solving strategies. CBT is typically conducted in groups, often utilizing discussion, modeling, and role-playing (with feedback and reinforcement from the leader) to aid in skill development. While several studies have documented the positive effects of CBT in treating aggressive youth, the combination of CBT and BPT is often more effective than either intervention alone (Kazdin et al. 2005).

Considerable research has examined the limitations of BPT and CBT, as well as moderating factors. A recent meta-analysis suggests that although both treatments are effective, BPT is superior for preschool and school-age children (McCart et al. 2006). However, one review (Nock and Ferriter 2005) concludes that age does not moderate outcomes in BPT. Comorbid psychiatric disorders in children appear not to

moderate the effectiveness of BPT, but there are few comparable data for CBT. Youth with greater dysfunction, higher levels of parental psychopathology, greater family dysfunction, and/or more difficult life circumstances often do poorly with either treatment. Motivation and other attitudinal factors likely affect treatment attendance, the ability to learn new skills, and the willingness to use skills learned in treatment. Adherence to treatment is particularly salient for BPT, as up to 40%–60% of parents drop out. Unfortunately, the families most likely to discontinue BPT are the ones at highest risk for persistence of aggressive/antisocial behavior, who need treatment the most.

Given the limitations of single interventions for youth with the greatest severity of aggression risk, multimodal approaches are often necessary. Substantial evidence supports the efficacy of Multisystemic Treatment (MST) (Henggeler et al. 2002) and Multidimensional Treatment Foster Care (MTFC) (Leve and Chamberlain 2005) for high-risk youth with aggressive, antisocial behavior—many of whom are also at risk for out-of-home placement and involvement with the juvenile justice system. MST and MTFC utilize well-established, developmentally appropriate strategies to target risk and support youth competence, in a manner that is highly intensive and tailored to the needs of the individual child and family. Both treatments reduce rates of recidivism, arrest, criminal offenses, substance-related offenses, and out-of-home placement—even in the highest risk youth. Importantly, despite offering intensive, multimodal interventions, both MST and MTFC have been shown to be cost-effective compared to alternative methods (e.g., psychiatric hospitalization).

Pharmacological Treatments

Pharmacotherapy of aggressive behavior should be considered as an adjunct to psychosocial treatment or to augment pharmacological and/or psychosocial treatment of underlying psychiatric disorders. It is generally considered preferable to address the underlying psychiatric condition first in attempting to ameliorate the aggressive behavior. However, when aggression is severe and frequently occurring, it is often necessary to implement a symptom-based approach targeting aggression directly.

There is limited evidence from controlled clinical trials to devise algorithms for the pharmacological treatment of aggression, especially since currently available treatments are mainly palliative. Nevertheless, the preponderance of hospitalized children and adolescents are treated for aggression using pharmacotherapy—with 40% receiving two or more medications, most commonly including an atypical antipsychotic medication (Pappadopulos et al. 2003). Similarly, 18% of all child and adolescent psychiatric visits in 2002 were for the administration and/or management of an atypical antipsychotic agent, with the largest proportion of these visits for the management of disruptive behavior disorders and/or aggression (Olfson et al. 2006).

Second-generation atypical neuroleptics have shown significant efficacy in decreasing aggression and regulating mood in youth. Risperidone is the best studied of these agents; positive findings from controlled trials of risperidone efficacy in the treatment of aggression in children with pervasive developmental disorders (Aman et al. 2002; McDougle et al. 2005) led to approval by the U.S. Food and Drug Administration for this indication. (Note: This is the only medication approved for the treatment of aggression in any diagnostic group.) In addition to improvement in aggressive behavior, risperidone produces robust improvement in impulsivity, social interactions, explosivity, self-injury, sleep, and hygiene. New York State and Columbia University, in partnership with leading investigators nationwide, produced consensus Treatment Recommendations for the Use of Antipsychotics for Aggressive Youth (TRAAY) (Pappadopulos et al. 2003; Schur et al. 2003). Key aspects of the TRAAY algorithm are to treat the primary disorder with first-line treatments first, to use monotherapy whenever possible, to first use psychosocial and behavioral treatments for aggression, and if/when these interventions fail, to add an atypical antipsychotic.

Other agents used in the treatment of aggression in children and adolescents include lithium; mood-stabilizing anticonvulsants; stimulants; selective serotonin reuptake inhibitors; anxiolytics; alpha-adrenergic agonists; beta-blockers; and sedatives (note that all are off-label for this indication). Stimulants are effective in treating both overt and covert aggression—certainly in the context of ADHD and possibly independent of ADHD. Treating underlying ADHD is an important, although sometimes overlooked, approach (Connor et al. 2002); it is considerably safer than many of the treatment alternatives and can be rapidly implemented. Nevertheless, severely aggressive youth often require additional or other interventions. Studies using lithium carbonate in hospitalized aggressive children with CD have yielded positive results (Malone et al. 2000), although the beneficial effects of this medication have varied across studies (Campbell et al. 1995). Initial double-blind, controlled studies with lithium found it to be as effective as haloperidol and superior to placebo in treating aggressive CD. However, subsequent studies found the benefits of lithium to be less substantial than initial data indicated. The anticonvulsant divalproex has also been shown to be effective in treating impulsive aggression (Steiner et al. 2003). Divalproex reduces the explosive aggression associated with bipolar disorder and CD and has fewer side effects and drug interactions than many other agents used for these conditions. Like the atypical antipsychotics, divalproex and other anticonvulsant mood stabilizers potentially have a dual role in the treatment of aggression—as interventions for a primary underlying disorder (e.g., bipolar and psychotic disorders) and as symptom-based treatments for aggression. There is considerable interest in the alpha-2 adrenergic agonists clonidine and guanfacine, although there are few published controlled trials. A new, long-acting guanfacine formulation has been studied for ADHD, and if approved, it could be available by late 2009. However, use of this agent for aggression would be off-label. Finally, beta-blockers have been used to treat aggression in patients with organic brain dysfunction (often requiring higher doses) and disruptive behavior disorders (often in combination with stimulants), but data are limited and use is otherwise infrequent.

Research Directions

Although we know a great deal about the psychological, interpersonal, and biological bases of aggression—and have several evidence-based psychosocial and pharmacological interventions for this condition—few of our "successes" have translated into meaningful changes in prevalence and treatment. There is an urgent need to identify effective, broadly accessible interventions that engage and retain youth and families in treatment in order to maximize outcomes. An important corollary is to study these interventions in relevant demographic and clinical groups, with a focus on community-based settings. Unfortunately, the most difficult patients to engage and treat are precisely the ones who need treatment the most. More important would be to improve primary and secondary prevention efforts. However, substantively changing risk for aggression will require major changes in social policy and allocation of resources, in addition to new developments in clinical science, as it is impossible to overstate the contribution of poverty and its consequences to the development and maintenance of aggression. Finally, while it is likely that psychopharmacological interventions will remain second-line interventions for aggression, research that more accurately elucidates the neurobiological bases and mechanisms of aggression holds promise for the development of safer, more effective, and more specific treatments.

References

Aman MG, De Smedt G, Derivan A, et al: Double-blind, placebo-controlled study of risperidone for the treatment of disruptive behaviors in children with subaverage intelligence. Am J Psychiatry 159:1337–1346, 2002

Barkley RA: Attention Deficit Hyperactivity Disorder: A Handbook for Diagnosis and Treatment, 3rd Edition. New York, Guilford, 2006

Barkley RA, Edelbrock C: Assessing situational variation in children's problem behaviors: the Home and School Situations Questionnaires, in Advances in Behavioral Assessment of Children and Families. Edited by Prinz R. Greenwich, CT, JAI Press, 1987

Brestan EV, Eyberg SM: Effective psychosocial treatments of conduct-disordered children and adolescents: 29 years, 82 studies, and 5,272 kids. J Clin Child Psychol 27:180–189, 1998

Buss AH, Durkee A: An inventory for assessing different types of hostility. J Consult Clin Psychol 21:343–349, 1957

Buss AH, Perry M: The aggression questionnaire. J Pers Soc Psychol 63:452–459, 1992

Button TM, Scourfield J, Martin N, et al: Do aggressive and nonaggressive antisocial behaviors in adolescents result from the same genetic and environmental effects? Am J Med Genet B Neuropsychiatr Genet 129B:59–63, 2004

Cadoret RJ, Yates WR, Troughton E, et al: Genetic-environmental interaction in the genesis of aggressivity and conduct disorders. Arch Gen Psychiatry 52:916–924, 1995

Campbell M, Kafantaris V, Cueva J: An update on the use of lithium carbonate in aggressive children and adolescents with conduct disorder. Psychopharmacol Bull 31:93–102, 1995

Capaldi DM, Patterson G: Interrelated influences of contextual factors on antisocial behavior in childhood and adolescence for males, Progress in Experimental Personality and Psychopathology Research. Edited by Fowles D, Sutker P, Goodman S. New York, Springer, 1994, pp 165–198

Caspi A, Taylor A, Moffitt TE, et al: Neighborhood deprivation affects children's mental health: environmental risks identified in a genetic design. Psychol Sci 11:338–342, 2000

Caspi A, McClay J, Moffitt TE, et al: Role of genotype in the cycle of violence in maltreated children. Science 297:851–854, 2002

Centers for Disease Control and Prevention, National Center for Chronic Disease Prevention and Health Promotion: Assessing Health Risk Behaviors Among Young People: Youth Risk Behavior Surveillance System, At-a-Glance. Atlanta, GA, Centers for Disease Control and Prevention, 2000

Connor DF, Glatt SJ, Lopez ID, et al: Psychopharmacology and aggression, I: a meta-analysis of stimulant effects on overt/covert aggression–related behaviors in ADHD. J Am Acad Child Adolesc Psychiatry 41:253–261, 2002

Costello EJ, Keeler GP, Angold A: Poverty, race/ethnicity, and psychiatric disorder: a study of rural children. Am J Public Health 91:1494–1498, 2001

Dodge KA, Coie JD: Social-information-processing factors in reactive and proactive aggression in children's peer groups. J Pers Soc Psychol 53:1146–1158, 1987

Dodge KA, Bates JE, Pettit GS: Mechanisms in the cycle of violence. Science 250:1678–1683, 1990

Dodge KA, Lansford JE, Burks VS, et al: Peer rejection and social information-processing factors in the development of aggressive behavior problems in children. Child Dev 74:374–393, 2003

Donnellan MB, Trzesniewski KH, Robins RW, et al: Low self-esteem is related to aggression, antisocial behavior, and delinquency. Psychol Sci 16:328–335, 2005

Flory JD, Newcorn JH, Miller C, et al: Serotonergic function in children with attention-deficit hyperactivity disorder: relationship to later antisocial personality disorder. Br J Psychiatry 190:410–414, 2007

Halperin JM, McKay KE, Newcorn JH: Development, reliability, and validity of the Children's Aggression Scale—Parent Version. J Am Acad Child Adolesc Psychiatry 41:245–252, 2002

Halperin JM, McKay KE, Grayson RH, et al: Reliability, validity, and preliminary normative data for the Children's Aggression Scale—Teacher Version. J Am Acad Child Adolesc Psychiatry 42:965–971, 2003

Halperin JM, Kalmar JH, Schulz KP, et al: Elevated childhood serotonergic function protects against adolescent aggression in disruptive boys. J Am Acad Child Adolesc Psychiatry 45:833–840, 2006

Henggeler SW, Clingempeel WG, Brondino MJ, et al: Four-year follow-up of multisystemic therapy with substance-abusing and substance-dependent juvenile offenders. J Am Acad Child Adolesc Psychiatry 41:868–874, 2002

Kazdin AE, Marciano PL, Whitley MK: The therapeutic alliance in cognitive-behavioral treatment of children referred for oppositional, aggressive, and antisocial behavior. J Consult Clin Psychol 73:726–730, 2005

Kruesi MJ, Casanova MF, Mannheim G, et al: Reduced temporal lobe volume in early-onset conduct disorder. Psychiatry Res 132:1–11, 2004

Leve LD, Chamberlain P: Association with delinquent peers: intervention effects for youth in the juvenile justice system. J Abnorm Child Psychol 33:339–347, 2005

Malone RP, Delaney MA, Luebbert JF, et al: A double-blind placebo-controlled study of lithium in hospitalized aggressive children and adolescents with conduct disorder. Arch Gen Psychiatry 57:649–654, 2000

Marks DJ, Miller SR, Schulz KP, et al: The interaction of psychosocial adversity and biological risk in childhood aggression. Psychiatry Res 151:221–230, 2007

McCart MR, Priester PE, Davies WH, et al: Differential effectiveness of behavioral parent-training and cognitive-behavioral therapy for antisocial youth: a meta-analysis. J Abnorm Child Psychol 34:527–543, 2006

McDougle CJ, Scahill L, Aman MG, et al: Risperidone for the core symptom domains of autism: results from the study by the autism network of the research units on pediatric psychopharmacology. Am J Psychiatry 162:1142–1148, 2005

McKay KE, Halperin JM: ADHD, aggression, and antisocial behavior across the lifespan: interactions with neurochemical and cognitive function. Ann NY Acad Sci 931:84–96, 2001

McKay MM, Harrison ME, Gonzales J, et al: Multiple-family groups for urban children with conduct difficulties and their families. Psychiatr Serv 53:1467–1468, 2002

Miczek KA, de Almeida RM, Kravitz EA, et al: Neurobiology of escalated aggression and violence. J Neurosci 27:11803–11806, 2007

Miller LS, Klein RG, Piacentini J, et al: The New York Teacher Rating Scale for disruptive and antisocial behavior. J Am Acad Child Adolesc Psychiatry 34:359–370, 1995

Miller-Johnson S, Coie JD, Maumary-Gremaud A, et al: Peer rejection and aggression and early starter models of conduct disorder. J Abnorm Child Psychol 30:217–230, 2002

Monuteaux MC, Faraone SV, Michelle Gross L, et al: Predictors, clinical characteristics, and outcome of conduct disorder in girls with attention-deficit/hyperactivity disorder: a longitudinal study. Psychol Med 37:1731–1741, 2007

Murakami S, Rappaport N, Penn JV: An overview of juveniles and school violence. Psychiatr Clin North Am 29:725–741, 2006

Mytton JA, DiGuiseppi C, Gough DA, et al: School-based violence prevention programs: systematic review of secondary prevention trials. Arch Pediatr Adolesc Med 156:752–762, 2002

Nock MK, Ferriter C: Parent management of attendance and adherence in child and adolescent therapy: a conceptual and empirical review. Clin Child Fam Psychol Rev 8:149–166, 2005

Olfson M, Blanco C, Liu L, et al: National trends in the outpatient treatment of children and adolescents with antipsychotic drugs. Arch Gen Psychiatry 63:679–685, 2006

Pappadopulos E, Macintyre J, Crismon M, et al: Treatment recommendations for the use of antipsychotics for aggressive youth (TRAAY), part II. J Am Acad Child Adolesc Psychiatry 42:145–161, 2003

Patterson GR, DeBaryshe BD, Ramsey E: A developmental perspective on antisocial behavior. Am Psychol 44:329–335, 1989

Schur S, Sikich L, Findling R, et al: Treatment recommendations for the use of antipsychotics for aggressive youth (TRAAY), part I: a review. J Am Acad Child Adolesc Psychiatry 42:132–144, 2003

Sorgi P, Ratey J, Knoedler DW, et al: Rating aggression in the clinical setting: a retrospective adaptation of the Overt Aggression Scale: preliminary results. J Neuropsychiatry Clin Neurosci 3:S52–S56, 1991

Stadler C, Sterzer P, Schmeck K, et al: Reduced anterior cingulate activation in aggressive children and adolescents during affective stimulation: association with temperament traits. J Psychiatr Res 41:410–417, 2007

Steiner H, Petersen ML, Saxena K, et al: Divalproex sodium for the treatment of conduct disorder: a randomized controlled clinical trial. J Clin Psychiatry 64:1183–1191, 2003

Teplin LA, Abram KM, McClelland GM: Prevalence of psychiatric disorders among incarcerated women, I: pretrial jail detainees. Arch Gen Psychiatry 53:505–512, 1996

Weiss B, Caron A, Ball S, et al: Iatrogenic effects of group treatment for antisocial youths. J Consult Clin Psychol 73:1036–1044, 2005

Yudofsky SC, Silver JM, Jackson W, et al: The Overt Aggression Scale for the objective rating of verbal and physical aggression. Am J Psychiatry 143:35–39, 1986

Zhang TY, Parent C, Weaver I, et al: Maternal programming of individual differences in defensive responses in the rat. Ann NY Acad Sci 1032:85–103, 2004

Genetics

Fundamentals Relevant to Child and Adolescent Psychiatry

James J. McGough, M.D.
Stanley F. Nelson, M.D.

Psychiatry has always struggled with the relative importance of nature versus nurture (McGuffin and Southwick 2003). In recent decades, advances in neuroscience have transformed debate over whether mental illness is biological or behavioral to an understanding that all behavior is biological and that this biology arises from genes, environments, and their interactions. Basic concepts in psychiatric genetics inform our current understanding of the biological basis of behavioral disorders and ongoing efforts to identify improved approaches to treatment. A glossary of common genetics terms is provided in Table 38–1.

The Molecular Basis of Heredity

In humans, the genome comprises approximately 3 billion nucleotide base pairs, with each individual ef-fectively encoded by 6 billion bases. The actual protein coding sequence in humans makes up less than 1.5% of the genome. While some of the genome encodes for elements that direct how genes should be expressed (promoters or enhancers), most consist of noncoding *junk DNA*, which appears to reflect our evolutionary history and possibly serves to increase genetic variability within the species. Originally, because of the genome's size, it was thought that humans had over 100,000 functional genes. However, estimates derived after completion of the Human Genome Project suggest that humans have between 20,000 and 25,000 functional genes, a remarkably small number given the complexity of the human species (Stein 2004). It is likely that this estimate will be revised further as we understand more about the actual structure of genes.

Nucleic Acids

Nucleic acids are large molecules of linked nucleotide chains that convey genetic information (Figure 38–1).

TABLE 38–1. Glossary of common genetics terms

Term	Definition
Allele	Alternative form or variant of a DNA marker.
Centimorgan (cM)	Unit of genetic map distance defined as the distance between two loci with a 1% probability of recombination, corresponding to approximately 1 million base pairs (1 Mb).
Complex traits	Phenotypes arising from the effects of multiple genes and their interactions with the environment.
Diploid	Cell containing two copies (2N) of each chromosome.
Epistasis	Phenomenon by which genes interact with each other, as when translated products of one gene serve as regulator agents at the promoter regions of other genes.
Exons	Portions of the gene that express mature RNA and proteins.
Gene	Segment of DNA that encodes functional products.
Genetic anticipation	When increasing numbers of trinucleotide repeats over successive generations create increased risk for illness.
Genome	Sum of heritable material found in an individual's DNA.
Genomics	Study of the function and structure of the genome.
Haploid	Cell containing one copy (N) of each chromosome.
Haplotype	Particular pattern of inherited alleles at multiple DNA markers in close proximity within a chromosomal region.
Insertion/deletion	Polymorphisms resulting from addition /removal of nucleotides from a gene.
Introns	Regions of the gene that code nucleic acid segments that are interspersed between exons and excised prior to RNA translation.
Law of equal segregation	Mendel's postulate that each sperm or egg receives one allele per gene from each parent, with an equal chance of receiving one or the other of the parents' two alleles.
Law of independent assortment	Mendel's postulate that the segregation of allele pairs for one trait into separate eggs or sperm is independent from the segregation of other traits.
Locus	Fixed position on a chromosome.
Mendelian inheritance	Inheritance following Mendel's laws of equal segregation and independent assortment. Applies to nonlinked simple traits in which alleles demonstrate dominant or recessive effects.
Mutation	Alteration in DNA nucleotide base sequence that results from copying errors or exposure to environmental toxins.
Nucleotide	Molecule comprising a nucleotide base, five-carbon sugar, and one to three phosphate groups, that when linked in a chain forms the basic structural unit of DNA and RNA.
Point mutation	Single nucleotide changes within a gene.
Polymorphism	Allele variant or mutation occurring in >1% of a population.
Population stratification	Differences in allele frequencies among different racial and ethnic groups.
Simple trait	Phenotypes arising from changes in single genes.
Single nucleotide polymorphism (SNP)	Single nucleotide base that varies among individuals in a population, resulting from random mutations over human history.
Trinucleotide repeat insertions	Repetitions of three nucleotide base pair units within a gene.
Variable number tandem repeat (VNTR)	Common polymorphism in which a base pair insertion repeats itself a variable number of times.

The most common nucleic acids are double-stranded *deoxyribonucleic acid (DNA)* and single-stranded *ribonucleic acid (RNA)*. *Nucleotides* are three-part structures composed of 1) a nitrogen-containing base—either a *pyrimidine* or *purine*; 2) a five-carbon sugar—*deoxyribose* for DNA and *ribose* for RNA; and 3) a phosphate group. The pyrimidines, *cytosine (C)* and *thymine (T)* or *uracil (U)*, contain one carbon ring. Thymine is only found in DNA, and uracil is only found in RNA. The purines, *adenine (A)*

and *guanine (G)*, contain two carbon rings. In humans, genes comprised of DNA encode for single-stranded RNA. DNA activity is limited to a cell's nucleus. RNA is synthesized within the nucleus and transported to other areas of the cell to facilitate protein synthesis.

Nucleic acids are formed by bonds between alternating sugar and phosphate groups linked at the number 5 and 3 carbon positions within each nucleotide's sugar molecule. The synthesis of a new DNA strand

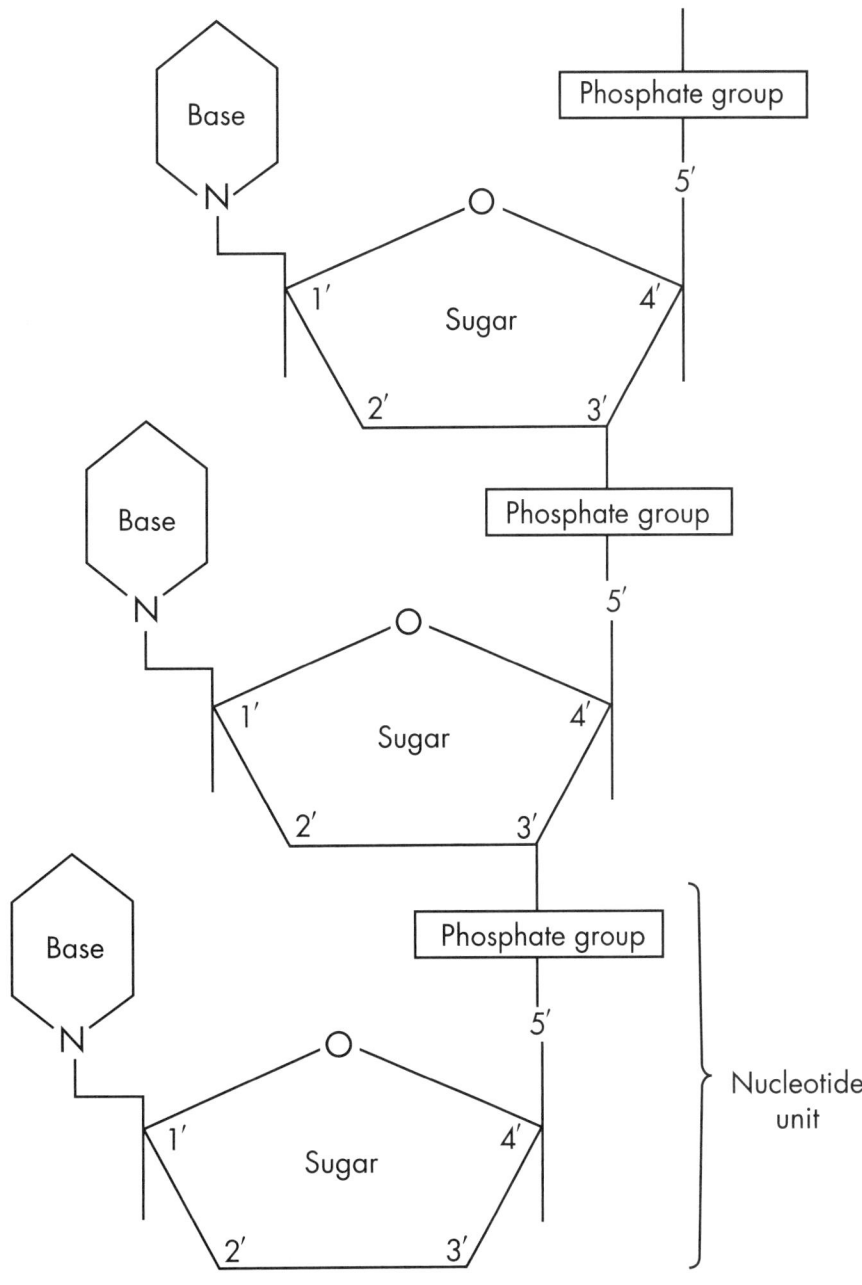

FIGURE 38–1. Basic structure of nucleic acids.
Nucleotides are three-part structures composed of a nitrogen-containing base, a five-carbon sugar, and a phosphate group. Chains of nucleic acid are formed by phosphate bonds between the 5′ and 3′ carbons of alternating nucleotide sugar molecules.

568

{=html}

cc _Dulcan's Textbook of Child and Adolescent Psychiatry_

proceeds with addition of new nucleotide to the 5′ carbon group of the sugar-phosphate backbone, proceeding in the 5′ to 3′ direction. Nucleotides are identified according to their respective nucleotide bases, which are linked to the 1′ sugar carbon. Each base is able to form an electrostatic bond with its complementary base—A with T or U; C with G. This allows two complementary single strands of DNA to form a double-helix, with each strand running in opposite directions around an axis. This complementary nucleotide bonding is the foundation of DNA replication, RNA synthesis, and protein transcription. Nucleic acid length is measured in numbers of bases for RNA or _base pairs (bp)_ for DNA. Bases are further quantified in multiples of thousands (_kilobases, Kb_) or millions (_megabases, Mb_).

DNA Damage and Repair

Mutations occur normally at a rate of 1 per each 1,000 bp in every replication cycle but can increase following exposure to environmental stressors such as radiation, chemical toxins, or viruses. Somatic cell mutations increase risk for malignancy. Germ cell mutations increase risk for genetic abnormalities or spontaneous abortions in offspring. If left unchecked, these errors would significantly damage an organism's ability to sustain itself or reproduce. Numerous enzyme mechanisms have evolved to monitor and repair DNA replication errors. Some mutations persist in the replicated DNA. Most have no effect because large areas of the genome do not contain functioning genes. Furthermore, duplicate copies of many functional genes provide backup if genetic damage remains unrepaired. Mutations within active genes can have no effect or can lead to either decreases or increases in protein synthesis with associated changes in cell function.

Genetic Polymorphisms

Nonharmful changes in DNA can be passed on to subsequent generations. Unless a DNA change causes an advantage or disadvantage in a particular environment, the mutation's frequency will vary randomly in the population from generation to generation in a phenomenon known as _genetic drift_. Most mutations randomly disappear over time. However, the frequency of some mutations within populations can increase solely by chance. When a given mutation occurs in more than 1% of a population, it is called a _polymorphism_. Over time, the frequencies of different alleles within the same gene exhibit relative stability, called _Hardy-Weinberg equilibrium_. Polymorphisms can be de-

fined as major or minor alleles according to their population frequency.

Single nucleotide polymorphisms (SNPs) are found in both coding and noncoding genomic regions, and each reflects a mutation that probably occurred once during human evolution. Consequently, SNPs usually have two variants, and the degree to which two individuals share common SNPs provides a measure of relatedness. SNPs have been particularly useful in mapping genes and locating genes that contribute susceptibility to disease.

Copy Number Variants

Although relatively uncommon, some genes contain large insertions or deletions that range from a few Kb to over 2 Mb. These mutations can encompass multiple copies of entire genes. As such, individuals can carry fewer or more-than-expected copies of a given gene, with concomitant differences in levels of protein transcription. These copy number variants (CNVs) are being actively explored in relation to psychiatric illnesses, as gene dosage over a lifetime can have substantial impact on psychiatric phenotypes or metabolism of psychiatric medications.

Chromosomes

Chromosomes comprise large molecules of DNA and associated proteins that package genomic material within the nucleus. DNA makes up less than one-third of chromosomal mass, with the remainder comprised of histone proteins that package DNA and facilitate RNA synthesis. The human genome consists of 22 pairs of autosomal chromosomes, numbered 1–22 in order of decreasing size, and a pair of sex chromosomes—XY in males or XX in females. The shorter arms of each chromosome are designated "p" (for petit), and the longer arms are designated "q" (for the next letter in the alphabet). Figure 38–2 shows the structure of a chromosome.

An ordered list of loci within a particular genome provides a genetic map. Locations on the map are specified by convention that includes the chromosome number, followed by an indication of arms p or q, and numbers to signify the regions, bands, and subbands seen when a stained chromosome is viewed under the microscope. For example, the chromosomal locus of the _DRD4_ gene is identified by 11p15.5, which signifies the first region, fifth band, and fifth subband of the short arm of chromosome 11. Although this terminology is still in common usage, more accurate assign-

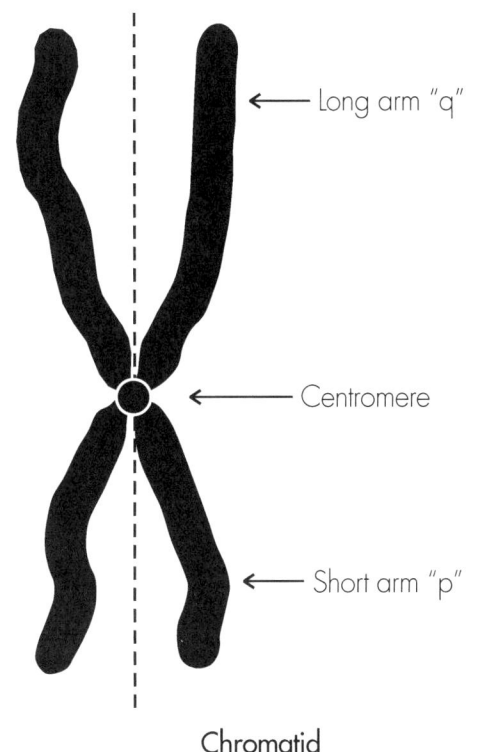

Long arm "q"

Centromere

Short arm "p"

Chromatid

FIGURE 38–2. Chromosome structure.
During cell division, chromosomal material becomes tightly compacted and individual chromosomes become visible as four-armed structures joined at a common centromere. Between cell divisions, chromosomal material is dispersed within the nucleus in a seemingly disorganized mass of DNA and protein.

ment and less ambiguous locations can now be specified by the exact base position relative to the consensus human genome.

Chromosome Division

During interphase, the period between cell divisions, each strand of chromosomal DNA replicates to form two identical sister chromatids. Both strands of DNA unwind and resynthesize their respective complementary strands via the enzymatic activity of *DNA-dependent DNA polymerase*. Somatic cells with diploid DNA divide to form two identical somatic cells in the process of *mitosis* (Figure 38–3). In *meiosis*, diploid sex cells initially divide to form two diploid germ cells followed by a second meiotic division leading to four haploid germ cells (eggs or sperm). In the course of mitosis, each of the 46 chromosomes aligns along the central cell axis prior to separation of two sets of identical chromatids into the daughter cells. In contrast, during meiosis matching pairs of chromosomes align together along the central cell axis prior to cell division. During

this period of alignment, homologous arms of corresponding chromatids intertwine and exchange genetic material, in processes known as *crossing over* and *recombination* (Figure 38–4).

Haplotypes

Haplotypes reflect patterns of genetic variation within populations and arise because certain combinations of alleles commonly occur near one another and because recombination rates vary across the genome. The International HapMap Project has mapped millions of sequences across the genome and determined their relationships between different populations (International HapMap Consortium 2003). Haplotypes reduce the genotyping effort required to find associations between diseases and genetic variants, since given sets of SNPs within specific haplotypes are known to occur together.

Chromosomal Disorders

Cell division can lead to several types of chromosomal abnormalities. *Nondisjunction* occurs when chromosomes fail to segregate properly, leaving daughter cells with either too many or too few chromosomes. The risk for nondisjunction in meiosis increases with maternal age, leading to a concomitant rise in chromosomal disorders in offspring of older mothers. Nondisjunction can also occur after fertilization, leading to chromosomal mosaics, where some cells have normal chromosomes while others are abnormal. *Translocation* occurs when DNA from one chromosome is transferred to a nonhomologous chromosome, resulting in an *insertion* on the recipient chromosome or a *deletion* on the contributing chromosome. Reciprocal translocations occur in approximately 1 of 600 births and are usually harmless, although individuals with these genotypes are usually infertile. A second type of translocation arises when 2 chromosomes fuse together, leading to a decrease in cell chromosome number. These individuals generally appear normal but are at increased risk for being infertile or having children with genetic abnormalities. Translocations can also occur in somatic cells, and if not corrected by cell machinery, they can lead to cancer.

Genes and Gene Function

Genes are coding regions within the genome that ultimately control protein synthesis. A simplified schematic of a typical gene appears in Figure 38–5. The two strands of DNA that comprise an individual gene are

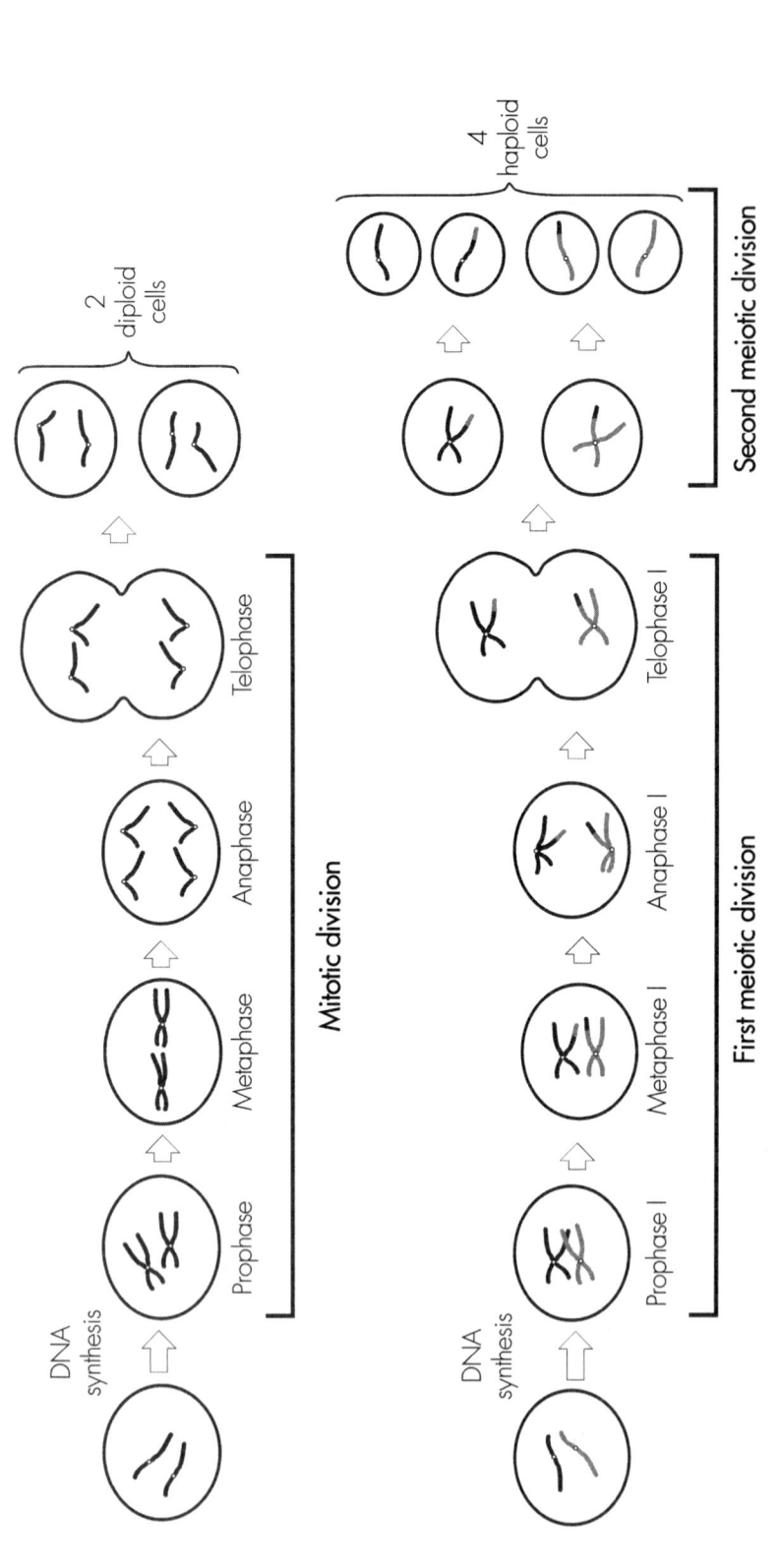

FIGURE 38–3.   Mitosis and meiosis.

In mitosis, somatic cells proceed through stages of prophase, metaphase, anaphase, and telophase resulting in two identical daughter cells. In meiosis, germ cells initially follow the same stages of division resulting in two identical daughter cells, followed by a second meiotic division, during which stages of prophase, metaphase, anaphase, and telophase are repeated but result in four haploid germ cells.

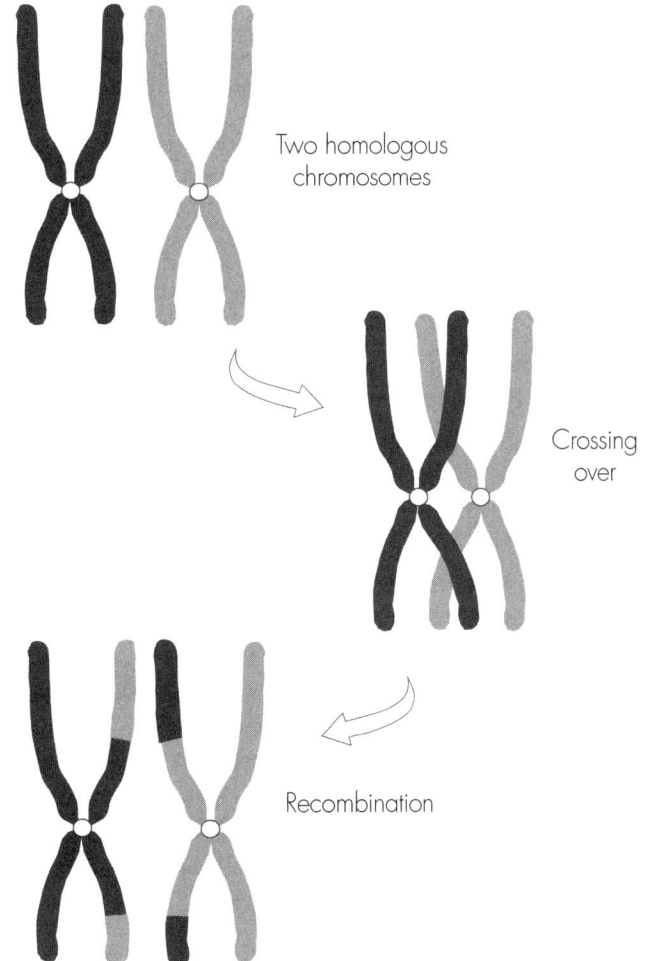

Two homologous chromosomes

Crossing over

Recombination

FIGURE 38–4. Crossing over and recombination.
During prophase of the first meiotic division, homologous arms of chromosome pairs become intertwined, in a process known as *crossing over*, and can undergo *recombination*, or exchange of DNA segments. Recombination serves to increase the genetic variability within chromosomes prior to segregation of homologous pairs into separate haploid daughter cells.

known as the template strand and the sense strand. *Transcription*, the synthesis of RNA from DNA, occurs only at the template strand, while the sense strand serves to preserve the official genetic code.

Base sequences within genes are arranged in three-nucleotide units, or *codons*, which specify the encoding of particular amino acids. The nonsense codons UAA, UAG, and UGA terminate translation and indicate the stopping point in protein chain synthesis. These nonsense codons also serve to abort the reading of RNA molecules initiated at an improper reading frame. Template DNA codons specify complementary *messenger RNA (mRNA)* codons, which pair with complementary *transfer RNA (tRNA)* anticodons and ultimately dictate the addition of a specified amino acid within a growing protein. Since the template DNA strand is complementary to the genetic code preserved in the sense strand, mRNA reflects the original genetic sequence, with the exception that uracil is substituted for thymine.

DNA Transcription

DNA sequences are copied through the enzymatic activity of *DNA-dependent RNA polymerase* to produce complementary strands of RNA in a process known as transcription. DNA transcription is the first step leading to *translation* of the genetic code through mRNA into functional cell products. As with DNA replication, synthesis of mRNA proceeds in a 5′ to 3′ direction. The *transcriptional unit* begins with a regulatory sequence, or *promoter*, that lies upstream to the 5′ end of the gene and extends downstream to a termination signal at the 3′ end. Nucleotides in the promoter are not transcribed but provide a binding site for *transcriptional factors*—proteins that serve to promote or inhibit

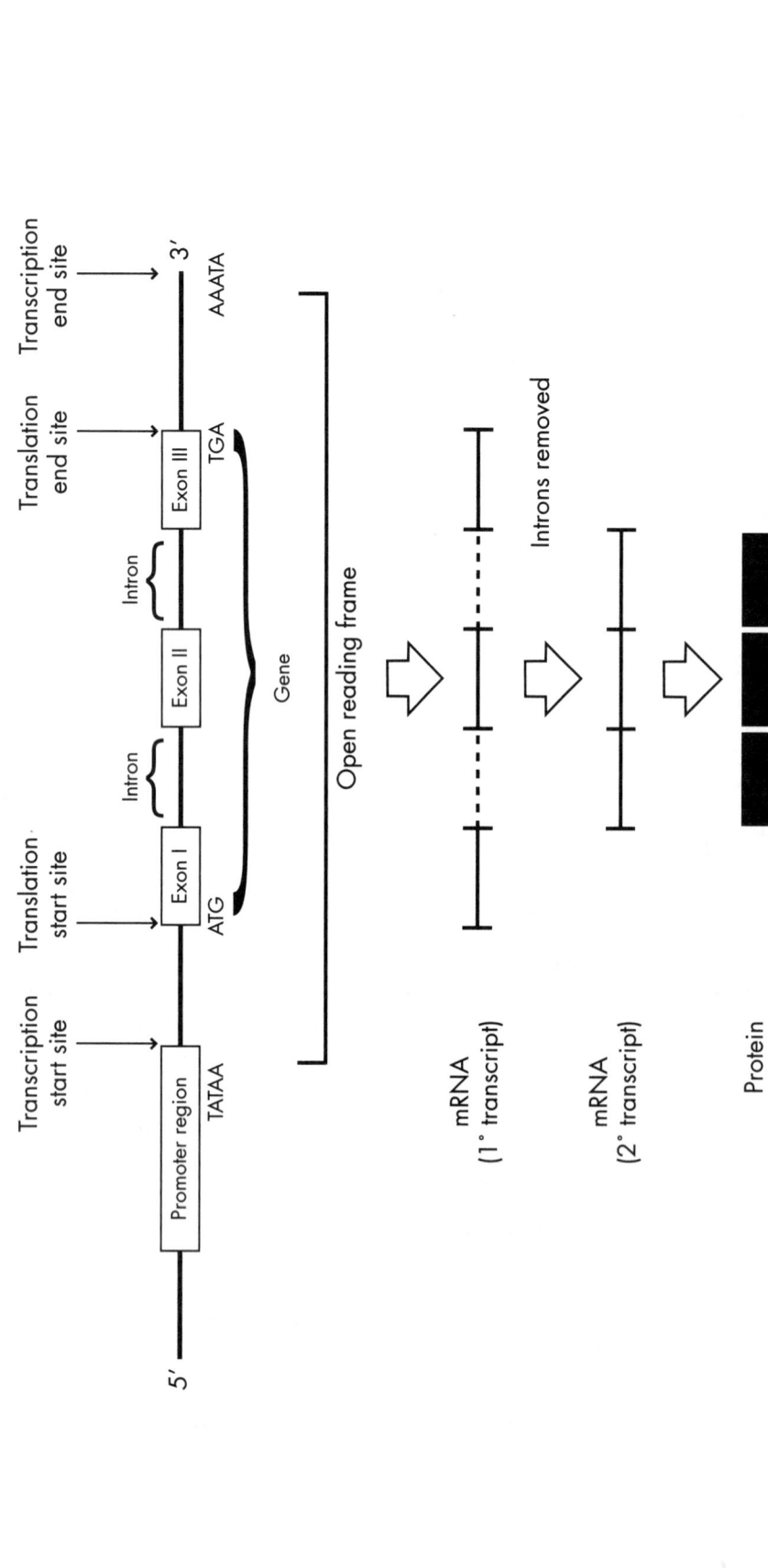

FIGURE 38–5.   A "typical" gene and steps in polypeptide synthesis.

DNA transcription is initiated at the 5′ end of the gene and proceeds in a 3′ direction, beginning at the promoter region. Transcribed precursor mRNA undergoes subsequent modifications into mature RNA prior to release in the cytoplasm where it serves to translate cell proteins.

transcription—and RNA polymerase. Transcription occurs within the cell's nucleus and comprises three stages: initiation, elongation, and termination.

Most transcription is initiated at the promoter when transcription factors and RNA polymerase bind an AT-nucleotide-rich sequence called the TATA box. The starting point for RNA synthesis is signaled by an ATG sequence on the sense strand that lies downstream to the promoter. Initiation of transcription at an ATG sequence ensures that nucleotide triplets are read within a proper frame. Elongation of the mRNA chain continues until terminated by the presence of the stop codon TGA, after which the RNA molecule is cleaved from the DNA template.

Initially, a very long mRNA molecule is made that consists of a nonprotein-coding 5' upstream sequence termed the *5' UTR* (for UnTranslated Region), all of the exons and introns of the entire gene, and a 3' UTR sequence. This huge RNA molecule, frequently many-fold larger than what will be used to make the protein sequence, is edited by cell machinery to remove all of the introns to create a mature mRNA molecule ready for translation.

RNA Processing and Translation

Following transcription, precursor mRNA is modified by several processes prior to transport into the cytoplasm. These changes include capping at the 5' end, cleavage at the 3' end followed by addition of a poly-adenosine tail, and removal of introns from the mature mRNA molecule. Additional processes, such as *RNA splicing, editing,* and *silencing,* further modify mRNA structure and function. Alternative splicing of identical RNA sequences contributes to the diversity of human proteins.

Ribosomes are organelles that consist of protein and ribosomal RNA (rRNA) and provide sites for mRNA-mediated protein synthesis within the cytoplasm. Ribosomes align successive mRNA codons with complementary anticodons on tRNA, which is bound to corresponding individual amino acids. RNA translation involves initiation, elongation, and termination, and it proceeds in a 5' to 3' direction. Protein synthesis begins at an initiation codon located toward the 5' end of the mRNA molecule. Synthesis proceeds by using tRNAs to align each successive amino acid until a termination codon, UAG, is reached at the 3' end. The resultant polypeptide requires further modification to be functional, possibly including proper folding, binding to other polypeptides, and binding to a heavy metal. Additionally, numerous processes, particularly phosphorylation of amino acid side-chains, lead to posttranslational modifications of cellular proteins. These modifications allow cells to respond to intracellular and extracellular signals and increase the functional versatility of cell products.

Regulation of Gene Expression

Each of an individual's nucleated cells (other than eggs or sperm) contains the same DNA and associated genes. Mechanisms that regulate gene expression enable this finite set of genes to control all the body's diverse functions. Gene transcription can be induced or silenced by transcription factors. Genes can be induced by other products synthesized within the cell or by exposure to exogenous compounds such as hormones or bacterial antigens. Changes in chromatin structure control the accessibility of genomic regions for DNA transcription. Histone acetylation facilitates the interaction of genomic sequences with gene regulator proteins and RNA polymerase, leading to enhanced DNA transcription. DNA methylation prevents the interaction of genomic regions with transcriptional factors and subsequently silences transcription.

Epigenetics are heritable changes in gene function that are not due to mutations or other changes in the genetic sequence. Modifications in genetic expression resulting from histone acetylation or DNA methylation can survive ensuing cell divisions and ultimately lead to cell differentiation. One specific epigenetic mechanism is *imprinting*, in which a small number of genes are expressed differently according to their parental origin (Fergusson-Smith and Surani 2001). For example, only the paternal allele for insulin-like growth factor II is expressed, while the maternally inherited allele remains inactive (DeChiara et al. 1991). Among psychiatric disorders, Prader-Willi syndrome results from a deletion in the paternally inherited long arm of chromosome 15, whereas Angelman's syndrome results from the same deletion in the maternal line (Cassidy et al. 2000). During female embryogenesis, random imprinting of one or the other X chromosome leads to permanent deactivation and avoids double expression of X chromosome genes compared with males (Reik and Lewis 2005). Genetic imprints are erased in germ cell lines and reprogrammed during formation of sperm and eggs to identify the parent of origin (Reik and Walter 2001).

Approaches to Psychiatric Genetics

Simple traits arise from changes in single genes and usually follow Mendelian patterns of inheritance. Genes encoding for simple traits are considered genes of major effect and usually result in the presence or absence of a disease state. For example, Huntington's disease is inherited as an autosomal dominant disorder stemming from an abnormal triplet repeat CAG within a gene on chromosome 4 (Roses 1996). Polymorphisms in genes coding for the amyloid precursor protein, presenilin 1, and presenilin 2 have been associated with Alzheimer's disease (Liddell et al. 2002), although both dominant and recessive patterns of inheritance have been proposed. Rett syndrome is caused by a mutation in the gene encoding methyl-CpG-binding protein-2 located on the X chromosome. Most cases of Rett syndrome arise from sporadic mutations, but patterns in family pedigrees suggest X-linked dominant inheritance in females and lethality in males (Schanen et al. 1997). Cystic fibrosis results from recessive mutations in the CF gene located on chromosome 7 (Riordan et al. 1989).

Complex traits arise from the interplay of multiple genes, usually with varying small degrees of effect, and the environment. Almost all psychiatric disorders represent complex traits and are not explained by Mendelian patterns of inheritance. Approaches in classical genetics were created to uncover genes of major effect but have not proven useful in complex disorders. Alternative strategies for gene discovery have been necessary to identify genetic contributions to psychiatric disorders.

Complex traits, also known as *quantitative traits*, vary continuously across a population, as opposed to being *qualitative* (i.e., present or absent). Height, intelligence, blood pressure, blood cholesterol, inattention, irritability, and novelty seeking are examples of complex traits that might or might not exceed a threshold associated with pathology (Falconer 1965). Genes that contribute to these complex systems are called *quantitative trait loci (QTL)*. A QTL is one of many genes that shift a phenotype toward one direction along a continuum. QTL analysis is used to identify genes with varying effects on a complex trait (Grisel 2000). Qualitative, or *categorical*, definitions of disorders, such as those found in DSM, often describe sets of behaviors that are too heterogeneous to facilitate gene discovery. Psychiatric genetics employs both qualitative and quantitative approaches for gene identification.

Genetic Epidemiology

Family, adoption, and twin studies are the foundation of psychiatric genetics. These epidemiological approaches provide a basis to determine whether individual susceptibility to specific disorders is due to family or genetic factors. *Family studies* identify disorders across extended pedigrees and can demonstrate whether shared environmental or genetic effects appear to influence disease risk. *Adoption studies* compare patterns of occurrence among biological and adopted relatives and disentangle the separate effects of environmental and genetic contributions to susceptibility. *Twin studies*, which compare disorder rates in monozygotic versus dizygotic siblings, allow for estimates of *heritability*, the proportion of phenotypic variation in the population attributable to genetic variability. Twin studies have demonstrated significant genetic contributions to numerous psychiatric disorders, including bipolar disorder, schizophrenia, autism, and attention-deficit/hyperactivity disorder (ADHD) (McGuffin and Southwick 2003). Genetic epidemiology provides a basis for subsequent molecular investigations (Kendler 2005).

Molecular Genetic Studies

While epidemiological studies demonstrate the genetic basis of psychiatric disorders, molecular genetic studies seek to identify the actual genes and allele variants that create increased risk for observed behaviors. Advances in molecular studies have been dependent on technological accomplishments, such as mapping the human genome, and the increasing ease and decreasing cost of genotyping. There are two basic strategies for gene discovery in complex disorders. Linkage studies make no a priori hypotheses concerning which genes encode specific traits but identify regions of the genome that segregate more commonly with the traits of interest. In contrast, association studies test whether particular polymorphisms of prespecified genes occur more frequently in individuals with the disease than would be expected by chance. Variations on these basic approaches, such as use of denser marker sets or genome-wide association studies, increase the likelihood of identifying significant genes.

Linkage Studies

Linkage studies examine the relationship between a phenotype and a genetic locus. During meiosis, genes on separate chromosomes have a 50% probability of being segregated together into a single egg or sperm as predicted by Mendel's Law of Independent Assortment. Similarly, if two genes lie on opposite ends of the same chromosome, there is a 50% probability that they will be inherited together, due to crossing over and recombination. Genes that lie more closely together are less vulnerable to crossing over and recombination and would be expected to segregate together more frequently. In classical genetics, family pedigrees were examined to determine which traits co-occurred to a greater degree than the 50% predicted by chance. These traits were assumed to be *linked*, and lower frequencies of independent assortment implied smaller distances between the genes on a given chromosome.

With development of powerful computer programs and identification of genetic markers scattered throughout the genome, multiple family pedigrees can be analyzed to assess the potential co-occurrence of marker polymorphisms with phenotypic traits (Pauls 1999). Linkage is demonstrated when traits and markers occur together more frequently than expected by independent assortment. Linkage analysis of multiple family pedigrees in which large numbers of individuals suffered from psychiatric illness initially led to claims of single gene findings for bipolar disorder and schizophrenia (Asherson and Curran 2001). However, it was subsequently recognized that these discoveries represented rare mutations in atypical family presentations and not the common genes that contribute to common presentations of these disorders (Risch 2000). Analyses were complicated by the incorrect assumption that these disorders followed Mendelian patterns of inheritance.

Subsequent linkage studies in psychiatry have addressed these limitations by emphasizing investigations with sibling pairs, small nuclear families, and population isolates (Risch 2000). In pairs of siblings with the same disorder, it is hypothesized that individuals share the risk allele inherited from one parent more frequently than the 50% sharing expected by chance. By comparing the degree of allele sharing over hundreds of markers in many families with multiple affected siblings, linkage peaks are identified within the genome that are likely to harbor genes conferring increased susceptibility for the disorder. These regions identify target areas for additional fine-mapping with denser marker sets that could potentially pinpoint areas in tight linkage with the susceptibility gene. This approach requires no assumptions about inheritance patterns but requires large numbers of affected pairs to identify genes of small to moderate effect.

The degree of linkage is expressed by a *lod score*, which is a log ratio reflecting the frequency of recombination between two markers divided by the expected frequency with independent assortment. In order to provide a common point of discussion between researchers, lod scores >2 are suggestive of linkage, lod scores >3 are considered evidence of linkage, and lod scores >4 are evidence of strong linkage with a gene of major effect (Lander and Kruglyak 1995). While linkage studies have proven useful, there have been few definitive findings in psychiatry, probably due to the heterogeneity of categorical clinical diagnosis (Dean 2003). QTL analysis, which examines genetic contributions on continuous variables, has greater power to detect effects than categorical variables if the trait varies continuously in the population. Analysis of *endophenotypes*—heritable neurophysiological, endocrinological, neuroanatomical, or neurophysiological traits that presumably identify more homogeneous subsets of patients (Gottesman and Gould 2003)—has been proposed to decrease genetic heterogeneity and to directly measure effects of susceptibility genes on underlying neurobiology (Hariri and Weinberger 2003; Prathikanti and Weinberger 2005). Endophenotypes are particularly well suited for QTL analysis and are being actively explored in a wide variety of psychiatric conditions.

Candidate Gene Studies

Candidate gene, or association, studies examine the relationship between specific allele variants and phenotypic traits. These studies presume that single point mutations through recombination over successive generations reach *linkage equilibrium* with other markers in the genome. Linkage disequilibrium occurs when a marker polymorphism lies so close to the disease susceptibility gene, possibly within the gene itself, that there is no recombination, even when the mutation occurred in a distant ancestor. Since the distances between candidate polymorphisms and susceptibility genes are much smaller than required for linkage studies, linkage disequilibrium studies have significantly greater power to detect genes of small effect (Risch and Merikangas 1996).

Whereas linkage studies make no a priori assumptions about specific markers, candidate gene studies presume some understanding of the biology of the disorder and test whether specific polymorphisms contribute to disease risk. For example, the understanding that stimulants used in ADHD treatment had effects on catecholaminergic systems led to candidate gene investigations of various catecholaminergic genes and consistently replicated findings that several of these genes confer small, but significantly increased, risk for the disorder (Faraone et al. 2005).

Case-control-based association studies.

Association studies contrast the frequencies of a given polymorphism in individuals with and without a particular trait. These studies are straightforward, employ simple statistics, and have no need to recruit and assess subjects' family members. These studies do require the recruitment of a genetically matched control population without the disorder of interest. However, association studies often lead to conflicting results or fail to replicate. This results in part from a failure to match subjects and controls on other clinical variables, particularly race and ethnicity, which can lead to global population genetic differences between groups that are unrelated to the phenotype in question.

Family-based association studies.

Family-based, or allele-sharing, studies provide an alternative to case-based association designs. The transmission disequilibrium test (TDT; Speilman and Ewens 1996) rests on the assumption that alleles that are not related to the phenotype in question will be randomly inherited from each parent 50% of the time. For the TDT, both parents and the affected offspring (trios) are genotyped to determine if one allele form is inherited more frequently by affected individuals than the 50% expected by chance. The TDT has high power to detect polymorphisms of small effect, but its power is highly dependent on the baseline frequencies of candidate alleles in the population and can require very large numbers of families. Only transmission of alleles from parents with two different alleles can be assessed. With the family-based method, problems with control groups and potential population stratification are avoided, since parents and their offspring presumably share genes associated with race and ethnicity.

Genome-Wide Association Studies

With recent technological advances, it has become possible to test virtually all common alleles within the human genome for association with any trait. This is an extension of the candidate gene approach but allows the power of association testing without the limits of identifying specific likely candidates. While there are many millions of polymorphisms within the human genome, and it would be theoretically possible to test them all for genome-wide association analysis, this is both economically prohibitive for typical studies and generally not needed due to human population history. Instead, it has been recognized that there is a large amount of linkage

disequilibrium within the human genome, and thus association studies are possible using haplotype blocks. These haplotypes are genomic intervals, typically 1–30 Kb, that can be identified by testing only a subset of the SNPs within the block. Thus, it now appears that testing 300,000 SNPs permits strong assessment of about 65% of the genome. Testing 1 million SNPs permits robust assessment of about 90% of the human genome. Statistical methods have been devised to analyze sliding windows of haplotype combinations with TDT analysis or case-control designs, which have considerable power to detect large and small genetic effects without the need for a priori hypotheses (Lin et al. 2004). A major issue in these studies is that since hundreds of thousands of genetic tests are performed simultaneously, the stringency of the statistical analysis must be set very high to avoid identification of a large number of false positives. It is anticipated that genome-wide association studies, a natural extension of candidate gene association studies, will ultimately detect most of the common polymorphisms contributing risk for common complex disorders (Dean 2003). However, the current study sizes of a few hundred or thousand individuals are inadequately powered to identify reliably all of the common allele contributions. An example of this is a study that attempted to detect disease associations in seven common disorders using about 2,000 cases with bipolar disorder (Wellcome Trust Case Control Consortium 2007). No statistically significant loci were identified for bipolar disorder, but one to three meaningful loci were identified in the other six disorders. Ultimately, successful genome-wide association studies will call for involving tens or hundreds of thousands of patients as well as unaffected individuals from the general population. In addition, these genetic studies will require careful attention to appropriate phenotyping to result in a more complete understanding of a number of neuropsychiatric conditions. Once investigators determine that a particular phenotype is associated with a specific haplotype, subsequent efforts to conduct high-density SNP mapping in the haplotype are likely to identify the functional disease loci.

Genetic Interactions

In disorders with Mendelian patterns of inheritance, single genes contribute major effects toward phenotype risk. For complex disorders, it is presumed that multiple genes interact with each other and the environment to increase susceptibility for illness.

Of equal or greater importance in psychiatric disorders are genetic interactions with the environment. Even among disorders with high heritability, concordance rates for monozygotic twins are less than 100%, suggesting that ultimate disease expression is not dependent on genetic variation alone (Craddock et al. 2005). Nonetheless, the most typical approach in psychiatric genetics assumes a straightforward relationship between genotype and phenotype. An alternative holds that environmental factors cause disorders, with genetic variants moderating susceptibility to environmental influences (Caspi and Moffit 2006). This view arose from observations that environmental variables independently predict risk for some disorders and that individuals vary in their responses to those environmental effects (Moffit et al. 2005).

Several preliminary reports support this hypothesis. A seminal report demonstrated that abused children with polymorphisms for decreased expression of monoamine oxidase A more frequently developed conduct disorder, antisocial personality, and violent behavior than those with increased monoamine oxidase A expression (Caspi et al. 2002). A second report found that individuals with two copies of the "short" allele found in the promoter region of the serotonin transporter gene developed depression more frequently after stressful life events than individuals with at least one copy of the "long" allele (Caspi et al. 2003). Several studies have found that the link between antenatal risk factors (e.g., maternal nicotine and alcohol use, low birth weight) and subsequent development of ADHD is mediated by polymorphisms in dopamine system genes (Brooks et al. 2005; Kahn et al. 2003; Neuman et al. 2007; Thapar et al. 2005). Innovative approaches to analysis of longitudinal data, including latent class modeling (Bartels et al. 2007) and factor mixture modeling (Muthen et al. 2006), are increasingly able to parse genetic, environmental, and gene-by-environment interactive effects.

Clinical Applications

The most likely clinical application of psychiatric genetics will be in enhanced patient education and decreased stigma as the general public recognizes the biological basis of behavioral disorders. Some researchers have suggested that diagnostic categories in future editions of DSM be organized around genetic findings (Kendler 2006). However, this is not likely to prove feasible in the short term, as genes associated with psychiatric disorders contribute small effects on disease risk, and many of the same genes are implicated in different disorders. This situation might im-

prove with much more detailed information from whole genome association studies on vast patient samples. However, it is unlikely that genetic testing will prove useful as the foundation for psychiatric diagnosis, in spite of great public interest in diagnosing psychiatric illness with "objective" laboratory measures. It is likely that genetic counselors will play an increasing role in patient care, as specific genetic and environmental risk factors for behavioral disorders are understood (Finn and Smoller 2006).

Pharmacogenetics and pharmacogenomics seek to optimize patient response to medication therapy on the basis of individual genetic variability. For example, polymorphisms in the cytochrome P450 isozyme system are responsible for up to 200-fold variations in the metabolic rates of over 100 drugs, including many used in psychiatric disorders (Xie et al. 2001). Approximately 20% of whites and varying percentages of other racial groups contain a polymorphism in the P450 2D6 isozyme that results in very slow metabolism and concomitantly elevated serum blood levels. Commercial testing of P450 2D6 alleles is already available. Other preliminary reports suggest that DNA testing might predict symptom response or risk of side effects with certain medications. For example, polymorphisms in the serotonin receptor 5-HT$_{2A}$ predict response to clozapine (Arranz et al. 2000); antidepressant response to serotonin reuptake inhibitors is mediated by polymorphisms in the serotonin transporter (Serretti et al. 2001); and numerous genes in the catecholamine system have predicted symptom reduction and medication tolerability in stimulant treatment of ADHD (McGough 2005; McGough et al. 2006). These findings require replication in large groups of patients before they are proven clinically useful.

Research Directions

Future research will make greater use of haplotypes and genome-wide association studies in large numbers of subjects and controls. Newly identified susceptibility genes will provide innovative targets for drug discovery. Ongoing efforts in pharmacogenetics will seek to identify genetic factors that will help physicians individually tailor medication regimens based on patients' individual genotypes. Further advances are expected in unraveling the relative contributions of genes, environmental variables, and their interactive effects in increasing risk for psychiatric disorders. Potential opportunities for primary prevention will emerge as clinical studies assess psychosocial interventions in individuals with known genetic predispositions for emotional or behavioral impairment. In addition, the translation of these research findings will require continuing integration with the traditional approaches to clinical assessment and care, including sensitivity to patients' psychological, family, and social needs (Owen et al. 2002).

Summary Points

- Simple traits or disorders are caused by mutations in single genes and generally follow Mendelian patterns of inheritance.

- Complex traits or disorders arise from the interplay of multiple genes, each contributing small effects, and the environment. Almost all psychiatric disorders represent complex traits and are not explained by Mendelian patterns of inheritance.

- Linkage studies make no a priori hypotheses concerning which genes encode specific traits, but they identify regions of the genome that segregate more commonly with the traits of interest.

- Candidate gene association studies test whether specified polymorphisms occur more frequently in individuals with the disease than would be expected by chance.

- Whole genome association studies test whether any polymorphism is associated with a trait, but they require large population samples and rigorous selection of genetically matched control groups to be valid.

- Environmental factors play a critical role in moderating genetic risk for most psychiatric disorders, even for those conditions that are highly heritable.

References

Arranz MJ, Munro J, Birkett J, et al: Pharmacogenetic prediction of clozapine response. Lancet 355:1615–1616, 2000

Asherson P, Curran S: Approaches to gene mapping in complex disorder and their application in child psychiatry and psychology. Br J Psychiatry 179:122–128, 2001

Bartels M, van Beijsterveldt CE, Derks EM, et al: a longitudinal multiple informant study of problem behavior. Twin Res Hum Genet 10:3–11, 2007

Brooks KJ, Mill J, Guindalini C, et al: A common haplotype of the dopamine transporter gene associated with attention-deficit/hyperactivity disorder and interacting with maternal use of alcohol during pregnancy. Arch Gen Psychiatry 63:74–81, 2005

Caspi A, Moffitt TE: Gene-environment interactions in psychiatry: joining forces with neuroscience. Nat Rev Genet 7:583–590, 2006

Caspi A, McClay J, Moffit TE, et al: Role of genotype in the cycle of violence in maltreated children. Science 297:851–854, 2002

Caspi A, Sugden, Moffit TE, et al: Influence of life stress on depression: moderation by a polymorphism in the 5-HTT gene. Science 301:386–389, 2003

Cassidy SB, Dykens E, Williams CA: Prader-Willi and Angelman syndromes: sister imprinted disorders. Am J Med Genet 97:136–146, 2000

Craddock N, O'Donovan MC, Owen MF: The genetics of schizophrenia and bipolar disorder: dissecting psychosis. J Med Genet 42:193–204, 2005

Dean M: Approaches to identify genes for complex human diseases: lessons from Mendelian disorders. Hum Mutat 22:261–274, 2003

DeChiara TM, Robertson EJ, Efstratiadis A: Parental imprinting of the mouse insulin-like growth factor II gene. Cell 64:849–859, 1991

Falconer DS: The inheritance of liability to certain diseases estimated from the incidence among relatives. Ann Hum Genet 29:51–76, 1965

Faraone SV, Perlis RH, Doyle AE, et al: Molecular genetics of attention-deficit/hyperactivity disorder. Biol Psychiatry 57:1313–1323, 2005

Fergusson-Smith AC, Surani MA: Imprinting and the epigenetic asymmetry between parental genomes. Science 293:1086–1089, 2001

Finn CT, Smoller JW: Genetic counseling in psychiatry. Harv Rev Psychiatry 14:109–121, 2006

Gottesman II, Gould TD: The endophenotype concept in psychiatry: etymology and strategic intentions. Am J Psychiatry 160:636–645, 2003

Grisel JE: Quantitative trait locus analysis. Alcohol Res Health 24:169–174, 2000

Hariri AR, Weinberger DR: Imaging genomics. Br Med Bull 65:259–270, 2003

International HapMap Consortium: The International HapMap Project. Nature 426:789–796, 2003

Kahn RS, Khoury J, Nichols WC, et al: Role of dopamine transporter genotype and maternal prenatal smoking in childhood hyperactive-impulsive, inattentive, and oppositional behaviors. J Pediatr 143:104–110, 2003

Kendler KS: Psychiatric genetics: a methodologic critique. Am J Psychiatry 162:3–11, 2005

Kendler KS: Reflections on the relationship between psychiatric genetics and psychiatric nosology. Am J Psychiatry 163:1138–1146, 2006

Lander E, Kruglyak L: Genetic dissection of complex traits: guidelines for interpreting and reporting linkage results. Nat Genet 11:241–247, 1995

Liddell MB, Williams J, Owen MJ: The dementias, in Psychiatric Genetics and Genomics. Edited by McGuffin P, Owen MJ, Gottesman II. New York, Oxford University Press, 2002, pp 341–397

Lin S, Chakravarti A, Cutler DJ: Exhaustive allelic transmission disequilibrium tests as a new approach to genome-wide association studies. Nat Genet 36:1181–1188, 2004

McGough JJ: Attention-deficit/hyperactivity disorder pharmacogenomics. Bio Psychiatry 57:1367–1373, 2005

McGough JJ, McCracken JT, Swanson J, et al: Pharmacogenetics of methylphenidate response in preschoolers with ADHD. J Am Acad Child Adolesc Psychiatry 45:1314–1322, 2006

McGuffin P, Southwick L: Fifty years of the double helix and its impact on psychiatry. Aust N Z J Psychiatry 37:657–661, 2003

Moffit TE, Caspi A, Rutter M: Strategy for investigating interactions between measured genes and measured environments. Arch Gen Psychiatry 62:473–481, 2005

Muthen B, Asparouhov T, Rebollo I: Advances in behavioral genetics modeling using Mplus: applications of factor mixture modeling to twin data. Twin Res Hum Genet 9:313–324, 2006

Neuman RJ, Lobos E, Reich W, et al: Prenatal smoking exposure and dopaminergic genes interact to cause a severe ADHD subtype. Biol Psychiatry 61:1320–1328, 2007

Owen MJ, McGuffin P, Gottesman I: The future of postgenomic psychiatry, in Psychiatric Genetics and Genomics. Edited by McGuffin P, Owen MJ, Gottesman II. New York, Oxford University Press, 2002, pp 463–480

Pauls D: Genetics of childhood disorders, IV: linkage analysis. J Am Acad Child Adolesc Psychiatry 38:932–934, 1999

Prathikanti S, Weinberger DR: Psychiatric genetics—the new era: genetic research and some clinical implications. Br Med Bull 73:102–122, 2005

Reik W, Lewis A: Co-evolution of X-chromosome inactivation and imprinting in mammals. Nat Rev Genet 6:403–410, 2005

Reik W, Walter J: Genomic imprinting: parental influence on the genome. Nat Rev Genet 2:21–32, 2001

Riordan JR, Rommens JM, Kerem B, et al: Identification of the cystic fibrosis gene: cloning and characterization of complementary DNA. Science 245:1066–1073, 1989

Risch N: Searching for genetic determinants in the new millennium. Nature 405:847–856, 2000

Risch N, Merikangas K: The future of genetic studies of complex human diseases. Science 273:1516–1589, 1996

Roses AD: From genes to mechanisms to therapies: lessons to be learned from neurological disorders. Nature Med 2:267–269, 1996

Schanen NC, Dahle EJ, Capozzoli F, et al: A new Rett syndrome family consistent with X-linked inheritance expands the X chromosome map. Am J Hum Genet 61:634–641, 1997

Serretti A, Zanardi R, Rossini D, et al: Influence of tryptophan hydroxylase and serotonin transporter genes on fluvoxamine antidepressant activity. Mol Psychiatry 6:586–592, 2001

Speilman RS, Ewens WJ: The TDT and other family-based tests for linkage disequilibrium and association. Am J Hum Genet 59:983–989, 1996

Stein LD: Human genome: end of the beginning. Nature 431:915–916, 2004

Thapar A, Langley K, Fowler T, et al: Catechol-O-methyltransferase gene variant and birth weight predict early-onset antisocial behavior in children with attention-deficit/hyperactivity disorder. Arch Gen Psychiatry 62:1275–1278, 2005

Wellcome Trust Case Control Consortium: Genome-wide association study of 14,000 cases of even common diseases and 3,000 shared controls. Nature 447:661–678, 2007

Xie HG, Kim RB, Wood AJ, et al: Molecular basis of ethnic differences in drug disposition and response. Annu Rev Pharmacol Toxicol 41:815–850, 2001

PART IX

SPECIAL CLINICAL CIRCUMSTANCES

Chapter 39

Psychiatric Emergencies

D. Richard Martini, M.D.

Children and adolescents with psychiatric disorders are presenting in the emergency department (ED) at ever increasing rates. Some of this is due to the limited availability of inpatient psychiatric beds and the subsequent growth of emergent care facilities (Christodulu et al. 2002). These young patients stress the system by placing unique demands on pediatric and mental health clinicians. Frequently, the emergency contact is their first visit with psychiatric services. Despite a lack of familiarity and information, the mental health team must safely, carefully, and in a culturally and developmentally appropriate manner, manage these cases. Patients may present with adults who are not the child's primary caregivers and who are unfamiliar with the psychiatric history. In addition, these children are more likely to be aggressive and dangerous, requiring more time and resources (see Table 39–1 for an assessment summary). Psychiatric symptoms may be the result of an intercurrent medical illness, which is more likely in patients who present with new-onset, acute psychiatric complaints (Olshaker et al. 1997). Each patient presenting for emergent care should, therefore, receive a medical history and a full medical evaluation. Identification

and treatment of psychiatric emergencies in children and adolescents are essential parts of the "safety net" that must be available for children in crisis and for those who have not been able to appropriately access mental health services.

Common Clinical Presentations

Suicidal Behavior

The assessment of pediatric patients for self-injurious behavior is based on the review of three basic questions:

- Is the patient likely to commit suicide in the future?
- Is the patient likely to make a suicide attempt in the future?
- Will the patient follow through on a psychiatric referral based on this evaluation? Suicide attempts are typically impulsive acts with little premeditation.

TABLE 39–1. Causes of aggression and agitation in the emergency department

Disruptive behavior disorders

  Attention-deficit/hyperactivity disorder

  Oppositional defiant disorder

  Conduct disorder

  Mental retardation

Anxiety-provoked aggression

  Separation anxiety disorder

  Panic disorder

  Obsessive-compulsive disorder

  Acute phobic hallucinations (especially in children ages 2–6 years)

Organic delirium

  Medical illness

    Fever

    Electrolyte imbalance

    Central nervous system infection, tumor, trauma, or vascular accident

    Seizures

    Endocrine or autoimmune disorder

    Hypoxia

    Metabolic disorder

  Adverse reaction to prescribed or over-the-counter medication

  Toxic ingestion

  Reaction to illicit substance

    Acute intoxication or toxic reaction

    Flashback

    Psychotic reaction to chronic drug use

Schizophrenia

Mania

Abuse or neglect

Epidemiology

Details on the characteristics of suicidal adolescents are provided in Chapter 35, "Youth Suicide." In emergency settings, there is a range of behaviors in adolescents at varying levels of severity. However, there are no known factors that predict either reattempts or completed suicide, which is important to remember when formulating a disposition from the emergency room (Centers for Disease Control and Prevention 2007). Possible risk factors for a suicide attempt are listed in Table 39–2.

Assessment

The mental health clinician in the emergency room can evaluate the suicidal adolescent (under age 18 in all but four states) without parental consent. The Emergency Medical Treatment and Active Labor Act states that every patient presenting to an ED is entitled to assessment and treatment in order to prevent death, disability, or pain and suffering (Sullivan 1993). Safety is a primary concern in the ED assessment that begins at the time of admission. Patients are searched, their clothing is removed, and they are dressed in hospital gowns. The evaluation takes place in an area away from other patients, potentially lethal substances, and medical instruments. The ED staff approaches the patient with compassion and educates the patient and family about what to expect from the admission. These contacts are particularly important because adherence to outpatient treatment following an assessment of suicidality in the ED depends upon the quality of staff interactions with the patient and family and the expectations of treatment and notions about suicide maintained by the patient and family at the conclusion of the evaluation (Spirito et al. 2002).

The psychiatric assessment includes a careful physical examination, including mental status. Evidence of an organic illness that may cause delirium, signs of previous suicide attempts (e.g., scars from cutting, bruises on the neck from attempted asphyxiation), indicators of physical or sexual abuse, and evidence of possible substance use are included. Patients who are delirious typically present with dramatic changes in behavior and mental status that are related to the appearance or treatment of a physical illness. Dangerousness is related to the presence of mood lability as well as cognitive and perceptual distortions. A urine toxicology screen and a pregnancy test for adolescent girls are also considerations. Additional tests, including liver enzymes and drug and alcohol screens, depend upon the method of suicide and resulting physical complications. Medical illnesses can cause a variety of psychiatric symptoms, and the evaluation should screen for neurological, endocrine, gastrointestinal, autoimmune, and infectious diseases when indicated.

The assessment of the suicidal patient focuses on two aspects of the behavior: lethality and intent. In adolescents, medical lethality is not necessarily related to severity of the attempt. Patients may accidentally ingest lethal amounts of a substance or overestimate the toxicity of a small amount while making an attempt with serious intent. The latter is common among adolescent attempters and is usually followed by a trend

TABLE 39–2. Risk factors for a suicide attempt

Patient history

Verbalization or threats regarding suicide

Substance abuse

Poor impulse control

A recent loss or other severe stressor

Previous suicide attempt(s)

A friend or family member who has committed suicide

Exposure to recent news stories or movies about suicide

Poor social supports

Victim of physical or sexual abuse

Nature of the attempt

Accidental discovery (vs. attempt in view of others or telling others immediately)

Careful plans to avoid discovery

Hanging or gunshot

Family

Wishes to be rid of child or adolescent

Does not take child's problems seriously

Is overly angry and punitive

Depression or suicidality is present in a family member

Is unwilling or unable to provide support and supervision

Mental status examination

Depression

Hopelessness

Regret at being rescued

Belief that things would be better for self or others if dead

Wish to rejoin a dead loved one

Belief that death is temporary and pleasant

Unwillingness to promise to call before attempting suicide

Psychosis

Intoxication

toward more lethal means. Young patients typically have limited access to methods with a high mortality rate. They do, however, have access to drugs, both prescription and over the counter, and choose overdose as the preferred approach. Clinicians should be aware of local preferences among children and adolescents and inquire about the patient's familiarity and previous experiences with these methods during both psychiatric

and pediatric assessments. The assessment of intent tends to focus on several important questions. Why was this method chosen? What were the expectations from the attempt (did the patient think that the attempt was going to kill him or her)? How reversible was the attempt? If possible, could the patient change his or her mind and quickly recover from the attempt? Does the patient demonstrate any ambivalence about living? How strong was the patient's intent to die? Was there evidence of premeditation, including preparations and precautions against discovery (Spirito et al. 1994)? The answers to these questions are not only found in the interview but also in the details of the patient's behavior. Incidents that immediately precede the attempt may provide clues about motivation and intent. In an ingestion, for example, does the patient take a large number of pills or perhaps all of the pills that are available? Does the patient tell anyone about the ingestion, particularly responsible caregivers? What does the patient do immediately after taking the pills? Does she seek help or does she simply disregard the danger of the ingestion and go to bed? When the patient experiences the physical consequences of an overdose (i.e., nausea, vomiting, abdominal pain) and is discovered, does she acknowledge her suicidal behavior or continue to hide the reasons for her discomfort?

The clinician should realize that there are precipitants of the suicide attempt and that a primary purpose of the assessment is to uncover and address those issues as well as predisposing factors. Adolescents experience relationship problems with friends, family, and boyfriends or girlfriends—or school failures in academics, sports, or the arts—that produce high levels of frustration and occasionally narcissistic injury leading to suicidal behavior. Children and adolescents, regardless of age, may express a real desire to die as a means of obtaining relief or of escaping from a difficult situation. These patients are more likely to suffer from symptoms of depression and have strong perfectionistic tendencies.

Treatment

For the clinician trying to determine relative risk, the likelihood of successful follow-up is critically important. Studies that examine this issue do not paint an optimistic picture. Approximately 14% of patients evaluated in an emergency setting for suicidal behavior never attend an outpatient mental health appointment. Thirty-three percent attend only one or two sessions, and 24% appear three or four times. A history of previous hospitalization improves outpatient follow-through, probably due to the individual and family interventions that identify the relative risk of suicidal behavior, the underlying psychiatric issues, and the need for subsequent therapy. As a further indication of the relationship between severity and treatment compliance, patients with higher levels of suicidal behavior and depression are more likely to attend outpatient appointments (Spirito et al. 1992, 2002). Family factors also play a role. Children of mothers with health and drug and alcohol problems are more likely to attend sessions, as are children of families in higher socioeconomic groups. The relationship between high lethality and subsequent treatment also suggests that caregivers are influenced by the life-threatening nature of the behavior and the underlying psychopathology. The clinician can improve the likelihood of attendance by first educating both the patient and caregiver about the nature of suicidal behavior and the importance of treatment. As appropriate, comorbid psychiatric disorders and the role that substance use plays in escalating the lethality of self-destructive behavior are reviewed. Families should understand the nature and importance of the therapeutic process in both treating the underlying psychiatric disorder and preventing a recurrence of suicidal behavior. Clinicians should be aware of the obstacles to effective service delivery, beginning with the ED contact. Parents of young psychiatric patients treated in a medical ED frequently complain that they are ignored or avoided when presenting their child for assessment and care. Waiting times may be long for evaluation and then for disposition. Efforts should be made by ED staff to increase the number and frequency of positive interactions with family members, even while orienting them to the surroundings, procedures, and hectic pace that is typical in a medical setting. When necessary, translation services for patients and families should be immediately available to assist the clinician throughout the assessment and disposition. Families must also negotiate the idiosyncrasies of insurance coverage and the frustration of long treatment waiting lists that accompany a psychiatric referral.

A recommendation for psychiatric hospitalization is made when the patient actively voices suicidal ideation with intent. These are patients who typically have frequent thoughts about suicide that occur over long periods of time. They describe specific plans that are not only well conceived and potentially lethal but also feasible in their home environment. The clinician should recommend that firearms be removed from the home and that access to medications and sharp objects be prevented to decrease risk. Clinicians should be particularly concerned when during the course of the inter-

view, the idea of suicide seems perfectly acceptable to the patient. In addition, suicidal patients who present with a history of psychiatric diagnoses unsuccessfully treated in an outpatient or day hospital setting should be admitted to an inpatient unit. Youth who are intoxicated at the time of assessment or who have an active history of substance abuse are strongly considered for admission. Lack of available social support may indicate a need for inpatient psychiatric admission in order to guarantee appropriate psychiatric follow-up and a reduction in the patient's level of dangerousness. This is a much stronger indicator for admission in children than in adults. Medical hospitalization may follow a suicide attempt, and when the patient is medically stable but remains dangerous, a transfer directly to an inpatient psychiatric facility is necessary. Outpatient treatment is appropriate for patients who exhibit low levels of suicidal behavior and who are prepared to participate in outpatient sessions with the support of their caregivers. Studies do not support the validity of "no-suicide contracts" created as part of the assessment and as an indicator of future dangerousness. It is a valuable exercise, however. Clinicians should be more concerned when a patient is unwilling to sign or even consider such a contract. Physicians should not prescribe medications with overdose potential to suicidal adolescents until the patient is considered stable and cooperative with treatment.

Eating Disorders

Less than 30% of children and adolescents who have behavior that may be classified as an eating disorder tell their physicians (Kaye et al. 2000). The problem is frequently uncovered when the medical consequences of the behavior prompt an emergency room visit. Patients present with profound weight loss and even evidence of starvation. They can also appear fatigued with a general malaise that suggests both illness and depression. Parents and family members are typically baffled and repeat their belief that their child is eating normally. They may not realize that the patient is dieting when not at home, is exercising excessively, or is repeating restricting, bingeing, and purging cycles that prohibit healthy weight gain.

Identifying an eating disorder in the ED requires an understanding of the nature and variety of physiological consequences. Changes in physiology are among the best indicators of disease severity and the need for inpatient admission. Patients experience low rates of metabolism with evidence of lanugo, hypothermia, and cyanotic extremities. The clinical picture is consistent with symptoms of hypothyroidism. Abnormalities in glucose metabolism lead to episodes of hypoglycemia and ketoacidosis. Patients who fall into patterns of bingeing and purging in desperate attempts to manage their weight experience elevated glucose levels. Adolescents with diabetes learn that by avoiding insulin, controlling intake, and burning fat rather than carbohydrates they can lose weight. The dangerous consequences of ketoacidosis are ignored. Patients experience electrolyte changes as a consequence of fluid restriction and sudden water intoxication. Bradycardia, hypotension, and cardiac arrhythmias result from restricted intake or chronic electrolyte disturbances. Gastrointestinal disturbances can be dramatic and include constipation, obstipation, and severe abdominal pain secondary to superior mesenteric syndrome. Dental caries and parotitis are telltale signs of bulimia. Calluses appear on their fingers (Russell's sign) secondary to repetitive gagging. Long-term starvation leads to loss of gray and white matter on computed tomography or magnetic resonance imaging without signs or symptoms of a neurological disorder. Eating disorder patients are susceptible to osteoporosis and osteopenia due to poor nutrition and are subsequently at risk for fractures. More information on the physiological consequences of eating disorders are covered in Chapter 26, "Anorexia Nervosa and Bulimia Nervosa."

Substance Abuse

Adolescents who are drug or alcohol abusers have an injury rate 10% higher than control populations. A study of 667 adolescent ED patients noted that 25% of the sample was alcohol positive by breathalyzer test, with a higher percentage of these patients treated for injury secondary to assaults and self-inflicted wounds than for illness or other forms of injury (Kelly et al. 2004). Clinicians do not recognize alcohol use in as many as 50% of the patients who eventually test positive in the ED. The inability to identify these patients is due not only to a reluctance to pursue this issue aggressively but also to the absence of a quick and effective means of identification in most settings. Concise screening instruments such as the Drug Abuse Screening Test (DAST) or the CRAFFT must accompany the use of laboratory studies in the ED (Burke et al. 2005; Yudko et al. 2007). Substance use should be suspected when there is a sudden change in behavior. Warning signs include a decline in academic or social functioning. Patients may use substances in physically dangerous situations. Legal problems begin to mount after multiple run-ins with police and the courts. Caregivers begin to notice evidence of dependence including tolerance, withdrawal, unsuccessful attempts to control access and intake, and physical or psychological consequences. Consequences range from hepatic and gastrointestinal disease to the loss of friendships and alienation from peers. If the goal is a treatment partnership with the adolescent, the assessment of substance abuse requires support rather than recrimination. The clinician should listen and gather information from the patient before reaching a conclusion. An appearance in the ED frequently indicates a medical complication that alerts the patient and caregivers about the need for treatment. This is a "critical period" for insight and change individually for the patient and within the family system (Meyers et al. 1999). Patients with substance abuse disorders frequently experience comorbid psychiatric disorders, particularly depression. The relationship between substance abuse and suicidal behavior is well known and is assessed in young patients along with dysphoric mood, disinhibition, impaired judgment, and an increased level of impulsivity. Parental involvement is an essential part of successful treatment. Parental supervision may motivate adolescents to change their behavior. In addition, the relationship between substance abuse and the need for subsequent medical treatment encourages parental participation. Parents and caregivers play important roles when seeking to improve assessment and treatment compliance in the adolescent (Barnett et al. 2002; Spirito et al. 2001). Medical professionals should be aware of community resources for young patients with substance abuse problems.

Pervasive Developmental Disorders

Children with pervasive developmental disorders typically present with delays in language and communication; restricted, repetitive, and stereotypic patterns of behaviors, interests, and activities; deficits in socialization; and a presentation that parallels those seen in patients with severe and profound mental retardation. Unfortunately, their lack of verbal skills is not compensated for by other forms of communication. It is, therefore, important to complete a thorough physical examination for signs of the results of aggression, agitation, or self-abuse. In addition, the exacerbation of emotional or behavioral symptoms may be the result of pain or discomfort from otitis media, dental caries, or any other physical disorder. The ED is typically an anxiety-provoking environment for these patients and their parents alike. The sights and sounds are frequently unsettling, and there is a steady stream of medical personnel either caring for the child or monitoring his or her behavior. The patient's behavior in the ED may not simply be a reflection of the pervasive developmental disorder but rather a response to a chaotic and stressful medical setting. ED staff should provide a safe and quiet environment away from traffic where the door can close and the family be given privacy. The parent or primary caregiver understands how best to communicate with the child and establish a level of cooperation that allows for assessment and treatment. The parent should also be the primary source of information on the patient's needs during the ED admission and define the parameters of calm and safe surroundings for the child. They are a resource for the clinician and can, therefore, assist in the medical management of these patients, particularly the urgent administration of medications. Clinical staff should routinely check in on the patients while they wait for an examination as a method of ensuring their safety and preventing unforeseen complications. For autistic patients, these interruptions can be unsettling. A small and consistent group of clinicians soothes the patient by encouraging the development of simple yet familiar routines during even brief stays in the ED.

Children and adolescents with pervasive developmental disorders have heterogeneous responses to medications. Drug regimens should not be started without a specific plan for follow-up. For example, benzodiazepines (0.5–1.0 mg of lorazepam) may produce paradoxical reactions that further complicate care. High potency neuroleptics (0.5–2 mg of haloperidol) may induce extrapyramidal side effects leading to a preference for atypical antipsychotics to effectively manage behavior.

Delirium

Delirium is characterized by a serious decline in functioning that develops over a short period of time and is typically the consequence of a medical condition, substance use or withdrawal, or toxin exposure. The most common symptoms in pediatric patients include disorientation, irritability, inattention, memory loss, diffuse cognitive deficits, and "clouded consciousness" (Turkel and Tavaré 2003). Children and adolescents less frequently present with disorganized thinking, language abnormalities, and disturbances in sleep-wake cycle. Young patients in the ED with the sudden

appearance of delusions, visual or auditory hallucinations, illusions, and affective lability are typically experiencing these acute mental status changes as a consequence of a physical illness. Critically ill patients in the ED are vulnerable to delirium secondary to the direct physiological effects of the disease, including metabolic abnormalities, changes in oxygen saturation, and volume depletion. The relative risk of the disorder is related to illness severity.

Diagnosing delirium in children and adolescents is challenging for a variety of reasons. Physicians typically do not conduct objective screening for acute mental status changes in young patients, and when they do so, symptoms are described in ambiguous diagnostic terminology. The clinical significance of the disorder for the comfort and welfare of the patient is not well understood. Delirium may prolong hospitalization and increase complication rates because patients are unable to actively participate in treatment. Clinicians more easily identify the "hyperactive" form of delirium that manifests with irritability, agitation, disorientation, and abnormalities of thought and perception. Although these patients may be considered simply oppositional management problems early in the course of their treatment, the extent of their symptomatology eventually leads to a psychiatric consultation. The "hypoactive" presentation is less well recognized and understood. These patients are quietly confused and anxious and are often misdiagnosed as depressed. Delirium typically presents with fluctuating levels of severity with lucid intervals followed by periods of confusion and agitation. Serial assessments are, therefore, required in order to adequately diagnose the disorder. Eliminating the organic cause of delirium is the most effective treatment. Quite often, patients present with multifactorial causes that are not easily identified or controlled.

Delirium originates with an acute insult to the central nervous system (CNS) that can manifest in the ED with infectious, traumatic, circulatory, neoplastic, degenerative, or toxic etiology. Illnesses may indirectly affect the CNS through a variety of mechanisms. *Hepatic encephalopathy*, for example, causes a decrease in acetylcholine synthesis, increased levels of serotonin and dopamine, and an increase in γ-aminobutyric acid (GABA) activity leading to a hypoactive-hypoalert presentation. *Burn injury* creates a hypermetabolic state with an increased turnover of glucose and inconsistent insulin secretion. The result can be either hypo- or hyperglycemia. Hemodynamic, metabolic, and hypothalamic changes in these children affect brain functioning. Children are more susceptible than adults to symptoms of delirium due to their small surface area and developing brains. Several case studies document acute changes in mental status in pediatric patients with *seizure disorders* (Benson and Klein 2001; Zorc and Ludwig 2004). Children experience confusion, lethargy, emotional lability, and disorientation before losing consciousness. Among the more common etiologies for acute mental status change following the sudden onset of a seizure disorder are viral infections and cerebral vasculitis. Delirium may be the initial indication of *systemic lupus erythematosus.* Patients present with changes in behavior, mood, and personality with evidence of social withdrawal, confusion, noncompliance, bizarre and disorganized behavior, and sleep continuity disorders. There may also be evidence of abnormalities of thought and perception including auditory, visual, and tactile hallucinations. Delirium following *steroid administration* was initially described in the 1950s. There is no dose-response relationship, but symptoms appear in a bimodal distribution, either after 4 days or after 15–25 days of treatment (Sirois 2003). Physicians misinterpret symptoms of delirium as indicators of inadequate pain management and aggressively treat these patients with narcotics. Unfortunately, these medications may cause a further deterioration in mental status. In a retrospective review, nondelirious adult patients received most of their pain medications during the day. Delirious patients received their medications for "breakthrough pain" at night, at a time when they typically experience an exacerbation of their symptoms in a presentation characterized as "sundowning" (Gagnon et al. 2001).

A study by Kakuma et al. (2003) described outcomes in a geriatric population evaluated and discharged from an ED and demonstrated the importance of adequate diagnosis and treatment. Both the geriatric and pediatric populations are considered vulnerable to acute mental status change, and so the results may be relevant to children as well. There was a 50% nondetection rate among older adult patients in the ED based on patient interviews and retrospective chart reviews. When misdiagnosed and discharged from the ED, delirious patients had a higher mortality in the first 6 months than nondelirious patients. Subjects who were appropriately diagnosed with delirium did not demonstrate a shorter survival.

The most effective treatment for delirium is the correction of the underlying medical cause of the disorder. When that is not possible, the clinician treats the symptoms in order to ease the distress of the patient and family and improve the medical outcome (American Psychiatric Association 1999). Serial assessments should be performed, given the waxing and waning nature of the disorder. The diagnosis is explained to the family as a consequence of the medical illness or its treatment. The patient is oriented frequently by consistent caregivers in the family or on the clinical staff. The environment in the examination room should neither over- nor understimulate the patient. Antipsychotic medications are recommended when the symptoms are persistent, severe, and affect the child's medical outcome. High potency neuroleptics are known to be effective, based on controlled trials in adults using standardized assessments. Haloperidol is administered at a low dose of 1 mg and titrated up by 0.25 mg to 0.5 mg increments (Tabet and Howard 2001). Atypical antipsychotics are now recommended in the adult literature, primarily because of the lower risk of extrapyramidal side effects (Preval et al. 2004; Sipahimalani and Masand 1998). Benzodiazepines alone are rarely effective in children and may complicate or exacerbate symptoms of delirium.

Management of the Aggressive Pediatric Patient

Violent behavior increases the likelihood that the patient will present in the ED. Payment for psychiatric hospitalization by both private and public organizations is based on the level of dangerousness rather than on the need for treatment. The system, therefore, supports the referral of aggressive patients to the ED for admission. The circumstances in the ED often dictate the course of treatment and the techniques used to manage the patient (American Academy of Child and Adolescent Psychiatry 2002). When evaluating children and adolescents, ED clinicians may not be aware of premorbid psychiatric histories and therefore may make decisions that affect the safety of the patient and staff based solely on the urgency of the situation. In addition, there are no evidence-based guidelines on how to best manage the dangerous patient in the ED. Children and adolescents supported by public aid are more likely to present with psychiatric emergencies. This interaction is an indication of the relationship between social and family functioning, the availability of mental health services, and the development of emergent psychiatric conditions. In addition, the ED has become the primary treatment site for many patients with chronic and severe mental illness. Agitated patients require more time and attention from the ED staff in order to identify the behaviors that trigger the patient's loss of control.

During the assessment, it is wise to inform the patient of the impact of his or her behavior on others and the fear he is eliciting among staff members, including the interviewer. Denying the impact of the patient's behavior on others may be perceived as a provocative challenge and result in an escalation of the aggressive symptoms. Irritable adolescents and children should be carefully assessed and approached in a calm and solicitous manner that avoids potentially antagonistic positions. The clinician negotiates with the patient in an attempt to meet his or her immediate needs. This assistance could include voluntary medications to calm the agitation. If the child or adolescent does not respond to a verbal reassurance, it may be necessary to provide a "show of force." This conveys a message to the patient that some external control will be placed on his or her behavior. Hospital security staff can effectively deter acting-out behaviors simply by being visible in sufficient numbers. Security's involvement may not necessarily be accompanied by any recommendations for action unless the patient engages in behaviors that are obviously a danger to himself or herself or to others. At this point, the staff should be prepared to initiate more direct interventions in the event that the patient's aggressive behavior rapidly escalates.

The child or adolescent should not be left alone but should instead remain in the company of a family member, caregiver, or ED staff member. When alone, the aggressive patient may ruminate about incidents that led to the admission and become increasingly anxious about the assessment and disposition from the ED. This increases the risk of escalation, physical aggression, and injury to staff, family, and patient. Behavior that is considered dangerous to the patient and others in the ED may require the administration of medication or the use of physical restraints or seclusion.

Seclusion and Restraint

Emphasis on the appropriate use of seclusion and restraint began with an exposé in the *Hartford Courant* (Weiss et al. 1998), stating that over a 10-year period, 142 people died during or after restraint or seclusion in local psychiatric facilities, mental retardation centers, or group homes. A disproportional number of these deaths occurred in children (15% of the sample, but 26% of the deaths). Some investigators questioned the validity of the statistical methods used in the study to determine these figures, but the story prompted a strong response from patient advocacy groups, the

Centers for Medicare and Medicaid Services (CMS), and the Joint Commission on Accreditation of Healthcare Organizations (JCAHO; now known as The Joint Commission). The result was a demand for specific guidelines for the initiation, use, and monitoring of seclusion and restraint.

The routine use of seclusion and restraint reflects the limited options available to staff when caring for the aggressive and unstable patient. Therefore, according to opponents, seclusion and restraint are legitimized within facilities without question or without evidence of effectiveness. Studies examined the use of restraint in medical and psychiatric settings and noted that physical or mechanical restraints were more likely to follow assaults against staff members than other patients (Garrison et al. 1989). The fear in these scenarios is that clinicians will use their own anger and frustration as indications for restraint. This is coupled with a general concern by patient advocates that physicians may abuse their "police" power and unnecessarily impose these controls on patients.

The definition of agitation, aggression, or psychiatric emergency varies by location and sometimes by clinician. In critical care settings, the reasons cited for restraint emphasize accident prevention and controlling interference with medical treatments. The Joint Commission and the CMS allow for medical immobilization—restrictive procedures that are necessary in order to facilitate healing and support a level of compliance that is beyond the developmental capabilities of the young patient. The remaining situations require appropriate neuropsychiatric assessments to identify the etiology of the aggressive and agitated behavior and determine an appropriate treatment course. When staff are trained on the management of circumstances that both precede and accompany seclusion and restraint, these interventions are used less frequently, and there are fewer incidents of patient and staff injury (Bower et al. 2003; Busch and Shore 2000). CMS defines the use of restraints as follows: "Managing behavioral emergencies is allowed only when all less restrictive measures have failed and unanticipated severely aggressive or destructive behavior places the patient or others in imminent danger." *Physical restraint* involves the use of physical force by one or more staff members to restrict the movement of the patient. *Chemical restraint* is the use of medications to either restrict patient movement or to control the normal functioning of at least part of the body. *Interventions* are defined as seclusion when the patient is placed alone in a room under the following circumstances: 1) the patient is behind a locked door, 2) the door is either held by staff members or locked with a spring-loaded latch, 3) free movement of the patient is inhibited in any manner, and 4) the patient is actively separated and taken to a specific location away from the group.

With the implementation of new guidelines from The Joint Commission, trends in the use of seclusion and restraint became more relevant. Allen and Currier (2004) noted that these interventions are used more frequently in hospitals based in large urban areas with populations greater than one million. There is less familiarity with the patients, less information available on the psychiatric and medical histories, and a more impersonal approach, particularly in the ED. The risk of assault from the patients is three times higher for nurses than for physicians. The use of restraints, therefore, is not simply to maintain an orderly environment but to protect staff members, a high percentage of them probably female, from attack and possible injury. There are obvious racial and ethnic trends as well. African American and Hispanic patients are more likely to experience seclusion and restraint during hospitalization than white youth. For African American children and adolescents, the rate is nearly double that of whites. Younger patients, between the ages of 5 and 11 years, are secluded and restrained more often than adolescents, suggesting that smaller and less intimidating patients are easier targets (D'Orio et al. 2004). These trends can also be at least partially explained by patterns in the provision of health care. Minorities are less likely to use psychiatric outpatient services. In fact, they are half as likely as whites to receive treatments from any community source. Therefore, when assessment and treatment are necessary, the behavior is severe enough to require emergency services and the most restrictive levels of care. These situations present significant potential for discrimination. Biased perceptions of assault risk exist when patient groups (racial, ethnic, socioeconomic) are unfamiliar to professional staff. This also demonstrates the need for cultural competence and sensitivity among the clinical staff when employing these interventions.

The guidelines for the application of seclusion and restraint are thoroughly outlined by The Joint Commission (Table 39–3). A continuation of seclusion and restraint can be ordered by a qualified and trained individual authorized by the hospital or treatment facility. Restraint does not include "therapeutic holds" that last for 30 minutes or less. The Joint Commission allows the licensed independent practitioner to delegate tasks to physician's assistants and advanced practice nurses. Recently, The Joint Commission modified the guidelines and allowed more flexibility in their appli-

TABLE 39–3. The Joint Commission guidelines for the use of seclusion and restraint

1. Restraint/seclusion is initiated by an individual order from a licensed independent practitioner
2. The family is notified of the initiation of restraint or seclusion
3. The licensed independent practitioner sees and evaluates the patient when restraint or seclusion is initiated
   a. Within 4 hours of initiation for patients 18 years or older
   b. Within 2 hours of initiation for patients 17 years and younger
   c. Within 24 hours of initiation if the patient is no longer in restraint or seclusion
4. Written and verbal orders are time limited
   a. 4 hours for patients 18 years of age or older
   b. 2 hours for children ages 9–17
   c. 1 hour for children under age 9
5. Patients in seclusion or restraint are routinely reevaluated
   a. Every 4 hours for patients 18 years of age or older
   b. Every 2 hours for children ages 9–17
   c. Every 1 hour for children under age 9
6. Patients in seclusion or restraint are continuously monitored
7. Qualified nurses can now initiate restraint and seclusion without the presence of a licensed independent practitioner
8. Patients and staff participate in a debriefing session after the restraint or seclusion is complete
9. Staff document all aspects of seclusion and restraint in a manner consistent with hospital policy

Source. Joint Commission on Accreditation of Healthcare Organizations 2006.

cation. Qualified nurses can now initiate restraint and seclusion without the presence of a licensed independent practitioner (Joint Commission on Accreditation of Healthcare Organizations 2006).

Following the publication and implementation of The Joint Commission guidelines for seclusion and restraint, studies examined the impact of these regulations on patient care. Among the positive findings are decreases in the number of episodes per patient and decreases in the duration of each episode. There is, however, an increase in the proportion of events associated with patient injuries and an increase in the use of prn medications (D'Orio et al. 2004). Both are indicators of escalating aggression. One possible explanation is that staff members are avoiding the use of seclusion or restraint until its application is inevitable due to the threatening nature of the patient's behavior.

Chemical Restraints

Chemical restraint is loosely defined as the use of medications for the sole purpose of behavioral control rather than as part of a plan of care for a diagnosable condition. This intervention is difficult to consistently identify in a medical setting primarily because accompanying documentation on the target behaviors and the underlying psychopathology is frequently inadequate. This issue is particularly true in the pediatric emergency room where every treatment decision, even those made abruptly to control aggression, is considered therapeutic by the clinical staff. To further illustrate this point, a survey of ED adult psychiatrists reports a belief that any medication administered in a behavioral health emergency setting is a form of treatment (Allen et al. 2003). In order to avoid chemical restraint, the patient should be appropriately assessed and medications prescribed in a manner consistent with the diagnosis. This includes medication prescribed on an as-needed (prn) basis for disruptive behavior. Pharmacological management of aggression is preferable to the use of restraints, particularly when considering the time and potential complications. In surveys of adult ED clinicians, oral medications are most commonly used in these situations, specifically lorazepam, haloperidol, and a variety of atypical antipsychotics, including risperidone with lorazepam, or olanzapine alone (Binder and McNiel 1999; Lukens et al. 2006). The atypical antipsychotics present a lower risk of extrapyramidal side effects than high potency medications and are effective for the treatment of aggression and self-injurious behavior in mentally retarded and developmentally delayed patients, as well as children with pervasive developmental disorder. Newer oral preparations that quickly dissolve in the mouth and are swallowed have become an option for agitated and uncooperative patients. Benzodiazepines are considered at least as effective in adults as haloperidol alone, but few studies are available in children. In the adult literature, intramuscular medications are recommended only in cases that involve uncooperative patients who refuse to take oral preparations. Oral risperidone is just as effective as intramuscular

haloperidol with similar onsets of action. Intramuscular ziprasidone with or without lorazepam is the treatment of choice followed by haloperidol plus lorazepam (Hilt and Woodward 2008). A study that surveyed pediatric emergency medicine fellowship training directors identified benzodiazepines, haloperidol, and antihistamines as the drugs most commonly used to treat agitation in their programs (Dorfman and Kastner 2004). The combination of benzodiazepines with either a typical or atypical antipsychotic may produce greater efficacy for symptoms of arousal as well as faster onset of action (Yildiz et al. 2003). There is, however, no consensus on the most appropriate medication strategy for the pediatric emergency psychiatry patient. Some simple recommendations can improve the quality of the patient's care:

- Administer repeated low-dose medications rather than a single high dose when titrating the drug.
- Combined treatments should be applied with caution and care.
- Use low-dose benzodiazepines carefully due to concerns about paradoxical reactions.

Use of Physical Restraints

Practical recommendations for the safe application of seclusion and restraint also followed the application of The Joint Commission guidelines. Restraint devices should only be those that are designed specifically for this purpose. This includes limb holders, abdominal belts, and vests. Makeshift restraints are always contraindicated because the devices are typically difficult to apply, are frequently tied too tightly but ineffectively, and are often uncomfortable and dangerous for the patient. The emergency team should anticipate the need for seclusion and restraint and identify roles for clinical personnel. This avoids confusion and encourages more efficient decision making in times of crisis. For example, the service identifies who makes the decision to initiate the restraint, who physically puts the patient in restraints, and who performs face-to-face assessments to evaluate the need for continued intervention. When applying a restraint, the prone position is initially safer for both patient and clinician. There is a lower risk of asphyxiation and of biting injury. Patients with medical considerations are restrained supine with their arms at their sides. Keep in mind that there are no randomized trials on the most appropriate method or position for restraint. No clinical trials demonstrate the most effective way to release a patient from restraints either. The process is best approached as an ongoing negotiation, with the clinician constantly communicating and reassuring the patient. Restraints are gradually released one step at a time, but the patient should never be left with one limb tied down. It provides too much mobility, and should the patient suddenly become combative, the situation may rapidly escalate into a dangerous incident.

Summary

Psychiatric emergencies in children and adolescents are occurring with increasing frequency in medical and mental health settings. Caregivers often do not work proactively to identify and treat behavioral and emotional disorders at the earliest stages, and even when

they do, services are not readily available. Symptoms progress and the severity of the clinical presentation escalates until the situation demands attention. As a consequence, these patients exhibit high levels of dangerousness to themselves and others. In emergency assessments, the clinician is often unfamiliar with the patient and must obtain details about psychiatric history and social environment from an agitated child and an anxious parent. The formulation and treatment recommendations are typically based on the current crisis and the need to ensure a safe environment for the patient and staff. The pediatric and mental health clinician should be familiar with features that identify the most problematic cases and be able to safely and effectively triage these young patients to the most appropriate care.

Summary Points

- The demand for emergency psychiatric care of children and adolescents is increasing along with the challenges of assessing and treating dangerous and volatile populations.

- Suicidal behavior can be characterized by lethality and intent, and disposition recommendations are based on risk factors for dangerousness.

- The emergent nature of eating disorders is frequently based on the presence of concomitant medical complications along with a history of failed outpatient treatment.

- Substance abuse is underrecognized in the ED, indicating a need for assessment and intervention whenever substance use is suspected.

- The ED is often a threatening and anxiety-provoking setting for a young patient with pervasive developmental disorder.

- Delirium should be suspected in patients who experience a sudden change in behavior as a consequence of a medical condition, substance use or withdrawal, or toxin exposure.

- Management of the agitated and aggressive child should take into account the safety of the patient and staff and follow the guidelines outlined by The Joint Commission.

References

Allen MH, Currier GW: Use of restraints and pharmacotherapy in academic psychiatric emergency services. Gen Hosp Psychiatry 26:42–49, 2004

Allen MH, Currier GW, Hughes DG, et al: Treatment of behavioral emergencies: a summary of the Expert Consensus Guidelines. J Psychiatr Pract 9:16–38, 2003

American Academy of Child and Adolescent Psychiatry: Practice Parameter for the prevention and management of aggressive behavior in child and adolescent psychiatric institutions, with special reference to seclusion and restraint. J Am Acad Child Adolesc Psychiatry 41:4s–25s, 2002

American Psychiatric Association: Practice guideline for the treatment of patients with delirium. Am J Psychiatry 156(suppl):1–20, 1999

Barnett NP, Lebeau-Craven R, O'Leary TA, et al: Predictors of motivation to change after medical treatment for drinking-related events in adolescents. Psychol Addict Behav 16:106–112, 2002

Benson PJ, Klein EJ: New-onset absence status epilepsy presenting as altered mental status in a pediatric patient. Ann Emerg Med 37:402–405, 2001

Binder RL, McNiel DE: Emergency psychiatry: contemporary practices in managing acutely violent patients in 20 psychiatric emergency rooms. Psychiatr Serv 50:1553–1554, 1999

Bower FL, McCullough CS, Timmons ME: A synthesis of what we know about the use of physical restraints and seclusion with patients in psychiatric and acute care settings: 2003 update. Sigma Theta Tau International 10:1, 2003

Burke PJ, O'Sullivan J, Vaughan BL: Adolescent substance use: brief interventions by emergency care providers. Pediatr Emerg Care 21:770–776, 2005

Busch AB, Shore MF: Seclusion and restraint: a review of recent literature. Harv Rev Psychiatry 8:261–270, 2000

Centers for Disease Control and Prevention: Mortality tables, in National Center for Health Statistics Data Warehouse. Atlanta, GA, Centers for Disease Control and Prevention, 2007. Available at: http://www.cdc.gov/nchs/datawh/statab/unpubd/mortabs.htm. Accessed September 2007.

Christodulu KV, Lichenstein R, Weist MD, et al: Psychiatric emergencies in children. Pediatr Emerg Care 18:268–270, 2002

D'Orio BM, Purselle D, Stevens D, et al: Reduction of episodes of seclusion and restraint in a psychiatric emergency service. Psychiatr Serv 55:581–583, 2004

Dorfman K, Kastner B: The use of restraint for pediatric psychiatric patients in emergency departments. Pediatr Emerg Care 20:151–156, 2004

Gagnon B, Lawlor PG, Mancini IL, et al: The impact of delirium on the circadian distribution of break through analgesia in advanced cancer patients. J Pain Symptom Manage 22:826–833, 2001

Garrison WT, Ecker B, Friedman M, et al: Aggression and counter aggression during child psychiatric hospitalization. J Am Acad Child Adolesc Psychiatry 29:242–250, 1989

Hilt RJ, Woodward TA: Agitation treatment for pediatric emergency patients. J Am Acad Child Adolesc Psychiatry 47:132–138, 2008

Joint Commission on Accreditation of Healthcare Organizations: Comprehensive Accreditation Manual for Hospitals: The Official Handbook. Oakbrook Terrace, IL, Joint Commission on Accreditation of Healthcare Organizations, 2006

Kakuma R, Galbaud du Fort G, Arsenault L, et al: Delirium in older emergency department patients discharged home: effect on survival. J Am Geriatr Soc 51:443–450, 2003

Kaye WH, Frank GK, Strober M: Anorexia and bulimia nervosa. Annu Rev Med 51:299–313, 2000

Kelly TM, Donovan JE, Cornelius JR, et al: Predictor of problem drinking among older adolescent emergency department patients. J Emerg Med 27:209–218, 2004

Lukens T, Wolf S, Edlwo JA, et al: Clinical policy: critical issues in the diagnosis and management of the adult psychiatric patients in the emergency department. Ann Emerg Med 47:79–99, 2006

Meyers K, Hagan TA, Zaniz D, et al: Critical issues in adolescent substance use assessment. Drug Alcohol Depend 55:235–246, 1999

Olshaker JS, Browne B, Jerrard DA, et al: Medical clearance and screening of psychiatric patients in the emergency department. Acad Emerg Med 4:124–128, 1997

Preval H, Klotz SG, Southard R, et al: Rapid-acting IM ziprasidone in a psychiatric emergency service: a naturalistic study. Gen Hosp Psychiatry 27:140–144, 2004

Sipahimalani A, Masand PS: Olanzapine in the treatment of delirium. Psychosomatics 39:422–430, 1998

Sirois F: Steroid psychosis. Gen Hosp Psychiatry 25:27–33, 2003

Spirito A, Plummer B, Gispert M, et al: Adolescent suicide attempters: outcomes at follow-up. Am J Orthopsychiatry 62:464–468, 1992

Spirito A, Lewander W, Levy S, et al: Emergency department assessment of adolescent suicide attempters: factors related to short-term follow-up outcome. Pediatr Emerg Care 20:6–12, 1994

Spirito A, Barnett NP, Lewander W, et al: Risks associated with alcohol-positive status among adolescents in the emergency department: a matched case-control study. J Pediatr 139:694–699, 2001

Spirito A, Boergers J, Donaldson D, et al: An intervention trial to improve adherence to community treatment by adolescents following a suicide attempt. J Am Acad Child Adolesc Psychiatry 41:435–442, 2002

Sullivan DJ: Minors and emergency medicine. Emerg Med Clin North Am 11:841–851, 1993

Tabet N, Howard R: Optimizing management of delirium: patients with delirium should be treated with care. BMJ 322:1602–1603, 2001

Turkel SB, Tavaré CJ: Delirium in children and adolescents. J Neuropsychiatry Clin Neurosci 15:431–435, 2003

Weiss EM, Altamira D, Blinded DF, et al: Deadly restraint: a Hartford Courant investigative report. Hartford Courant (serial online), October 11–15, 1998

Yildiz A, Sachs GS, Turgay A: Pharmacological management of agitation in emergency settings. Emerg Med J 20:339–346, 2003

Yudko E, Lozhkina O, Fouts A: A comprehensive review of the psychometric properties of the Drug Abuse Screening Test. J Subst Abuse Treat 32:189–198, 2007

Zorc JJ, Ludwig S: A 12 year-old girl with altered mental status and a seizure. Pediatr Emerg Care 20:613–616, 2004

Chapter 40

Family Transitions

Challenges and Resilience

Froma Walsh, Ph.D.

This chapter addresses the challenges posed by major family transitions for child, adolescent, and family functioning. A brief overview places family transitional dilemmas in broad societal context. Normative and nonnormative family developmental transitions are examined, with focus on the effects of highly disruptive transitions with death; divorce and stepfamily formation; immigration; multicrisis families; and foster care. Clinical guidelines are offered to buffer stresses and strengthen resilience in youth and their families for optimal adaptation.

Family Transformations in a Changing Society

In the midst of social, economic, and political upheavals over recent decades, families have been becoming more diverse and complex (Walsh 2003b). It is useful to highlight the following trends: 1) varied family structures and changing gender roles; 2) increasing cultural diversity and economic disparity; and 3) varying, expanded family life course.

Changing Family Structures and Gender Roles

The 1950s-model family—white, middle-class, intact nuclear household, headed by a breadwinner father and a homemaker mother—is now only a narrow band on the wide spectrum of families (Coontz 1997). Family structures today encompass two-earner households; divorced, single-parent, and stepfamilies; extended kinship care; and families headed by gay and lesbian parents.

Economic pressures, career aspirations, and divorce have brought over 70% of all mothers into the workforce (Barnett and Hyde 2001). Two-earner and single parents must juggle job, household, childrearing, and elder care challenges. The assumption that mothers' work outside the home harms children has fueled maternal guilt and blame but has not been supported in research. What matters most is stable, quality care. While some families, particularly recent immigrants, hold a traditional patriarchal model and role division, most couples strive for an egalitarian partnership and shared involvement in childrearing. Most men carry more household and child care responsibilities than their own fathers did, although still much less than their wives' share (Lamb 2004).

Divorce rates, after rising in recent decades, have leveled off at around 45% for first marriages. Most children in divorced families undergo further transition with parental remarriage and stepfamily formation. Difficulties in combining households and forging new step-relationships contribute to the high divorce rate (near 60%) for remarriages (Visher et al. 2003). Nearly half of all children, and over 60% of poor, ethnic minority children, live for some time in one-parent households (nearly 90% headed by divorced or unmarried mothers) (Anderson 2003). Unwed teen parenting holds high risk for long-term poverty and for health and psychosocial problems for both mothers and children. Children generally fare well in financially secure and stable one-parent homes with strong parental functioning. Kinship care, particularly with grandparents, is increasingly common when parents are working or unable to provide care (Ehrle and Green 2002; Johnson-Garner and Meyers 2003; Messing 2006).

Increasing numbers of gay and lesbian single parents and couples are raising children. Research clearly shows that their children fare as well as those with heterosexual parents, although challenged by social stigma (Green 2004; Stacey and Biblarz 2001). Adoptive families have also been increasing for couples and single parents, gay and straight (Rampage et al. 2003). Most adoptions are now open, based on findings that children benefit developmentally if they know who their birth families are, have the option for contact, and in biracial and international adoption are encouraged to develop bicultural identities and connections.

Preconceptions of "the normal family" compound a sense of deficiency and failure for families in transition that don't conform to the intact nuclear family model. The term "single-parent family" can blind clinicians to the important role of a nonresidential parent or a caregiving grandparent and kin network. A stepparent or adoptive parent may feel inherently deficient when seen as not the "real" or "natural" parent.

Cultural Diversity and Socioeconomic Disparity

Growing numbers of children and families are multiethnic, biracial, and multifaith (McGoldrick et al. 2005; Walsh 2009). Therefore, clinicians must be attuned to the diverse beliefs and practices in families, their views of healthy development and dysfunction, and their preferred pathways in solving their problems. Strong kinship bonds foster resilience, particularly for African Americans, American Indians, and immigrants struggling to overcome conditions of poverty and discrimination (Boyd-Franklin 2004; Falicov 1998).

The gap of inequality between the rich and poor has widened. Many families are struggling anxiously through uncertain times. Those with limited education, job skills, and employment opportunities have been hit hardest. Declining economic conditions and job dislocation have a devastating impact on family stability and well-being (McLanahan et al. 2003). Persistent unemployment or recurring job transitions can fuel substance abuse, family conflict and violence, marital dissolution, homelessness, and an increase in poor single-parent households. Conditions of discrimination, neighborhood decay, poor schools, crime, violence, and inadequate health care worsen life chances.

Varying, Extended Family Life Course

With greater life expectancy, four- and five-generation families are increasingly common (Bengston 2001), as are two or more committed relationships over time, with periods of cohabitation and single living. Children and their parents are likely to transition in and out of several household and kinship arrangements over the life course. Some adults become first-time parents at the age when others become grandparents. Some start second families at midlife, with children even a generation apart. Our view of the family life cycle must be expanded to the varied life course that makes each family unique. For resilience, families need to buffer transitions and learn how to live successfully in complex arrangements.

Given the diversity of family structures, cultural and socioeconomic influences, and the timing of nodal events, no single model or life trajectory is essential for healthy child development (Walsh 2003b). There is abundant evidence that children can be raised well in a variety of family structures (Amato and Fowler 2002;

Lansford et al. 2001), yet disruptive family transitions are distressing, and highly unstable relationships increase the risk for child maladaptation. What matters most for healthy child development and resilience are caring committed relationships and effective family processes through stressful transitions.

Family Systems–Oriented Practice

Family systems practice approaches are guided by a developmental, multisystemic perspective on human problems and processes of change, attending to the family and social context of dysfunction and resilience (Rolland and Walsh 2008). This biopsychosocial orientation addresses the complex interplay of individual, family, and social influences, including school, workplace, court, and health care systems. It attends to cultural, spiritual, and socioeconomic influences, including the impact of racism and other forms of discrimination. Regardless of the origin of problems, families can play a key role for optimal child development.

The family is viewed as a transactional system evolving over the life course and across the generations (Carter and McGoldrick 1999). Individual and family development are intertwined, with each phase posing new challenges. Shifts in family organization, roles, and boundaries are required with relationship changes and with the addition and loss of members. Child distress often occurs around major family transitions, including both predictable, normative stresses and unexpected disruptions. Stressful transitions affect the family as a functional unit, with reverberations for all members and their relationships. In turn, family processes can heighten risk or foster positive adaptation (Walsh 2003a). Thus, the family is an essential partner in assessment and treatment.

A systemic lens is required to identify key members in the family system, including all household members, nonresidential parents and steprelations, the extended kin network, and other significant relationships (e.g., intimate partner, informal kin, and caregivers). Pets can also be vital resources (Walsh, in press). The *genogram* and timeline (McGoldrick et al. 2008) are essential tools to map the family system, noting relationship information and tracking system patterns to guide intervention planning. A resilience-oriented assessment (Walsh 2003a, 2006) searches for positive influences and potential resources alongside

problematic patterns (e.g., substance abuse, relational conflicts, or cutoffs).

Family functioning is assessed in the context of the multigenerational system over time. A timeline is useful to note the sequence of critical events or pileup of stressors and presenting problems. For instance, a son's drop in school grades may be precipitated by family tensions around his father's recent job loss. Because family members may not mention, or even notice, such connections, the genogram and timeline can guide inquiry and reveal patterns to explore. Clinicians need to inquire about family organizational shifts and coping strategies in response to anticipated, recent, and past stressors, particularly disruptive transitions. Family strain increases exponentially if a current crisis, such as a threatened separation, reactivates past trauma or loss (Carter and McGoldrick 1999). Families may conflate the situations, generating catastrophic fears. It is important to identify processes that promote resilience, such as active coping and perseverance, and to draw out stories of positive adaptation in facing other life challenges.

Childrearing Phases: Expectable Developmental Transitions

Anticipated family developmental transitions are more manageable than unexpected changes, yet they are stressful because family structures must adapt to meet emerging needs and priorities (Combrinck-Graham 2005). Symptoms often coincide with family developmental transitions. Families need to counterbalance continuity and change to provide stability through disruption and to maintain ongoing connections.

Transition to Parenthood and Early Childrearing

With the birth or adoption of a child, parents must reorganize their lives. For the development of secure attachments, they must be emotionally engaged and consistently attentive to innumerable demands. Raising two or more children requires even more juggling of time and resources. With the first child, transformations take place in a couple's relationship as they expand their bond from dyad to triad (Cowan and Cowan 2003; Falicov 1988). Each partner's identity and focus shift in new parental roles and the formation of a shared parental coalition. All life patterns are altered for new parents: time and space, money, work schedules, and leisure. Couples need to negotiate workplace-family strains and relational imbalances as well as childrearing values and practices, such as discipline. In many ethnic groups, as in Latino families, parent–child bonds commonly take precedence as the dominant dyad, which can generate tensions in the couple relationship (Falicov 1998). To prevent conflictual triangles, couples need to maintain their intimate bonds and establish generational boundaries with children.

Single parents function best when they can draw on practical, emotional, and financial resources in kin and social networks. When grandparents provide support, intergenerational tensions can arise over issues of authority, especially in a shared household. Problematic triangles occur when a mother and grandmother compete for a child's loyalty, affection, or obedience. Grandparents with financial or health concerns may become overburdened and resentful. Most functional is a caring, collaborative relationship, with clear coordination and communication.

Transitions With Adolescence

Family transitions with adolescence are particularly disruptive, requiring flexible shifts in family roles, rules, and relationships to fit needs for greater autonomy, separate space, and peer involvement. Parents often confront stresses on both generational sides, with financial, practical, and emotional support of their teenagers and their own aging parents. In one case, a mother's escalating conflict with her "out of control" teenage son was fueled by her anxiety that she could not provide care for her mother, whose worsening dementia was now "out of control." In other cases, past family-of-origin issues are reactivated. A close father-son relationship became stormy as the launching transition approached, replicating the father's unresolved conflict with his own father around leaving home.

Highly Disruptive Family Transitions

Nonnormative family transitions—unanticipated and untimely—are highly disruptive in family life, height-

ening risk for child and adolescent emotional and behavioral problems. The loss of a breadwinner's job or a parent's life-threatening illness can generate anxiety and family upheaval. The impact of death and loss will be considered first, followed by transitions with divorce and stepfamily formation, immigration, multicrisis families, and foster care, all of which require attention to loss for positive adaptation.

Adaptation to Death and Loss

Coming to terms with loss through death is the most difficult challenge a family must confront. From a family systems perspective, the transactional process involves those who die and all who survive in a shared life cycle, recognizing both the finality of death and the continuity of life (Walsh and McGoldrick 2004). A death in the family involves multiple losses: the person, the meaning of a relationship for each member, family role functions (e.g., breadwinner, caregiving grandmother), and special position (e.g., only child). Survivors experience the loss of their intact family and the loss of hopes and dreams for the future. A traumatic loss often is accompanied by "shattered assumptions" in family members' worldviews, such as predictability, security, and trust (Walsh 2007).

Variables in Child and Family Risk

The *nature and circumstances of loss* can increase risk for child and family dysfunction. Such situations include the following:

1. *Sudden death* leaves the child and family without time to prepare for the loss, to say good-byes, or to deal with unfinished business.
2. *Lingering death,* such as after a long illness, depletes family resources and generates both relief and guilt that a prolonged ordeal is over.
3. *Ambiguous loss* occurs when there is lack of clarity about the fate of a loved one who is missing or when there is psychological and relational loss of a loved one who is still alive, as in dementia (Boss 1999).
4. *Disenfranchised losses,* with socially unacknowledged losses (such as miscarriage, pet loss) or stigmatized deaths (as with HIV/AIDS or suicide), produce secrecy, guilt, and estrangement.
5. *Violent deaths,* such as a fatal accident, homicide, or suicide, generate lingering anger, guilt, or remorse and forgiveness issues.

The particular *timing of a loss* in the family life cycle may heighten risk for dysfunction; these types of risk include the following:

1. *Untimely loss,* especially early loss of a parent or death of a child.
2. *Concurrence of death with other loss, stressors, or transitions,* which may overload families and pose incompatible demands (e.g., grieving and attachment)
3. *Past traumatic loss and complicated mourning,* which intensify reactions to other transitions, especially with attachment and separation

Transgenerational anniversary reactions can be triggered by a current developmental transition. In each situation, the state of relationships and role functions lost will interact in effects. Unresolved conflicts and cutoffs have long-lasting reverberations for survivors. Reconnection and repair foster resilience.

Death of a Parent

Children who lose a parent or primary caretaker are at risk for long-term complications, such as difficulty in forming intimate attachments or catastrophic fears of separation and abandonment (Worden 2002). The kin network needs to provide support, structure, and reassurance that children will be cared for and not suffer further loss. Adolescents, with their own developmental thrust for separation, may minimize the meaning of the loss and withdraw, rebuffing family efforts for closeness and mutual support. If there has been conflict over autonomy and control issues, adolescents may develop guilt or long-term patterns of conflict with authority figures. Reactions are also influenced by peer models of acting-out behavior to escape pain, such as drinking, drug use, stealing, eating disorders, sexual activity, and pregnancy. For a surviving parent, financial and childrearing demands can interfere with mourning processes. Mourning can also be blocked if children suppress their grief to support the parent or if well-meaning relatives push for premature closure and precipitous replacement of a spouse/parent.

Death of a Child or Sibling

The death of a child is especially tragic, reversing generational life cycle expectations. Families often struggle with a sense of injustice and shattering of hopes and dreams for their child. Because parents are responsible for their children's well-being, their guilt and blame can be especially strong in accidental or ambiguous deaths. Miscarriages and perinatal losses, often minimized by others, involve the loss of a desired child and fear of future pregnancy complications. Well-intentioned relatives may push couples to try to have another child before they have grieved, complicating the new attachment.

Bereaved fathers commonly minimize their grief and vulnerability; too often only mothers attend support groups. The loss of a child places the parents' relationship at risk for conflict and divorce if they withdraw, grieve separately, or blame each other. Brief couples therapy or support groups can facilitate mourning, recovery, and mutual support.

With the illness and death of a child, the needs of siblings may suffer in parental preoccupation with caregiving or their own grief. In some cases, parents withdraw to avoid further vulnerability to loss or they become anxiously overprotective of surviving children and may have difficulty with later normative transitions of separation and launching. Survivor guilt, common for siblings and parents, can block life pursuits. A sibling may be inducted into an undifferentiated replacement role for the family, sacrificing his or her own developmental needs and unique qualities. Attempts at separation and individuation can disrupt the family equilibrium and precipitate intense delayed grief in parents. When a child is in crisis, it is particularly important to note other deaths at the same age and life cycle transition.

Case Example

After a suicide attempt, Dan, age 13, remained silent, and his parents were unable to comprehend his actions. They made no mention of an older deceased brother. A family genogram revealed that Dan's older brother had died of leukemia at age 13. Over the years, the parents never talked about their loss, to avoid their grief. Yet Dan, aware of their loss, had tried to assuage their sadness by taking his brother's place, wearing his clothes, and combing his hair to look like his photos. Now turning 14 and changing physically with adolescence, he didn't know "who to be," so he decided to join his brother in heaven.

The death of an adolescent can be agonizing for family members. The most common adolescent deaths are from accidents, suicide, and homicide. In cases of impulsive, risk-taking behavior, as with substance abuse or reckless driving, family members commonly carry intense anger, frustration, and despair about the senseless loss of life and future potential. Stigma and blame can block comprehension, communication, and social support. It is crucial to explore possible connections to other traumatic losses in the family and peer network. Inner-city violence takes a tragic toll on young lives, particularly in poor, blighted neighborhoods. The frequency of early violent death, especially for young males, contributes to a foreshortened expectation of their life chances and to a present focus, high-risk sex, and self-destructive substance abuse.

Facilitating Adaptation to Loss

Family adaptation to loss involves sharing grief, gaining meaning and perspective, and moving ahead with life. Bereavement has no orderly sequence, timetable, or final resolution. Facets of the grief process can resurface at such nodal points as birthdays and anniversaries. The multiple meanings of any death are transformed over the life cycle and integrated with other life experiences, particularly losses. Work with families facing loss requires respect for diverse cultural and spiritual preferences. Families may need help in tolerating members' varied reactions, coping styles, and pace. Four core family tasks facilitate immediate and long-term adaptation for children and strengthen the family as a functional unit (Walsh and McGoldrick 2004):

1. *Share acknowledgment of the reality of death and loss*: Information; communication.
2. *Share experience of loss*: Memorial rituals; empathic sharing of feelings and meaning-making.
3. *Reorganize family system*: Restabilize; realign relationships and role functions to provide continuity, cohesion, and adaptive flexibility.
4. *Reinvest in relationships and life pursuits, and transform bonds with deceased* from living presence to spiritual connections, memories, and legacies.

Divorce and Stepfamily Formation

Family transitions with divorce pose a series of challenges over time and are especially painful and disruptive through the first year. However, claims that divorce inevitably damages children have been refuted by longitudinal research (Greene et al. 2003; Hetherington and Kelly 2002). Despite some reports of a higher rate of problems for children of divorced parents than those in intact families, fewer than one in four children from divorced families shows serious or lasting difficulties. Financial strain and unreliable contact and support by the nonresidential parent heighten risk. However, the vast majority adjust reasonably well, and a third do remarkably well. In high-conflict families, children whose parents divorce tend to do

better than those whose families remain intact. Although grown children may have painful memories of the divorce, most have no greater difficulty developing committed intimate relationships than those whose parents stayed unhappily married. What matters most for adaptation is the quality of relationships with parents and between the parents before and after divorce (Ahrons 2004).

Longitudinal studies have tracked family processes associated with successful adaptation versus dysfunction: from an escalation of tensions in the predivorce climate, through separation, legal divorce processes, and subsequent reorganization of households, roles, and relationships (Hetherington and Kelly 2002). Divorce mediation and collaborative divorce counseling are recommended, except in extreme cases such as abusive relationships. Joint custody works well when parents can cooperate in decision making, child contact, financial support, and shared responsibilities. With serious conflict, sole custody and a primary residence are advised, with clear guidelines for support and visitation by the nonresidential parent (Bauserman 2002; Kelly 2007). The term "single-parent family" may blind clinicians to the potential significance of nonresidential parents. If barriers can be surmounted and a child's safety is protected, nonresidential parents often can become more involved in supporting their child's positive development.

Divorce adaptation is complicated by ambiguous loss: the family unit is dissolved, but parents move on in separate lives, forming new attachments, marriages, and families. Continuing contact between parents around child-related issues and events can arouse painful feelings. In contrast to the idealization and sorrow common in widowhood, divorce tends to highlight hurts and injustices, with anger and resentment often stoked by lengthy litigation and custody battles. Parents may need help not to disparage the other parent or triangulate a child in disputes or tugs for loyalty (Bernstein 2007).

Research on risk and resilience with divorce can inform efforts to help parents plan separation decisions and custody, residential and visitation options, as well as postdivorce transitions, such as changes in residence or remarriage and stepfamily formation. Clinicians need to explore previous family units, the timing and nature of transitions, and future anticipated changes. In particular, recent or impending changes in membership or household composition may precipitate a crisis related to presenting problems. Focusing only on the current household can result in tunnel vision.

Case Example

A single-parent father with custody of his two children, Matt, age 14, and Maggie, age 12, sought help for Maggie's stormy behavior with him. The therapist initially focused on the father-daughter relationship and parenting skills, without success. A developmental, systemic inquiry revealed that the father had divorced the mother 2 years earlier after learning of her infidelity. He won a bitter custody fight and continued to demonize her to the children, severely restricting their contact. He plunged into a new relationship with a divorced woman with two children, who was now pressing him to get married. Maggie was angry at having been turned against her mother, upset by her loss of contact, and resentful of the "replacement" mom in the wings. The father, in an individual session, then expressed his own anxiety about remarriage, rooted in his unresolved emotional divorce, shattered trust, and sense of betrayal. These issues required therapeutic work before moving on to consider remarriage and the complications of new steprelations.

Immigration Challenges

Immigration poses multiple challenges in navigating disruptive transitions and losses and adapting to a new culture and way of life. Immigrants often experience a profound loss of kin and social networks and a sense of rootlessness: between two worlds and belonging to neither. Ongoing stresses can be overwhelming—meeting practical challenges of housing, jobs, schools, and language barriers; navigating immigration laws, cultural rules, and customs; and experiencing marginalization and loss of identity and status.

Falicov (2007) has developed a multilevel model for prevention and intervention with transnational families, integrating three contexts in risk and resilience: the relational, the community, and the cultural-sociopolitical. The relational level deals with marital and parent-child interaction patterns that are a product of the migration experience. The community level addresses the loss of social networks and the reconstitution of new and old community bonds. The sociopolitical level attends to issues of cultural diversity and to encounters with prejudice and discrimination that affect adaptation.

It is crucial to assess the fit of children and their families with their sociocultural contexts. Family processes that may have been functional in their homeland may not fit adaptive norms and challenges in their new setting. Families and their children do best over time when they not only acculturate to "fit into" their new world but also preserve valued connections with their kin,

community, ethnic, and spiritual roots. If a parent finds it too painful to maintain contact with children left behind, those children's feelings of abandonment complicate later reunions. Divided loyalties can occur if the parent forms a new family in the United States. Resilience is fostered by weaving together a bicultural identity, sustaining cultural continuities, regular contact, and affective bonds that bolster health and mental health when coping with migration stresses. Stories and rituals that sustain links to cultural heritage are especially valuable for recent immigrant families, whose members can too easily lose their identity and pride in the pressures for assimilation to the dominant culture (Falicov 1998, 2003).

Spiritual beliefs and practices should also be explored. In many immigrant families, indigenous beliefs about spirit possession or traditional faith healing practices may not be mentioned unless a therapist inquires respectfully about them (Falicov 1998; Walsh 2009). Inquiry about family migration experiences should attend both to traumas and losses family members suffered and to the sources of resilience that enabled them to survive, regenerate, and make their way in a new world.

Intergenerational tensions are common between immigrant parents and adolescents born and/or raised in the United States. Frequently there is a clash of gender and cultural norms (for instance, for teenage daughters in traditional Middle Eastern families who want to date and socialize). Conflict often arises around authority and autonomy.

Case Example

Stavros, an Eastern European immigrant, brought his 17-year-old only son, Stavros Jr., for therapy to "straighten him out." He was furious that his son was hanging around with "no-good" friends and wanted to quit school. Steve (as the son preferred to be called) defended his friends and said he felt constantly pressured by his father to succeed academically. He looked down on his father's work as a janitor and felt badgered to make up for the father's "failure" in life.

The therapist encouraged Stavros to share his migration story with his son. He described the brutal military regime that he had fled, leaving school at 17 to escape being drafted. In the United States he took the only work he could find, adding odd jobs to send money back to his parents. In a hushed voice, he revealed his shame at his humble position and his poor English. Like many immigrants, he struggled tenaciously to enable his children to have a better life, putting away a few dollars whenever he could for his son's college education. He was so proud to have such a smart son. How could Steve not care about his future?

Despite initial disinterest in his father's story, Steve listened intently. Coming to realize his hardships and courage, his view of his father as a failure and a tyrant shifted to admiration and appreciation. Having felt only his father's disapproval, he became aware of his father's pride in him. The sessions also helped his father gain tolerance for his friends and activities as he came to understand Steve's differences less as rejection and more about finding himself and his place in American culture. He reflected that in demanding that Steve do everything *his* way, he had become like the dictator he had fled. Therapy helped to rebalance their relationship. Steve still needed his father's support in making his own choices for a good life. Cast in a new light, the very possibility of choice meant that Stavros had truly succeeded in his dream of a better life for his son, giving him the gift of freedom.

In this resilience-oriented approach, the therapist drew out the father's life story to help the son gain compassion for his father's struggles and appreciate his loving intentions. Reaching greater mutual understanding, the father became less controlling and more accepting of his son's autonomous strivings. In turn, the son became less likely to make bad choices for himself out of angry defiance.

Refugee families face myriad additional challenges, particularly overcoming experiences of physical and psychosocial trauma and loss. Many have fled persecution, brutal atrocities, or harsh conditions and have endured multiple relocations, with uncertainty about their future. Many have suffered traumatic losses of loved ones, homes, and communities. Marital and intergenerational tensions common in migration can be intensified by posttraumatic distress. Survivor guilt and anxieties about the safety of loved ones left behind can add to suffering. Refugees commonly do not use mental health services, feeling pathologized and stigmatized by labels of symptoms as mental illness. Most immigrants respond well to family-centered, community-based approaches. Resilience-oriented multifamily groups provide a respectful, supportive context to share their full experience of loss and suffering, as well as positive strivings for adaptation (Weine et al. 2004).

Multicrisis Families: Chronic Disruption and Instability

Family vulnerability is heightened by a pileup of stressors and disruptive transitions. Multiple traumas, losses, and dislocations can overwhelm coping efforts. Recurrent crises and persistent demands drain resources, especially for single parents. Family organization, patterns of interaction, and relationships can become fragmented and chaotic, contributing to abuse and neglect, youth substance abuse, and conduct disorder. When leadership is erratic and boundaries are weak, a child may be drawn into a parentified role to fill the void, such as "man of the house," or a child may be sexually abused. Constant stress and frustration can spark intense conflict. With inconsistent limit setting and discipline, frustration can trigger violence or threat of abandonment.

Families in poor communities, disproportionately minorities, are most likely to be destabilized by frequent crises, traumatic losses, abrupt transitions, and chronic stresses of unemployment, housing, discrimination, and health care. With neighborhood crime, violence, and drugs, parents worry constantly for their children's safety (Garbarino 1997). Bleak life prospects make it hard to break the cycle of poverty and despair, leaving parents defeated by repeated frustration and failure. High instability in their lives and relationships increases youth adjustment problems (Amato and Fowler 2002). Intertwined family and environmental stresses contribute to school dropout, gang activity, and teen pregnancy.

Even in brief therapy, it is crucial to understand how symptoms and catastrophic fears are fueled by a pileup of stresses, trauma, and losses. When therapy is overly problem-focused, it grimly replicates the patient's problem-saturated experience. A resilience-oriented perspective seeks to empower multicrisis families to manage their stress-laden lives. Interventions that enhance positive interactions, support coping efforts, and build resources are more effective in reducing stress and enhancing pride and more effective functioning. A compassionate understanding of struggles can engage parents in efforts to break dysfunctional cycles and raise their children well. All parents want a better life for their children, even when a myriad of difficulties blocks their ability to act on these intentions. They often know what they need to change in their lives and will take active steps if clinicians value their potential and support their best efforts (Walsh 2006).

By strengthening the family, the home becomes a more solid foundation for at-risk youth. If parents are unable to provide this structure, it is important to recruit positive models and mentoring relationships in the kin network to nurture their resilience (Ungar 2004). Seeing the whole family together may not be feasible in overstressed or fragmented families. Maintaining a family focus involves a systemic view that addresses their problems, repairs and strengthens bonds, and supports efforts for positive growth (Madsen 2006; Minuchin et al. 2006).

A strengths-oriented assessment lays the groundwork for therapist-family collaboration by prioritizing areas of concern and identifying potential resources in kin and community networks (see Chapter 56, "Family Therapy"). Genograms and timelines are essential to diagram and plan interventions with complex family systems, such as those with unstable households, multiple fathers, foster placements, or extended kin care. Seeing everyone on the same "family tree" can bring a sense of coherence for children in fragmented families.

With a family in perpetual crisis, therapists can get caught up in a reactive mode, responding to the latest crisis. Well-structured family interviews facilitate planning and proactive interventions to anticipate, avert, and buffer problem situations before they spiral out of control. The therapeutic priorities are to strengthen the family structure, stability, and leadership to provide nurturance, guidance, and protection. It is important to build positive connections in shared mealtime and pleasurable activities. Action-oriented, concrete approaches work best, with clear objectives and small manageable steps to build on successes. Tasks are designed to reduce stress and to strengthen cohesion and functioning. Therapy is present- and future-focused yet draws on each family's past. A parent may have been powerless as a child in a troubled family but can learn from that experience to become a better parent. Building on their potential, families gain hope and confidence that they can rise above persistent adversity.

Families and Foster or Kinship Care

When children are removed from their home to protect them from abuse or neglect, too often this transition is abrupt and traumatic, with complete cutoff from contact with parents and extended family members. Siblings may lose a vital bond when separated.

Traditional approaches to foster care—rescuing children from dysfunctional families—set up parents and foster caregivers as adversaries (i.e., the bad parents vs. the good parents).

In a collaborative resilience-oriented approach, family assessment expands beyond the risk posed by an offender to potential resources in the kin network. By involving family members in placement decisions, they are more likely to support the best arrangement for children. A family council—much like a tribal council—can be convened, rallying key members (e.g., a grandparent, aunts, uncles, or godparent) whose input

could be valuable. Together with professionals, they consider various options, taking stock of kin and community resources. This process reduces the sense that children are being removed by outside forces beyond family control, such as arbitrary court decisions. Decisions for child placement are made without robbing parents of humanity and dignity, and with hope that they can turn their lives around. Involving key family members also promotes their cooperation with a foster arrangement, ongoing contact with children, and investment in a successful placement experience.

With placement, maintaining the continuity of significant relationships for children is a priority. Planning should determine how they can be nurtured and protected from abuse *and* at the same time maintain some connections with their family network and their cultural and spiritual roots. Loss issues too often go unaddressed, particularly with multiple placements. Children are less likely to feel abandoned and unloved when ways are found to sustain vital bonds through monitored contact with parents, visits with relatives, phone calls, e-mail, cards, and letters. When direct contact isn't feasible (as with a parent's incarceration), photos and keepsakes, such as a favorite scarf, can be precious during separation. Upon the child's return to parents, photos, scrapbooks, and occasional contact (such as birthday greetings) from a former foster family help the child integrate the experience. Children can be encouraged to make drawings and keep journals to record their experiences, memories, and future hopes and dreams.

Recidivism in child placements is high. It is critical to plan the transition back to parents carefully and to link them with foster parents (Minuchin et al. 2006). Clinicians need to address the disruption and shifts in role relations.

Case Example

Terrell, age 8, was seen in therapy for anxiety and poor concentration in school soon after he and three siblings were returned to their mother's custody following her recovery from drug addiction. They had been living with their maternal grandmother for 2 years. In regaining their mother, the children had now lost their grandmother. The mother cut off all contact between the children and grandmother, still angry that the grandmother had initiated the court-ordered transfer of the children. Now becoming overwhelmed by job and child care demands, the mother risked losing custody again.

A systemic approach was needed to guide intervention efforts. Sessions with the mother and grandmother were held to calm the transitional upheaval, repair their strained relationship, and negotiate their changing role relations. The therapist facilitated their collaboration across households, with the mother in charge as primary parent. It was crucial to reframe the grandmother's role—not rescuing the children from a deficient mother, but supporting her daughter's best efforts to succeed with her children and her job. The children's vital bond with their grandmother was renewed in her after-school child care.

Follow-up sessions are crucial. Often, after an initial "honeymoon" period in family relationships, risk increases toward the end of the first year, with substance abuse relapses, return of an abusive partner, or a pileup of stresses. Periodic sustaining contacts can solidify gains and prevent recurrence of serious problems.

Clinical Approaches With Family Transitions

Brief family intervention is useful when the chief complaint is a focal problem involving a family transition. A preventive, early intervention consultation with a family can avert a major crisis or spiraling of distress. More intensive family therapy may be needed with multiple, chronic stressors or complications of past trauma and losses. Family members involved may include 1) those affected by a stressful transition, 2) those involved in problem maintenance, and 3) those who can contribute to positive adaptation and resilience.

Family psychoeducational models (Rolland and Walsh 2008) are finding useful application with families facing disruptive transitions and multistress conditions. Multifamily groups provide practical information, social support, and guidelines for stress reduction, management, and problem solving through transitional crises and stressful periods. Formats may include family consultations and brief or ongoing multifamily groups. Intervention "modules" can be timed with critical transitions to provide a psychosocial road map for navigating a long-term coping process, such as the initial crisis or chronic, terminal, or bereavement phases of a life-threatening illness (Rolland 1994). Stressors can be approached as ongoing processes with landmarks, transitions, and changing demands. Each phase poses challenges that may require varied family strengths. A brief transitional crisis demands immediate mobilization; afterwards, a family may resume accustomed patterns in living. In a transition with long-term ramifications, such as divorce, the family must grieve the loss of its precrisis identity and alter familiar patterns, as well as hopes and dreams, to accommodate a new set of circumstances. This framework can guide consultations and periodic family "psychosocial checkups" to strengthen family capacity to manage stress-related crises and to sustain efforts over time.

Summary Points

- Major family transitions are disruptive for all members and relationships; family processes can heighten risk or promote resilience for children and adolescents.

- A systemic approach addresses symptoms in the context of family and sociocultural influences and in relation to developmental challenges.

- A genogram and timeline are useful tools to note the influence of family transitional stresses in manifesting problems and to identify potential resources for resilience.

- Therapists work collaboratively with key family members to repair and strengthen vital bonds and tap resources for positive adaptation and resilience.

References

Ahrons C: We're Still Family. New York, HarperCollins, 2004

Amato PR, Fowler F: Parenting practices, child adjustment, and family diversity. J Marriage Fam 64:708–716, 2002

Anderson CM: The diversity, strengths, and challenges of single-parent households, in Normal Family Processes: Growing Diversity and Complexity, 3rd Edition. Edited by Walsh F. New York, Guilford, 2003, pp 121–152

Barnett RC, Hyde J: Women, men, work, and family: an expansionist theory. Am Psychol 56:781–796, 2001

Bauserman R: Child adjustment in joint-custody versus sole-custody arrangements: a meta-analytic review. J Fam Psychol 16:91–102, 2002

Bengston VG: Beyond the nuclear family: the increasing importance of multigenerational bonds. J Marriage Fam 63:1–16, 2001

Bernstein A: Re-visioning, restructuring, and reconciliation: clinical practice with complex postdivorce families. Fam Process 45:67–78, 2007

Boss P: Ambiguous Loss. Cambridge, MA, Harvard University Press, 1999

Boyd-Franklin N: Black Families in Therapy: A Multi-Systems Approach, 2nd Edition. New York, Guilford, 2004

Carter B, McGoldrick M (eds): The Expanded Life Cycle: Individual, Family, and Social Perspectives, 3rd Edition. Needham Heights, MA, Allyn and Bacon, 1999

Combrinck-Graham L: Children in Families at Risk: Maintaining the Connections, 2nd Edition. New York, Guilford, 2005

Coontz S: The Way We Really Are: Coming to Terms With America's Changing Families. New York, Basic Books, 1997

Cowan PA, Cowan CP: Normative family transitions, normal family processes, and healthy child development, in Normal Family Processes, 3rd Edition. Edited by Walsh F. New York, Guilford, 2003, pp 424–459

Ehrle J, Green R: Children Cared for by Relatives: Identifying Service Needs. Washington, DC, Urban Institute, National Survey of American Families, 2002

Falicov CJ (ed): Family Transitions: Continuity and Change Over the Life Cycle. New York, Guilford, 1988

Falicov CJ: Latino Families in Therapy: A Guide to Multicultural Practice. New York, Guilford, 1998

Falicov CJ: Immigrant family processes, in Normal Family Processes: Growing Diversity and Complexity, 3rd Edition. Edited by Walsh F. New York, Guilford, 2003, pp 280–300

Falicov CJ: Working with transnational immigrants: expanding meanings of family, community and culture. Fam Process 46:157–172, 2007

Garbarino J: Raising Children in a Socially Toxic Environment. San Francisco, CA, Jossey-Bass, 1997

Green RJ: Risk and resilience in lesbian and gay couples. J Fam Psychol 18:290–292, 2004

Greene S, Anderson E, Hetherington EM, et al: Risk and resilience after divorce, in Normal Family Processes, 3rd Edition. Edited by Walsh F. New York, Guilford, 2003, pp 96–120

Hetherington EM, Kelly J: For Better or For Worse: Divorce Reconsidered. New York, WW Norton, 2002

Johnson-Garner MY, Meyers SA: What factors contribute to the resilience of African-American children within kinship care? Child and Youth Care Forum 32:255–269, 2003

Kelly JB: Children's living arrangements following separation and divorce: insights from empirical and clinical research. Fam Process 46:35–52, 2007

Lamb ME (ed): The Role of the Father in Child Development, 4th Edition. New York, Wiley, 2004

Lansford JE, Ceballo R, Abby A, et al: Does family structure matter? A comparison of adoptive, two-parent biological, single-mother, stepfather, and stepmother households. J Marriage Fam 63:840–851, 2001

Madsen WC: Collaborative Therapy With Multi-Stressed Families, 2nd Edition. New York, Guilford, 2006

McGoldrick M, Giordano, Garcia-Preto N (eds): Ethnicity and Family Therapy, 3rd Edition. New York, Guilford, 2005

McGoldrick M, Gerson R, Petry S: Genograms: Assessment and Intervention, 3rd Edition. New York, WW Norton, 2008

McLanahan S, Garfinkel I, Reichman N, et al: The Fragile Families and Child Wellbeing Study: Baseline National Report. Princeton, NJ, Center for Research on Child Wellbeing, Princeton University, 2003

Messing JT: From the child's perspective: a qualitative analysis of kinship care placements. Child Youth Serv Rev 28:1415–1434, 2006

Minuchin P, Colapinto J, Minuchin S: Working With Families of the Poor, 2nd Edition. New York, Guilford, 2006

Rampage C, Eovaldi M, Ma C, et al: Adoptive families, in Normal Family Processes: Growing Diversity and Complexity, 3rd Edition. Edited by Walsh F. New York, Guilford, 2003, pp 210–232

Rolland JS: Families, Illness, and Disability: An Integrative Treatment Model. New York, Basic Books, 1994

Rolland JS, Walsh F: Family systems theory and practice, in Textbook of Psychotherapeutic Treatments. Edited by Gabbord G. Washington, DC, American Psychiatric Publishing, 2008, pp 499–531

Stacey J, Biblarz TJ: How does the sexual orientation of parents matter? Am Sociol Rev 66:159–183, 2001

Ungar M: The importance of parents and other caregivers to the resilience of high-risk adolescents. Fam Process 43:23–41, 2004

Visher E, Visher JS, Pasley K: Remarriage families and stepparenting, in Normal Family Processes: Growing Diversity and Complexity, 3rd Edition. Edited by Walsh F. New York, Guilford, 2003, pp 153–175

Walsh F: Family resilience: a framework for clinical practice. Fam Process 42:1–18, 2003a

Walsh F (ed): Normal Family Processes: Growing Diversity and Complexity, 3rd Edition. New York, Guilford, 2003b

Walsh F: Strengthening Family Resilience, 2nd Edition. New York, Guilford, 2006

Walsh F: Traumatic loss and major disasters: strengthening family and community resilience. Fam Process 46:207–227, 2007

Walsh F: Human-animal bonds: the role of pets in family systems and family therapy. Fam Process, in press

Walsh F (ed): Spiritual Resources in Family Therapy, 2nd Edition. New York, Guilford, 2009

Walsh F, McGoldrick M (eds): Living Beyond Loss: Death in the Family, 2nd Edition. New York, WW Norton, 2004

Weine S, Muzurovic N, Kulauzovic Y, et al: Family consequences of refugee trauma. Fam Process 43:147–160, 2004

Worden WJ: Grief Counseling and Grief Therapy, 3rd Edition. New York, Springer, 2002

Chapter 41

Psychiatric Aspects of Chronic Physical Disorders

D. Richard Martini, M.D.
John V. Lavigne, Ph.D., A.B.P.P.

Approximately 10–20 million children in the United States experience a medical condition that requires periodic intervention (Wallander et al. 2003). For most of these children, the condition is mild and requires routine, periodic intervention, but approximately 10% of these children and adolescents have conditions that affect them nearly every day (Wallander et al. 2003). Advances in medicine have improved survival to such an extent that nearly 90% of children whose conditions were at one time considered terminal are now living into adulthood (Thompson and Gustafson 1996). While some of these individuals will experience a full recovery, the number of people who must live with a chronic condition will continue to increase.

Psychological Adjustment

Most children with chronic physical illnesses are not affected emotionally, behaviorally, or developmentally by their condition (American Academy of Pediatrics 1993). There is evidence, however, that children and adolescents with chronic illnesses are at increased risk for emotional adjustment problems (Wallander et al. 2003). These patients are more likely to have internalizing syndromes, including depressive and anxiety disorders that appear early and persist over time (Breslau and Marshall 1985; Stuber 1996; Thompson et al. 1990).

Differences in the rates of psychological problems associated with various illnesses may be due to disease-related or family- and child-related factors. In general, disease-related factors seem to play a relatively small part in affecting the child's psychological adjustment. While illness severity might be expected to affect psychological adjustment to a chronic condition, in fact its significance is relatively minor and much less than family factors, such as parental mental health (Lavigne and Faier-Routman 1993).

Of greater significance than severity of the disorder in affecting the child's adjustment is the degree to which the central nervous system (CNS) is involved in the disease process. Disorders affecting CNS functioning (e.g., epilepsy, cerebral palsy, hydrocephalus) show higher rates of psychological problems than other disorders (DeMaso et al. 1990; Lavigne and Faier-Routman 1992; Noeker et al. 2005). Numerous studies have found that among conditions not involving the brain (e.g., cystic fibrosis, diabetes mellitus, or asthma), there is no relationship between disease severity and psychosocial adjustment (Campis et al. 1995; DeMaso et al. 1991, 1995; Shaw and DeMaso 2006). Exceptions may be found in cases where adolescents must cope with multiple chronic physical conditions (Newacheck et al. 1991) and/or long-term physical disability (Holmbeck et al. 2003). These patients are at greater risk for psychiatric disorder.

Models of Adaptation and Coping

Understanding the biopsychosocial factors associated with psychological adjustment and the development of psychiatric disorder among healthy children is a daunting task that becomes even more formidable when adding the biological, psychological, and social issues that accompany physical health problems. As a result, it should not be surprising that a variety of models of the effects of chronic illness on adjustment have been proposed.

Early Models

One of the earliest models was proposed by Beatrice Wright (1960). Wright's model posited a central role for the effects of chronic illness on the self-system, including body image, and on the individual's values. Wright argued that the self-system is not a unitary phenomenon but is organized in a systematic, hierarchical fashion, with some concepts more central than others. For example, most of us have a sense of ourselves as workers, and our sexuality is more central to our self-concept than, say, our ballroom dancing skills. Similarly, some aspects of our bodies are more important than others—e.g., our facial appearance is usually more central than

how our hands look. Wright argued that the impact of a chronic physical condition would be greater if it had an impact on something central or peripheral to self-concept or body image. Wright also noted that illness can have an impact on the individual's values. For example, the typical healthy individual highly values work performance and intimate relationships and tends to take health for granted, directing his or her attention and energy into the highly valued areas. The individual with a chronic illness, on the other hand, may value having a physical status "like everyone else" as a high priority. Because this is unattainable, it may affect his or her emotional state and lead to less investment in areas that could be more beneficial.

Wright's model was innovative, but regrettably, generated little research. Pless and Pinkerton (1975), however, integrated her work on self-concept with early work by coping researchers to advance the notion that both the self-system and coping processes were central to the adjustment of children and adolescents to chronic illness.

Recent Integrative Models

More recently, better articulated and integrative models of adaptation to pediatric illnesses (Thompson 1985; Thompson and Gustafson 1996; Wallander and Varni 1992) have been developed that emphasize the interplay between child and parent adaptation in adjustment. The ecological systems theory relies on a transactional model of stress and coping. Successful adaptation to the chronic illness by the patient and family is dependent upon an interaction between the disease and a variety of biomedical, developmental, and psychosocial factors (Wallander et al. 2003). The transactional model emphasizes the interplay between chronic illness and exposure to negative life events in the etiology of adjustment disorders. These adverse events may be a direct consequence of the illness and the way it alters life's expectations, or they may simply be the result of life's natural course (Wallander et al. 2003).

Factors Affecting Adaptation to Illness
Coping Style

An individual's approach to illness is affected by the cognitive, emotional, and behavioral responses that characterize coping style. For example, a method that directly handles the stressor and the subsequent emotional response is considered "approach-oriented." An "avoidance-oriented" style seeks to control upset by evading the stressor (Hubert et al. 1988). Patients and families may also deal with distress by taking a practical approach and focusing primarily on the problems at hand. Others struggle to maintain emotional control and cope by regulating their emotional responses (Folkman and Lazarus 1988).

The child with an acute or chronic medical illness should be encouraged to take advantage of the coping style that he or she identifies as most comfortable (Shaw and DeMaso 2006). There is no single preferred method, although some evidence suggests that a problem-focused coping style may be more effective in cases of chronic pediatric illness (Band and Weisz 1988). With increasing age, children are better able to choose from a variety of coping strategies based on the circumstances and their level of flexibility (Thompson and Gustafson 1996).

Developmental Factors

Adaptation to physical illness and the ability to garner the necessary coping resources depend on a variety of developmental factors. The understanding and use of medical information, the sense of illness causality and personal responsibility, and the need for compliance with treatment are all addressed in the context of the child's developmental level (Shaw and DeMaso 2006; Thompson and Gustafson 1996). For example, preschool children cannot grasp the complicated explanations that accompany medical diagnosis and treatment. Their adjustment is, therefore, affected by a fear of the unknown and the unanticipated (Melamed et al. 1982; Simeonsson et al. 1979). School-age children can recall and comprehend information about medical diagnosis and treatment. They worry over loss of control and an inability to protect themselves from harm. Assigning responsibility, and consequently blame, becomes an important element of emotional adjustment, particularly when directed at parents or themselves. Adolescents typically strive for independence, a sense of autonomy, body integrity, and identity. Physical illness is frequently an assault on these priorities, particularly when it involves loss of function and/or a change in appearance. When the illness is chronic, the age and developmental level of patients do not have a significant effect on the development of behavioral or emotional problems (Wallander et al. 2003).

History of Illness and Medical Experience

Children may be traumatized by difficult and painful medical procedures, some that recur as part of a treatment regimen and others that are repeated when clinicians are unsuccessful in their initial attempts. The patient anxiously anticipates similar experiences during subsequent hospital or clinic visits (Dahlquist et al. 1986). As a result, both child and family may begin to avoid contact with medical professionals for fear of re-experiencing these situations and the emotional aftermath. Medical care suffers because the patient does not receive routine services, increasing the likelihood of unforeseen medical complications that require aggressive attention and possibly invasive procedures.

Temperament

A child's temperament can influence the choices he or she makes in response to acute and chronic medical illness (Rudolph et al. 1995). Anxious children avoid medical interventions and in the process become more noncompliant. Children who are less affected by the illness are more likely to participate actively in treatment and inquire about their care and prognosis. Young patients with certain temperamental styles, such as slow-to-warm-up children or children with difficult temperaments, are more likely to suffer long-term behavioral and emotional complications (Wallander et al. 2003).

Parent and Family Factors

Anxious parents are more likely to be distressed by procedures and the uncertainty that frequently accompanies medical diagnoses. Unfortunately, their personal preoccupations leave them less available for their children's emotional needs. They cannot, for example, help their children generate appropriate coping strategies and deal with the immediate and long-term effects of the illness (Melamed 1993; Shaw and DeMaso 2006). Studies of parental psychopathology find that maternal depression and anxiety play an important role in long-term emotional adjustment (DeMaso et al. 1991, 1995, 2004; Wallander et al. 2003).

Families adapt to physical illness in three distinct developmental phases: crisis, chronic, and terminal (Rolland and Walsh 2006). The crisis or acute phase occurs immediately before and after the diagnosis of an illness, when most energy is spent to understand and manage the symptoms while coping with the grief that accompanies the loss of a healthy child. Medical disorders may be stable, progressive, or episodic in nature. The family adjusts to these characteristics during the chronic phase, with an emphasis on maintaining family stability, minimizing the impact of the illness, and providing appropriate medical care. The terminal phase follows the death of the child and involves managing and processing the feelings and responses that result.

Comorbidity of Medical and Psychiatric Conditions: Somatopsychic and Psychosomatic Relationships

There is a constant interplay between organic and functional factors in an illness, and it is difficult, therefore, to simply classify cases as either medical or psychiatric. Patients' symptoms evolve over time in a relationship that is clearly bidirectional. The inability to recognize psychiatric disorder in a physically ill child may prolong and unnecessarily complicate the treatment course. Psychiatric disorders in physically ill children include those conditions that existed prior to or following the onset of the medical illness and those that develop as a direct consequence of the disease. The former can be classified as coincidental comorbidity and the latter as causal comorbidity. An example of coincidental comorbidity may involve the care of a patient with preexisting attention-deficit/hyperactivity disorder who is diagnosed with diabetes. An example of causal comorbidity is the development of depression in patients with Addison's disease, because a deficiency in cortisol can lead to symptoms of mood disorder. Recurrent physical complaints that do not correlate with the medical findings are characteristic of mood, anxiety, and psychosomatic disorders. A good example is the patient with functional abdominal pain who also presents with panic disorder (Shaw and DeMaso 2006).

Psychiatric disorder not only affects the child's medical compliance, lifestyle, and adjustment to the illness, but there is also the direct impact on physiology and the disease process. For example, children with diabetes are at greater risk for depressive disorders (Kovacs et al. 1997). Young diabetics with comorbid depression who do not follow the treatment regimen are hospitalized more frequently and experience more disease-related complications (Garrison et al. 2005; Kovacs et al. 1995). Young asthmatics frequently suffer from depressive symptoms, and for inner-city children, mood disorder is associated with a worse prognosis (Waxmonsky et al. 2006). Dysfunctional and chaotic families exacerbate the child's depression and increase asthma symptom severity (Wood et al. 2006).

Categorical and Noncategorical Approaches

The psychological adjustment to illness is typically considered in the context of either a categorical (diagnosis-specific) experience or a broader noncategorical experience (Knapp and Harris 1998; Lavigne and Faier-Routman 1993; Thompson and Gustafson 1996; Wallander et al. 2003). Within a categorical approach, each illness is thought to differ from others in important ways psychologically. For example, asthma, diabetes, and recurrent abdominal pain are identified as medical diagnoses with characteristic patterns of behavior and reasonably well-understood interactions between the psychological and physiological aspects of illness. Therefore, from a categorical viewpoint, it is important to take a diagnosis-specific approach and consider these factors when planning treatment for certain aspects of these disorders (Campo et al. 2004; Hocking and Lochman 2005; Wamboldt et al. 1998).

A noncategorical approach identifies common aspects of the illness experience (e.g., visible/invisible, fatal/nonfatal, stable/unpredictable) when evaluating the child's response to a disease (Knapp and Harris 1998; Shaw and DeMaso 2006). For example, posttraumatic stress symptoms may appear following a number of medical interventions in both diagnostic and treatment settings (Stuber and Shemesh 2006). Developmentally, young patients who are paraplegic as a result of traumatic injury or congenital malformation frequently experience symptoms of anxiety and depression when faced with the expectations of self-sufficiency during adolescence and young adulthood. The family dimensions of cohesion, flexibility, affection, and expressiveness are important factors in determining patient outcome regardless of medical illness (Fisher and Weihs 2000; Lewis and Vitulano 2003; Vitulano 2003). The general illness models discussed above are applicable across disease groups and tend to be noncategorical in their approach. The models recognize that individual differences might affect outcomes—e.g., children with certain temperamental styles may do better than others in dealing with an illness, and presumably that would be true across types of illness. The general models posit, however, that key aspects of adjusting to a chronic illness are the same across disorders and that it is not necessary to conceptualize the psychological aspects of each disorder differently.

Impact of Chronic Illness on the Family

Most families with a medically ill child are well adjusted and productive. Individual members, however, are more likely to experience symptoms of irritability, anxiety, depression, and somatic complaints than the general population (Jacobs 2000). Shaw and DeMaso (2006) suggest that the amount of disability, predictability of the disease course and prognosis, any stigma associated with the disorder, and how much monitoring is required may affect the family's experience of, and adjustment to, the disorder. Parental behavior must also be understood in the context of family beliefs and prior experience with illness and death (Shaw and DeMaso 2006).

Along with providing the instrumental care and emotional support their child needs, parents must also deal with their own feelings about being unable to protect their child from disease and their loss of control over their child's life. Forced to rely upon professional help, parents are obliged to surrender certain degrees of control and may need to forsake their traditional roles. While successful coping may require parents to develop a good understanding of their child's illness, parents can become overly concerned with medical information and neglect both their child's and family's psychosocial needs.

The demands of caring for an ill child may affect the parents' marital relationship (Kazak et al. 2003). Parents may be highly supportive of one another and even be drawn closer to one another, but there is a risk that the marital relationship may be weakened, particularly if marital problems existed before the child's illness developed. When genetic factors are known contributors to the illness, a parent blaming himself or the other parent is not uncommon.

Parental response to illness can have both a beneficial and deleterious effect on the behavior of the physically ill child (see Shaw and DeMaso 2006 for review). In addition, family factors play a larger role in the child's adjustment to illness than do illness-related factors (Lavigne and Faier-Routman 1993). Both inappropriate responses (e.g., threats, punishment, relinquishing control to the child) and overresponding to the child (via excessive parental attention, reassurance, empathy, and apologies) can interfere with the child's ability to cope with his or her illness (Frank et al. 1995; Logan and Scharff 2005). Generally, a calm supportive response, the continuation of familiar "family rules," and appropriate limit setting are important for helping the child adjust to his or her illness (Peterson and Harbaugh 1995).

Siblings

Siblings of chronically ill children also show increased levels of emotional and behavioral difficulties, including increased shyness or anxiety when compared to control subjects (Kazak et al. 2003; Siemon 1984; Shaw and DeMaso 2006).

Depending on the illness severity, siblings may be somewhat "frozen out" of families preoccupied with meeting the demands imposed by the child's illness, occasionally becoming emotionally disengaged from busy parents, less able to engage in activities with the affected child, jealous of the attention directed toward the ill child, and feeling guilt about not being affected. Roles can change if a sibling's achievements surpass those of the child who is now limited by the physical illness. At times, siblings take on a parental role for the other siblings and do more caretaking for the ill child.

General Considerations in Psychiatric Management

Psychopharmacology

Psychotropic medications may be effective in the management of emotional and behavioral problems that accompany medical illness. Frequently, psychopharmacological interventions are instituted when the medical team believes that the psychiatric symptoms in the child are affecting the patient's care. The diagnosis of a psychiatric disorder is rarely made in these situations, and the treatment targets specific symptoms rather than syndromes (Shaw and DeMaso 2006). For example, a stem cell transplant patient becomes despondent and discouraged as she suffers through treatment complications and medication side effects. Members of the oncology team notice her lack of participation, social isolation, minimal eye contact with staff, and pessimistic assessment of her prognosis. They fear that she is depressed and that her mood problems are complicating an already difficult hospital course. A decision is made to start the patient on a combination of stimulants (short-acting methylphenidate) and a selective serotonin reuptake inhibitor (SSRI). The stimulant almost immediately improves her level of participation in treatment and her compliance on the transplant unit. The antidepressant gradually takes effect over the course of 3–4 weeks, improving her mood and her relationships with family and medical staff. With her progress on the antidepressant, the methylphenidate is eventually discontinued, and she is maintained on the SSRI alone.

Before starting the patient on a medication, the clinician should be aware of possible interactions between the illness and the treatment. Patients and caregivers should provide information on any alternative treatments or over-the-counter preparations taken by the patient as well as current medication regimens. Psychotropic drugs may have a variety of effects on the pharmacokinetic and pharmacodynamic properties of other medications, and these factors should be considered in treatment planning.

Young patients are affected by illnesses that impair organ systems and change drug metabolism—particularly those patients with hepatic, gastrointestinal, renal, and cardiac diseases. It is, therefore, wise to follow the axiom "start low, go slow" when initiating medication. Drug levels for psychotropic medications are not reliable indicators of efficacy or toxicity. In medically ill children, it is best to use one medication at a time and choose a drug with a short half-life that can be administered in single doses and that quickly reaches a therapeutic level. The medically ill child and caregiver are already overwhelmed with complicated therapeutic regimens. Simple and direct psychopharmacological recommendations will improve adherence.

Pharmacokinetics

Pharmacokinetics involves the absorption, distribution, and metabolism of medications (Robinson and Owen 2005). Medical illness, particularly as it affects organ systems, alters pharmacokinetics. Most psychotropic medications, with the exception of lithium, venlafaxine, divalproex sodium, methylphenidate, gabapentin, and topiramate are bound to protein at a rate of 80%–90%. The unbound drug is considered "active." Patients with chronic diseases of the liver and kidney lose protein and as a result are likely to have more unbound active drug. Most psychotropic medications are absorbed in the gastrointestinal tract, metabolized in the liver and gastrointestinal tract, and excreted through the kidneys. Diseases of these organ systems require dose reductions in order to prevent toxicity. In addition, any medication or illnesses that reduce hepatic metabolism, renal excretion, or blood flow to these organs should be considered when choosing a drug or medication dose (Shaw and DeMaso 2006).

Pharmacodynamics

Pharmacodynamics involves changes in the drug's effectiveness as a consequence of drug-drug interactions or modifications in drug receptor site binding. For example, the hepatic cytochrome P450 (CYP450) system is responsible for most drug metabolism and interactions. Clinicians should be aware of medications that either potentiate or inhibit the CYP450, particularly in medically ill patients on multiple drug regimens. In these situations, drug metabolism is altered and drug-drug interactions are more likely (Shaw and DeMaso 2006).

Medication Use in Specific Illnesses

Hepatic Disease

Hepatic disease lowers the first-pass extraction and biotransformation of medications. In the presence of liver failure, there is a greater risk for medication side effects, particularly after oral administration and with drugs that have a narrow therapeutic index (like tricyclic antidepressants [TCAs]). Liver disease affects the ability of medications to bind to proteins and affects the metabolism of most antidepressants, benzodiazepines like diazepam, and neuroleptics including haloperidol. With chronic liver failure, there should be a 25%–50% reduction in dosage because medications that are not bound to protein are more active. In cases of acute hepatic disease, alterations in drug dose are not necessary. When choosing an antidepressant medication, citalopram and fluvoxamine are less protein bound and therefore more effective than other SSRIs. Clinicians should avoid carbamazepine, valproate, nefazodone, and the phenothiazines due to hepatotoxicity. Intravenous drug administration avoids first-pass metabolism by the CYP450 system and may allow medication doses more typical for patients with normal hepatic function (Beliles 2000; Shaw and DeMaso 2006).

Gastrointestinal Disease

Drug absorption is affected by gastrointestinal mucosal integrity and motility, particularly when medications are given orally. Motility is altered by medications, including psychotropic agents (particularly those with anticholinergic side effects), and a variety of medical conditions including colitis and diabetes. Delays in gastric emptying or diseases of the small bowel (Crohn's) that affect the integrity of the intestine lead to poor absorption. This may also inhibit protein binding, leading to uneven drug distribution. Extended-release preparations generally produce less gastrointestinal upset because of the gradual exposure to the medication and the slower increase in plasma levels (Beliles 2000).

Renal Disease

Renal disease does not generally affect the metabolism of medications, with the exception of lithium, gabapentin, methylphenidate, venlafaxine, divalproex sodium, and topiramate. Lithium is excreted unchanged in the urine, and toxicity in the presence of renal disease is associated with a decrease in renal concentration ability. Occasionally, patients have nephrogenic diabetes insipidus with lithium toxicity. These problems are typically reversible but can become permanent if uncorrected. Significant dosage adjustments should be made in these cases. Clinicians should generally decrease doses and increase dosage intervals in the presence of renal failure. A good general rule is to decrease the dose by one-third in patients with renal disease. Hemodialysis initially lowers the plasma blood concentrations, followed by a rebound when the drug moves from the periphery to the circulation. Protein-bound medications are not typically cleared by hemodialysis.

Cardiac Disease

Cardiovascular disease affects perfusion of the liver and kidneys and the volume of distribution for the medication. This is particularly true with congestive heart failure and the associated fluid retention. Psychotropic medications may have direct effects on the cardiovascular system. TCAs cause both blood pressure and heart rate increases and are class I antiarrhythmics with quinidine-like properties. TCAs are potentially fatal in overdose due to the risk of arrhythmia. These medications are contraindicated in patients with heart disease and in patients with a history of suicidal behavior. SSRIs are associated with a moderate slowing of the heart rate but are not contraindicated in patients with heart disease. Bupropion increases blood pressure in adults, but similar changes are not documented in children. Lithium occasionally causes sinus node dysfunction and arrhythmias. Episodes of syncope with T wave flattening and inversion (typically benign) are also possible. Clonidine decreases systolic blood pressure and decreases cardiac output and heart rate although the medication does not cause clinically significant hypotension. Low-potency antipsychotics (e.g., chlorpromazine, thioridazine) with anticholinergic, antihista-

minic, and alpha-adrenergic blocking effects may cause hypotension. In addition, the medications have quinidine-like effects on conduction with QT prolongation. These side effects are also found in some atypical antipsychotics (risperidone). Haloperidol, administered parenterally in high doses, is associated with lengthening of the QT interval, torsades de pointes, and multifocal ventricular tachycardia. Stimulant medication is used with caution in patients with preexisting heart disease, including postoperative tetralogy of Fallot, coronary artery abnormalities, subaortic stenosis, or hypertrophic cardiomyopathy (Pliszka and AACAP Work Group on Quality Issues 2007). Children and adolescents with a history of syncope, chest pain, and palpitations are considered at risk for sudden cardiac death, particularly with a positive family history. In these cases, the patient should receive a thorough cardiac evaluation before beginning treatment (Alexander et al. 2005; Pliszka and AACAP Work Group on Quality Issues 2007; Shaw and DeMaso 2006).

Pulmonary Disease

Hypoxia and hypercarbia can affect pharmacokinetics of psychoactive medications by changing pH and affecting drug absorption and distribution. Patients in respiratory distress may experience symptoms of anxiety and panic in a direct response to increasing levels of carbon dioxide. Use of anxiolytics, particularly benzodiazepines, requires great caution if used in patients with respiratory disease because of their tendency to decrease respiratory drive. Should benzodiazepines be required, as in cases when it is necessary to alleviate anxiety in a patient in critical care as he or she is being weaned from a ventilator, doses must be titrated carefully. SSRIs can effectively treat anxiety in patients with comorbid respiratory disease. Buspirone is also considered an anxiolytic that is not associated with respiratory depression and may have mild respiratory stimulant effects.

Epilepsy

Psychotropic medications should be used with caution in patients with epilepsy, not only because of the seizure risk but also because of drug interactions. First- and second-generation antipsychotics can be used judiciously, with the exception of chlorpromazine, loxapine, and clozapine. Haloperidol has a low seizure risk. SSRIs generally do not present a significant risk; neither does trazodone nor the alpha-agonists. Bupropion is contraindicated because it lowers the seizure threshold. Lithium is considered a proconvulsant but can be used with care in appropriate cases. The U.S. Food and Drug Administration (FDA) states that stimulants are contraindicated in patients with comorbid seizure disorders, but data suggest that the medications can be used safely, particularly when the seizures are well controlled (Gucuyener et al. 2003; Hemmer et al. 2001). Benzodiazepines are administered as anticonvulsants but can cause seizures if withdrawn too quickly.

Psychosocial Interventions

Individual Psychotherapy

Psychotherapy provides the child with an opportunity to discuss his or her concerns and feelings about dealing with the illness or disability (Shaw and DeMaso 2006). While Wright (1960) emphasized the role of the self-system and altering inappropriate values in counseling with individuals with chronic illness, more recently, a bereavement model has been found to be useful in conceptualizing the process of adaptation to a physical illness as well as guiding treatment (Shaw and DeMaso 2006). The child's emotional responses to a physical illness or disability may be viewed as a process beginning with shock and denial and moving toward an assimilation of illness information and adjustment (Shaw and DeMaso 2006). There are several models of individual psychotherapies used with physically ill children.

In supportive treatment, the therapist seeks to provide a climate of understanding and acceptance through which the child can relate his or her experiences, begin to manage the strong feelings he or she feels, and get help improving the coping mechanisms needed to deal with the chronic illness experience (Green 2000).

In applying principles of psychodynamic psychotherapy, the therapist seeks to help the individual understand the emotional conflicts that contribute to the problem behaviors while adjusting to the chronic illness or disability. As Shaw and DeMaso (2006) note, this therapy is often limited by patients' diminished cognitive skills due to the illness itself and the limited time often available for therapy in the pediatric setting.

Narrative therapy, a relatively recent advance in treating children with chronic illness, allows children and their families the opportunity to share, organize, and validate their experiences and physical condition. Studies have shown significant benefits to patients given the opportunity to "tell their stories" (Adler 1997; Clark and Standard 1997). Cognitive-behavioral

therapy (CBT) attempts to help the child alter maladaptive patterns of thinking that lead to excessive feelings of anxiety, depression, or anger; improve problem solving and coping skills; and in some instances, modify physiological responses to disorders such as asthma (Spirito and Kazak 2006; Szigethy et al. 2007). Using cognitive restructuring, behavioral activation, and problem-solving skills, CBT attempts to change the maladaptive cognitions that are producing exaggerated or inappropriate emotional responses.

Behavior therapy may be used to improve the child's functional ability and decrease unwanted, negative behaviors (Spirito and Kazak 2006). Behavioral programs with appropriate incentives and an effective system of monitoring and rewards can be used to reinforce desired behaviors such as medication adherence. Biofeedback, relaxation training, and hypnosis may play a role in reducing emotional distress and autonomic arousal and, in some instances, improving the child's physical condition (e.g., asthma, diabetes mellitus, headache, hypertension) (McQuaid and Nassau 1999).

Individual therapy with medically ill children and adolescents frequently incorporates aspects of several therapeutic modalities. An adolescent with spina bifida, for example, may enter into therapy because of a sense of dependency and hopelessness for the future that leads to recurrent bouts of anxiety and depression. Therapy encourages the patient to recount the challenges of his disability while providing support, perspective, and practical solutions. Behavioral interventions are structured for the patient and family as a means of encouraging progress and clarifying the goals of treatment.

Family Therapy

Clearly, a child's illness is a total family experience. While the physically ill child who develops behavioral or emotional problems may enter treatment as the identified patient, providing all family members the opportunity to tell their stories about their experience with the illness can be important. Parents' emotional health and functioning play a major role in helping the child maintain his or her emotional well-being and can affect adherence to medical regimens. Family therapy can play a critical role in helping with the child's, parent's, and sibling's adjustment to the illness (see Shaw and DeMaso 2006 and Spirito and Kazak 2006 for reviews).

Group Therapy

Group therapy has been used with patients experiencing a variety of physical diagnoses (Eccleston et al.

2003; Shaw and DeMaso 2006; Stauffer 1998). Group therapy can take the form of support groups or psychoeducational groups providing information to participants about the diagnosis, treatment, and psychosocial aspects of a particular disorder, while other groups may focus on decreasing physical symptoms (Shaw and DeMaso 2006).

Adherence

As many as 33% of patients with acute conditions and 55% of those with chronic illnesses do not adhere to recommended treatment plans (Sabaté 2003; Shaw et al. 2003), making nonadherence a significant health issue (La Greca and Bearman 2003; Sabaté 2003). Children are at greater risk for noncompliance when they have a history of psychological distress, including symptoms of depression, oppositional behavior, and poor impulse control. These tend to be patients who deny the significance of the medical illness and have a history of nonadherence. Families have high levels of conflict and low levels of cohesion, communication, support, and parental responsibility. Low socioeconomic status further complicates the situation. Illnesses that require long periods of follow-up with little optimism generate lower levels of adherence. Similarly, patients are less likely to comply with treatments that are complex, invasive, and expensive, without strong evidence of efficacy. Interventions typically involve increasing parental participation in care and treatment, the education of patient and family on the need for adequate medical supervision and follow-up, and the initiation of behavioral, individual, and family therapies (Shaw et al. 2003). Spirito and Kazak (2006) recommend specific family therapy techniques that address noncompliance by normalizing adolescent rebellion, improving family communication, and implementing family problem-solving strategies.

Pain Management

Pain management in pediatric patients is affected by developmental as well as physiological factors. Young patients may not communicate their needs effectively and are frightened by the hospital environment and the physical intensity of their symptoms. Caregivers may either inadvertently reinforce the pain symptoms with continuous attention or become frustrated and angry over the child's complaints and physical limitations (Shaw and DeMaso 2006; Spirito and Kazak 2006). Clinicians should avoid decisions based on a need to better "manage" the patient without properly assessing the presence, extent, and degree of pain. In these in-

stances, children may be considered anxious or manipulative, prompting either inadequate pain treatment or oversedation. Pain should be treated early and aggressively in the patient's treatment course with family, behavioral, and pharmacological interventions (Shaw and DeMaso 2006). Clinicians should assess the child's level of pain, address the reasons for his or her requests or objections, and prescribe symptomatic treatment appropriately. Pain management is typically handled through a multidisciplinary team of medical and mental health professionals.

Procedural Preparation and Play Strategies

Children with chronic illnesses or disabilities may experience many invasive medical procedures. Prevention strategies have focused either on identifying risk factors for emotional distress (DeMaso et al. 1995) or on preparing patients for procedures or hospitalizations (Kain et al. 1996). Procedures designed to reduce the anxiety or pain associated with an invasive medical procedure tend to provide information relevant to the illnesses or treatment that might reduce unfamiliarity with the child's situation in hospital (e.g., preadmission programs, bibliotherapy, or support groups) and provide coping models who express anticipatory anxiety and then master it (Fielding and Duff 1999; Kain et al. 1996). During a painful procedure, a distraction involving video games can be useful. Their use requires minimal staff participation and costs are low (Vasterling et al. 2003). Various resources are available to help parents and professionals in the use of such procedures (DeMaso 2007; Stuber et al. 2006; Van Horn and DeMaso 2003).

Coping strategies such as breathing, deep muscle relaxation, distraction, behavioral rehearsal, positive reinforcement, modeling, visual imagery, and hypnosis can be used during procedures (Blount et al. 2003; Spirito and Kazak 2006) and have been shown to reduce procedural distress. Local anesthetics can play a useful role in needle-related procedures (e.g., EMLA cream).

Psychosocial Interventions With Specific Disorders: Empirical Support

There are too many chronic physical disorders to review the psychological treatment literature for all of them. Instead, we have chosen to examine the treatment of four conditions: asthma, diabetes, cancer, and juvenile rheumatoid arthritis. Asthma was chosen because of its prevalence and status as a chronic condition that has attracted research designed to alter symptoms of the disease as well as overall psychological adjustment. Diabetes is a chronic disorder with a wide range of psychological issues involved in its treatment. Cancer represents disorders that, while life expectancy has improved, nonetheless remain a life-threatening condition. Delirium is an example of the neurological sequelae that may be associated with a variety of chronic physical disorders.

Asthma

Studies of psychological intervention with asthma have attempted to reduce the symptom of the disease, reduce the impact of disease (e.g., "morbidity," such as school absences), improve adherence to the medication regimen, improve psychological adjustment of asthma patients, or some combination of these problems. Drotar's (2006) review found that there are some indications that psychological interventions can have an impact in each of these areas for asthma.

A review by McQuaid and Nassau (1999) concluded that frontalis electromyographic biofeedback was probably efficacious for reducing asthma symptoms, relaxation training was probably efficacious, and family therapy was a promising treatment. Lemanek et al. (2001) concluded that interventions emphasizing behavioral and educational strategies improved both adherence and health outcome, such as peak flow rate and asthma symptoms. Perrin et al. (1992) demonstrated that a multicomponent intervention using education, stress management, and coping interventions improved the adjustment of children with asthma compared to controls, reflected in fewer behavior problems and fewer internalizing symptoms. A large, multisite study compared a group of inner-city children with asthma to nontreated controls, with the treated-group participants assigned a case manager who provided education and intervention for behavior management, training in ways to reduce allergen exposure, and help getting access to health care. Over a 2-year period, the treated group showed fewer days with symptoms and fewer hospitalizations (Evans et al. 1999).

Diabetes

Numerous studies of psychological interventions for insulin-dependent diabetes mellitus have been conducted over the years. While studies vary in quality, the available systematic reviews suggest that these interventions have an impact in several areas. Hampson et al. (2000, 2001) reviewed behavioral interventions with adolescents with type 1 diabetes. Larger effect sizes (around .39) were noted for studies designed to reduce psychological adjustment problems and somewhat lower effect sizes for improving blood glucose control (around .33), while effect sizes were lowest for improving diabetic self-management (.15). Delamater et al. (2001) found that psychoeducational intervention improved glycemic control. Multicomponent interventions emphasizing self-management skills have been described as probably efficacious (Lemanek et al. 2001).

Cancer

The research literatures on psychological treatments of pediatric cancer have most commonly addressed ways to reduce procedural pain and distress. Kuppenheimer and Brown (2002) found that CBT had some success in the treatment of procedure pain, although a variety of methodological problems limit the generalization of results. In other areas, psychological interventions with pediatric cancer patients have shown effects in improving social skills of children with brain tumors (Barakat et al. 2003) and improving school adjustment upon reentry to school (Katz et al. 1988).

Juvenile Rheumatoid Arthritis

Compared to the literature on diabetes, asthma, and cancer, there have been relatively few studies of psychological interventions for juvenile rheumatoid arthritis. Small-scale studies show promising results for reducing pain associated with juvenile rheumatoid arthritis (Lavigne et al. 1992; Walco and Ilowite 1992; Walco et al. 1992). Single-subject designs show that behavioral interventions (e.g., behavioral monitoring, verbal feedback reinforcement) can improve adherence.

Delirium

Delirium is characterized by impairments in attention and orientation, deficits in language and visuospatial skills, and deterioration in cognition not explained by an underlying dementia (Murphy 2000). Symptoms tend to fluctuate throughout the day and the onset appears as a consequence of an illness or its treatment. Patients should be evaluated several times over an extended period before making the diagnosis. Pediatric patients seem to be especially vulnerable to delirium following toxic, metabolic, or traumatic CNS insults and fever regardless of the etiology. The most common causes of delirium are CNS infections (e.g., meningitis) or medication toxicity. The evaluation of young patients for the presence of delirium is affected by the developmental limitations of the child, particularly in the areas of communication and cognition. Only the most severe cases are identified and the remainder are either ignored or mismanaged under incorrect diagnoses. In one such case, a 14-year-old girl had a 4-week history of irritability, aggression, disorganization, and paranoia in a presentation consistent with bipolar disorder. The pediatrician immediately referred the case to a psychiatrist and informed the family that she would require long-term therapy and possibly medications. The child and adolescent psychiatrist elicited a history of a viral illness immediately preceding the mental status change. There was no family history of mood disorder, and the patient's symptoms were exacerbated when given diphenhydramine for sleeplessness. The psychiatrist suspected delirium secondary to viral encephalitis, treated the patient symptomatically, and told the family that she would gradually improve without symptom recurrence.

The adult literature cites increasing complication rates and longer hospital stays in delirious patients, but few studies examine delirium in pediatric patients. The effect of the diagnosis on pediatric care is poorly understood; thus, clinicians are less motivated to assess or treat the disorder. Hypoactive delirium is often misdiagnosed as depression when children appear distant, unresponsive, and isolative. Psychiatric consultations are more frequently recommended for patients with paranoia, hallucinations, and aggression. Unfortunately, these patients are often considered oppositional and defiant and are labeled as behavior problems. Cases can also be very complicated with multifactorial causes of delirium that include aspects of treatment as well as illness (Lawlor and Bruera 2002). The most effective treatment for delirium is the identification and management of the cause. When this is not immediately possible, care involves environmental changes that orient and calm the patient with the addition of pharmacotherapy (antipsychotic medications) when necessary (Breitbart et al. 1996; Martini 2005).

Research Directions

While there has been considerable progress in our understanding of the psychiatric aspects of chronic physical conditions in the last few decades, a considerable amount of work remains to be done. While it is clear that children with physical disorders are at increased risk for psychological adjustment problems, the mechanisms involved in producing the increased risk need to be delineated more clearly. Certain risk factors, such as maternal depression, family conflict, and life stresses, are known to contribute to psychological adjustment in healthy children. Chronic illness may serve as a moderator for such relationships, such that the presence of a chronic illness may increase the impact of such common risk factors in a multiplicative fashion, thereby accelerating the rates of emotional or behavioral problems among children with chronic illness. If this occurs, then it makes sense to adapt interventions for healthy children displaying those risk factors for use with children with chronic illnesses. There may be processes specific to chronic illness, however, that contribute to the development of emotional or behavioral problems in children with chronic illness; in such circumstances, interventions need to be designed specifically for children with chronic illness that address such problems. This would occur, for example, if there were concerns about pain, changes in self-concept, or problems with adherence that influenced psychological adjustment beyond the effects of common risk factors. More research on factors contributing to psychological adjustment problems will inform future interventions for these children. Presently, many types of interventions, both psychosocial and pharmacological, have not been adequately tested; in other instances, studies have not been conducted to try to replicate existing results. It is, perhaps, not surprising that research is slow to be executed in a field that involves special groups of children treated in centers where available samples are small and many years may be needed to accumulate sample sizes required for randomized clinical trials. Nonetheless, meeting the challenges of conducting such trials will be critical to improving the care of children with chronic illness and physical disabilities in the future.

Summary Points

- Children and adolescents with chronic illness are at increased risk for emotional adjustment problems, particularly from internalizing syndromes including depressive and anxiety disorders that appear early and persist over time.

- The young patient's ability to cope with physical illness is affected by the interplay of personal, psychosocial, and biological factors, as well as the exposure to negative life events.

- Adaptation to illness is also determined by the patient's developmental level, history of medical illness, and temperament, in addition to parental and family factors.

- Psychiatric disorders in physically ill children can affect compliance, lifestyle, and adjustment to illness and can have a direct impact on physiology and the disease process.

- Family members may be affected individually with higher rates of irritability, anxiety, depression, and somatic complaints than the general population and may become overinvolved in aspects of medical care at the expense of family needs. The demands of caring for an ill child can change relationships between parents and among parents, patient, and siblings.

- Psychopharmacological interventions are instituted when the medical team believes that the psychiatric symptoms in the child are affecting the patient's care. The physician should be aware of possible interactions between the illness and the treatment.

- Psychosocial interventions, including individual, group, and family therapies, provide an opportunity for the patient and family to express their concerns and feelings about the illness or disability.

- When treating the child with chronic physical illness, the mental health clinician should routinely address adherence, pain management, and procedural preparation.

References

Adler HM: The history of present illness as treatment: who's listening, and why does it matter? J Am Board Fam Pract 10:28–35, 1997

Alexander M, Vaughan B, Urion D, et al: Adderall use in children and adolescents. Children's Hospital Boston Pediatric Views, May 2005. Available at: http://www.childrenshospital.org/views/june05/adderall_p.html. Accessed May 4, 2009.

American Academy of Pediatrics Committee on Children With Disabilities and Committee on Psychosocial Aspects of Child and Family Health: Psychosocial risks of chronic health conditions in childhood and adolescence. Pediatrics 92:876–878, 1993

Band EB, Weisz JR: How to feel better when it feels bad: children's perspectives on coping with everyday stress. Dev Psychol 24:247–253, 1988

Barakat LP, Hetzke J, Foley B, et al: Evaluation of a social-skills training group intervention with children treated for brain tumors: a pilot study. J Pediatr Psychol 28:299–307, 2003

Beliles KE: Psychopharmacokinetics in the medically ill, in Psychiatric Care of the Medical Patient, 2nd Edition. Edited by Stoudemire A, Fogel BS, Greenberg DB. Oxford, England, Oxford University Press, 2000, pp 272–394

Blount RL, Piira T, Cohen LL: Management of pediatric pain and distress due to medical procedures, in Handbook of Pediatric Psychology, 3rd Edition. Edited by Roberts MC. New York, Guilford, 2003, pp 216–233

Breitbart W, Marotta R, Platt MM, et al: A double-blind trial of haloperidol, chlorpromazine, and lorazepam in the treatment of delirium in hospitalized AIDS patients. Am J Psychiatry 153:231–237, 1996

Breslau N, Marshall IA: Psychological disturbance in children with physical disabilities: continuity and change in a 5-year follow-up. J Abnorm Child Psychol 12:199–216, 1985

Campis LB, DeMaso DR, Twente AW: The role of maternal factors in the adaptation of children with craniofacial disfigurement. Cleft Palate Craniofac J 32:55–61, 1995

Campo JV, Bridge J, Ehmann M, et al: Recurrent abdominal pain, anxiety, and depression in primary care. Pediatrics 113:817–824, 2004

Clark MC, Standard PL: The caregiving story: how the narrative approach informs caregiving burden. Issues Ment Health Nurs 18:87–97, 1997

Dahlquist L, Gil K, Armstrong D, et al: Preparing children for medical examinations: the importance of previous medical experience. Health Psychol 5:249–259, 1986

Delamater AM, Jacobsen MD, Anderson B, et al: Psychosocial therapies in diabetes: report of the Psychosocial Therapist Working Group. Diabetes Care 23:1286–1292, 2001

DeMaso DR (ed): The Experience Journals. Boston, MA, Children's Hospital Boston, 2007. Available at: http://www.experiencejournal.com. Accessed May 4, 2009.

DeMaso DR, Beardslee WR, Silbert AR, et al: Psychological functioning in children with cyanotic heart defects. J Dev Behav Pediatr 11:289–294, 1990

DeMaso DR, Campis LK, Wypij D, et al: The impact of maternal perceptions and medical severity on the adjustment of children with congenital heart disease. J Pediatr Psychol 16:137–149, 1991

DeMaso DR, Twente AW, Spratt EG, et al: The impact of psychological functioning, medical severity, and family functioning in pediatric heart transplantation. J Heart Lung Transplant 14:1102–1108, 1995

DeMaso DR, Kelley SD, Bastardi H, et al: The longitudinal impact of psychological functioning, medical severity, and family functioning in pediatric heart transplantation. J Heart Lung Transplant 23:473–480, 2004

Drotar D: Psychological Interventions in Childhood Chronic Illness. Washington, DC, American Psychological Association, 2006

Eccleston C, Malleson PN, Clinch J, et al: Chronic pain in adolescents: evaluation of a programme of interdisciplinary cognitive behaviour therapy. Arch Dis Child 88:881–885, 2003

Evans R, Gergen PJ, Mitchell H, et al: A randomized clinical trial to reduce asthma morbidity among inner-city children: results of the National Cooperative Inner City Asthma Study. J Pediatr 135:332–338, 1999

Fielding D, Duff A: Compliance with treatment protocols: interventions for children with chronic illness. Arch Dis Child 80:196–200, 1999

Fisher L, Weihs KL: Can addressing family relationships improve outcomes in chronic disease? Report of the National Working Group on Family-Based Intervention in Chronic Disease. J Fam Pract 49:561–566, 2000

Folkman S, Lazarus RS: The relationship between coping and emotion: implications for theory and research. Soc Sci Med 26:309–317, 1988

Frank NC, Blount RL, Smith AJ, et al: Parent and staff behavior, previous child medical experience, and maternal anxiety as they relate to child procedural distress and coping. J Pediatr Psychol 20:277–289, 1995

Garrison MM, Katon WJ, Richard LP: The impact of psychiatric comorbidities on readmissions for diabetes in youth. Diabetes Care 28:2150–2154, 2005

Green SA: Principles of medical psychotherapy, in Psychiatry Care of the Medical Patient. Edited by Stoudemire A, Fogel BS, Greenberg DB. Oxford, England, Oxford University Press, 2000, pp 3–15

Gucuyener K, Erdemoglu AK, Senol S, et al: Use of methylphenidate for attention-deficit hyperactivity disorder in patients with epilepsy or electroencephalographic abnormalities. J Child Neurol 18:109–112, 2003

Hampson SE, Skinner TC, Hart J, et al: Behavioral interventions with adolescents with Type 1 diabetes. Diabetes Care 23:1416–1422, 2000

Hampson SE, Skinner TC, Hart J, et al: Effects of educational and psychosocial interventions for adolescents with diabetes mellitus: a systematic review. Health Technol Assess 5:1–78, 2001

Hemmer SA, Pasternak JF, Zecker SG, et al: Stimulant therapy and seizure risk in children with ADHD. Pediatr Neurol 24:99–102, 2001

Hocking MC, Lochman JE: Applying the transactional stress and coping model to sickle cell disorder and insulin-dependent diabetes mellitus: identifying psychosocial variables related to adjustment and intervention. Clin Child Fam Psychol Rev 8:221–246, 2005

Holmbeck GN, Westhoven VC, Phillips WS, et al: A multi-method, multi-informant, multidimensional perspective on psychosocial adjustment in preadolescents with spina bifida. J Consult Clin Psychol 71:782–796, 2003

Hubert NC, Jay SM, Saltoun M, et al: Approach-avoidance and distress in children undergoing preparation for painful medical procedures. J Clin Child Psychol 17:194–202, 1988

Jacobs J: Family therapy in chronic medical illness, in Psychiatric Care of the Medical Patient, 2nd Edition. Edited by Stoudemire A, Fogel BS, Greenberg DB. Oxford, England, Oxford University Press, 2000, pp 31–39

Kain ZN, Mayes LC, Caramico LA: Preoperative preparation in children: a cross-sectional study. J Clin Anesth 8:508–514, 1996

Katz ER, Rubenstein CL, Hubert NC, et al: School and social reintegration of children with cancer. J Psychol Oncol 6:123–140, 1988

Kazak AE, Rourke MT, Crump TA: Families and other systems in pediatric psychology, in Handbook of Pediatric Psychology, 3rd Edition. Edited by Roberts MC. New York, Guilford, 2003, pp 159–175

Knapp PK, Harris ES: Consultation-liaison in child psychiatry: a review of the past 10 years. Part I: clinical findings. J Am Acad Child Adolesc Psychiatry 37:17–25, 1998

Kovacs M, Mukerji P, Drash A, et al: Biomedical and psychiatric risk factors for retinopathy among children with IDDM. Diabetes Care 18:1592–1599, 1995

Kovacs M, Obrosky DS, Goldston D, et al: Major depressive disorder in youths with IDDM: a controlled prospective study of course and outcome. Diabetes Care 2:45–51, 1997

Kuppenheimer WG, Brown RT: Painful procedures in pediatric cancer: a comparison of interventions. Clin Psychol Rev 22:753–786, 2002

La Greca A, Bearman KJ: Adherence to pediatric treatment regimens, in Handbook of Pediatric Psychology, 3rd Edition. Edited by Roberts MC. New York, Guilford, 2003, pp 119–140

Lavigne JV, Faier-Routman J: Psychological adjustment to pediatric physical disorders: a meta-analytic review. J Pediatr Psychol 17:133–157, 1992

Lavigne JV, Faier-Routman J: Correlates of psychological adjustment to pediatric physical disorders: a meta-analytic review and comparison to existing models. J Dev Behav Pediatr 14:117–123, 1993

Lavigne JV, Ross CK, Berry SL, et al: Evaluation of a psychological treatment package for treating pain in juvenile rheumatoid arthritis. Arthritis Care Res 5:101–110, 1992

Lawlor DA, Bruera ED: Delirium in patients with advanced cancer. Hematol Oncol Clin North Am 16:701–714, 2002

Lemanek KL, Kamps J, Chung NB: Empirically supported treatments in pediatric psychology: regimen adherence. J Pediatr Psychol 26:253–275, 2001

Lewis M, Vitulano LA: Biopsychosocial issues and risk factors in the family when the child has a chronic illness. Child Adolesc Psychiatr Clin N Am 12:389–399, 2003

Logan DE, Scharff L: Relationships between family and parent characteristics and functional abilities in children with recurrent pain syndromes: an investigation of moderating effects on the pathway from pain to disability. J Pediatr Psychol 30:698–707, 2005

Martini DR: Commentary: the diagnosis of delirium in pediatric patients. J Am Acad Child Adolesc Psychiatry 44:395–398, 2005

McQuaid EL, Nassau JH: Empirically supported treatments of disease-related symptoms in pediatric psychology: asthma, diabetes, and cancer. J Pediatr Psychol 24:305–328, 1999

Melamed BG: Putting the family back in the child. Behav Res Ther 31:239–247, 1993

Melamed BG, Robbins RL, Fernandez J: Factors to be considered in psychological preparation for surgery, in Advances in Developmental and Behavioral Pediatrics. Edited by Routh D, Wolraich M. New York, JAI, 1982, pp 51–72

Murphy BA: Delirium. Emerg Med Clin North Am 18:243–252, 2000

Newacheck PW, McManus MA, Fox HB: Prevalence and impact of chronic illness among adolescents. Am J Dis Child 145:1367–1373, 1991

Noeker M, Haverkamp-Krois A, Haverkamp F: Development of mental health dysfunction in childhood epilepsy. Brain Dev 27:5–16, 2005

Perrin JM, MacLean WE, Gortmaker SL, et al: Improving the psychological status of children with asthma: a randomized controlled trial. J Dev Behav Pediatr 13:241–247, 1992

Peterson C, Harbaugh BL: Children's and adolescents' experiences while undergoing cardiac catheterization. Mat Child Nurs J 23:15–25, 1995

Pless IB, Pinkerton P: Chronic Childhood Disorder: Promoting Patterns of Adjustment. Chicago, IL, Henry Kimpton, 1975

Pliszka S, AACAP Work Group on Quality Issues: Practice parameter for the assessment and treatment of children and adolescents with attention-deficit/hyperactivity disorder. J Am Acad Child Adolesc Psychiatry 46:894–921, 2007

Robinson MD, Owen JA: Psychopharmacology, in The American Psychiatric Press Textbook of Psychosomatic Medicine. Edited by Levenson JL. Washington, DC, American Psychiatric Publishing, 2005, pp 871–922

Rolland JS, Walsh F: Facilitating family resilience with childhood illness and disability. Curr Opin Pediatr 18:527–538, 2006

Rudolph KD, Dennig MD, Weisz JR: Determinants and consequences of children's coping in the medical setting: conceptualization, review, and critique. Psychol Bull 118:328–357, 1995

Sabaté E (ed): Adherence to Long-Term Therapies: Evidence for Action. Geneva, Switzerland, World Health Organization, 2003

Shaw RJ, DeMaso DR: Clinical Manual of Pediatric Psychosomatic Medicine: Mental Health Consultation With Physically Ill Children and Adolescents. Washington, DC, American Psychiatric Publishing, 2006

Shaw RJ, Palmer L, Blasey C, et al: A typology of nonadherence in pediatric renal transplant recipients. Pediatr Transplant 7:489–493, 2003

Siemon M: Siblings of the chronically ill or disabled child: meeting their needs. Nurs Clin North Am 19:295–307, 1984

Simeonsson RJ, Buckley L, Munson L: Conceptions of illness causality in hospitalized children. J Pediatr Psychol 4:77–84, 1979

Spirito A, Kazak AE: Effective and Emerging Treatments in Pediatric Psychology. Oxford, England, Oxford University Press, 2006

Stauffer MH: A long-term psychotherapy group for children with chronic medical illness. Bull Menninger Clin 62:15–32, 1998

Stuber ML: Psychiatric sequelae in seriously ill children and their families. Psychiatr Clin North Am 19:481–493, 1996

Stuber ML, Shemesh E: Posttraumatic stress response to life-threatening illnesses in children and their parents. Child Adolesc Psychiatr Clin N Am 15:597–609, 2006

Stuber ML, Schneider S, Kassam-Adams N, et al: The medical traumatic stress toolkit. CNS Spectr 11:137–142, 2006

Szigethy E, Kenney E, Carpenter J, et al: Cognitive-behavioral therapy for adolescents with inflammatory bowel disease and subsyndromal depression. J Am Acad Child Adolesc Psychiatry 46:1290–1298, 2007

Thompson RJ: Coping with the stress of chronic childhood illness, in Management of Chronic Disorders of Childhood. Edited by O'Quinn AN. Boston, MA, GK Hall, 1985, pp 11–41

Thompson RJ, Gustafson KE: Adaptation to Chronic Childhood Illness. Washington, DC, American Psychological Association, 1996

Thompson RJ, Hodges K, Hamlett KW: A matched comparison of adjustment in children with cystic fibrosis and psychiatrically, 1990

Van Horn M, DeMaso DR: Helping your child with medical experiences: a practical parent guide, in The Experience Journals. Boston, MA, Children's Hospital Boston, 2003. Available at: http://www.experiencejournal.com/cardiac/clinic/parentguide.pdf. Accessed May 4, 2009.

Vasterling J, Jenkins RA, Tope DM, et al: Cognitive distraction and relaxation training for the control of side effects due to cancer chemotherapy. J Behav Med 16:65–80, 2003

Vitulano LA: Psychosocial issues for children and adolescents with chronic illness: self-esteem, school functioning and sports participation. Child Adolesc Psychiatr Clin N Am 12:585–592, 2003

Walco GA, Ilowite NT: Cognitive-behavioral intervention for juvenile primary fibromyalgia syndrome. J Rheumatol 19:1617–1619, 1992

Walco GA, Varni JW, Ilowite NT: Cognitive-behavioral pain management in children with juvenile rheumatoid arthritis. Pediatrics 89:1075–1079, 1992

Wallander JL, Varni JW: Adjustment in children with chronic physical disorders: programmatic research on a disability-stress-coping model, in Stress and Coping in Child Health. Edited by La Greca AM, Siegel LJL, Wallander JL, et al. New York, Guilford, 1992, pp 279–299

Wallander JL, Thompson RJ, Alriksson-Schmidt A: Psychosocial adjustment of children with chronic physical conditions, in Handbook of Pediatric Psychology, 3rd Edition. Edited by Roberts MC. New York, Guilford, 2003, pp 141–158

Wamboldt MZ, Fritz G, Mansell A, et al: Relationship of asthma severity and psychological problems in children. J Am Acad Child Adolesc Psychiatry 37:943–950, 1998

Waxmonsky J, Wood BL, Stern T, et al: Association of depressive symptoms and disease activity in children with asthma: methodological and clinical implications. J Am Acad Child Adolesc Psychiatry 45:945–954, 2006

Wood BL, Miller BD, Lim J, et al: Family relational factors in pediatric depression and asthma: pathways of effect. J Am Acad Child Adolesc Psychiatry 45:945–954, 2006

Wright B: Physical Disability: A Psychosocial Approach. New York, Harper and Row, 1960

Chapter 42

Children of Parents With Psychiatric and Substance Abuse Disorders

William R. Beardslee, M.D.
Jacqueline L. Martin, Ph.D.

In clinical practice, it is common to encounter parents with either medical or psychiatric illness or both. Working with parents with such illnesses provides an important opportunity to help both parents and their children. In this chapter, we address two areas. First, we discuss parental mental illness that places families at higher risk for the development of disorder in children and at the same time provides an important opportunity for preventive intervention. Using children of parents with depression as a model, we specifically discuss risk factors, protective factors, and resilience and review prevention programs. We outline prevention programs that have been developed for families with anxiety disorders and substance abuse disorders. Second, we address directly what clinicians can do when they encounter parents with mental illness in their practice, based on both clinical experience and the research on preventive intervention. We have not focused on medical illness, although we believe many of the same principles apply, given many studies include parents who have both mental and physical illness.

Clinical Presentation

Parents with mental illness come to the attention of clinicians in one of three ways:

1. For clinicians who work with children, it is not uncommon to encounter difficulties in parents when children are seen for evaluation or treatment of

psychiatric or developmental problems. The clinician may become aware of a parent's illness through obtaining a psychiatric history of the family, through the parent volunteering the information at some point during the child's treatment, or through interacting in a way that suggests psychiatric symptoms. The child might mention a parent's problem, or it can become evident if parents struggle with getting children to appointments or implementing programs at home.

2. Adult mental health practice often involves working with adults who have children, but parents' concerns about their children and their parenting role are often not addressed. Many clinicians trained to work with adults are uncomfortable asking about children, especially if they might possibly have psychiatric illness, and this agenda has not been a focus either in training or practice.

3. Parents involved in treatment have contact for other reasons with health care professionals, who may discover mental illness.

   For example, because depression is common, there has been a strong effort to increase recognition and treatment (Olson et al. 2005). Depression often emerges as the explanatory construct for other difficulties. In studies of parents on public assistance, it is often parents with depression who are least able to obtain food stamps or other benefits (Seifert et al. 2000). Another study found that depressed parents were less able to adhere to asthma treatment regimens at home (Bartlett et al. 2004). Given the high rates of depression and other mental illnesses, clinicians working in a variety of settings need to be alert to parental difficulties, to inquire about the children, and where appropriate, to evaluate and treat the children or make suitable referrals.

   Unfortunately, many such parents remain unidentified and receive no treatment. The Surgeon General has estimated that only one-third of those with depression receive adequate treatment (U.S. Department of Health and Human Services 2000).

Eisenberg's (1984) distinction between the disease process and the experience of the illness is important. Clinical training focuses on psychopathology and the disease process, but it is the conscious felt experience of the illness that is most vivid for the patient and family. Listening to the story of the illness—and understanding the illness experience of the parent, the spouse, and the children—can be therapeutic, and at the same time, can ground intervention strategies.

Similarly, it is helpful to ask what the parents are concerned about and address those concerns. Providing information about treatment and assuring that the parent receives treatment are essential.

Children of parents with mental illness will have the same hopes and expectations of their parents as do all children and are likely to view their parents as powerful, positive forces in their lives. Understanding what the child has experienced, the child's perspective, and his or her needs and questions is an important part of helping parents who struggle with mental illness or related difficulties to be effective parents.

A Prevention Intervention Perspective

Research on preventive interventions for families at high risk due to parental mental illness and associated factors has shown considerable positive effects. While the application of a particular prevention program requires specific training, understanding the core principles allows them to be applied in daily clinical practice and can help both families and clinicians.

Specific work on prevention in high-risk families takes place against a much larger backdrop of rapid progress over the past 20 years in prevention intervention methodology and design and in substantive efficacy and effectiveness trials (Albee and Gulotta 1997; Hosman et al. 2004; Mrazek and Haggerty 1994). Repeatedly, national and international commissions have called for the development of programs for children at risk for mental illness. The Institute of Medicine Committee on Prevention supports the following system of classification of prevention programs (Mrazek and Haggerty 1994; Munoz et al. 1996):

1. *Indicated prevention programs*—Target at-risk individuals who already have symptoms or a biological marker but do not meet full diagnostic criteria.
2. *Selective prevention programs*—Target individuals presumed to be at high risk for the development of a disorder. Prevention programs that target children of parents with mental illness are selective preventions, while those that target children who themselves have symptoms are a combination of selective and indicated programs.
3. *Universal prevention programs*—Target entire populations, regardless of risk factors.

Risk

Children who grow up with parents with a psychiatric illness are at significantly higher risk of developing a mental disorder at some point in their life compared to those who have parents without mental illness. The rates and types of child disorder vary according to the specific parental disorder, but this is a high-risk group of children. Data from the Netherlands Mental Health Survey and Incidence Study suggest a lifetime prevalence of psychiatric disorders in approximately 50% of children when one parent has a history of psychiatric disorder. The risk increases substantially when both parents are ill (Bijl et al. 2002). Numerous studies have documented that the children of depressed parents are at two to four times higher risk for developing depression in adolescence. They are also at risk for interpersonal difficulties, school dropout, and a variety of other psychiatric difficulties (Beardslee et al. 1998). Parental substance abuse disorder increases risk for a variety of poor outcomes, including substance abuse disorder in offspring (Cuijpers et al. 1999; Steinhausen 1995). A variety of investigators have examined the effect of other parental disorders on children's well-being—e.g., anxiety disorder (Beidel and Turner 1997; Biederman et al. 2001), bipolar disorder (DelBello and Geller 2001), eating disorder (Park et al. 2003), and personality disorder (Coolidge et al. 2001). Each of these studies found an increased risk of psychopathology in the children, giving evidence that parental mental disorder is a major risk factor for children (Beardslee et al. 2007).

Mechanisms of risk may operate differently depending on the type of parental psychopathology, but several general principles apply. First, it is important both in research and clinical work with families to recognize that the parental mental illness often is a marker of a constellation of risk factors, and it is likely the latter that place the children at increased risk (Beardslee et al.

2007). Children, and sometimes entire families, of mentally ill parents may require prevention services, but their needs may be related to factors other than their parents' illness (e.g., recent immigration, lack of community support, or recent loss). Therefore, it is important to characterize all the risk factors that are present and gauge their effects on children. Often a variety of different mechanisms operate at once. Some disorders, such as depression or alcoholism, have a genetic vulnerability. Having parents and grandparents with the illness may predispose offspring to the illness. In a classic study of monozygotic twins reared apart whose parent had a mood disorder, when one twin developed bipolar disorder, approximately 70% of the time the other twin did also. For severe unipolar depression, the rate was about 40% (Beardslee et al. 2003). Thus, the impact of nongenetic factors may be substantial and varies depending on the type of mood disorder.

Several general principles apply to preventive approaches, whatever the particular psychiatric condition. There are several well-established risk factors for depression and other disorders for which there is empirical justification (Table 42–1). Studies show that children raised in poverty have higher lifetime rates of depression. In the New Haven Epidemiologic Catchment Area Study, poverty was a potent risk factor for the onset of depression in adults in the year following initial assessment (Bruce et al. 1991). Poverty is associated with a variety of other negative outcomes. Exposure to violence is well documented to be associated with an increased prevalence of anxiety disorders, posttraumatic stress disorder (PTSD), and depression (Felitti et al. 1998; MacMillan 1997; McAlister-Groves et al. 1993). Social isolation has long been associated with increased rates of depression.

Parent-child interaction patterns characteristic of parents with certain psychiatric disorders can also be a risk factor for children. Depressed mothers have been shown to have greater negative feelings toward their

TABLE 42–1. Specific and nonspecific risks for depression and other disorders

Specific risks for depression	Nonspecific risks for depression and other disorders
Extensive family history of depression, especially parents	Exposure to trauma
	Poverty
Prior history of depression	Social isolation
Depressogenic cognitive style	Job loss
Bereavement	Unemployment
	Family breakup
	Loss of community
	Dislocation/immigration
	Historical trauma

children and exhibit less warmth and greater use of psychological control (Cornish et al. 2006; Cummings et al. 2005). Parents of children with anxiety disorders (who might have anxiety disorders themselves) have been found to be more likely to discourage autonomy, model fear, reinforce child avoidance, and overprotect the child (Chorpita et al. 1996; Dadds et al. 1996; Hirshfeld-Becker and Biederman 2002; Hirshfeld et al. 1997; Siqueland et al. 1996).

Thus, one broad implication for clinical practice is the importance of assessing the range of risk factors that are present when a parent has mental illness.

Developmental Transactions

Two constructs underlie the evolving studies of risk and resilience. The cornerstone of prevention is bolstering protective factors, but their study has been relatively neglected. It is helpful to understand resilience as defined by Luthar et al. (2000), who emphasize it is a "dynamic developmental construct" that leads to competence in the face of adversity. Others have argued that the developmental transactional framework is the most useful perspective in understanding children at risk (Cicchetti and Schneider-Rosen 1986; Sameroff and Chandler 1987). In this framework, risk factors pose difficulty and may start out as static. However, the processes that lead either to psychopathology or to health are dynamic and strongly influenced by changes across the life span. Moreover, systems and individuals influence one another. A close bond between a caregiver and an infant is fostered by the caregiver's anticipation of the child's needs and a match between the caregiver's expectations and the temperament of the child. Zeanah et al. (1997) document that developmental risk factors are mediated by the caregiving context in early childhood. In adolescence also, genetic risk factors for depression can be mediated by specific parenting practices (Reiss et al. 2000). Such fluid developmental transactions between parents and children are likely to be more clearly understood as knowledge is gained concerning the interplay between genetics, development, and environment. It is crucial to remember the important possibilities of developmental plasticity. The relationship between risk factors and later outcome for children is probabilistic, not deterministic (Beardslee et al. 2005). Developmental events continually influence the relationship between risk and outcome (Eisenberg 1995).

An equally important conceptual framework that operates for risk and protective factors is the additive, interactive, and cumulative nature of such factors (Cicchetti and Cohen 1995; Sameroff et al. 1998). The Rochester Longitudinal Study examined in parents with a variety of mental illnesses a series of risk factors for poor child outcome: type of parental mental illness, minority status, stressful life events, family size, various domains of family support, and social class. A single risk factor did not increase the likelihood of disorder, but as the number of risk factors grew, the overall functioning of the child decreased and the likelihood of a psychiatric illness increased (Sameroff et al. 1998). It was not the diagnostic category of the parent but the chronicity, severity, and amount of impairment that were associated with effects on the child. Sameroff observed that children from poor families with parents with minimal education fared more poorly than youngsters living in advantaged homes, even those with a parent with mental illness. Social context is crucially important.

In the years to come, as more is learned about factors such as how gene expression varies depending on environmental and other conditions, there will undoubtedly be further definitions of risk and opportunities for prevention. It is also important to remember that a family history of psychopathology does not necessarily imply only a genetic mechanism. Children and parents experience the same adversities, which may precipitate both episodes of parent illness and have direct effects on children. Exposure to violence or bereavement are examples. Adversities may also affect children because such stressors interfere with parenting.

Resilience

Counterbalancing risk factors is the presence of buffering protective influences. It is striking how many of these children do well despite parental mental illness. The study of resilience is rapidly evolving (Luthar 2006; Luthar et al. 2000). While there are conceptual and definitional issues still to be resolved, it is clear that understanding the protective resources and strengths within a child, a parent, or a family is crucial to mounting effective prevention programs. In one study of children of parents with mood disorders, investigators examined a subset of resilient children from a larger group of children at risk (Beardslee and Podorefsky 1988). Using a combination of structured and semistructured interviews, 18 children (from 14 families) who exhibited good functioning were interviewed. Three domains robustly characterized these youngsters. First, they were active in pursuing and accomplishing age-appropriate developmental tasks—e.g., going to school, excelling academically, being committed to outside activities, and dedicated to religious and community activities. Their activity formed a striking contrast to the withdrawn and passive behavior of their depressed parent. Second, they were deeply committed to relationships and had strong friendships and good relationships within families and often with teachers and mentors. Third, they reported that understanding that their parents had an illness and that they were not to blame was crucial in their being able to move on with their own lives. As we describe later, enhancing these three qualities forms the basis of an effective preventive intervention for children of depressed parents. Correspondingly, in parents, an intense commitment to parenting despite depression and openness to self-reflection were important qualities that fostered their children's resilience. These parents reported being very worried about their children and not having anyone to talk to about these concerns.

The study of resilience has identified protective factors at the individual, family, school, and community levels (Luthar 2006; Masten et al. 1990). Within the individual, the capacity for religious faith and the presence of unusual talents such as writing ability or other creativity are protective. Within the environment, the presence of good schools, positive peer influences, and mentors are crucially important. Good physical health; a sense of purpose, hope, and optimism; thoughtfulness; spirituality; and the capacity for intimacy were found to be important and evolve over time (Beardslee 2002). A clinical inference from this literature is to help parents discover and recognize the strengths and resilience within their youngsters.

Clinical Implications

For any given disorder, practitioners need to consider two important points. When dealing with a parent with a mental or medical illness, in addition to managing the situation in the moment, it is useful to reflect on what risk and protective factors are present and what mechanisms of transmission for both factors exist. A second question is how to enlist resources to foster a healthy developmental outcome. Parents are likely very worried about the effects of the illness on their

children, in particular, whether they have harmed their children by having the illness and whether their children are likely to develop the illness. Understanding these concerns leads naturally to providing parents with educational resources and knowledge and helping them promote the healthy development of their children.

Prevention Approaches in Families With Parental Depression

Two programs that illustrate different prevention approaches in families where parents have depression are described: one is an indicated program and the other a selective program. Common principles in these programs are applicable to preventive intervention and treatment.

Based on social learning models of depression, Clarke and Lewinsohn (1995) developed a Coping With Stress psychoeducational group program that targets adolescents at risk for the development of depressive disorders. This program is a modification of their Coping With Depression course that was developed for use with clinically depressed adolescents. It aims to help vulnerable adolescents gain control over negative moods, learn new ways to resolve conflicts, and handle thought patterns that lead to negative or self-blaming strategies. The program also encourages positive thinking and offers anticipatory guidelines about how to deal with stressful situations. In the original study, the program was designed for children ages 13–18 years and it was administered by skilled therapists. Fifteen 1-hour group sessions were conducted over an 8-week period. The initial study took place in schools and included youngsters with some depressive symptoms. Significant outcome differences were found between the group that received the preventive intervention and the control group.

In a randomized clinical trial, Clarke et al. (2001) recruited adolescents whose parents were depressed and who themselves were manifesting symptoms of depression. The criteria used for parent inclusion were two separate prescriptions for an antidepressant in the previous year or two mental health visits within the previous year. Adolescents were assessed and divided into three groups: those who were demoralized with subdiagnostic levels of depressive symptoms or high self-report depressive scores (invited to participate), those who were depressed and met criteria for major depressive disorder (referred for treatment), and those who were described as resilient, with no history of depressive disorder and no present symptoms (not offered any services). There was blind assessment pre- and postintervention and careful attention to fidelity in the delivery of the manual-based preventive intervention. Demoralized youngsters were randomly assigned to either the experimental group, in which they participated in 15 one-hour group sessions, or usual care. Youth in either condition were allowed to continue or initiate any type of mental health care service during the study. These services constituted the care of youth in the usual care condition. Parents of children in both groups were invited to three separate informational and psychoeducational meetings during the early, middle, and later sessions of the youth groups. On self-report measures and diagnostic interview at follow-up, the experimental group experienced significantly less depression. Survival analysis over a 15-month period indicated a rate of depression of 9% in the experimental group vs. 28% in the control group. Involvement in parent groups did not make a difference.

The Boston Prevention Project developed public health interventions for families in which parents were depressed (Beardslee et al. 2003), based on Rutter's observation that the risk of transmission occurs primarily through negative interactions between parents and children (Rutter 1990). This model emphasizes increasing positive parent-child interactions, decreasing negative interactions, and reducing factors that interfere with effective parenting. Parents are taught to be self-reflective about parenting and learn problem-solving skills to deal with depression. The approach emphasizes a strong psychoeducational orientation involving the family as a whole and building strengths and resilience in youngsters. Based on the resilience work mentioned above, youth were encouraged to build strength in three specific areas: activities outside the home, involvement in relationships, and development of the capacity for self-understanding. The intervention is a public health approach, designed to be useful to all families with depressed parents. Thus, youth with and without depressive symptoms were included in the assessment and intervention phases of the study. For experimental purposes, youth who were already acutely depressed and receiving treatment were provided the intervention but excluded from the assessment phases. The principles were incorporated in two different interventions: public health lectures and a six-session clinician-led family intervention. The latter intervention included a family meeting co-led by the parents and

the clinician to talk with the children about depression and strategies for how it would be overcome. Both interventions were effective and led to sustained gains and changes in behaviors and attitudes toward the illness. After the fourth assessment point, 2.5 years following enrollment of over 100 families with little sample loss, sustained parent behavior and attitude changes were found. Importantly, there were sustained increases in children's understanding of parents' depression and related issues. Most strikingly, regardless of the intervention to which they were assigned, parents who showed the greatest behavior and attitude change had youngsters who showed the greatest increase in understanding the parental depression. Recently, these findings have been replicated through the sixth assessment point, approximately 4.5 years after enrollment. In both study conditions, parents and children showed increases in positive family functioning, and children's internalizing symptoms decreased (Beardslee et al. 2007).

Three processes that occur in families who deal effectively with an illness were identified by the research team. First, the sustained behavior and attitude changes reflected the fact that the families had ongoing conversations about depression. Families reported that they were more likely to seek care in the early stages of a depressive episode. This phenomenon was called the "emergence of the healer within." Parents also found that as the children matured through late adolescence and left home, they expressed the need for more complex explanations of depression and related family adversities. Also, many families experienced further episodes of parental illness. Taken together, this led to the continued need for "understanding depression anew." Finally, as parents were able to be effective in their parenting role despite depression, they often were able to reemerge into community and religious life and to feel that their lives could go on despite depression. This progression was called "making peace and moving on."

These families had many other adversities in addition to depression: high rates of comorbid illness, particularly anxiety disorder and alcoholism; a fair amount of marital strife with about 20% of the families having undergone divorce; and medical illness. Features of the intervention make it suitable to a wide variety of presenting problems. The presentation of psychoeducational information and linking such information to the life experience of the families can be useful in many situations. Perhaps most importantly, the long-term follow-up of the families emphasized that the presence of parental mental illness requires a long-term perspective on intervention, not necessarily a long-term intervention. Issues regarding the illness and the children will continue to arise; therefore, provision to address those is needed. The effects of the long-term follow-up were not directly tested, but families noted it was of value to them. Thus, another basic clinical principle is planning for follow-up over the long-term. Because parental depression had a major impact on families, the intervention drew on healing resources from many different areas. In fact, healing from depression is not unlike healing from other illnesses, such as medical disorders.

Prevention of Anxiety Disorders in Children

Negative parenting behaviors associated with anxiety suggest the importance of parent psychoeducation and involvement in prevention programs. In addition, parents with anxiety disorders, especially when untreated, arguably may have difficulty helping their children to learn how to manage anxiety. Although prevention programs for childhood anxiety developed to date usually do not target children of parents with anxiety disorders, this is potentially an important referral source and would allow prevention programs to target children at an early age. There are relatively few available prevention programs for children at risk for anxiety disorders, despite a strong argument for their importance. Pediatric onset of anxiety is common, and the problems can be quite debilitating for children (Beidel and Turner 1997; Hirshfeld-Becker and Biederman 2002; March 1995). If left untreated, pediatric anxiety disorders can extend into adulthood and are associated with impaired functioning and comorbid problems (Costello and Angold 1995).

Prevention programs developed to date in the area of anxiety disorders are for the most part indicated preventions in which the children's anxiety symptoms, as opposed to the presence of parental anxiety disorder, instigate the referral mechanism (Foa et al. 2005). Anxiety prevention interventions typically focus on psychoeducation and cognitive-behavioral therapy (CBT) skill development. Many of the available programs and studies have been conducted in Australia. Both parent-focused (e.g., LaFreniere and Capuano 1997; Rapee 2002) and child-focused (e.g., Dadds et al. 1997, 1999) preventive interventions have been developed and studies show positive results. One universal prevention program, FRIENDS, developed in Australia, is a school-based CBT program

that can be delivered by teachers or psychologists (www.friendsinfo.net). It is delivered to all students over a 10-week period, followed by booster sessions (Barrett and Turner 2001; Lowry-Webster et al. 2001). Study results indicated lower child self-rated anxiety in children receiving the FRIENDS program and no significant differences between results if teacher- or psychologist-delivered. FRIENDS has also been used with a group of culturally diverse children in Australia (e.g., Yugoslav, Chinese, mixed) and similar, promising effects were found (Barrett et al. 2003).

As with other populations, early intervention with children at risk for anxiety disorders is important, and an important referral mechanism includes identification through parents' symptoms (Hirshfeld-Becker and Biederman 2002). The authors propose the following components of an effective prevention protocol for preschoolers:

1. A way to identify at-risk children (e.g., children of parents with anxiety disorders and depression, children with behavioral inhibition, children showing anxiety symptoms)
2. A means of addressing parents' concerns and ensuring parental involvement
3. A protocol that incorporates efficacious CBT techniques (e.g., psychoeducation regarding anxiety management, coping strategies, and parenting an anxious child; principles of graduated exposure; relapse prevention)

Thus, as with prevention programs for depression, it is important to impart psychoeducational information about anxiety and its management to children and parents and improve parent-child interactions.

Prevention Programs for Children of Parents With Substance Abuse Disorders

Prevention interventions in the area of substance abuse often are indicated programs that target early emerging behavior problems in children. This group is targeted because the prevalence of later substance use disorders in such children is "nearly ubiquitous" (Beardslee et al. 2005). Also, common genetic factors have been found between adult antisocial behavior, childhood conduct disorder, drug dependence, and alcohol dependence (Hicks et al. 2004). Thus, it makes sense to target this population for prevention programs. In general, family-centered care and psychoeducation are important components of prevention programs in the domain of substance abuse (e.g., Nurse-Family Partnership; Olds 2002). Two strong programs that target families with a parent with substance abuse problems are discussed below.

The Strengthening Families Program (SFP) is a 14-session family skills training program with multiple components that was originally developed for children of parents with alcohol or drug addiction (Kumpfer et al. 2003). Booster sessions occur at 6- and 12-month follow-up with the goal of maintaining intervention gains. There are three components to the intervention: parent skills training, child skills training, and family life-skills training. Parents and children meet at a convenient community site (e.g., church, school) and first participate in a meal. Parents and children then take part in separate skills-focused 1-hour groups. In the second hour, parents and children come together again and practice family playtime, family communication, family meetings, and effective discipline. Weekly sessions take approximately 2.5 hours and require four trainers. The SFP program has been found to improve parenting skills, children's social skills and peer relationships, and family relationships. It has been shown to be effective in many replications including cultural adaptations. A shortened 7-session version has been developed for use in junior high schools (Kumpfer et al. 2003).

The Family Check-up Preventive Intervention (FCU; Dishion and Kavanagh 2003) targets early starter pathways to antisocial behavior and substance abuse through inclusion of families with environmental adversity (low socioeconomic status), maternal depression and/or substance abuse, and child conduct problems. It is described as an ecological approach to child and family interventions and represents an initial step to reduce behavior problems and increase emotional well-being in children and families. The FCU was first developed for adolescents with substance abuse (Adolescent Transitions Program) and now focuses on the toddler years. The intervention is based on motivational interviewing techniques and modeled after the Drinker's Check-up program. The FCU is a three-session intervention that contains a get-to-know-you meeting with the family, a broad assessment of the family context and parenting practices, and a formal feedback session that uses motivational interviewing. Some families are provided additional support on managing child behavior and family context issues. In a recent study that included 120 families with boys ages 2–4 years, the FCU resulted in reductions in disruptive

behavior and greater maternal involvement. The effects were particularly strong for children at greater risk for conduct problems (Shaw et al. 2006).

Thus, two ways to find children at risk for substance abuse that may benefit from prevention interventions are through parents with substance abuse disorders and children displaying early conduct problems. In both situations, children are at risk for developing later substance abuse problems. As noted earlier, before conducting prevention work with children and families, parents' illnesses must first be treated and adverse family contexts addressed. Following this initial step, clinical interventions include parent management training and skills development for children. Motivational interviewing helps to engage parents who might be resistant to engaging in interventions to help their children and improve family functioning.

Clinical Implications: Addressing the General Concerns of Parents, Parent and Child Skill Development, and Improving Family Communication

On the basis of both clinical experience and review of prevention intervention programs, there are important clinical implications to consider when working with adults who are parents. After the clinical needs of parents have been directly addressed through appropriate referrals or provision of treatment, there are a number of interventions that provide assistance to children and families:

1. First, it is important to ask parents their concerns about their children. Unfortunately, clinicians treating adults for physical or mental illness rarely ask about these patients' children. Consistently in our experience, adult patients who are parents are deeply concerned about their children. Inquiry about children's functioning and whether parents have concerns about their children are good starting points.

   In turn, common questions that parents ask include, "Is my illness going to be transmitted to my children?" and "Has my having an illness already damaged them?" In most instances, it is true to say there is an increased risk of transmission of the illness but also that the majority of children will not develop the illness and that it is highly unlikely that children are already irrevocably damaged.

2. Some children may already have symptoms of illness or distress and need further evaluation. These concerns can be directly addressed by asking the parent how the child is doing in important life domains of family, school, and peer relations and gaining an understanding of symptoms that may be present. Meeting individually with the child is also helpful, and sometimes necessary, to gain further information about the child's functioning and perspective. In doing so, it is important to recognize both the value of the child's perspective and the possible parental fear that talking directly to the child may reveal something about the parent's illness or the child's frustration with the parent. Reassurance to the parent, honesty, and openness about the domains of inquiry and support usually make such interventions work well. When symptoms are discovered or distress identified, a decision needs to be made about referral for further evaluation. Thus, access to both treatment and prevention services for children is necessary when working with mentally ill parents.

   As mentioned, adequate treatment for parents makes a large difference for children. For example, in a recent report based on the STAR*D study, children whose mothers were depressed and treated to remission were compared with children whose mothers were depressed and not treated to remission. Over a 3-month follow-up period, the children whose parents were treated to remission had significantly fewer symptoms and better functioning (Weissman et al. 2006).

3. It is essential to also recognize that families may have very important concerns about school; family events such as bereavement, job loss, or divorce; or other matters that affect family functioning but may not be directly relevant to the parent's medical or mental illness.

4. Another priority is to gain understanding of the parent's history with the child, and in particular, whether the illness has changed or disrupted the structure of the household, routines, or the time parents have with their children. For example, the illness might have resulted in separation due to hospitalization, and such departures from regular family functioning are likely to be of concern to

both parent and child. In our experience, with careful support, it is useful for parents to be able to discuss both the illness and these larger experiences that the child remembers.

5. It is important to note that risk factors experienced by parents (e.g., exposure to trauma or poverty) may be either directly or indirectly experienced by their children, as these risk factors affect the parent.

6. Parents' interactions with their children might have been disrupted by the illness, in particular the functions of support and monitoring. Inquiry in this domain often leads to understanding another crucial dimension for both parent and child: other supports in the child's life. In two-parent families, often the well parent can step in and provide the necessary support and monitoring. In single-parent families, finding support is more difficult but by no means impossible. Some attempt must be made to maintain the routines that are vital for the child and some explanation of the effects of the illness must be given.

7. In addition to addressing parents' concerns, psychoeducation about the illness and about how families can build resilience in their children is likely of high value. Teaching should impart information about diagnosis, treatment, prevention, and ways of destigmatizing the illness. Individualized psychoeducation for parents and children that directly deals with their experiences and concerns is key. Similarly, it is important to emphasize the accomplishment of age-appropriate developmental tasks that include building relationships, self-understanding, and understanding of the parent's illness (Beardslee 2002). The material should be carefully presented and enough time set aside to make sure that the parents have understood the information. It is also crucial to allow ample time for parents to ask their own questions. Parents may profit from general skill development regarding coping with depression (e.g., problem solving, recognizing negative cognitions, behavioral activation) and improvement of communication skills with family and others.

8. Just as the concept of resilience is essential, actualizing it in the lives of families through activities is equally important. Parents and children will be aided through guidance on how to promote resilience, in particular through encouragement of involvement in activities, friendships, and gaining understanding of the illness. Helping parents plan conversations with their children is valuable as well (Beardslee et al. 2003). If children exhibit symptoms

of the parent's disorder (e.g., depression, anxiety), teaching the child coping strategies and building a tool kit of skills are important (e.g., exposure to feared situations, cognitive restructuring). A range of intervention options needs to be available, as different approaches may be needed over time as new issues arise. It is also helpful to adopt a long-term perspective on prevention that includes scheduled follow-up sessions. This gives families the ability to easily gain assistance if future challenges arise (Beardslee 2002; Beardslee et al. 2007).

Perhaps most important, in addition to these specific intervention elements, is recognizing that depression often attacks a sense of optimism and hope for the future. Providing hope for families by helping parents find concrete actions they can take to protect their children, get treatment themselves, and foster understanding in the family must be an essential part of any engagement with parents with mental illness.

Research Directions

There is evidence of a developing area of quality research on prevention interventions for children of parents with mental and physical illnesses, but more work is needed. Compared to treatment interventions, there is a paucity of prevention-focused interventions, especially for certain populations, and likewise few large-scale studies have been conducted. For example, prevention programs in the area of depression have received much attention, but despite the overlapping populations, relatively little work has been done on prevention of anxiety disorders. As in the domain of treatment development and evaluation, more attention to cultural diversity and developmental issues is key in the area of prevention (Spoth et al. 2002). Most prevention research has focused on efficacy studies, but Drs. Garber, Clarke, Beardslee, and Brent are currently conducting a four-site effectiveness study using the Coping With Stress prevention program. This study will shed important light on whether the positive findings of the randomized study (Clarke et al. 2001; discussed earlier in the section "Prevention Approaches in Families With Parental Depression") are present in an effectiveness trial.

Finally, prevention programs often target children universally, or children displaying symptoms of disorders, but rarely target children of parents with mental illness. As noted in this chapter, this is another important avenue to reach populations who can profit from prevention.

Summary Points

- There is an enormous need for prevention interventions for children and families of parents with mental and physical illness.

- Psychiatric training programs often neglect instruction on how to care for the child and family needs of parents with psychiatric disorders.

- Although there are fewer prevention studies in comparison to intervention studies, prevention of depression in children has received more attention than many other psychiatric conditions (e.g., anxiety disorders) and shows promising findings.

- Prevention programs must include psychoeducation for parents and children concerning the effects of the illness on the family. Time must be allowed for parents to voice their concerns about their children and to ask questions about their children and the impact of the illness on their children's lives. Providing psychoeducation about children's resilience and helping families increase resilience are essential components of prevention programs.

- Building a toolbox of coping skills and improving communication in parents and children are important components.

- Programs need to also include information and strategies for dealing with comorbidity as it is often present in parents with mental illness.

- Future research directions for prevention work in families of parents with psychiatric disorders include broadening target populations to include other major psychiatric conditions, such as parental anxiety disorders; conducting large-scale efficacy and effectiveness trials, including diverse cultural populations; and striving to have greater understanding of developmental factors—all of which can better inform prevention strategies.

References

Albee GW, Gulotta TP: Primary Prevention Works. Thousand Oaks, CA, Sage, 1997

Barrett PM, Turner C: Prevention of anxiety symptoms in primary school children: preliminary results from a universal school-based trial. Br J Clin Psychol 40:399–410, 2001

Barrett PM, Sonderegger R, Xenos S: Using FRIENDS to combat anxiety and adjustment problems among young migrants to Australia: a national trial. Clin Child Psychol Psychiatry 8:241–260, 2003

Bartlett SJ, Krishnan AJ, Reikert KA, et al: Maternal depressive symptoms and adherence to therapy in inner-city children with asthma. Pediatrics 113:229–237, 2004

Beardslee WR: When a Parent Is Depressed: How to Protect Your Children From the Effects of Depression in the Family. Boston, MA, Little, Brown, 2002

Beardslee WR, Podorefsky D: Resilient adolescents whose parents have serious affective and other psychiatric disorders: the importance of self-understanding and relationships. Am J Psychiatry 145:63–69, 1988

Beardslee WR, Versage E, Gladstone TRG: Children of affectively ill parents: a review of the past ten years. J Am Acad Child Adolesc Psychiatry 37:1134–1141, 1998

Beardslee WR, Gladstone TRG, Wright, EJ, et al: A family-based approach to the prevention of depressive symptoms in children at risk: evidence of parental and child change. Pediatrics 112:119–131, 2003

Beardslee WR, Boris N, Compton W, et al: The Prevention of Mental Disorders in General Psychiatric Practice: Implications for Assessment, Intervention and Research: A Report Submitted by the Task Force on Prevention to the Council on Research. Washington, DC, American Psychiatric Association, 2005

Beardslee WR, Wright EJ, Gladstone TRG, et al: Long-term effects from a randomized trial of two public health preventive interventions for parental depression. J Fam Psychol 21:703–713, 2007

Beidel DC, Turner SM: At risk for anxiety, I: psychopathology in the offspring of anxious parents. J Am Acad Child Adolesc Psychiatry 36:918–924, 1997

Biederman J, Faraone SV, Hirshfeld-Becker DR, et al: Patterns of psychopathology and dysfunction in high-risk children of parents with panic disorder and major depression. Am J Psychiatry 158:49–57, 2001

Bijl RV, Cuijpers P, Smit F: Psychiatric disorders in adult children of parents with a history of psychopathology. Soc Psychiatry Psychiatr Epidemiol 37:7–12, 2002

Bruce ML, Takeuchi DT, Leaf PJ: Poverty and psychiatric status: longitudinal evidence from the New Haven Epidemiologic Catchment Area Study. Arch Gen Psychiatry 48:470–474, 1991

Chorpita B, Albano A, Barlow D: Cognitive processing in children: relation to anxiety and family influences. J Clin Child Psychol 25:170–176, 1996

Cicchetti D, Cohen DJ (eds): Developmental psychopathology: Risk, disorder, and adaptation, Vol 2. New York, Wiley, 1995

Cicchetti D, Schneider-Rosen K: An organizational approach to childhood depression, in Depression in Young People: Developmental and Clinical Perspectives. Edited by Rutter M, Izard CE, Read PB. New York, Guilford, 1986, pp 71–134

Clarke GN, Lewinsohn PM: Instructor's Manual for the Adolescent Coping With Stress Course. Portland, OR, Kaiser Permanente Center for Health Research, 1995

Clarke GN, Hornbrook M, Lynch F, et al: A randomized trial of a group cognitive intervention for preventing depression in adolescent offspring of depressed parents. Arch Gen Psychiatry 58:1127–1134, 2001

Coolidge FL, Thede LL, Jang KL: Heritability of personality disorders in childhood: a preliminary investigation. J Pers Disord 15:33–40, 2001

Cornish AM, McMahon CA, Ungerer J, et al: Maternal depression and the experience of parenting in the second postnatal year. J Reprod Infant Psychol 24:121–132, 2006

Costello EJ, Angold A: Epidemiology, in Anxiety Disorders in Children and Adolescents. Edited by March JS. New York, Guilford, 1995, pp 109–124

Cuijpers P, Langendoen Y, Bijl RV: Psychiatric disorders in adult children of problem drinkers: prevalence, first onset and comparison with other risk factors. Addiction 94:1489–1498, 1999

Cummings EM, Keller PS, Davies PT: Towards a family process model of maternal and paternal depressive symptoms: exploring multiple relations with child and family functioning. J Child Psychol Psychiatry 46:479–489, 2005

Dadds MR, Barrett PM, Rapee RM, et al: Family process and child anxiety and aggression: an observational analysis. J Abnorm Child Psychol 24:715–735, 1996

Dadds MR, Spence SH, Holland DE, et al: Prevention and early intervention for anxiety disorders: a controlled trial. J Consult Clin Psychol 65:627–635, 1997

Dadds MR, Holland DE, Laurens KR, et al: Early intervention and prevention of anxiety disorders in children: results at 2-year follow-up. J Consult Clin Psychol 67:145–150, 1999

DelBello MP, Geller B: Review of studies of child and adolescent offspring of bipolar parents. Bipolar Disord 3:325–334, 2001

Dishion TJ, Kavanagh K: Intervening in Adolescent Problem Behavior: A Family Centered Approach. New York, Guilford, 2003

Eisenberg L: Prevention, rhetoric and reality. J R Soc Med 77:268–280, 1984

Eisenberg L: The social construction of the human brain. Am J Psychiatry 152:1563–1575, 1995

Felitti V, Anda RF, Nordenberg D, et al: Relationship of childhood abuse and household dysfunction to many of the leading causes of death in adults. Am J Prev Med 14:245–258, 1998

Foa EB, Costello EJ, Franklin M, et al: Prevention of anxiety disorders, in Treating and Preventing Adolescent Mental Health Disorders: What We Know and What We Don't Know: A Research Agenda for Improving the Mental Health of Our Youth. Edited by Evans DL, Foa EB, Gur RE, et al. Oxford, England, Oxford University Press, 2005, pp 222–246

Hicks BM, Krueger RJ, Iacono WG, et al: Family transmission and heritability of externalizing disorders: a twin-family study. Arch Gen Psychiatry 61:922–928, 2004

Hirshfeld DR, Biederman J, Brody L, et al: Associations between expressed emotion and child behavioral inhibition and psychopathology: a pilot study. J Am Acad Child Adolesc Psychiatry 36:205–213, 1997

Hirshfeld-Becker DR, Biederman J: Rationale and principles for early intervention with young children at risk for anxiety disorders. Clin Child Fam Psychol Rev 5:161–172, 2002

Hosman C, Jané-Llopis E, Saxena S: Prevention of Mental Disorders: Effective Interventions and Policy Options: A Summary Report. Geneva, Switzerland, World Health Organization, 2004

Kumpfer KL, Alvadaro R, Whiteside HO: Family-based interventions for substance use and misuse prevention. Subst Use Misuse 38:1759–1787, 2003

LaFreniere PJ, Capuano F: Preventive intervention as a means of clarifying direction of effects in socialization: anxious-withdrawn preschoolers case. Dev Psychopathol 9:551–564, 1997

Lowry-Webster HM, Barrett PM, Dadds MR: A universal prevention trial of anxiety and depressive symptomatology in childhood: preliminary data from an Australian study. Behav Change 18:36–50, 2001

Luthar SS: Resilience in development: a synthesis of research across five decades, in Developmental Psychopathology: Risk, Disorder, and Adaptation, 2nd Edition. Edited by Cicchetti D, Cohen DJ. New York, Wiley, 2006, pp 739–795

Luthar SS, Cicchetti D, Becker B: The construct of resilience: a critical evaluation and guidelines for future work. Child Dev 71:543–562, 2000

MacMillan HL: Child sexual abuse: an overview (part II). Canadian Child Psychiatric Bulletin 5:90–94, 1997

March J: Cognitive-behavioral psychotherapy for children and adolescents with OCD: a review and recommendations for treatment. J Am Acad Child Adolesc Psychiatry 34:7–18, 1995

Masten AS, Best KM, Garmezy N: Resilience and development: contributions from the study of children who overcome adversity. Dev Psychopathol 2:425–444, 1990

McAlister-Groves BM, Zuckerman B, Marans S, et al: Silent victims: children who witness violence. JAMA 269:262–264, 1993

Mrazek PJ, Haggerty RJ: Reducing Risks for Mental Disorders. Washington, DC, Institute of Medicine, National Academy Press, 1994

Munoz RF, Mrazek PJ, Haggerty RJ: Institute of Medicine report on prevention of mental disorders: summary and commentary. Am Psychol 51:1116–1122, 1996

Olds DL: Prenatal and infancy home visiting by nurses: from randomized trials to community replication. Prev Sci 3:153–172, 2002

Olson AL, Dietrich AJ, Prazar G, et al: Two approaches to maternal depression screening during well child visits. Dev Behav Pediatr 26:169–176, 2005

Park RJ, Senior R, Stein A: The offspring of mothers with eating disorders. Eur Child Adolesc Psychiatry 12:1110–1119, 2003

Rapee RM: The development and modification of temperamental risk for anxiety disorders: prevention of a lifetime of anxiety. Biol Psychiatry 52:947–957, 2002

Reiss D, Neiderhiser J, Hetherington EM, et al: The relationship code: deciphering genetic and social patterns in adolescent development. Cambridge, MA, Harvard University Press, 2000

Rutter M: Commentary: some focus and process considerations regarding effects of parental depression on children. Dev Psychol 26:60–67, 1990

Sameroff AJ, Chandler MJ: Reproductive risk and the continuum of caretaking casualty, in Review of Child Developmental Research, Vol 4. Edited by Horowitz FD, Hetherington M, Scarr-Salopatek S. Chicago, IL, University of Chicago Press, 1987, pp 187–244

Sameroff A, Bartko WT, Baldwin A, et al: Family and social influences on the development of child competence, in Families, Risk, and Competence. Edited by Feiring C, Lewis M. Mahwah, NJ, Lawrence Erlbaum Associates, 1998, pp 161–185

Seifert K, Bowman PJ, Heflin CM, et al: Social and environmental predictors of maternal depression in current and recent welfare recipients. Am J Orthopsychiatry 70:510–522, 2000

Shaw DS, Dishion TJ, Supplee L, et al: Randomized trial of a family centered approach to the prevention of early conduct problems: 2-year effects of the family check-up in early childhood. J Consult Clin Psychol 74:1–9, 2006

Siqueland L, Kendall P, Steinberg L: Anxiety in children: perceived family environments and observed family interaction. J Clin Child Psychol 25:225–237, 1996

Spoth RL, Kavanagh KA, Dishion TJ: Family centered preventive intervention science: toward benefits to larger populations of children, youth, and families. Prev Sci 3:145–152, 2002

Steinhausen H: Children of alcoholic parents. Eur Child Adolesc Psychiatry 4:143–152, 1995

U.S. Department of Health and Human Services: Mental Health: A Report of the Surgeon General. Washington, DC, U.S. Department of Health and Human Services, 2000. Available at: http://www.surgeongeneral.gov/library/mentalhealth/home.html. Accessed July 23, 2009.

Weissman MM, Pilowsky DJ, Wickramartne PJ, et al: Remissions in maternal depression and child psychopathology: a STAR*D-child report. JAMA 295:1389–1398, 2006

Zeanah CH, Boris NW, Larrieu JA: Infant development and developmental risk: a review of the past 10 years. J Am Acad Child Adolesc Psychiatry 36:165–178, 1997

Chapter 43

Legal and Ethical Issues

John B. Sikorski, M.D.
Anlee D. Kuo, J.D., M.D.

Clinicians working at the interface of child and adolescent psychiatry and the law are aware of the evolving nature of both science and evidence-based medicine and the evolving and complex nature of the law and related ethical considerations. This warrants proceeding with thoughtful caution, maintaining a current knowledge base in the areas of clinical work, developing systems of maintaining awareness of relevant legal developments in the local jurisdiction, and when in doubt, consulting with experienced colleagues or seeking the advice of one's own counsel.

It is the intent of this chapter to 1) provide a framework for understanding the current status of rights of children and ethical issues and behavior in clinical practice and research and 2) provide an overview of legal issues involved in the clinical practice of child and adolescent psychiatry, including divorce and child custody, child abuse and neglect, and civil litigation involving minors and school-related legal issues.

Evolving Concepts of the Status of Children

From the tradition of Roman law and English common law through to the eighteenth century, children were considered the chattel or property of their families, particularly their fathers, who were entitled to the child's labor in exchange for what was viewed as the child's needs for care and protection. If the child was orphaned or abandoned, the child might come under the authority of the state under the concept of *parens patriae* derived from the notion that the crown or the state had guardianship over individuals unable to legally act for themselves. By the end of the nineteenth century, child labor laws began to limit the exploitation of children in the mines and factories. At that time, children who were charged with criminal offenses were tried in adult courts and when convicted sent to adult jails. By 1875, the first case of child abuse was brought to court in New York by the Society for Prevention of Cruelty to Animals (Schetky 2002).

In a practical sense, we can consider a *right* to be a claim for an individual's freedom of action or for money, goods, or services that is enforceable by a court of competent jurisdiction. It has been observed that "law typically follows rather than leads social change" (Kay 2000). Current concepts and interpretations of civil rights, privacy rights, rights of minors (children and adolescents), and family and dependency law are legislative enactments or appellate court interpretations and opinions that have evolved in the context of vast technological, demographic, and sociocultural changes in American society during the twentieth century. The introduction of the new technology of birth control pills brought changes to the traditional status and roles of women, enlivening the women's movement of the 1960s and subsequent family and law reforms in the 1970s. While the civil rights movement of the 1950s and 1960s was focused primarily on the adult status and due process, there was growing social concern about the well-being, health, education, and the age-appropriate needs and rights of minors. As noted in her landmark review of "Children Under the Law," Hillary Rodham (1973) stated, "Children's rights cannot be secured until some particular institution has recognized them and assumed responsibility for enforcing them."

A consensus regarding children's rights and needs was developed at the White House Conference on Children convened in 1970, asserting specific rights essential to a child's well-being (U.S. Government Printing Office 1971):

1. The right to grow in a society that respects the dignity of life and is free of poverty, discrimination, and other forms of degradation
2. The right to be born and to be healthy and wanted through childhood
3. The right to grow up nurtured by affectionate parents
4. The right to be a child during childhood; to have meaningful choices in the process of maturation and development, and to have a meaningful voice in the community
5. The right to be educated to the limits of one's capacity and through processes designed to elicit one's full potential
6. The right to have social mechanisms to enforce the foregoing rights

While these principles have served as lofty sounding pronouncements, legislation at both federal and state levels has been contentious and slow in meaningfully enacting them. Most advances in recognizing the rights of minors have been downward extrapolations of the rights of adults—e.g., rights of emancipated minors as defined by each state or the establishment of rights regarding children's special needs, i.e., free appropriate public education for all handicapped children (Education for All Handicapped Children Act of 1975).

It is also of particular interest to note that the United States has not ratified the U.N. Convention on the Rights of the Child of November 20, 1989 (United Nations 1989). The U.S. government's rationale for the refusal to ratify this convention on the rights of the child is based on its perceived conflict with the rights of the parents, U.S. sovereignty, and state and local laws.

Since the 1960s, states have defined the age of majority at age 18, providing the usual range of adult rights and responsibilities at that age except for the purchase of alcoholic beverages, which is usually age 21. However, states vary widely in their provisions for specific rights of minors for emancipation; marriage; obtaining a driver's license; and access and consent to health care, including physical, mental, sexually related conditions, and substance abuse–related health care. States also vary in their provisions for rights of minors in educational services, in paid employment, and in contractual obligations, particularly in arts, entertainment, and professional sports. In these regards, clinical practitioners should familiarize themselves with the specific statutes in their respective states. For example, information regarding California laws related to minors can be found in Kauble (2008).

Our contemporary society's perception and treatment of minors continues to fluctuate between the legal doctrines of parens patriae and "the best interests of the child." Parens patriae traditionally has empowered state initiatives to protect persons who are unable to care for or protect themselves—and also has allowed state agencies to interfere with parental prerogatives when there is evidence of neglect, inability to perform their parental responsibilities, or evidence of abuse of minors.

The interface between children's rights and needs has continued to fluctuate and evolve in both clinical practice and the law as the U.S. Supreme Court noted in *Santosky v. Kramer* (1982), "So long as the child is part of a viable family his own interests are merged with those of the other members. Only after the family fails in its functions should the child's interests become a matter for state intrusion."

The best interests of the child is the legal standard. Prioritizing children's needs evolved at the turn of the century and was articulated by Judge Benjamin Cardozo as specifying the court's role to serve as parens patriae and do "what is in the best interests of the child" (*Finlay v. Finlay* 1925).

As the legal standard for clinical decision making, the best interests of the child was extensively studied at the Yale Child Study Center (Goldstein et al. 1996), initially focusing on child placement conflicts requiring value preferences and clinical judgment in determining in each case what is in the child's best interest.

This standard became codified in various forms in various states as the standard for child custody determination and family law. It has been criticized as too vague and imprecise and a rationalization for adult decision makers to project their prejudices and judgments about children's futures.

It has also been advocated as providing a rational framework for judgments involving the multiple factors and issues in the tension and balance between a) parental values and responsibilities and b) children's rights and needs.

Ethical Issues in Clinical Practice

Ethics can be defined as the study of moral principles and values that guide and determine the conduct of individuals in particular, usually professional circumstances and relationships.

The awareness of ethical values and duties in the practice of medicine dates back to the time of the Hippocratic oath. These include the concepts of doing no harm, using the physician's best ability and judgment to help the patient, keeping professional confidences, and not abusing one's professional role and relationship. Ethical guidelines are evolving to highlight several principle issues: respect for the patient's autonomy, beneficence, and justice. The concept of respect for the person's autonomy includes informed consent in treatment and research, including maintaining appropriate professional boundaries and confidences, as well as factual honesty and avoidance of misrepresentations. The concept of beneficence expands the "do no harm" concept to include acting in the patient's best interests and minimizing risks and maximizing benefits in professional judgments and relationships.

The concept of justice has more recently come into ethical consideration in the biomedical arena, having to do with social justice in the allocation of resources and fair and equitable distribution of risks and benefits.

Psychiatric disorders may adversely affect the individual's autonomy, decision-making ability, and ability to provide informed consent. The "Principles of Medical Ethics With Annotations Especially Applicable to Psychiatry" has been revised and published in the form of an ethics primer (American Psychiatric Association 2001). This document provides the framework and guidelines for ethical considerations in decision making in the practice of psychiatry. Chapter 2, "Children, Adolescents, and Families," of the ethics primer discusses the special ethical considerations involved in the practice of child and adolescent psychiatry. The American Academy of Child and Adolescent Psychiatry has developed and adopted a Code of Ethics (American Academy of Child and Adolescent Psychiatry 1995) that expands on the ethical issues and tensions particularly relevant to the practice of child and adolescent psychiatry.

These ethical tensions derive from the evolving developmental stages of the child or adolescent, the family structure, and treatment contexts. There may also be overlapping and potentially conflicting rights and responsibilities for the child and for the child's parents or guardians. The nature of clinical work with children interfaces with agencies external to the family—such as schools, courts, and specialized treatment, educational, or recreation programs that may have responsibility or authority for the child—and may require exchange of information or consultative or collateral professional work.

In addition, the clinician has an ethical duty to maintain current knowledge of the state of the art and science regarding treatment efficacy and risk and benefit considerations relevant to their clinical practice and professional responsibilities.

The more common ethical dilemmas in child and adolescent mental health practice involve informed consent, confidentiality, conflict of interest, and role and boundary confusions or violations.

The ethical duty for the clinician is to provide sufficient relevant and factual information regarding the patient's condition, prognosis, risks and benefits of types of treatments available, and recommendations, so that the patient can provide informed consent to the diagnostic procedures and treatment process.

Clinical work with children and adolescents poses additional complications to the clinician because their minority age status usually requires parent or legal guardian informed consent for consultation, evaluation, and treatment. *Consent* refers to the legal authority to provide permission, which resides with the parent or legal guardian. Nevertheless, the development of trust in the treatment relationship usually requires that the child have sufficient information as he can understand at his level of development, so that he can assent and agree to participate in the clinical work or research protocol.

The ethical principle of confidentiality is considered the cornerstone for building trust and honest communication in the physician-patient relationship. This principle obligates the clinician to hold in confidence the communications with the patient, as the patient, even if a minor, is the holder of the right to confidentiality and must give consent for the release of that information. However, as with all children under legal age of maturity, the legal consent must be made by the parents or legal guardian, except where there are specific statutory exceptions, such as the mandatory child abuse reporting laws, or where the child is an imminent danger to self or others.

In clinical practice with children and parents, the clinician strives to articulate the issues involved in confidentiality and informed consent with the child and the parents or legal guardian during the beginning of the evaluation process, taking into account the child's level of understanding and ability to assent to participate in the process and the treatment planning.

Circumstances may arise in civic and social situations where the clinician meets the patient or the patient's family or where the clinician is active in other contexts such as school consultation, civic board responsibilities, or by chance at a social gathering. It remains the clinician's ethical responsibility to maintain his or her professional role with its implied confidentiality and not violate or exploit the professional relationship for personal advantage or to the detriment of the patient. In addition, transference and countertransference phenomena in the professional relationship may develop to blur the appropriate role and boundary, leading to inappropriate advocacy for or exploitation of the patient. Vigilance in one's usual and customary practice and consultation with one's peers is helpful in maintaining professional roles and boundaries and minimizing conflicts of interest.

Ethical Issues in Research

The deficiency of the scientific knowledge base and need for research has generated a need to further develop ethical principles relevant to research (Munir and Earls 1992).

The interests of the subject have priority over the interests of science and society, and voluntary informed consent is essential. In response to federal requirements, research and educational institutions have developed local institutional review boards (IRBs) to insure legal and ethical conduct in human subject research. IRBs are made up of researchers, clinicians, members of the public, patient advocates, and experts in relevant law and ethics.

Children and adolescents, especially if they are mentally disabled, are particularly vulnerable because they cannot provide informed consent to volunteer as research subjects, and the parent or guardian of such a child may have a conflict of interest in providing for the legal consent. Federal regulations state in part: "The IRB shall determine that adequate provisions are made for soliciting the assent of children when in the judgment of the IRB, children are capable of providing assent. In determining whether children are capable of assenting, the IRB shall take into account the ages, maturity, and psychological state of the children involved" (U.S. Department of Health and Human Services 1991).

Ethical standards in clinical practice, in research, and in medical education have taken on a global dimension. The International Association for Child and Adolescent Psychiatry and Allied Professions (2006) has adopted guidelines and principles of ethics in child and adolescent mental health.

Legal Issues in Clinical Practice
Confidentiality, Privilege, and Duty

Confidentiality and privilege are two distinct ethical and legal duties protected by state statutes to promote communication and trust between the physician and patient. *Privilege* refers to the patient's right to prevent disclosure of information obtained during treatment in judicial or quasi-judicial proceedings. The term *confidentiality* is broader and refers to the clinician's obligation to avoid disclosure of the patient's information to any person other than the patient.

The legal and ethical rights of confidentiality and privilege belong to the patient and can be waived only by the patient except as provided for by certain statutory exceptions. For example, the right of confidentiality is automatically waived when the patient is a threat to herself or others or when a reportable condition is revealed such as sexual abuse, neglect, maltreatment, or physical abuse. Frequent exceptions to privileged communications include commitment proceedings, will contests, child custody cases, and criminal matters (Macbeth 2002). In these types of proceedings, the court may mandate the disclosure of confidential or privileged communication, such as when a client puts his or her own mental condition at issue in a lawsuit (Bernet 1998). States are not uniform in these rules and exceptions to confidential and privileged communication, so clinicians should familiarize themselves with the relevant statutes in their jurisdiction.

Confidentiality becomes more complicated when it involves the legal status of minors and raises the issue as to who holds the right. In general, the parent who is legally entitled to authorize treatment for the child holds the legal right to confidentiality for the child (Macbeth 2002). Some jurisdictions allow minors to hold the right to confidentiality based on their age or their ability to consent to certain treatments on their own. The law has increasingly given adolescents the right and responsibilities of adults, so psychiatrists should be familiar with the statutory exceptions specific to each state.

Informed Consent and Competence

Minors are generally not deemed competent to give legal consent to psychiatric evaluation, treatment, or the release of information. The consent of the parent or guardian is required unless statutory exceptions exist or the minor is emancipated. The consent must also be based on an informed choice—i.e., the patient (or parent/guardian) must have the cognitive capacity and mental competence to adequately understand the nature of the condition, the recommended treatment, and the potential risks, benefits, and alternatives of the treatment. Furthermore, the patient choice must be voluntary and not coerced. The informed consent from the parent or legal guardian should be clearly documented in the medical records.

States provide various statutory exceptions to the general requirement of parental consent. For example, emancipated minors can consent to their own treatment. This group includes minors who are older than age 15, living away from parents, and economically self-sufficient; married minors; minors on active duty in the U.S. armed services; and minors who have been emancipated through a specific court order. Courts can also determine that a minor is "mature" and able to appreciate the nature, extent, and consequences of a medical treatment.

State legislatures have allowed more minors to consent to treatment such as care related to sexual behavior and time-limited outpatient mental health treatment. This trend raises increasing concern about the lack of sufficient maturity, understanding, and experience in minors to make an informed judgment about a procedure. Clinicians should always explain relevant information at a level that is developmentally appropriate.

Civil Commitment

Parents, legal guardians, and state agencies may occasionally need to hospitalize a seriously disturbed child or adolescent, and this necessity may conflict with the child's or adolescent's desire for autonomy and self-determination. American Academy of Child and Adolescent Psychiatry (1989) has published guidelines regarding this issue and listed the following factors to consider: 1) a qualified psychiatrist's evaluation; 2) diagnosis by DSM criteria; 3) severity of impairment in two or more areas of daily functioning; 4) likelihood of benefit from the proposed treatment; 5) prior consideration of less restrictive treatment procedures and the judgment that they are inappropriate or inadequate to meet the patient's needs; 6) encouragement of the child to voluntarily participate in the admission, treatment planning, and discharge process; and 7) the parent's full information about and participation in the hospitalization and treatment planning decisions.

In the governing U.S. Supreme Court case on this issue, *Parham v. J.R.* (1979), the Supreme Court granted substantial autonomy to parents in making decisions about placing their children in mental health facilities. However, an independent medical review must confirm the nature of the illness and the likelihood of benefit from the proposed treatment, and the youth may request periodic reviews of the treatment and confinement necessity. States have addressed this situation by implementing exceptions to the general rule of parental consent (Horowitz 2002).

Professional Liability

In the past few decades, child psychiatrists are increasingly subject to malpractice suits based on matters such as abandonment of patients, battery, breach of confidentiality or duty, failure to follow standards of care, failure to report or protect against abuse or harassment of patients, negligence, improper treatment, harmful effects of medications, or other alleged violations of federal or state laws regarding professional practice.

These suits are based on principles of tort law or civil wrongful behavior, in which the practitioner may be liable for the unintended consequences of alleged harm or injury to the patient or to a third party that could have or should have been prevented by the practitioner's action. The four elements of a claim of professional negligence are as follows:

1. *Duty*—a duty of care was owed to the patient by the physician
2. *Dereliction*—the duty of care was breached
3. *Damages*—the patient experienced actual damage due to the breach of duty
4. *Direct causation*—the dereliction was the direct cause of the damages

The plaintiff must demonstrate to the court the existence of these elements according to the standard of care in the community at the time. In civil cases, the standard of proof is the preponderance of evidence (i.e., more likely than not).

One area of increasing ethical and legal vulnerability involves the conflict between independent clinical judgment of attending physicians and the cost containment purposes of managed care agencies. When a managed care company denies coverage for a service for "lack of medical necessity," the physician has four duties (*Wickline v. California* 1986): 1) appeal the decision, 2) discuss the issues raised by the managed care company with the patient, 3) treat the patient in an emergency even without payment, and 4) develop alternative treatment plans.

Responding to a Subpoena

A *subpoena* is a legal order requiring the appearance at a specified proceeding or the production of certain documents or both. The subpoena may be issued to a practitioner if either party in a legal proceeding believes that the clinician may possess information relevant to the legal dispute. If a clinician receives a subpoena, he should immediately inform the patient of the facts of the subpoena and discuss with the patient the possible responses. If the patient provides consent for the release of information, the clinician must respond or run the risk of being held in contempt. If the patient does not provide consent for release of the in-

formation requested by the subpoena, the clinician should consult with his own attorney. In special circumstances, the clinician can request to have the records reviewed in private chambers by the judge to determine their relevance to the case at hand. However, in no circumstances should a clinician ignore a valid subpoena. In institutional practice, the clinician should always immediately contact the risk management and/or legal department.

Overview of the Legal System

Structurally, the legal system is divided into two main courts: state courts and federal courts. State courts adjudicate both civil and criminal cases arising under state law. They consist of lower courts (i.e., trial courts), higher courts (i.e., appellate courts), and the state's supreme court. The appellate and supreme courts play a supervisory role over the trial courts. Some specialized courts exercise jurisdiction over specific types of cases. For example, juvenile courts deal with juvenile delinquency and abuse and neglect. Family courts have jurisdiction over matters involving divorce and child custody issues. Probate courts handle wills and administer decedent's estates.

The federal court system presides over civil and criminal cases arising under the U.S. Constitution and federal statutes. It can also adjudicate civil actions if the parties are residents of different states. This system consists of federal trial courts, 13 U.S. Courts of Appeal, and the U.S. Supreme Court. The appellate courts hear appeals from the trial courts and the U.S. Supreme Court hears appeals from the federal appellate courts and exercises discretionary jurisdiction to grant review in other cases by writ of certiorari.

The courts of general jurisdiction preside over two types of legal proceedings: civil and criminal cases. Civil cases include breach of contract disputes; property and financial disputes; and torts, including injury, negligence, professional liability, libel, and slander. Torts are the most common civil action where a plaintiff asserts that a defendant owed her a "duty of care" and acted in a negligent manner, causing the plaintiff a foreseeable harm, loss, or injury.

The standard of proof is the level of certainty required for a certain judicial outcome, which varies depending on the type of legal proceeding. For example, the standard of a preponderance of evidence is used in most civil proceedings. The intermediate standard of "clear and convincing evidence" is required in cases where a deprivation of fundamental rights or liberty is at stake, such as deprivation of parental rights. The highest standard of proof, "beyond a reasonable doubt," is used in criminal proceedings as well as juvenile court and delinquency proceedings. Physicians who testify in court typically state their opinions within a reasonable degree of medical certainty. This standard reflects the level of certainty equivalent to what a physician uses when making a diagnosis and starting treatment (Rappeport 1985).

Child Psychiatrist as Expert Witness

Child psychiatrists are increasingly being called upon to testify as experts in various types of legal proceedings. In the emerging subspecialty field of forensic psychiatry, the child psychiatrist applies her clinical and scientific expertise to legal issues in legal contexts. This role is distinguished from the role of treating clinician by the absence of a doctor-patient relationship. The psychiatrist's opinion may even ultimately result in harm to the child. For example, the child may be waived to an adult court or taken away from her parents in a dependency hearing. As an expert witness, a child psychiatrist will draw upon her specific body of knowledge to form an opinion about a legal issue. No treatment is rendered, and the usual medical, legal, and ethical principles between a physician and patient do not apply. The psychiatrist's client is the attorney or judge who is hiring her to render an expert opinion. Acting as an expert witness, the psychiatrist is typically asked to read legal documents, conduct some interview and then write a report, provide depositions, and/or testify in court.

When an attorney or the court calls upon the psychiatrist's expertise for child custody evaluations, the expert typically assists the court in determining a custody and visitation schedule in accordance with the best interests of the child (Goldstein et al. 1996). In child abuse and neglect cases, the forensic evaluator often conducts assessments on the nature and extent of harm to a child, evaluates parental fitness, and makes recommendations regarding placement, treatment, or termination of parental rights (American Academy of Child and Adolescent Psychiatry 1997b). These assessments are used in dependency and guardianship pro-

ceedings, custodial disputes, termination of parental right, and criminal and civil litigation (Barnum 1997). Child psychiatrists can also conduct assessments on adolescents in the juvenile and adult criminal courts. In these cases, they are often called on to evaluate and provide testimony regarding the juvenile's degree of dangerousness and amenability to treatment or rehabilitation and discuss potential disposition options. One topic of increasing concern involves the juvenile's competence to stand trial or waive Miranda rights (Grisso and Schwartz 2000). Finally, the child psychiatrist can be called to evaluate children in legal issues related to special education such as compliance with state and federal disability statutes.

Practice guidelines have been developed for assessing children and youth in many of these legal proceedings (American Academy of Child and Adolescent Psychiatry 1997a, 1997b; Deprato and Hammer 2002).

Forensic Aspects of Child Custody and Divorce

With approximately half of marriages in the United States ending in divorce, legal and ethical considerations are increasingly encountered in forensic aspects of child custody and divorce work (American Academy of Child and Adolescent Psychiatry 1997a).

One of the most important ethical concepts to understand in this line of work involves role clarification by the child psychiatrist. Unlike a clinician who acts as the child's advocate for the purpose of treatment, the forensic evaluator is a neutral expert who can draw upon objective facts and data to arrive at impartial and informed opinions for the family court. The evaluator should clearly communicate her role to the parent and child prior to the assessment and avoid the mistake of "wearing two hats"—i.e., acting as both clinician and forensic expert (Schetky 2007). Clarification of the role and avoidance of boundary blurring will protect the objectivity of the evaluation and prevent the client from being misled or deceived in the interview process.

Forensic evaluations in child custody and divorce cases involve communications between the forensic expert and the child and parent that are not confidential. The information obtained from the interview will be used in a report, deposition, or testimony that is available to the judge, attorneys, and other involved legal personnel. The evaluee should have a clear understanding of this lack of confidentiality in the forensic setting. The potential evaluator should also be careful about bias and conflict of interest pitfalls. Prior involvement with either party may unduly influence the evaluator and jeopardize the objectivity of the assessment. Similarly, conducting a unilateral evaluation with the assessment of the child interacting with only one parent inherently leads to biased opinions (Herman 2002).

The prevailing legal doctrine of the best interests of the child is the guiding principle in deciding child custody disputes. Although the concept remains ambiguous, some clarification has been achieved through legislation and statutes. The Uniform Marriage and Divorce Act, promulgated by the National Conference of Commissioners on Uniform State Laws and approved by the American Bar Association in 1974, established the language and definition regarding the best-interests criteria and includes factors such as the wishes of the parent and child; the interactions of the child with those who may significantly affect his or her best interests; the child's adjustment to his or her home, school, and community; and the mental and physical health of all individuals involved (Group for the Advancement of Psychiatry 1980). The majority of states have adapted their statutes from the concept and language of this act.

The two main legal outcomes of a child custody dispute are joint or sole custody. In joint legal custody, both parents have legal decision-making power for the child. In sole legal custody, only one parent has the authority. For clinicians providing treatment for a child, this concept is important because in joint custody situations, treatment and medication administration must first be approved by both parents. In joint physical custody, both parents share physical custody of the child and the child typically lives in both homes, each for a percentage of the time. Again, in clinical work, comprehension of the physical custody arrangement is important for understanding the child's daily routine and the stresses he or she endures living in two different environments. For the forensic evaluator, understanding the meaning of these different outcomes is critical for making a recommendation to the courts.

To minimize the risks of the expert providing unwarranted conclusions and to promote uniformity and maintain standards of care, several guidelines have been published by organizations and practitioners (American Academy of Child and Adolescent Psychiatry 1997a; American Association of Family and Conciliation Courts 1994; Herman 2002; Judicial Council of California 2004; Stahl 1999).

Forensic Aspects of Child Abuse and Neglect

Child mental health professionals are increasingly involved in the assessment and treatment of children who have been abused. Since the passage of the Child Abuse Prevention and Treatment Act in 1974 and implementation of federally mandated guidelines, all states have passed laws mandating designated persons, such as child mental health professionals, to report child abuse and neglect. Failure to do so can result in civil liabilities and criminal penalties.

Forensic aspects of child abuse and neglect cases can involve a broad range of functions, such as assessment of the extent of physical and emotional harm to the child, parental fitness evaluations, and recommendations regarding placement, treatment, and/or termination of parental rights (American Academy of Child and Adolescent Psychiatry 1997b). These assessments may be used in a variety of legal proceedings, including divorce and custody disputes, civil and criminal proceedings, and in dependency, guardianship, and termination of parental right actions. Several guidelines are available to help assist the child mental health professional conduct an appropriate forensic assessment of a child who may have been abused (American Academy of Child and Adolescent Psychiatry 1997b; Barnum 1997, 2002; Quinn 2002).

Child as Witness

Due to a frequent lack of sufficient physical evidence in cases of sexual abuse allegations, a child's testimony is often critical in determining the likelihood of truth behind an allegation of abuse. With the increase in allegations of child sexual abuse over the past several decades and the importance of a child's testimony in these legal cases, a large body of information has developed regarding children's competency, memory, suggestibility, and credibility (Bruck and Ceci 2002; Bruck et al. 1998; Clark 2002; Corelli et al. 1997).

A child's competency to act as a witness essentially refers to his or her ability to testify in court in a reliable and meaningful manner. In general, competence is determined by four criteria: the capacity to register an event, the ability to accurately recall and recount the event, the ability to distinguish truth from falsehood, and the capacity to communicate based on personal knowledge of the facts.

A large body of research has explored the accuracy of children's memory and suggestibility. Studies indicate that memory and retention generally begin to exist at about age 3 and continue to improve with age. The literature also shows that children are highly suggestible, with preschool children being more suggestible than older children or adults (Loftus 1997; Loftus and Pickrell 1995; Poole and Lindsay 1995).

The credibility of a child refers to the child's truthfulness and accuracy and is ultimately determined by the judge or jury. Forensic experts can assist the judge and jury in the determination through expert testimony. Several authors have examined the factors relevant to determining the issue of credibility (American Academy of Child and Adolescent Psychiatry 1997b; Benedek and Schetky 1987a, 1987b; Green 1986; Raskin and Esplin 1991). Some of the factors that enhance the likelihood of accuracy in allegations include spontaneity and consistency in statements and the use of age-appropriate terminology. However, these factors are not definitive in assessing credibility, since suggestive interviewing techniques and other more complicated aspects of memory can contaminate the information.

The child's own testimony as a witness may be required in criminal proceedings as well as in civil litigation against the perpetrator. The evaluation of the child in these cases may subject her to multiple assessments in the home, school, clinical, or police settings and lead to increasing concern about the effect of the process on the child witness.

The U.S. Supreme Court has decided a number of cases that balanced the best interests and the cognitive and emotional capabilities of a child witness against the constitutional rights of defendants. These rights include protection against self-incrimination (Fifth Amendment), the right to confront and cross examine witnesses (Sixth Amendment), and due process (Fourteenth Amendment.) In *White v. Illinois* (1992), the U.S. Supreme Court recognized what amounts to a specific hearsay exception: The testimony of a physician was admitted and did not violate the defendant's Sixth Amendment rights because the child's statement to the physician was a "spontaneous declaration" made to the physician for the purpose of medical diagnosis and treatment. This area of law continues to evolve, and clinicians should be aware of current standards of assessment and legal guidelines related to their particular case.

Civil Litigation

Civil lawsuits involving children and adolescents are frequently brought by their parents or guardians in the form of a tort, which is 1) a claim that a wrong has been done by the negligence or intention of another person or entity and 2) a demand for compensation for the damage suffered by the victim (Schetky and Guyer 2002). The majority of civil litigation involving children alleging psychic trauma is the result of accidental injury, dog bites, burns, battery and violence, negligence by caregivers or product manufacturers, and toxic exposure. Aside from assessing the physical injuries the child may have sustained, the child psychiatrist or other mental health professional is called upon for clinical diagnosis and treatment or for forensic examination and testimony as an expert witness (American Academy of Child and Adolescent Psychiatry 1998).

If the same clinician provides both the clinical work and the forensic expert evaluation and testimony, an ethical violation based on conflict of interest and dual agency would result. The forensic evaluation, by a court-appointed expert or forensic expert hired by a party in the lawsuit, has a different set of professional and ethical duties and responsibilities from those of the treating clinician. These include understanding and defining the clinician's role in the evaluation and legal proceedings including the limits on confidentiality, striving for honesty and objectivity, and maintaining one's competence and qualifications (American Academy of Psychiatry and the Law 2005).

School-Related Legal Issues

Until the latter half of the twentieth century, the Federal government played no role in the public education of children. However, the landmark U.S. Supreme Court decision, *Brown v. Board of Education,* ended segregation as a legal policy in public schools (*Brown v. Board of Education* 1954). Included in the Rehabilitation Act of 1973, Section 504, Congress established the cornerstone of civil rights for the handicapped, stating in part, "No otherwise qualified handicapped individual in the United States…shall solely by reason of her or his handicap be excluded from participation in, be denied benefits of, or be subject to discrimination under any program or activity receiving federal financial assistance." The Americans With Disabilities Act of 1990 expanded the articulation of these rights of the handicapped and serves as a basis for accommodations in school curriculum, procedures, and school-based activities. Title IX of the Education Amendments of 1972) also prohibits sex discrimination in any educational institution receiving federal funding.

In the landmark Education for All Handicapped Children Act of 1975, Congress stated that the purpose of the act was to ensure that "All handicapped children have available to them a free appropriate public education which emphasizes special education, and related services, designed to meet their unique needs." This law provided federal definitions of such conditions, such as learning disabilities, serious emotional disturbance, mental retardation, and speech and language disorders. The law also defined processes and procedures to be followed in special education services, including "free and appropriate public education," "related services," "individual educational plan," and "least restrictive environment," along with numerous rights and procedural safeguards.

In 1991, Congress amended and changed the name of this act to Individuals With Disabilities Education Act (IDEA). This act, defining processes and procedures for special education for states and school districts, is modified and reauthorized every 5–6 years, the latest being 2004 (Individuals With Disabilities Education Improvement Act 2004).

Clinicians working with children involved in school district special education programs should be aware that the Department of Education definitions of various mental and emotional disorders may be different from DSM-IV-TR (American Psychiatric Association 2000) diagnoses and that school districts are required to follow Department of Education diagnostic criteria and procedures.

Each state must develop its own implementing regulations. Therefore, clinicians should familiarize themselves with the state-mandated criteria, as well as with the DSM-IV-TR criteria.

The American Academy of Child and Adolescent Psychiatry "Practice Parameter for Psychiatric Consultation to Schools" (Walter and Berkovitz 2005) provides the clinician with recent comprehensive descriptions and references to school mental health consultation and services.

Summary Points

- Children's rights as a legal concept developed during the twentieth century and are reflective of continuously changing sociocultural values.

- The best interest of the child is the legal standard for decision making regarding children's needs and placement.

- Ethical guidelines for clinical practice include respect for the patient's autonomy, beneficence, and justice balanced with traditional concepts of parents' rights and responsibilities.

- The principle of confidentiality requires the clinician to hold in confidence the patient's privileged communication.

- Psychiatric evaluation, treatment, and release of information require informed consent from the parent or legal guardian of a minor except in cases that involve emancipated or mature minors or where there are specific statutory exceptions.

- Clinicians are vulnerable to malpractice suits that are based on principles of tort law.

References

American Academy of Child and Adolescent Psychiatry: Policy Statement: Inpatient Hospital Treatment of Children and Adolescents. Washington, DC, American Academy of Child and Adolescent Psychiatry, 1989
American Academy of Child and Adolescent Psychiatry: Annotation to American Academy of Child and Adoles-
cent Psychiatry Ethics Code With Special References to Evolving Healthcare Delivery and Reimbursement Systems. Washington, DC, American Academy of Child and Adolescent Psychiatry, 1995
American Academy of Child and Adolescent Psychiatry: Practice parameters for child custody evaluations. J Am Acad Child Adolesc Psychiatry 36:57S–67S, 1997a
American Academy of Child and Adolescent Psychiatry: Practice parameters for the forensic evaluation of children and adolescents who may have been physically or

sexually abused. J Am Acad Child Adolesc Psychiatry 36:423–442, 1997b

American Academy of Child and Adolescent Psychiatry: Practice parameters for the assessment and treatment of children and adolescents with posttraumatic stress disorder. J Am Acad Child Adolesc Psychiatry 37(suppl):4S–22S, 1998

American Academy of Psychiatry and the Law: Ethical Guidelines for the Practice of Forensic Psychiatry. Bloomfield, CT, American Academy of Psychiatry and the Law, 2005

American Association of Family and Conciliation Courts: Model Standards of Practice for Child Custody Evaluations. Madison, WI, American Association of Family and Conciliation Courts, 1994

American Psychiatric Association: Diagnostic and Statistical Manual of Mental Disorders, 4th Edition, Text Revision. Washington, DC, American Psychiatric Association, 2000

American Psychiatric Association: Ethics Primer of the American Psychiatric Association. Washington, DC, American Psychiatric Association, 2001

American Psychological Association: Guidelines for child custody evaluations in divorce proceedings. Am Psychol 49:677–680, 1994

Americans With Disabilities Act of 1990, P.L. 101-336, 42 U.S.C. §12101 et. seq.

Barnum R: A suggested framework for forensic consultation in cases of child abuse and neglect. J Am Acad Psychiatry Law 25:581–593, 1997

Barnum R: Parenting assessment in cases of neglect and abuse, in Principles and Practice of Child and Adolescent Forensic Psychiatry. Edited by Schetky D, Benedek E. Washington, DC, American Psychiatric Publishing, 2002, pp 81–96

Benedek EP, Schetky DH: Problems in validating allegations of sexual abuse, 1: factors affecting perception and recall of events. J Am Acad Child Adolesc Psychiatry 26:912–915, 1987a

Benedek EP, Schetky DH: Problems in validating allegations of sexual abuse, 2: clinical evaluation. J Am Acad Child Adolesc Psychiatry 26:916–921, 1987b

Bernet W: The child and adolescent psychiatrist and the law, in Handbook of Child and Adolescent Psychiatry. Edited by Adams P, Bleiberg E. New York, Wiley, 1998, pp 438–468

Brown v Board of Education 347 U.S. 483 (1954)

Bruck M, Ceci SJ: Reliability and suggestibility of children's statements, in Principles and Practice of Child and Adolescent Forensic Psychiatry. Edited by Schetky D, Benedek E. Washington, DC, American Psychiatric Publishing, 2002, pp 137–145

Bruck M, Ceci SJ, Hembrooke H: Reliability and credibility of young children's reports. Am Psychol 53:136–149, 1998

Clark BK: Developmental aspects of memory in children, in Principles and Practice of Child and Adolescent Forensic Psychiatry. Edited by Schetky D, Benedek E. Washington, DC, American Psychiatric Publishing, 2002, pp 129–135

Corelli TB, Hoag MJ, Howell RJ: Memory, repression and child sexual abuse: forensic implications for the mental health professional. J Am Acad Psychiatry Law 25:31–45, 1997

Deprato DK, Hammer JH: Assessment and treatment of juvenile offenders in psychiatry, in Principles and Practice of Child and Adolescent Forensic Psychiatry. Edited by Schetky D, Benedek E. Washington, DC, American Psychiatric Publishing, 2002, pp 267–278

Education Amendments of 1972, Title IX. 20 U.S.C. Sect. 1681 et. seq.

Education for All Handicapped Children Act, P.L. 94-142, sec. 611, 88 Stat. 579, et. seq., 1975

Finlay v. Finlay, 148 N.E. 624 (N.Y. ct. app. 1925)

Goldstein J, Solnut AJ, Goldstein S: In the Best Interests of the Child. New York, Free Press, 1996

Green AH: True and false allegations of sexual abuse in child custody disputes. J Am Acad Child Psychiatry 25:449–456, 1986

Grisso T, Schwartz RG: Youth on Trial: A Developmental Perspective on Juvenile Justice. Chicago, IL, The University of Chicago Press, 2000

Group for the Advancement of Psychiatry: Divorce, Child Custody and the Family. New York, Mental Health Materials, 1980

Herman SP: Child custody evaluations, in Principles and Practice of Child and Adolescent Forensic Psychiatry. Washington, DC, American Psychiatric Publishing, 2002, pp 69–78

Horowitz R: Legal rights of children. Child Adolesc Psychiatr Clin N Am 11:705–717, 2002

Individuals With Disabilities Education Act, P.L. 102–119, 1991

Individuals With Disabilities Education Improvement Act, P.L. 108–446, 2004

International Association for Child and Adolescent Psychiatry and Allied Professions: IACAPAP Ethics 2006. Melbourne, Australia, International Association for Child and Adolescent Psychiatry and Allied Professions, 2006

Judicial Council of California: Court Ordered Child Custody Evaluations. California Rules of Court, Rule 5.220, 2004

Kauble PD: California Laws Relating to Minors. Los Angeles, CA, Legal Books Distributing, 2008

Kay HH: Symposium on Law in the Twentieth Century: From the Second Sex to the Joint Venture: An Overview of Women's Rights and Family Law in the United States During the Twentieth Century, 88 Cal. L. Rev. 2017, 2091 (2000)

Loftus E: Creating false memories. Sci Am 277:70–75, 1997

Loftus E, Pickrell J: The formation of false memories. Psychiatr Ann 25:720–725, 1995

Macbeth J: Legal issues in the treatment of minors, in Principles and Practice of Child and Adolescent Forensic Psychiatry. Edited by Schetky D, Benedek, E. Washington, DC, American Psychiatric Publishing, 2002, pp 309–323

Munir K, Earls F: Ethical principles governing research in child and adolescent psychiatry. J Am Acad Child Adolesc Psychiatry 31:408–414, 1992

Parham v. J.R., 422 U.S. 584, 99 S. Ct. 2493, 61 L. Ed. 2d 101 (1979)

Poole DA, Lindsay DS: Interviewing preschoolers: effects of nonsuggestive techniques, parental coaching and leading questions on reports of nonexperienced events. J Exp Child Psychol 60:129–154, 1995

Quinn KM: Interviewing children for suspected sexual abuse, in Principles and Practice of Child and Adolescent Forensic Psychiatry. Edited by Schetky D, Benedek EP. Washington, DC, American Psychiatric Publishing, 2002, pp 149–159

Rappeport JR: Reasonable medical certainty. Bull Am Acad Psychiatry Law 13:5, 1985

Raskin D, Esplin P: Statement validity assessment: interview procedures and content analysis of children's statements of sexual abuse. Behav Assess 13:265–291, 1991

Rehabilitation Acts of 1973, Sect. 504. 29 U.S.C. Sect. 794

Rodham H: Children under the law, in The Rights of Children. Harv Educ Rev 43:487–514, 1973

Santosky v Kramer, 455 U.S. 745 (1982)

Schetky DH: History of child and adolescent forensic psychiatry, in Principles and Practice of Child and Adolescent Forensic Psychiatry. Edited by Schetky D, Benedek E.

Washington, DC, American Psychiatric Publishing, 2002, pp 3–6

Schetky DH: Ethics, in Lewis's Child and Adolescent Psychiatry: A Comprehensive Textbook, 4th Edition. Edited by Martin A, Volkmar FR. Philadelphia, PA, Lippincott Williams & Wilkins, 2007, pp 17–22

Schetky DH, Guyer MJ: Psychic trauma and civil litigation, in Principles and Practice of Child and Adolescent Forensic Psychiatry. Edited by Schetky D, Benedek E. Washington, DC, American Psychiatric Publishing, 2002, pp 355–364

Stahl P: Complex Issues in Child Custody Evaluations. Thousand Oaks, CA, Sage Publications, 1999

United Nations: Convention on the Rights of the Child, 20 November 1989. New York, United Nations, 1989

U.S. Department of Health and Human Services, Protection of Human Subjects, C.F.R. Title 45, Part 46, 1991

U.S. Government Printing Office: Report to the President: White House Conference on Children. Washington, DC, U.S. Government Printing Office, 1971

Walter HJ, Berkovitz IH: Practice parameter for psychiatric consultation to schools. J Am Acad Child Adolesc Psychiatry 44:1068–1083, 2005

White v Illinois, 112 S. Ct. 736 (1992)

Wickline v California, 192 Cal. App. 3d 1630, 239 Cal Rptr 810 (1986)

Chapter 44

Telepsychiatry

Kathleen Myers, M.D., M.P.H., M.S.
Sharon Cain, M.D.

Advances in technology affect many aspects of daily life, and health care is no exception. A report by the Institute of Medicine (2001), *Crossing the Quality Chasm: A New Health System for the 21st Century,* has identified health information technology as one of the critical forces that could significantly improve clinical decision-making, patient safety, and overall quality of health care in the United States. The President's New Freedom Commission on Mental Health 2003 report *Achieving the Promise: Transforming Mental Health Care in America* has recommended telecommunications technologies as one of the most promising means of improving access to specialty mental health care. Many new technologies now contribute to increasing access to mental health services and to improving the quality of that care. Telepsychiatry is one of these new technologies that uses interactive videoteleconferencing, or televideo, to allow a psychiatrist and patient in different locations to interact in real time for the provision of care that usually is delivered in person. Child and adolescent telepsychiatry could substantially change psychiatric practice by bringing services not only to underserved communities but also to naturalistic settings like schools and day care, and potentially into patients' homes. Here, we provide an overview of the development, applications, and future of child and adolescent telepsychiatry.

Technical Aspects of Telepsychiatry

The technology underlying telepsychiatry is inherently interesting and complicated, but a comprehensive understanding of the technology is not critical to its use. The technology is a vehicle to deliver clinical services. A brief summary of the basic terminology used in the telehealth literature is provided in Table 44–1. Table 44–2 reviews the different types of connectivity, or protocols, used to establish a televideo link between sites. More information can be found at the Web site for the Telemedicine Information Exchange (http://tie.telemed.org), the Web site for the American Telemedicine Association (www.americantelemed.org), and in Simmons et al. (2003).

Development of Child and Adolescent Telepsychiatry

History and Literature Review

Telepsychiatry was first reported with children and adolescents in 1976 in New York City at Mount Sinai

School of Medicine. There was then little activity until the 1990s, when technological improvements led to a rapid growth of telemedicine programs nationally and internationally. Accurate data on the number of telepsychiatry programs are difficult to obtain. Review of reimbursement records suggests that at least 27 states include telemedicine in their Medicaid services (Brown 2006; Center for Telemedicine Law and the Office for the Advancement of Telehealth 2007; Centers for Medicare and Medicaid Services 2007a, 2007b), and 64 states have reported reimbursement by private payers (American Telemedicine Association and AMD Telemedicine, Inc. 2004; Brown 2006; Whitten and Buis 2007). Many of these payers include mental health services. The Telemedicine Information Exchange Web site (http://tie.telemed.org) lists 125 telemedicine programs in the United States and identifies 65 of these as including mental health programs. How many of these programs include child and adolescent psychiatric services is unclear.

TABLE 44–1. Technical terms relevant to telepsychiatry practice

Technical term	Definition
E-health	Health services provided from a clinician to a patient or the lay public through any electronic medium, in real time or store-and-forward modality, including the Internet, telephone, or facsimile.
Interactive televideo (ITV) communication	The interaction of two or more individuals in real time to share information through electronic media.
Telemedicine	The use of ITV to deliver medical care that is usually delivered in person
Telepsychiatry	The application of telemedicine to psychiatry.
Patient site and provider site	Participants at each end of the ITV link. Multiple other terms have been used (Centers for Medicare and Medicaid Services 2007a), such as "originating site," "distant site," spoke, hub, and remote site.
Bandwidth	The theoretical maximum rate that data can travel through a network in a fixed period of time. Bandwidth is often expressed in units of kilobits per second (kb/sec). The higher the bandwidth, the greater amount of data that can be transmitted. Standard telephones that transmit audio signals are low-bandwidth devices; cable television and telecommunications lines that transmit audio and video signals simultaneously are high-bandwidth devices. Most health care applications use bandwidths at or above 384 kb/sec, often referred to as "virtually live" or "80% television quality."
Telecommunication technology or connectivity	The technical methods, or protocols, used to establish an ITV connection. Brief definitions, advantages, disadvantages, and applications are summarized in Table 44–2. More information can be found at the Web site for the Telemedicine Information Exchange (http://tie.telemed.org).
Frame rate	The rate of display of the multiple still images (or frames) that comprise a video signal. This rate is determined by the bandwidth as well as by quality of the camera and monitor. Each second of broadcast-quality video has 25–30 frames per second. A lower rate produces pixilation and may be suboptimal for assessing features such as facial movements and affect.

TABLE 44–2. Telecommunications technologies

Connectivity	Bandwidth	Advantages	Disadvantages	Applications
Plain old telephone system (POTS) Videophones (analog, public-switched, telephone network in use over the world)	64 kbits/sec	Low cost, low bandwidth, low-end technology, and easy use allow for diverse applications in multiple settings, including in-home.	Low bandwidth and low resolution produce considerable auditory lag, visual pixilation, and asynchrony between audio and video transmission. May not be HIPAA compliant. Will be replaced with computer videophones.	Has been used for many applications but most appropriate for clinical work not requiring diagnosis (e.g., in-home monitoring and contact between regular sessions). May be especially helpful for youth who cannot be easily transported for in-clinic care.
Integrated services digital network (ISDN) lines	128–768 kbits/sec	Use existing telephone lines that are universally available. Predictable bandwidth. Sets of two channels provide 128 kbits/sec bandwidth, which are then combined into higher bandwidth depending on application needs. Secure point-to-point transmission is HIPAA compliant.	Costs for initial line installation and ongoing line fees. Line fees vary, similar to those for phone calls. Long-distance calling makes ISDN expensive and unpredictable. Infrastructure maintenance.	Most psychiatric applications including diagnostic assessment, initial appointments. Excellent for educational, training, and conferencing activities. Universal availability of ISDN lines allows good-quality televideo to be set up outside of major organizational settings (e.g., to allow in-office or in-home telepsychiatry practice).
T1 or T3 lines; fractional T1 line (digitally multiplexed telecommunications carrier systems)	384 kbits/sec to 45 Mbits/sec	Leased lines are at set cost. Monthly expenses are contracted with leasing company and are therefore expectable. Predictable high to very high bandwidth available. Secure point-to-point transmission is HIPAA compliant.	Costs of initial line installation and other costs. Infrastructure maintenance. Placement of T1 lines may not be universally available.	Most psychiatric applications including diagnostic assessment, initial appointments. Excellent for educational, training, and conferencing activities.
Internet protocol	>1 Mbit/sec	Universal availability from desktop. Lower cost than ISDN or T1 lines.	Available bandwidth not predictable. Requires encryption to be HIPAA compliant if using public Internet.	Most psychiatric applications if HIPAA compliance can be ensured. Universal availability allows in-office or in-home telepsychiatry practice.

Note. HIPAA = Health Insurance Portability and Accountability Act.

652 Dulcan's Textbook of Child and Adolescent Psychiatry

Initially, telepsychiatry programs were developed by major medical centers to provide specialty services to rural communities. Telepsychiatry services have rapidly evolved to include subspecialty services, high intensity services, crisis intervention, and management of chronic illnesses to various underserved populations. Child and adolescent telepsychiatry programs are now sited in diverse settings such as community medical centers (Alicata et al. 2008; Myers et al. 2004), community mental health centers (Cain and Spaulding 2006), urban day care (Cain and Spaulding 2006), rural schools (Adelsheim and Mattison 2008; Alicata et al. 2006; Harper 2006), corrections facilities (Myers et al. 2006), residential settings (Storck 2007), and private practice (Cassidy and Glueck 2008; George 2007; Glueck 2007). Youth with special challenges, such as developmental impairments, have also been served through telepsychiatry (Szeftel et al. 2008). Finally, telepsychiatry has been used successfully with minority youth, such as African Americans (Cain and Spaulding 2006), Hispanics (Adelsheim and Mattison 2008; Harper 2006), American Indians (Savin et al. 2006, 2008), and Hawaiians (Alicata et al. 2006).

There is a small but growing literature examining telepsychiatry with children and adolescents. In a randomized investigation of 23 youth evaluated in telepsychiatry and in-person sessions, 96% of the diagnoses and treatment recommendations were comparable as was family satisfaction (Elford et al. 2000, 2001). In an equivalency trial, 28 depressed children were randomly assigned to telemental health or in-person cognitive-behavioral therapy with comparable improvements over several weeks (Nelson et al. 2003). A retrospective assessment of 3-month outcomes with a convenience sample of 41 youth found improvements in the Affect and Oppositional domains of the Child Behavior Checklist (Yellowlees et al. 2008). The demographic and clinical comparability of telepsychiatry patients (N=159) to those evaluated in usual in-person care (N=210) has been demonstrated in a descriptive study that showed the same profile of gender, age, payer status, and diagnoses for these two groups (Myers et al. 2004). A single descriptive study has reported pharmacotherapy (Myers et al. 2006). Functional behavioral analysis of developmentally impaired children conducted through telepsychology led to effective classroom interventions (Barretto et al. 2006). Telepsychiatry with children and adolescents has been shown to be feasible, acceptable, and sustainable in consultation to primary care clinicians (Myers et al. 2007). Most studies have measured satisfaction (Elford et al. 2000, 2001; Kopel et al. 2001; Myers et al.

2004, 2006; Pesamaa et al. 2004) and have found that providers (Myers et al. 2007), families (Myers et al. 2008), and youth (Myers et al. 2006) are very satisfied with their care. Although satisfaction does not equate to efficacy, it implies perception of improvement and informs future direction for systematic investigation. Several case reports have described the ability to conduct treatment through telepsychiatry (Alessi 2002; Goldfield and Boachie 2003; Hilty et al. 2000; Savin et al. 2006). However, most reports have simply described successes and challenges of program implementation. Table 44–3 summarizes clinical work published since 2000.

Despite these successes and the increasing demand for telepsychiatry services, there is little scientific evidence of their efficacy. A reasonable conclusion from the limited evidence is that telepsychiatry is a viable option when usual in-person psychiatric care is not available. Cost effectiveness also remains to be demonstrated. Savings may result from the elimination of travel, but technology expenses may drive costs even higher. In future investigations, efficacy, cost effectiveness, and benefits to both children and their communities should be considered together to obtain a full perspective of the value of telepsychiatry.

Information resources are available for readers interested in keeping up with this rapidly evolving field, including a professional organization, the American Telemedicine Association (ATA); dedicated journals such as *Telemedicine and e-Health* and the *Journal of Telemedicine and Telecare*; and published books (Wootton and Batch 2005; Wootton et al. 2003).

Factors Promoting Child and Adolescent Telepsychiatry

As psychiatry relies predominantly on conversation and observation, it has become one of the most widely adopted disciplines in telemedicine (Hersh et al. 2006). Many factors in the current health care system converge with new technologies to promote child and adolescent telepsychiatry (Wootton et al. 2003; Yellowlees 2003).

Clinically, telepsychiatry fits well with the shift in treatment philosophy to a more patient-focused system of care by bringing the treatment to the patient's setting. Families generally take a more proactive role in their children's treatment to produce an informed patient, or informed family. *Socially,* families and health care providers are increasingly demanding quality care for all society. Telepsychiatry can reduce barriers to care by redistributing clinical expertise and providing earlier interventions for youth at risk. *Educationally,* many schools are seeking to understand how mental health needs affect students' learning. Their K-12 videoconferencing systems offer an opportunity to readily obtain telepsychiatric consultation and to upgrade teachers' skills. *Systemically,* the health care system is moving away from episodic care to continuity of care, especially for patients with chronic disease, and from an individual approach to a team approach. This shift makes care at a distance more possible and attractive as patients' participation in their care is emphasized, and other clinicians or paraprofessionals assume intermediary roles. Telepsychiatry can bring a missing piece to teams in distant communities. *Professionally,* child psychiatrists can pursue new venues for their practices without incurring the disadvantages of leaving their families and offices. Advantages for local mental health professionals include access to consultation with distant experts. Finally, *institutionally,* major medical centers interested in building referral networks can reach out to distant clinicians and communities with a range of needed services.

Clinical Practice of Telepsychiatry

Developmental and Clinical Considerations

Applications of telepsychiatry have been described across development and most diagnostic categories. Children as young as 3 years old have been treated (Elford et al. 2000; Myers et al. 2004). School-age children comprise the modal age group (Broder et al. 2004; Hockey et al. 2004; Nelson et al. 2003; Pesamaa et al. 2004), and attention-deficit/hyperactivity disorder is the most commonly treated disorder, although most diagnostic groups have been treated (Myers et al. 2004, 2007). Developmentally impaired children may not be able to provide their own perspectives, but school records, parents' records, and telepsychiatrist's observations can readily facilitate treatment planning. Children who are uncooperative pose challenges, but they can be treated with assistance at the patient site. The appropriateness of a youth for telepsychiatry should be individualized to developmental considerations, parents' preferences, supports at the patient site, and the telepsychiatrist's resourcefulness.

Optimizing the Virtual Clinical Encounter

The key to successful telepsychiatry is not the technology, but effective clinical care. The clinical encounter will be affected by the arrangement of the space at both the provider and patient sites and factors affecting the virtual relationship that develops between a clinician and a patient (Godleski et al. 2003; Onor and Misan 2005).

Interview Room

The room at the patient site should provide privacy and be large enough to include a clinical staff member, the youth, and at least one parent. It is also preferable if the room can accommodate another person whom the parent might invite, such as a teacher. The room should be large enough to evaluate children's motor skills, play, and exploration (American Academy of Child and Adolescent Psychiatry 1997a, 1997b). A table allows the child to draw or play but should not interfere with viewing motor skills. The room should be away from clinic and street noise as the microphones are very sensitive, and extraneous noises can interfere with the session.

Lighting and visual contrasts are crucial (Godleski et al. 2003; Onor and Misan 2005). Incandescent lighting provides a more natural appearance, and ideally should emanate from behind the camera to avoid shadows. Pastel colors optimize visual transmission while white coats or dark or very bright colors adversely affect contrast. Patterns, particularly horizontal stripes, distort the image.

Camera placement poses a problem. The camera is typically mounted above the monitor, causing individuals to appear to be looking downward. Conversely, a camera placed below the monitor will make the individual appear to be looking upward. These views might falsely convey difficulties in relatedness or impede rapport. Therefore, the telepsychiatrist should alternate his or her gaze from camera to monitor to provide sufficient eye contact to convey optimal relatedness. To address this shortcoming clinically, telepsychiatrists should query parents about the child's relatedness. Two technological approaches address this issue. If a laptop is used, placing the camera slightly behind the laptop just above the center of the screen can approximate the appearance of direct eye contact. Also, a new technology termed *Telepresence* places a camera in the middle of a monitor in back of a projecting surface and surrounded by a series of re-

TABLE 44–3. Published reports and studies in child and adolescent telepsychiatry

Citation	Title	Specific disorders	Sample size	Findings
Elford et al. 2000	A randomized controlled trial of child psychiatric assessments conducted using videoconferencing	Diagnostic spectrum	25	96% concordance between VTC and FTF evaluations; no differences in satisfaction.
Hilty et al. 2000	Telepsychiatric consultation for ADHD in the primary care setting	ADHD	1	ADHD symptoms responded well to telepsychiatry treatment.
Elford et al. 2001	A prospective satisfaction study and cost analysis of a pilot child telepsychiatry service in Newfoundland	NA	30	Shows high satisfaction of children, teens, parents, and providers with TMH.
Kopel et al. 2001	Evaluating satisfaction with a child and adolescent psychological telemedicine outreach service	NA	136	High satisfaction of families and rural health workers in New South Wales, Australia.
Alessi 2002	Telepsychiatric care of a depressed adolescent	Depression and disruptive behaviors	1	Medication, individual therapy, and family therapy over 12 sessions led to clinical improvements in teen's depression.
Goldfield and Boachie 2003	Delivery of family therapy in the treatment of anorexia nervosa using telehealth	Anorexia nervosa	1	Weight increased in girls with anorexia; family relationships stabilized.
Nelson et al. 2003	Treating childhood depression over videoconferencing	Depression	28	Controlled study comparing TMH with FTF treatment in the psychotherapy of depressed children: comparable outcomes.
Pesamaa et al. 2004	Videoconferencing in child and adolescent telepsychiatry: a systematic review of the literature	NA	NA	Review article describes status of child and adolescent TMH; generally good outcomes per satisfaction ratings.
Myers et al. 2004	Telepsychiatry with children and adolescents: are patients comparable to those evaluated in usual outpatient care?	Diagnostic spectrum	159	TMH patients were demographically and clinically representative of the usual outpatient child and adolescent psychiatry population.

TABLE 44–3. Published reports and studies in child and adolescent telepsychiatry *(continued)*

Citation	Title	Specific disorders	Sample size	Findings
Barretto et al. 2006	Using telemedicine to conduct behavioral assessments	Developmental disabilities	2	Describes use of standard clinical assessment tools through TMH to elucidate children's behavioral patterns.
Myers et al. 2006	Telepsychiatry with incarcerated youth	Diagnostic spectrum	115	Describes large series of incarcerated youth, including medication management.
Savin et al. 2006	Telepsychiatry for treating rural American Indian youth	Reactive attachment disorder; Asperger's disorder	2	Describes TMH with a preschooler and young teen, leading to clarification of diagnoses and needs; well accepted by American Indian community.
Myers et al. 2007	Feasibility, acceptability, and sustainability of telepsychiatry for children and adolescents	Diagnostic spectrum	172 patients and 387 visits	Describes telepsychiatry services in four sites, high satisfaction of primary care physicians, and reimbursement of services; pediatricians more satisfied than family physicians.
Myers et al. 2008	Child and adolescent telepsychiatry: utilization and satisfaction	Diagnostic spectrum	172 patients and 387 visits	Describes utilization of telepsychiatry by families and their high satisfaction with initial and return visits; less satisfied with care for adolescents than for younger children.
Yellowlees et al. 2008	A retrospective analysis of a child and adolescent e-mental health program	Diagnostic spectrum	41	A retrospective assessment of 3-month outcomes with a convenience sample found improvements in the Affect and Oppositional domains of the Child Behavior Checklist.

Note. ADHD=attention-deficit/hyperactivity disorder; FTF=face-to-face; NA=not available; TMH=telemental health; VTC=videoteleconferencing.

flecting surfaces to refocus gaze and better approximate eye contact. This new technology also approximates a three-dimensional image that provides participants a more lifelike experience.

The Virtual Relationship and Videoconferencing Etiquette

Most telepsychiatry work has emphasized the technical dimensions or clinical processes, such as diagnosis and treatment, which have been good (Myers et al. 2004, 2007, 2008; Yellowlees et al. 2003). Less studied is the interpersonal dimension such as the social and psychological aspects of treatment, particularly the doctor-patient relationship. The virtual relationship depends upon screen presence (Cruz et al. 2005; Godleski et al. 2003; Onor and Misan 2005). The image of a newscaster showing the telepsychiatrist from head to waist is a good model. Interpersonal style is adjusted to overcome limitations imposed by the technology. For example, more animation is generally demonstrated with broader hand gestures; however, if these gestures occur too fast, pixilation will occur. Verbal communications are more deliberate to adjust for the slight auditory lag and to clearly indicate when the telepsychiatrist has finished speaking and to facilitate reciprocity in communication.

Rapport is established within a space that does not physically exist, and participants do not have access to all aspects of the other's presentation to decipher nuances of communication (Werner 2004). It is unknown how this lack of physical presence affects the relationship, but emerging information suggests a more casual style optimizes rapport (Godleski et al. 2003; Onor and Misan 2005). Rapport building can also be facilitated by showing youth their image on the full screen or in the "picture-in-picture" box on the screen and teaching them how to manipulate the camera to obtain "close-ups" of themselves and their parents, or to scan the telepsychiatrist's room.

The Clinical Session

Clinical care via telepsychiatry should be consistent with the practice parameters of the American Academy of Child and Adolescent Psychiatry. The Practice Parameters for the Psychiatric Assessment of Children and Adolescents (American Academy of Child and Adolescent Psychiatry 1997a) recommends that some time be spent interviewing the youth alone. Older children with good impulse control, adequate verbal skills, and the ability to separate can be interviewed alone. Younger, developmentally impaired, or impul-

sive youth need a modified approach. Traditional play sessions (American Academy of Child and Adolescent Psychiatry 1997a) may be challenging. The child may be observed interacting with staff in a structured or free play session. Some limited play with the child may be possible over the telemonitor (e.g., drawing pictures and then discussing themes or developing a play scenario with puppets).

In assessing toddlers, it is helpful to set up several scenarios to observe the child in developmentally appropriate interactions (American Academy of Child and Adolescent Psychiatry 1997b). This should include the child's interactions with his or her parent(s) and preferably with an unfamiliar adult, perhaps a staff member. The telepsychiatrist should also attempt direct interaction with the child, with the parent and/ or a staff member in the room. This might be done by giving the child simple tasks—e.g., to distinguish colors, to point to body parts, or to count. As it may be difficult to appreciate the young child's level of attunement, pleasure in the interaction, or spontaneity in play, it is helpful to have an adult present to comment on these aspects of the mental status.

Pharmacotherapy

Pharmacotherapy is the most commonly requested telepsychiatry service and should comply with existing practice parameters (American Academy of Child and Adolescent Psychiatry, in press). Different approaches to medication management have been used depending on the system in which the telepsychiatrist is working. Medication may be prescribed directly by the telepsychiatrist, by a collaborating midlevel clinician, or by the referring primary care physician. Whichever approach is used, clear procedures should be communicated regarding the method for obtaining initial prescriptions and refills and for managing complications between sessions.

Care Between Sessions

Families receiving ongoing services will need guidelines about interim care. Nonscheduled care is helpful to patients and communities, but it is difficult to arrange. If nonscheduled care is offered, patients should be informed of how to access such services. If not offered, then alternatives should be identified, especially for crises. Some telepsychiatrists recommend e-mail contact (Hilty et al. 2006b). Procedures for interim care should emphasize the importance of integrating telepsychiatry into a system of care so that other components can be accessed according to the youth's needs and the family's resources, and to reduce confusion for families and the burden for clinicians (American Academy of Child and Adolescent Psychiatry 2007).

Telepsychiatry in a System of Care

The telepsychiatry services provided will depend in part on other services available in the child's community. Some telepsychiatry interventions might be possible in a community providing a comprehensive system of care but are not possible in a less well-developed system. With increasing emphasis on providing evidence-based mental health care, new models of service delivery and of training therapists in remote areas will be needed. Telepsychiatry combined with other forms of information technology may bring evidence-based services to communities. A psychiatrist or team of specialists can be telecommuted to the patient's community, or the system of care can choose from a menu of services at the provider's site. The telepsychiatrist can readily collaborate in the child's care by virtually meeting on demand with local team members, such as school personnel. Alternatively, a telepsychiatrist might train local therapists in evidence-based treatments. This is an underexplored application of telepsychiatry.

Starting a Telepsychiatry Practice

The following is a brief overview of issues that potential telepsychiatrists should address in determining whether telepsychiatry is relevant to their clinical practice.

Determine Whether Telepsychiatry Is Feasible and Sustainable

Feasibility of a telepsychiatry program is predicated on an accurate needs assessment. The needs assessment should include what services the requesting site needs, whether telepsychiatry is a feasible option for meeting those needs, whether telepsychiatry complements existing services, and whether telepsychiatry would be acceptable to the stakeholders. For example,

if a site requests crisis management services, does the telepsychiatrist or provider site have the flexibility that such services require, and will there be a backup system at the patient site? Sustainability of telepsychiatry should be determined within the larger context of the community's needs. For example, telepsychiatry may not be the most cost-efficient approach for a local medical center that seeks to provide mental health services, but the medical center might profit from lower use of emergency room services. A community might profit from lower use of correctional services, or the school might benefit from lower staffing for children with mental health challenges. If the provider site is at a major medical center, it might elect to absorb disadvantageous financial arrangements in order to develop referral networks or capture greater market share for other clinical specialties.

Assessment of sustainability should consider costs of the technology at both sites, its upkeep, other infrastructure, additional staffing, and payment mechanisms. Grant funding is helpful during start-up, especially if it covers equipment purchase, but it will not sustain a service. Contracts that reimburse a set rate for the psychiatrist's time and cover the ancillary costs (e.g., line charges, office management) appear to be the most beneficial for the provider. Third-party payment, or fee-for-service, will likely not cover videoconferencing costs or infrastructure. It will also not cover additional staffing that might be needed. Staffing might be minimal—e.g., if the patient's local therapist attends the session—or considerable, if providing crisis service. Billing codes are the same as usual care, with a modifier code added to specify telepsychiatry. If fee-for-service billing is sought, it is helpful to prepare a statement of "intent to bill" to open discussions with the payer. The Centers for Medicare and Medicaid Services address coverage (2007a) and billing (2007b), which vary by state (www.cms.hhs.gov/Manuals/IOM/list.asp). The American Telemedicine Association Web site (www.americantelemed.org) provides more information about reimbursement.

Identify the Population and Model of Care

The patients to be served should be identified and may be determined by the site, such as all patients at a mental health center, primary care practice, or school. Patient inclusion and exclusion criteria should be based upon needs of the referring clinicians, judgment of the telepsychiatrist, and resources at the patient site, including the site's ability to attend to acutely suicidal or agitated patients (Wootton et al. 2003). The telepsychiatrist should have appropriate on-site backup in order to safely conduct an evaluation (Godleski et al. 2003). At a minimum, protocols should address the management of emergencies, use of crisis services, and the telepsychiatrist's role within the continuum of services. Exclusionary criteria may include factors such as youth without accompanying guardians, patients without a primary care physician, or patients with a primary care physician who is uncomfortable resuming care for psychiatric patients. If the telepsychiatrist is to treat youth with psychotic or bipolar disorders in a consultative model, the primary care physician must be comfortable prescribing neuroleptics and mood stabilizers.

Several models of care have been used in telepsychiatry (Hilty et al. 2006a) as summarized in Table 44–4. A core issue relates to whether new patients will be evaluated over televideo or in person. A requirement for in-person initial evaluation dilutes the value of telepsychiatry for communities and families (Godleski et al. 2003; Wootton et al. 2003). Another core issue is whether urgent and emergency care will be provided (Godleski et al. 2003; Moehr et al. 2006; Sorvaniemi et al. 2005). Such care is valuable to communities but requires considerable resources and flexibility by the provider site. The available system of care at the patient site for managing crises will likely guide decisions about offering urgent and emergent care. For example, a telepsychiatrist might be more willing to provide urgent care if a community has effective wraparound and follow-up services to help in managing the patient.

Most programs focus on consultation (Cruz et al. 2005), but ongoing care is most helpful to communities, referring clinicians, and patients, especially for complicated pharmacotherapy (Cain and Spaulding 2006; Cruz et al. 2005; Myers et al. 2004, 2007). If ongoing care is offered, a primary care physician should be identified to provide care when the telepsychiatrist is unavailable and to resume care when the patient becomes stable.

Finally, the telepsychiatrist should decide whether a staff person should remain in the room to assist with the interview, operate equipment, help with disruptive children, and provide communication about the session with the referring physician. In small communities, families may feel that their privacy is not protected if local staff are present. Thus, such arrangements should be addressed in the initial needs assessment and then individually for each family.

Evaluating a Telepsychiatry Service

The demand for telepsychiatry services has outstripped the evidence base supporting its efficacy, and more outcome data are needed. All telepsychiatrists are encouraged to collect process and outcome data for their telepsychiatry practices. Most programs measure utilization and the satisfaction of families, referrers, and providers, which has been consistently high (Broder et al. 2004; Elford et al. 2001; Hockey et al. 2004; Kopel et al. 2001; Myers et al. 2004, 2007, 2008). Satisfaction ratings typically cover technical and clinical aspects of care. Technical items address video quality, sound quality, and privacy. Clinical aspects include the patient's ability to understand and have confidence in the provider, whether the family would return, and whether telepsychiatry is comparable to an in-person appointment. Adolescents' own satisfaction should be included (Myers et al. 2006). It is also helpful to know whether the referring clinician perceives greater ease in patient management and improved patient functioning (Myers et al. 2007). Clinical outcome indicators may include rating scales, interviews, and functional assessments. Utilization outcomes may include adverse events, hospitalization, adherence to the treatment plan, and equipment failures, as well as changes in caregiver burden, clinicians' practices, school staffing, and barriers to care.

Regulatory and Ethical Issues

At the national level, Medicare and the Joint Commission for the Accreditation of Healthcare Organizations (JCAHO; now known as The Joint Commission) have regulations applicable to telemedicine. More extensive regulations are determined by state laws. For example, most states require telepsychiatrists to be licensed in both the state in which they practice and in the state where the patient receives care. Laws regarding involuntary commitment and reporting child maltreatment may vary across jurisdictions. Other factors to consider include the patient's privacy and compliance of the televideo transmission with the Health Insurance Portability and Accountability Act (HIPAA). Informed consent for treatment generally includes an additional consent for telepsychiatry with review of its potential limitations (American Academy of Child and Adolescent Psychiatry 2008; Godleski et al. 2003). Until nationally accepted telepsychiatry care guide-

TABLE 44–4. Models of care in child and adolescent telepsychiatry

Model	Advantages	Disadvantages	Clinical applications
Consultee-centered consultation (PCP attends session with patient)	Empowers PCPs and provides opportunity for PCPs' learning. PCP retains responsibility for all patient care and thus ensures continuity of care. Optimal communication between PCP and telepsychiatrist. Convenient for patient.	Referring PCP must take time from practice. Minimizes opportunities for repeated sessions, which are often necessary to understand needs. Unclear patient comfort with both physicians attending the session.	Helpful for emergent and urgent care and to augment PCP practice. Mostly practiced in international sites (e.g., Canada).
Client-centered consultation (PCP does not attend session with patient)	Expert consultation. Families can present problems in their own manner for expert opinion. Provides optimal privacy. Variable number of sessions to adequately cover the data base. Helpful to communities for crisis care.	Typical 1–2 session consultation does not offer longitudinal perspective to understand complicated cases. Timely communication with referring clinician is crucial. PCP may not have resources to implement telepsychiatrist's recommendations. Providing crisis care can be challenging for the provider.	Useful for crisis care. Best to implement routine telepsychiatry services before implementing crisis services. Most common outpatient telepsychiatry model.
Ongoing direct care	Most consistent with in-person model of care. Offers most expert care and greatest privacy. Most helpful to PCPs and patients.	If limited number of telepsychiatrist hours per month are available, this model may not be able to provide adequate frequency of follow-up or will preclude services to the maximum number of youth. Potential for suboptimal communication with referring PCP.	Ongoing outpatient care; correctional care. Must decide whether initial session will occur through telepsychiatrist or in person and who will prescribe medication. Need procedure for interim care. Pharmacotherapy is most requested telepsychiatry service.
Collaboration with a midlevel professional (e.g., nurse practitioner or physician assistant)	Midlevel professional can provide continuity of care, including crises and medications; optimizes communication between providers. Opportunity for midlevel professional to obtain supervision.	May only be available at mental health centers although could be addressed during contracting. Could be more expensive for agency. In some rural areas, families do not want to include a member of the community in mental health sessions.	Patients in a system of mental health care, especially mental health centers.

TABLE 44–4. Models of care in child and adolescent telepsychiatry (*continued*)

Model	Advantages	Disadvantages	Clinical applications
Comprehensive telemental health (direct clinical services and wraparound services)	Child receives spectrum of services from multiple providers. Care can all be provided at provider site or by combination of services at the provider and patient sites. Offers opportunity to integrate telepsychiatry into a youth's system of care.	Families and/or other clinicians and administrators at the patient site may find this model too alien if all services are offered through the provider site. Sometimes difficult to find personnel at patient site to collaborate in such models.	Youth with psychiatric disorders that impact their functioning across multiple domains.
System consultation	Telepsychiatry offers neutral mediation and guidance to a system struggling to meet youth's needs.	Some communities may not like an "outsider" intervening in systems issues, especially when the outsider is intervening virtually, not firsthand.	Schools are major utilizers, but this model also is helpful to agencies such as foster care and juvenile justice.

Note.   PCP=primary care physician.

lines are available, telepsychiatrists should adhere to existing procedures for in-person care (American Academy of Child and Adolescent Psychiatry 2008).

care. Thus, mainstream telepsychiatry awaits a new breed of child and adolescent psychiatrists who embrace technological approaches to clinical care.

Obstacles

Telepsychiatry is not yet part of mainstream clinical practice. The most obvious obstacles are financial, related to start-up costs of equipment and technology assistance, but also related to ongoing factors such as reimbursement. The Telemedicine Information Exchange (http://tie.telemed.org/funding/) and other organizations are actively pursuing legislation that will reimburse telemedicine services with parity to in-person care. Patients and families have readily accepted telepsychiatry. A major obstacle is psychiatrists' reluctance to adopt this approach to providing

Research Directions

Outcome studies are needed to demonstrate that telepsychiatry is comparable to in-person psychiatric care and superior to care rendered in primary care. With efficacy demonstrated, it will be important to examine optimal models of care. Studies are also needed to show whether telepsychiatry can be used to disseminate evidence-based treatments. Finally, studies of the virtual relationship may help us to understand how and why this mode of service delivery works, as well as to understand the therapeutic relationship in all venues of care.

Summary Points

- Child and adolescent telepsychiatry has been practiced in diverse settings, for most psychiatric disorders, across development, with youth of various ethnicities.

- Efficacy studies are needed to establish an evidence base for telepsychiatry.

- While efficacy studies are being awaited, telepsychiatric care should adhere to evidence-based guidelines and best practices as summarized in the practice parameters of the American Academy of Child and Adolescent Psychiatry.

- Telepsychiatrists should use the highest bandwidth that is financially and technologically feasible to optimize the clinical experience.

- Before a telepsychiatry practice is established, a careful assessment of need, sustainability, the existing system of care, and stakeholders' interests will best insure success.

- The Centers for Medicare and Medicaid Services, The Joint Commission, and state laws have established regulatory guidelines for telepsychiatry that should be consulted in establishing a telepsychiatry practice.

References

Adelsheim S, Mattison R: Telepsychiatry with rural school-based health centers in New Mexico. Clinical perspectives presentation at the 55th Annual Meeting of the American Academy of Child and Adolescent Psychiatry, Chicago, IL, October 28–November 2, 2008

Alessi N: Telepsychiatric care of a depressed adolescent. J Am Acad Child Adolesc Psychiatry 41:894–895, 2002

Alicata D, Saltman D, Ulrich D: Child and adolescent telepsychiatry in rural Hawaii. Presented at the 53rd Annual Meeting of the American Academy of Child and Adolescent Psychiatry, San Diego, CA, October 2006

Alicata D, Koyanagi C, Guerrero A, et al: Telepsychiatry in rural Hawaii: The Big Island Telepsychiatry Initiative. Clinical perspectives presentation at the 55th Annual Meeting of the American Academy of Child and Adolescent Psychiatry, Chicago, IL, October 28–November 2, 2008

American Academy of Child and Adolescent Psychiatry: Practice parameters for the psychiatric assessment of children and adolescents. J Am Acad Child Adolesc Psychiatry 36(suppl):4S–20S, 1997a

American Academy of Child and Adolescent Psychiatry: Practice parameters for the psychiatric assessment of infants and toddlers (0–36 months). J Am Acad Child Adolesc Psychiatry 36(suppl):21S–36S, 1997b

American Academy of Child and Adolescent Psychiatry: Practice parameter on child and adolescent mental health care in community systems of care. J Am Acad Child Adolesc Psychiatry 46:284–299, 2007

American Academy of Child and Adolescent Psychiatry: Practice parameter for telepsychiatry with children and adolescents. J Am Acad Child Adolesc Psychiatry 47:1468–1483, 2008

American Academy of Child and Adolescent Psychiatry: Practice parameter on the use of psychotropic medication in children and adolescents. J Am Acad Child Adolesc Psychiatry, in press

American Telemedicine Association and AMD Telemedicine, Inc: Private Payer Reimbursement Information Directory, 2004. Available at: http://www.amdtelemedicine.com/private_payer/index. cfm. Accessed August 13, 2007.

Barretto A, Wacker DP, Harding J, et al: Using telemedicine to conduct behavioral assessments. J Appl Behav Anal 39:333–340, 2006

Broder E, Manson E, Boydell K, et al: Use of telepsychiatry for child psychiatric issues: first 500 cases. CPA Bull 36:11–15, 2004

Brown NA: State Medicaid and private payer reimbursement for telemedicine: an overview. J Telemed Telecare 12(suppl):S32–S39, 2006

Cain S, Spaulding R: Telepsychiatry: lessons from two models of care. Presented at the 53rd Annual Meeting of the American Academy of Child and Adolescent Psychiatry, San Diego, CA, October 2006

Cassidy L, Glueck D: Private practice telepsychiatry. Workshop presentation at the 55th Annual Meeting of the American Academy of Child and Adolescent Psychiatry, Chicago, IL, October 28–November 2, 2008

Center for Telemedicine Law and Office for the Advancement of Telehealth: Telemedicine Reimbursement Report, 2007. Available at: http://www.hrsa.gov/telehealth/pubs/reimbursement.htm. Accessed August 13, 2007.

Centers for Medicare and Medicaid Services: Covered medical and other health services, section 270: telehealth services, in Medicare Benefit Policy Manual, Pub No 100-02. Baltimore, MD, Centers for Medicare and Medicaid Services, 2007a. Available at: http://www.cms.hhs.gov/manuals/Downloads/bp102c15.pdf. Accessed August 13, 2007.

Centers for Medicare and Medicaid Services: Physician/Nonphysician Practitioners, section 190: Medicare payment for telehealth services, in Medicare Claims Processing Manual, Pub No 100-04. Baltimore, MD, Centers for Medicare and Medicaid Services, 2007b. Available at: http://www.cms.hhs.gov/manuals/downloads/clm104c12.pdf. Accessed August 13, 2007.

Cruz M, Krupinski EA, Lopez AM, et al: A review of the first five years of the University of Arizona telepsychiatry programme. J Telemed Telecare 11:234–239, 2005

Elford R, White H, Bowering R, et al: A randomized, controlled trial of child psychiatric assessments conducted using videoconferencing. J Telemed Telecare 6:73–82, 2000

Elford R, White H, St John K, et al: A prospective satisfaction study and cost analysis of a pilot child telepsychiatry service in Newfoundland. J Telemed Telecare 7:73–81, 2001

George R: A private practice model of telepsychiatry for residential treatment. Presented at the 54th Annual Meeting of the American Academy of Child and Adolescent Psychiatry, Boston, MA, October 2007

Glueck D: Telepsychiatry and the Adolescent Treatment Outcomes Module. Presented at the 54th Annual Meeting of the American Academy of Child and Adolescent Psychiatry, Boston, MA, October 2007

Godleski L, Darkins A, Lehmann L: Telemental Health Toolkit. Field Work Group of the Veterans' Health Administration. Washington, DC, U.S. Department of Veterans Affairs, 2003

Goldfield GS, Boachie A: Delivery of family therapy in the treatment of anorexia nervosa using telehealth. Telemed J E Health 9:111–114, 2003

Harper RA: Telepsychiatry consultation to schools and mobile clinics in rural Texas. Presented at the 53rd Annual Meeting of the American Academy of Child and Adolescent Psychiatry, San Diego, CA, October 2006

Hersh WR, Hickman DH, Severance SM, et al: Diagnosis, access and outcomes: update of a systematic review of telemedicine services. J Telemed Telecare 12(suppl):S3–S31, 2006

Hilty DM, Sison JI, Nesbitt TS, et al: Telepsychiatric consultation for ADHD in the primary care setting. J Am Acad Child Adolesc Psychiatry 39:15–16, 2000

Hilty DM, Yellowlees PM, Cobb HC, et al: Models of telepsychiatric consultation-liaison service to rural primary care. Psychosomatics 47:152–157, 2006a

Hilty DM, Yellowlees PM, Cobb HC, et al: Use of secure e-mail and telephone: psychiatric consultations to accelerate rural health service delivery. Telemed J E Health 12:490–495, 2006b

Hockey AD, Yellowlees PM, Murphy S: Evaluation of a pilot second-opinion child telepsychiatry service. J Telemed Telecare 10(suppl):48–50, 2004

Institute of Medicine, Committee on Quality of Health Care in America. Crossing the Quality Chasm: A New Health System for the 21st Century. Washington, DC, National Academies Press, March 2001. Available at: http://www.iom.edu/Object.File/Master/27/184/Chasm-8pager.pdf. Accessed August 4, 2009.

Kopel H, Nunn K, Dossetor D: Evaluating satisfaction with a child and adolescent psychological telemedicine outreach service. J Telemed Telecare 7(suppl):35–40, 2001

Moehr JR, Schaafsma J, Anglin C, et al: Success factors for telehealth: a case study. Int J Med Inform 75:755–763, 2006

Myers KM, Sulzbacher S, Melzer SM: Telepsychiatry with children and adolescents: are patients comparable to those evaluated in usual outpatient care? Telemed J E Health 10:278–285, 2004

Myers K, Valentine J, Melzer SM, et al: Telepsychiatry with incarcerated youth. J Adolesc Health 38:643–648, 2006

Myers KM, Valentine JM, Melzer SM: Feasibility, acceptability, and sustainability of telepsychiatry for children and adolescents. Psychiatr Serv 58:1493–1496, 2007

Myers KM, Valentine JM, Melzer SM: Child and adolescent telepsychiatry: utilization and satisfaction. Telemed J E Health 14:131–137, 2008

Nelson EL, Barnard M, Cain S: Treating childhood depression over videoconferencing. Telemed J E Health 9:49–55, 2003

Onor MS, Misan MD: The clinical interview and the doctor-patient relationship in telemedicine. Telemed J E Health 11:102–105, 2005

Pesamaa L, Ebeling H, Kuusimaki ML, et al: Videoconferencing in child and adolescent telepsychiatry: a systematic review of the literature. J Telemed Telecare 10:187–192, 2004

President's New Freedom Commission on Mental Health: Achieving the Promise: Transforming Mental Health Care in America. Final Report (DHHS Publ No SMA-03-3832). Rockville, MD, 2003. Available at: http://www.mentalhealthcommission.gov/reports/Final Report/toc.html. Accessed August 4, 2009.

Savin D, Garry MT, Zuccaro P, et al: Telepsychiatry for treating rural American Indian youth. J Am Acad Child Adolesc Psychiatry 45:484–488, 2006

Savin D, Garry MT, Zuccaro P, et al: Telepsychiatry for treating American Indian youth while training local providers. Clinical perspectives presentation at the 55th Annual Meeting of the American Academy of Child and Adolescent Psychiatry, Chicago, IL, October 28–November 2, 2008

Simmons SC, West VL, Chimiak WJ: Telecommunications and videoconferencing for psychiatry, in Telepsychiatry and E-Mental Health. Edited by Wooten R, Yellowlees P, McLaren P. London, Royal Society of Medicine Press, 2003, pp 15–28

Sorvaniemi M, Ojanen E, Santamaki O: Telepsychiatry in emergency consultations: a follow-up study of sixty patients. Telemed J E Health 11:439–441, 2005

Storck M: Bringing the community to the state hospital through teleconferencing. Presented at the 54th Annual Meeting of the American Academy of Child and Adolescent Psychiatry, Boston, MA, October 2007

Szeftel R, Hakak R, Meyer S, et al: Training residents and fellows in a telepsychiatry developmental disabilities clinic. Clinical perspectives presentation at the 55th Annual Meeting of the American Academy of Child and Adolescent Psychiatry, Chicago, IL, October 28–November 2, 2008

Werner P: Willingness to use telemedicine for psychiatric care. Telemed J E Health 10:286–292, 2004

Whitten P, Buis L: Private payer reimbursement for telemedicine services in the United States. Telemed J E Health 13:15–23, 2007

Wootton R, Batch J: Telepediatrics: Telemedicine and Child Health. London, Royal Society of Medicine Press, 2005

Wootton R, Yellowlees P, McLaren P (eds): Telepsychiatry and E-Mental Health. London, Royal Society of Medicine Press, 2003

Yellowlees P: E-Mental health in the future, in Telepsychiatry and E-Mental Health. Edited by Wooten R, Yellowlees P, McLaren P. London, Royal Society of Medicine Press, 2003, pp 306–316

Yellowlees P, Miller EA, McLaren P, et al: Introduction, in Telepsychiatry and E-Mental Health. Edited by Wooten R, Yellowlees P, McLaren P. London, Royal Society of Medicine Press, 2003, pp 3–14

Yellowlees P, Hilty DM, Marks SL, et al: A retrospective analysis of a child and adolescent e-mental health program. J Am Acad Child Adolesc Psychiatry 47:103–107, 2008

PART X

SOMATIC TREATMENTS

Chapter 45

Principles of Psychopharmacology

Noah L. Miller, M.D.
Robert L. Findling, M.D.

When clinicians contemplate the therapeutic options for psychiatric disorders, psychopharmacotherapy is often one of those options. However, there are many considerations in thinking about treatment for a youngster with a psychiatric disorder. These considerations differ from those for adults with a psychiatric disorder or for children with pediatric disorders. Factors that make psychopharmacotherapy in children and adolescents distinct from both psychopharmacotherapy in adults and pharmacotherapy for general medical conditions in children include the following:

- Differences between children and adults in drug metabolism
- Differences in psychotropic drug efficacy and tolerability between young people and adults

- Limitations of current psychiatric nosology when diagnosing psychiatric disorders in the young
- Relative paucity of research data on pediatric psychopharmacology
- Involvement of outside parties in treatment planning (e.g., parents, other relatives, teachers, counselors, therapists, pediatricians, neurologists)
- Multidisciplinary nature of most child and adolescent psychiatric treatment
- Chronic nature of most childhood psychiatric illnesses

Despite pediatric psychopharmacology's unique challenges, the use of psychotropic medication is a therapeutic option worthy of consideration for the treatment of a substantial number of children and adolescents who present with psychiatric illnesses. This consideration is primarily based on the rationale that the potential risks of untreated psychiatric illnesses in the young are generally worse than the known and potentially unknown risks and side effects of many psychotropic medications (Vitiello 2008).

Although numerous potential benefits of treatment with psychotropic medication for some children and adolescents exist, there is still a need for clinicians to be thoughtful and cautious when prescribing psychiatric medication for their young patients. Such diligence can be achieved by looking beyond the principles of pharmacokinetics and pharmacodynamics and considering other clinically important principles such as child and adolescent development, drug efficacy and safety, regulatory issues, ethical issues, and treatment adherence when treating these vulnerable youth. Clinicians can then thoughtfully review with patients and their parents whether or not a psychiatric medication should be prescribed. This decision is usually based on the results of a thorough assessment using current evidence-based practice guidelines (when available) and using a biopsychosocial approach to the treatment of youth and their families. Assessment of each developmental period is covered in the first two sections of this text.

Brief History of Pediatric Psychopharmacology

Many consider the field of child and adolescent psychopharmacology to have begun in the late 1930s, when Charles Bradley published a landmark study on the salutary effects of racemic amphetamine (Benzedrine) in children with behavioral disturbances (Bradley 1937). Over the next 50 years, with the exception of the psychostimulants for treatment of attention-deficit/hyperactivity disorder (ADHD), there were few studies pertaining to psychopharmacology in pediatric populations. Clinicians were frequently obliged to rely primarily on adult psychopharmacology research when treating psychiatric disorders in the young. Treating children and adolescents with psychotropics was at times problematic, with pediatric data pertaining to dosing, safety, and efficacy seldom available.

By the mid-1980s, the treatment of early-onset psychiatric disorders in addition to ADHD began to be investigated more frequently in children and adolescents and included pervasive developmental disorders, de-

pressive disorders, bipolar disorder, obsessive-compulsive disorder, schizophrenia, and conduct disorder. Improved experimental design and assessment methods paved the way for this increase in pediatric psychopharmacology research. In 1997, U.S. federal legislation further promoted the study of drugs in children by providing new financial incentives to pharmaceutical companies for studying drugs in pediatric populations. As a result, by the end of the 1990s, pediatric psychopharmacology grew into a substantial and independent field of study (Connor and Meltzer 2006).

General Principles of Psychopharmacological Assessment, Diagnosis, and Treatment

The clinical implementation of child and adolescent psychopharmacology differs from the clinical practice of adult psychopharmacology. The initial steps that clinicians take in completing this evaluation generally include performing a complete psychiatric assessment of the patient and the family, arriving at a psychiatric diagnosis, crafting a biopsychosocial case formulation, and developing an evidence-based comprehensive treatment plan.

Psychiatric Assessment

The first step in the psychiatric treatment of a child or adolescent is the completion of a thorough assessment of the patient. This initial assessment has several goals, one of which is for the clinician to identify psychiatric symptoms that may indicate one or more underlying psychiatric disorders. The clinician can then decide which elements of these disorders might be best addressed by psychopharmacological treatments, which might be best treated with psychosocial treatments and/or environmental interventions, and which elements might deserve a combination therapy approach. Another goal of the psychiatric assessment is to uncover relevant patient and family historical information that may determine which modalities of psychiatric treatment or which psychotropic medications might be most suitable for this patient.

During the initial assessment, the clinician becomes acquainted with the patient while trying to understand the patient's concerns and functioning in multiple contexts, including the patient's family, school, and peer group. This evaluation is also a time during which the clinician can begin to develop a rapport with the patient and patient's parents, which can eventually develop into an effective therapeutic alliance. Good rapport between the clinician, patient, and patient's parents is generally beneficial to all three participants, as the patient and parents may share important information more openly and the family may be more likely to adhere to psychiatric treatment and follow-up.

Sources of Assessment Information

The primary source of information is usually the patient and his or her family. Typically, a psychiatric assessment requires a face-to-face interview of both the patient and the patient's family. If the patient is less than 18 years of age, then the patient's parents or legal guardians (hereafter referred to as "parents") generally need to be present and consent to the evaluation. However, some state laws allow exceptions to this rule for substance abuse treatment, brief counseling, and emergency situations.

Additional sources of information may include other people who spend time with the patient, such as classroom teachers, relatives, and babysitters. Other providers of medical or mental health care, such as therapists, counselors, and pediatricians or neurologists, can also provide valuable information. These individuals can be contacted with the written permission of the patient's parents (and depending on age and state law, the patient).

To supplement the information gathered during the assessment interview, psychiatric rating scales are typically used (see Chapter 8, "Rating Scales"). These questionnaires can be completed by the patient, teachers, and/or parents before the assessment, allowing clinicians to review the results during the interview. A commonly used rating scale that has been found to be valid and reliable is the Child Behavior Checklist (CBCL) (Achenbach and Rescorla 2001; Ivanova et al. 2007). Another frequently used group of psychometric assessments is the Conners 3rd Edition (Conners 3) rating scales (Conners 2008). These scales can screen for multiple types of psychopathology. The CBCL and the Conners 3 allow for the calculation of a standardized score. Therefore, these scales allow for the comparison of symptoms reported by or about the patient to symptoms noted in youth of the same sex and age who are not suffering from a psychiatric disorder. While these psychometric scales were not designed to diagnose psychiatric disorders per se, they can supplement clinical psychiatric diagnoses by providing information about symptom severity.

Assessment Interview

During the assessment interview, a clinician asks questions and gathers information about key aspects of a patient's history and presentation (Table 45–1). As clinicians gather this clinical information, they typically concentrate on the data that will help establish the psychiatric diagnosis and determine the best options for treatment, including possible psychopharmacotherapy.

Interviewing pediatric patients can be challenging, owing to the distinct psychological and cognitive characteristics of children and adolescents. For example, younger children may have relatively limited verbal abilities and may be less experienced than adults at recognizing their emotions and feelings. Thus, children may have difficulty talking about their mood or thoughts. It is not until late childhood or early adolescence that children generally become more proficient at recognizing their emotions and feelings and verbally communicating that information to others. Younger children may also have difficulty estimating lengths of periods of time. For this reason, it can be useful for clinicians to reference concrete landmarks of time (e.g., holidays or birthdays) and significant life experiences (e.g., the birth of a sibling, a move to a new house, a specific year in school) when asking a child about the timing of certain events.

While older children typically have better verbal skills, they may not understand psychiatric terms such as "irritability," "euphoria," or "paranoia." Similarly, clinicians and adolescents may use different words or phrases to describe certain concepts. To prevent an incorrect assumption, a clinician can always ask a young patient "What do you mean?" to clarify what the patient is saying. A clinician may improve communication with an adolescent patient by taking note of the patient's language skills and vocabulary. For instance, if a patient uses a lot of slang language, a clinician may similarly use more slang and less technical language in order to improve the patient's understanding of what is being said.

Lastly, it can be helpful for clinicians to remember that the act of a pediatric patient answering a clinician's question does not necessarily signify that the patient understands the question. If a clinician suspects that a patient does not comprehend what is being discussed, the clinician can inquire about the patient's understanding and present the information again using different language or examples if necessary.

TABLE 45–1. Selected areas of the psychiatric assessment that are important to pediatric psychopharmacology

Area of psychiatric assessment	Relevance to pediatric psychopharmacology
Chief complaint	The parents' principal areas of concern help define the goals for psychiatric pharmacotherapy.
History of present illness	Certain psychiatric symptoms and responses to psychosocial stressors may be amenable to psychopharmacological treatment. Target symptoms can be identified and monitored to determine drug effectiveness.
Psychiatric review of systems	Comorbid disorders may require modified psychopharmacological treatment.
Past psychiatric history	Information on past psychotropic medication trials (reason prescribed, highest dose achieved, effectiveness, side effects, duration of treatment, and reason for discontinuation) can guide future medication choices and dosing. Current psychotropic medications may need to be adjusted or discontinued if new medications are initiated in order to prevent toxicity or drug-drug interactions.
Suicidality and homicidality history	Past and current safety concerns may require certain precautions as pharmacotherapy is initiated (choosing drugs that are less toxic in overdose, prescribing limited amounts of medication, or monitoring patient particularly closely for behavioral changes).
Substance abuse and chemical dependency history	Past chemical dependency may necessitate caution when prescribing controlled substances. Current abuse of medications, illicit drugs, or alcohol can cause drug-drug interactions with psychotropic medications. Current chemical dependency may require detoxification. Comprehensive chemical dependency treatment may be necessary before psychopharmacotherapy for comorbid psychiatric disorders is initiated.
Developmental and early childhood history	A history of maternal drug or alcohol abuse may theoretically be associated with alterations in the effects of psychotropic medications. A patient's slow growth may raise concern over potential negative effects on stature associated with the long-term use of certain psychotropic medications.
General medical history	Known drug allergies may limit psychopharmacotherapy options. Past and current medical conditions may affect choice of psychotropic medications (avoiding psychostimulants in youth with cardiac problems, valproic acid in children with hepatic disease, or lithium in youth with renal insufficiency).
Family history	Psychotropic medication that is effective for a patient's close relative may be more effective for the patient than other medication choices.
School history	Younger children or older children with low intellectual functioning may require increased parental monitoring of psychotropic medication. The timing of a child's ADHD symptoms throughout the school day may require certain adjustments in dosing the child's psychostimulant medication. Adverse medication effects such as sedation may interfere with academic performance.
Social history	Peer relationships and attitudes may affect a youth's adherence to psychotropic medication. Adverse medication effects such as sedation may interfere with leisure activities.

Mental Status Examination

While assessing a child or adolescent patient, clinicians typically conduct a mental status examination by observing the key features of a patient's appearance, behavior, speech, language, mood, affect, thought process, thought content, cognition, and social relatedness. These observations, when added to the data from the patient interview, can help the clinician establish a diagnosis and decide on possible pharmacological treatment options. Also, certain psychiatric symptoms that are observed during the mental status exam may be used by the clinician as a baseline to subsequently assess the effectiveness of a patient's response to psychopharmacotherapy.

Variability in mental status is common in children and adolescents. An appreciation of such variability is important because various circumstances can influence a patient's mood or behavior during the initial psychiatric assessment. For example, a child with ADHD symptoms that are typically well controlled with a psychostimulant may appear to have problems with hyperactivity or concentration during the mental status examination if he or she did not receive medication that day. Or a child with untreated ADHD may appear to have good attention and concentration in the office at the first visit with a new clinician, owing to the unfamiliarity and novelty of the encounter. Similarly, a youth who is experiencing symptoms of an upper respiratory infection may present with low energy and irritable mood, which to a clinician may appear to be symptoms of depression. Thus, it is advisable for clinicians to consider any suspected influences on a patient's mental status exam as the diagnosis and options for possible psychopharmacological treatment are being considered.

Physical Evaluation

Not only is a mental status examination conducted during a psychiatric assessment, but a patient's physical condition is also typically assessed (see Chapter 9, "Pediatric Evaluation and Laboratory Testing," and Chapter 10, "Neurological Examination, Electroencephalography, and Neuroimaging"). The clinician's decisions about which components to include in this focused physical evaluation depend on the patient's general physical health and the type of psychotropic medication that the clinician is considering prescribing. There are several key reasons to evaluate a young patient's physical health prior to definitively ascribing a psychiatric diagnosis or making treatment recommendations. One reason is that general medical conditions may manifest with psychiatric symptomatology. For instance, depressive symptoms in a patient may be either caused or exacerbated by hypothyroidism. Additionally, the presence of certain general medical conditions might substantively influence decisions about the prescription of psychotropic agents. For example, the decision whether or not to prescribe a psychostimulant to a patient with ADHD might be considered with greater caution if the patient has a structural cardiac abnormality.

Examining the physical well-being of patients and measuring selected physical parameters prior to the initiation of pharmacotherapy also provide a baseline with which subsequent evaluations can be compared. Therefore, obtaining pretreatment information may facilitate the assessment of possible adverse effects that occur as a result of treatment with psychotropic medication.

It is also desirable for mental health clinicians to collaborate with the patient's primary medical doctor throughout the patient's psychiatric care. This collaboration is valuable, as the mental health clinician is thus able to stay informed of changes in the patient's general medical status or nonpsychotropic medications that are being prescribed. Conversely, communication between the mental health clinician and the general medical physician provides the general medical physician an appraisal of changes in the child's diagnosis and psychiatric care.

Physical examination.

Ideally, a pediatric patient will have been seen by his or her primary medical doctor for a physical examination within the year prior to the psychiatric assessment. If the patient has not had a general medical examination within the past year, it is often advisable that the patient receive one before psychotropic medication is administered.

Other physical parameters.

Clinicians may check a patient's vital signs, height, and weight during the psychiatric assessment in order to screen for any immediate medical concerns such as obesity or hypertension prior to possibly initiating psychotropic medication. Comparison of such baseline measurements to future physical parameters can aid clinicians in monitoring for potential adverse medication effects, including changes in patients' growth. Monitoring for potential growth effects is advisable since, with the exception of psychostimulants, there are relatively few data available on the long-term effects of psychopharmacotherapy on children's growth and development.

Laboratory tests.

These tests can supplement the data gathered from the physical examination and other diagnostic procedures. The additional information can help a clinician rule out certain underlying medical conditions, which in turn may guide the clinician's choice of possible psychotropic medication. Furthermore, establishing certain baseline laboratory values prior to initiating psychotropic medications can aid in monitoring for potential adverse medication effects. Common tests that a clinician may choose are included in Table 45–2 (Zametkin et al. 1998; see Chapter 9, "Pediatric Evaluation and Laboratory Testing").

Electrocardiogram and other diagnostic procedures.

In patients with a history or symptoms of cardiovascular illness or a family history of heart disease, clinicians may elect to obtain a baseline electrocardiogram (ECG) to assess for the presence of cardiac illness before initiating psychotropic medication. Certain medications may either prolong the QTc interval or substantively affect cardiovascular functioning at therapeutic doses. These psychotropic medications include (McNally et al. 2007):

- Alpha-2-adrenergic agonists such as clonidine or guanfacine
- First-generation antipsychotics (neuroleptics) such as thioridazine and pimozide
- Atypical (second-generation) antipsychotics such as clozapine and ziprasidone
- Tricyclic antidepressants
- Lithium

Additional diagnostic procedures that clinicians may wish to obtain for certain pediatric patients prior to psychopharmacotherapy include an electroencephalogram (EEG) and a computed tomography (CT) or magnetic resonance imaging (MRI) scan of the brain (see Chapter 10, "Neurological Examination, Electroencephalography, and Neuroimaging"). An EEG may be considered for patients who have a history of seizure disorder and are being considered for pharmacotherapy with psychotropic medications that potentially lower the seizure threshold (e.g., antipsychotics such as clozapine, tricyclic antidepressants, or lithium). Clinicians may decide to obtain a CT or MRI of the brain to either confirm or refute the presence of an anatomic abnormality that may be a potential etiology of psychiatric symptoms in certain young patients.

Diagnosis

Following the psychiatric assessment, the clinician is next faced with the task of identifying the primary psychiatric diagnosis (if one exists), as well as recognizing any comorbid disorders. An accurate psychiatric diagnosis is important because it helps identify appropriate treatment options. The psychiatric diagnosis is the basis for evidence-based treatment guidelines that have been developed for many disorders.

The *Diagnostic and Statistical Manual of Mental Disorders,* Fourth Edition, Text Revision (DSM-IV-TR; American Psychiatric Association 2000) recognizes constellations of emotional, thought, and behavioral symptoms and classifies these sets of symptoms into various categories of psychiatric disorders. Diagnostic classifications generally improve the ability of clinicians to agree on patients' psychiatric diagnoses and communicate clinical information with one another (see Chapter 5, "Classification of Psychiatric Disorders"). A significant limitation in the current nosology for diagnosing psychiatric disorders in the young is that disorders such as ADHD and mood disorders may manifest differently in children than in adults. Since many mental illnesses first manifest during childhood, the challenges of accurately diagnosing disorders in children are important for clinicians to consider as they make plans for potential psychopharmacotherapy.

It is important for clinicians to successfully identify any comorbid diagnoses since psychiatric comorbidity can influence pharmacological management. Though there are more data on the treatment of individual psychiatric disorders than the treatment of comorbid psychiatric disorders, clinicians can consult empirically based treatment guidelines while adhering to the general principles of pediatric psychopharmacology to safely initiate treatment with psychotropic medication.

It is important to discuss the patient's diagnoses with the patient and parents because a well-informed family can better make educated and responsible decisions about psychiatric treatment. Patients and their parents frequently have questions about the diagnoses, including possible causes of the disorders, typical symptoms associated with the disorders, treatment options for the primary disorder and its comorbidities, and expected prognosis. After answering these questions, clinicians may refer families to sources of information, such as reputable books and Web sites. A good starting point for families is the Web site for the American Academy of Child and Adolescent Psychiatry (www.aacap.org).

TABLE 45–2. Laboratory tests to check during the psychopharmacological assessment of a pediatric patient

Laboratory test	Psychopharmacological reasons for obtaining test
Complete blood count with differential	Screening for anemia, which can cause decreased energy; baseline for drugs that may affect blood counts
Serum electrolytes	Screening for purging or restricting of food for patients in whom an underlying eating disorder is suspected
Blood urea nitrogen, creatinine	Screening for renal dysfunction, which may alter psychopharmacotherapy options; baseline for lithium treatment
"Liver function tests" (aspartate aminotransferase, alanine aminotransferase, alkaline phosphatase, bilirubin)	Screening for hepatic problems, which may affect psychopharmacotherapy options; baseline and for subsequent monitoring
Fasting glucose level	Screening for metabolic syndrome and/or diabetes mellitus, especially if second-generation antipsychotics are being considered
Fasting lipid profile (high-density and low-density cholesterol, triglycerides)	Screening for hyperlipidemia and/or hypercholesterolemia, especially if weight-gain-inducing agents are being considered
Urinalysis	Screening for renal disease and/or diabetes mellitus
Urine toxicology screen	Screening for illicit drug abuse
Thyroid-stimulating hormone (TSH) level	Screening for thyroid dysfunction, which can contribute to symptoms of depression, anxiety, and psychosis; baseline for lithium treatment
Urine pregnancy test	Screening for pregnancy in females of reproductive age
Serum lead level	Screening for lead toxicity, especially in children under 7 years of age

Biopsychosocial Formulation and Treatment Planning

Factors other than a DSM-IV-TR diagnosis can affect a youth's emotions and behaviors and include comorbid medical conditions, level of development, psychological distress, family relationships, social relationships, environmental stressors, and educational functioning. A biopsychosocial formulation supplements the diagnosis by describing the predisposing, precipitating, perpetuating, and protective factors that have shaped the patient's clinical presentation.

The next task for the clinician, patient, and family is to develop a treatment plan. Treatment planning for young patients typically involves multiple people, including parents, relatives, teachers, and pediatricians. A multidisciplinary and multimodal treatment approach is commonly used, which may include pharmacotherapy as well as individual psychotherapy, group psychotherapy, family psychotherapy, parental counseling, or educational interventions. Psychopharmacological treatment should generally not be initi-

ated without the consideration of accompanying psychotherapeutic interventions.

Treating Psychiatric Disorders Rather Than Target Symptoms

It is important to note that clinical guidelines do not recommend psychiatric pharmacotherapy solely to address specific target psychiatric symptoms. Rather, clinicians generally treat psychiatric syndromes with medications and then measure treatment response by tracking specified target symptoms. This principle is not unique to child and adolescent psychiatry but is one that occurs in general pediatric practice as well. For instance, fever is not necessarily treated with antibiotics. However, bacterial pneumonia is treated with antibiotics, and fever is one of several parameters that may be monitored to see if the antibiotic treatment is being helpful. Fever may also be treated symptomatically while the underlying cause receives specific treatment or resolves spontaneously. As an example in child and adolescent psychiatry, it is not generally recommended that a specific agent be prescribed to a child with a dysfunctionally irritable mood. This is because there are multiple potential causes of irritability in children. A few of these causes include major depressive disorder, dysthymic disorder, bipolar disorder, generalized anxiety disorder, and posttraumatic stress disorder, as well as developmental, cognitive, medical, or environmental causes. Addressing irritability depends on the accurate identification of the most likely cause. Once an accurate diagnosis and assessment are made, the success of the selected course of treatment can be monitored by tracking the patient's level of irritability.

Therapeutic Alliance

In order to reach an agreement with the parents on a treatment plan, a clinician may use certain styles of presenting the information and answering the family's questions. The style chosen can generally be either authoritative (presenting the options and asking the family to choose one) or authoritarian (being more directive with the family regarding which option or options they should choose). In many treatment settings, it is advisable for clinicians to take an authoritative approach to the family. By being thorough and comprehensive in the assessment and diagnosis of a patient, a clinician can develop a positive rapport and strong therapeutic alliance with the patient and parents. Furthermore, by making reasonable and appropriate treatment recommendations and by taking the time to adequately answer the family's questions, a clinician can help provide a sense of confidence to the patient and the patient's family. A family may be more likely to agree to and remain adherent with the treatment recommendations of such a positively regarded authoritative clinician.

There are some instances, however, when a family may agree with treatment recommendations from an authoritarian clinician. This approach may be necessary when the patient's parents are either having difficulty making treatment choices or requesting treatment approaches that may result in harm to the patient or others.

Selecting Psychopharmacological Agents

Clinicians typically rely on several principles when selecting and dosing psychotropic medications for children and adolescents. These considerations include the differences in drug metabolism between children and adults, data on the efficacy and safety of psychotropic medication in children, regulatory issues associated with the off-label use of psychotropic medications, and ethical issues surrounding the psychopharmacological treatment of children and adolescents.

Drug Metabolism and Disposition

Children are not merely "little adults" when it comes to the metabolism of drugs. This fact is a result of physiological differences between youth and adults that affect drug dosing, therapeutic effect, and safety.

Pharmacokinetics

The primary differences in drug metabolism between children and adults are a result of two key pharmacokinetic factors:

1. Youth have proportionally more liver tissue than adults, when adjusted for body weight. As a result, youth may have more rapid hepatic drug metabolism than adults, possibly resulting in more rapid elimination of drugs that use hepatic pathways (Kearns et al. 2003).
2. When adjusted for body weight, children may have higher glomerular filtration rates than adults, possibly resulting in more rapid excretion of drugs that use renal pathways (Chen et al. 2006).

As a result of these pharmacokinetic differences, children may require larger weight-adjusted doses of psychiatric medications than adults in order to attain comparable serum drug levels. In addition, youth may also benefit from more frequent drug dosing in order to compensate for shorter drug half-lives (Jatlow 1987).

Drugs may also be absorbed and distributed differently in children's bodies. As a result, some drugs may require further dosing adjustments when compared to dosing for adults. These pharmacokinetic differences in comparison to adults include the following (Kearns et al. 2003):

- Children have proportionally more extracellular and total-body water than adults, which may lead to lower plasma concentrations of hydrophilic drugs. As a result, some drugs (e.g., lithium) may require higher weight-based dosing in youth.
- Children have proportionally less fat tissue than adults, so higher plasma concentrations of some li-

pophilic drugs (e.g., paroxetine) may be expected in children.

- The functioning of the gastrointestinal tract does not fully mature until 10–12 years of age. This phenomenon may lead to greater variability of oral drug absorption in the young when compared to adults.

The differences in drug disposition in children when compared to adults appear to gradually diminish throughout childhood, with an abrupt decline typically occurring during puberty. At approximately age 15 years, children's pharmacokinetic characteristics begin to become more adult-like in nature. Accordingly, clinicians can generally assume that adult drug doses may be employed in youth once they reach mid-adolescence (Jatlow 1987).

Pharmacodynamics

Some psychiatric medications do not have the same efficacy or tolerability in children and adolescents as in adults. For example, the tricyclic class of antidepressants, which is an effective treatment for depression in adults, has repeatedly been found to be ineffective for depressed children and adolescents (Hazell et al. 2002). One factor that may be responsible for age-related differences seen in drug effect and tolerability is the relative immaturity of certain neurotransmitter systems in the young. The serotonin and catecholamine (norepinephrine, epinephrine, and dopamine) networks of the central nervous system play important roles in regulating mood, thinking, and behavior. As such, these networks are also the primary targets of psychiatric medications. However, these neural pathways are not fully developed in the young and do not fully acquire adult functionality until the third decade of life (Murrin et al. 2007).

Drug Efficacy and Safety

As outlined earlier in this chapter, there are historical reasons for the current paucity of pediatric drug efficacy data, including limitations in experimental design and assessment methods prior to the 1980s. There are also practical limitations to conducting psychopharmacological research in children, which include the greater level of difficulty that is generally associated with conducting research in children as compared to adults, the scarcity of available funding to

support psychopharmacological research in children, and the ethical issues that surround clinical research in children. Much of the currently available pediatric psychopharmacology data address the efficacy of pharmacotherapy for the acute phases of psychiatric illnesses. However, fewer data exist documenting long-term efficacy. Since many psychiatric disorders first manifest during childhood and are chronic in nature, there is a great need for more information about the effectiveness and risks of the long-term pharmacological management of these disorders.

The safety of medications is an important consideration. Safety is a comparative notion, as the risks of pharmacotherapy are not considered individually but rather are measured against the risks of untreated psychiatric illness. All medications carry some risk of adverse events. It is important for clinicians to educate young patients and their parents about not only the risks of a drug's potential side effects but also the potential benefits of effective intervention.

Most psychotropic medications have warnings, precautions, and contraindications that are included in each drug's labeling information. Some psychotropic medications have more serious warnings, commonly referred to as black box warnings. A black box warning that has greatly affected the practice of pediatric psychopharmacotherapy is the "increased suicidality in children and adolescents" warning that was added to all antidepressants by the U.S. Food and Drug Administration (2004). A similar warning has been added to the labeling for anticonvulsants (U.S. Food and Drug Administration 2008). Clinicians must be aware of these safety warnings and discuss safety issues with patients and their parents. Specific safety issues are covered in Chapter 46, "Medications Used for Attention-Deficit/Hyperactivity Disorder"; Chapter 47, "Antidepressants"; Chapter 48, "Mood Stabilizers"; Chapter 49, "Antipsychotic Medications"; Chapter 50, "Alpha-Adrenergics, Beta-Blockers, Benzodiazepines, Buspirone, and Desmopressin"; and Chapter 51, "Medications Used for Sleep."

Clinicians should also be aware of potentially dangerous drug-drug interactions. Clinicians should take a careful inventory of all of a patient's prescription and over-the-counter medications, vitamins, and herbal preparations during the assessment interview and throughout treatment. In addition, the prescribing physician should review potentially dangerous drug-drug interactions with patients and their guardians prior to and during pharmacotherapy.

Regulatory Considerations

Because a large percentage of psychotropic medications have not been adequately studied in youth, many of these compounds do not have U.S. Food and Drug Administration (FDA)–approved indications for pediatric patients. Therefore, medications are frequently used in children and adolescents in an off-label fashion. The FDA does not regulate physician prescribing practices and therefore does not prohibit the off-label use of medication. However, as FDA-approved indications are generally the result of methodologically stringent evidence, clinicians may desire to first consider FDA-approved medication options, when available, rather than prescribe agents for off-label indications.

One key means by which the dearth of research in pediatric drugs is being addressed is through U.S. federal legislation on drug studies in children and adolescents. The U.S. Food and Drug Administration Modernization Act of 1997 (FDAMA) gave pharmaceutical companies greater financial incentives to voluntarily conduct clinical trials of medications in children and adolescents. In 2002, the Best Pharmaceuticals for Children Act renewed the financial incentives previously provided by the FDAMA while authorizing the National Institutes of Health (NIH) to fund pediatric studies of older off-patent medications. More recently, the Pediatric Research Equity Act of 2003 required pharmaceutical companies to begin conducting pediatric studies of drugs in development if those drugs had potential for use in the young. Since the passage of these federal laws, there has been an increase in the number of pediatric clinical studies. This increase has resulted in improved data about the efficacy of several medications in children and may lead to less off-label drug use as more medications become FDA approved for use in pediatric patients. Data derived from these multicenter studies have also led to a better characterization of these agents' tolerability profile, and in some instances, have led to new warnings pertaining to drug safety.

Ethical Issues

Since children and adolescents are a particularly vulnerable population, certain ethical principles guide the practice of pediatric psychopharmacotherapy, including obtaining informed consent and assent prior to prescribing psychotropic medications and continuing discussions with the patient and family about the treatment over time.

Informed Consent and Assent

As treatment options are presented to the patient and parents, the clinician provides education to help the family understand the purpose of the therapeutic interventions and the potential risks and benefits associated with each treatment option. This initiates both an informed consent process with the parents and an assent process with the patient that generally occur before beginning psychopharmacological treatment. Informed consent to initiate or continue a psychotropic medication generally requires the patient's parents to be competent, to demonstrate adequate knowledge about the proposed medication, and to make the treatment decision freely, without coercion. "Adequate knowledge" about a psychotropic medication usually includes an understanding of the nature of the patient's psychiatric disorder; the potential risks, benefits, and side effects of the proposed psychopharmacological treatment; the possible alternatives to the proposed treatment; and the patient's expected prognosis both with and without the proposed treatment.

Children generally have a limited capacity to fully understand the issues surrounding medical treatment, which is why decisions about medical treatment are usually made by a child's parents. However, many children can still provide assent for their psychopharmacological treatment. Informed assent generally requires a child to demonstrate an age-appropriate awareness of the psychiatric diagnosis and both an understanding and acceptance of the recommended psychopharmacological treatment (including possible diagnostic procedures). Once the general requirements for informed consent are met, the parents can then decide whether to begin or eschew the proposed psychopharmacological treatment.

Explaining Psychotropic Medication to Children and Adolescents

When prescribing psychotropic medication to a pediatric patient, clinicians are encouraged not only to discuss the medication with the patient to properly obtain informed assent but also to help the patient feel like a participant in the treatment planning process and help the patient feel a greater sense of control in treatment. The patient can thus become an active participant in treatment, monitoring the effects of psychotropic medication on psychiatric symptoms, providing information about internal experiences such as mood and thought content, and watching for possible adverse side effects. Active participation can be a positive experience for many youth, especially adolescents who are typically dealing with developmental issues of autonomy. Thus, encouraging a pediatric patient's active participation in treatment can strengthen the patient's therapeutic alliance and possibly improve future treatment adherence.

Management of Psychopharmacotherapy

Psychopharmacotherapy generally consists of three phases: initiation of psychotropic medication, medication maintenance, and discontinuing the medication (if there are clinical indications to do so). Throughout these phases of psychopharmacological treatment, a clinician may encounter various medication-related issues, such as adverse side effects and insufficient therapeutic effect. Also, clinicians may encounter challenges in the management of psychopharmacotherapy in children and adolescents, such as the treatment of comorbid psychiatric conditions and treatment nonadherence.

Initiating and Titrating Psychotropic Medication

The first task after selecting a specific psychotropic medication is to select the starting dose. It is generally recommended that psychotropic medication be started using evidence-based dosing. Frequently this means starting treatment at relatively low doses. After the initial dose's tolerability has been determined, the amount of drug that is prescribed can then be titrated upwards to a level that is expected to be therapeutic. For any given medication, the rate at which it is increased, its target dose, and the maximum total daily dose should all be based as much as possible on extant scientific evidence from patients of similar age. As both side effects and benefits are frequently increased at higher doses, patients should generally be treated with the dose that provides for them the best balance of symptom amelioration and tolerability.

Symptom Response

The effectiveness of psychopharmacological treatment is typically measured by the patient, family, clinician, and other involved observers, who all monitor for improvement in selected target symptoms. Various symptom rating scales can be used to assist in assessing psychiatric symptom improvement or worsening. Additionally, serum levels of certain psychotropic medications (such as lithium and valproic acid) can be measured to guide the clinician in choosing a therapeutic dose while avoiding drug toxicity.

Side Effects

Side effects may occur at any time during psychotropic treatment. For instance, some side effects (such as sedation or appetite increase) may become apparent soon after medication initiation, while others (such as tardive dyskinesia) may occur later in the course of treatment. The monitoring of certain adverse effects may require the serial measurement of various physical parameters such as vital signs, laboratory tests, and ECGs. For example, a pediatric patient who is taking medication that can cause weight gain may require periodic checks of fasting glucose level and lipid profile in order to monitor for the onset of metabolic syndrome or diabetes mellitus.

When side effects do occur, several courses of action may be taken, including lowering the drug dose or changing the drug dosing schedule to minimize side effects. For example, a once-a-day medication given in the morning that is sedating to a patient during the first few hours after each dose may instead be given at bedtime in an attempt to decrease the patient's daytime sedation. Other adverse effects may improve after the coadministration of an additional agent. For instance, if a patient is experiencing extrapyramidal muscular side effects due to an antipsychotic medication, the addition of an anticholinergic drug may alleviate these symptoms. Proper management of adverse effects may prevent a patient from discontinuing a psychopharmacological treatment that has been otherwise effective.

Medication Maintenance

If the medication has been adequately effective and well-tolerated, the patient next enters the maintenance phase of psychopharmacotherapy. The primary goal of maintenance treatment is to prevent a recurrence of symptoms. As the majority of psychiatric disorders are chronic in nature, the maintenance of psychotropic medication for prolonged periods of time may be necessary in order to reduce the risk of symptom recurrence. The continuation of psychotropic medications, sometimes for years, can help optimize a patient's functioning throughout adolescence and into adulthood.

Adequacy of a Medication Trial

A common mistake made by clinicians is to discontinue a psychotropic medication for lack of effectiveness before a trial of the medication at an adequate dose for an adequate length of time has been completed. The dose and length of treatment required for an adequate trial depend on both the drug being used and the condition being treated. For example, for a disorder such as ADHD, only a few weeks of psychostimulant treatment are needed on a trial basis, while for a diagnosis such as major depressive disorder, up to 2–3 months of antidepressant treatment may be required before making the final determination of whether psychopharmacological treatment is effective. If the medication in question is found to be ineffective after an adequate trial, the medication may be discontinued and a new psychotropic medication and/or other treatment options may be considered. It is generally not wise to just add another medication.

Changing Medications

When a psychotropic medication is not effective or causes intolerable side effects, a clinician may recommend replacing the currently prescribed drug with a new psychotropic agent, weighing the empirical evidence when choosing which psychotropic medication to try next. Although a different drug from the same therapeutic family may be considered, a trial of a medication from a different therapeutic family may be warranted. In instances in which treatment with a psychotropic medication results in a partial therapeutic response, augmentation with an additional psychotropic agent may be considered. However, data on combination medication treatment strategies for psychiatric disorders are generally limited, particularly in children and adolescents.

Discontinuing Psychotropic Medication

At some point, it may become clinically indicated or medically necessary to discontinue a psychotropic medication. For example, a child's ADHD symptoms may naturally improve as the child matures into an adolescent, or side effects may limit a drug's dosing to subtherapeutic levels. Prior to discontinuing a psychotropic medication, a clinician generally discusses with a patient and parents the possible risks (psychiatric symptom recurrence) and benefits (decreased risk of medication-related side effects) associated with medication discontinuation. Drugs that are more rapidly metabolized or medications that can result in drug tolerance may require a gradual taper of the dose in order to prevent "rebound" effects or withdrawal syndromes, respectively.

Challenges in Pediatric Psychopharmacotherapy

Treatment of Comorbid Diagnoses

The psychotropic treatment of comorbid psychiatric disorders presents challenges because there are very limited supporting treatment strategies for various psychiatric comorbidities in pediatric patients. Clinicians may choose to treat certain comorbidities (e.g., ADHD and oppositional defiant disorder) with a single psychotropic agent. In other instances, comorbid disorders (e.g., mania and ADHD) may require a stepwise approach, where a clinician first treats the primary (or more disabling) psychiatric disorder with one psychotropic medication and then addresses the remaining comorbid disorder with a second psychotropic agent.

Treatment Adherence

Nonadherence to psychopharmacological treatment is a commonly observed problem. Reasons may include the result of the patient or parent perceiving a lack of drug efficacy, the patient experiencing adverse drug effects, misperceptions about the possible effects of psychotropic medications, peer pressure to avoid taking psychiatric medication, social stigma associated with mental illness, pressure from relatives, or the patient's oppositional behavior toward following directions from his or her parents and other adults. A positive rapport among the clinician, patient, and child's parents may reduce the likelihood of treatment nonadherence by facilitating the communication of educational information to the family and the patient.

Research Directions

Recently, there has been a substantial increase in psychopharmacology research in pediatric patients. However, most of these studies are acute single-drug efficacy trials, and long-term safety data generally do not exist beyond 6 months. In order to better define potential tardive medication effects, longer-term data pertaining specifically to safety and tolerability would be beneficial. In addition, there appears to be very few head-to-head studies that have compared different agents within the same therapeutic class. Such clinical trials might be very informative to clinicians. Finally, as combination drug approaches appear to be commonly used in clinical practice, medication trials that rigorously and meticulously scrutinize this form of intervention are needed.

Summary Points

- Psychopharmacological treatment of children and adolescents begins with a meticulous diagnostic assessment.

- Differences in drug biodisposition in children and adolescents when compared to adults may substantively affect drug dosing in the young.

- Psychotropic medications that are safe and effective in adults may be neither effective nor well tolerated in pediatric patients.

- Fastidious measurement of target symptoms and thoughtful monitoring of side effects can facilitate rational drug therapy.

- Clinicians should employ evidence-based treatments, as they are available, in the clinical practice of pediatric psychopharmacology.

- The risk-benefit deliberations associated with psychopharmacological treatment decisions in children should include a consideration of the risks associated with untreated psychiatric illnesses.

References

Achenbach TM, Rescorla LA: Manual for the ASEBA School-Age Forms and Profiles. Burlington, University of Vermont, Research Center for Children, Youth, and Families, 2001

American Psychiatric Association: Diagnostic and Statistical Manual of Mental Disorders, 4th Edition, Text Revision. Washington, DC, American Psychiatric Association, 2000

Bradley C: The behavior of children receiving Benzedrine. Am J Orthopsychiatry 94:577–585, 1937

Chen N, Aleksa K, Woodland C, et al: Ontogeny of drug elimination by the human kidney. Pediatr Nephrol 21:160–168, 2006

Conners CK: Conners 3rd Edition. North Tonawanda, NY, Multi-Health Systems, 2008

Connor D, Meltzer B: A brief history of the field, in Pediatric Psychopharmacology Fast Facts. New York, WW Norton, 2006, pp 4–6

Hazell P, O'Connell D, Heathcote D, et al: Tricyclic drugs for depression in children and adolescents. Cochrane Database of Systematic Reviews 2002, Issue 2. Art. No.: CD002317. DOI: 10.1002/14651858.CD002317

Ivanova MY, Dobrean A, Dopfner M, et al: Testing the 8-syndrome structure of the Child Behavior Checklist in 30 societies. J Clin Child Adolesc Psychol 36:405–417, 2007

Jatlow PI: Psychotropic drug disposition during development, in Psychiatric Pharmacosciences of Children and Adolescents. Edited by Popper C. Washington, DC, American Psychiatric Press, 1987, pp 27–44

Kearns GL, Abdel-Rahman SM, Alander SW, et al: Developmental pharmacology: drug disposition, action, and therapy in infants and children. N Engl J Med 349:1157–1167, 2003

McNally P, McNichols F, Oslizlok P: The QT interval and psychotropic medications in children: recommendations for clinicians. Eur Child Adolesc Psychiatry 16:33–47, 2007

Murrin LC, Sanders JD, Bylund DB: Comparison of the maturation of the adrenergic and serotonergic neurotransmitter systems in the brain: implications for differential drug effects on juveniles and adults. Biochem Pharmacol 73:1225–1236, 2007

U.S. Food and Drug Administration: Public Health Advisory: Suicidality in Children and Adolescents Being Treated with Anti-depressant Medications. October 15, 2004. Available at: http://www.fda.gov/Safety/MedWatch/SafetyInformation/SafetyAlertsforHumanMedicalProducts/ucm155488.htm. Accessed June 23, 2009.

U.S. Food and Drug Administration: Safety Alerts for Human Medical Products: Antiepileptic Drugs. January 31, 2008. Available at: http://www.fda.gov/Safety/MedWatch/SafetyInformation/SafetyAlertsforHumanMedicalProducts/ucm074939.htm. Accessed June 23, 2009.

Vitiello B: Developmental aspects of pediatric psychopharmacology, in Clinical Manual of Child and Adolescent Psychopharmacology. Edited by Findling RL. Washington, DC, American Psychiatric Publishing, 2008, pp 1–31

Zametkin AJ, Ernst M, Silver R: Laboratory and diagnostic testing in child and adolescent psychiatry: a review of the past 10 years. J Am Acad Child Adolesc Psychiatry 37:464–472, 1998

Chapter 46

Medications Used for Attention-Deficit/Hyperactivity Disorder

Thomas J. Spencer, M.D.
Joseph Biederman, M.D.
Timothy E. Wilens, M.D.

Attention-deficit/hyperactivity disorder (ADHD) is one of the major clinical and public health problems in the United States in terms of morbidity and disability in children and adolescents. It is estimated to affect at least 5% of school-age children. Its impact on society is enormous in terms of the financial cost, the stress to families, the impact on schools, and the damaging effects on self-esteem.

Pathophysiology

ADHD is a heterogeneous disorder of unknown etiology. An emerging neuropsychological and neuroimaging literature suggests that abnormalities in frontal networks or frontostriatal dysfunction is the disorder's underlying neural substrate, and catecholamine dysregulation is its underlying pathophysiology. The pattern of neuropsychological deficits found in children with ADHD implicates executive functions and working memory. This pattern is similar to what has been found among adults with frontal lobe damage, which suggests that the frontal cortex or regions projecting to the frontal cortex are dysfunctional in at least some subjects with ADHD.

The emerging neuroimaging literature points to abnormalities in frontal networks in ADHD (frontostriatal dysfunction), and it is these networks that control attention and intentional motor behavior.

Zametkin and Rapoport (1987) postulated that "inhibitory influences of frontal cortical activity, predominantly noradrenergic, (act) on lower (striatal) structures that are driven by…dopamine agonists." The frontosubcortical pathways are rich in catecholamines. In addition, catecholamines are implicated in ADHD because of the mechanism of action of stimulants. Notably, in both childhood and adulthood, ADHD symptoms respond favorably to drugs that block either the dopamine transporter or the norepinephrine transporter. Yet, human studies of the catecholamine hypothesis of ADHD have produced conflicting results, perhaps due to the insensitivity of peripheral measures.

Data from family genetic, twin, and adoption studies as well as segregation analysis suggest a genetic origin for some forms of the disorder (Biederman et al. 1992). Although the results are still tentative, molecular genetic studies suggest that some genes may increase the susceptibility to ADHD: the D_4 dopamine receptor gene, the dopamine transporter gene, and the D_2 dopamine receptor gene (Faraone 2000). Increasingly, there has been recognition that ADHD is highly heterogeneous with high levels of psychiatric, cognitive, and social disability comorbidity.

Psychopharmacology

Stimulant Treatments

Stimulant drugs are the first class of compounds reported as effective in the treatment of the behavioral disturbances that are evident in children with ADHD. Stimulants are sympathomimetic drugs structurally similar to endogenous catecholamines. The most commonly used compounds in this class include methylphenidate (Ritalin and others), d-methylphenidate (Focalin), d-amphetamine (Dexedrine), and a mixed amphetamine product (Adderall). These drugs have been shown to enhance dopaminergic and noradrenergic neurotransmission in the central nervous system and peripherally (Volkow et al. 2001). Since the various stimulants have somewhat different mechanisms of action, some patients may respond preferentially to one or another (Greenhill et al. 1998).

Stimulant Dosing

The usual daily dose range is 0.3–2 mg/kg/day for methylphenidate and approximately half of that for dextromethylphenidate and amphetamine compounds since they are roughly twice as potent as methylphenidate (Table 46–1). Due to their short half-life, the short-acting, immediate-release stimulants (methylphenidate and dextroamphetamine) are given in divided doses throughout the day, typically 4 hours apart. The starting dose is generally 2.5–5 mg/day, given in the morning, with the dose being increased if necessary every few days by 2.5–5 mg in a divided dose schedule. Due to the anorexogenic effects of the stimulants, it may be beneficial to administer the medicine after meals. Mixed amphetamine salts can last up to 6 hours; thus, for full coverage they are typically given twice daily (such as 8:00 A.M. and 2:00 P.M.) in dosages of 1–1.5 mg/kg/day. Typically, stimulants have a rapid onset of action so that clinical response will be evident when a therapeutic dose has been obtained.

Stimulant Efficacy

An extensive literature has clearly documented the short-term efficacy of methylphenidate treatment, mostly in latency-age white boys (Spencer et al. 1997). A much more limited literature exists for stimulants at other ages, for females, and for ethnic minorities. Despite small numbers, the few studies of stimulants in adolescents reported rates of response highly consis-

TABLE 46–1. Stimulants

Medication	Daily dose, mg/kg	Daily dosage schedule
Dextroamphetamine (Dexedrine)	0.3–1.0	Two or three times
Mixed salts of levoamphetamine and dextroamphetamine (Adderall)	0.5–1.5	Once or twice
Methylphenidate (Ritalin, Methylin, others)	1.0–2.0	Two or three times
Dexmethylphenidate (Focalin)	0.5–1.0	Once or twice

Note. Doses are general guidelines. All doses must be individualized with appropriate monitoring. Weight-corrected doses are less appropriate for obese children. FDA-approved total daily dosages: methylphenidate, 60 mg; dexmethylphenidate, 20 mg; mixed amphetamine salts, 30 mg.

tent with those seen in latency-age children. In contrast, the few studies on preschoolers appear to indicate that young children respond less well to stimulant therapy, suggesting that in preschoolers ADHD may be more treatment refractory.

A large multicenter controlled trial (the Preschool ADHD Treatment Study [PATS]) investigated the efficacy and safety of immediate-release methylphenidate (MPH-IR), given tid to children ages 3–5.5 years with ADHD (Greenhill et al. 2006a). The 8-phase, 70-week PATS protocol included two double-blind, controlled phases and a crossover titration trial followed by a placebo-controlled parallel trial. Of 303 preschoolers enrolled, 165 were randomly assigned the titration trial. Compared with placebo, significant decreases in ADHD symptoms were found on MPH-IR at 2.5 mg ($P<0.01$), 5 mg ($P<0.001$), and 7.5 mg ($P<0.001$) tid doses, but not for 1.25 mg ($P<0.06$) doses. The mean optimal MPH-IR total daily dosage for the entire group was 14.2±8.1 mg/day (0.7±4 mg/kg/day). For the preschoolers later randomly assigned to the parallel phase ($n=114$), only 21% on best-dose MPH-IR and 13% on placebo achieved the categorical criterion for remission (as defined by the Multimodal Treatment Study of Children With ADHD [MTA]) for school-age children with ADHD. Thirty percent of parents spontaneously reported moderate to severe adverse events in all study phases after baseline (Wigal et al. 2006). These included emotional outbursts, difficulty falling asleep, repetitive behaviors/thoughts, appetite decrease, and irritability. During maintenance treatment, trouble sleeping and appetite loss persisted and other MPH-related adverse events decreased. There were transient one-time pulse and blood pressure elevations in five children. Twenty-one children (11%) discontinued treatment because of drug-attributed adverse events. Of the serious adverse events reported, only one was possibly related to MPH.

The literature clearly documents that treatment with stimulants improves not only abnormal behaviors of ADHD but also self-esteem and cognitive, social, and family function, thus supporting the importance of treating patients with ADHD beyond school or work hours to include evenings, weekends, and vacations. Controlled clinical trials have documented the efficacy of methylphenidate and amphetamine in adults with ADHD (Spencer et al. 1995; Wilens et al. 1999a).

Treatment with stimulants improves a wide variety of cognitive abilities (Barkley 1977; Gittelman-Klein 1987; Rapport et al. 1988), increases school-based productivity (Famularo and Fenton 1987), and improves performance in academic testing (Scheffler et al. 2009).

However, despite these beneficial cognitive effects, it is important to be aware that patients with ADHD can manifest additional learning disabilities that are not responsive to pharmacotherapy (Bergman et al. 1991) but may respond to educational remediation.

The early concern that optimal clinical efficacy is attained at the cost of impaired learning ability has not been confirmed (Gittelman-Klein 1987). In fact, the majority of studies indicate that both behavior and cognitive performance improve with stimulant treatment in a dose-dependent fashion (Barr et al. 1999; Douglas et al. 1988; Gittelman-Klein 1987; Kupietz et al. 1988; Pelham et al. 1985; Rapport et al. 1987, 1989). The literature on the association between clinical benefits in ADHD and plasma levels of stimulants has been equivocal and complicated by large inter- and intraindividual variability in plasma levels at constant oral doses (Gittelman-Klein 1987).

Stimulant Side Effects and Risks

The U.S. Food and Drug Administration (FDA) recently reviewed the prescribing information on stimulants in an effort to clarify risks and benefits. After this careful review, the only black box warning for stimulants concerns their abuse potential. While misuse for treating fatigue can be accomplished by oral administration, abuse for euphoria typically requires insufflation, and thus there is greater risk in immediate-release formulations that can be crushed. Despite the concern that ADHD may increase the risk of drug abuse in adolescents and young adults (or their associates), to date there is no clear evidence that stimulant-treated youth with ADHD abuse prescribed medication when they are appropriately diagnosed and carefully monitored. Moreover, the most commonly abused substance in adolescents and adults with ADHD is marijuana and not stimulants (Biederman et al. 1995b). Furthermore, there is naturalistic evidence that the use of stimulants and other pharmacological treatments for ADHD is associated with significantly decreased risk for subsequent substance use disorders in youth with ADHD (Biederman et al. 1999).

The most commonly reported side effects associated with the administration of stimulant medication are appetite suppression and sleep disturbances. Delay of sleep onset is commonly reported and usually accompanies late afternoon or early evening administration of the stimulant medications. Preexisting sleep disturbance is common, due to oppositional defiant disorder (ODD), separation anxiety, environmental overstimulation, and so forth. Less commonly reported are mood disturbances ranging from increased tearfulness and social withdrawal to a full-blown major depression–like syndrome (Wilens and Biederman 1992). Other fairly common side effects include headaches and abdominal discomfort, and more rarely, increased lethargy and fatigue.

Regarding adverse cardiovascular effects of stimulants, studies have consistently documented mild increases in pulse and blood pressure of unclear clinical significance (Brown et al. 1984). Recent concerns about cardiovascular safety led to the temporary removal of Adderall-XR from the Canadian market. The FDA issued the following statement:

> The Canadian action was based on U.S. postmarketing reports of sudden deaths in pediatric patients.... When one considers the rate of sudden death in pediatric patients treated with Adderall products based on the approximately 30 million prescriptions written between 1999 and 2003 (the period of time in which these deaths occurred), it does not appear that the number of deaths reported is greater than the number of sudden deaths that would be expected to occur in this population without treatment. For this reason, the FDA has not decided to take any further regulatory action at this time. (www.fda.gov/cder/drug/advisory/adderall.htm)

However, because it appeared that patients with underlying heart defects might be at increased risk for sudden death, the labeling for all stimulants was changed to include a warning that these patients might be at particular risk and that these patients should ordinarily not be treated with stimulants. While at this time there is limited concern about the general cardiovascular safety of psychostimulants, the American Heart Association (AHA) issued guidelines stating that caution should be used in the treatment of patients presenting with a family history of early cardiac death or arrhythmias or a personal history of structural abnormalities, chest pain, palpitations, shortness of breath, or fainting episodes of unclear etiology, especially during exercise or during treatment with stimulants (Gutgesell et al. 1999). Before initiating treatment, patients should have a careful history to assess for the presence of preexisting cardiac disease. In such cases, consultation with a cardiologist is recommended. Stimulant cardiovascular risk guidelines were recently reviewed by the AHA (Vetter et al. 2008). Recommendations were unchanged from the 1999 report except for a new recommendation for routine use of electrocardiograms (ECGs) in prescreening. A subsequent clarification was issued by the AHA:

> It is reasonable for a physician to consider obtaining an ECG as part of the evaluation of children being considered for stimulant drug therapy, but this should be at the physician's judgment, and it is not mandatory to obtain one. (http://circ.ahajournals.org/cgi/content/full/CIRCULATIONAHA.107.189473/DC1)

In addition, the American Academy of Pediatrics published a policy statement that an ECG is not routinely indicated prior to stimulant treatment in otherwise healthy youth (Perrin et al. 2008). Although less of an immediate clinical concern in pediatric care, blood pressure and pulse should be monitored with stimulant treatment and may be of greater clinical significance in the treatment of adults with ADHD.

Stimulant-associated toxic psychosis has been very rarely observed, usually in the context of either a rapid rise in the dose or very high doses. This reported psychosis in children resembles a toxic phenomenon (i.e., visual hallucinosis) and is dissimilar to the exacerbation of psychotic symptoms present in schizophrenia. The development of psychotic or manic symptoms in a child exposed to stimulants requires careful evaluation to rule out the presence of a preexisting psychotic or bipolar disorder. Aggressive behavior is often observed in children or adolescents with ADHD, and stimulants are often effective treatments for aggression in that context (Connor et al. 2002). However, all patients beginning treatment should be monitored for the appearance or worsening of aggressive behavior or hostility.

Early reports indicated that children with a personal or family history of tic disorders were at greater risk for developing a tic disorder when exposed to stimulants (Lowe et al. 1982). However, more recent work has increasingly challenged this view. In a controlled study of 34 children with ADHD and tics, Gadow et al. (1995) reported that methylphenidate effectively suppressed ADHD symptoms with only a weak effect on the frequency of tics. In addition, in a study of 128 boys with ADHD, Spencer et al. (1999) reported no evidence of earlier onset, greater rates, or worsening of tics in the subgroup exposed to stimulants. Moreover, a multisite placebo-controlled trial of methylphenidate in children with ADHD found that the proportion of individual subjects reporting a worsening of tics as an adverse effect was no higher in those treated with MPH (20%) than those being administered placebo (22%) (Tourette's Syndrome Study Group 2002). Although this work is reassuring, clearly more information is needed in a larger number of subjects over longer periods of time to obtain closure on this issue. Until more is known, it seems prudent to weigh risks and benefits in individual cases with appropriate discussion with the child and family about the benefits and pitfalls of the use of stimulants in children with ADHD and tics.

Persistent concerns remain about the effects of stimulants on growth in children. To address this issue, Faraone et al. (2008) published a meta-analysis of growth effects in a large number of longitudinal stimulant studies. These studies provide strong evidence that for most patients, treatment with stimulant medication into adolescence leads to, at worst, modest delays in growth. Weight deficits were greater than height deficits, and the two were only modestly associated with one another. This effect is greatest for taller and heavier children and is greater for children compared with adolescents. The studies reviewed suggest these deficits attenuate over time, even with continued treatment, and do not differ between methylphenidate and amphetamine or between long- and short-acting formulations. Some studies suggest that ADHD itself, and not its treatment, is associated with dysregulation of growth and that final adult height is not affected (Klein and Mannuzza 1988; Spencer et al. 1998b). Thus, although treatment with stimulants can lead to some reductions in expected growth velocity in height and weight, these reductions are, on average, small, attenuate with time, and do not cause a greater proportion of children to become extremely short or thin.

While growth does need to be monitored in children treated with stimulants, the data on growth would not support the routine practice of "drug holidays" in ADHD children. However, it seems prudent in children suspected of stimulant-associated growth deficits to provide them with unmedicated periods or alternative treatment. This recommendation should be carefully weighed against the risk for exacerbation of symptoms due to drug discontinuation. In some children, transient behavioral deterioration can occur upon the abrupt discontinuation of stimulant medications. The prevalence of this phenomenon and the etiology are unclear. Rebound phenomena can occur in some children between doses or following the final dose of the day, creating an uneven, often disturbing clinical course. In those cases, consideration should be given to alternative or supplementary treatments.

New-Generation Stimulants

Stimulant stereo-enantiomers.
Methylphenidate has four optical isomers: d-threo, l-threo, d-erythro, and l-erythro. There is stereoselectivity in receptor site binding and its relationship

to response. The standard preparation is comprised of the threo, d, l racemate. Recent data suggest that the d-methylphenidate isomer is the active form. In a positron emission tomography (PET) study, d-threo-methylphenidate was found to bind specifically to the basal ganglia, rich in dopamine transporter receptors, whereas l-threo-methylphenidate was widely distributed with only nonspecific binding (Ding et al. 1995). This has led to the development of a purified d, threo-methylphenidate compound, Focalin. Studies have documented similar pharmacokinetic profiles of d-threo-methylphenidate and d, l-threo-methylphenidate when given in equimolar doses. Thus the time to maximum concentration (T_{max}), the maximum concentration of d-threo-methylphenidate (C_{max}), and the half-life were the same between d and d, l-threo-methylphenidate.

The efficacy of Focalin was established in two controlled studies. In the first trial, 132 children and adolescents were randomly assigned to receive d-threo-methylphenidate; d, l-threo-methylphenidate; or placebo at 8:00 A.M. and noon for 4 weeks. At week 4, teacher ratings on the Swanson, Nolan, and Pelham Rating Scale (SNAP) revealed robust improvement in both active treatments. The average improvement from baseline was equivalent to one standard deviation on the SNAP, a magnitude of change that is clinically important. Parent ratings on the SNAP revealed superiority of both treatments to placebo 3 hours after dosing, but superiority of only d-methylphenidate and not d, l-methylphenidate 6 hours after dosing (Wigal et al. 2004). In a second controlled study, investigators tested the specificity of response to d-threo-methylphenidate (Arnold et al. 2004). Patients were treated openly with d-threo-methylphenidate (*N*=116) to determine the optimal dose. At the end of 6 weeks, 75 responders were randomly assigned to blinded treatment with d-threo-methylphenidate or placebo over 2 weeks. Subjects randomly assigned to placebo had a high rate (62%) of relapse compared to those who continued on d-threo-methylphenidate (17%). In addition, the parent SNAP ratings indicated persistent effect of d-threo-methylphenidate 6 hours after dosing. In both studies, adverse effects of d-threo-methylphenidate were consistent with those of d, l-threo-methylphenidate. These studies have shown Focalin to be as effective as the racemate at half the dosage. Focalin is available in 2.5, 5, and 10 mg to approximate 5, 10, and 20 mg of d, l-methylphenidate.

Long-acting stimulant formulations.
A new generation of highly sophisticated, well-developed, safe and effective, long-acting preparations of

stimulant drugs has reached the market and revolutionized the treatment of ADHD (Table 46–2). These compounds employ novel delivery systems to overcome acute tolerance termed *tachyphylaxis* and allow a reduced number of doses per day. In a number of these medications, an analogue classroom paradigm was used to test the fine-grained pharmacodynamic and pharmacokinetic profiles of these medications. Developed by Swanson and colleagues, these settings simulate real-life demands and distractions of a typical classroom (Swanson et al. 2000). Hour-by-hour ratings are made by trained observers recording frequency counts of behaviors as well as academic production and accuracy. Sequential serum sampling (using venous catheters) allows correlation of blood levels to behavioral activity.

The first of these medications developed was Concerta, which uses an osmotic pump mechanism to create an ascending level of methylphenidate in the blood. This provides effective extended treatment that approximates tid dosing of MPH-IR. Concerta is available in 18, 27, 36, and 54 mg to approximate 5, 7.5, 10, and 15 mg tid dosing of MPH-IR. A laboratory classroom study of 68 children found that a single morning dose of Concerta was effective for 12 hours on social and on-task behaviors, as well as academic performance (Pelham et al. 2001).

A large multicenter randomized clinical trial was used to determine the safety and efficacy of Concerta in an outpatient setting (Wolraich et al. 2001). Children with ADHD (ages 6–12 years; $N=282$) were randomly assigned to placebo, MPH-IR tid, or Concerta once a day in a double-blind, 28-day trial. Children in the Concerta and MPH-IR groups showed significantly greater reductions in core ADHD symptoms than did children on placebo throughout the study. Concerta was well tolerated, with mild appetite suppression but no sleep abnormalities.

Metadate CD is a capsule with a mixture of immediate- and delayed-release beads containing methylphenidate, 30% of which are immediate release and 70% delayed. It is designed to provide effective treatment for 6–8 hours. The efficacy and safety of Metadate CD were tested in a multicenter randomized, double-blind, placebo-controlled trial conducted at 32 sites on 316 children with ADHD. There was a 1-week single-blind, placebo run-in, followed by a 3-week double-blind titration and treatment period. Improve-

TABLE 46–2. Long-acting stimulants

Medication	Daily dose, mg/kg	Daily dosage schedule	Duration of behavioral effect	Comments
Methylphenidate	1.0–2.0	Once or twice		
Concerta			10–12 hours	Ascending profile, OROS technology Capsules with immediate-release (IR) and delayed-release (DR) beads
Ritalin LA			8–9 hours	50:50 ratio (IR:DR)
Metadate CD			6–8 hours	30:70 ratio (IR:DR)
Focalin XR			10–12 hours	50:50 ratio (IR:DR)
Daytrana			12 hours with 9-hour wear-time	Patch with variable wear-time
Mixed salts of levoamphetamine and dextroamphetamine (Adderall XR)	0.5–1.5	Once or twice	10–12 hours	Capsule with IR and DR beads 50:50 ratio (IR:DR)
Lisdexamfetamine (Vyvanse)	0.5–1.5	Once	12 hours	Prodrug; continuous conversion of nonactive prodrug to active d-amphetamine

Note. Doses are general guidelines. All doses must be individualized with appropriate monitoring. Weight-corrected doses are less appropriate for obese children. FDA-approved total daily dosages: methylphenidate, 60 mg; OROS, 72 mg; dexmethylphenidate, 20 mg; amphetamine salts, 30 mg; lisdexamfetamine, 70 mg.

ment with treatment versus placebo was equally good morning and afternoon as rated by teachers on the Conners' Global Index. The medication was well tolerated, with relatively low rates of decreased appetite (9.7% vs. 2.5%) and insomnia (7.1% vs. 2.5%) in active treatment versus placebo. Metadate CD is available in 10, 20, 30, 40, 50, and 60 mg capsules (Greenhill et al. 2002). The bioavailability and tolerability of Metadate CD are not altered when the capsule is opened and the beads are sprinkled on food (Pentikis et al. 2002). This is useful for children who do not swallow capsules.

Ritalin LA has been developed to provide effective methylphenidate treatment for 8–9 hours. It uses a bi-modal release system that produces pharmacokinetic characteristics that in single-dose administration, re-semble those of two doses of Ritalin tablets adminis-tered 4–5 hours apart. Ritalin LA consists of a mixture of immediate- and delayed-release beads in a 50:50 ratio. The delayed-release beads are coated with an absorption-delaying polymer. Ritalin LA is available in 10, 20, 30, and 40 mg capsules to approximate 10, 15, and 20 mg bid dosing of MPH-IR. Ritalin LA may be used as a sprinkle preparation for children unable to swallow pills. An analogue classroom study evaluated the pharmacodynamic (efficacy) profile, safety, and tolerability of Ritalin LA (Spencer et al. 2000). One-time administration of Ritalin LA was effective rela-tive to placebo in improving classroom behavior and academic productivity over the subsequent 9-hour pe-riod. Ritalin LA had a rapid onset of effect, and the im-provement relative to placebo was statistically signifi-cant during both the morning (0–4 hours after dosing) and the afternoon (4–9 hours after dosing).

Ritalin LA was further tested in a multicenter double-blind trial of 160 children (Biederman et al. 2003). There was an initial 2–4 week titration to optimal dose followed by a 1-week placebo washout period. Subjects with persistent ADHD symptoms during the washout (*n*=137) were randomly assigned to Ritalin LA or placebo. Children on Ritalin LA were rated as greatly improved over placebo by teachers and parents on the Conners' ADHD/DSM-IV Scale (CADS). Improvements were equally robust in the subscales of inattention and hyperactivity. Significant drug-specific improvement was also noted by clinicians on the Clinical Global Impressions Scale—Improvement (CGI-I). Ritalin LA was well tolerated with minimal side effects. Rates of mild appetite suppression and mild insomnia were both low (3.1%).

Adderall XR is a capsule with a 50:50 ratio of immediate- to delayed-release beads designed to release drug content in a time course similar to that of Adder-

all given bid (0 and 4 hours). Adderall XR is available in 5, 10, 15, 20, 25, and 30 mg capsules. An analogue classroom study compared various doses of Adderall XR to Adderall bid and placebo (McCracken et al. 2003). Behavioral and academic improvement were documented to 12 hours postdose. The efficacy and safety of Adderall XR were further tested in a multi-center randomized, double-blind, placebo-controlled trial conducted at 47 sites (Biederman et al. 2002). Children with ADHD (*N*=584) were randomly assigned to receive single daily morning doses of placebo or Adderall XR 10 mg, 20 mg, or 30 mg for 3 weeks. Continuous significant improvement in morning and afternoon assessments was found by teachers and in morning, afternoon, and late afternoon assessments by parents on the Conners' Global Index Scale for Teachers and Parents. All active treatment groups showed significant dose-related improvement in behavior from baseline. The medication was well tolerated with rates of adverse events similar for active treatments and placebo. A 1-year follow-up of 411 children on Adderall XR examined long-term safety and efficacy (McGough et al. 2005). Efficacy was maintained for 12 months as measured by the Conners' Global Index Scale. The medication was safe and well tolerated with a low frequency of mild adverse events and no evidence of untoward cardiovascular effects.

A new extended-release dosage form of Focalin (Focalin XR) has been developed to provide effective methylphenidate treatment for 10 to 12 hours. Focalin XR uses the same bimodal release system as Ritalin LA, producing pharmacokinetic characteristics that in single-dose administration resemble those of two doses of Focalin tablets administered 4–5 hours apart. Similarly, Focalin XR consists of a mixture of immediate- and delayed-release beads in a 50:50 ratio. The delayed-release beads are coated with an absorption-delaying polymer. Focalin XR is available in 5, 10, and 20 mg capsules. Focalin XR was found to be effective in children, adolescents, and adults and is FDA approved for all three age groups.

Focalin XR was tested in a multicenter random-ized, double-blind, study of 103 patients ages 6–17 years (Greenhill et al. 2006b). They were flexibly dosed to receive 5–30 mg capsules or placebo once daily for 7 weeks. Doses were titrated to optimal levels during the first 5 weeks and maintained for the final 2 weeks. Efficacy was evaluated weekly at school and at home using the CADS. Drug-specific improvement was doc-umented on each scale. At final visit, 67.3% of patients receiving Focalin XR and 13.3% receiving placebo were "very much improved" or "much improved" on the CGI-I (*P*<. 001) scale. Focalin XR was well tolerated, with adverse event rates similar to those reported with immediate-release dexmethylphenidate.

A transdermal delivery system for methylphenidate has been developed (methylphenidate transdermal system—MTS). Methylphenidate is contained within a multipolymeric adhesive layer attached to a transparent backing. Patches are applied once daily and deliver a consistent amount of methylphenidate during the time the patch is worn. The drug does not go through first-pass metabolism in the liver; therefore, more methylphenidate is bioavailable. Transdermal delivery of methylphenidate might represent a useful treatment option for patients who have difficulty swallowing or tolerating oral formulations (e.g., nausea) or for patients who need flexible duration of medication effect. An initial randomized, double-blind study of MTS (Pelham et al. 2005b) was conducted in a summer treatment program that demonstrated significant improvement on measures of social behavior in recreational settings, classroom functioning, and parent ratings of evening behavior. However, patch wear-times of at least 12 hours resulted in insomnia for many of the participants. Ensuing trials (Pelham et al. 2005a) used MTS with a wear-time of 9 hours. A classroom analogue study (McGough et al. 2006) demonstrated effectiveness over 12 hours for a wear-time of 9 hours.

A large 5-week randomized, double-blind multicenter study of MTS and OROS methylphenidate was conducted in children ages 6–12 years diagnosed with ADHD (*n*=282; Findling et al. 2008). Treatment with MTS was effective at reducing the symptoms of ADHD as assessed by clinicians, teachers, and parents and was generally well tolerated. Skin redness or itching at the application site is common and does not necessitate discontinuation. More severe rashes, as indicated by swelling, bumps, or blisters around the application site, may indicate a skin allergy to MTS and may necessitate discontinuation. Due to differences in bioavailability, a 10 mg MTS patch is approximately equivalent to 5 mg of MPH-IR tid, and 20 mg MTS to about 10 mg MPH-IR. MTS is available in dose strengths of 10, 15, 20, and 30 mg.

Lisdexamfetamine dimesylate (LDX) is a novel prodrug in which *d*-amphetamine is covalently bound to the amino acid L-lysine. This chemical bond renders the amphetamine component therapeutically inactive. Following oral administration, LDX is converted in the body to the active *d*-amphetamine after enzymatic hydrolysis in a rate-limited manner, at or following absorption. The saturable rate-limited hydrolysis releases active amphetamine slowly, creating predictable long-acting delivery of active drug (d-amphetamine). Saturation of enzymatic hydrolysis at supratherapeutic doses suggests that LDX may be associated with diminished risk for abuse and toxicity. LDX dose strengths of 30 mg, 50 mg, and 70 mg were developed to provide an amphetamine base approximately equivalent to mixed amphetamine salts—10 mg, 20 mg, and 30 mg, respectively. While adequately powered comparison studies have not been done, in a classroom analogue study, these doses of LDX were at least as effective and long-lasting as the comparable mixed amphetamine salts doses (Biederman et al. 2007a). In a large 4-week double-blind study of children (ages 6–12) with ADHD (*N*=290), single daily dosages of LDX (30 mg, 50 mg, or 70 mg) were effective and well tolerated (Biederman et al. 2007b). Improvements were observed throughout the day up to 6:00 P.M. The tolerability profile was similar to currently marketed extended-release stimulants. LDX is available in 20, 30, 40, 50, 60, and 70 mg.

Specific Norepinephrine Reuptake Inhibitors

Atomoxetine is one of a new class of compounds, known as specific norepinephrine reuptake inhibitors (Table 46–3). Initial encouraging results in an adult trial (Spencer et al. 1998a), coupled with extensive safety data, fueled efforts in developing this compound in the treatment of pediatric ADHD. An open-label dose-ranging study of this compound in pediatric ADHD documented strong clinical benefits with excellent tolerability, including a safe cardiovascular profile, and provided dosing guidelines for further controlled studies (Spencer et al. 2001).

Atomoxetine Efficacy

Further controlled trials have led to FDA approval of atomoxetine for children and adults with ADHD. In the first pediatric controlled studies, 291 children ages 7–13 with ADHD were randomly assigned in two trials (combined: atomoxetine, *n*=129; placebo, *n*=124; and methylphenidate, *n*=38) (Spencer et al. 2002b). The acute treatment period was 9 weeks. The stimulant-naive stratum patients were randomly assigned to double-blind treatment with atomoxetine, placebo, or methylphenidate. Stimulant-prior-exposure stratum (prior exposure to any stimulant) patients were randomly assigned to double-blind treatment with atomoxetine or placebo. Atomoxetine significantly re-

TABLE 46–3. Specific noradrenergic reuptake inhibitor

Medication	Daily dose, mg/kg/day	Daily dosage schedule	Main indications	Common adverse effects/Comments
Atomoxetine (Strattera)	0.5–1.4	Once or twice	ADHD ADHD+ Enuresis TIC ANX	Mechanism of action: noradrenergic-specific reuptake inhibitor Mild/moderate appetite decrease Gastrointestinal symptoms Mild initial weight loss Cardiovascular effects (mild increase in blood pressure, pulse) No ECG conduction or repolarization delays Not abusable Rare serious hepatotoxicity Uncommon increase in suicidal thoughts

Note. Doses are general guidelines. All doses must be individualized with appropriate monitoring. Weight-corrected doses are less appropriate for obese children. When high doses are used, serum levels may be obtained in order to avoid toxicity. FDA-approved total daily dose: 1.4 mg/kg ($\leq$100 mg).
ADHD=attention-deficit/hyperactivity disorder; ANX=anxiety disorders; ECG=electrocardiogram; TIC=tic disorder.

duced total scores on an investigator-rated DSM-IV ADHD rating scale. The definition of response was a $\geq$25% decrease in the ADHD rating scale, and the response rates were greater on atomoxetine than placebo (61.4% vs. 32.3%, respectively; $P<.05$). In the stimulant-naive stratum, 69.1% of atomoxetine patients, 73% of methylphenidate patients, and 31.4% of placebo patients were considered responders.

In an additional controlled study, 297 children and adolescents were randomly assigned to different doses of atomoxetine or placebo for 8 weeks (Michelson et al. 2001). Atomoxetine was associated with a graded dose response. Response was best at 1.2 or 1.8 mg/kg/day and superior to 0.5 mg/kg/day, which was superior to placebo. In close parallel was found a dose-dependent enhancement of social and family function. The Child Health Questionnaire was used to assess the well-being of the child and family. Parents of children on atomoxetine reported less emotional difficulties and behavioral problems as well as greater self-esteem in their children and less emotional worry and less limitation in their own personal time.

Atomoxetine Side Effects and Risks

Atomoxetine was well tolerated in pediatric studies (Spencer et al. 2002b). Mild appetite suppression was reported in 22% on atomoxetine versus 32% on methylphenidate and 7% on placebo. Compared to methylphenidate, there was less insomnia on atomoxetine (7.0% vs. 27.0%; $P<.05$). Mild increases in diastolic blood pressure and heart rate were noted in the atom-

oxetine treatment group with no significant differences between atomoxetine and placebo in laboratory parameters and ECG intervals.

A year-long open follow-up of atomoxetine-treated children and adolescents (N=325) found that atomoxetine treatment continued to be effective and well tolerated. The acute mild increases in diastolic blood pressure and heart rate persisted without worsening. Growth in height and weight was normal, and there were no significant differences between atomoxetine and placebo in laboratory parameters or ECG intervals (Kratochvil et al. 2001; Spencer et al. 2005).

Two cases of severe liver injury were reported in a denominator of greater than 3 million patients who have taken atomoxetine since approval. Both patients have recovered with normal liver function after discontinuing the medication. While this was rare and both cases recovered, severe drug-related liver injury might progress to acute liver failure resulting in death or the need for a liver transplant. Eli Lilly added a bolded warning to the product label for atomoxetine (www.lilly.com), which indicates that the medication should be discontinued in patients with jaundice (yellowing of the skin or whites of the eyes) or laboratory evidence of liver injury. Patients on atomoxetine are cautioned to contact their doctor immediately if they develop pruritus, jaundice, dark urine, upper right-sided abdominal tenderness, or unexplained "flu-like" symptoms. It will be important to remain current on any new information on this risk.

There is now a boxed warning for the increased risk of suicidal ideation with atomoxetine use in children and adolescents. Pooled analyses of short-term (6–18 weeks) placebo-controlled trials of atomoxetine in children and adolescents (a total of 12 trials involving over 2,200 patients, including 11 trials in ADHD and 1 trial in enuresis) revealed a greater risk of suicidal ideation early during treatment in those receiving atomoxetine compared to placebo. The average risk of suicidal ideation in patients receiving atomoxetine was 0.4% (5/1,357 patients), compared to none in placebo-treated patients (851 patients). No suicides occurred in these trials.

Atomoxetine Dosing

Current dosing guidelines recommend that atomoxetine be initiated at 0.5 mg/kg/day for 2 weeks and increased to a target dosage of 1.2 mg/kg/day with a recommended maximum dosage of 1.4 mg/kg/day or 100 mg/day. While higher doses are not FDA approved, clinicians familiar with the medication have reported further improvement at dosages up to 1.8 mg/kg/day, a dosage maximum reported in both the juvenile and adolescent studies. While atomoxetine is effective at once-a-day dosing, twice-a-day dosing can provide a better tolerability profile and potentially a more robust effect later in the day. Since atomoxetine is metabolized by the hepatic 2D6 enzymatic system, care should be taken with coadministration with medications that inhibit 2D6 (e.g., fluoxetine, paroxetine). In addition, atomoxetine has been shown to have low abuse potential (Heil et al. 2002).

Nonstimulants

While there is no doubt that the stimulants are effective in the treatment of ADHD, it is estimated that at least 30% of affected individuals do not adequately respond to or cannot tolerate stimulant medication (Barkley 1977; Gittelman 1980; Spencer et al. 1996). In addition, immediate-release stimulants are short-acting drugs that require multiple administrations during the day, with their attendant impact on compliance and need to take treatment during school or work hours. Although the problem of multiple doses may be offset by the use of long-acting stimulants, this class of drugs may adversely affect sleep, making use in the evening hours difficult when symptom control is still needed. The fact that stimulants are controlled substances continues to fuel worries in children, families, and the treating community that inhibit their use. These fears are based on lingering concerns about the abuse potential of stimulant drugs by the child, family

member, or associates; the possibility of diversion; and safety concerns regarding the use of a controlled substance by patients who are impulsive and may have antisocial tendencies (Goldman et al. 1998). Similarly, the controlled nature of stimulant drugs poses medicolegal concerns to the treating community that further increase the barriers to treatment.

Antidepressants

Of nonstimulants, noradrenergic and dopaminergic compounds, including monoamine oxidase inhibitors (MAOIs) (Zametkin et al. 1985), secondary amine tricyclic antidepressants (TCAs) (Biederman et al. 1989; Donnelly et al. 1986; Wilens et al. 1993), and bupropion (Barrickman et al. 1995; Casat et al. 1989; Conners et al. 1996), have been found to be superior to placebo in controlled clinical trials. Possible advantages of these compounds over stimulants include a longer duration of action without symptom rebound or insomnia, the option of monitoring plasma drug levels, and minimal risk of abuse or dependence as well as the potential treatment of comorbid internalizing symptoms and tics (Table 46–4).

Tricyclic antidepressants.

Efficacy. Historically, the first nonstimulant treatments for ADHD that were extensively evaluated were the TCAs. Out of 33 studies (21 controlled, 12 open) evaluating TCAs in children and adolescents ($N=1,139$) and adults ($N=78$), 91% reported positive effects on ADHD symptoms (Spencer et al. 1997). Imipramine and desipramine are the most studied TCAs, followed by a handful of studies on other TCAs.

In the largest controlled study of a TCA in children, our group reported favorable results with desipramine in 62 clinically referred ADHD children, most of whom had previously failed to respond to psychostimulant treatment (Biederman et al. 1989). The study was a randomized, placebo-controlled, parallel-design, 6-week clinical trial. Clinically and statistically significant differences in behavioral improvement were found for desipramine over placebo, at an average daily dosage of 5 mg/kg. Although the presence of comorbidity increased the likelihood of a placebo response, neither comorbidity with conduct disorder, depression, or anxiety nor a family history of ADHD yielded differential responses to desipramine treatment. In addition, desipramine-treated ADHD patients showed a substantial reduction in depressive symptoms compared with placebo-treated patients.

In a prospective placebo-controlled discontinuation trial, we demonstrated the efficacy of nortriptyline in dosages of up to 2 mg/kg daily in 35 school-age youth with ADHD (Prince et al. 2000). ADHD youth receiving nortriptyline also were found to have more modest but statistically significant reductions in oppositionality and anxiety. Nortriptyline was well tolerated, with some weight gain. Weight gain is frequently considered to be a desirable side effect in this population.

Studies of TCAs have consistently reported a robust rate of response in ADHD subjects with comorbid tic disorders (Dillon et al. 1985; Hoge and Biederman 1986; Riddle et al. 1988; Singer et al. 1994; Spencer et al. 1993a, 1993b). For example, in a controlled study, Spencer et al. (2002a) replicated data from a retrospective chart review indicating that desipramine had a beneficial effect on ADHD and tic symptoms.

The mechanism of action of the antidepressants appears to be due to various effects on pre- and postsynaptic receptors impacting the release and reuptake of brain neurotransmitters, including norepinephrine, serotonin, and dopamine. Although these agents have variable effects on various pre- and postsynaptic neurotransmitter systems, their effect and adverse effect profiles differ greatly among the various classes of antidepressant drugs. Since a substantial interindividual variability in metabolism and elimination has been demonstrated in children, dose should always be individualized.

Dosing. The TCAs include the tertiary (imipramine and amitriptyline) and the secondary (desipramine and nortriptyline) amine compounds. Treatment with a TCA should be initiated with a 10 mg or 25 mg dose and increased slowly every 4–5 days by 20%–30%. When a daily dosage of 3 mg/kg (or a lower effective dose) or 1.5 mg/kg for nortriptyline is reached, steady-state serum levels and an ECG should be obtained. Typical dose ranges for the TCAs are 2.0–5.0 mg/kg (1.0–3.0 mg/kg for nortriptyline).

Side effects and risks. Common short-term adverse effects of the TCAs include anticholinergic effects, such as dry mouth, blurred vision, and constipation. However, there are no known deleterious effects associated with chronic administration of these drugs. Gastrointestinal symptoms and vomiting may occur when these drugs are discontinued abruptly; thus, slow tapering of these medications is recommended. Since the anticholinergic effects of TCAs limit salivary flow, they may promote tooth decay.

Evaluations of short- and long-term effects of therapeutic doses of TCAs on the cardiovascular system in children have found TCAs to be generally well tolerated with only minor ECG changes associated with

TCA treatment in daily oral dosages as high as 5 mg/kg. TCA-induced ECG abnormalities (conduction defects) have been consistently reported in children at doses higher than 3.5 mg/kg (Biederman et al. 1989) (1.0 mg/kg for nortriptyline). Although of unclear hemodynamic significance, the development of conduction defects in children receiving TCA treatment merits closer ECG and clinical monitoring, especially when relatively high doses of these medicines are used. In the context of cardiac disease, conduction defects may have potentially more serious clinical implications. When in doubt about the cardiovascular state of the patient, a more comprehensive cardiac evaluation is suggested, including 24-hour ECG and cardiac consultation, before initiating treatment with a TCA to help determine the risk-benefit ratio of such an intervention.

Several case reports in the 1980s of sudden death in children being treated with desipramine raised concern about the potential cardiotoxic risk associated with TCAs in the pediatric population (Riddle et al. 1991). Despite uncertainty and imprecise data, an epidemiological evaluation of this issue (Biederman et al. 1995a) suggested that the risk of desipramine-associated sudden death may be slightly elevated but not much greater than the baseline risk of sudden death in children not on medication. Nevertheless, treatment with a TCA should be preceded by a baseline ECG, with serial ECGs at regular intervals throughout treatment. Because of the potential lethality of TCA overdose, parents should be advised to carefully store the medication in a place inaccessible to the children or their siblings.

Bupropion.

Efficacy. Bupropion hydrochloride is a novel-structured antidepressant of the aminoketone class related to the phenylisopropylamines but pharmacologically distinct from known antidepressants. Although its specific site or mechanism of action remains unknown, bupropion seems to have an indirect mixed agonist effect on dopamine and norepinephrine neurotransmission. Bupropion has been shown to be effective for ADHD in children in a controlled multisite study ($N=72$) (Casat et al. 1987, 1989; Conners et al. 1996) and in a comparison with methylphenidate ($N=15$) (Barrickman et al. 1995). A double-blind, controlled clinical trial of bupropion in adults with ADHD documented superiority over placebo (Wilens et al. 1999c, 2005), with an effect size highly consistent with the pediatric trials.

Dosing, side effects, risks, and formulations. Bupropion is rapidly absorbed, with peak plasma levels usually achieved after 2 hours, with an average

TABLE 46–4. Antidepressants

Drug, generic/brand	Daily dose, mg/kg	Daily dosage schedule	Main indications	Common adverse effects/Comments
Tricyclic antidepressants (TCAs) *Tertiary amines* Imipramine (Tofranil) *Secondary amines* Desipramine (Norpramin) Nortriptyline (Aventyl, Pamelor)	2.0–5.0 (1.0–3.0 for nortriptyline) Dose adjusted according to serum levels (therapeutic window for nortriptyline)	Once or twice	ADHD ADHD+ Enuresis TIC ?ANX	Mixed mechanism of action (noradrenergic/serotonergic) Secondary amines more noradrenergic Clomipramine primarily serotonergic Narrow therapeutic index Overdoses can be fatal Anticholinergic effects (dry mouth, constipation, blurred vision) Weight loss Cardiovascular effects (mild increase in diastolic blood pressure and ECG conduction parameters with daily dosages >3.5 mg/kg) Treatment requires serum levels and ECG monitoring No known long-term side effects Withdrawal effects can occur (severe gastrointestinal symptoms, malaise) Risk of seizures
Monoamine oxidase inhibitors (MAOIs) Phenelzine (Nardil) Tranylcypromine (Parnate) Selegiline (Carbex, Eldepryl)	0.5–1.0 0.5–1.0 0.2–0.4	Two or three times	?ADHD	Difficult medicines to use in juveniles Reserved for refractory cases Severe dietary restrictions (high tyramine foods) Drug-drug interactions Hypertensive crisis with dietetic transgression or with certain drugs Weight gain Drowsiness Changes in blood pressure Insomnia Liver toxicity (remote)
Bupropion SR (Wellbutrin SR) Bupropion XR (Wellbutrin XR)	3–6 3–6	Twice Once	?ADHD ?ADHD+ ?DEP CESS ?CRV ?BP DEP	Mixed mechanism of action (dopaminergic/noradrenergic) Irritability Insomnia Drug-induced seizures (in doses >6 mg/kg) Contraindicated in bulimia patients

TABLE 46–4. Antidepressants *(continued)*

Drug, generic/brand	Daily dose, mg/kg	Daily dosage schedule	Main indications	Common adverse effects/ Comments
Venlafaxine XR (Effexor XR)	1–3	Once	?ADHD ?ADHD+ ?DEP ANX ?OCD	Mixed mechanism of action (serotonergic/noradrenergic) Similar to SSRIs Irritability Insomnia Gastrointestinal symptoms Headaches Potential withdrawal symptoms Blood pressure changes

Note. Doses are general guidelines. All doses must be individualized with appropriate monitoring. Weight-corrected doses are less appropriate for obese children. When high doses are used, serum levels may be obtained in order to avoid toxicity.
ADHD=attention-deficit/hyperactivity disorder; ANX=anxiety disorders; BP DEP=bipolar depression; CESS=smoking cessation; CRV=anticraving effects; DEP=depression; ECG=electrocardiogram; OCD=obsessive-compulsive disorder; SSRIs=selective serotonin reuptake inhibitors; TIC=tic disorder.

elimination half-life of 14 hours (8–24 hours). The usual dosage range is 4.0–6.0 mg/kg/day in divided doses. Side effects include irritability, anorexia, insomnia, and rarely, edema, rashes, and nocturia. Exacerbation of tic disorders also has been reported with bupropion. While bupropion has been associated with a slightly increased risk (0.4%) for drug-induced seizures relative to other antidepressants, this risk has been linked to high doses, a previous history of seizures, and eating disorders. Bupropion has been formulated into long-acting preparations (SR, XR) that can be administered twice daily.

Monoamine oxidase inhibitors: efficacy, dosing, side effects, and risks.

Although a small number of studies suggested that MAOIs may be effective in juvenile and adult ADHD, their potential for hypertensive crisis associated with dietetic transgressions and drug interactions seriously limits their use. The MAOIs include the hydrazines (phenelzine) and nonhydrazines (tranylcypromine) compounds. Daily doses should be carefully titrated based on response and adverse effects and range from 0.5 to 1.0 mg/kg. Short-term adverse effects include orthostatic hypotension, weight gain, drowsiness, and dizziness. However, major limitations for the use of MAOIs in children and adolescents are the severe dietetic restrictions of tyramine-containing foods (e.g., most cheeses), pressor amines (e.g., sympathomimetic substances), and severe drug interactions (e.g., most cold medicines, amphetamines), which can induce a hypertensive crisis and a serotonergic syndrome.

Venlafaxine: efficacy and side effects.

The usefulness of mixed serotonergic/noradrenergic atypical antidepressant venlafaxine in the treatment of ADHD is uncertain. While a 77% response rate was reported in completers in four open studies of ADHD adults (N=61 combined), 21% dropped out due to side effects (Adler et al. 1995; Findling et al. 1996; Hornig-Rohan and Amsterdam 1995; Reimherr et al. 1995). Additionally, a single open study of venlafaxine in 16 ADHD children reported a 50% response rate in completers with a 25% rate of dropout due to side effects, most prominently increased hyperactivity.

Selective serotonin reuptake inhibitors.

At present, expert opinion does not support the usefulness of selective serotonin reuptake inhibitors (SSRIs) in the treatment of core ADHD symptoms (National Institute of Mental Health 1996). Nevertheless, because of the high rates of comorbidity in ADHD, these compounds are frequently combined with effective anti-ADHD agents. Since many psychotropics are metabolized by the cytochrome P450 system (Nemeroff et al. 1996), which in turn can be inhibited by the SSRIs, caution should be exercised when combining agents, such as the TCAs with SSRIs.

Noradrenergic modulators: clonidine, guanfacine, guanfacine extended release.

See Chapter 50, "Alpha-Adrenergics, Beta-Blockers, Benzodiazepines, Buspirone, and Desmopressin," for discussion.

Beta-adrenergic agents: pindolol, nadolol.

Beta, noradrenergic blockers also have been studied for use in ADHD. In a controlled study of pindolol in 52 ADHD children, symptoms of behavioral dyscontrol and hyperactivity were improved with less apparent cognitive benefit. However, prominent adverse effects such as nightmares and paresthesias led to discontinuation of the drug in all test subjects. An open study of nadolol in aggressive developmentally delayed children with ADHD symptoms reported effective diminution of aggression with little apparent effect on ADHD symptoms (Connor et al. 1997).

Other Compounds

Modafinil.

Modafinil is an antinarcoleptic agent that is structurally and pharmacologically different from other agents approved to treat ADHD (Table 46–5). While the mechanism of action is unknown, it may improve symptoms of ADHD via the same mechanism by which it improves wakefulness. Preclinically, modafinil selectively activates the cortex without causing widespread central nervous system (CNS) stimulation (Engber et al. 1998). Modafinil does not appear to activate areas of the brain that mediate reward and abuse and has a low potential for abuse (Myrick et al. 2004).

Efficacy and dosing. While initial studies demonstrated significant improvement in ADHD symptoms, recent studies reported increased efficacy with higher dosages (340–425 mg/day) in children and adolescents (Swanson et al. 2006). A concentrated form of modafinil was developed to produce a small tablet that would ease administration of these doses in the pediatric population. A 9-week randomized, double-blind, placebo-controlled, flexible-dosage trial evaluated the efficacy and tolerability of this new formulation of modafinil in once-daily dosing (Biederman et al. 2005). Medication was titrated to an optimal dose based on efficacy and tolerability (range: 170–425 mg once daily). Patients ($N=246$) were treated with modafinil ($n=164$) or placebo ($n=82$). Significant improvements were observed with modafinil treatment on the ADHD-RS-IV School Version at week 1, with an effect size of 0.69 by final visit. At the final visit, 48% of modafinil-treated patients were rated as "much" or "very much" improved in overall clinical condition compared with 17% of placebo-treated patients (CGI-I).

Side effects and risks. The most commonly reported adverse events in the modafinil group were insomnia (29%), headache (20%), and decreased appetite (16%). While these findings are evidence of the effectiveness of modafinil in ADHD, modafinil was not FDA approved for ADHD because of concerns about a few potentially serious Stevens-Johnson-like rashes in these trials. When used off-label for ADHD in children, the risk-benefit evaluation should take into account the possibility of a rash of this type.

Nonbenzodiazepine anxiolytics: buspirone.

An open study of 12 children with ADHD reported that the nonbenzodiazepine anxiolytic buspirone at 0.5 mg/kg/day improved both ADHD symptoms and psychosocial function in ADHD youth (Malhotra and Santosh 1998). Buspirone has a high affinity to 5-HT$_{1A}$ receptors, both pre- and postsynaptic, as well as a modest effect on the dopaminergic system and alpha-adrenergic activity. However, results from a multisite controlled clinical trial of transdermal buspirone failed to separate it from placebo in a large sample of children with ADHD (unpublished data, Bristol-Myers Squibb).

Typical antipsychotics.

While an old literature suggested that typical antipsychotics were effective in the treatment of children with ADHD, their spectrum of adverse effects, both short-term (extrapyramidal reactions) and long-term (tardive dyskinesia), greatly limits their usefulness.

Anticonvulsants: carbamazepine.

A meta-analysis pooling data from 10 studies provided preliminary evidence that carbamazepine may have activity in ADHD (Silva et al. 1996), although it has an unacceptable side-effect profile for clinical use in ADHD.

Research Directions: Cholinergic Agents

In recent years, evidence has emerged that nicotinic dysregulation may contribute to the pathophysiology of ADHD. This is not surprising, considering that nicotinic activation enhances dopaminergic neurotransmission (Mereu et al. 1987; Westfall et al. 1983). Independent lines of investigation have documented that ADHD is associated with an increased risk and earlier age at onset of cigarette smoking (Milberger et al. 1997; Pomerleau et al. 1996), that maternal smoking during pregnancy increases the risk for ADHD in the offspring, and that in utero exposure to nicotine in animals confers a heightened risk for an ADHD-like syn-

TABLE 46–5. Modafinil

Drug, generic/brand	Daily dose, mg/kg	Daily dosage schedule	Main indications	Common adverse effects/ Comments
Modafinil (Provigil)	0.3–1.0	Once (in the A.M.)	? ADHD	Insomnia, headache, decreased appetite Limited abuse liability Rare, potentially serious Stevens-Johnson-like rash

Note. For noradrenergic modulators (clonidine, guanfacine), see Chapter 50, "Alpha-Adrenergics, Beta-Blockers, Benzodiazepines, Buspirone, and Desmopressin."
ADHD=attention-deficit/hyperactivity disorder.

drome in the newborn (Fung 1988; Fung and Lau 1989; Johns et al. 1982; Milberger et al. 1996). In non-ADHD subjects, central nicotinic activation has been shown to improve temporal memory (Meck and Church 1987), attention (Jones et al. 1992; Peeke and Peeke 1984; Wesnes and Warburton 1984), cognitive vigilance (Jones et al. 1992; Parrott and Winder 1989; Wesnes and Warburton 1984), and executive function (Wesnes and Warburton 1984).

Although a controlled clinical trial of nicotine in adults with ADHD (Levin et al. 1996) documented that the commercially available transdermal nicotine patch resulted in significant improvement of ADHD symptoms, working memory, and neuropsychological functioning, the trial was very short (2 days) and included only a handful of patients. ABT-418 is a central nervous system cholinergic, nicotinic-activating agent with structural similarities to nicotine. Phase I studies of this compound in humans indicated its low abuse liability, as well as adequate safety and tolerability in elderly adults (Abbott Laboratories, unpublished

data). A double-blind, placebo-controlled, randomized crossover trial comparing a transdermal patch of ABT-418 (75 mg/day) to placebo in adults with DSM-IV ADHD (American Psychiatric Association 1994) showed a significantly higher proportion of ADHD adults to be very much improved while receiving ABT-418 than when receiving placebo (40% vs. 13%; McNemar χ^2=5.3, P=.021) (Wilens et al. 1999b). Although preliminary, these results suggest that nicotinic analogues may have activity in ADHD.

Conclusion

ADHD is a heterogeneous disorder with a strong neurobiological basis that afflicts millions of individuals of all ages worldwide. Although the stimulants remain the mainstay of treatment for this disorder, a new generation of nonstimulant drugs is emerging that provides viable alternatives for patients and families.

Summary Points

- There is a substantial body of literature documenting the efficacy of multiple unrelated pharmacological agents in individuals with ADHD.
- Pharmacological treatment leads to improvement not only on core behavioral (ADHD, ODD) symptoms but also on associated impairments including cognition, social skills, and family function.
- Anti-ADHD compounds include not only the stimulants but also a specific norepinephrine reuptake inhibitor (atomoxetine), several antidepressants, and alpha-adrenergic agents (clonidine and guanfacine).
- Effective pharmacological treatments for ADHD seem to share noradrenergic and dopaminergic mechanisms of action.
- Despite great progress, less is known about the treatment of ADHD in preschoolers, adolescents, adults, females, and minorities.

- There are limited data on the differential response of medications in comorbid ADHD, the effects of combined pharmacotherapy, or the effects of combined pharmacotherapy and psychotherapy.
- Risks of stimulant use include their abuse potential, (rare) cardiac risk in individuals with preexisting structural cardiac abnormalities, and precipitation or exacerbation of anxiety, agitation, aggression, manic symptoms, and psychotic symptoms.
- Risks of atomoxetine use include possible suicidal ideation, (rare) risk of severe liver injury, (rare) cardiac risk in individuals with preexisting structural cardiac abnormalities, and precipitation or exacerbation of agitation, aggression, manic symptoms, and psychotic symptoms.

References

Adler L, Resnick S, Kunz M, et al: Open-Label Trial of Venlafaxine in Attention Deficit Disorder. Orlando, FL, New Clinical Drug Evaluation Unit Program, 1995

American Psychiatric Association: Diagnostic and Statistical Manual of Mental Disorders, 4th Edition. Washington, DC, American Psychiatric Association, 1994

Arnold LE, Lindsay RL, Conners CK, et al: A double-blind, placebo-controlled withdrawal trial of dexmethylphenidate hydrochloride in children with attention deficit hyperactivity disorder. J Child Adolesc Psychopharmacol 14:542–554, 2004

Barkley RA: A review of stimulant drug research with hyperactive children. J Child Psychol Psychiatry 18:137–165, 1977

Barr CL, Wigg K, Malone M, et al: Linkage study of catechol-O-methyltransferase and attention-deficit hyperactivity disorder. Am J Med Genet 88:710–713, 1999

Barrickman L, Perry P, Allen AJ, et al: Bupropion versus methylphenidate in the treatment of attention-deficit hyperactivity disorder. J Am Acad Child Adolesc Psychiatry 34:649–657, 1995

Bergman A, Winters L, Cornblatt B: Methylphenidate: effects on sustained attention, in Ritalin: Theory and Patient Management. Edited by Greenhill L, Osman B. New York, Mary Ann Liebert, 1991, pp 223–231

Biederman J, Baldessarini RJ, Wright V, et al: A double-blind placebo controlled study of desipramine in the treatment of ADD, I: efficacy. J Am Acad Child Adolesc Psychiatry 28:777–784, 1989

Biederman J, Faraone SV, Keenan K, et al: Further evidence for family genetic risk factors in attention deficit hyperactivity disorder: patterns of comorbidity in probands and relatives in psychiatrically and pediatrically referred samples. Arch Gen Psychiatry 49:728–738, 1992

Biederman J, Thisted R, Greenhill LL, et al: Estimation of the association between desipramine and the risk for sudden death in 5- to 14-year-old children. J Clin Psychiatry 56:87–93, 1995a

Biederman J, Wilens T, Mick E, et al: Psychoactive substance use disorder in adults with attention deficit hyperactivity disorder: effects of ADHD and psychiatric comorbidity. Am J Psychiatry 152:1652–1658, 1995b

Biederman J, Wilens T, Mick E, et al: Pharmacotherapy of attention-deficit/hyperactivity disorder reduces risk for substance use disorder. Pediatrics 104:e20, 1999

Biederman J, Lopez FA, Boellner SW, et al: A randomized, double-blind, placebo-controlled, parallel-group study of SLI381 (Adderall XR) in children with attention-deficit/hyperactivity disorder. Pediatrics 110:258–266, 2002

Biederman J, Quinn D, Weiss M, et al: Efficacy and safety of Ritalin LA, a new, once-daily, extended-release dosage form of methylphenidate hydrochloride, in children with ADHD. Paediatr Drugs 5:833–841, 2003

Biederman J, Swanson J, Wigal SB, et al: Efficacy and safety of modafinil film-coated tablets in children and adolescents with attention-deficit/hyperactivity disorder: results of a randomized, double-blind, placebo-controlled, flexible-dose study. Pediatrics 116:e777–e784, 2005

Biederman J, Boellner SW, Childress A, et al: Lisdexamfetamine dimesylate and mixed amphetamine salts extended-release in children with ADHD: a double-blind, placebo-controlled, crossover analog classroom study. Biol Psychiatry 62:970–976, 2007a

Biederman J, Krishnan S, Zhang Y, et al: Efficacy and tolerability of lisdexamfetamine dimesylate (NRP-104) in children with attention-deficit/hyperactivity disorder: a phase III, multicenter, randomized, double-blind, forced-dose, parallel-group study. Clin Ther 29:450–463, 2007b

Brown RT, Wynne ME, Slimmer LW: Attention deficit disorder and the effect of methylphenidate on attention, behavioral, and cardiovascular functioning. J Clin Psychiatry 45:473–476, 1984

Casat CD, Pleasants DZ, Van Wyck Fleet J: A double-blind trial of bupropion in children with attention deficit disorder. Psychopharmacol Bull 23:120–122, 1987

Casat CD, Pleasants DZ, Schroeder DH, et al: Bupropion in children with attention deficit disorder. Psychopharmacol Bull 25:198–201, 1989

Conners K, Casat C, Gualtieri CT, et al: Bupropion hydrochloride in attention deficit disorder with hyperactivity. J Am Acad Child Adolesc Psychiatry 35:1314–1321, 1996

Connor D, Ozbayrak K, Benjamin S, et al: A pilot study of nadolol for overt aggression in developmentally delayed individuals. J Am Acad Child Adolesc Psychiatry 36:826–834, 1997

Connor D, Glatt SJ, Lopez ID, et al: Psychopharmacology and aggression, I: a meta-analysis of stimulant effects on overt/covert aggression-related behaviors in ADHD. J Am Acad Child Adolesc Psychiatry 41:253–261, 2002

Dillon DC, Salzman IJ, Schulsinger DA: The use of imipramine in Tourette's syndrome and attention deficit disorder: case report. J Clin Psychiatry 46:348–349, 1985

Ding Y, Fowler J, Volkow ND, et al: Carbon-11-d-threo-methylphenidate binding to dopamine transporter in baboon brain. J Nucl Med 36:2298–2305, 1995

Donnelly M, Zametkin AJ, Rapoport JL, et al: Treatment of childhood hyperactivity with desipramine: plasma drug concentration, cardiovascular effects, plasma and urinary catecholamine levels, and clinical response. Clin Pharmacol Ther 39:72–81, 1986

Douglas VI, Barr RG, Amin K, et al: Dosage effects and individual responsivity to methylphenidate in attention deficit disorder. J Child Psychol Psychiatry 29:453–475, 1988

Engber TM, Koury EJ, Dennis SA, et al: Differential patterns of regional c-Fos induction in the rat brain by amphetamine and the novel wakefulness-promoting agent modafinil. Neurosci Lett 241:95–98, 1998

Famularo R, Fenton T: The effect of methylphenidate on school grades in children with attention deficit disorder without hyperactivity: a preliminary report. J Clin Psychiatry 48:112–114, 1987

Faraone SV: Genetics of childhood disorders, XX. ADHD, Part 4: is ADHD genetically heterogeneous? J Am Acad Child Adolesc Psychiatry 39:1455–1457, 2000

Faraone SV, Biederman J, Morley CP, et al: The effect of stimulants on height and weight: a review of the literature. J Am Acad Child Adolesc Psychiatry 47:994–1009, 2008

Findling R, Schwartz M, Flannery DJ, et al: Venlafaxine in adults with ADHD: an open trial. J Clin Psychiatry 57:184–189, 1996

Findling RL, Bukstein OG, Melmed RD, et al: A randomized, double-blind, placebo-controlled, parallel-group study of methylphenidate transdermal system in pediatric patients with attention-deficit/hyperactivity disorder. J Clin Psychiatry 69:149–159, 2008. Erratum in: J Clin Psychiatry 69:329, 2008

Fung YK: Postnatal behavioural effects of maternal nicotine exposure in rats. J Pharm Pharmacol 40:870–872, 1988

Fung YK, Lau YS: Effects of prenatal nicotine exposure on rat striatal dopaminergic and nicotinic systems. Pharmacol Biochem Behav 33:1–6, 1989

Gadow K, Sverd J, Sprafkin J, et al: Efficacy of methylphenidate for attention-deficit hyperactivity disorder in children with tic disorder. Arch Gen Psychiatry 52:444–455, 1995 (published erratum appears in Arch Gen Psychiatry 52:836, 1995)

Gittelman R: Childhood disorders, in Drug Treatment of Adult and Child Psychiatric Disorders. Edited by Klein D, Quitkin F, Rifkin A, et al. Baltimore, MD, Williams & Wilkins, 1980, pp 576–756

Gittelman-Klein R: Pharmacotherapy of childhood hyperactivity: an update, in Psychopharmacology: The Third Generation of Progress. Edited by Meltzer HY. New York, Raven, 1987, pp 1215–1224

Goldman L, Genel M, Bezman RJ, et al: Diagnosis and treatment of attention-deficit/hyperactivity disorder in children and adolescents. JAMA 279:1100–1107, 1998

Greenhill L, Halperin J, Abikoff H: Stimulant medications. J Am Acad Child Adolesc Psychiatry 38:503–512, 1998

Greenhill L, Findling RL, Swanson JM, et al: A double-blind, placebo-controlled study of modified-release methylphenidate in children with attention-deficit/hyperactivity disorder. Pediatrics 109:E39, 2002

Greenhill L, Kollins S, Abikoff H, et al: Efficacy and safety of immediate-release methylphenidate treatment for preschoolers with ADHD. J Am Acad Child Adolesc Psychiatry 45:1284–1293, 2006a

Greenhill L, Muniz R, Ball RR, et al: Efficacy and safety of dexmethylphenidate extended-release capsules in children with attention-deficit/hyperactivity disorder. J Am Acad Child Adolesc Psychiatry 45:817–823, 2006b

Gutgesell H, Atkins D, Barst R, et al: Cardiovascular monitoring of children and adolescents receiving psychotropic drugs: a statement for healthcare professionals from the Committee on Congenital Cardiac Defects, Council on Cardiovascular Disease in the Young, American Heart Association. Circulation 99:979–982, 1999

Heil SH, Holmes HW, Bickel WK, et al: Comparison of the subjective, physiological, and psychomotor effects of atomoxetine and methylphenidate in light drug users. Drug Alcohol Depend 67:149–156, 2002

Hoge SK, Biederman J: A case of Tourette's syndrome with symptoms of attention deficit disorder treated with desipramine. J Clin Psychiatry 47:478–479, 1986

Hornig-Rohan M, Amsterdam J: Venlafaxine vs. Stimulant Therapy in Patients With Dual Diagnoses of ADHD and Depression. Orlando, FL, New Clinical Drug Evaluation Unit Program, 1995

Johns JM, Louis TM, Becker RF, et al: Behavioral effects of prenatal exposure to nicotine in guinea pigs. Neurobehav Toxicol Teratol 4:365–369, 1982

Jones GM, Sahakian BJ, Levy R, et al: Effects of acute subcutaneous nicotine on attention, information processing and short-term memory in Alzheimer's disease. Psychopharmacology 108:485–494, 1992

Klein R, Mannuzza S: Hyperactive boys almost grown up, III: methylphenidate effects on ultimate height. Arch Gen Psychiatry 45:1131–1134, 1988

Kratochvil CJ, Bohac D, Harrington M, et al: An open-label trial of tomoxetine in pediatric attention deficit hyperactivity disorder. J Child Adolesc Psychopharmacol 11:167–170, 2001

Kupietz SS, Winsberg BG, Richardson E, et al: Effects of methylphenidate dosage in hyperactive reading-disabled children, I: behavior and cognitive performance effects. J Am Acad Child Adolesc Psychiatry 27:70–77, 1988

Levin ED, Conners CK, Sparrow E, et al: Nicotine effects on adults with attention-deficit/hyperactivity disorder. Psychopharmacology 123:55–63, 1996

Lowe TL, Cohen DJ, Detlor J, et al: Stimulant medications precipitate Tourette's syndrome. JAMA 247:1168–1169, 1982

Malhotra S, Santosh P: An open clinical trial of buspirone in children with attention-deficit/hyperactivity disorder. J Am Acad Child Adolesc Psychiatry 37:364–371, 1998

McCracken JT, Biederman J, Greenhill LL, et al: Analog classroom assessment of a once-daily mixed amphetamine formulation, SLI381 (ADDERALL XR), in children with ADHD. J Am Acad Child Adolesc Psychiatry 42:673–683, 2003

McGough JJ, Biederman J, Wigal SB, et al: Long-term tolerability and effectiveness of once-daily mixed amphetamine salts (Adderall XR) in children with ADHD. J Am Acad Child Adolesc Psychiatry 44:530–538, 2005

McGough JJ, Wigal SB, Abikoff H, et al: A randomized, double-blind, placebo-controlled, laboratory classroom assessment of methylphenidate transdermal system in children with ADHD. J Atten Disord 9:476–485, 2006

Meck WH, Church RM: Cholinergic modulation of the content of temporal memory. Behav Neurosci 101:457–464, 1987

Mereu G, Yoon K, Boi V, et al: Preferential stimulation of ventral tegmental area dopaminergic neurons by nicotine. Eur J Pharmacol 141:395–399, 1987

Michelson D, Faries D, Wernicke J, et al: Atomoxetine in the treatment of children and adolescents with attention-deficit/hyperactivity disorder: a randomized, placebo-controlled, dose-response study. Pediatrics 108:E83, 2001

Milberger S, Biederman J, Faraone SV, et al: Is maternal smoking during pregnancy a risk factor for attention deficit hyperactivity disorder in children? Am J Psychiatry 153:1138–1142, 1996

Milberger S, Biederman J, Faraone SV, et al: Attention deficit hyperactivity disorder is associated with early initiation of cigarette smoking in children and adolescents. J Am Acad Child Adolesc Psychiatry 36:37–44, 1997

Myrick H, Malcolm R, Taylor B, et al: Modafinil: preclinical, clinical, and postmarketing surveillance: a review of abuse liability issues. Ann Clin Psychiatry 16:101–109, 2004

National Institute of Mental Health: Alternative Pharmacology of ADHD, 1996

Nemeroff C, DeVane L, Pollock BG: Newer antidepressants and the cytochrome P450 system. Am J Psychiatry 153:311–320, 1996

Parrott AC, Winder G: Nicotine chewing gum (2 mg, 4 mg) and cigarette smoking: comparative effects upon vigilance and heart rate. Psychopharmacology 97:257–261, 1989

Peeke SC, Peeke HV: Attention, memory, and cigarette smoking. Psychopharmacology 84:205–216, 1984

Pelham WE, Bender ME, Caddell J, et al: Methylphenidate and children with attention deficit disorder. Arch Gen Psychiatry 42:948–952, 1985

Pelham WE, Gnagy EM, Burrows-Maclean L, et al: Once-a-day Concerta methylphenidate versus three-times-daily methylphenidate in laboratory and natural settings. Pediatrics 107:E105, 2001

Pelham WE, Burrows-Maclean L, Gnagy EM, et al: Transdermal methylphenidate, behavioral, and combined treatment for children with ADHD. Exp Clin Psychopharmacol 13:111–126, 2005a

Pelham WE, Manos MJ, Ezzell CE, et al: A dose-ranging study of a methylphenidate transdermal system in children with ADHD. J Am Acad Child Adolesc Psychiatry 44:522–529, 2005b

Pentikis HS, Simmons RD, Benedict MF, et al: Methylphenidate bioavailability in adults when an extended-release multiparticulate formulation is administered sprinkled on food or as an intact capsule. J Am Acad Child Adolesc Psychiatry 41:443–449, 2002

Perrin JM, Friedman RA, Knilans TK, et al: Cardiovascular monitoring and stimulant drugs for attention-deficit/hyperactivity disorder. Pediatrics 122:451–453, 2008

Pomerleau O, Downey K, Stelson FW, et al: Cigarette smoking in adult patients diagnosed with ADHD. J Subst Abuse 7:373–378, 1996

Prince JB, Wilens TE, Biederman J, et al: A controlled study of nortriptyline in children and adolescents with attention deficit hyperactivity disorder. J Child Adolesc Psychopharmacol 10:193–204, 2000

Rapport MD, Jones JT, DuPaul GJ, et al: Attention deficit disorder and methylphenidate: group and single-subject analyses of dose effects on attention in clinic and classroom settings. J Clin Child Psychol 16:329–338, 1987

Rapport MD, Stoner G, DuPaul GJ, et al: Attention deficit disorder and methylphenidate: a multilevel analysis of dose-response effects on children's impulsivity across settings. J Am Acad Child Adolesc Psychiatry 27:60–69, 1988

Rapport MD, DuPaul GJ, Kelly KL: Attention deficit hyperactivity disorder and methylphenidate: the relationship between gross body weight and drug response in children. Psychopharmacol Bull 25:285–290, 1989

Reimherr F, Hedges D, Strong R, et al: An Open Trial of Venlafaxine in Adult Patients With Attention Deficit Hyperactivity Disorder. Orlando, FL, New Clinical Drug Evaluation Unit Program, 1995

Riddle MA, Hardin MT, Cho SC, et al: Desipramine treatment of boys with attention-deficit hyperactivity disorder and tics: preliminary clinical experience. J Am Acad Child Adolesc Psychiatry 27:811–814, 1988

Riddle MA, Nelson JC, Kleinman CS, et al: Sudden death in children receiving Norpramin: a review of three reported cases and commentary. J Am Acad Child Adolesc Psychiatry 30:104–108, 1991

Scheffler RM, Brown TT, Fulton BD, et al: Positive association between attention-deficit/hyperactivity disorder medication use and academic achievement during elementary school. Pediatrics 123:1273–1279, 2009

Silva R, Munoz D, Alpert M: Carbamazepine use in children and adolescents with features of attention-deficit hyperactivity disorder: a meta-analysis. J Am Acad Child Adolesc Psychiatry 35:352–358, 1996

Singer S, Brown J, Quaskey S, et al: The treatment of attention-deficit hyperactivity disorder in Tourette's syndrome: a double-blind placebo-controlled study with clonidine and desipramine. Pediatrics 95:74–81, 1994

Spencer T, Biederman J, Kerman K, et al: Desipramine in the treatment of children with tic disorder or Tourette's syndrome and attention deficit hyperactivity disorder. J Am Acad Child Adolesc Psychiatry 32:354–360, 1993a

Spencer T, Biederman J, Wilens T, et al: Nortriptyline in the treatment of children with attention deficit hyperactivity disorder and tic disorder or Tourette's syndrome. J Am Acad Child Adolesc Psychiatry 32:205–210, 1993b

Spencer T, Wilens T, Biederman J, et al: A double-blind, crossover comparison of methylphenidate and placebo in adults with childhood-onset attention-deficit hyperactivity disorder. Arch Gen Psychiatry 52:434–443, 1995

Spencer T, Biederman J, Wilens T, et al: Pharmacotherapy of attention deficit hyperactivity disorder across the lifecycle: a literature review. J Am Acad Child Adolesc Psychiatry 35:409–432, 1996

Spencer T, Biederman J, Wilens T: Pharmacotherapy of ADHD: a life span perspective, in American Psychiatric Press Review of Psychiatry, Vol 16. Edited by Dickstein LJ, Riba MB, Oldham JM. Washington, DC, American Psychiatric Press, 1997, pp IV87–IV127

Spencer T, Biederman J, Wilens T, et al: Effectiveness and tolerability of atomoxetine in adults with attention deficit hyperactivity disorder. Am J Psychiatry 155:693–695, 1998a

Spencer T, Biederman J, Wilens T: Growth deficits in children with attention deficit hyperactivity disorder. Pediatrics 102:501–506, 1998b

Spencer T, Biederman J, Coffey B, et al: The 4-year course of tic disorders in boys with attention-deficit/hyperactivity disorder. Arch Gen Psychiatry 56:842–847, 1999

Spencer T, Swanson J, Weidenman M, et al: Pharmacodynamic profile of Ritalin LA, a new extended-release dosage form of Ritalin, in children with ADHD. Presented at the 47th annual meeting of the American Academy of Child and Adolescent Psychiatry, New York, October 2000

Spencer T, Biederman J, Heiligenstein J, et al: An open-label, dose-ranging study of atomoxetine in children with attention deficit hyperactivity disorder. J Child Adolesc Psychopharmacol 11:251–265, 2001

Spencer T, Biederman J, Coffey B, et al: A double-blind comparison of desipramine and placebo in children and adolescents with chronic tic disorder and comorbid attention-deficit/hyperactivity disorder. Arch Gen Psychiatry 59:649–656, 2002a

Spencer T, Heiligenstein J, Biederman J, et al: Results from 2 proof-of-concept, placebo-controlled studies of atomoxetine in children with attention-deficit/hyperactivity disorder. J Clin Psychiatry 63:1140–1147, 2002b

Spencer T, Newcorn J, Kratochvil CJ, et al: Effects of atomoxetine on growth after 2-year treatment in pediatric patients with ADHD. Pediatrics 116:e74–e80, 2005

Swanson J, Agler D, Fineberg E, et al: University of California, Irvine, laboratory school protocol for pharmacokinetic and pharmacodynamic studies, in Ritalin: Theory and Practice, 2nd Edition. Edited by Greenhill L, Osman BB. Larchmont, NY, Mary Ann Liebert, 2000, pp 405–430

Swanson JM, Greenhill LL, Lopez FA, et al: Modafinil film-coated tablets in children and adolescents with attention-deficit/hyperactivity disorder: results of a randomized, double-blind, placebo-controlled, fixed-dose study followed by abrupt discontinuation. J Clin Psychiatry 67:137–147, 2006

Tourette's Syndrome Study Group: Treatment of ADHD in children with tics: a randomized controlled trial. Neurology 58:527–536, 2002

Vetter VL, Elia J, Erickson C, et al: Cardiovascular monitoring of children and adolescents with heart disease receiving stimulant drugs: a scientific statement from the American Heart Association Council on Cardiovascular Disease in the Young Congenital Cardiac Defects Committee and the Council on Cardiovascular Nursing. Circulation 117:2407–2423, 2008

Volkow ND, Wang G, Fowler JS, et al: Therapeutic doses of oral methylphenidate significantly increase extracellular dopamine in the human brain. J Neurosci 21:RC121, 2001

Wesnes K, Warburton DM: The effects of cigarettes of varying yield on rapid information processing performance. Psychopharmacology 82:338–342, 1984

Westfall TC, Grant H, Perry H, et al: Release of dopamine and 5-hydroxytryptamine from rat striatal slices following activation of nicotinic cholinergic receptors. Gen Pharmacol 14:321–325, 1983

Wigal S, Swanson JM, Feifel D, et al: A double-blind, placebo-controlled trial of dexmethylphenidate hydrochloride and d,l-threo-methylphenidate hydrochloride in children with attention-deficit/hyperactivity disorder. J Am Acad Child Adolesc Psychiatry 43:1406–1414, 2004

Wigal T, Greenhill L, Chuang S, et al: Safety and tolerability of methylphenidate in preschool children with ADHD. J Am Acad Child Adolesc Psychiatry 45:1294–1303, 2006

Wilens T, Biederman J: The stimulants. Psychiatr Clin North Am 15:191–222, 1992

Wilens T, Biederman J, Geist DE, et al: Nortriptyline in the treatment of attention deficit hyperactivity disorder: a chart review of 58 cases. J Am Acad Child Adolesc Psychiatry 32:343–349, 1993

Wilens T, Biederman J, Spencer T, et al: Controlled trial of high doses of pemoline for adults with attention-deficit/hyperactivity disorder. J Clin Psychopharmacol 19:257–264, 1999a

Wilens T, Biederman J, Spencer T, et al: A pilot controlled clinical trial of ABT-418, a cholinergic agonist, in the treatment of adults with attention deficit hyperactivity disorder. Am J Psychiatry 156:1931–1937, 1999b

Wilens T, Spencer T, Biederman J, et al: A Controlled Trial of Bupropion SR for Attention Deficit Hyperactivity Disorder in Adults. Boca Raton, FL, New Clinical Drug Evaluation Unit Program, 1999c

Wilens T, Haight BR, Horrigan JP, et al: Bupropion XL in adults with ADHD: a randomized, placebo-controlled study. Biol Psychiatry 57:793–801, 2005

Wolraich M, Greenhill LL, Pelham W, et al: Randomized, controlled trial of oros methylphenidate once a day in children with attention-deficit/hyperactivity disorder. Pediatrics 108:883–892, 2001

Zametkin A, Rapoport JL: Noradrenergic hypothesis of attention deficit disorder with hyperactivity: a critical review, in Psychopharmacology: The Third Generation of Progress. Edited by Meltzer HY. New York, Raven, 1987, pp 837–842

Zametkin A, Rapoport JL, Murphy DL, et al: Treatment of hyperactive children with monoamine oxidase inhibitors, I: clinical efficacy. Arch Gen Psychiatry 42:962–966, 1985

Chapter 47

Antidepressants

Graham J. Emslie, M.D.
Paul Croarkin, D.O.
Taryn L. Mayes, M.S.

Antidepressants are widely used in children and adolescents for a variety of disorders, with significant increases over the past 20 years. Primarily, antidepressants have been used for the same disorders as in adults (depression, anxiety), with additional potential use for attention-deficit/hyperactivity disorder (ADHD), repetitive behaviors (e.g., autism spectrum disorders), and reactive aggression. Newer antidepressants, particularly selective serotonin reuptake inhibitors (SSRIs), have demonstrated efficacy and safety in children and adolescents, with the greatest effect seen in obsessive-compulsive disorder (OCD) and anxiety disorders, followed by major depressive disorder (MDD). Yet, limited data are available on pharmacokinetics and dosing in this age group. For example, it is not known whether lower doses may be equally efficacious in children or whether this age group does, in fact, require adult dosing. Theoretically, children may metabolize medications more quickly due to their proportionally larger liver mass.

Prior to 1995, less than 250 children and adolescents with depression had been studied in randomized controlled trials (RCTs). Clearly, widespread use of antidepressants despite lack of evidence of efficacy or safety was a major concern. To address the issue, the U.S. Food and Drug Administration (FDA), through the U.S. Food and Drug Administration Modernization Act of 1997 (U.S. Food and Drug Administration 1997), began requiring an increase in pediatric data for new compounds that were likely to be used in the pediatric population and encouraging pediatric research on adult-approved medications that were commonly used for youth. This process substantially increased the amount of research in pediatric pharmacology in general, and with antidepressants in particular. However, problems with the new data included limited re-

701

search infrastructure (trials included sites with limited pediatric psychiatry experience) and uncertain methodology for optimal trials. Furthermore, many of these earlier studies were conducted with short timelines because of limited remaining medication patent time; thus, the incentive was simply to complete the trials, with less emphasis on proving efficacy. Regardless of these limitations, there is now substantial information on use of antidepressants in the pediatric age group, with over 5,300 children and adolescents participating in antidepressant RCTs by 2009.

Evaluating Antidepressant Studies

It has become increasingly clear that extrapolating from adult data to determine effectiveness and safety of antidepressants in the pediatric population is not possible. In evaluating efficacy in the pediatric age group, there appears to be continuity between the child and adult versions of the same disorder in, for example, OCD. This has allowed effectiveness of antidepressants to be proven based on extrapolating from adults and conducting only one bridging study in children (though issues still remain about dosing). Similarly, the effect size and treatments of pediatric anxiety disorders with antidepressants have generally been large (Bridge et al. 2007). However, the lack of efficacy of tricyclic antidepressants (TCAs; the previous gold standard in adults) raised questions about extrapolating from adult efficacy data for MDD in spite of continuity across the life span based on phenomenology and pathophysiology (Birmaher et al. 1996). Thus, in MDD, two positive trials are required in the pediatric population for the medication to receive an FDA indication.

Pharmacodynamics

Pediatric drug development needs to move beyond the concept of children just being "little adults," particularly regarding dosing. The majority of pediatric antidepressant trials were conducted with limited preliminary data on dosing for children. Doses for trials were often determined by adjusting from adult doses based on weight. It is possible that some differences seen between antidepressants in children reflect wrong choice of doses for the trial rather than different levels of effec-

tiveness. Because antidepressants are metabolized primarily in the liver and children have a proportionately large liver mass, half-lives of antidepressants are generally shorter in children. In addition, clinical trials frequently use forced titration of medication, so it remains unclear whether equal effectiveness can be achieved at a lower dose.

Outcome Assessments

Use of outcome assessments as part of routine clinical care is increasingly recommended in adults. However, adult rating scales are not appropriate for children. Thus, child- and adolescent-specific outcome measures have been developed to assess efficacy. For clinicians to interpret clinical trial data, it is necessary to have some familiarity with what is being measured and whether the criterion (e.g., 25% decrease in the Yale-Brown Obsessive Compulsive Scale—Child version [CY-BOCS]) is a clinically meaningful change.

Safety

RCTs are the gold standard for assessing not only efficacy but also safety. Without a placebo control, it is very difficult to identify whether adverse events are related to the medication, especially if they occur relatively frequently (e.g., headaches). In large clinical trials of newer antidepressants (both SSRIs and atypical antidepressants) in children and adolescents, rates of discontinuation due to adverse events have generally been low, especially compared to older antidepressants. For example, in the paroxetine adolescent trial, discontinuation from the study was equivalent in the paroxetine and placebo groups (9.7% and 6.9%, respectively) but was substantially higher in the imipramine group (31.5%) (Keller et al. 2001).

To assume that antidepressant adverse events are the same in children and adolescents as adults would be erroneous. It appears, for example, that increased rates of suicidality reported in children and adolescents treated with antidepressants relative to placebo (Hammad et al. 2006) extend only to age 25 (Friedman and Leon 2007).

The controversy around increases in suicidality in children and adolescents treated with antidepressants also highlighted problems in assessing adverse effects in clinical trials. When the initial reports suggesting increased activation, agitation, and suicidal behavior became available, it became evident that the process of eliciting these events (spontaneous report) and definition of the events (what constitutes a suicide attempt or increased suicidal ideation) were inconsistent across trials and across sites. This resulted in the FDA requesting an independent reanalysis of the adverse event data. Even with the reanalysis and the findings that suicidality (not suicide) occurred in 4% of children on antidepressants compared to 2% on placebo based on spontaneous report, the prospectively collected rating scales from those studies did not demonstrate any difference in suicidality between active treatment and placebo (Bridge et al. 2007; Hammad et al. 2006). In addition to assessing previous and ongoing suicidality, the FDA recommended monitoring for "associated symptoms," including anxiety, agitation, panic, insomnia, irritability, hostility, impulsivity, akathisia, hypomania, and mania.

The recent controversies have highlighted the need to assess antidepressant-specific adverse events before and during treatment. Systematic review of body systems elicits more adverse events than spontaneous reports obtained through general inquiry (Greenhill et al. 2004). Attempts are being made to develop validated questionnaires to assess adverse events, and a large registry of adverse events on SSRIs is being conducted as part of the Child and Adolescent Psychiatry Trials Network (March et al. 2004). Such advances will hopefully provide more information on the safety of antidepressants in the pediatric age group.

Selective Serotonin Reuptake Inhibitors

As a class, the primary mode of action for SSRIs is thought to be presynaptic inhibition of serotonin reuptake. Chronic treatment also downregulates serotonin receptors in most cases and modulates serotonergic transmission. However, mechanisms extend further than this and vary among SSRIs. For example, some SSRIs inhibit dopamine and norepinephrine transporters as well. They also have differences in antagonism at a variety of receptor sites. SSRIs display a lower side-effect profile than TCAs and monoamine oxidase inhibitors (MAOIs), are relatively safe in overdose, and are easily absorbed from the gastrointestinal tract. Table 47–1 provides the formulations and dosing of SSRIs.

General Side Effects

Most side effects manifest within the first few weeks of treatment with an SSRI, but many of these adverse effects will resolve with time. Known side effects of SSRIs include nausea, vomiting, diarrhea, headaches, dizziness, bruxism, somnolence, vivid or strange dreams, changes in appetite, weight loss, weight gain, tremors, akathisia, skin rashes, increased sweating, and mania; however, there is a great deal of individual variation among patients. SSRIs may increase the risk of bleeding, especially in patients taking aspirin or nonsteroidal anti-inflammatory medications. Sexual side effects are also common, including decreased libido, anorgasmia, and erectile dysfunction. As noted, SSRIs, along with all antidepressants, carry a risk of increased suicidal thinking and behaviors. Therefore, careful monitoring of suicidality, especially during initial stages of treatment and following dose adjustments, is necessary.

Discontinuation symptoms similar to flulike symptoms (e.g., headache, diarrhea, nausea, vomiting, chills, dizziness, fatigue) may occur when suddenly stopping SSRI medications, and this is more common in agents with short half-lives. Fortunately, SSRIs also have a higher margin of safety in overdoses compared to TCAs and MAOIs. However, deaths have been reported with large ingestions of SSRIs (either alone or in combination with other medications).

Contraindications

SSRIs should not be taken with any of the MAOIs, as this combination may lead to confusion, high blood pressure, tremor, and hyperactivity. In addition, tryptophan can cause headaches, nausea, sweating, and dizziness when taken with an SSRI. Patients taking pimozide also should not take SSRIs. Although rare, coadministration with tramadol hydrochloride (a centrally acting analgesic sometimes used for chronic pain) can cause seizures.

Efficacy

SSRIs are the first-line medication treatment for youth with MDD, OCD, and other anxiety disorders (Birmaher et al. 2007; Cheung et al. 2007; Connolly and Bernstein 2007; Hughes et al. 2007). In a meta-analysis of all newer antidepressants, Bridge and colleagues found that pooled benefit-risk difference favored SSRIs for MDD (11%; [95% confidence interval {CI}, 6%–15%]), OCD (19.8%; [95% CI, 13%–26.6%]), and other anxiety

TABLE 47–1.   Formulations and dosing for selective serotonin reuptake inhibitors

Medication	Formulations	Initial dose, mg	Target dose, mg		Maximum dose, mg
			Children	Adolescents	
Citalopram	Tablet: 10 mg, 20 mg, 40 mg Solution: 10 mg/5 mL	10	20–40	20–40	60
Escitalopram	Tablet: 5 mg, 10 mg, 20 mg Solution: 5 mg/5 mL	5–10	10–20	10–20	30
Fluoxetine	Capsule: 10 mg, 20 mg, 40 mg Tablet: 10 mg Solution: 20 mg/5 mL	10	20	20–40	60
Fluvoxamine	Tablet: 25 mg, 50 mg, 100 mg	25	50–200	50–200	200 300
Paroxetine	Tablet: 10 mg, 20 mg, 30 mg, 40 mg Tablet CR: 12.5 mg, 25 mg, 37.5 mg Suspension: 10 mg/5 mL	10	10–30	20–40	50
Sertraline	Tablet: 25 mg, 50 mg, 100 mg Solution: 20 mg/mL	12.5–25	50–200	50–200	200

Note.   CR=controlled release.

disorders (40%; [95% CI, 31%–48%]) (Bridge et al. 2007). Table 47–2 lists the approved indications for SSRIs. SSRIs also have potential utility in several other areas, including OCD spectrum disorders, autism spectrum disorders, aggression, eating disorders, and psychiatric symptoms related to medical conditions. However, few controlled trials have been conducted in these areas. Table 47–3 provides an overview of the available RCTs with SSRIs in children and adolescents.

Information on specific SSRI antidepressants is detailed below.

Citalopram

Chemical Structure and Pharmacology

Citalopram is a racemic bicyclic phthalane derivative. Its structure is chemically unrelated to other antidepressants, and it is the most selective of all SSRIs. It has a greater than 3,000-fold potency for inhibiting serotonin reuptake as compared to norepinephrine and a greater than 20,000-fold potency compared to dopamine reuptake (Hyttel et al. 1995). Citalopram's S-(+) enantiomer inhibits serotonin reuptake. Its R-(–) enantiomer is inactive. In animal studies, there is an increase in extracellular serotonin following administration. This, in turn, activates serotonin type 1A (5-HT$_{1A}$) autoreceptors. It is thought that this leads to a feedback inhibition of the raphe nuclei, and downregulations of autoreceptors, with an increase in serotonergic activity.

Pharmacokinetics

Citalopram is easily absorbed after oral intake with a bioavailability of 80%. Food does not affect its absorption. Peak plasma levels are achieved after 2–4 hours with single or multiple doses (Bezchlibnyk-Butler et al. 2000). The mean peak plasma concentration (C$_{max}$) with a dosage of 40 mg daily at steady state is 311 nmo/L. Its volume of distribution (V$_d$) is 12–16 L/kg. Citalopram is estimated to be 80% protein bound, which is less than other SSRIs. Citalopram is thought to have a low liability for drug interactions via protein-binding interactions, P-glycoprotein, or renal clearance. It is also believed to have a wide margin of safety if plasma levels rise. It is affected little by first-pass metabolism and drug-drug interactions involving protein binding (Baumann and Larsen 1995). Table 47–4 provides the pharmacodynamic and pharmacokinetic data for citalopram and other SSRIs.

There are two pharmacokinetic studies of citalopram in children and adolescents, with varying results. The first study, which compared the pharmacokinetic data of adolescents and adults, found that citalopram's half-life was 38.4 hours in adolescents and 44 hours in adults. A second study, which included children and adolescents (ages 9–17), displayed a half-life of 16.9 hours after a 20 mg dose and 19.2 hours after multiple doses, which were substantially smaller than previous studies of adult half-lives. Investigators have questioned whether twice daily

TABLE 47–2. U.S. Food and Drug Administration (FDA) indications for selective serotonin reuptake inhibitors

Medication	FDA-approved indication	Indication age range
Citalopram (Celexa)	Depression	Adults
Escitalopram (Lexapro)	Depression	Adults
Fluoxetine (Prozac)	Depression	8 years to adult
	OCD	7 years to adult
	Bulimia	Adults
Fluvoxamine (Luvox)	OCD	8 years to adult
Paroxetine (Paxil)	Depression	Adults
	OCD	Adults
	PD	Adults
	SOC	Adults
	GAD	Adults
	PTSD	Adults
Sertraline (Zoloft)	Depression	Adults
	OCD	6 years to adult
	PMDD	Adults
	PD	Adults

Note. GAD=generalized anxiety disorder; OCD=obsessive-compulsive disorder; PD=panic disorder; PMDD=premenstrual dysphoric disorder; PTSD=posttraumatic stress disorder; SOC=social anxiety disorder.

dosing for youth may improve efficacy, although this has not yet been studied (Findling et al. 2006a).

Adverse Effects Profile

Citalopram is generally safe and well tolerated at doses of 20–60 mg per day. Due to its low liability for drug interactions, it is an ideal choice for patients requiring multiple medications. However, use with any other serotonergic agent should be undertaken only with caution given the potential for serotonin syndrome. Citalopram is relatively safe with large ingestions, although fatal ingestions of 840 to 4,000 mg have been reported in adults (Luchini et al. 2005; Ostrom et al. 1996). Convulsions can develop with doses exceeding 600 mg, and ventricular fibrillation occurred in a 2 gram ingestion (Personne et al. 1997).

Efficacy

Two RCTs have been conducted in pediatric patients with MDD, with inconsistent findings. Wagner et al. (2004b) reported greater improvement of depressive symptoms with citalopram compared to placebo as early as week 1, which persisted throughout the study. A second study, however, showed no difference between citalopram and placebo on any outcome measures. In this study, which was conducted internationally, both inpatients and outpatients were enrolled in

the study, suggesting a potentially more severe population. In addition, approximately two-thirds of subjects were receiving psychotherapy during the study. Although not powered to detect a significant difference in the subgroup of subjects who did not receive psychotherapy, citalopram treatment showed greater response than placebo (41% vs. 25%). On the other hand, in subjects receiving psychotherapy, there was no significant difference between active medication and placebo (44% vs. 53%). The results are difficult to interpret due to the limited available data, the fact that both inpatients and outpatients were used, and inclusion of psychotherapy for most patients (von Knorring et al. 2006).

No double-blind RCTs of citalopram have been conducted in any other pediatric population.

Escitalopram

Chemical Structure and Pharmacology

Escitalopram is the active (S)-enantiomer of citalopram, which has been shown to be twice as potent as citalopram with respect to serotonin inhibition (Aronson and Delgado 2004). With oral administration of 10 mg, it is rapidly and almost entirely absorbed, and achieves peak plasma concentrations of 10–30 ng/mL in approximately 2–6 hours (Table 47–3) (Rao 2007). Its

TABLE 47–3. Pediatric randomized controlled trials for selective serotonin reuptake inhibitors

Individual study	Disorder	N	Age	Duration, wks	Primary outcome	Secondary outcomes	Funding source	Comments
Citalopram								
Wagner et al. 2004b	MDD	174	7–17	8	+	−	Forest	Two studies combined
Von Knorring et al. 2006	MDD	233	13–18	12	−	−	Forest	Included inpatients and outpatients; therapy allowed
Escitalopram								
Wagner et al. 2006	MDD	264	6–17	8	−	−	Forest	Adolescents positive
Emslie et al. 2009	MDD	312	12–17	8	+	+	Forest	
Fluoxetine								
Simeon et al. 1990	MDD	40	13–18	8	−	−		Incompletely described methods
Emslie et al. 1997	MDD	96	7–18	8	+	+	NIMH	
Emslie et al. 2002	MDD	219	8–18	9	−	+	Eli Lilly	
Treatment for Adolescents With Depression Study 2004	MDD	439	12–17	12	+	+	NIMH	
Riddle et al. 1992	OCD	14	8–15	8	+	−		
Geller et al. 2001	OCD	103	7–17	13	+	+	Eli Lilly	
Liebowitz et al. 2002	OCD	43	6–18	8–16	+	+	NIMH	Outcomes positive at 16 weeks, but not 8 weeks
Black and Uhde 1994	SM + SOC	15	6–11	12	+	+		Most subjects still symptomatic
Birmaher et al. 2003	GAD, SAD, SOC	74	7–17	12	+	+		Positive for GAD and SOC only
Hollander et al. 2005	ASD (repetitive behavior)	45	5–17	8	+	+	NIH, FDA	Low doses of liquid fluoxetine
Fluvoxamine								
Riddle et al. 2001	OCD	120	8–17	10	+	+		
Research Unit on Pediatric Psychopharmacology et al. 2001	GAD, SAD, SOC	128	6–17	8	+	+	NIMH	

TABLE 47–3. Pediatric randomized controlled trials for selective serotonin reuptake inhibitors *(continued)*

Individual study	Disorder	N	Age	Duration, wks	Primary outcome	Secondary outcomes	Funding source	Comments
Fluvoxamine (*continued*)								
Abikoff et al. 2005	ADHD + ANX	25	6–17	8	–	–	NIMH	
Paroxetine								
Keller et al. 2001	MDD	275	12–18	8	–	+	SKB (now GSK)	
Berard et al. 2006	MDD	275	13–18	12	–	+	GSK	Positive for subjects ages ≥16 years
Emslie et al. 2006	MDD	203	7–17	8	–	–	GSK	High dropout rate due to AEs in children
Geller et al. 2004	OCD	207	7–17	10	+	+	GSK	High dropout rate due to AEs in children
Wagner et al. 2004a	Social anxiety	319	8–17	16	+	+	GSK	
Sertraline								
Wagner et al. 2003	MDD	376	6–17	10	+	+	Pfizer	Greater difference in adolescents
March et al. 1998	OCD	187	6–17	12	+	+	Pfizer	High dropout rate due to AEs
Pediatric OCD Treatment Study 2004	OCD	112	7–17	12	+	–	NIMH	
Rynn et al. 2001	GAD	22	5–17	9	+	+	NIMH	
Cohen et al. 2007	PTSD	24	10–17	12	–	+	NIMH	All subjects in CBT
Walkup et al. 2008	ANX	488	7–17	12	+	+	NIMH	

Note. +=positive outcome; –=negative outcome; ADHD=attention-deficit/hyperactivity disorder; AEs=adverse events; ANX=anxiety disorders; ASD=autism spectrum disorders; CBT=cognitive-behavioral therapy; FDA=U.S. Food and Drug Administration; GAD=generalized anxiety disorder; GSK=GlaxoSmithKline; MDD=major depressive disorder; NIH=National Institutes of Health; NIMH=National Institute of Mental Health; OCD=obsessive-compulsive disorder; PTSD=posttraumatic stress disorder; SAD= separation anxiety disorder; SKB=SmithKline Beecham; SM=selective mutism; SOC=social phobia.

TABLE 47–4. Pharmacodynamics and pharmacokinetics of selective serotonin reuptake inhibitors

Medication	Half-life	Time to steady state	CYP enzyme inhibited	Kinetics
Citalopram	20 hours	6–10 days	2D6 (weak)	Linear
Escitalopram	27–32 hours	7 days	2D6 (weak)	Linear
Fluoxetine	4–6 days	>4 weeks	1A2 (weak) 2B6 (moderate) 2C9 (moderate) 3A4 (moderate) 2C19 (potent) 2D6 (potent)	Nonlinear
Fluvoxamine	15 hours	10 days	2D6 (weak) 3A4 (moderate) 2C9 (moderate) 2B6 (moderate) 2C19 (moderate) 1A2 (potent)	Nonlinear
Paroxetine	21 hours	7–14 days	1A2 (weak) 2C9 (weak) 2C19 (weak) 3A4 (moderate) 2B6 (potent) 2D6 (potent)	Nonlinear
Sertraline	26 hours	5–7 days	1A2 (weak) 3A4 (moderate) 2B6 (moderate) 2D6 (moderate at low doses, potent at high doses)	Linear

Note. CYP=cytochrome P450.

affinity for dopamine and norepinephrine receptors is negligible. Like citalopram, escitalopram inhibits serotonin reuptake. Radioligand single-photon emission computed tomography (SPECT) studies with patients receiving escitalopram or citalopram indicate that serotonin transporter occupancy in the midbrain was higher with escitalopram (N. Klein et al. 2007).

Pharmacokinetics

The pharmacokinetics of escitalopram are very similar to citalopram. Pharmacokinetic studies in pediatrics are limited. One study with a single dose of 10 mg given to 11 teenagers and 12 adults found that the half-life of escitalopram was 19 hours in adolescents and 28.9 hours in adults. Total blood levels were 15% greater in adults than adolescents as well (Findling et al. 2006a).

Adverse Effects Profile

Escitalopram's adverse event profile is similar to that of other SSRIs. It is relatively safe with large ingestions, and there have been no deaths or adverse events in published reports of overdoses up to 300 mg (LoVecchio et al. 2006).

Efficacy

Two RCTs have been conducted with escitalopram in youth with MDD. Although the first study, which included children and adolescents, was negative, there was some evidence of efficacy for the adolescent subgroup on several secondary outcomes (Wagner et al. 2006). As a result of the potential utility in adolescents, a trial of adolescents only (N=312) was recently completed. Results demonstrated positive efficacy on several outcomes (Emslie et al. 2009). No placebo-controlled RCTs of escitalopram have been conducted in any other pediatric psychiatry disorders. Escitalopram was FDA approved for treatment of depression in adolescents in 2009.

Fluoxetine

Chemical Structure and Pharmacology

Fluoxetine's chemistry is similar to diphenhydramine, but its pharmacological activity is very different. Its structure is unique among other antidepressants. However, like other SSRIs, fluoxetine appears to target the serotonin transporter, thereby inhibiting serotonin reuptake. Fluoxetine's inhibition decreases further release of serotonin, inhibits firing in the dorsal raphe nuclei, downregulates serotonin autoreceptors, and increases serotonergic transmission in the hippocampus. Fluoxetine does not have clinically significant noradrenergic or dopaminergic activity. Its binding at muscarinic, histaminergic, and alpha-1 adrenergic receptors is minimal and much less than that of TCAs (DeVane 1998).

Pharmacokinetics

Fluoxetine is almost totally absorbed with oral administration. Food can decrease the rate but not the degree of absorption. Its bioavailability is less than 90% due to first-pass effect. It is lipophilic and has a volume of distribution of 14–100 L/kg. This surpasses all other SSRIs. Fluoxetine's long half-life (Table 47–4) makes withdrawal or discontinuation effects unlikely but requires an extensive washout period before starting medications with drug-drug interactions (e.g., 5 weeks for MAOIs). Patients with renal failure have little difficulty metabolizing this drug; however, liver damage reduces plasma clearance of fluoxetine (Hiemke and Hartter 2000).

One pharmacokinetic study of 10 children (ages 6–12) and 11 adolescents (ages 13–18) with OCD or MDD demonstrated higher concentrations of fluoxetine and norfluoxetine in children than adolescents. After correcting for weight, this difference was not significant. Population analysis also indicated that oral clearance, absorption rate constant, and volume of distribution were not significantly different from adults (Findling et al. 2006a).

Adverse Effects Profile

Overall, fluoxetine is well tolerated, and side effects parallel other SSRIs. Fluoxetine has a high margin of safety in overdose. One patient ingested 8 grams and survived. However, deaths have been reported in patients ingesting as little as 520 mg. The largest known pediatric ingestion is 3 grams (patient recovered).

Fluoxetine should not be used in combination with any MAOI, or within a minimum of 14 days of discontinuing an MAOI. Furthermore, fluoxetine should be discontinued for at least 5 weeks before starting an MAOI.

Efficacy

To date, three large RCTs in pediatric MDD have been conducted with fluoxetine, with all three demonstrating superiority over placebo (Emslie et al. 1997, 2002; Treatment for Adolescents With Depression Study 2004). It is the only antidepressant to demonstrate efficacy in more than one RCT of MDD in the pediatric age group. Only one small RCT of fluoxetine ($n=40$) has failed to demonstrate a positive response over placebo. However, the results of this study are difficult to interpret because of the small sample size and incompletely described methodology (Simeon et al. 1990).

Unlike with some of the other SSRIs, fluoxetine appears to be equally effective in the younger age group (<12). Random regression of the Children's Depression Rating Scale, Revised (CDRS-R), showed a treatment group by age group interaction ($f_{1,338}=4.10$, $P=.044$), indicating that the treatment effect was significantly more pronounced in children than adolescents (Mayes et al. 2007). Bridge et al. (2007) confirmed this in their meta-analysis, indicating that in children younger than age 12 with MDD, only fluoxetine showed benefit over placebo.

Fluoxetine has also been studied in three RCTs of children and adolescents with OCD, totaling 160 subjects (Geller et al. 2001; Liebowitz et al. 2002; Riddle et al. 1992). In the largest of the three studies ($n=103$), response was significantly greater with fluoxetine compared to placebo (49% vs. 25%; $P=0.03$) (Geller et al. 2001).

Two RCTs of other anxiety disorders have also demonstrated efficacy for fluoxetine in youth. In a small trial ($n=15$) of selective mutism plus social phobia in 6- to 11-year-olds, fluoxetine was more efficacious than placebo in improving anxiety and mutism (Black and Uhde 1994). In a larger study of generalized anxiety disorder (GAD), social phobia, or separation anxiety in 74 children and adolescents, fluoxetine led to greater response rates than placebo for GAD (67% vs. 36%; $P=0.04$) and social phobia (76% vs. 21%; $P<0.001$) but not for separation anxiety (54% vs. 41%; NS). Across all disorders, fluoxetine was superior to placebo (61% vs. 35%; $P=0.03$) (Birmaher et al. 2003).

Finally, liquid fluoxetine was superior to placebo in reducing repetitive behaviors in 45 children and adolescents with autism in a double-blind, placebo-controlled crossover study (Hollander et al. 2005).

Thus, fluoxetine is the only antidepressant to have more than one positive RCT for MDD, OCD, and anxiety disorders. It is the only antidepressant FDA approved for treatment of depression in both children and adolescents and is one of three antidepressants indicated for treatment of pediatric OCD. It may also be beneficial in improving OCD symptoms associated with other disorders (e.g., repetitive symptoms associated with autism).

Fluvoxamine

Chemical Structure and Pharmacology

Fluvoxamine maleate is a 2-aminoethyl oxime ether of aralkylketone with a structure that is unique among other SSRIs and TCAs. Fluvoxamine's mechanism of action is similar to other SSRIs. It inhibits the presynaptic reuptake of serotonin in brain neurons, thereby enhancing serotonergic transmission. Fluvoxamine has no clinically significant affinity for histaminergic, alpha- or beta-adrenergic, muscarinic, or dopaminergic receptors.

Pharmacokinetics

After oral ingestion, fluvoxamine is easily, and more than 90%, absorbed. Food does not affect its bioavailability, which is approximately 53% due to fast and extensive first-pass effect. Nearly 100% of orally administered fluvoxamine is excreted in the urine, but only minute amounts are unchanged. Gender differences in metabolism have been reported at doses of 100 mg/day, with the blood levels significantly increased in female subjects. This effect attenuates if the daily dose is doubled (Hiemke and Hartter 2000). Multiple-dose studies of children and adolescents indicate that steady-state plasma concentrations are significantly higher in children than adolescents. Peak plasma concentrations are significantly higher in female children compared to male children, but there are no gender differences in adolescents. Thus, female children may need lower doses, although this has not yet been studied. In adolescents, steady-state concentrations of fluvoxamine are similar to adults with 300 mg (Labellarte et al. 2004).

Fluvoxamine has multiple cytochrome P450 interactions. Clinicians should consult references for drug-drug interactions frequently and maintain a high index of caution.

Adverse Effects Profile

The most common side effects of fluvoxamine are sleep disturbances (either somnolence or insomnia).

Fluvoxamine is thought to have the lowest incidence of sexual side effects of all the SSRIs. Its cytochrome P450 inhibition should be considered when coadministering with other agents. Otherwise, its side-effect profile is similar to other SSRIs. In overdoses, fluvoxamine appears to have a wide margin of safety as patients ingesting up to 9 grams have had mild symptoms and a complete recovery (Henry 1991).

Efficacy

Fluvoxamine is FDA approved for the treatment of childhood OCD. In a multicenter RCT, fluvoxamine-treated subjects showed statistically significant improvements compared to placebo on the primary outcome (CY-BOCS) at weeks 1, 4, 6, and 10. The active treatment group also displayed significantly greater improvement than placebo in secondary efficacy measures (National Institute of Mental Health Global Obsessive-Compulsive Scale and Clinical Global Impressions Scale) at all postrandomization visits (Riddle et al. 2001). Fluvoxamine has also demonstrated greater reduction in anxiety symptoms compared to placebo in a study of youth with social phobia, separation anxiety, or GAD (Research Unit on Pediatric Psychopharmacology et al. 2001). However, a pilot trial of sequential treatment for 25 children with comorbid ADHD and anxiety showed no benefit in adding fluvoxamine to subjects on stimulants with stable ADHD symptoms but with ongoing anxiety (Abikoff et al. 2005).

Most studies of pervasive developmental disorders in children have not been promising (McDougle et al. 2000). However, one study suggested that genetic polymorphisms of the serotonin transporter gene promoter region (5-HTTLPR) may affect response to fluvoxamine in young autistic patients (Sugie et al. 2005).

Fluvoxamine has not been studied in pediatric depression.

Paroxetine

Chemical Structure and Pharmacology

Paroxetine hydrochloride is a salt of a phenylpiperidine compound, is structurally unrelated to other antidepressants, and is a pure enantiomer. Among the SSRIs, it is the most potent serotonin and norepinephrine reuptake inhibitor. Its muscarinic acetylcholine antagonism also rivals that of TCAs and surpasses desipramine and maprotiline. However, it has minimal affinity for histamine, alpha-1, alpha-2, beta-adrenergic, dopamine (D_1 or D_2), and serotonin (5-HT_1 and 5-HT_2) receptors (Hiemke and Hartter 2000).

Pharmacokinetics

Paroxetine is easily and almost completely absorbed after oral administration. Calculations of bioavailability range from 50% to 100% in normal volunteers (DeVane 1992). Food does not affect absorption. Paroxetine is subject to first-pass metabolism. At least one-third of paroxetine is excreted through feces, with less than 1% of this amount being unaffected drug. Paroxetine is highly lipophilic, at least 95% protein bound, and has a large volume of distribution (2–12 L/kg). Unlike fluoxetine and sertraline, paroxetine's metabolites have no activity related to monoamine reuptake (DeVane 1992; Hiemke and Hartter 2000).

Like other SSRIs, paroxetine's effects are thought to relate to its inhibition of serotonin transporter leading to increased synaptic serotonin levels. It differs from other SSRIs in that it has the most potent serotonergic blockade, and it has antagonistic activity at the norepinephrine transporter as well (DeVane 1992; Hiemke and Hartter 2000).

Paroxetine pharmacokinetics in children have been examined in two studies. The first was a single-dose (10 mg) study of 30 depressed subjects (ages 6–17). The average half-life was 11.1 hours, with a wide range of variability. Investigators also found that metabolism correlated with CYP2D6 phenotype. Subsequently, blood levels were collected weekly during 8 weeks of treatment. Most children and adolescents remained on 10 mg of paroxetine. Eight of these subjects had a dose increase, which led to nearly a 7-fold increase in paroxetine blood levels (Findling et al. 1999, 2006b). Another study involved a 6-week trial of patients with MDD or OCD with 27 children (ages 7–11) and 35 adolescents (ages 12–17). This study also supported the idea that paroxetine has nonlinear kinetics and that optimal treatment for younger children may involve smaller doses (Findling et al. 2006b).

Adverse Effects Profile

Paroxetine's side effects are similar to other SSRIs. Due to its short half-life in children, its discontinuation symptoms are thought to be more severe than other SSRIs. Thus, slow tapering is recommended to avoid psychological or somatic discontinuation symptoms. Paroxetine is relatively safe with large ingestions. Ingestions of 100–800 mg of paroxetine have been reported in children, with no resultant deaths or serious sequelae (Myers and Krenzelok 1997).

Efficacy

Three RCTs have been conducted in pediatric MDD with inconsistent findings. A study of adolescents only (*N*=275) demonstrated positive efficacy on some outcomes, although the primary outcome was negative (Keller et al. 2001). Two other RCTs of paroxetine, however, were negative on all outcome measures. In one of these studies, older adolescents (≥16 years) showed greater response to active treatment than placebo, suggesting that the older age group may be more responsive to the medication (Berard et al. 2006). In addition, in the study of both children and adolescents, children had significantly higher dropout rates due to adverse events with paroxetine than with placebo. Due to the high dropout rates in the younger age group, it is difficult to interpret efficacy outcomes for this subgroup. It is possible that smaller doses may be beneficial in prepubertal children (Emslie et al. 2006).

One multicenter RCT of paroxetine has been conducted in pediatric OCD. The mean difference between paroxetine and placebo for CY-BOCS decrease showed statistically significant superiority for paroxetine. Further, three of six secondary efficacy measures showed statistically significant improvement with paroxetine. However, similar to the pediatric MDD trial, 10% of the paroxetine-treated patients withdrew early due to adverse events (Geller et al. 2004). Unlike fluoxetine, fluvoxamine, and sertraline, which all received an FDA indication following one positive RCT, paroxetine is not yet approved for treatment of OCD.

One multicenter RCT has examined paroxetine in children and adolescents with social anxiety disorder and reported greater improvement with paroxetine over placebo at all time points (Wagner et al. 2004a).

Sertraline

Chemical Structure and Pharmacology

Sertraline is the second most potent SSRI (second to paroxetine) and the only SSRI with affinity for dopamine receptors. It is similar to paroxetine in that it has two chiral centers. The marketed preparation of this drug contains only the more potent enantiomer (1S, 4S). It has no clinically relevant affinity for beta-adrenergic, histaminergic, γ-aminobutyric acid (GABA), or benzodiazepine receptors. However, its alpha-1 antagonism is at least 10 times greater than other SSRIs. This antagonism apparently causes no significant cardiac effects such as hypotension or tachycardia (DeVane et al. 2002; Hiemke and Hartter 2000).

Pharmacokinetics

Unlike other SSRIs, food intake significantly increases sertraline's maximum plasma levels (by approximately 25%) and reduces time to peak plasma concentrations. Sertraline is 98% protein bound (DeVane et al. 2002; Hiemke and Hartter 2000).

One pharmacokinetic study of 29 children (ages 6–12) and 32 adolescents (ages 13–17) with OCD and MDD suggested that at daily doses of 200 mg, half-lives were similar to adults (26 hours for children and 27 hours for adolescents). Children appeared to have higher peak plasma concentrations, but this was likely due to body weight differences. Studies suggest that lower dosages of sertraline will have decreased half-lives in adolescents. Hence twice-daily dosing may be considered in dosages less than 200 mg (Axelson et al. 2002; Findling et al. 2006a).

Adverse Effects Profile

Sertraline's side effects are similar to other SSRIs. It appears to be relatively safe in large overdoses, although death has been reported with some adult patients with large doses.

Efficacy

Two identical RCTs were conducted to compare sertraline and placebo in children and adolescents with MDD. Although the two studies individually did not demonstrate significant differences between sertraline and placebo, when combined, sertraline was superior to placebo on improving MDD symptoms. Of interest is that greater differences were noted in adolescents than in children (Wagner et al. 2003).

In a large RCT involving 187 children and adolescents with OCD (ages 6–17), sertraline led to greater improvement in OCD symptoms over placebo at week 3, which persisted through the remaining 9 weeks of the study (March et al. 1998). Based on this study, sertraline received FDA approval for the treatment of pediatric OCD.

Sertraline has also been examined as part of the Pediatric OCD Treatment Study (POTS), which compared sertraline alone, cognitive-behavioral therapy (CBT) alone, combined sertraline and CBT, or pill placebo for 12 weeks. Combined treatment, CBT, and sertraline displayed statistically meaningful benefit versus placebo, with combined treatment being superior to each individual modality. Individual sertraline and CBT treatments did not display statistically significant differences compared to each other. These investigators concluded that initial treatment for children and

adolescents with OCD should consist of sertraline and CBT or individual CBT (Pediatric OCD Treatment Study 2004).

Most recently, 488 children and adolescents (ages 7–17) with anxiety disorders (separation anxiety disorder, generalized anxiety disorder, or social phobia) were randomly assigned to CBT, sertraline, combination CBT plus sertraline, or a placebo drug for 12 weeks. Combination treatment was more effective than both monotherapies and placebo, with 80.7% responding. Response rates were also higher for both CBT (59.7%) and sertraline alone (54.9%) than placebo (23.7%) (Walkup et al. 2008).

Unlike in the above two studies, sertraline in conjunction with trauma-focused CBT (TF-CBT) was no more effective than TF-CBT plus placebo in a pilot study of 24 female subjects (ages 10–17) with posttraumatic stress disorder (PTSD) related to a history of sexual abuse. Although the study was underpowered, the authors conclude that for children with PTSD, evidence suggests that an initial trial of an evidence-based psychotherapy is warranted prior to treatment with an SSRI (Cohen et al. 2007).

Finally, a small study of 22 children and adolescents with GAD demonstrated some superiority of sertraline over placebo, although this study warrants replication with a larger sample (Rynn et al. 2001).

Atypical Antidepressants

The atypical antidepressants listed below (bupropion, duloxetine, mirtazapine, trazodone, and venlafaxine) have unique mechanisms. Although they are widely used in clinical practice and FDA approved for some adult disorders (Table 47–5), limited data are available for use in children and adolescents. Table 47–6 describes the formulations and recommended dosing for the atypical antidepressants used in children and adolescents. Of note, nefazodone (a mixed serotonin antagonist and reuptake inhibitor) is also an atypical antidepressant; however, because Serzone has been taken off the market in the United States due to the risk of hepatotoxicity, nefazodone is not recommended for children and adolescents, and therefore it will not be reviewed in this chapter.

General Side Effects

These novel antidepressants display a lower side-effect profile than TCAs and MAOIs. Generally, these medi-

TABLE 47–5. U.S. Food and Drug Administration (FDA) indications for atypical antidepressants

Medication	Drug class	FDA-approved indication (adults only)
Bupropion (Wellbutrin)	NDRI	Depression
Duloxetine (Cymbalta)	SSNRI	Depression; GAD
Mirtazapine (Remeron)	NaSSA	Depression
Trazodone (Desyrel)	SARI	Depression
Venlafaxine (Effexor)	SSNRI	Depression; GAD

Note. GAD=generalized anxiety disorder; NaSSA=noradrenergic and specific serotonergic antidepressant; NDRI=norepinephrine-dopamine reuptake inhibitor; SARI=serotonin agonist and serotonin reuptake inhibitor; SSNRI=selective serotonin-norepinephrine reuptake inhibitor.

cations have no sexual side effects (except trazodone), but otherwise share similar untoward effects as the SSRIs. Most side effects manifest within the first few weeks of treatment, and while there is a great deal of individual variation, most resolve with time. Ideally, atypical antidepressants are tapered slowly to avoid discontinuation symptoms. These symptoms are most pronounced with venlafaxine. These novel antidepressants have a higher margin of safety in overdoses compared to TCAs and MAOIs. However, in some cases deaths have been reported with large ingestions.

Contraindications

These antidepressants should not be taken with any of the MAOIs (or within 2 weeks of beginning or discontinuing MAOIs), as these combinations may lead to confusion, high blood pressure, tremor, hyperactivity, and death. In addition, tryptophan can cause head-

aches, nausea, sweating, and dizziness when taken concurrently with these antidepressants. Although rare, coadministration with tramadol hydrochloride can cause seizures. Bupropion should not be given to patients with eating disorders, epilepsy, or high risk for seizures. Blood pressure must be monitored closely in patients taking venlafaxine or duloxetine.

Efficacy

These agents are FDA approved for the treatment of major depressive disorder in adults. Currently, there are no approved indications for children and adolescents, and data supporting their efficacy are limited (Table 47–7). However, based on current guidelines from the Texas Children's Medication Algorithm Project for childhood MDD, bupropion, venlafaxine, mirtazapine, and duloxetine are stage 3 interventions. This means that depressed children should have failed

TABLE 47–6. Formulations and dosing for atypical antidepressants

Medication	Formulations	Initial dose, mg	Target dose, mg Children	Target dose, mg Adolescents	Maximum dose, mg
Bupropion, Bupropion SR	Tablet: 75 mg, 100 mg Tablet ER: 100 mg, 150 mg, 200 mg	100	150–300	300	300
Bupropion XL	Tablet ER: 150 mg, 300 mg	150	150–300	450	450
Duloxetine	Capsule: 20 mg, 30 mg, 60 mg	20 bid	40–60	40–60	60
Mirtazapine	Tablet: 15 mg, 30 mg, 45 mg Tablet (dissolving): 15 mg, 30 mg, 45 mg	7.5–15	15–45	15–45	45
Trazodone	Tablet: 50 mg, 100 mg, 150 mg, 300 mg	25–50	100–150	100–150	150
Venlafaxine XR	Capsule: 37.5 mg, 75 mg, 150 mg	37.5	150–225	150–225	300

Note. bid=twice a day; ER=extended release; SR=sustained release; XL=extended release; XR=extended release.

at least two adequate trials of SSRIs prior to treatment with these novel agents (Hughes et al. 2007). In a meta-analysis of all newer antidepressants, Bridge and colleagues found that the pooled benefit-risk difference favored antidepressants for MDD (including SSRIs and atypical antidepressants), OCD, and anxiety disorders. Of note, for depression this analysis included one trial of nefazodone, two trials of mirtazapine, and two venlafaxine trials. The anxiety disorder analysis also included one trial for venlafaxine in GAD and one venlafaxine trial for social anxiety disorder (Bridge et al. 2007). Table 47–7 describes pharmacokinetics for atypical antidepressants (further information on specific atypical antidepressants is provided in the sections below). Table 47–8 reviews the available evidence for novel antidepressants in child and adolescent psychiatric disorders.

Bupropion

Chemical Structure and Pharmacology

Bupropion is a structurally novel antidepressant that resembles diethylpropion and is related to phenylethylamine. It is classified as a monocyclic phenylbutylamine aminoketone and is highly lipophilic. Bupropion was originally synthesized with the hopes of creating a compound with antidepressant activity but divergent pharmacology from TCAs and MAOIs. Bupropion is a norepinephrine and dopamine reuptake inhibitor. Its effects on serotonin are negligible. It does not have cholinergic activity and is not sympathomimetic (DeVane 1998). It is marketed in immediate-, sustained-, and extended-release forms.

Pharmacokinetics

Bupropion has rapid absorption after oral administration. It is 80% protein bound, has a bioavailability of 90%, and a volume of distribution of 27–60 L/kg. Administration with food has no clinically significant effects on absorption or metabolism. Hepatic impairment appears to extend the half-life of this drug. The effects of renal disease are unknown, but this could likely delay elimination as well (DeVane 1998).

Pharmacokinetic studies have been conducted with adolescent smokers. No differences were found between smoking and nonsmoking adolescents in a study of 75 subjects. However, female adolescents had significantly higher blood levels, a larger volume of distribution, and longer half-lives than males. Bupropion clearance normalized with body weight and did not differ with gender. Although the pharmacokinetics of bupropion in adolescents and adults are similar, studies involving its metabolite, hydroxybupropion, have shown significant differences in adults and adolescents (Daviss et al. 2006a; Hsyu et al. 1997; Stewart et al. 2001).

Adverse Effects Profile

Seizures have occurred with bupropion and are thought to be dose related. At 300 mg/day, the risk for seizure is 0.1%. This increases to 0.4% at doses of 400 mg/day. Bupropion is contraindicated in patients with epilepsy, eating disorders, or other individuals at

TABLE 47–7. Pharmacodynamics and pharmacokinetics of atypical antidepressants

Medication	Half-life	Time to steady state	CYP enzyme inhibited	Kinetics
Bupropion	Biphasic: 1.5 hours 14 hours	8 days	2D6 (potent)	Linear
Bupropion SR	21 hours	8 days	2D6 (potent)	Linear
Duloxetine	12.5 hours	3 days	1A2 (potent) 2D6 (potent)	Linear
Mirtazapine	20–40 hours	4 days	No known inhibition substrate for 1A2, 2D6, 3A4	Linear
Trazodone	Biphasic: 3–6 hours 5–9 hours	Unknown	No known inhibition substrate for 3A4, 2D6	Nonlinear
Venlafaxine XR	10.3 hours	3 days	2D6 (weak) 3A4 (weak)	Linear

Note. CYP=cytochrome P450; SR=sustained release; XR=extended release.

TABLE 47–8. Pediatric randomized controlled trials for atypical antidepressants[a]

Study	Disorder	N	Age	Duration, wks	Primary outcome	Secondary outcomes	Funding source	Comments
Mirtazapine								
Cheung et al. 2005[b]	MDD		7–17		–	–	Organon	2 identical studies
Trazodone								
Battistella et al. 1993	Migraines	40	7–18	12 and 24	–	+		
Venlafaxine								
Mandoki et al. 1997	MDD	33	8–17	6	–	–		All subjects in therapy
Emslie et al. 2007	MDD	334	7–17	8	–	–	Wyeth	2 studies; positive for adolescents; increase in suicidal ideation with venlafaxine
Rynn et al. 2007	GAD	320	6–17	8	+	+	Wyeth	2 studies
March et al. 2007	SOC	293	8–17	16	+	Not reported	Wyeth	

Note. += positive outcome; – = negative outcome; GAD = generalized anxiety disorder; MDD = major depressive disorder; SOC = social phobia.
[a]No studies are available to date for bupropion or duloxetine.
[b]Review of antidepressant studies.

risk for seizures. In addition, coadministration with tramadol hydrochloride can cause seizures. This medication can also precipitate mania, but this may be at a lower rate than SSRIs. Large overdoses of bupropion appear to be nonlethal.

Efficacy

No double-blind, placebo-controlled RCTs of bupropion for anxiety disorders or depression have been conducted in pediatric psychiatry. However, an open trial of bupropion in 24 adolescents (ages 11–16) with ADHD and depression was promising (Daviss et al. 2001), and a small open trial suggested that higher plasma levels of bupropion were associated with treatment response in depressed youth ($n=16$) (Daviss et al. 2006b). For additional information on the use of bupropion for ADHD, see Chapter 46, "Medications Used for Attention-Deficit/Hyperactivity Disorder."

Duloxetine
Chemical Structure and Pharmacology

Duloxetine is a selective serotonin-norepinephrine reuptake inhibitor with comparably high affinity for neurotransmitter systems. It has less potent dopaminergic reuptake inhibition and has minimal affinity for serotonergic, adrenergic, cholinergic, histaminergic, opioid, dopamine, glutamate, and GABA receptors. Duloxetine does not affect monoamine oxidase. These properties are thought to confer less risk for side effects compared to TCAs and MAOIs. Its multiple metabolites do not appear to have relevant pharmacological activity (Hunziker et al. 2005).

Pharmacokinetics

Duloxetine has extensive absorption after oral administration and reaches peak blood levels in approximately 6 hours. Food intake does not appear to have any effect on bioavailability. This drug is not recommended in patients with severe or end-stage renal disease, but mild to moderate renal insufficiency does not appear to impact its clearance. Duloxetine is not recommended for patients with hepatic failure, as metabolism and elimination are decreased (Hunziker et al. 2005). At this time, there are no pharmacokinetic studies of duloxetine in children and adolescents.

Adverse Effects Profile

Small increased heart rate and blood pressure have been reported with duloxetine. In clinical trials, dulox-

etine increased transaminase levels in some patients. Small but significant weight gain (1.4–1.9 kg) has been reported in trials lasting 6 months. Patients treated with duloxetine should be monitored by a physician carefully, and blood pressure should be monitored during treatment. Duloxetine should be given with caution in patients with epilepsy. At this time, there is limited data on safety in large-dose ingestions.

Efficacy

Duloxetine was released in 2004, and there are currently no pediatric trials (RCT or open-label) on duloxetine for any disorder. Two case reports have suggested that duloxetine may improve experience of pain and depressive symptoms in three cases of adolescent females with chronic or severe pain and depressive symptoms (Desarkar et al. 2006; Meighen 2007).

Mirtazapine
Chemical Structure and Pharmacology

Mirtazapine is a piperazino-azepine with a unique pharmacological profile in that it is a noradrenergic and specific serotonergic antidepressant (NaSSA). It is a racemic mixture with potent serotonergic antagonism at 5-HT$_2$ and 5-HT$_3$ receptors but has no affinity for 5-HT$_{1A}$ and 5-HT$_{1B}$ receptors. Mirtazapine is also a central alpha-2-adrenergic and peripheral alpha-1-adrenergic antagonist. Its 5-HT$_2$ and 5-HT$_3$ antagonism is thought to modulate serotonergic neurotransmission by an increase in 5-HT$_{1A}$ activity. It is also a potent histamine (H$_1$) antagonist. Mirtazapine also has some antagonism for muscarinic receptors. It has no affinity for dopamine receptors and does not block serotonin reuptake (Kent 2000).

Pharmacokinetics

Mirtazapine absorption is rapid and complete after oral intake, and food does not appear to affect its absorption. Of note, mirtazapine's pharmacokinetics appear to vary with enantiomers, with the R-enantiomer having higher plasma levels and a longer half-life. Females and elderly patients appear to have higher blood levels than males and young people. Liver and renal failure can decrease mirtazapine clearance by 30%–50% (Timmer et al. 2000).

Pharmacokinetic data in children and adolescents come from a study of one single 15-mg dose for 16 subjects (ages 7–17) with depression. Half-life increased significantly (ranging from 17.8 to 48.4 hours) with increased weight, and maximum plasma concentration decreased with increased age (Findling et al. 2006a).

Adverse Effects Profile

Mirtazapine has fewer side effects than other antidepressants and generally is well tolerated, although the substantial weight gain noted with mirtazapine should be considered when prescribing to youth. Mirtazapine can lead to hypotension, elevated liver enzymes, and leukopenia with a flulike syndrome. Mirtazapine appears to not have any untoward effects on the seizure threshold or cardiovascular system. It appears to have a high margin of safety in overdose. Reported deaths have always involved polydrug ingestions. Nonfatal, single-dose ingestions of 900–1,500 mg have been reported (Kirkton and McIntyre 2006).

Efficacy

Two multicenter trials of children and adolescents (ages 7–17) with MDD were conducted to compare mirtazapine (15–45 mg/day) and placebo, with no significant differences on any of the outcome variables in either study (Cheung et al. 2005). No studies of mirtazapine in other psychiatric disorders in youth have been reported.

Trazodone

Chemical Structure and Pharmacology

Trazodone is a triazolopyridine derivative with a structure unique to other antidepressants. However, it does resemble side-chain groups of phenothiazines and TCAs. Its triazole moiety is thought to confer antidepressant properties. Trazodone blocks presynaptic reuptake of serotonin with lower potency than SSRIs. It is relatively specific and has negligible effects on dopamine or norepinephrine reuptake. Other serotonergic effects of this drug are complex and include serotonin receptor antagonism, particularly 5-HT$_2$. Its major active metabolite, *m*-chlorophenylpiperazine (m-CPP), is a potent serotonin agonist. Thus, trazodone is a serotonin reuptake inhibitor and a mixed serotonergic agonist and antagonist.

Pharmacokinetics

Trazodone is almost completely absorbed after oral administration and reaches peak plasma concentrations in approximately 1 hour on an empty stomach (2 hours if taken with food). Age and food do not appear to alter bioavailability. Trazodone is approximately 90%–95% protein bound. It has biphasic elimination with half-lives of 3–6 hours for the first phase and 5–9 hours for the second phase.

Adverse Effects Profile

Side effects with trazodone can be immediate, but usually wane with time. Trazodone has an association with priapism. In approximately one-third of these cases, surgery is required. Sometimes erectile functioning is permanently compromised. Patients and families must be educated about this risk. Males with prolonged erections should be instructed to seek emergency medical care. Trazodone can be lethal when combined with alcohol or other drugs. Other antidepressants, such as SSRIs, can increase trazodone's blood level.

Efficacy

No placebo-controlled RCTs have examined trazodone for treatment of pediatric depressive or anxiety disorders. One double-blind, crossover trial evaluated trazodone for treatment of migraines in pediatric patients. Although both the active treatment and placebo groups improved initially, only those on trazodone during the second phase of the study continued to show improvement in migraines (Battistella et al. 1993).

Despite the frequent use of trazodone to improve sleep disturbance, no studies have been conducted to examine the effects of trazodone on sleep. One retrospective chart review suggested that trazodone treatment led to faster improvement in sleep disturbance compared to fluoxetine (2 days vs. 4 days). However, the difference, although statistically significant, was not considered clinically significant by the authors (Kallepalli et al. 1997).

Venlafaxine

Chemical Structure and Pharmacology

Venlafaxine is a novel bicyclic phenylethylamine derivative that inhibits presynaptic serotonin and norepinephrine reuptake. It is a weak inhibitor of dopamine. Venlafaxine's major active metabolite, O-desmethylvenlafaxine (ODV), has similar actions. Venlafaxine and ODV have no clinically meaningful affinity for cholinergic, histaminergic, or alpha-adrenergic receptors. This drug has one chiral center and is a racemic mixture. Its R-enantiomer confers dual inhibition of serotonin and norepinephrine reuptake. The S-enantiomer primarily inhibits serotonin. Other minor metabolites with lower potencies include N-demethylvenlafaxine and N,O-didemethylvenlafaxine. Venlafaxine is marketed in immediate- and extended-release formulations (Horst and Preskorn 1998).

Pharmacokinetics

Venlafaxine is easily absorbed with oral administration. It is subjected to extensive hepatic metabolism to form ODV. Food can slow the rate of absorption but does not decrease its absolute bioavailability (which is 45%). Among antidepressants, venlafaxine has a favorable side-effect profile with regard to the cytochrome P450 system.

There is one multiple-dose pharmacokinetic study of venlafaxine in children and adolescents. This involved 6 children and 6 adolescents on daily doses near 2 mg/kg. Investigators concluded that exposure to venlafaxine and ODV was lower in children and adolescents than observed in adults with similar dosing regimens (Findling et al. 2006a).

Adverse Effects Profile

In clinical trials of this medication, dropout rates are high. Venlafaxine has caused ECG changes and blood pressure elevations, so blood pressure should be monitored regularly. Treatment-emergent suicidal thinking and agitation in children and adolescents may be more common with venlafaxine than with other antidepressants. In the safety analyses conducted by the FDA, venlafaxine was the only individual antidepressant to have significantly more suicide-related adverse events than placebo, which was primarily driven by increased suicidal ideation (Hammad et al. 2006). Patients require close monitoring when initiating and taking this medication. A fatal 30 g overdose of venlafaxine has been reported (Mazur et al. 2003).

Efficacy

Three double-blind, controlled trials of venlafaxine have been conducted in children and adolescents with MDD, none of which demonstrated efficacy of venlafaxine over placebo (Emslie et al. 2007; Mandoki et al. 1997). Emslie et al. (2007) combined the two large studies—and although there was still no difference between active treatment and placebo in the overall sample, only the subgroup of adolescents found greater improvement in depression with venlafaxine over placebo, suggesting that adolescents may show more response to venlafaxine treatment than younger children.

As a result of limited acute efficacy support and the increased risk of emergent suicidal thinking, venlafaxine is currently a third-line treatment option for youth with treatment-resistant MDD. However, recently,

Brent and colleagues (2008) reported on 334 adolescents with depression who had not responded to SSRI treatment and were subsequently randomly assigned to an alternative SSRI or venlafaxine (both medications with or without CBT). No differences were found between the two medication options, although adding CBT improved outcomes. Thus, in youth who do not improve with initial SSRI treatment, switching to an alternative SSRI or venlafaxine is equally effective.

Venlafaxine has also been examined for GAD and social phobia. In the report on GAD, two RCTs were combined to evaluate venlafaxine in 320 children and adolescents (ages 6–17), with venlafaxine demonstrating greater improvements in reduction of anxiety symptoms than placebo. On the individual studies, one study was positive on the primary and secondary outcomes, while the second study was only positive on some secondary outcomes (Rynn et al. 2007).

The RCT of venlafaxine for social phobia also showed superiority of venlafaxine in reducing anxiety symptoms (March et al. 2007). Thus, venlafaxine appears to be more efficacious for pediatric anxiety disorders than depression.

Tricyclic Antidepressants

TCAs include tertiary amines (amitriptyline, clomipramine, and imipramine) and secondary amines (such as desipramine and nortriptyline). Tertiary amines are serotonin and norepinephrine reuptake inhibitors, while secondary amines (which are the metabolites of tertiary amines) primarily inhibit the norepinephrine transporter. The use of these agents in children has fallen out of favor with the advent of newer antidepressants and case reports of sudden death in children taking TCAs. Table 47–9 lists the pharmacokinetics of TCAs.

Adverse effects of TCAs involve anticholinergic side effects, such as dry mouth, blurred vision, and constipation. Long-term use may be associated with weight gain. Documented cardiovascular effects include tachycardia, hypertension, arrhythmias, and impaired conduction. Children may be more susceptible to these effects as they are presumed to have increased metabolism to the desmethyl forms of some TCAs, which are more cardiotoxic. This risk appears to be greatest for children under the age of 12.

TCAs have been employed for the treatment of depression, ADHD, enuresis, OCD, separation anxiety disorder, and pervasive developmental disorders in children and adolescents. Meta-analyses of TCAs have shown no significant differences from placebo in de-

TABLE 47–9. Pharmacodynamics and pharmacokinetics of tricyclic antidepressants

Medication	Half-life	Time to steady state	CYP enzyme inhibited	Kinetics
Tertiary amines				
Amitriptyline	10–40 hours	4–10 days	2D6 (weak) 2C19 (moderate)	Linear
Clomipramine	16–36 hours	3–4 weeks	2D6 (weak)	Linear
Imipramine	11–25 hours	2–5 days	2D6 (weak) 2C19 (moderate)	Linear
Secondary amines				
Desipramine	12–76 hours	2–11 days	2D6 (weak)	Nonlinear
Nortriptyline	16–90 hours	4–19 days	2D6 (moderate)	Linear

Note. CYP=cytochrome P450.

pressed youth (Maneeton and Srisurapanont 2000). However, TCAs may be more efficacious for anxiety disorders. Three small controlled studies of clomipramine for OCD demonstrated positive benefit (De-Veaugh-Geiss et al. 1992; Flament et al. 1985; Leonard et al. 1989). However, clomipramine did not show benefit compared to placebo in an RCT for school refusal (Berney et al. 1981). Three RCTs of imipramine for school phobia have demonstrated efficacy (Bernstein et al. 1990, 2000; Gittelman-Klein and Klein 1973). One other study of imipramine for separation anxiety did not demonstrate efficacy (R.G. Klein et al. 1992).

Thus, the unfavorable side-effect profile of TCAs and limited evidence of efficacy makes it difficult to determine the role of TCAs in pediatric psychopharmacology. They might be considered in cases where multiple agents have failed or when other family members have had a positive response, but they are not considered a first-line treatment option for any disorder.

Monoamine Oxidase Inhibitors

MAOIs (such as phenelzine, isocarboxazid, tranylcypromine, selegiline, moclobemide, and brofaromine) modulate the concentration of monoamines in the central nervous system (CNS) by inhibiting either MAO-A or MAO-B isoforms. These medications are seldom used in children and adolescents due to requisite dietary restrictions, concern of multiple side effects, and multiple dangerous (possibly fatal) drug-drug interactions. No research has been conducted on any of these medications in the pediatric population.

Alternative Antidepressant Treatments

The use of alternative or complementary medicine is popular among pediatric patients despite little empirical evidence. The most commonly used remedies for depressive and anxiety disorders are St. John's wort, omega-3 fatty acid, and S-adenosylmethionine.

In open studies of St. John's wort, a daily dose between 300 mg to 1,800 mg was well tolerated by children. No RTCs of St. John's wort in pediatric depression or anxiety disorders have been published.

One small controlled study with pediatric depression has been done with omega-3 fish oil. Nemets and colleagues (2006) reported the data on 20 Israeli children with depression randomized to omega-3 fish oil or placebo for 16 weeks. Of children who received a 1,000 mg daily dose of omega-3 fish oil, 70% responded versus 0% in the placebo group. The omega-3 fish oil was well tolerated and no significant side effects were reported. No studies of omega-3 fish oil have been reported in pediatric anxiety disorder.

No pediatric studies in pediatric depressive or anxiety disorders have been done for S-adenosylmethionine.

Research Directions

Little research has been done on the long-term impact of antidepressants on children and adolescents. For example, how does treatment with antidepressants affect the developing brain? It is unknown if these medications lead to permanent changes in the brain, either positively or negatively. Additional studies are needed not only on the efficacy of these medications but also on their safety (both short- and long-term). Additional data are also still needed on pharmacokinetics and dosing specific to this age group.

Summary Points

- SSRIs are generally well tolerated in children and adolescents and have demonstrated efficacy in depression and anxiety disorders.
- SSRIs are considered the first-line pharmacological treatment for both MDD and anxiety disorders.
- Fluoxetine is the only antidepressant with an FDA indication for treatment of both children and adolescents with MDD. Escitalopram has an FDA indication for adolescents with MDD. Fluoxetine, sertraline, and fluvoxamine have an FDA indication for treatment of pediatric OCD.
- No non-SSRIs have demonstrated efficacy for acute MDD, but some appear efficacious in anxiety disorders. Non-SSRIs may be beneficial for youth who do not respond to SSRIs, although only one study of treatment-resistant MDD has been conducted to examine this strategy.
- Dose-finding studies are needed.

References

Abikoff H, McGough J, Vitiello B, et al: Sequential pharmacotherapy for children with comorbid attention-deficit/hyperactivity and anxiety disorders. J Am Acad Child Adolesc Psychiatry 44:418–427, 2005

Aronson S, Delgado P: Escitalopram. Drugs Today (Barc) 40:121–131, 2004

Axelson DA, Perel JM, Birmaher B, et al: Sertraline pharmacokinetics and dynamics in adolescents. J Am Acad Child Adolesc Psychiatry 41:1037–1044, 2002

Battistella PA, Ruffilli R, Cernetti R, et al: A placebo-controlled crossover trial using trazodone in pediatric migraine. Headache 33:36–39, 1993

Baumann P, Larsen F: The pharmacokinetics of citalopram. Reviews in Contemporary Pharmacotherapy 6:271–285, 1995

Berard R, Fong R, Carpenter DJ, et al: An international, multicenter, placebo-controlled trial of paroxetine in adolescents with major depressive disorder. J Child Adolesc Psychopharmacol 16:59–75, 2006

Berney T, Kolvin I, Bhate SR, et al: School phobia: a therapeutic trial with clomipramine and short-term outcome. Br J Psychiatry 138:110–118, 1981

Bernstein GA, Garfinkel BD, Borchardt CM: Comparative studies of pharmacotherapy for school refusal. J Am Acad Child Adolesc Psychiatry 29:773–781, 1990

Bernstein GA, Borchardt CM, Perwien AR, et al: Imipramine plus cognitive-behavioral therapy in the treatment of school refusal. J Am Acad Child Adolesc Psychiatry 39:276–283, 2000

Bezchlibnyk-Butler K, Aleksic I, Kennedy SH: Citalopram: a review of pharmacological and clinical effects. J Psychiatry Neurosci 25:241–254, 2000

Birmaher B, Ryan N, Williamson DE, et al: Childhood and adolescent depression: a review of the past 10 years, part I. J Am Acad Child Adolesc Psychiatry 35:1427–1439, 1996

Birmaher B, Axelson DA, Monk K, et al: Fluoxetine for the treatment of childhood anxiety disorders. J Am Acad Child Adolesc Psychiatry 42:415–423, 2003

Birmaher B, Brent D, Bernet W, et al: Practice parameter for the assessment and treatment of children and adolescents with depressive disorders. J Am Acad Child Adolesc Psychiatry 46:1503–1526, 2007

Black B, Uhde TW: Treatment of elective mutism with fluoxetine: a double-blind, placebo-controlled study. J Am Acad Child Adolesc Psychiatry 33:1000–1006, 1994

Brent D, Emslie G, Clarke G, et al: Switching to another SSRI or to venlafaxine with or without cognitive behavioral therapy for adolescents with SSRI-resistant depression: the TORDIA randomized controlled trial. JAMA 299:901–913, 2008

Bridge JA, Iyengar S, Salary CB, et al: Clinical response and risk for reported suicidal ideation and suicide attempts in pediatric antidepressant treatment: a meta-analysis of randomized controlled trials. JAMA 297:1683–1696, 2007

Cheung A, Emslie GJ, Mayes TL: Review of the efficacy and safety of antidepressants in youth depression. J Child Psychol Psychiatry 46:735–754, 2005

Cheung A, Zuckerbrot RA, Jensen PS, et al: Guidelines for Adolescent Depression in Primary Care (GLAD-PC), II:

treatment and ongoing management. Pediatrics 120:e1313–e1326, 2007

Cohen JA, Mannarino AP, Perel JM, et al: A pilot randomized controlled trial of combined trauma-focused CBT and sertraline for childhood PTSD symptoms. J Am Acad Child Adolesc Psychiatry 46:811–819, 2007

Connolly SD, Bernstein GA: Practice parameter for the assessment and treatment of children and adolescents with anxiety disorders. J Am Acad Child Adolesc Psychiatry 46:267–283, 2007

Daviss WB, Bentivoglio P, Racusin R, et al: Bupropion sustained release in adolescents with comorbid attention-deficit/hyperactivity disorder and depression. J Am Acad Child Adolesc Psychiatry 40:307–314, 2001

Daviss WB, Perel JM, Birmaher B, et al: Steady-state clinical pharmacokinetics of bupropion extended-release in youths. J Am Acad Child Adolesc Psychiatry 45:1503–1509, 2006a

Daviss WB, Perel JM, Brent DA, et al: Acute antidepressant response and plasma levels of bupropion and metabolites in a pediatric-aged sample: an exploratory study. Ther Drug Monit 28:190–198, 2006b

Desarkar P, Das A, Sinha VK: Duloxetine for childhood depression with pain and dissociative symptoms. Eur Child Adolesc Psychiatry 15:496–499, 2006

DeVane CL: Pharmacokinetics of the selective serotonin reuptake inhibitors. J Clin Psychiatry 53(suppl):13–20, 1992

DeVane CL: Differential pharmacology of newer antidepressants. J Clin Psychiatry 59(suppl):85–93, 1998

DeVane CL, Liston HL, Markowitz JS: Clinical pharmacokinetics of sertraline. Clin Pharmacokinet 41:1247–1266, 2002

DeVeaugh-Geiss J, Moroz G, Biederman J, et al: Clomipramine hydrochloride in childhood and adolescent obsessive-compulsive disorder: a multicenter trial. J Am Acad Child Adolesc Psychiatry 31:45–49, 1992

Emslie GJ, Rush AJ, Weinberg WA, et al: A double-blind, randomized, placebo-controlled trial of fluoxetine in children and adolescents with depression. Arch Gen Psychiatry 54:1031–1037, 1997

Emslie GJ, Heiligenstein JH, Wagner KD, et al: Fluoxetine for acute treatment of depression in children and adolescents: a placebo-controlled, randomized clinical trial. J Am Acad Child Adolesc Psychiatry 41:1205–1215, 2002

Emslie GJ, Wagner KD, Kutcher S, et al: Paroxetine treatment in children and adolescents with major depressive disorder: a randomized, multicenter, double-blind, placebo-controlled trial. J Am Acad Child Adolesc Psychiatry 45:709–719, 2006

Emslie GJ, Findling RL, Yeung PP, et al: Venlafaxine ER for the treatment of pediatric subjects with depression: results of two placebo-controlled trials. J Am Acad Child Adolesc Psychiatry 46:479–488, 2007

Emslie GJ, Ventura D, Korotzer A, et al: Escitalopram in the treatment of adolescent depression: a randomized placebo-controlled multisite trial. J Am Acad Child Adolesc Psychiatry 48:721–729, 2009

Findling RL, Reed MD, Myers C, et al: Paroxetine pharmacokinetics in depressed children and adolescents. J Am Acad Child Adolesc Psychiatry 38:952–959, 1999

Findling RL, McNamara NK, Stansbrey RJ, et al: The relevance of pharmacokinetic studies in designing efficacy trials in juvenile major depression. J Child Adolesc Psychopharmacol 16:131–145, 2006a

Findling RL, Nucci G, Piergies AA, et al: Multiple dose pharmacokinetics of paroxetine in children and adolescents with major depressive disorder or obsessive-compulsive disorder. Neuropsychopharmacology 31:1274–1285, 2006b

Flament MF, Rapoport JL, Berg CJ, et al: Clomipramine treatment of childhood obsessive-compulsive disorder: a double-blind controlled study. Arch Gen Psychiatry 42:977–983, 1985

Friedman RA, Leon AC: Expanding the black box: depression, antidepressants, and the risk of suicide. N Engl J Med 356:2343–2346, 2007

Geller DA, Hoog SL, Heiligenstein JH, et al: Fluoxetine treatment for obsessive-compulsive disorder in children and adolescents: a placebo-controlled clinical trial. J Am Acad Child Adolesc Psychiatry 40:773–779, 2001

Geller DA, Wagner KD, Emslie GJ, et al: Paroxetine treatment in children and adolescents with obsessive-compulsive disorder: a randomized, multicenter, double-blind, placebo-controlled trial. J Am Acad Child Adolesc Psychiatry 43:1387–1396, 2004

Gittelman-Klein R, Klein DF: School phobia: diagnostic considerations in the light of imipramine effects. J Nerv Ment Dis 156:199–215, 1973

Greenhill LL, Vitiello B, Fisher P, et al: Comparison of increasingly detailed elicitation methods for the assessment of adverse events in pediatric psychopharmacology. J Am Acad Child Adolesc Psychiatry 43:1488–1496, 2004

Hammad TA, Laughren T, Racoosin J: Suicidality in pediatric patients treated with antidepressant drugs. Arch Gen Psychiatry 63:332–339, 2006

Henry JA: Overdose and safety with fluvoxamine. Int Clin Psychopharmacol 6(suppl):41–45; discussion 45–47, 1991

Hiemke C, Hartter S: Pharmacokinetics of selective serotonin reuptake inhibitors. Pharmacol Ther 85:11–28, 2000

Hollander E, Phillips A, Chaplin W, et al: A placebo controlled crossover trial of liquid fluoxetine on repetitive behaviors in childhood and adolescent autism. Neuropsychopharmacology 30:582–589, 2005

Horst WD, Preskorn SH: Mechanisms of action and clinical characteristics of three atypical antidepressants: venlafaxine, nefazodone, bupropion. J Affect Disord 51:237–254, 1998

Hsyu PH, Singh A, Giargiari TD, et al: Pharmacokinetics of bupropion and its metabolites in cigarette smokers versus nonsmokers. J Clin Pharmacol 37:737–743, 1997

Hughes CW, Emslie GJ, Crismon ML, et al: Texas Children's Medication Algorithm Project: update from Texas Consensus Conference Panel on Medication Treatment of Childhood Major Depressive Disorder. J Am Acad Child Adolesc Psychiatry 46:667–686, 2007

Hunziker ME, Suehs BT, Bettinger TL, et al: Duloxetine hydrochloride: a new dual-acting medication for the treatment of major depressive disorder. Clin Ther 27:1126–1143, 2005

Hyttel J, Arnt J, Sanchez C: The pharmacology of citalopram. Reviews in Contemporary Pharmacotherapy 6:271–285, 1995

Kallepalli BR, Bhatara VS, Fogas BS, et al: Trazodone is only slightly faster than fluoxetine in relieving insomnia in adolescents with depressive disorders. J Child Adolesc Psychopharmacol 7:97–107, 1997

Keller MB, Ryan N, Strober M, et al: Efficacy of paroxetine in the treatment of adolescent major depression: a randomized, controlled trial. J Am Acad Child Adolesc Psychiatry 40:762–772, 2001

Kent JM: SNaRIs, NaSSAs, and NaRIs: new agents for the treatment of depression. Lancet 355:911–918, 2000

Kirkton C, McIntyre IM: Therapeutic and toxic concentrations of mirtazapine. J Anal Toxicol 30:687–691, 2006

Klein N, Sacher J, Geiss-Granadia T, et al: Higher serotonin transporter occupancy after multiple dose administration of escitalopram compared to citalopram: an [123I]ADAM SPECT study. Psychopharmacology (Berl) 191:333–339, 2007

Klein RG, Koplewicz HS, Kanner A: Imipramine treatment of children with separation anxiety disorder. J Am Acad Child Adolesc Psychiatry 31:21–28, 1992

Labellarte MJ, Biederman J, Emslie GJ, et al: Multiple-dose pharmacokinetics of fluvoxamine in children and adolescents. J Am Acad Child Adolesc Psychiatry 43:1497–1505, 2004

Leonard HL, Swedo SE, Rapoport JL, et al: Treatment of obsessive-compulsive disorder with clomipramine and desipramine in children and adolescents: a double-blind crossover comparison. Arch Gen Psychiatry 46:1088–1092, 1989

Liebowitz MR, Turner SM, Piacentini J, et al: Fluoxetine in children and adolescents with OCD: a placebo-controlled trial. J Am Acad Child Adolesc Psychiatry 41:1431–1438, 2002

LoVecchio F, Watts D, Winchell J, et al: Outcomes after supratherapeutic escitalopram ingestions. J Emerg Med 30:17–19, 2006

Luchini D, Morabito G, Centini F: Case report of a fatal intoxication by citalopram. Am J Forensic Med Pathol 26:352–354, 2005

Mandoki MW, Tapia MR, Tapia MA, et al: Venlafaxine in the treatment of children and adolescents with major depression. Psychopharmacol Bull 33:149–154, 1997

Maneeton N, Srisurapanont M: Tricyclic antidepressants for depressive disorders in children and adolescents: a meta-analysis of randomized-controlled trials. J Med Assoc Thai 83:1367–1374, 2000

March JS, Biederman J, Wolkow R, et al: Sertraline in children and adolescents with obsessive-compulsive disorder. JAMA 280:1752–1756, 1998

March JS, Silva S, Compton SN, et al: The Child and Adolescent Psychiatry Trials Network (CAPTN). J Am Acad Child Adolesc Psychiatry 43:515–518, 2004

March JS, Entusah AR, Rynn M, et al: A randomized controlled trial of venlafaxine ER versus placebo in pediatric social anxiety disorder. Biol Psychiatry 62:1149–1154, 2007

Mayes TL, Tao R, Rintelmann JW, et al: Do children and adolescents have differential response rates in placebo-controlled trials of fluoxetine? CNS Spectr 12:147–154, 2007

Mazur JE, Doty JD, Krygiel AS: Fatality related to a 30-g venlafaxine overdose. Pharmacotherapy 23:1668–1672, 2003

McDougle CJ, Kresch LE, Posey DJ: Repetitive thoughts and behavior in pervasive developmental disorders: treatment with serotonin reuptake inhibitors. J Autism Dev Disord 30:427–435, 2000

Meighen KG: Duloxetine treatment of pediatric chronic pain and comorbid major depressive disorder. J Child Adolesc Psychopharmacol 17:121–127, 2007

Myers LB, Krenzelok EP: Paroxetine (Paxil) overdose: a pediatric focus. Vet Hum Toxicol 39:86–88, 1997

Nemets H, Nemets B, Apter A, et al: Omega-3 treatment of childhood depression: a controlled, double-blind pilot study. Am J Psychiatry 163:1098–1100, 2006

Ostrom M, Eriksson A, Thorson J, et al: Fatal overdose with citalopram. Lancet 348:339–340, 1996

Pediatric OCD Treatment Study: Cognitive-behavior therapy, sertraline, and their combination for children and adolescents with obsessive-compulsive disorder: the Pediatric OCD Treatment Study (POTS) randomized controlled trial. JAMA 292:1969–1976, 2004

Personne M, Persson H, Sjoberg E: Citalopram toxicity. Lancet 350:518–519, 1997

Rao N: The clinical pharmacokinetics of escitalopram. Clin Pharmacokinet 46:281–290, 2007

Research Unit on Pediatric Psychopharmacology, Walkup JT, Labellarte MJ, et al: Fluvoxamine for the treatment of anxiety disorders in children and adolescents. The Research Unit on Pediatric Psychopharmacology Anxiety Study Group. N Engl J Med 344:1279–1285, 2001

Riddle MA, Scahill L, King RA, et al: Double-blind, crossover trial of fluoxetine and placebo in children and adolescents with obsessive-compulsive disorder. J Am Acad Child Adolesc Psychiatry 31:1062–1069, 1992

Riddle MA, Reeve EA, Yaryura-Tobias JA, et al: Fluvoxamine for children and adolescents with obsessive-compulsive disorder: a randomized, controlled, multicenter trial. J Am Acad Child Adolesc Psychiatry 40:222–229, 2001

Rynn MA, Siqueland L, Rickels K: Placebo-controlled trial of sertraline in the treatment of children with generalized anxiety disorder. Am J Psychiatry 158:2008–2014, 2001

Rynn MA, Riddle MA, Yeung PP, et al: Efficacy and safety of extended-release venlafaxine in the treatment of generalized anxiety disorder in children and adolescents: two placebo-controlled trials. Am J Psychiatry 164:290–300, 2007

Simeon JG, Dinicola VF, Ferguson HB, et al: Adolescent depression: a placebo-controlled fluoxetine treatment study and follow-up. Prog Neuropsychopharmacol Biol Psychiatry 14:791–795, 1990

Stewart JJ, Berkel HJ, Parish RC, et al: Single-dose pharmacokinetics of bupropion in adolescents: effects of smoking status and gender. J Clin Pharmacol 41:770–778, 2001

Sugie Y, Sugie H, Fukuda T, et al: Clinical efficacy of fluvoxamine and functional polymorphism in a serotonin transporter gene on childhood autism. J Autism Dev Disord 35:377–385, 2005

Timmer CJ, Sitsen JM, Delbressine LP: Clinical pharmacokinetics of mirtazapine. Clin Pharmacokinet 38:461–474, 2000

Treatment for Adolescents With Depression Study: Fluoxetine, cognitive-behavioral therapy, and their combination for adolescents with depression: Treatment for Adolescents With Depression Study (TADS) randomized controlled trial. JAMA 292:807–820, 2004

U.S. Food and Drug Administration: Guidance for Industry: Industry Supported Scientific and Educational Activities. Fed Regist 62:64093–64100, 1997

von Knorring AL, Olsson GI, Thomsen PH, et al: A randomized, double-blind, placebo-controlled study of citalopram in adolescents with major depressive disorder. J Clin Psychopharmacol 26:311–315, 2006

Wagner KD, Ambrosini PJ, Rynn M, et al: Efficacy of sertraline in the treatment of children and adolescents with major depressive disorder: two randomized controlled trials. JAMA 290:1033–1041, 2003

Wagner KD, Berard R, Stein MB, et al: A multicenter, randomized, double-blind, placebo-controlled trial of paroxetine in children and adolescents with social anxiety disorder. Arch Gen Psychiatry 61:1153–1162, 2004a

Wagner KD, Robb AS, Findling RL, et al: A randomized, placebo-controlled trial of citalopram for the treatment of major depression in children and adolescents. Am J Psychiatry 161:1079–1083, 2004b

Wagner KD, Jonas J, Findling RL, et al: A double-blind, randomized, placebo-controlled trial of escitalopram in the treatment of pediatric depression. J Am Acad Child Adolesc Psychiatry 45:280–288, 2006

Walkup JT, Albano AM, Piacentini J, et al: Cognitive behavioral therapy, sertraline, or a combination in childhood anxiety. N Engl J Med 359:2753–2766, 2008

Chapter 48

Mood Stabilizers

Robert A. Kowatch, M.D., Ph.D.
Arman Danielyan, M.D.

The mood stabilizers lithium and valproate have been used to treat children and adolescents with mood and seizure disorders for many years. Lithium was first used over 40 years ago to treat "manic-depressive" illness in children (Annell 1969). Since then, a variety of "mood stabilizing" agents have been used to treat psychiatric disorders in children and adolescents. The mood stabilizers can be divided into the traditional agents—lithium, valproate, and carbamazepine—and the newer or "novel" agents. The novel mood stabilizers include lamotrigine, oxcarbazepine, topiramate, and gabapentin (Weisler et al. 2006). These agents have migrated from pediatric neurology to child psychiatry after clinicians noticed their behavioral effects. All of these drugs have been used to treat children and adolescents with mood and/or behavior problems, and all of these agents, except lithium, are used to treat seizure disorders. Now that six atypical antipsychotics are available in the United States, these mood stabilizers

are not prescribed as often as they once were. Lithium and valproate are still often used to treat bipolar disorder in children and adolescents, and the evidence base for the safety and efficacy of these two mood stabilizers as well as the newer antiepileptic agents in children and adolescents is steadily increasing (Kowatch and DelBello 2006; Pavuluri et al. 2005).

Lithium

Lithium carbonate is the most well-studied mood stabilizer in children and adolescents and is the only mood stabilizer approved by the U.S. Food and Drug Administration (FDA) for the treatment of "manic episodes of manic-depressive illness" in patients ages 12 years and older. Lithium carbonate is a naturally occurring salt that was discovered in 1937 to have mood-stabilizing properties by the Australian urologist, Joseph Cade (1949). Lithium has multiple complex effects in the central nervous system (CNS), particularly at the second messenger level. These effects include 1) blocking the activity of inositol polyphosphatase 1-phosphatase and inositol second messenger systems; 2) inhibiting adenyl cyclase by competing with magnesium in this second messenger system; 3) down-regulating hippocampal serotonin (5-HT$_{1A}$) receptors; 4) increasing the proportion of low-affinity β receptors; 5) inducing subsensitivity of α$_2$ receptors; and 6) increasing dopamine levels in tuberoinfundibular pathways (Alessi et al. 1994). In addition, recent data suggest that lithium, along with valproate, may have neurotrophic effects via indirectly regulating a number of factors involved in cell survival pathways, including cAMP response element-binding protein, brain-derived neurotrophic factor, bcl-2, and mitogen-activated protein kinases (Manji and Zarate 2002).

Disorders in Which Lithium May Be Useful

Lithium has been used for many years in children and adolescents to treat child- and adolescent-onset mania (Brumback and Weinberg 1977; Campbell et al. 1984; Dyson and Barcai 1970; Varanka et al. 1988); recently for bipolar depression (Patel et al. 2006); for aggressive behavior in hospitalized children with conduct disorder (Campbell et al. 1972, 1995a, 1995b; Malone et al. 2000); for the treatment of bipolar adolescents with comorbid substance use disorders (Geller et al. 1998a); and for manic symptoms secondary to traumatic brain injury in children (Cohn et al. 1989).

Lithium may also be useful for the prevention of mood episodes in children and adolescents with bipolar disorder. Strober et al. (1990) prospectively evaluated 37 adolescents whose mood had been stabilized with lithium while hospitalized. After 18 months of naturalistic follow-up, 35% of these patients had discontinued lithium; of those who discontinued, 92% subsequently relapsed as compared to 38% of those who were lithium compliant, suggesting the potential utility of lithium for maintenance treatment for bipolar disorder in adolescents.

Evidence for Efficacy

There have been six older "controlled" trials of lithium in bipolar children and adolescents. Of these six studies, four (DeLong and Nieman 1983; Gram and Rafaelsen 1972; Lena 1979; McKnew et al. 1981) used a

crossover design, which is not ideal for assessing outcome in an illness whose inherent nature is to wax and wane. The average number of subjects in each of these older studies was 18, and response rates ranged from 33%–80%, reflecting the heterogeneity of the sample and the differences among study designs. Several open-label studies suggest that approximately 40%–50% of manic children and adolescents with bipolar disorder will improve symptomatically with lithium monotherapy (Findling et al. 2003; Kowatch et al. 2000; Youngerman and Canino 1978).

In a small ($n=25$), prospective, placebo-controlled trial of lithium in children and adolescents with bipolar disorders and comorbid substance abuse, subjects treated with lithium for 6 weeks showed a significant improvement in global assessment of functioning (46% response rate in the lithium-treated group vs. 8% response rate in the placebo group) (Geller et al. 1998a). There was also a statistically significant decrease in positive urine toxicology screens following lithium treatment. But this was a small study, not all of these subjects met full criteria for bipolar I disorder (some were "bipolar with 'predictors'"), and no specific mania rating scales were used.

In an open, prospective study of 100 adolescents ages 12–18 years with an acute manic episode treated with lithium, 63 adolescents met response criteria and 26 achieved remission of manic symptoms at the week 4 assessment (Kafantaris et al. 2003). Prominent depressive features, age at first mood episode, severity of mania, and comorbidity with attention-deficit/hyperactivity disorder (ADHD) did *not* distinguish responders from nonresponders to lithium. Kafantaris et al. (2004) subsequently reported the results of a placebo-controlled, discontinuation study of lithium in adolescents with mania. There were 40 subjects in this study with a mean age of 15 years. During the first part of this study, subjects received open treatment with lithium at therapeutic serum levels (mean 0.99 mEq/L) for at least 4 weeks. Responders to lithium were then randomly assigned to continue or discontinue lithium during a 2-week double-blind, placebo-controlled phase. Of these subjects, 58% experienced a clinically significant symptom exacerbation during the 2-week double-blind phase. However, the slightly lower exacerbation rate in the group maintained on lithium (53%) versus the group switched to placebo (62%) did not reach statistical significance. This study did not appear to support a large effect for lithium continuation treatment of adolescents with acute mania, but with only a 2-week discontinuation period, it is hard to draw definitive conclusions about the efficacy of lithium in adolescents with mania. It is very possible that if the discontinuation period had been longer, a clear separation between the lithium and placebo groups would have been observed.

Recently, Patel et al. (2006) evaluated the use of lithium in 27 adolescents (12–18 years old) with an episode of depression associated with bipolar disorder, type I. These patients received open-label lithium, which was adjusted to achieve a therapeutic serum level (1.0–1.2 mEq/L). The mean scores of the Childhood Depression Rating Scale, Revised (CDRS-R), in these patients decreased significantly from baseline to endpoint, resulting in a large effect size of 1.7. The findings of this study suggest that lithium is effective for the treatment of an acute episode of depression in adolescents with bipolar disorder, although controlled trials are needed.

Several studies have demonstrated the usefulness of lithium for aggressive behaviors in the context of conduct disorder. In 1972, Campbell and colleagues reported that lithium was effective in "hyperactive severely disturbed young children" (Campbell et al. 1972). Subsequent controlled studies by Campbell and others have demonstrated the efficacy of lithium for children and adolescents with aggression and conduct disorder (Campbell et al. 1995a; Malone et al. 2000).

Baseline Assessments

Baseline studies prior to initiating treatment with lithium should include a general medical history and physical examination; serum electrolytes; creatinine, serum urea nitrogen, and serum calcium levels; thyroid function tests; electrocardiogram (ECG); complete blood count with differential; and a pregnancy test for sexually active females (Danielyan and Kowatch 2005). Renal function should be tested every 2–3 months during the first 6 months of treatment and thyroid function should be tested during the first 6 months of treatment (McClellan et al. 2007). Thereafter, renal and thyroid functions should be checked every 6 months or when clinically indicated. Chronic treatment with lithium can cause hyperparathyroidism, therefore serum calcium levels should be checked once a year (Bendz et al. 1996a, 1996b).

Contraindications

Lithium should be administered cautiously and serum levels monitored carefully in patients with significant renal, cardiovascular, or thyroid disease or severe dehydration. Lithium is associated with an increased rate of cardiac abnormalities in fetuses and should not be used in pregnant or potentially pregnant females (Cohen et al. 1994).

Side Effects

Lithium is not always easy for pediatric patients to tolerate. It has a very narrow therapeutic window (0.8–1.2 mEq/L) and patients may develop signs of lithium toxicity when this window is exceeded. The signs of lithium toxicity include nausea, vomiting, slurred speech, and dyscoordination. With blood levels above 3.0 mEq/L, patients may develop more serious neurological symptoms, including seizures, coma, and death (Gelenberg et al. 1989). Common side effects in children and adolescents include nausea, diarrhea, abdominal distress, sedation, tremor, polyuria, weight gain, enuresis, and acne. Adherence with lithium treatment is a major problem in adolescents who find the possibility of weight gain and acne to be disincentives for continued treatment. Very young children (less than age 6 years) are more prone to develop neurological side effects, especially during the initiation phase of lithium treatment (Hagino et al. 1998).

Lithium may occasionally affect cardiac conduction, causing first-degree atrioventricular block, irregular sinus rhythms, and increased premature ventricular contractions (Gelenberg et al. 1989). Reversible conduction abnormalities have been reported in children (Campbell et al. 1984). It is recommended that a baseline ECG be obtained and another ECG once a therapeutic level has been reached.

There is a concern over the effect of long-term lithium use on renal function in children and adolescents. Long-term lithium use in adults is associated with clinically significant reduction in the glomerular filtration rate and in the maximum urinary concentrating capacity (Bendz et al. 1994). In addition, due to lithium's action on antidiuretic hormone on the distal tubules and collecting ducts, some cases of diabetes insipidus following treatment with lithium have been reported. This symptom was reversible if lithium was discontinued (Gelenberg et al. 1989). Focal glomerulosclerosis has occasionally been reported in children taking lithium, but in most cases this will remit once lithium is discontinued (Sakarcan et al. 2002). There have been case reports of youth who developed hypothyroidism, goiter, and thyroid autoantibodies while taking lithium (Alessi et al. 1994; DeLong and Aldershof 1987). In one sample of children and adolescents treated with lithium and valproate for a bipolar disorder, one-quarter of them showed thyroid-stimulating hormone (TSH) elevations of at least 10 mU/L within an average exposure to lithium of less than 3 months (Gracious et al. 2004). The factors associated with elevation in TSH in these lithium-treated subjects included a higher baseline TSH level and a higher lithium level. Close monitoring of thyroid function in children and adolescents taking lithium is recommended.

Another area of concern in children and adolescents treated with lithium is its possible effect on cognitive functioning. One double-blind, placebo-controlled study of lithium in 91 hospitalized children diagnosed with conduct disorder with severe aggressiveness and explosiveness suggested that some children would develop cognitive impairment at low plasma levels (Campbell et al. 1991). Adequate birth control measures must be followed in adolescent females taking lithium, as lithium is associated with an increased rate of cardiac abnormalities following fetal exposure (Cohen et al. 1994).

Table 48–1 lists management tactics for the common side effects of lithium.

Drug Interactions

Medications that increase lithium level include several antibiotics (e.g., ampicillin and tetracycline), nonsteroidal anti-inflammatory agents (e.g., ibuprofen), angiotensin-converting enzyme inhibitors, calcium channel blockers, antipsychotic agents, propranolol, and serotonin-specific reuptake inhibitors (e.g., fluoxetine).

Clinical Use

Lithium is a fairly good mood stabilizer and one that all child psychiatrists should be comfortable prescribing. Lithium is readily absorbed from the gastrointestinal system with peak levels occurring 2–4 hours after each dose. Lithium is excreted by the kidneys, and the serum half-life in children and adolescents is estimated to be approximately 18 hours (Vitiello et al. 1988). Serum lithium levels in the range of 0.8–1.2 mEq/L are typically necessary for mood stabilization, although these levels are based on studies of adults with bipolar disorder. In general, lithium should be titrated to a dose of 30 mg/kg/day in two to three divided doses, which typically results in a therapeutic serum level of 0.8–1.2 mEq/L.

Valproate

Valproate (valproate sodium) is a simple branched-chain fatty acid that was first introduced in the United States in 1978 as an antiseizure agent. It is currently approved by the FDA for the treatment of partial-com-

plex seizures, migraines, and manic episodes of bipolar illness in adults.

Disorders in Which Valproate May Be Useful

In children and adolescents, valproate may be effective in the treatment of mania, aggression, and migraine headaches.

Evidence for Efficacy

For many years valproate has been used to treat adults with mania. A review of the five controlled studies of valproate for the acute treatment of mania in adults showed an average response rate of 54%, demonstrating efficacy for valproate versus placebo (McElroy and Keck 2000). In many of these studies, positive results were obtained even though patients were selected from a population previously refractory to lithium treatment and were characterized by rapid cycling, mixed affective states, and irritability. There have been several case reports and open prospective trials suggesting the effectiveness of valproate for the treatment of children and adolescents with bipolar disorders (Deltito et al. 1998; Kastner and Friedman 1992; Kastner et al. 1990; Papatheodorou and Kutcher 1993; Papatheodorou et al. 1995; West et al. 1994, 1995; Whittier et al. 1995). Wagner et al. (2002) published the results of an open-label study of valproate in 40 children and adolescents (ages 7–19 years) with bipolar disorder. In the initial open-label phase of this study, subjects were given the initial dose of 15 mg/kg/day of divalproex. The mean final dose was 17 mg/kg/day. Twenty-two subjects (61%) showed ≥50% improvement in Mania Rating Scale scores during the open-label phase of treatment.

Findling et al. (2005) published the results of a discontinuation trial of lithium and divalproex to determine whether divalproex was superior to lithium in the maintenance monotherapy of youth diagnosed with bipolar disorder who had been previously stabilized on the combination of lithium and divalproex. Subjects with bipolar I or II disorder with a mean age of 10.8±3.5 years ($N = 139$) were initially treated with lithium and divalproex for a mean duration of 10.7±5.4 weeks initially. Patients meeting remission criteria for 4 consecutive weeks were then randomly assigned in a double-blind fashion to treatment with either lithium ($n = 30$) or divalproex ($n = 30$) for up to 76 weeks. At the end of the study, the lithium and divalproex treatment groups did not differ in either 1) survival time until

TABLE 48–1. Management of common lithium side effects

System	Side effect	Tactic
Central nervous system	Tremor, sedation, headache	Use a slow-release formulation; dose twice daily.
Dermatological	Acne	Collaborate with primary care physician for management of acne.
Endocrine	Hypothyroidism	Consult with endocrinologist; augment with triiodothyronine.
Gastrointestinal	Nausea, diarrhea	Split into 2–3 daily doses. Use a slow-release formulation.
Metabolic	Weight gain	Encourage diet and exercise. Consider a trial of metformin (Klein et al. 2006).
Renal	Polyuria, decreases in renal function	Write note to school that allows the patient to go to the bathroom as needed during school; monitor serum creatinine or creatinine clearance, serum urea nitrogen, and urine osmolality every 6 months.

emerging symptoms of relapse or 2) survival time until discontinuation for any reason. The authors concluded that lithium was not found to be superior to divalproex as maintenance treatment in youth who had stabilized on combination lithium and divalproex pharmacotherapy. The mean survival time in this trial for both agents was 113 days. This trial also demonstrated that monotherapy was not sufficient for maintenance treatment of children and adolescents with bipolar disorder.

Recently, the results of a large, randomized, placebo-controlled, double-blind, multicenter study designed to evaluate the safety and efficacy of Depakote ER in the treatment of bipolar I disorder, manic or mixed episode, in children and adolescents ages 10–17 years were released (Abbott Laboratories 2006). During this trial, 150 subjects with a current clinical diagnosis of bipolar I disorder, in a manic or mixed episode, were enrolled at 20 study sites. Subjects were outpatients with a manic or mixed episode with a Young Mania Rating Scale (YMRS) score ≥20 at screening and baseline. Subjects were randomly assigned in a 1:1 ratio to receive active study medication (250 mg and/or 500 mg tablets of Depakote ER) or matching placebo tablets. The duration of this study was 6 weeks, including a screening period lasting 3–14 days, a 4-week treatment period, and an optional 1-week taper period. There was no statistically significant treatment difference between valproate and placebo on any of the efficacy variables, primary or secondary. This trial may have been negative because the active treatment period of 4 weeks was not long enough or because the serum levels of divalproex were not high enough.

Kowatch et al. (2007) presented the results of a large National Institute of Mental Health (NIMH)–funded, controlled trial of lithium versus divalproex versus placebo in subjects ages 7–17 years with bipolar I disorder. In this trial, 153 outpatient subjects were randomly assigned in a double-blind manner to treatment with lithium, divalproex, or placebo in a 2:2:1 ratio. Subjects were diagnosed using the Washington University at St. Louis Kiddie Schedule for Affective Disorders and Schizophrenia (WASH-U-KSADS), and the primary outcome measures were weekly YMRS and Clinical Global Impression (CGI) Scale—Improvement ratings (Geller et al. 1998b). The total trial length for each subject was 24 weeks. During the first 8 weeks, subjects were treated with lithium, divalproex, or placebo in a double-blind fashion, and no other psychotropic medications were allowed other than for short-term "rescue" agents. The mean age of these subjects was 10.6±2.7 (range of 7–17). Eighty-six percent of these subjects were male. At the end of 8 weeks, divalproex demonstrated efficacy on both a priori outcome measures whereas lithium did not. The response rates based on a CGI-Improvement Score of "1 or 2" (much or very much improved) were divalproex, 54%; lithium, 42%; and placebo, 29%. There was a definite trend toward efficacy for lithium but it did not clearly separate from placebo on the primary outcome measures.

Steiner et al. (2003) conducted a randomized controlled trial of divalproex sodium (Depakote) with 71 incarcerated youth with conduct disorder. Subjects were randomly assigned into high- and low-dose (subtherapeutic) conditions and were openly managed by a clinical team with subjects and independent outcome raters blind to which treatment condition the subjects were assigned. Self-reported weekly impulse control was significantly better in the high-dose condition. This is the only controlled study of divalproex sodium in conduct disorder and further controlled studies are needed in this population.

Baseline Assessments

Baseline studies prior to initiating treatment with valproate in children and adolescents should include general medical history and physical examination with height and weight, liver function tests, complete blood count with differential and platelets, and a pregnancy test for sexually active females. A complete blood count with differential, platelet count, and liver functions should be checked every 6 months or when clinically indicated as divalproex can cause liver dysfunction and lower platelet counts.

Contraindications

Valproate should be administered cautiously and serum level and liver functions monitored carefully in patients with significant liver dysfunction (Asconape 2002) or in patients with inborn errors of ammonia metabolism (Konig et al. 1994; Treem 1994).

Side Effects

Common side effects of valproate in children and adolescents include nausea, increased appetite, weight gain, sedation, thrombocytopenia, transient hair loss, tremor, and vomiting. Rarely, pancreatitis (Sinclair et al. 2004;

Werlin and Fish 2006) and liver failure (Ee et al. 2003; Konig et al. 1994; Treem 1994) can occur in children treated with valproate. Fetal exposure to valproate is associated with an increased rate of neural tube defects.

Valproate-induced hyperammonemia has been observed in children and adolescents treated with valproate for psychiatric disorders (Carr and Shrewsbury 2007; Raskind and El-Chaar 2000). It can present as lethargy, disorientation, and reversible cognitive deficits, which may progress to marked sedation, coma, and even death. It is a transient and asymptomatic phenomenon but can become chronic if undetected.

There are increasing concerns about the possible association between valproate and polycystic ovarian syndrome (PCOS). PCOS is an endocrine disorder characterized by ovulatory dysfunction and hyperandrogenism, affecting 3%–5% of women who are not taking psychotropic medications (Rasgon 2004). Common symptoms of PCOS include irregular or absent menstruation, lack of ovulation, weight gain, hirsutism, and/or acne. The initial reports of the association between PCOS and divalproex exposure were in women with epilepsy. The association was particularly strong if their exposure was during adolescence (Isojarvi et al. 1993). In a report on adults with bipolar disorder, there was a sevenfold increased risk of new-onset oligoamenorrhea with hyperandrogenism in women who were treated with valproate (Joffe et al. 2006). All females who are treated with valproate should have a baseline assessment of menstrual cycle patterns and have continued monitoring for menstrual irregularities, weight gain, hirsutism, and/or acne that may develop during valproate treatment. If symptoms of PCOS develop, referral to an endocrinologist should be considered.

Table 48–2 lists management tactics for the common side effects of valproate.

TABLE 48–2. Management of common valproate side effects

System	Side effect	Tactic
Central nervous system	Tremor, headache, sedation	Use a slow-release formulation; split the dose.
Endocrine	Polycystic ovary syndrome	Check for weight gain, abnormal menstrual periods, and hirsutism. Consult with endocrinologist about management/labs.
Gastrointestinal	Nausea, stomach pains	Take with food. Use a slow-release formulation.
Hematological	Leukopenia, thrombocytopenia	Consult with hematologist. Consider switching to a different mood stabilizer.
Hepatic	Elevated liver function enzymes or pancreatic enzymes	Recheck lab values. Consult with gastroenterologist.

Drug Interactions

Valproate is metabolized in the liver by cytochrome P450 enzymes and has interactions with several medications that also are metabolized by this system. Medications that will increase valproate levels include erythromycin, selective serotonin reuptake inhibitors (SSRIs), cimetidine, and salicylates. Valproate may increase the levels of phenobarbital, primidone, carbamazepine, phenytoin, tricyclics, and lamotrigine.

Clinical Use

Valproate is readily absorbed from the gastrointestinal system with peak levels occurring 2–4 hours after each dose. But if valproate is given with meals to decrease nausea, peak levels may not be reached for 5–6 hours. Valproate is highly protein bound. It is metabolized in the liver and has a serum half-life of 8–16 hours in children and young adolescents (Cloyd et al. 1993). A starting dose of divalproex sodium of 15 mg/kg/day in 2–3 divided doses in children and adolescents will produce serum valproate levels in the range of 50–60 µg/mL. Once, this low serum level is attained, the dose is usually titrated upwards depending upon the subject's tolerance and response. It is optimal to measure serum valproate levels 12 hours after the last dose. Optimum serum levels for treating mania in adults are between 85–110 µg/mL, and the same is thought to be true in children and adolescents (Bowden et al. 1996).

Carbamazepine

Carbamazepine is an anticonvulsant agent structurally similar to imipramine that was first introduced in the United States in 1968 for the treatment of seizures. Carbamazepine is metabolized by the P450 hepatic system to an active metabolite, carbamazepine-10,11-epoxide. Carbamazepine induces its own metabolism and this "autoinduction" is complete 3–5 weeks after achieving a fixed dose. Initial carbamazepine serum half-lives range from 25–65 hours and then decrease to 9–15 hours after autoinduction of the P450 enzymes (Wilder 1992).

Disorders in Which Carbamazepine May Be Useful

In children and adolescents, carbamazepine may be useful for mania and conduct disorder.

Evidence for Efficacy

Two controlled studies of a long-acting preparation of carbamazepine in adults with bipolar disorder demonstrated efficacy for carbamazepine as monotherapy for mania (Weisler et al. 2006). There have been no controlled studies of carbamazepine for the treatment of children and adolescents with bipolar disorder, and the majority of reports in the literature concern its use in children and adolescents with ADHD or conduct disorder (Cueva et al. 1996; Evans et al. 1987; Kafantaris et al. 1992; Puente 1975). Pleak et al. (1988) reported the worsening of behavior in 6 of 20 child and adolescent patients treated with carbamazepine for ADHD and conduct disorder. There is not good evidence to support the use of carbamazepine as a first-line agent for bipolar children and adolescents, and this drug's numerous P450 drug interactions make its clinical use difficult.

Baseline Assessments

Complete pretreatment blood counts, including platelets, should be obtained at baseline prior to treatment. If a patient in the course of treatment exhibits low or decreased white blood cell or platelet counts, the patient's counts should be monitored closely.

Serious and sometimes fatal dermatological reactions, including toxic epidermal necrolysis (TEN) and Stevens-Johnson syndrome, have been reported with carbamazepine treatment. The risk of these events is estimated to be about 1 to 6 per 10,000 new users in countries with mainly white populations. Retrospective case-control studies have found that in patients of Chinese ancestry, there is a strong association between the risk of developing Stevens-Johnson syndrome or TEN with carbamazepine treatment and the presence of an inherited variant of the HLA-B gene, HLA-B*1502. HLA-B*1502 is largely absent in individuals not of Asian origin (e.g., whites, African Americans, Hispanics, and American Indians). It is recommended that before starting carbamazepine, testing for HLA-B*1502 should be performed in patients of Chinese ancestry.

Contraindications

Carbamazepine should not be used in patients positive for HLA-B*1502 unless the benefits clearly outweigh the risks. Carbamazepine should not be used in patients with a history of previous bone marrow depression, hypersensitivity to the drug, or known sensitivity to any of the tricyclic compounds.

Side Effects

Common side effects of carbamazepine in children and adolescents include sedation, ataxia, dizziness, blurred vision, nausea, and vomiting. Uncommon side effects of carbamazepine include aplastic anemia, hyponatremia, TEN, and Stevens-Johnson syndrome (Devi et al. 2005; Keating and Blahunka 1995). The risk of these events is estimated to be about 1 to 6 per 10,000 new users in countries with mainly white populations. Carbamazepine should be discontinued at the first sign of a serious rash, unless the rash is clearly not drug-related. If signs or symptoms suggest Stevens-Johnson syndrome or TEN, carbamazepine should not be resumed. Carbamazepine can cause fetal harm and is therefore contraindicated during pregnancy.

Drug Interactions

Due to its stimulation of the hepatic P450 isoenzyme system, carbamazepine has many clinically significant drug interactions. Carbamazepine decreases lithium clearance and increases the risk of lithium toxicity. Medications that will increase carbamazepine levels include erythromycin, cimetidine, fluoxetine, verapamil, and valproate. Carbamazepine may increase the levels of the following medications: oral contraceptives, phenobarbital, primidone, phenytoin, tricyclics, and lamotrigine (Ciraulo et al. 1995). Carbamazepine decreases the serum levels of many of the atypical antipsychotics (Besag and Berry 2006), leading to symptomatic relapses in some patients.

Clinical Use

In patients 6–12 years of age, a reasonable starting dose of carbamazepine is 100 mg twice daily and in patients ages 12 and older, 100 mg three times daily. Carbamazepine serum levels 8–11 mg/mL are necessary for seizure control; however, the level for therapeutic effects in bipolar youth are unknown. The maximum daily dose of carbamazepine should not exceed 1,000 mg/day in children ages 6–12 years and 1,200 mg/day in patients ages 13 years and older.

Table 48–3 provides mood stabilizer dosing and monitoring guidelines.

Lamotrigine

Lamotrigine is an antiseizure agent indicated as adjunctive therapy for partial seizures, the generalized seizures of Lennox-Gastaut syndrome, and primary generalized tonic-clonic seizures in adults and pediatric patients over 2 years of age. It works by blocking voltage-sensitive sodium channels and secondarily inhibiting the release of excitatory neurotransmitters, particularly glutamate and aspartate (Ketter et al. 2003). Lamotrigine also inhibits serotonin reuptake, suggesting it might possess antidepressant properties. The FDA has approved lamotrigine for the maintenance treatment of bipolar I disorder in adults to delay the time to occurrence of mood episodes (e.g., depression, mania, hypomania, mixed episodes) in patients treated for acute mood episodes with standard therapy.

Disorders in Which Lamotrigine May Be Useful

Lamotrigine is used to treat seizure disorders and it may be useful for bipolar depression.

Evidence for Efficacy

Several prospective studies in adults with bipolar disorder (bipolar I, II, and not otherwise specified) suggest that lamotrigine may be beneficial for the treatment of mood (especially depressive) symptoms in bipolar disorder (Bowden et al. 2003; Calabrese et al. 1999). Chang et al. recently published an 8-week, open-label trial of lamotrigine alone or as adjunctive therapy for the treatment of 20 adolescents ages 12–17 years (mean age 15.8 years) with bipolar disorder (bipolar I, II, and not otherwise specified), who were experiencing a depressive or mixed episode (Chang et al. 2006). The mean final dose was 131.6 mg/day. Of these subjects, 84% were rated as much or very much improved on the CGI. Larger, placebo-controlled studies of lamotrigine in bipolar children and adolescents are needed.

Baseline Assessments

Prior to starting lamotrigine, a patient's complete blood cell count, differential, platelet count, and liver function tests should be checked.

TABLE 48–3. Mood stabilizer dosing and monitoring guidelines

Generic name	U.S. trade name	How supplied (mg)	Starting dose	Target dose	Therapeutic serum level	Cautions
Carbamazepine Carbamazepine XR	Tegretol Tegretol XR Equetro	100, 200 100, 200, 400	Outpatients: 7 mg/kg/day 2–3 daily doses	Based on response and serum levels	8–11 mg/L	Monitor for P450 drug interactions
Gabapentin	Neurontin	100, 300, 400	100 mg bid or tid	Based on response	NA	Watch for behavioral disinhibition
Lamotrigine	Lamictal	25, 100, 200	12.5 mg qd	Increase weekly based on response	NA	Monitor carefully for rashes, serum sickness
Lithium carbonate Lithium carbonate Lithium citrate	Lithobid Eskalith Cibalith-S	300 (and 150 generic) 300 or 450 CR 5 cc=300 mg	Outpatients: 25 mg/kg/day 2–3 daily doses	30 mg/kg/day 2–3 daily doses	0.8–1.2 mEq/L	Monitor for hypothyroidism Avoid in pregnancy
Oxcarbazepine	Trileptal	150, 300, 600	150 mg bid	20–29 kg: 900 mg/day 30–39 kg: 1,200 mg/day >39 kg: 1,800 mg/day	NA	Monitor for hyponatremia
Topiramate	Topamax	25, 100	25 mg qd	100–400 mg/day	NA	Monitor for memory problems, kidney stones
Valproic acid Divalproex sodium	Depakene Depakote	125, 250, 500	15 mg/kg/day 2 daily doses	20 mg/kg/day 2–3 daily doses	85–110 µg/mL	Monitor liver functions and for pancreatitis Monitor for polycystic ovary syndrome in females Avoid in pregnancy

Note.   bid=twice a day; CR=controlled release; qd=once a day; tid=three times a day; XR=extended release.

Contraindications

Lamotrigine is contraindicated in patients who have demonstrated hypersensitivity to it.

Side Effects

The most common side effects of lamotrigine are dizziness, tremor, somnolence, nausea, asthenia, and headache. Cases of lupus, leukopenia, agranulocytosis, hepatic failure, and multiorgan failure associated with lamotrigine treatment have been reported (reviewed in Sabers and Gram 2000). However, lamotrigine has been well tolerated as long-term treatment in pediatric patients with epilepsy.

Benign rashes develop in 12% of adult patients, typically within the first 8 weeks of lamotrigine therapy (Calabrese et al. 2002). Rarely, severe cutaneous reactions such as Stevens-Johnson syndrome and TEN have been described. The risk of developing a serious rash is approximately three times greater in children and adolescents less than 16 years old compared with adults. The FDA has issued a black box warning which states, "Lamictal is not indicated for use in patients below the age of 16 years." The frequency of serious rash associated with lamotrigine (defined as rashes requiring hospitalization and discontinuation of treatment), including Stevens-Johnson syndrome, is approximately 1/100 (1%) in children ages less than 16 years and 3/1,000 (0.3%) in adults (GlaxoSmithKline 2001). Lamotrigine crosses the placenta and is excreted in breast milk.

Drug Interactions

Lamotrigine is primarily eliminated by hepatic metabolism through glucuronidation processes (Sabers and Gram 2000). The glucuronidation of lamotrigine is inhibited by valproic acid and is induced by carbamazepine. The addition of carbamazepine to lamotrigine decreases lamotrigine blood levels by 50%. Concomitant treatment with valproate increases lamotrigine blood levels; therefore, it is advisable to use lower lamotrigine doses and proceed very cautiously when coadministering these medications. Patients on oral contraceptives may require increased lamotrigine doses since estrogen induces the metabolism of lamotrigine. If the contraceptives are discontinued or the patient is postpartum, the dose of lamotrigine should be decreased since lamotrigine levels may double for a given dose (Reimers et al. 2005).

Clinical Use

The starting dose of lamotrigine for an adolescent not on valproate is 25 mg/day for 2 weeks, with a gradual titration to 200–400 mg/day. If the patient is on valproate, then the starting dose of lamotrigine is 25 mg every other day for 2 weeks. It is important to follow the current dosing guidelines recommended by GlaxoSmithKline for lamotrigine to avoid serious rashes. For patients less than age 12 years, the dosing of lamotrigine is weight based, and these guidelines can be found at http://www.lamictal.com/epilepsy/hcp/dosing/pediatric_dosing.html.

Gabapentin

Gabapentin is an antiseizure agent approved for the treatment of partial seizures in patients over 12 years of age and postherpetic neuralgia in adults. It is structurally similar to γ-aminobutyric acid (GABA), increases GABA release from glia, and may modulate sodium channels. Gabapentin is eliminated from the systemic circulation by renal excretion as it is not appreciably metabolized in humans. The half-life of gabapentin in children is on the average 4.7 hours.

Disorders in Which Gabapentin May Be Useful

In children and adolescents, gabapentin may be useful as a second- or third-line treatment for anxiety disorders comorbid with bipolar disorder.

Evidence for Efficacy

Adult double-blind controlled studies of gabapentin as adjunctive therapy to lithium or valproate and as monotherapy suggest it is no more effective than placebo for the treatment of mania (Pande et al. 2000); however, gabapentin may be useful in combination with other mood-stabilizing agents for the treatment of comorbid anxiety disorders in individuals with bipolar disorder (Keck et al. 2006).

Baseline Assessments

There are no specific laboratory tests necessary prior to starting gabapentin.

Contraindications

Gabapentin is contraindicated in patients who have demonstrated hypersensitivity to it.

Side Effects

Gabapentin has a relatively benign side-effect profile. The most common side effects in studies involving bipolar patients are sedation, dizziness, tremor, headache, ataxia, fatigue, and weight gain. Gabapentin has been reported to sometimes cause behavioral disinhibition in younger children (Lee et al. 1996; Tallian et al. 1996).

Drug Interactions

Gabapentin is not metabolized or protein bound and does not alter hepatic enzymes or interact with other anticonvulsants.

Clinical Use

The effective dose of gabapentin in children and adolescents is 600–1,800 mg/day given in divided doses (three times a day), with a starting dose of 50–100 mg three times a day. Gabapentin has a saturable absorption, and patients may benefit from administration in divided doses. The bioavailability of gabapentin is decreased by 20% with concomitant use of aluminum/magnesium hydroxide antacids.

Topiramate

Topiramate is indicated for monotherapy in patients 10 years of age and older with partial onset or primary generalized tonic-clonic seizures and in adults for the prophylaxis of migraine headache. It is a sulfamate-substituted monosaccharide, with several potential mechanisms of action, including blockade of voltage-gated sodium channels, antagonism of the kainate/AMPA subtype of glutamate receptor, enhancement of GABA activity, and carbonic anhydrase inhibition. Pediatric patients have a 50% higher clearance of topiramate and consequently a shorter elimination half-life than adults.

Topiramate is a weak inducer of cytochrome P450 enzymes and therefore is potentially associated with a risk of oral contraceptive failure (particularly, low-dose estrogen oral contraceptives). Topiramate is associated with limb agenesis in rodents and should be used with caution in females of childbearing potential.

Disorders in Which Topiramate May Be Useful

Topiramate has been shown to be moderately effective in causing weight loss in adult and adolescent patients with psychotropic-induced obesity (McElroy et al. 2007; Tramontina et al. 2007). It has not been shown to be an effective mood stabilizer.

Evidence for Efficacy

DelBello et al. (2005) published the results of an industry-funded, double-blind, placebo-controlled study of topiramate monotherapy for acute mania in children and adolescents with bipolar disorder type I. This trial was unfortunately discontinued early by the pharmaceutical company after several adult mania trials with topiramate failed to show efficacy. During the pediatric trial, 56 children and adolescents (ages 6–17 years) with a diagnosis of bipolar disorder type I were randomly assigned in a double-blinded fashion to topiramate (52%) or placebo (48%). The mean final dose of topiramate was 278 ± 121 mg/day. The reduction on the primary outcome variable, the mean YMRS score from baseline to final visit, was not statistically different between the topiramate group and the placebo group. This is considered a negative trial with the caveat that the results are largely inconclusive because of premature termination resulting in a limited sample size.

Baseline Assessments

Measurement of baseline and periodic serum bicarbonate during topiramate treatment is recommended.

Contraindications

Topiramate is contraindicated in patients who have demonstrated hypersensitivity to it.

Side Effects

The side effects of topiramate include sedation, fatigue, impaired concentration, and psychomotor slowing. In patients with epilepsy, there is a 1%–2% rate of nephrolithiasis because of carbonic anhydrase inhibition. Word-finding difficulties have been reported in up to one-third of adult patients treated with topiramate, and this also has been reported in children.

Drug Interactions

Topiramate is a weak inducer of cytochrome P450 enzymes, and therefore is potentially associated with a risk of oral contraceptive failure (particularly, low-dose estrogen oral contraceptives). Topiramate decreases the serum levels of risperidone and valproate.

Clinical Use

Topiramate can be started at 25 mg twice daily and titrated to 100–200 mg/day over 3–4 weeks. A lower starting dose and slower titration may decrease some of the side effects of topiramate.

Oxcarbazepine

Oxcarbazepine is indicated for use as monotherapy or adjunctive therapy in the treatment of partial seizures in adults and as monotherapy in the treatment of partial seizures in children. It is the 10-keto analogue of carbamazepine that is biotransformed by hydroxylation to its active metabolite 10,11-dihydro-10-hydroxy carbamazepine (MHD). MHD is the primary active metabolite and accounts for its antiseizure properties.

Wagner et al. (2006) reported the results of an industry-sponsored, multisite, randomized, double-blind, placebo-controlled study in children and adolescents with bipolar disorder. During this study, 116 youth with bipolar disorder (mean age 11.1±2.9 years) were randomly assigned to receive either oxcarbazepine or placebo. Between the treatment groups, the difference in the primary outcome variable—change in YMRS mean scores—was neither statistically nor clinically significant. This single negative trial does not support the use of oxcarbazepine as monotherapy in the treatment of mania in children and adolescents, but further controlled trials are needed. Whether this medication may be useful for the treatment of hypomania, bipolar disorder not otherwise specified, or cyclothymia is unknown.

Suicide and Mood Stabilizers

At a joint meeting in July 2008, members of the FDA peripheral and CNS and psychopharmacology advisory committees voted in favor of adding warnings and precautions about the suicidality risk to the package inserts of all antiepileptic drugs—but not in the form of a black box warning. Recently, the FDA analyzed almost 200 studies of 11 antiseizure drugs, some that have been on the market for decades. The studies tracked almost 28,000 people given the medications and another 16,000 given dummy pills. Very rarely were suicidal thoughts or behavior reported. Still, the FDA found that drug-treated patients did face about twice the risk: 0.43% of drug-treated patients experienced suicidal thoughts or behavior, compared with 0.22% of placebo takers. Overall, four people in the drug-treated groups committed suicide, and none in the placebo groups. This means that for every 1,000 patients, about 2 more drug-treated patients experienced suicidal thoughts than placebo takers, the FDA concluded. Antiseizure drugs are used for a variety of illnesses in addition to epilepsy, including migraines, certain nerve pain disorders, and psychiatric diseases such as bipolar disorder, which themselves carry a risk of suicide. The FDA found that drug-treated patients were at increased risk no matter their diagnosis, but the risk was highest for epilepsy subjects. The 11 drugs included in the analysis were carbamazepine, divalproex sodium, felbamate, gabapentin, lamotrigine, levetiracetam, oxcarbazepine, pregabalin, tiagabine, topiramate, and zonisamide. Clinicians who prescribe any of the agents should:

- Balance the risk with the patients' need for the drug.
- Tell patients and their families about the risk so they can be aware of changes in mood.
- Make sure patients and families know to contact a doctor if someone experiences common suicide warning signs, such as talking or thinking about hurting oneself; becoming preoccupied with death; withdrawal; becoming depressed or experiencing worsening depression; and giving away prized possessions.

Maintenance Treatment

The question of how long to continue a mood stabilizer is difficult to answer because there have been few pediatric studies longer than several months with these agents. It is reasonable to maintain a child or adolescent with bipolar disorder who has had a single manic episode on a mood-stabilizing agent for several years; then if the patient is euthymic and asymptomatic, slowly taper the mood-stabilizing agent over several months. If mood symptoms recur, the mood-stabilizing agent(s) should be reintroduced. If a bipolar child or adolescent has been psychotic, he or she should be maintained on an antipsychotic (typical or atypical) for a minimum of 1 month, even if the psychosis has resolved (Kafantaris et al. 2001).

Research Directions

There have been several large controlled adult studies that have demonstrated the efficacy of combining mood stabilizers like lithium or valproate with several atypical antipsychotics in adults with bipolar disorder. Similar trials are needed in children and adolescents with bipolar disorder. There is also emerging evidence that the traditional mood stabilizers, lithium

and valproate, may be "neuroprotective" in the CNS (Chuang 2004; Rowe and Chuang 2004). The mechanisms of these possible neuroprotective effects are complex but appear to involve changes at the level of the genome (Zhou et al. 2005). The positive and negative long-term effects of these agents on brain, social, and cognitive development need additional study.

Future Directions

Both the traditional and novel mood stabilizers may be effective in the treatment of children and adolescents with mood and behavior disorders. The evidence is strongest for lithium, somewhat strong for valproate, and weaker for the other agents. What is clear from emerging studies in pediatric bipolar disorder is that the atypical antipsychotics are more powerful and work faster than mood stabilizers (DelBello et al. 2006). Recently, risperidone and aripiprazole were given FDA indications for the short-term (risperidone) and long-term (aripiprazole) treatment of acute manic or mixed episodes associated with bipolar I disorder in children and adolescents ages 10–17 years. In the very near future the mood stabilizers will be regulated to a second-line treatment of many child and adolescent psychiatric disorders because of the broad range and power of the atypical antipsychotics.

Summary Points

- The traditional and novel mood stabilizers are widely used to treat pediatric patients with bipolar disorders, conduct disorders, seizure disorders, migraine headaches, and other disorders.

- Lithium is a good mood stabilizer with a moderate clinical effect size. In some patients, it may take as long as 6–8 weeks to get a full response to lithium. The side effects of weight gain, enuresis, and exacerbation of acne may limit lithium's use in some patients. There are still unanswered concerns about lithium's long-term effect on renal function.

- Valproate is usually better tolerated than lithium and works faster, generally between 4–6 weeks, in patients with bipolar disorder.

- Carbamazepine is considered a third-line agent after lithium and valproate because of its numerous P450 drug interactions.

References

Abbott Laboratories: A Double-Blind, Placebo-Controlled Trial to Evaluate the Safety and Efficacy of Depakote ER for the Treatment of Mania Associated with Bipolar Disorder in Children and Adolescents. Abbott Park, IL, Abbott Laboratories, 2006. Available at: http://pdf.clinicalstudyresults.org/documents/company-study_1561_0.pdf. Accessed May 20, 2009.

Alessi N, Naylor MW, Ghaziuddin M, et al: Update on lithium carbonate therapy in children and adolescents. J Am Acad Child Adolesc Psychiatry 33:291–304, 1994

Annell AL: Manic-depressive illness in children and effect of treatment with lithium carbonate. Acta Paedopsychiatr 36:292–301, 1969

Asconape JJ: Some common issues in the use of antiepileptic drugs. Semin Neurol 22:27–39, 2002

Bendz H, Aurell M, Balldin J, et al: Kidney damage in long-term lithium patients: a cross-sectional study of patients with 15 years or more on lithium. Nephrol Dial Transplant 9:1250–1254, 1994

Bendz H, Sjodin I, Aurell M: Renal function on and off lithium in patients treated with lithium for 15 years or more: a controlled, prospective lithium-withdrawal study. Nephrol Dial Transplant 11:457–460, 1996a

Bendz H, Sjodin I, Toss G, et al: Hyperparathyroidism and long-term lithium therapy: a cross-sectional study and the effect of lithium withdrawal. J Intern Med 240:357–365, 1996b

Besag FM, Berry D: Interactions between antiepileptic and antipsychotic drugs. Drug Saf 29:95–118, 2006

Bowden CL, Janicak PG, Orsulak P, et al: Relation of serum valproate concentration to response in mania. Am J Psychiatry 153:765–770, 1996

Bowden CL, Calabrese JR, Sachs G, et al: A placebo-controlled 18-month trial of lamotrigine and lithium maintenance treatment in recently manic or hypomanic patients with bipolar I disorder. Arch Gen Psychiatry 60:392–400, 2003

Brumback RA, Weinberg WA: Mania in childhood, II: therapeutic trial of lithium carbonate and further description of manic-depressive illness in children. Am J Dis Child 131:1122–1126, 1977

Cade JF: Lithium salts in the treatment of psychotic excitement. Med J Aust 36:349–352, 1949

Calabrese J, Bowden C, Sachs G, et al: A double-blind placebo-controlled study of lamotrigine monotherapy in outpatients with bipolar I depression. J Clin Psychiatry 60:79–88, 1999

Calabrese JR, Sullivan JR, Bowden CL, et al: Rash in multicenter trials of lamotrigine in mood disorders: clinical relevance and management. J Clin Psychiatry 63:1012–1019, 2002

Campbell M, Fish B, Korein J, et al: Lithium and chlorpromazine: a controlled crossover study of hyperactive severely disturbed young children. J Autism Child Schizophr 2:234–263, 1972

Campbell M, Perry R, Green WH: Use of lithium in children and adolescents. Psychosomatics 25:95–101, 105–106, 1984

Campbell M, Silva RR, Kafantaris V, et al: Predictors of side effects associated with lithium administration in children. Psychopharmacol Bull 27:373–380, 1991

Campbell M, Adams PB, Small AM, et al: Lithium in hospitalized aggressive children with conduct disorder: a double-blind and placebo-controlled study. J Am Acad Child Adolesc Psychiatry 34:445–453, 1995a

Campbell M, Kafantaris V, Cueva JE: An update on the use of lithium carbonate in aggressive children and adolescents with conduct disorder. Psychopharmacol Bull 31:93–102, 1995b

Carr RB, Shrewsbury K: Hyperammonemia due to valproic acid in the psychiatric setting. Am J Psychiatry 164:1020–1027, 2007

Chang K, Saxena K, Howe M: An open-label study of lamotrigine adjunct or monotherapy for the treatment of adolescents with bipolar depression. J Am Acad Child Adolesc Psychiatry 45:298–304, 2006

Chuang DM: Neuroprotective and neurotrophic actions of the mood stabilizer lithium: can it be used to treat neurodegenerative diseases? Crit Rev Neurobiol 16:83–90, 2004

Ciraulo DA, Shader RJ, Greenblatt DJ, et al (eds): Drug Interactions in Psychiatry. Baltimore, MD, Williams & Wilkins, 1995

Cloyd JC, Fischer JH, Kriel RL, et al: Valproic acid pharmacokinetics in children, IV: effects of age and antiepileptic drugs on protein binding and intrinsic clearance. Clin Pharmacol Ther 53:22–29, 1993

Cohen LS, Friedman JM, Jefferson JW, et al: A reevaluation of risk of in utero exposure to lithium. JAMA 271:146–150, 1994

Cohn JB, Collins G, Ashbrook E: A comparison of fluoxetine imipramine and placebo in patients with bipolar depressive disorder. Int Clin Psychopharmacol 4:313–322, 1989

Cueva JE, Overall JE, Small AM, et al: Carbamazepine in aggressive children with conduct disorder: a double-blind and placebo-controlled study. J Am Acad Child Adolesc Psychiatry 35:480–490, 1996

Danielyan A, Kowatch RA: Management options for bipolar disorder in children and adolescents. Paediatr Drugs 7:277–294, 2005

DelBello MP, Findling RL, Kushner S, et al: A pilot controlled trial of topiramate for mania in children and adolescents with bipolar disorder. J Am Acad Child Adolesc Psychiatry 44:539–547, 2005

DelBello MP, Kowatch RA, Adler CM, et al: A double-blind randomized pilot study comparing quetiapine and divalproex for adolescent mania. J Am Acad Child Adolesc Psychiatry 45:305–313, 2006

DeLong GR, Nieman MA: Lithium-induced behavior changes in children with symptoms suggesting manic-depressive illness. Psychopharmacol Bull 19:258–265, 1983

DeLong GR, Aldershof AL: Long-term experience with lithium treatment in childhood: correlation with clinical diagnosis. J Am Acad Child Adolesc Psychiatry 26:389–394, 1987

Deltito JA, Levitan J, Damore J, et al: Naturalistic experience with the use of divalproex sodium on an in-patient unit for adolescent psychiatric patients. Acta Psychiatr Scand 97:236–240, 1998

Devi K, George S, Criton S, et al: Carbamazepine: the commonest cause of toxic epidermal necrolysis and Stevens-Johnson syndrome: a study of 7 years. Indian J Dermatol Venereol Leprol 71:325–328, 2005

Dyson WL, Barcai A: Treatment of children of lithium-responding parents. Curr Ther Res Clin Exp 12:286–290, 1970

Ee LC, Shepherd RW, Cleghorn GJ, et al: Acute liver failure in children: a regional experience. J Paediatr Child Health 39:107–110, 2003

Evans RW, Clay TH, Gualtieri CT: Carbamazepine in pediatric psychiatry. J Am Acad Child Adolesc Psychiatry 26:2–8, 1987

Findling RL, McNamara NK, Gracious BL, et al: Combination lithium and divalproex sodium in pediatric bipolarity. J Am Acad Child Adolesc Psychiatry 42:895–901, 2003

Findling RL, McNamara NK, Youngstrom EA, et al: Double-blind 18-month trial of lithium versus divalproex maintenance treatment in pediatric bipolar disorder. J Am Acad Child Adolesc Psychiatry 44:409–417, 2005

Gelenberg AJ, Kane JM, Keller MB, et al: Comparison of standard and low serum levels of lithium for maintenance treatment of bipolar disorder. N Engl J Med 321:1489–1493, 1989

Geller B, Cooper TB, Sun K, et al: Double-blind and placebo-controlled study of lithium for adolescent bipolar disorders with secondary substance dependency. J Am Acad Child Adolesc Psychiatry 37:171–178, 1998a

Geller B, Warner K, Williams M, et al: Prepubertal and young adolescent bipolarity versus ADHD: assessment and validity using the WASH-U-KSADS, CBCL, and TRF. J Affect Disord 51:93–100, 1998b

GlaxoSmithKline: Lamictal (lamotrigine) product information, in Physicians Desk Reference, 56th Edition. Research Triangle Park, NC, Thomson Healthcare, 2001

Gracious BL, Findling RL, Seman C, et al: Elevated thyrotropin in bipolar youths prescribed both lithium and divalproex sodium. J Am Acad Child Adolesc Psychiatry 43:215–220, 2004

Gram LF, Rafaelsen OJ: Lithium treatment of psychotic children and adolescents: a controlled clinical trial. Acta Psychiatr Scand 48:253–260, 1972

Hagino OR, Weller EB, Weller RA, et al: Comparison of lithium dosage methods for preschool- and early school-age children. J Am Acad Child Adolesc Psychiatry 37:60–65, 1998

Isojarvi JI, Laatikainen TJ, Pakarinen AJ, et al: Polycystic ovaries and hyperandrogenism in women taking valproate for epilepsy. N Engl J Med 329:1383–1388, 1993

Joffe H, Cohen LS, Suppes T, et al: Valproate is associated with new-onset oligoamenorrhea with hyperandrogenism in women with bipolar disorder. Biol Psychiatry 59:1078–1086, 2006

Kafantaris V, Campbell M, Padron-Gayol MV, et al: Carbamazepine in hospitalized aggressive conduct disorder children: an open pilot study. Psychopharmacol Bull 28:193–199, 1992

Kafantaris V, Dicker R, Coletti DJ, et al: Adjunctive antipsychotic treatment is necessary for adolescents with psychotic mania. J Child Adolesc Psychopharmacol 11:409–413, 2001

Kafantaris V, Coletti DJ, Dicker R, et al: Lithium treatment of acute mania in adolescents: a large open trial. J Am Acad Child Adolesc Psychiatry 42:1038–1045, 2003

Kafantaris V, Coletti DJ, Dicker R, et al: Lithium treatment of acute mania in adolescents: a placebo-controlled discontinuation study. J Am Acad Child Adolesc Psychiatry 43:984–993, 2004

Kastner T, Friedman DL: Verapamil and valproic acid treatment of prolonged mania. J Am Acad Child Adolesc Psychiatry 31:271–275, 1992

Kastner T, Friedman DL, Plummer AT, et al: Valproic acid for the treatment of children with mental retardation and mood symptomatology. Pediatrics 86:467–472, 1990

Keating A, Blahunka P: Carbamazepine-induced Stevens-Johnson syndrome in a child. Ann Pharmacother 29:538–539, 1995

Keck PE Jr, Strawn JR, McElroy SL: Pharmacologic treatment considerations in co-occurring bipolar and anxiety disorders. J Clin Psychiatry 67(suppl):8–15, 2006

Ketter TA, Wang PW, Becker OV, et al: The diverse roles of anticonvulsants in bipolar disorders. Ann Clin Psychiatry 15:95–108, 2003

Klein DJ, Cottingham EM, Sorter M, et al: A randomized, double-blind, placebo-controlled trial of metformin treatment of weight gain associated with initiation of atypical antipsychotic therapy in children and adolescents. Am J Psychiatry 163:2072–2079, 2006

Konig SA, Siemes H, Blaker F, et al: Severe hepatotoxicity during valproate therapy: an update and report of eight new fatalities. Epilepsia 35:1005–1015, 1994

Kowatch R, DelBello M: Pediatric bipolar disorder: emerging diagnostic and treatment approaches. Child Adolesc Psychiatr Clin N Am 15:73–108, 2006

Kowatch RA, Suppes T, Carmody TJ, et al: Effect size of lithium, divalproex sodium and carbamazepine in children and adolescents with bipolar disorder. J Am Acad Child Adolesc Psychiatry 39:713–720, 2000

Kowatch R, Findling R, Scheffer R, et al: Placebo controlled trial of divalproex versus lithium for bipolar disorder. Presented at the American Academy of Child and Adolescent Psychiatry 54th Annual Meeting, Boston, MA, October 2007

Lee DO, Steingard RJ, Cesena M, et al: Behavioral side effects of gabapentin in children. Epilepsia 37:87–90, 1996

Lena B: Lithium in child and adolescent psychiatry. Arch Gen Psychiatry 36:854–855, 1979

Malone RP, Delaney MA, Luebbert JF, et al: A double-blind placebo-controlled study of lithium in hospitalized aggressive children and adolescents with conduct disorder. Arch Gen Psychiatry 57:649–654, 2000

Manji HK, Zarate CA: Molecular and cellular mechanisms underlying mood stabilization in bipolar disorder: implications for the development of improved therapeutics. Mol Psychiatry 7(suppl):S1–S7, 2002

McClellan J, Kowatch R, Findling RL: Practice parameter for the assessment and treatment of children and adolescents with bipolar disorder. J Am Acad Child Adolesc Psychiatry 46:107–125, 2007

McElroy S, Keck PJ: Pharmacologic agents for the treatment of acute bipolar mania. Biol Psychiatry 48:539–557, 2000

McElroy SL, Frye MA, Altshuler LL, et al: A 24-week, randomized, controlled trial of adjunctive sibutramine versus topiramate in the treatment of weight gain in overweight or obese patients with bipolar disorders. Bipolar Disord 9:426–434, 2007

McKnew DH, Cytryn L, Buchsbaum MS, et al: Lithium in children of lithium-responding parents. Psychiatry Res 4:171–180, 1981

Pande AC, Crockatt JG, Janney CA, et al: Gabapentin in bipolar disorder: a placebo-controlled trial of adjunctive therapy. Bipolar Disord 2:249–255, 2000

Papatheodorou G, Kutcher SP: Divalproex sodium treatment in late adolescent and young adult acute mania. Psychopharmacol Bull 29:213–219, 1993

Papatheodorou G, Kutcher SP, Katic M, et al: The efficacy and safety of divalproex sodium in the treatment of acute mania in adolescents and young adults: an open clinical trial. J Clin Psychopharmacol 15:110–116, 1995

Patel NC, DelBello MP, Bryan HS, et al: Open-label lithium for the treatment of adolescents with bipolar depression. J Am Acad Child Adolesc Psychiatry 45:289–297, 2006

Pavuluri MN, Birmaher B, Naylor MW: Pediatric bipolar disorder: a review of the past 10 years. J Am Acad Child Adolesc Psychiatry 44:846–871, 2005

Pleak RR, Birmaher B, Gavrilescu A, et al: Mania and neuropsychiatric excitation following carbamazepine. J Am Acad Child Adolesc Psychiatry 27:500–503, 1988

Puente RM: The use of carbamazepine in the treatment of behavioural disorders in children, in Epileptic Seizures–Behavior–Pain. Edited by Birkmayer W. Baltimore, MD, University Park Press, 1975, pp 243–252

Rasgon N: The relationship between polycystic ovary syndrome and antiepileptic drugs: a review of the evidence. J Clin Psychopharmacol 24:322–334, 2004

Raskind JY, El-Chaar GM: The role of carnitine supplementation during valproic acid therapy. Ann Pharmacother 34:630–638, 2000

Reimers A, Helde G, Brodtkorb E: Ethinyl estradiol, not progestogens, reduces lamotrigine serum concentrations. Epilepsia 46:1414–1417, 2005

Rowe MK, Chuang DM: Lithium neuroprotection: molecular mechanisms and clinical implications. Expert Rev Mol Med 6:1–18, 2004

Sabers A, Gram L: Newer anticonvulsants: comparative review of drug interactions and adverse effects. Drugs 60:23–33, 2000

Sakarcan A, Thomas DB, O'Reilly KP, et al: Lithium-induced nephrotic syndrome in a young pediatric patient. Pediatr Nephrol 17:290–292, 2002

Sinclair DB, Berg M, Breault R: Valproic acid-induced pancreatitis in childhood epilepsy: case series and review. J Child Neurol 19:498–502, 2004

Steiner H, Petersen ML, Saxena K, et al: Divalproex sodium for the treatment of conduct disorder: a randomized controlled clinical trial. J Clin Psychiatry 64:1183–1191, 2003

Strober M, Morrell W, Lampert C, et al: Relapse following discontinuation of lithium maintenance therapy in adolescents with bipolar I illness: a naturalistic study. Am J Psychiatry 147:457–461, 1990

Tallian KB, Nahata MC, Lo W, et al: Gabapentin associated with aggressive behavior in pediatric patients with seizures. Epilepsia 37:501–502, 1996

Tramontina S, Zeni CP, Pheula G, et al: Topiramate in adolescents with juvenile bipolar disorder presenting weight gain due to atypical antipsychotics or mood stabilizers: an open clinical trial. J Child Adolesc Psychopharmacol 17:129–134, 2007

Treem WR: Inherited and acquired syndromes of hyperammonemia and encephalopathy in children. Semin Liver Dis 14:236–258, 1994

Varanka TM, Weller RA, Weller EB, et al: Lithium treatment of manic episodes with psychotic features in prepubertal children. Am J Psychiatry 145:1557–1559, 1988

Vitiello B, Behar D, Malone R, et al: Pharmacokinetics of lithium carbonate in children. J Clin Psychopharmacol 8:355–359, 1988

Wagner KD, Weller EB, Carlson GA, et al: An open-label trial of divalproex in children and adolescents with bipolar disorder. J Am Acad Child Adolesc Psychiatry 41:1224–1230, 2002

Wagner KD, Kowatch RA, Emslie GJ, et al: A double-blind, randomized, placebo-controlled trial of oxcarbazepine in the treatment of bipolar disorder in children and adolescents. Am J Psychiatry 163:1179–1186, 2006

Weisler RH, Cutler AJ, Ballenger JC, et al: The use of antiepileptic drugs in bipolar disorders: a review based on evidence from controlled trials. CNS Spectr 11:788–799, 2006

Werlin SL, Fish DL: The spectrum of valproic acid-associated pancreatitis. Pediatrics 118:1660–1663, 2006

West SA, Keck PE Jr, McElroy SL, et al: Open trial of valproate in the treatment of adolescent mania. J Child Adolesc Psychopharmacol 4:263–267, 1994

West SA, Keck PE Jr, McElroy SL: Oral loading doses in the valproate treatment of adolescents with mixed bipolar disorder. J Child Adolesc Psychopharmacol 5:225–231, 1995

Whittier MC, West SA, Galli VB, et al: Valproic acid for dysphoric mania in a mentally retarded adolescent. J Clin Psychiatry 56:590–591, 1995

Wilder BJ: Pharmacokinetics of valproate and carbamazepine. J Clin Psychopharmacol 12(suppl):64S–68S, 1992

Youngerman J, Canino IA: Lithium carbonate use in children and adolescents: a survey of the literature. Arch Gen Psychiatry 35:216–224, 1978

Zhou R, Gray NA, Yuan P, et al: The anti-apoptotic, glucocorticoid receptor cochaperone protein BAG-1 is a long-term target for the actions of mood stabilizers. J Neurosci 25:4493–4502, 2005

Chapter 49

Antipsychotic Medications

Christoph U. Correll, M.D.

Since their discovery in the 1950s, antipsychotics have become an important pharmacological treatment option for a number of severe mental disorders. In children and adolescents, antipsychotics are increasingly used (Olfson et al. 2006) for both psychotic and nonpsychotic disorders (Findling et al. 2005; Jensen et al. 2007). Emerging data from randomized controlled trials (RCTs) indicate that antipsychotics have significantly greater efficacy than placebo for pediatric bipolar disorder, schizophrenia, and irritability and aggression associated with autistic disorder. Due to physiological developmental differences between children and adults, higher antipsychotic doses per kilogram weight are generally required in pediatric patients to achieve similar serum levels and efficacy, and more frequent dosing per day may be required in younger children (Woods et al. 2002). In addition, pediatric patients appear to be more sensitive to several relevant antipsychotic adverse effects compared with adults (Correll et al. 2006), mandating careful treatment selection and adverse effect monitoring and management in this vulnerable group of patients.

Pharmacology

Pharmacokinetic Considerations

Table 49–1 shows the pharmacokinetic properties of selected second-generation antipsychotics (SGAs) and selected first-generation antipsychotics (FGAs). Knowledge about specific cytochrome P450 (CYP) enzymes that metabolize antipsychotics is important in predicting and managing potential drug-drug interactions. Six CYP enzymes located in the brain and the periphery are responsible for approximately 90% of all

This work was supported in part by The Zucker Hillside Hospital NIMH Advanced Center for Intervention and Services Research for the Study of Schizophrenia MH 074543–01, and the NSLIJ Research Institute NIH General Clinical Research Center MO1RR018535.

TABLE 49–1. Pharmacokinetic information for first- and second-generation antipsychotics

Antipsychotic	Principal liver enzyme target	Protein binding	Bioavailability	Half-life, h	Time to peak level, h	CHLOR dose equivalent, mg[a]	Typical PED starting dose, mg[a,b]	Typical PED titration interval[b]	Typical PED dose range, mg[b,c]	Maximum regulatory approved adult dose, mg[a]	Dose strength, mg	Route of administration/Formulation
Second-generation												
ARI	2D6>3A4	>99%	87%	50–72	3–5	7.5	2–5	To next higher available dose every third day when starting at 2 mg; every 7–14 days after steady state	10–30	30	Tablets: 2, 5, 10, 15, 20, 30 Diss: 10, 15 Liquid: 1 mg/mL (only 30 mg=25 mL)	po, im short, diss, liquid
CLO	1A2 (30%) >2C19 (24%) >3A4 (22%) >2C9 (12%) >2D6 (6%)	97%	70%	12	1–4	50	12.5	25 mg every day	50–600	900	25, 100	po
OLA	1A2, 2D6, 3A4	93%	60%	30	6	5	2.5–10	2.5–10 mg every 5–7 days	N/A	20	Tablets: 2.5, 5, 7.5, 10, 15, 20; Diss: 5, 10, 15, 20 im: 10	po, im short, diss
PAL	<10% hepatic clearance	74%	28%	21–30	24	3	3	3 mg every 5–7 days	3–12	12	3, 6, 9	po, ER
QUE	3A4	83%	<20%	6–7	2	75	25–100 IR 200–300 XR	25–100 mg every 1–2 days	150–750	800	25, 100, 200	po, XR
RIS	2D6>3A4	90%	70%	3	1–2	2	0.25–1	0.25–1 mg every 1–5 days	1–6	16	Tablets: 0.5, 1, 2, 3, 4 Diss: 0.5, 1, 2 Liquid: 1 mg/mL 30 mL bottle	po, im long, diss, liquid
ZIP	Aldehyde oxidase (2/3) >3A4 (1/3)	>99%	60%	7	5	60	20–40	20–40 mg every 1–2 days	80–160	160	Tablets: 20, 40, 60, 80 im: 20	po, im short

TABLE 49–1. Pharmacokinetic information for first- and second-generation antipsychotics *(continued)*

Antipsy-chotic	Principal liver enzyme target	Protein binding	Bioavail-ability	Half-life, h	Time to peak level, h	CHLOR dose equivalent, mg[a]	Typical PED starting dose, mg[a,b]	Typical PED titration interval[b]	Typical PED dose range, mg[b,c]	Maximum regulatory approved adult dose, mg[a]	Dose strength, mg	Route of administration/ Formulation
First-generation												
HAL	3A4	92%	60%–70%	3–6 po 10–20 im	24 po 21 im	2	0.25–1	0.25–1 mg at intervals of 5–7 days	1–6	100	Tablets: 0.5, 1, 2, 5, 10, 20 Liquid: 2, 10 mg/mL im: 5	po, im short, im long
MOL	2D6	76%	>80%	1.5	1.5	10	0.5–1 mg/kg/day divided in 3–4 doses	0.5–1 mg/kg every 1–2 days	20–140	225	5, 10, 25, 50	po
PER	2D6	>90%	40%	8–12	1–3	10	2–4	2–4 mg every 5–7 days	8–32	64	2, 4, 8, 16	po

Note. ARI=aripiprazole; CHLOR=chlorpromazine; CLO=clozapine; diss=dissolvable tablet; ER=extended release; HAL=haloperidol; IR=immediate release; MOL=molindone; N/A=not applicable; OLA=olanzapine; PAL=paliperidone; PED=pediatric; PER=perphenazine; QUE=quetiapine; RIS=risperidone; XR=extended release; ZIP=ziprasidone.

[a]CHLOR dose equivalents (i.e., dose given in the table is equivalent to 100 mg of CHLOR) based on Woods et al. 2002 and Haase 1983.

[b]Doses need to be individualized based on efficacy and tolerability.

[c]Average dose range provided for adolescents with schizophrenia or bipolar disorder; for prepubertal patients or those with other diagnoses, average dose may be approximately 33%–50% lower.

Source. Correll 2008a; package insert information for each medication.

the CYP activity (Meyer 2007). Whenever medications are metabolized by the same liver enzyme, the competition can lead to increased serum levels of both drugs. Conversely, medications, nutraceuticals, and smoking that can induce CYP enzyme production may lower antipsychotic serum levels. The CYP enzymes 3A4, 2D6, and 1A2 are most important for antipsychotic clearance. CYP3A4 is a low-affinity, high-capacity enzyme, making it relatively immune to saturation, unless very potent inhibitors are present. CYP3A4 is mainly relevant for haloperidol, quetiapine, and olanzapine clearance. The CYP2D6 is a high-affinity, low-capacity enzyme. It is very efficient and not readily inducible, but it can be saturated more easily (Meyer 2007). Moreover, most known genetic polymorphisms affect CYP2D6. Aripiprazole, molindone, perphenazine, and risperidone are predominantly cleared by CYP2D6. The CYP1A2 enzyme is also a low-affinity, high-capacity enzyme and is relevant for the clearance of clozapine and, to some degree, of olanzapine. The CYP2C19 and 2C9 are only relevant for clozapine clearance. In addition, the aldehyde oxidase system, which is neither saturable nor inhibitable, is responsible for 67% of ziprasidone's metabolism. Since <10% of paliperidone and only 33% of ziprasidone are undergoing CYP first-pass metabolism, the likelihood of drug-drug interactions is lowest with these two antipsychotics. Updated CYP450 interactions are available at: http://medicine.iupui.edu/flockhart/table.htm.

Knowledge about the half-life of antipsychotics can help predict how quickly steady state is achieved and how fast the body eliminates the drug. In general, it takes about five times the half-life of a drug for both steady state and elimination. As shown in Table 49–1, the half-life of antipsychotics differs considerably. Titration can be faster (daily) with drugs that achieve almost full steady state within 24 hours (e.g., quetiapine and ziprasidone), particularly beyond the initial titration phase when peripheral receptors responsible for early side effects are downregulated. Conversely, dose increases may have to be every 5–7 days with olanzapine and risperidone/paliperidone. For aripiprazole, a dose increase every 10–14 days is most rational after steady state has been reached. However, the initial titration of aripiprazole can be faster (e.g., every 3–5 days), as the lower starting dose seems to minimize early side effects that are likely due to partial D_2 agonism (i.e., nausea, vomiting, and psychomotor restlessness). Such a titration schedule was used in two randomized, placebo-controlled trials in children and adolescents with schizophrenia (Findling et al. 2008) and bipolar disorder (Chang et al. 2007), where doses were increased every third day, escalating from 2 mg to 5 mg, 10 mg (reached by day 5), and further to 15 mg, 20 mg, 25 mg, and 30 mg (reached by day 11 or 13, respectively). Nevertheless, it is important to note, that the half-life is measured via peripheral serum levels, not in cerebrospinal fluid or by functional regional receptor activity. Thus, it is possible that central nervous system (CNS) actions are more prolonged. Moreover, many antipsychotics have active metabolites about which less information is available and which may have a longer half-life than the parent drug.

The time until peak level can help to predict the rapidity of the onset of therapeutic action and side effects after a single dose. Again, antipsychotics differ considerably (see Table 49–1). Because antipsychotic peak levels are measured peripherally, time to maximum level and onset of action in the CNS may differ. Most likely, peripheral side effects are more closely related to time to peak levels. If the clinician wants to reduce peak level–related side effects during titration, splitting the dose or administration with fatty food (which slows down drug absorption) will reduce peak levels, leaving unaltered the total dose delivered (i.e., total area under the curve). Doses needed for sufficient dopamine blockade to reach antipsychotic, antimanic, and/or antiaggressive efficacy (see Table 49–1) depend in part on the affinity for the dopamine D_2 receptor that varies across antipsychotics. Table 49–1 provides the relative dose strengths expressed as chlorpromazine equivalents that allow estimating dose requirements during a switch from one antipsychotic to another. Dose equivalences are only approximations, however.

Pharmacodynamic Considerations

The central feature of all antipsychotics is their ability to block the dopamine D_2 receptor. This activity seems to be associated with the antipsychotic, antimanic, and antiaggressive effects of antipsychotic medications. The overall goal of treatment is to reduce the hyperactivity of pathways that at least in part mediate psychosis, mania, and aggression. Simultaneously, the pathways that regulate motor movements, prolactin secretion, and especially cognition and motivation need to be preserved. Antipsychotic drugs also bind to serotonin, alpha-adrenergic, histaminic, and muscarinic receptors, which can in part predict the therapeutic and adverse effects during therapy with a particular drug (Correll 2008a). Antipsychotics, which bind more tightly to receptors other than dopamine D_2 receptors, contain these effects in addition to the antidopaminergic efficacy. In the case of antipsychotics with relatively weak dopamine binding (e.g., chlorpromazine, clozapine, quetiapine), non–antidopaminergic effects can predominate at low doses. The tighter binding at nondopaminergic receptors can be beneficial, as in the tighter binding of SGAs to 5-HT$_2$ receptors, which seems to be associated with less propensity for extrapyramidal symptoms (EPS) and prolactin elevation. Conversely, the stronger binding to nondopaminergic receptors can also lead to lasting adverse effects of an antihistaminergic or anticholinergic nature (Table 49–2).

The dosage, degree of receptor occupancy, and intrinsic activity at the receptor to which the antipsychotic binds are all important determinants of therapeutic and adverse effects. With a full antagonist, approximately 60%–70% dopamine receptor occupancy is needed for antipsychotic efficacy. With a partial agonist (e.g., aripiprazole), receptor occupancy is not equivalent to blockade and a higher degree of occupancy (at least 80%–85%) is required to achieve the same level of blockade (Burris et al. 2002).

Pharmacokinetic and Pharmacodynamic Rebound Phenomena

Rebound effects that can diminish the initial therapeutic efficacy may occur during medication changes due to interactions between the previous medication and the new medication, particularly when the properties of the two antipsychotics vary greatly and when the change is very fast. Depending on the receptor system(s) involved, withdrawal or rebound symptoms can manifest as anxiety, insomnia, agitation, mania, psychosis, confusion, EPS, or akathisia, mimicking psychiatric worsening and primary inefficacy of the new agent (see Table 49–2). Pharmacokinetic rebound effects can be seen in the following circumstances:

- When a patient becomes nonadherent or when the new antipsychotic is relatively underdosed
- During switching (without adequate overlap) if the first antipsychotic has a relatively short half-life and is replaced by an antipsychotic with a much longer half-life that requires longer to achieve steady-state concentrations (e.g., aripiprazole)
- When the new antipsychotic requires slower titration (e.g., clozapine)

- When it is less absorbed unless given with food (e.g., ziprasidone)
- When it crosses the blood-brain barrier less readily, requiring higher doses to achieve equivalent levels (e.g., switching from risperidone to paliperidone)

Pharmacodynamic rebound effects are most likely when receptor binding profiles are very different between the first and second agent (Correll 2008a). This is especially likely when a patient goes off a strongly antihistaminic or anticholinergic drug, such as clozapine, olanzapine, or quetiapine. Histamine blockade is associated with anxiolytic, calming, sleep-inducing, and EPS-reducing effects (see Table 49–2, left column). Cholinergic blockade is associated with calming and anti-EPS effects (see Table 49–2, left column). During a rapid switch from a potently antihistaminergic or anticholinergic antipsychotic to one of the newer agents with less sedation and less anticholinergic blockade (e.g., aripiprazole, ziprasidone, and less so, risperidone or paliperidone), upregulated, sensitized receptors can promote the transmission of histaminergic and muscarinic activity. This can result in (transient) rebound agitation, insomnia, anxiety, restlessness, EPS, and akathisia (Table 49–2, right column). Similarly, switching from a strongly antidopaminergic drug—such as a high- or medium-potency FGA or risperidone or paliperidone—to a less tightly binding antipsychotic (such as clozapine or quetiapine) or to a partial D_2 agonist can result transiently in a relative lack of dopamine blockade in the presence of hypersensitive and upregulated D_2 receptors (unless the new antipsychotic is dosed high enough). Clinically, this can manifest as rebound psychosis, mania, agitation, aggression, akathisia, or withdrawal dyskinesia (Table 49–2, right column).

Rebound phenomena may be avoided in many cases by using an overlapping or "plateau" cross-titration (Correll 2006) or by treating withdrawal and rebound symptoms with time-limited, targeted use of benzodiazepines, antihistamines, anticholinergics, gabapentin, mirtazapine, or nonbenzodiazepine anxiolytics and sedatives.

Indications

Table 49–3 shows the clinical and regulatory indications for antipsychotics in adult and pediatric patients. As can be seen, antipsychotics are used clinically for far more indications than they have received an indication for from the U.S. Food and Drug Administration (FDA). As of June 2009, risperidone and ari-

TABLE 49–2. Therapeutic and adverse effects of antipsychotic receptor occupancy and abrupt withdrawal

Neuroreceptor	Blockade	Withdrawal/rebound
α_1-adrenergic	Postural hypotension, dizziness, syncope	Tachycardia, hypertension
α_2-adrenergic	Increased alertness; increase in blood pressure, antidepressant	Postural hypotension, dizziness, syncope
Dopamine D_2	Antipsychotic, antimanic, antiaggressive, EPS/akathisia, tardive dyskinesia, prolactin increase, sexual or reproductive system dysfunction	Psychosis, mania, agitation, akathisia, withdrawal dyskinesia
Histamine H_1	Anxiolytic, sedation, weight gain, anti-EPS/akathisia	Agitation, insomnia, anxiety, EPS
Muscarinic M_1 (central)	Memory, cognition, anti-EPS/akathisia	Agitation, confusion, psychosis, anxiety, insomnia, sialorrhea, EPS/akathisia
Muscarinic M_{2-4} (peripheral)	Dry mouth, constipation, urinary retention	Diarrhea, diaphoresis, nausea, vomiting, bradycardia, hypotension, syncope
Serotonin $5-HT_{1A}$ (partial agonism)	Anxiolytic, antidepressant, anti-EPS/akathisia (?)	EPS/akathisia
Serotonin $5-HT_{2A}$	Anti-EPS/akathisia, antipsychotic (?)	EPS/akathisia, possible psychosis

Note. EPS=extrapyramidal symptoms.

piprazole have FDA pediatric indications for bipolar disorder (ages 10–17) and schizophrenia (ages 13–17). Risperidone also received an indication for irritability associated with autistic disorder.

Efficacy From Randomized Controlled Trials

Early-Onset Schizophrenia

Eleven RCTs ($N=931$) showed superior efficacy of antipsychotic monotherapy for pediatric schizophrenia (Kumra et al. 2008b). The study and patient characteristics and main efficacy outcomes, including study-defined response and remission, are summarized in Table 49–4. A clinically useful measure for the difference between treatment groups is the number needed to treat (NNT), which is the number of patients who need to be exposed to a treatment until one additional positive event of interest occurs in excess of the rate in the comparator. In an older 4-week placebo-controlled trial (Pool et al. 1976), haloperidol and loxapine were associated with significantly greater reductions in Brief Psychiatric Rating Scale (BPRS) scores compared to

placebo, but there were no differences between the two active medication groups. In the other active-controlled studies with modest sample sizes not involving clozapine and lasting 4–8 weeks, antipsychotics did not show significant efficacy differences (Realmuto et al. 1984; Sikich et al. 2004, 2008). By contrast, in relatively small active-controlled trials, clozapine (mean dosage: 176–403 mg/day) was superior in several efficacy measures (especially negative symptoms) compared to haloperidol (Kumra et al. 1996), olanzapine (Shaw et al. 2006), and "high-dose" olanzapine (Kumra et al. 2008a). The NNTs for study-specific "response" in early-onset schizophrenia ranged from 5 to 8 with nonclozapine antipsychotics compared to placebo, and from 3 to 6 for clozapine compared to olanzapine.

Bipolar I Disorder, Manic or Mixed Episode

Seven recent RCTs ($N=1,220$) demonstrated efficacy of SGAs in pediatric patients with bipolar I disorder. Five RCTs in youth (ages 10–17, $N=1,081$) showed superior efficacy of antipsychotic monotherapy compared to placebo regarding reduction in the Young Mania Rating (YMRS) Scale score (Table 49–5). Furthermore,

TABLE 49–3. Indications for antipsychotic use in adults and in children and adolescents

Antipsychotic	SCZ	SCZ maintenance	Other psychotic disorders	Bipolar mania[a]	Bipolar DEP	Bipolar maintenance	Refractory unipolar DEP	Refractory OCD[d]	TIC[e]	Aggression/ irritability in autism[f]	DBD[f]	PTSD[d]
Second-generation												
Amisulpride	+A	+A	+	+	+	+		+	+	+	+	+
Aripiprazole	+A, C	+A	+	+A[b], C	+	+A [C[c]]	+A[d]	+	+	+	+	+
Clozapine	+[A]	+	+	+	+	+	+	+	+	+	+	+
Olanzapine	+A, [C]	+A	+	+A, [C]	+A	+A	+A	+	+	+	+	+
Paliperidone ER	+A	+	+	+	+	+	+	+	+	+	+	+
Quetiapine	+A	+A	+	+A[g], [C]	+A	+A	+[A[d,h]]	+	+	+	+	+
Risperidone	+A, C	+A	+	+A, C	+	+	+	+	+	+C	+	+
Ziprasidone	+A	+[A]	+	+A, [C]	+	+	+	+	+	+	+	+
First-generation												
Chlorpromazine	+A	+	+	+	–	+[i]	–	+	+	+	+	+
Haloperidol	+A, C	+	+	+	–	+[i]	–	+	+	+	+	+
Molindone	+A, |C|	+	+	+	–	+[i]	–	+	+	+	+	+
Perphenazine	+A	+	+	+	–	+[i]	–	+	+	+	+	+

Note. += clinically indicated based on open-label data, anecdotal evidence, and clinical practice; – = not generally used.
A = FDA indication in adults; [A] = at least one positive randomized, placebo-controlled trial in adults; C = FDA indication in pediatric populations; [C] = at least one positive randomized, placebo-controlled trial in pediatric populations; |C| = positive data available from one randomized, active-controlled trial in pediatric populations with similar efficacy as olanzapine and risperidone; DEP = depression; TIC = tic disorders.
DBD = disruptive behavior disorder; OCD = obsessive-compulsive disorder; PTSD = posttraumatic stress disorder; SCZ = schizophrenia.
a Including mixed mania and augmentation of mood stabilizer treatment, unless noted otherwise.
b Positive augmentation data only available from non-U.S. studies.
c Placebo-controlled maintenance data available from a 30-week double-blind extension trial but not in placebo-controlled discontinuation design required by the FDA for maintenance indication.
d As augmentation after antidepressant failure.
e Generally after failure of alpha-2 agonists.
f Generally after failure of nonpharmacological and/or stimulant treatment if comorbid attention-deficit/hyperactivity disorder.
g Mixed mania patients were excluded.
h In monotherapy.
i While preventing mania, it may induce depression.

TABLE 49–4. Double-blind, randomized, placebo-controlled and active-controlled trials of antipsychotics in children and adolescents with schizophrenia

Study	Design	Inclusion criteria	Drug	Mean dose, mg/day	N	Male, %	White, %	Age, mean (range)	Primary outcome	Response (as study-defined), %	NNT response	Remission (study-defined), %	NNT remission	≥7% Weight gain, %
Schizophrenia, placebo-controlled														
Pool et al. 1976	4-wk DB-RPCT	SCZ	Total		75				BPRS-C: ns (sign from baseline for all groups); CGI-S improved: 88 vs. 70 vs. 36% (P=.06)					
			LOX	87.5	26	39		15.6						
			HAL	9.8	25	72		15.7						
			Pbo	5.4	24	63		15.3 (13–18)						
Spencer et al. 1992	8-wk DB-RPCT	SCZ	Total		12	75		8.8 (5–12)	CGI-I and CGI-S: HAL >Pbo					
			HAL	2.02										
			Pbo											
Kryzhanovskaya et al. 2009	6-wk DB-RPCT	SCZ	Total		107				PANSS: OLA>Pbo					
			OLA	11.1	72	71	72	16.1		38	6			46[a]
			Pbo		35	69	71	16.3 (13–17)		26				15
Findling et al. 2008	6-wk DB-RPCT	SCZ	Total		302	57	59.9 (181)	15.5 (13–17)	PANSS: ARI 10 and ARI 30>Pbo					
			ARI	10 (9.5)	100					68	8	54	6	4
			ARI	30 (27.8)	102					71	6	58	5	5
			Pbo		100					54		36		1
Haas et al. 2007	6-wk DB-RPCT	SCZ	Total		160	36	53	15.6	PANSS: RIS 1–3 and RIS 4–6 >Pbo	65	6			15
			RIS	1–3 (2.6)	55	46	60	15.7		72	5			16
			RIS	4–6 (5.3)	51	28	47	15.7		35				2
			Pbo		54	65	50	15.5 (13–17)						
Schizophrenia, active-controlled														
Realmuto et al. 1984	4–6-wk SBRCT	SCZ	Total		21				BPRS-C and CGI-S: ns between groups					
			THIX	0.26	13			15.1						
			THIO	2.57	8			16.1 (11–18)						
Kumra et al. 1996	6-wk DB-RCT	Early-onset SCZ	Total		21				BPRS-C: CLO>HAL (P=.04)					
			CLO	176	10	50		14.4						
			HAL	16	11	54		13.73						

TABLE 49–4. Double-blind, randomized, placebo-controlled and active-controlled trials of antipsychotics in children and adolescents with schizophrenia *(continued)*

Study	Design	Inclusion criteria	Drug	Mean dose, mg/day	N	Male, %	White, %	Age, mean (range)	Primary outcome	Response (as study-defined), %	NNT response	Remission (study-defined), %	NNT remission	≥7% Weight gain, %
Schizophrenia, active-controlled *(continued)*														
Sikich et al. 2004	8-wk DB-RCT	SCZ spectrum d/o: 52%; affective d/o: 48%	Total		50	60	60	14.8	BPRS-C: ns (sign from baseline for all groups)					
			RIS	4.0	19	68	47	14.6		74	5			
			OLA	12.3	16	56	63	14.6		88	3			
			HAL	5.0	15	53	73	15.4 (8–19)		53				
Shaw et al. 2006	8-wk DB-RCT	SCZ, resistant to ≥2 APs	Total		25				SAPS, SANS, CGI-S: ns (sign from baseline for both groups)					
			CLO	327	12	67	58	11.7		33	6			
			OLA	18.1	13	54	54	12.8 (7–16)		15				
Kumra et al. 2008a	12-wk DB-RCT	SCZ, resistant to ≥2 APs	Total		39				BPRS-C: (sign from baseline for both groups)					
			CLO	403.1	18	44	13	15.8		67	3			
			OLA	26.2	21	62	29	15.5 (10–18)		33				
Sikich et al. 2008	8-wk DB-RCT	SCZ	Total		119				BPRS-C: (sign from baseline for all groups)					
			OLA	11.4	35					49				
			RIS	2.8	41					46				
			MOL	59.9	40					60				

Note. APs=antipsychotics; ARI=aripiprazole; BPRS-C=Brief Psychiatric Rating Scale for Children; CGI-I=Clinical Global Impressions Improvement Scale; CGI-S=Clinical Global Impressions Severity of Symptoms Scale; CLO=clozapine; DB-RCPT=double-blind, randomized, placebo-controlled trial; d/o=disorder; HAL= haloperidol; LOX=loxapine; MOL=molindone; NNT=number needed to treat; ns=not significant; OLA=olanzapine; PANSS=Positive and Negative Syndrome Scale; Pbo=placebo; RIS=risperidone; SANS=Schedule for the Assessment of Negative Symptoms; SAPS=Schedule for the Assessment of Positive Symptoms; SBRCT=single-blind, randomized controlled trial; SCZ=schizophrenia; THIO=thioridazine; THIX=thiothixene.
[a]Number needed to harm, ≥7% weight gain: 4.

TABLE 49–5. Double-blind, randomized, placebo-controlled trials of antipsychotics in children and adolescents with bipolar disorders

Study	Design	Inclusion criteria	Drug	Mean dose, mg/day	N	Male, %	White, %	Age, mean (range)	Primary outcome	Response (as study-defined), %	NNT response	Remission (study-defined), %	NNT remission	≥7% Weight gain, %
Bipolar disorder, placebo-controlled														
Chang et al. 2007; Correll et al. 2007	4-wk DB-RPCT	Bipolar I	Total ARI ARI Pbo	10 (9.5) 30 (28.5)	296 98 99 99	54	65	13.4 (10–17)	YMRS: ARI 10 and ARI 30>Pbo	45 64 26	6 3	25 48 5	5 3	3 9 3
Tohen et al. 2007	3-wk DB-RPCT	Bipolar disorder	Total OLA Pbo	8.9	161 107 54	57 44	66 76	15.1 15.4 (13–17)	YMRS: OLA>Pbo	49 22	4	35 11	5	42 2
DelBello et al. 2007	3-wk DB-RPCT	Bipolar I mania	Total QUE QUE Pbo	400 600	277 93 95 99	56 56 58 61	77 79 77 74	13.2 13.1 13.1 13.3 (10–17)	YMRS: QUE>Pbo	64 58 37	5 4	53 54 30	5 5	15 10 0
Pandina et al. 2007	3-wk DB-RPCT	Bipolar disorder	Total RIS RIS Pbo	0.5–2.5 3–6	169 50 61 58	49 56 43 48	77 70 82 78	13.0 (10–17)	YMRS: RIS 0.5–2.5 and RIS 3–6>Pbo	59 63 26	3 3			
DelBello et al. 2008	4-wk DB-RPCT	Bipolar I disorder[a]	Total ZIP Pbo	40–160	237 149 88			(10–17)	YMRS: ZIP>Pbo	62 35				7 4
DelBello et al. 2002	6-wk DB-RPCT	Bipolar I disorder[a]	Total QUE+DVP Pbo+DVP	432 102 µg/mL	30 15 15			14.3 (12–18)	YMRS: QUE+VPA>Pbo +VPA (P=.05)	87 53	3			
Bipolar disorder, active-controlled														
DelBello et al. 2006	4-wk DB-RPCT	Bipolar I disorder[a]	Total QUE DVP	412 101 µg/mL	50 25 25	42	26	15.0 (12–18)	YMRS: ns (but faster onset with QUE, P=.01)	60 28	4	55 17	3	

Note. ARI=aripiprazole; DVP=divalproex; NNT=number needed to treat; OLA=olanzapine; Pbo=placebo; QUE=quetiapine; RIS=risperidone; SIADH=syndrome of inappropriate antidiuretic hormone secretion; VPA=valproate; YMRS=Young Mania Rating Scale; ZIP=ziprasidone.
[a]Mixed or manic episode.

quetiapine (mean dosage: 432 mg/day) had superior efficacy for adolescents with bipolar mania when added to valproic acid compared to augmentation of valproic acid with placebo (DelBello et al. 2002). In a head-to-head study, quetiapine (mean dosage: 412 mg/day) had similar efficacy as valproic acid, although speed of response was faster and remission was more frequent with quetiapine (DelBello et al. 2006). In pediatric patients with bipolar disorder, NNTs compared to placebo for response (defined as at least a 50% reduction in the YMRS total score) and for remission (defined by a YMRS total score ≤12) ranged from 3 to 6 with aripiprazole, olanzapine, quetiapine, risperidone, and ziprasidone (Correll et al., in press).

Aggressive Behaviors Associated With Autism Spectrum Disorders, Disruptive Behavior Disorders, ADHD, and Mental Retardation/Subaverage IQ

Eight RCTs (*N*=423) showed superior efficacy of antipsychotics in pediatric patients with autism spectrum disorders in all adequately powered studies (four studies with <15 patients) (Table 49–6). NNTs for study-defined response in autism spectrum disorders ranged from 2 to 4 for risperidone and from 3 to 4 in patients treated with olanzapine.

In eight placebo-controlled studies (*N*=322), superiority of risperidone compared to placebo has been demonstrated for aggressive behaviors associated with conduct disorder, disruptive behavior disorders, attention-deficit/hyperactivity disorder (ADHD), and/or mental retardation/subaverage IQ (Table 49–7). In one additional, active-controlled trial, molindone was found to be superior to thioridazine for conduct disorder in youth. NNTs for study-defined "response" ranged from 2 to 5 for risperidone in patients with aggression due to disruptive behavior spectrum disorders. In addition, risperidone has been shown to be superior to placebo for relapse prevention of autism (Research Units on Pediatric Psychopharmacology Autism Network 2005) and disruptive behavior disorders (Reyes et al. 2006).

Tourette's Syndrome

Superiority of risperidone or ziprasidone compared to placebo was shown in two randomized, placebo-controlled trials of youth with Tourette's syndrome (*N*=54), with an NNT of 4 for risperidone (see Table 49–7).

Adverse Effects

Children and adolescents seem to be more sensitive to most antipsychotic adverse effects, including sedation, EPS (except for akathisia), withdrawal dyskinesia, prolactin abnormalities, weight gain, and metabolic abnormalities (Correll et al. 2006). On the other hand, adverse effects that require a longer time to develop (e.g., diabetes mellitus) and that are related to greater medication dose and lifetime exposure (e.g., tardive dyskinesia) are less prevalent in youth. However, there is concern that these later-onset adverse effects are not seen because of short follow-up periods and that they may emerge in vulnerable patients prematurely in adulthood the earlier antipsychotics are started in childhood. Table 49–8 summarizes general side-effect propensities across seven SGAs available in the United States and three selected FGAs.

Neuromotor Adverse Effects

Extrapyramidal Side Effects

In general, children and adolescents are more sensitive than adults to EPS associated with FGAs and SGAs (Correll et al. 2006). An RCT of 40 youth with psychotic disorders comparing haloperidol (mean dosage: 5 mg/day), risperidone (mean dosage: 4 mg/day), and olanzapine (mean dosage: 12 mg/day) found substantial EPS not only with haloperidol (67%) but also with olanzapine (56%) and risperidone (53%), although haloperidol-treated patients reported more severe EPS (Sikich et al. 2004). In another study of 119 pediatric patients with schizophrenia, molindone (mean dosage: 60 mg/day) was associated with greater benztropine use (48%) compared to risperidone (37%, mean dosage: 2.8 mg) and olanzapine (26%, mean dosage: 11 mg/day), even though patients randomly assigned to molindone received 0.5 mg benztropine bid prophylactically (Sikich et al. 2008). Clozapine and quetiapine appear to be associated with relatively low rates of EPS in pediatric patients (as in adults). For aripiprazole and ziprasidone, rates of EPS appear to increase with increasing dose.

Since reported rates of EPS are highly dependent on dose and elicitation method, results have to be interpreted within these limitations, especially as most of the risperidone trials had been conducted in prepubertal boys with aggressive spectrum disorders in whom low doses of risperidone (only around 1 mg/day) were used. Moreover, noticeable rates of EPS in the placebo arms of placebo-controlled trials suggest

TABLE 49–6. Double-blind, randomized, placebo-controlled and active-controlled trials of antipsychotics in children and adolescents with autism spectrum disorders

Study	Design	Inclusion criteria	Drug	Mean dose, mg/day	N	Male, %	White, %	Age, mean (range)	Primary outcome	Response (as study-defined), %	NNT response	Remission (study-defined), %	NNT remission	≥7% Weight gain, %
Autism spectrum disorders, placebo-controlled														
Hollander et al. 2006	8-wk DB-RPCT	PDD	Total OLA Pbo	10	11 6 5	82 100 60	64 50 80	9.0 9.3 8.9 (6–14)	OASS and CGI-S: ns	50 20	4			67[a] 20
RUPP Autism Network 2005; Anderson et al. 2007; Aman et al. 2005	8-wk DB-RPCT	Autistic disorder	Total RIS Pbo	1.8	101 49 52	81	66	8.8 (5–17)	ABC: RIS>Pbo	69 12	2			
Aman et al. 2004	6-wk DB-PCT	CD, ODD, or DBD-NOS with comorbid ADHD	Total RIS+Stim RIS Pbo+Stim Pbo		155 35 43 38 39	86 81 92 74	66 56 74 56	9.0 8.6 8.9 8.3 (5–12)	ABC and N-CBRF: RIS>Pbo					
Luby et al. 2006	6-mo DB-RPCT	Autism	RIS Pbo	1.14	11 12	82 67	91 92	4.1 4 (2–6)	CARS: ns					
Shea et al. 2004	8-wk DB-RPCT	Autism, PDD	Total RIS Pbo	1.48	79 40 39	73 82	67 72	7.6 7.3 (5–12)	ABC and N-CBRF: RIS>Pbo	54 18	4			
Nagaraj et al. 2006	6-mo DB-RPCT	Autism	Total RIS Pbo	1	39 19 20	87 84 90		4.8 5.3 (2–9)	CARS: RIS>Pbo	95 30	2			
Autism spectrum disorders, active-controlled														
Miral et al. 2008	12-wk DB-RCT	Autistic disorder	RIS HAL	2.6 2.6	15 15	87 73		10.9 10.0 (7–17)	ABC and Turgay DSM-IV PDD: RIS>HAL	60 85	4			
Malone et al. 2001	6-wk ROT	Autistic disorder	Total OLA HAL	7.9 1.4	12 6 6	67 67 67	58 50 68	7.8 8.5 7.3 (4–12)	CGI-I, CGI-S, and CPRS: ns	83 50	3			

Note. ABC = Aberrant Behavior Checklist; ADHD = attention-deficit/hyperactivity disorder; CARS = Childhood Autism Rating Scale; CD = conduct disorder; CGI-I = Clinical Global Impressions Improvement Scale; CGI-S = Clinical Global Impressions Severity of Symptoms Scale; DBD-NOS = disruptive behavior disorder not otherwise specified; DB-RPCT = double-blind, randomized, placebo-controlled trial; HAL = haloperidol; N-CBRF = Nisonger Child Behavior Rating Form; NNT = number needed to treat; OASS = Overt Agitation Severity Scale; ODD = oppositional defiant disorder; OLA = olanzapine; Pbo = placebo; PDD = pervasive developmental disorder; RIS = risperidone; ROT = randomized open trial; RUPP = Research Units on Pediatric Psychopharmacology; Turgay DSM-IV PDD = Turgay DSM-IV Pervasive Developmental Disorder Scale.
[a]Number needed to harm, ≥7% weight gain: 3.

that some rates could be inflated by carryover effects of prior antipsychotic treatment.

Akathisia

In youth, less is known regarding the risk for akathisia, which has been substantial with FGAs across age groups and which seems to be similar across antipsychotics in pediatric compared to adult patients. Incidence rates of akathisia from placebo-controlled RCTs in pediatric schizophrenia have been reported for aripiprazole (5% for placebo, 5% in the 10 mg/day group, and 11.8% in the 30 mg/day group) and risperidone (6% for placebo, 6% in the 1-3 mg/day group, and 10% in the 4-6 mg/day group), corresponding to the number needed to harm (NNH) of 14.7 to no risk for aripiprazole 30 mg/day and 5 mg/day, respectively, and NNH of 25 to no risk for risperidone 4-6 mg/day and 1-3 mg/day, respectively (Correll 2008b). In an RCT in pediatric bipolar disorder, akathisia rates varied at 2.1% for placebo, 8.2% for aripiprazole 10 mg/day, and 11.8% for aripiprazole 30 mg/day, with corresponding NNTs of 9.1 to 14.1, respectively (Correll 2008b). The relatively high akathisia rates for placebo, especially in the pediatric schizophrenia trials, suggest the potential presence of a relevant carryover effect from prior antipsychotic treatment or the possibility of withdrawal phenomena after a brief washout from antipsychotics and/or medications that can mitigate akathisia. In the Treatment of Early Onset Schizophrenia Spectrum Disorders (TEOSS) study, molindone, but not olanzapine or risperidone, was associated with a significant increase in the Barnes Akathisia Scale score (Sikich et al. 2008). However, in interpreting these results, the clinician needs to consider that the occurrence of akathisia may depend on dose and speed of titration and that the identification and differentiation of akathisia from agitation, restlessness, or anxiety can be quite difficult.

Withdrawal Dyskinesia

During FGA treatment, youth are at risk of developing withdrawal dyskinesias, yet unlike in adults, the dyskinesias are frequently reversible (Campbell et al. 1997). Withdrawal dyskinesia rates appear to be lower with SGAs compared to FGAs (Connor et al. 2001), although a switch from an antipsychotic with strong D_2 affinity (risperidone or aripiprazole) to one with less potent affinity (quetiapine or clozapine) may predispose to withdrawal dyskinesia.

Tardive Dyskinesia

A meta-analysis of 10 studies lasting at least 11 months reported on tardive dyskinesia (TD) rates in 783 patients ages 4–18 years (weighted mean: 10 years). Most patients were prepubertal (80%), male (82%), and white (79%). Across these studies, only 3 cases of TD were reported, resulting in an annualized incidence rate of 0.4% (Correll and Kane 2007). While this pediatric rate is approximately half of the risk found in a meta-analysis including 1,964 nonelderly adults (Correll et al. 2004), firm conclusions are precluded by the fact that none of the pediatric studies was designed specifically to detect TD, antipsychotic doses were low, and lifetime exposure was relatively short.

Neuroleptic Malignant Syndrome

Neuroleptic malignant syndrome (NMS) is a rare but potentially fatal complication of antipsychotic treatment. It has been suggested that SGAs may be associated less with NMS than FGAs and that SGAs are associated with a more benign course of NMS (Ananth et al. 2004), but this is unclear. In children and adolescents, several cases of NMS have been reported even with SGAs. Thus, clinicians should be vigilant and rule out NMS in antipsychotic-treated youth presenting with fever, tachycardia, and marked motor rigidity by measuring white cell count and creatine kinase levels, which would both be elevated—with creatine kinase levels typically found to be 1,000 or higher in cases of true NMS.

Weight Gain and Metabolic Adverse Effects

Weight Gain

Although pediatric data are still limited, youth with psychiatric disorders seem to be at increased risk for being overweight or obese (Patel et al. 2007), especially when exposed to antipsychotics for longer periods of time (Laita et al. 2007). Age-inappropriate weight gain is of particular concern in pediatric patients, due to its association with glucose and lipid abnormalities and cardiovascular morbidity/mortality (American Diabetes Association et al. 2004). Reasons for weight gain are complex and include psychiatric illness, unhealthy lifestyle, and treatment effects. A review of pediatric data suggested that the weight gain potential of SGAs follows roughly the same ranking order as found in adults (see Table 49–8) but that the magnitude is greater (Correll and Carlson 2006). Exceptions may be a greater rel-

TABLE 49–7. Double-blind, randomized, placebo-controlled trials of antipsychotics in children and adolescents with disruptive behavior disorders and Tourette's syndrome

Study	Design	Inclusion criteria	Drug	Mean dose, mg/day	N	Male, %	White, %	Age, mean (range)	Primary outcome	Response (as study-defined), %	NNT response	Remission (study-defined), %	NNT remission	≥7% Weight gain, %
Disruptive behavior disorders, placebo-controlled														
Aman et al. 2002	6-wk DB-RPCT	Disruptive behavior, subaverage IQ	RIS Pbo	1.16	55 63	85 79	51 62	8.7 8.1	ABC: RIS>Pbo	54 8	3			
Snyder et al. 2002	6-wk DB-RPCT	CD, DBD, subaverage IQ	Total RIS Pbo	0.98	110 53 57	77 74	77 74	8.6 8.8	ABC: RIS>Pbo	38 16	3			
Campbell et al. 1984	4-wk DB-RPCT	CD	Total HAL Lithium Pbo	2.95 1.166	20 21 20	93 90 100 90	16	8.9 (5–12)	CPRS, hyperactivity, hostility, aggression: HAL and lithium>Pbo					
Van Bellinghen et al. 2001	4-wk DB-RPCT	Behavioral disturbances, subaverage IQ	Total RIS Pbo	1.2	13 6 7	39 33 43		10.5 11.0 (6–14)	ABC: RIS>Pbo	83 0	2			
Buitelaar et al. 2001	6-wk DB-RPCT	Aggression, subaverage IQ	Total RIS Pbo	2.9	38 19 19	90 84		14.0 13.7	ABC: RIS>Pbo					
Armenteros et al. 2007	4-wk DB-RPCT	ADHD + aggressive behavior	Total RIS Pbo	1.08	25 12 13	83 92	50 46	7.3 8.8 (7–12)	CAS-P and CAS-T: ns	100 77	5			
Findling et al. 2000	10-wk DB-RPCT	CD	Total RIS Pbo	1.26	20 10 10	95	50	10.7 8.2 (5–15)	ABC and RAAPP: RIS>Pbo					
Disruptive behavior disorders, active-controlled														
Greenhill et al. 1985	8-wk DB-RCT	CD	Total MOL THIO	26.8 169.9	31 15 16	100	19	9.8 10.3 (6–11)	CGI-S: MOL>THIO					

TABLE 49–7. Double-blind, randomized, placebo-controlled trials of antipsychotics in children and adolescents with disruptive behavior disorders and Tourette's syndrome *(continued)*

Study	Design	Inclusion criteria	Drug	Mean dose, mg/day	N	Male, %	White, %	Age, mean (range)	Primary outcome	Response (as study-defined), %	NNT response	Remission (study-defined), %	NNT remis-sion	≥7% Weight gain, %
Tourette's syndrome, placebo-controlled														
Scahill et al. 2003	8-wk DB-RPCT	Tourette's syndrome	Total RIS Pbo	2.5	26 12 14	96		11.1	YGTSS: RIS>Pbo					
Sallee et al. 2000	8-wk DB-RPCT	Tourette's syndrome	Total ZIP Pbo	28.2	28 16 12	79 88 67		11.3 11.8 (7–17)	YGTSS: ZIP>Pbo					

Note. ABC=Aberrant Behavior Checklist; ADHD=attention-deficit/hyperactivity disorder; CAS-P=Children's Aggression Scale—Parent; CAS-T=Children's Aggression Scale—Teacher; CD=conduct disorder; CPRS=Conners' Parent Rating Scale; DBD=disruptive behavior disorder; DB-RPCT=double-blind, randomized, placebo-controlled trial; HAL=haloperidol; IQ=intelligence quotient; MOL=molindone; MR=mental retardation; PDD=pervasive developmental disorder; RAAPP=Rating of Aggression Against People and/or Property Scale; RIS=risperidone; THIO=thioridazine; YGTSS=Yale Global Tic Severity Scale; ZIP=ziprasidone.

TABLE 49–8. Adverse effect profiles of antipsychotics in children and adolescents

Adverse effect	Time course	Dose dependent	Second-generation antipsychotics							First-generation antipsychotics		
			ARI	CLO	OLA	PAL	QUE	RIS	ZIP	HAL	MOL	PER
Acute parkinsonism	Early	+++	+	0	+	++	0	++	+	+++	++	++
Akathisia	Early/intermediate	+++	++	+	+	+	+	+	+/++	+++	++	++
Stroke	?	0?	?[a,b]	?[a,b]	?[a,b]	?[a,b]	?[a,b]	?[a,b]	?[a,b]	?[a,b]	?[a,b]	?[a,b]
Diabetes mellitus	Late	0/+?	0/+[a]	+++	+++	+[a]	++	+	0/+[a]	0/+[a]	0/+[a]	+
Diabetes insipidus	Late	+?	0	0/+	0	0	0	0	0	0	0	0
↑ Lipids	Early/intermediate	0?	0/+[a]	++	++	+[a]	+/++	+	0/+[a]	0/+[a]	0/+[a]	+
Neutropenia	Mostly first 6 months	+?	0/+	++	0/+	0/+	0/+	0/+	0/+	0/+	0/+	0/+
Orthostasis	Early/titration	+++	0/+	+++	++	+	++[c]	+	0	0	+	+
↑ Prolactin/sexual dysfunction	Early, may improve	+++	0	0	+/++	+++	0	+++	+	++	++	++
↓ Prolactin	Early	+?	++	0	0	0	0	0	0	0	0	0
↑ QTc interval	Early/titration	0/+?	0/+[d]	+[d]	0/+[d]	+[d]	+[d]	+[d]	++[d]	0+[d]	+[d]	+[d]
Rash, serious: Stevens-Johnson syndrome	High starting dose, fast titration	++	0/+	0/+	0/+	0/+	0/+	0/+	0/+	0/+	0/+	0/+
Sedation	Early, may improve	+++	0/+	+++	++	+	++[c]	+	0/+	0/+	+	+
Seizures	During titration	+++	0/+	++[a]	0/+	0/+	0/+	0/+	0/+	0/+	0/+	0/+
Tardive dyskinesia	Late	++	0/+[a]	0	0/+[e]	0/+[a]	0/+[e]	0/+	0/+[e]	++	+/++	+/++
Hyponatremia/SIADH	Intermediate/late	+?	0	0	0	0	0	0	0	0	0	0
Hypothyroidism	Intermediate/late	++	0	0	0	0	0/+[f]	0	0	0	0	0
Hyperparathyroidism	Intermediate/late	0?	0	0	0	0	0	0	0	0	0	0
Withdrawal dyskinesia	Early during (fast) switch	+++	++	+++	+++	+	0/+	+	+	++	+/++	+/++
Weight gain	First 3–6 months	0?	+	+++	+++	+/++	++	++	+	+	0/+	++

Note. A large part of the data information is extrapolated from adult populations. Therefore, information contained in this table may change as more data from large pediatric populations become available.

↑=increased; ↓=decreased; 0=none; 0/+=minimal; +=mild; ++=moderate; +++=severe; ARI=aripiprazole; CLO=clozapine; HAL=haloperidol; MOL=molindone; OLA=olanzapine; PAL=paliperidone; PER=perphenazine; QUE=quetiapine; RIS=risperidone; SIADH=syndrome of inappropriate antidiuretic hormone secretion; ZIP=ziprasidone.
[a]Insufficient long-term data to fully determine the risk; [b]Unlikely due to low risk factors in childhood and adolescents and long lag time for cerebrovascular disease to develop disease; [c]Less at higher doses (? above 250 mg/day); [d]Relevance for the development of torsades de pointes not established; [e]Less than 1% per year in adults who were often pretreated with first-generation antipsychotics; [f]Of unclear clinical relevance.

ative weight gain propensity of risperidone (Safer 2004) and a greater likelihood of aripiprazole and ziprasidone to not be weight neutral in subgroups of pediatric patients. Of note, combined treatment with an SGA and a stimulant does not seem to attenuate SGA-induced weight gain (Aman et al. 2004; Calarge et al. 2009), whereas combined SGA plus mood stabilizer treatment seems associated with more weight gain than mood stabilizer monotherapy and even combined mood stabilizer treatment. However, due to absent data, it is uncertain if this is also true for the combination of lower-risk SGAs (e.g., aripiprazole, ziprasidone) with conventional mood stabilizers (Correll 2007).

In an 8-week RCT, patients ages 7–16 years taking either clozapine or olanzapine for refractory schizophrenia exhibited similar weight gain (3.8±6.0 kg vs. 3.6±4.0 kg, respectively) (Shaw et al. 2006). In another RCT involving youth ages 10–18 years with early-onset schizophrenia, clozapine and haloperidol produced similar weight gain (0.9±6.5 kg vs. 0.9±2.9 kg, respectively) (Kumra et al. 1996), although the amount was lower than the gain reported by Shaw et al. (2006). In an open label naturalistic study, olanzapine was associated with greater weight gain (4.6±1.9 kg) than clozapine (2.5±2.9 kg), which had a weight gain similar to that of risperidone (2.8±1.3 kg) (Fleischhacker et al. 2006). However, because clozapine is given only in the case of treatment-refractoriness, the lower weight gain potential in youth treated with clozapine could be attenuated by a previous antipsychotic exposure.

In an 8-week study, Sikich et al. (2004) found a higher weight gain in young patients ages 5–17 years with psychotic disorders taking olanzapine for 8 weeks (7.1±4.1 kg) than in those taking either risperidone (4.9±3.6 kg) or haloperidol (3.5±3.7 kg); all weight gain was severe and disproportionate to that expected from normal growth. Similarly, in an earlier 12-week study, Ratzoni et al. (2002) found similarly severe weight gain with olanzapine (7.2±6.3 kg) and risperidone (3.9±4.8 kg), yet finding that patients taking haloperidol experienced no significant change in average weight (1.1±3.3 kg). In this study, weight gain of at least 7% occurred in 90.3% of patients taking olanzapine, 42.9% taking risperidone, and 12.5% taking haloperidol. Moreover, even in preschool-age children (ages 4–6 years), high weight gain rates have been reported with olanzapine and risperidone, amounting to 12.9±7.1% and 10.1±6.1% of baseline body weight during only 8 weeks of treatment (Biederman et al. 2005).

However, the interpretation of these results is complicated by the effects of baseline weight, developmental stage and growth, past antipsychotic exposure, treatment duration and setting, comedications, etc., that varied across trials. Therefore, randomized head-to-head studies of antipsychotics in youth are needed to directly compare risk-benefit ratios. Moreover, mean weight change results are complicated by the fact that a relevant group of patients may gain a lot of weight, whereas another group may lose weight after a switch from an agent with greater weight gain potential to one with less weight gain potential. Therefore, it is important to assess the proportion of patients who gained ≥7% of their baseline weight in the available short-term RCTs with SGAs.

Results from three 6-week studies in adolescents with schizophrenia (see Table 49–4) suggest that the olanzapine group had the greatest risk for significant weight gain (Kryzhanovskaya et al. 2009), risperidone was associated with intermediate risk (Haas et al. 2007), and aripiprazole showed the lowest risk (Findling et al. 2008). Although the duration of the RCTs was only 3 weeks (olanzapine and quetiapine) and 4 weeks (aripiprazole and ziprasidone), results from trials in pediatric bipolar disorder largely confirmed this pattern for olanzapine (Tohen et al. 2007) and aripiprazole (Correll et al. 2007), providing an additional intermediate-risk estimate for quetiapine (DelBello et al. 2007) and a low-risk estimate for ziprasidone (DelBello et al. 2008) (see Table 49–5). The respective NNHs for ≥7% weight gain in adolescents with schizophrenia were 4 for olanzapine, 8 for risperidone, and 25–34 for aripiprazole (see Table 49–4; Correll 2008b). The corresponding NNHs for patients with pediatric bipolar disorder were 3 for olanzapine, 7–10 for quetiapine, and 16 to – 100 (i.e., less harm than with placebo) for aripiprazole (see Table 49–5; Correll 2008b).

Metabolic Adverse Effects

Whereas in adults the link between antipsychotics and adverse metabolic effects, such as dyslipidemia, hyperglycemia, diabetes, and metabolic syndrome, has been established (American Diabetes Association et al. 2004), the few pediatric studies (Biederman et al. 2005, 2007; Malone et al. 2007; Martin and L'Ecuyer 2002; Sikich et al. 2004) have produced mostly negative results. Interpretation of these findings is limited by the small sample size, varying treatment histories, and inclusion of nonfasting blood assessments. Case reports of new-onset diabetes in antipsychotic-treated youth and the known link between weight gain and metabolic abnormalities suggest that youth are at least as liable to develop metabolic abnormalities as adults. However, in pediatric RCTs, so far only olanzapine has been associated with significant increases in glucose, insulin, and lipids (Kryzhanovskaya et al. 2009; Sikich et al. 2008; Tohen et al. 2007). Nevertheless, the lack of reported significant metabolic abnormalities in the other short-term RCTs despite mostly significant weight gain needs to be interpreted with caution, as the negative findings could be due to the short-term trial duration, lack of strict fasting assessments, and order effects in patients with more extensive past antipsychotic exposure. The relevant effect of past antipsychotic exposure and study duration is suggested by preliminary results of relevant metabolic abnormalities in antipsychotic-naive youth from an ongoing prospective study (Correll and Carlson 2006), as well as by a small 6-month naturalistic study of 66 pediatric patients with psychotic disorders and less than 30 days of lifetime antipsychotic exposure treated with olanzapine ($N=20$), risperidone ($N=22$), or quetiapine ($N=24$) (Fraguas et al. 2008). In this nonrandomized, unmatched population, 6 months of treatment with olanzapine and with quetiapine were associated with significant increases in fasting total cholesterol.

Prolactin-Related Side Effects

FGAs and SGAs can elevate prolactin levels. Hyperprolactinemia can result in sexual side effects, although prolactin levels are not tightly correlated with these symptoms; these include amenorrhea or oligomenorrhea, erectile dysfunction, decreased libido, hirsutism, and breast symptoms such as enlargement, engorgement, pain, or galactorrhea (Correll and Carlson 2006). Data also suggest that hyperprolactinemia is dose dependent, reduces over time, and resolves after antipsychotic discontinuation. The relative potency of antipsychotic drugs in increasing prolactin levels is higher in adolescents than in adults but follows roughly the same pattern: paliperidone≥risperidone>haloperidol>olanzapine>ziprasidone>quetiapine≥clozapine>aripiprazole. To date, adequate long-term data are lacking to determine if hyperprolactinemia at levels found during antipsychotic therapy alters bone density, sexual maturation, or the risk for benign prolactinomas (Correll and Carlson 2006). Because aripiprazole is a partial agonist at the D_2 receptor, prolactin levels can decrease below baseline. To date, no adverse effects have been described that might be related to low prolactin. Complicating the interpretation of available studies in youth is the fact that sexual side effects may not be present or expressed in prepubertal or sexually inactive youth and that symptoms are infrequently asked about. Thus, more research is needed to determine long-term effects of prolactin-level changes during development.

Cardiac Side Effects

QTc Prolongation

Antipsychotics can differentially prolong the heart rate–corrected QT interval of the electrocardiogram (ECG), which may be associated with torsades de pointes, a potentially fatal arrhythmia (Blair et al. 2005). Even in adults, QTc prolongation is usually minimal compared to placebo, except for thioridazine. Among SGAs, ziprasidone has been associated with the greatest QTc prolongation (Glassman and Bigger 2001). QTc prolongation to >430 ms was described (Blair et al. 2005) in 3 of 20 youth treated prospectively with ziprasidone (mean peak QTc prolongation of 28 ± 26 ms, $P<0.01$), without relationship to ziprasidone dosage (mean: 30 ± 13 mg/day, range: 30–60 mg/day). In another study ($N=12$), Malone et al. (2007) also reported a statistically significant increase in QTc (15 ± 21 ms, $P=0.04$) at a mean ziprasidone dosage of 99 mg/day (range: 40–160 mg/day). However, QTc changes were nonsignificant in studies of 12 (McDougle et al. 2002), 16 (Sallee et al. 2000), and 21 (Biederman et al. 2007) patients at ziprasidone dosages of 57 mg/day (range: 20–120 mg/day), 28 mg/day (range: 5–40 mg/day), and 60 mg/day (range: 20–120 mg/day), respectively. Further, no patient in these studies reported cardiac side effects, such as dizziness, palpitations, or syncope. This indicates that the clinical relevance of this degree of QTc prolongation (not reaching the generally accepted pathological threshold of >500 ms or an increase in QTc over baseline of >60 ms [Glassman and Bigger 2001]) is unclear. Thus, theoretical concerns about QTc prolongation with ziprasidone need to be weighed against its more certain weight-related and metabolic benefits. However, ECGs may need to be obtained whenever there is a family history of early sudden death, prolonged QT syndrome, or a personal history of irregular heart beat, tachycardia at rest, shortness of breath, dizziness on exertion, or syncope. Only clozapine has been associated with a myocarditis risk that is greatest early in treatment. Clinical signs of acute myocarditis include palpitations, chest pain, shortness of breath, and syncope. Characteristic ECG changes include ectopic beats, atrioventricular block, atrial fibrillation or flutter, intraventricular conduction disturbance, ventricular tachycardia or fibrillation, and low QRS voltages. In youth, the incidence seems relatively low (Wehmeier et al. 2004).

Miscellaneous Adverse Effects

Sedation/Somnolence

Sedation is a frequent and often impairing antipsychotic side effect that usually is dose dependent, although tolerance may develop. An exception to the dose-dependent nature of sedation may be quetiapine, which seems to be less sedating at dosages above 200–300 mg/day where alpha-2 blockade sets in, increasing noradrenergic tone. Although limited by different methodologies, a comparison of adult FDA labeling trials with pediatric data suggested a similar rank order of sedation but increased rates in youth (Correll et al. 2006). Sedation rates were 0%–33% for aripiprazole, 42%–69% for ziprasidone, 25%–80% for quetiapine, 29%–89% for risperidone, 44%–94% for olanzapine, and 46%–90% with clozapine. These rates are of particular concern in youth due to the potential interference with learning and school performance.

Liver Enzyme Abnormality/Toxicity

Abnormal liver enzymes have been reported with pediatric antipsychotic use (Kumra et al. 1997; Sikich et al. 2004, 2008). In two RCTs of olanzapine (Kryzhanovskaya et al. 2009; Tohen et al. 2007), significantly more patients had abnormal liver function tests of greater than three times the norm than patients on placebo. Abnormal aspartate transaminase (AST) was present in 35% versus 7% and 22% versus 2% in patients with schizophrenia and bipolar disorder, respectively. Abnormal alanine transaminase was present in 48% versus 3% and 34% versus 2% in patients with schizophrenia and bipolar disorder, respectively. These frequencies translate into an NNH of 3–5 for abnormal liver function with olanzapine compared to placebo. In the TEOSS study, olanzapine, but not risperidone or molindone, increased transaminases, with a significant baseline to endpoint increase for AST (Sikich et al. 2008). Although the extent and significance of liver enzyme abnormalities are unclear, the combination of divalproex with antipsychotics, particularly olanzapine, may increase the risk of abnormal liver function (Gonzalez-Heydrich et al. 2003).

Neutropenia and Agranulocytosis

With the exception of clozapine, the antipsychotic-associated decrease in white blood cell counts is generally not clinically significant. In a chart review of 172 clozapine-treated pediatric patients (Gerbino-Rosen et al. 2005), the cumulative 1-year probability of an initial adverse hematological event was 16% (neutropenia:

13%; agranulocytosis: 0.6%). However, 48% of the 24 children and adolescents with newly emerging neutropenia were successfully rechallenged, and only 8 patients discontinued clozapine because of neutropenia (*n*=7) or agranulocytosis (*n*=1).

Adverse Effect Assessment and Monitoring

Adverse effect assessment and monitoring should be proactive, taking into consideration developmental norms and thresholds. Suggested baseline and follow-up assessments and intervals are detailed in Table 49–9.

Healthy Lifestyle

Healthy (or unhealthy) lifestyle behaviors related to diet, activity, sleep, and substance use should be inquired about and compared with recommendations in the pediatric (American Medical Association 2007) or psychiatric population (Correll and Carlson 2006). These recommendations are listed in Table 49–10.

Neuromotor Adverse Effects

Parkinsonian side effects and akathisia should be monitored at baseline, during titration, at 3 months, and annually, unless there are abnormalities noted. Dyskinetic movements should be assessed at least at baseline, 3 months, and annually, unless there are abnormalities noted. It can be useful to measure these adverse effects with widely available rating scales, such as the Simpson-Angus Scale for parkinsonian side effects, the Barnes Akathisia Rating Scale for akathisia, and the Abnormal Involuntary Movement Scale for TD.

Body Weight and Composition

Ideally, weight should be monitored at each clinical visit (see Table 49–9). Clinically, the most commonly used measures to monitor weight include absolute weight change (kg, lbs), percentage weight change (weight change/baseline weight), and change in body mass index (BMI). Although easily obtained and valid in adults, these measures are useful only for periods of ≤3 months in pediatric patients, as they do not account for normal growth. Therefore, age- and sex-adjusted BMI percentiles (used to determine weight category;

TABLE 49–9. Suggested monitoring strategies in children and adolescents treated with antipsychotic agents[a]

Assessment	Baseline	Each visit	During titration and at target dose	At 3 months	Every 3 months	Every 6 months	Annually
Lifestyle behaviors[b]	✓	✓	—	—	—	—	—
Sedation/somnolence	✓	✓	—	—	—	—	—
Height, weight (calculate BMI percentile, BMI z score)	✓	✓	—	—	—	—	—
Sexual/reproductive dysfunction	✓	—	✓	✓	✓	—	—
Fasting blood glucose and lipids	✓	—	—	✓	—	✓	—
Parkinsonism (SAS or ESRS), akathisia (AIMS or ESRS)	✓	—	✓	✓	—	—	✓
Tardive dyskinesia	✓	—	—	✓	—	—	✓
Blood pressure and pulse	✓	—	—	✓	—	—	✓
Personal and family medical history[c]	✓	—	—	—	—	—	✓
Liver function tests	If symptomatic or significant weight gain	—	—	✓	—	—	If symptomatic or significant weight gain
Electrolytes, full blood count, renal function	If symptomatic, regular blood counts if on clozapine	—	—	—	—	—	If symptomatic, regular blood counts if on clozapine
Electrocardiogram	If on ziprasidone or clozapine	—	✓ (If on ziprasidone) (only if symptomatic if on clozapine)	—	—	—	—
Prolactin[d]	If symptomatic	—	If symptomatic	If symptomatic	If symptomatic	If symptomatic	If symptomatic

Note. AIMS=Abnormal Involuntary Movement Scale (Guy 1976); BMI=body mass index; ESRS=Extrapyramidal Symptom Rating Scale (Chouinard et al. 1980); SAS=Simpson Angus Rating Scale (Simpson and Angus 1970).

[a]More frequent assessments of abnormalities occur or patient is at very high risk for specific adverse effects by personal or family history.

[b]Lifestyle behaviors=diet, exercise, smoking, substance use, sleep hygiene.

[c]Including components of the metabolic syndrome (obesity, arterial hypertension, diabetes, dyslipidemia), past medical history for coronary heart disease or coronary heart disease equivalent disorders (e.g., diabetes mellitus, peripheral arterial disease, abdominal aortic aneurysm, and symptomatic carotid artery disease), history of premature coronary heart disease in first-degree relatives (males <55 years and females <65 years), and past efficacy and adverse effect experiences in patients and/or family members.

[d]In case of abnormal sexual symptoms or signs; draw fasting in the A.M. and approximately 12 hours after the last antipsychotic dose.

TABLE 49–10. Healthy lifestyle recommendations for children and adolescents in the general and psychiatric populations

	American Medical Association 2007	Correll and Carlson 2006
Target group	General pediatric population ages 2–19 years; prevention and intervention for individuals who are overweight (≥85th BMI percentile) or obese (≥90th BMI percentile)	Pediatric patients <18 years receiving psychotropic medications associated with weight gain
Parenting style	Allow child to self-regulate meals; encourage authoritative parenting style[a] supporting increased physical activity and reduced sedentary behavior; provide tangible and motivational support; discourage overly restrictive parenting style[b]	–
Family involvement	Yes	Yes
Diet		
Sugar-containing beverages	No sugar-sweetened beverages; assess for excessive consumption of 100% fruit juice	Replace sugar-containing drinks, including "diet" drinks, with water or moderate amounts of unsweetened tea or milk
Meal frequency	Assess for meal frequency (including quality)	Four to less than six separate meals per day, with two meals or less in the evening or at night
Breakfast	Daily breakfast	Avoid skipping breakfast
Meal portions	Assess for consumption of excessive portion sizes for age	Promote serving small meal portions
Pacing of food consumption	–	Eat slowly and take second helpings only after a delay
Sugar content	Assess for excessive consumption of foods that are high in energy density	Preferentially eat food with a low glycemic index (i.e., of 55 or less; http://www.glycemicindex.com)
Fat content	Diet with balanced macronutrients (calories from fat, carbohydrate, and protein in proportions for age recommended by Dietary Reference Intakes)	Reduce saturated fat intake, but avoid extensive consumption of processed fat-free food items
Fiber content	Diet high in fiber; five or more servings of fruits and vegetables per day	At least 25–30 grams of soluble fiber per day
Snacks	Assess for snacking patterns (including quality); limit consumption of energy-dense foods	Avoid snacking in a satiety state, replacing high-fat, high-calorie snacks with fruits and vegetables
Outside meals/fast food	Limit meals outside the home, especially in fast-food restaurants; family meals at least 5–6 times/week	Limit fast food to no more than once per week
Activity		
Sedentary behavior	Two or fewer hours of screen time per day, and no television in the room where the child sleeps	Limit sedentary behaviors, such as watching TV or playing computer/video games, to less than 2 hours per day
Exercise	One hour or more of daily physical activity	Perform moderate-level physical activity for at least 30–60 minutes/day

[a]Authoritative parents are both demanding and responsive. "They monitor and impart clear standards for their children's conduct. They are assertive, but not intrusive and restrictive. Their disciplinary methods are supportive, rather than punitive. They want their children to be assertive as well as socially responsible, and self-regulated as well as cooperative" (American Medical Association 2007). [b]Restrictive parenting=heavy monitoring and controlling of a child's behavior (American Medical Association 2007).

Table 49–11) and BMI z scores (used for change over time) need to be calculated, using growth charts (www.cdc.gov/growthcharts/) or calculators (e.g., http://www.kidsnutrition.org/bodycomp/bmiz2.html). A BMI z score (standard deviations) of zero and the 50th BMI percentile represent the population mean. Continuation on the same BMI z score or percentile represents stable relative weight over time. Although in adults waist circumference is preferred over BMI as a metabolic syndrome criterion, it is not recommended as a routine assessment in youth, due to difficulty in accurate measurements and uncertainty of age-dependent cutoffs (American Medical Association 2007).

Blood Sugar and Insulin

To assess the risk for hyperglycemia and emerging diabetes (see Table 49–11), fasting blood glucose should be measured at baseline, 3 months, and every 6 months (see Table 49–9) (Correll 2008a). Families should be instructed that the patient must consume nothing but water for ≥8 hours prior to the blood draw. High-risk patients (e.g., family history of diabetes, nonwhite, BMI ≥95th percentile, weight gain >0.5 BMI z score) may require more frequent assessments. Patients should be asked at each visit about unintended weight loss, polyuria, and polydipsia to rule out emerging diabetes. Developing insulin resistance (i.e., increased insulin secretion) is more likely than diabetes in the context of weight gain as long as pancreatic beta cells are able to compensate for the decreased insulin sensitivity. A simple measure of insulin resistance is the homeostatic model assessment (HOMA-IR): insulin (μU/mL) x fasting glucose (mmol/L)/22.5. HOMA-IR of ≥4.4 represents insulin resistance in adolescents (Lee et al. 2006). Nevertheless, insulin levels are not currently recommended in clinical practice, as they are expensive and not subject to standardized assays in the United States. Moreover, HOMA-IR predominantly reflects hepatic insulin sensitivity, which determines fasting levels of glucose and insulin, whereas insulin resistance also occurs in skeletal muscle, particularly early on. The ratio of fasting triglycerides to high-density lipoprotein (HDL) cholesterol has also been proposed as a widely applicable and sensitive measure of insulin resistance, with 3.5 being discussed as the threshold predicting insulin resistance, yet this marker has not been evaluated in youth. Nonfasting or postprandial glucose or hemoglobin A1c levels are not recommended as screening tests for hyperglycemia or diabetes (Correll 2008a).

Blood Lipids

Like blood sugar, fasting serum lipids should be obtained at baseline, 3 months, and every 6 months (see Table 49–9), with shorter intervals in case of abnormal lipids or significant weight gain (Correll 2008a). The panel should include total cholesterol, HDL cholesterol, and triglycerides. Table 49–11 summarizes pediatric-specific blood lipid thresholds.

Blood Pressure

Blood pressure should be measured with a cuff large enough that 80% of the upper arm is covered. To assess for hypertension, the patient's height percentile has to be calculated (https://www.nutropin.com/patient/3_5_3_growth_charts.jsp). The measured blood pressure is compared with population norms from children of the same age, sex, and height (hypertension: ≥90th percentile for sex and age; see Table 49–11) (National High Blood Pressure Education Program Working Group on High Blood Pressure in Children and Adolescents 2004).

Prolactin and Sexual/ Reproductive System Side Effects

In case of hyperprolactinemia, common causes need to be ruled out (e.g., hormonal contraception or pregnancy, hypothyroidism, or renal failure) by measuring serum human chorionic gonadotropin (hCG), thyroid-stimulating hormone (TSH), or creatinine, respectively. To identify hyperprolactinemia-related hypogonadism, the clinician should inquire at baseline, during drug titration, and quarterly about menstruation, nipple discharge, breast enlargement, sexual functioning, and (if appropriate) pubertal development. Since the effects of subclinical prolactin elevations are unclear, current thinking dictates that prolactin levels only be measured if manifest clinical problems develop. Because prolactin undergoes diurnal variations and increases with exercise, stress, and food intake, it should be measured in the morning, after fasting, and 8–12 hours after the last medication dose. Prolactin thresholds are laboratory dependent and higher for postpubertal youth and females (upper level: ~20–30 ng/mL) than in males (upper level: ~11–15 ng/mL or age in years up until age 18).

Liver Enzymes

Liver enzyme testing to check for potential signs of fatty liver infiltration should be considered in patients who 1) have abdominal/gastrointestinal symptoms, 2) gain ≥7% of their baseline body weight over 3 months, or 3) have ≥0.5 BMI z scores when treated for >3 months. In patients with AST, alanine aminotransferase, or γ-glutamyl transferase levels three times the norm and without other medical causes, discontinuation of the antipsychotic or of possibly responsible comedications should be considered.

White Cell and Granulocyte Counts

The increased risk of agranulocytosis associated with clozapine requires enrollment in a central national database. Guidelines mandate weekly monitoring of the white blood cell count (WBC) and absolute neutrophil count (ANC) for the first 6 months. If the counts are normal (WBC >3,500 and ANC >2,000), intervals change to biweekly for the next 6 months and monthly thereafter. If there is a single drop or cumulative drop within 3 weeks of WBC ≥3,000/mm^3 or of ANC ≥1,500/mm^3, or if WBC is <3,500/mm^3 and ≥3,000/mm^3 or ANC is <2,000/mm^3 and ≥1,500/mm^3 (mild leukopenia/granulocytopenia), twice-weekly blood monitoring is to be initiated until WBC >3,500/mm^3 and ANC >2,000/mm^3, at which point the clinician may return to previous monitoring frequency. In case of moderate leukopenia/granulocytopenia (WBC <3,000/mm^3 and ≥2,000/mm^3 and/or ANC <1,500/mm^3 and ≥1,000/mm^3), clozapine is to be stopped, daily blood tests are required until WBC >3,000/mm^3 and ANC >1,500/mm^3, followed by twice-weekly blood tests until WBC >3,500/mm^3 and ANC >2,000/mm^3. Clozapine rechallenge is permitted when WBC >3,500/mm^3 and ANC >2,000/mm^3. However, if clozapine rechallenge is initiated, weekly monitoring is required for 1 year before returning to the usual monitoring schedule of every 2 weeks for 6 months and then every 4 weeks as long as results are normal. In case of WBC <2,000/mm^3 and/or ANC <1,000/mm^3, clozapine is to be discontinued and a rechallenge is not permitted.

Of note, the thresholds for discontinuing clozapine do not take into account ethnic variations. Considering ethnic variations is important, as a subgroup of patients with African descent (25%–50%) and some people of Middle Eastern origin have habitually low white counts in the absence of any infections—also called benign eth-

nic (or cyclic) neutropenia (Rajagopal 2005). African Americans have lower WBCs and ANCs than whites, and people of African descent have lower values than people of African American descent. Men have lower values than women, independent of ethnicity (Hsieh et al. 2007). Based on these findings and successful clozapine treatment in patients with benign ethnic neutropenia (Whiskey and Taylor 2007), adjusted thresholds for patients with habitually low white counts have been proposed (Rajagopal 2005) that are 500/mm^3 lower than in the general population for normal white cell/neutrophil count (≥3,000/≥1,500/mm^3 instead of ≥3,500/≥2,000/mm^3), mild leukopenia/neutropenia (≥2,500–3,000/≥1,000–1,500 mm^3 instead of ≥3,000–3,500/≥1,500–2,000/mm^3), and moderate leukopenia/neutropenia (<2,500 to >2,000/<1,000 to >500/mm^3 instead of <3,000 to >2,000/<1,500 to >1,000/mm^3).

Cardiac Conduction and Repolarization

Although a very uncommon complication of antipsychotic treatment, any QTc value of ≥500 ms, confirmed by manual reading, should lead to a discontinuation of the antipsychotic, unless other QT-prolonging agents can be discontinued instead or hypomagnesemia or hypokalemia is present that can be corrected.

Managing Adverse Effects

In addition to discussion in this section, Table 49–12 lists some suggested adverse effect management strategies in children and adolescents treated with antipsychotic agents.

Neuromotor Adverse Effects

Extrapyramidal adverse effects are dose and titration dependent. In milder cases, a dose reduction or slowing of the titration can bring relief. In cases of more severe parkinsonian side effects, oral or (especially for acute dystonia) intramuscular anticholinergics, antihistamines, or adjunctive benzodiazepines can be used. Once the patient is stabilized and on maintenance therapy, gradual withdrawal of the adjunctive treatments for the neuromotor adverse effects can be tried to reduce the potential cognitive burden that anticholinergics especially may have. Often, patients adapt to the dopamine blockade over time and do not require sustained

TABLE 49–11. Clinically relevant thresholds for body weight and metabolic parameters in adults and in children and adolescents

Variables	Children and adolescents	Adults
Body weight		
Underweight	BMI <5th percentile for sex and age[b]	BMI[a] <18.5
Normal weight	BMI 5th to <85th percentile for sex and age[b]	BMI[a] 18.5 to <25
Overweight (previously "at-risk for overweight" in pediatric patients)	BMI 85th to <95th percentile for sex and age[b]	BMI[a] 25 to <30
Obese (previously "overweight" in pediatric patients)	BMI ≥95th percentile for sex and age[b]	BMI[a] ≥30
Blood glucose		
Fasting hyperglycemia ("prediabetes")	100–125 mg/dL	100–125 mg/dL
2-hour postglucose load hyperglycemia ("impaired glucose tolerance")	140–199 mg/dL	140–199 mg/dL
Fasting diabetes (needs to be repeated)	≥126 mg/dL	≥126 mg/dL
2-hour postglucose load diabetes	≥200 mg/dL	≥200 mg/dL
Insulin and insulin resistance		
Fasting hyperinsulinemia	>20 μmol/L	?
Homeostatic model assessment (HOMA)[e]	≥4.4	?
Triglycerides:HDL-cholesterol ratio	? >3.5	>3.5
Blood lipids		
Total cholesterol	≥170 mg/dL	≥200 mg/dL
LDL cholesterol	≥130 mg/dL	Dependent on 10-year coronary heart disease risk calculation[c] and presence of coronary heart disease equivalents[d]
HDL cholesterol	<40 mg/dL in males and females	<40 mg/dL in males; <50 mg/dL in females
Triglycerides	≥110 mg/dL	≥150 mg/dL
Metabolic syndrome	≥ Three out of five criteria required	≥ Three out of five criteria required
Abdominal obesity criterion	Waist circumference ≥90th percentile, or BMI ≥95th percentile for sex and age[f]	Waist circumference >40 inches (102 cm) in males; >35 inches (88 cm) in females
Fasting triglycerides criterion	≥110 mg/dL	≥150 mg/dL
Fasting HDL cholesterol criterion	<40 mg/dL in males and females	<40 mg/dL in males; <50 mg/dL in females
Blood pressure criterion	≥90th percentile for sex and age[g]	≥130/85 mm/Hg

TABLE 49–11. Clinically relevant thresholds for body weight and metabolic parameters in adults and in children and adolescents *(continued)*

Variables	Children and adolescents	Adults
Metabolic syndrome *(continued)*		
Fasting glucose criterion	≥110 mg/dL	≥110 mg/dL
Adjusted fasting glucose criterion	≥100 mg/dL	≥100 mg/dL

Note. **Thresholds shown in boldface are specific for children and adolescents.**
BMI=body mass index; HDL=high-density lipoprotein; LDL=low-density lipoprotein.

[a]BMI (unadjusted=weight (kg)/height (m)^2; or weight (lbs) × 733/height (inches)).

[b]Sex- and age-adjusted BMI expressed in percentile (population norm: 50th BMI percentile) or BMI z scores (population norm: 0 BMI z score): Growth charts: www.cdc.gov/growthcharts/; or Web-based calculators: http://www.kidsnutrition.org/bodycomp/bmiz2.html, or http://www.gcrc.uci.edu/utilities/bmi2.cfm. Stable age- and sex-adjusted weight is indicated by absence of any change in BMI percentile and BMI z score over time.

[c]10-year coronary heart disease risk calculation based on Framingham Point Scoring System (Expert Panel on Detection, Evaluation, and Treatment of High Blood Cholesterol in Adults 2001).

[d]Coronary heart disease equivalents: peripheral arterial disease, abdominal aortic aneurysm, and symptomatic carotid artery disease.

[e]HOMA: homeostatic model assessment=fasting insulin (μmol/L) × glucose (mmol/L)/22.5; glucose mmol/L = glucose m/dL/17.979797 or fasting insulin (mg/dL) × glucose (mg/dL)/405.

[f]Sex- and age-adjusted waist circumference percentile tables (Fernandez et al. 2004).

[g]Sex- and age-adjusted blood pressure percentile tables (National High Blood Pressure Education Program Working Group on High Blood Pressure in Children and Adolescents 2004).

anticholinergic treatment. For akathisia, beta-blockers, benzodiazepines, dopamine agonists, or mirtazapine can be helpful. Unfortunately, unless the patient can be maintained without antipsychotic therapy, no evidence-based therapy for TD exists, but dose reduction (or dose increase to mask the movements) or a switch from an FGA to an SGA or to clozapine can be tried.

Weight and Metabolic Dysfunction

Medical health strategies for youth treated with antipsychotics were recently summarized (Correll 2008c). *Primary preventive strategies* include 1) educating about and maximizing adherence to healthy lifestyle behaviors (see Table 49–10) and 2) choosing an agent with the lowest likelihood of adverse effects on body composition and metabolic status. *Secondary preventive strategies* in overweight patients and those with mild baseline metabolic abnormalities, significant weight gain, or beginning metabolic abnormalities (see Table 49–11) during therapy include 1) intensification of healthy lifestyle instructions, 2) consideration of switching to a lower-risk agent, and 3) a nonpharmacological weight-loss treatment or adjunctive pharmacological intervention that targets normalization or reversal of weight abnormalities (see Table 49–12). *Tertiary preventive strategies* in patients who are obese or have clinically defined related abnormalities (e.g., hyperglycemia, diabetes, dyslipidemia, or hypertension; see Table 49–11) require intensified weight reduction interventions, attempts at changing to or initiating lower-risk medications for the underlying psychiatric condition, and targeted treatments of these suprathreshold metabolic or endocrine abnormalities, often in conjunction with a subspecialist.

Despite concern about age-inappropriate weight gain in pediatric patients, no consensus exists regarding the cutoff for clinically meaningful weight change. Rather, BMI ≥85th percentile (i.e., overweight or obese) is the accepted threshold for intervention (American Medical Association 2007; see Table 49–11). However, in psychiatric practice, where the underlying illness in conjunction with adverse treatment effects can lead to relevant and often rapid weight gain, clinicians require guidance regarding at what point to consider changing therapy or using adjunctive treatments. Clinically significant weight gain or abnormal weight status in psychiatrically ill patients requiring a reconsideration of the current treatment plan has been operationalized as follows (Correll and Carlson 2006):

1. >5% weight gain during 3 months; or
2. Any of the following three conditions at any time during treatment:
   a. ≥0.5 increase in BMI z score
   b. BMI percentile ≥85–94.9 plus one adverse health consequence (hyperglycemia, dyslipidemia, hyperinsulinemia, hypertension, or orthopedic, gallbladder, or sleep disorder)
   c. BMI ≥95th percentile or abdominal obesity (>90th percentile).

As outlined above, the treatment of choice for abnormalities in body weight or metabolic health includes healthy lifestyle education and modification strategies. While such strategies have been tested and shown to be successful to a certain degree in adults (Faulkner et al. 2007), the effects of healthy lifestyle programs have not yet been reported in antipsychotic-treated youth. The recent American Medical Association (2007) Expert Committee Stage 1 recommendations for healthy lifestyle behaviors in pediatric patients that can be implemented widely without significant training are summarized in Table 49–9. Progression to the *structured* Stage 2 weight management protocol is indicated if after 3–6 months no improvement in weight status has occurred and if the patient and family show readiness for change. Stage 2 interventions can be implemented by a primary care physician or allied health care provider highly trained in weight management and include the following:

1. Structured dietary and physical activity behaviors
   a. Plan development for a balanced macronutrient diet containing few energy-dense foods
   b. Structured daily meals and snacks
   c. Supervised active play of ≥60 minutes daily
   d. Screen time of ≤1 hour daily
2. Increased monitoring (e.g., of screen time, physical activity, dietary intake, restaurant logs) by provider, patient, or family
3. Goal setting of weight maintenance resulting in a decreasing BMI percentile as age and height increase

If no improvement in BMI percentile or weight occurs after 3–6 months, the patient should be advanced to Stage 3, consisting of a comprehensive protocol implemented by a multidisciplinary obesity care team and aiming at weight maintenance or gradual weight loss until BMI <85th percentile (American Medical Association 2007).

769 Antipsychotic Medications

TABLE 49–12. Suggested adverse effect management strategies in children and adolescents treated with antipsychotic agents

Assessment	Selected interventions for relevant abnormality
Unhealthy lifestyle behaviors[c]	Healthy lifestyle instruction or intervention program
Sedation/somnolence	Wait if tolerance develops, decrease dose (increase if on low-dose quetiapine, which may lead to less sedation at dosages ≥300 mg/day); switch to lower-risk drug; modafinil coadministration
Postural hypotension/dizziness/syncope	Slow down titration, reduce dose (increase if on low-dose quetiapine, which may lead to less orthostasis at dosages ≥300 mg/day); increase fluid intake; switch to lower-risk drug
Parkinsonism	Slow down titration, reduce dose; switch to lower-risk drug; add anticholinergic,[a] antihistamine,[a] benzodiazepine,[a,c] and so forth
Akathisia	Slow down titration, reduce dose; switch to lower-risk drug; add benzodiazepine,[a,b,c] beta-blocker,[b] antihistamine,[a] anticholinergic, and so forth
Tardive dyskinesia	Reduce dose; increase dose (masking); if possible, replace with non-antipsychotic; switch to clozapine; add vitamin E
Developmentally inappropriate weight gain	Switch to lower-risk drug; healthy lifestyle intervention; add weight-loss agents (metformin,[d] orlistat,[e] amantadine,[f,g] topiramate,[a] bupropion,[g] and the like)
Arterial hypertension/tachycardia	Switch to lower-risk drug; healthy lifestyle intervention; add weight-loss agents (metformin,[d] orlistat,[e] amantadine,[f,g] topiramate,[a] bupropion,[g] and the like; add antihypertensive
Hyperglycemia/diabetes	Switch to lower-risk drug; healthy lifestyle intervention; add weight-loss agents (metformin,[d] orlistat,[e] amantadine,[f,g] topiramate,[a] bupropion,[g] and the like; add antihyperglycemic agent
Dyslipidemia	Switch to lower-risk drug; healthy lifestyle intervention; add weight-loss agents (metformin,[d] orlistat,[e] amantadine,[f,g] topiramate,[a] bupropion,[g] and the like); add lipid-lowering agent
Clinically relevant abnormal electrolytes, full blood count, renal function	Switch to lower-risk drug; address specific abnormality as needed
Abnormally elevated liver enzymes (>2 upper limit)	Reassess need for medication, consider switch
Hyperprolactinemia	If asymptomatic, may wait if values normalize with time; reduce dose; switch to lower-risk drug if symptomatic Only if symptomatic hyperprolactinemia continues despite switch to a low-risk antipsychotic: obtain MRI of the sella turcica or bone density scan or add a full (e.g., bromocriptine,[f,g] amantadine,[f,g]) or partial (e.g., aripiprazole) dopamine agonist
Sexual/reproductive dysfunction	Reduce dose; switch to lower-risk drug; for performance: add bupropion,[g] sildenafil, and so forth
Clinically relevant ECG abnormalities	Reassess need for medication, consider switch

Note. ECG=electrocardiogram; MRI=magnetic resonance imaging.
[a]Can impair cognitive abilities; [b]Can cause bradycardia, dizziness, and syncope; [c]Can impair coordination; [d]Lactic acidosis and hypoglycemia no real risk in children; nausea, stomachache, flatulence, and diarrhea can occur; [e]Unless low-fat diet is observed, flatulence, diarrhea, and involuntary encopresis can occur; [f]Potential risk for exacerbation of psychosis; [g]Potential risk for exacerbation of mania.

If behavioral measures alone are insufficient, pharmacological weight loss interventions may be added. Data in nonpsychiatrically ill youth with obesity support the use of sibutramine (serotonin-norepinephrine reuptake inhibitor), orlistat (enteric lipase inhibitor), and metformin (insulin sensitizer) (Correll 2008c; Correll and Carlson 2006). Orlistat (e.g., 120 mg tid, paired with a low-fat diet to minimize gastric side effects) and sibutramine (e.g., 5–15 mg/day) are FDA approved for weight loss in adolescents. Sibutramine may increase blood pressure, should not be given together with other serotonin-enhancing drugs (e.g., antidepressants, stimulants, and lithium), and is approved only for patients ≥16 years old. Therapies that have had some success in producing weight loss in pediatric patients receiving antipsychotics include metformin (e.g., 250 mg/day tid if <50 kg, or 500 mg/day tid to 1,000 mg/day bid if ≥50 kg titrated over 3–4 weeks), topiramate (e.g., 25–400 mg/day), amantadine (e.g., 100 mg bid or tid), and orlistat (Correll and Carlson 2006). Dyslipidemia should be treated initially with dietary measures; if this is not sufficient, drug therapy may be given with a fibric acid derivative (e.g., gemfibrozil, fenofibrate), a statin, fish oil, or niacin, if appropriate. Diabetes may be treated with diet, oral hypoglycemic agents, or insulin as needed, but diabetes induced by atypical antipsychotic agents sometimes disappears when the drug is stopped or changed to a lower-risk agent (Correll and Carlson 2006). While medications used to mitigate or reverse antipsychotic-induced weight gain may be prescribed by psychiatric health care providers, medications used to treat dyslipidemia or hyperglycemia are likely managed by pediatricians or pediatric endocrinologists.

Hyperprolactinemia and Sexual/Reproductive System Side Effects

If serum prolactin is <200 ng/mL, management strategies include antipsychotic dose reduction or change to a prolactin-sparing drug, such as aripiprazole, quetiapine, or in treatment-resistant patients, clozapine (Correll and Carlson 2006). If serum prolactin is >200 ng/mL or is persistently elevated despite change to a prolactin-sparing drug, the clinician should obtain a magnetic resonance imaging (MRI) scan of the sella turcica to look for a pituitary adenoma or parasellar tumor. If the MRI scan is normal, sex steroids (e.g., oral contraceptives for women of menstrual age, testosterone for men) can be replaced to treat the hypogonad-

ism, or drugs such as bisphosphonates (alendronate, risedronate, and the like) can be given to treat and prevent osteoporosis. Prolactin levels can also be lowered by adding a dopamine agonist (e.g., amantadine, bromocriptine) or by adding a partial dopamine agonist (e.g., aripiprazole: 5–15 mg/day), which can be effective without worsening psychosis or mania (Shim et al. 2007). The beneficial effects on prolactin levels after a switch to a lower-risk agent or addition of a full or partial dopamine agonist can be evaluated at least five times the half-life after the offending drug is stopped and the new agent has been titrated to the target dose.

Neutropenia

Since neutropenia may follow a diurnal variation pattern, afternoon levels in patients with habitually low white blood counts should be obtained to reconsider clozapine initiation in such patients (Esposito et al. 2006). Moreover, lithium at low to medium doses (300–600 mg/day) may be used to increase white blood counts, which increase partly due to a shedding of white cells from the vascular walls, partly due to bone marrow stimulation (Sporn et al. 2003; Whiskey and Taylor 2007). In cases where agranulocytosis has developed, treatment with granulocyte colony-stimulating factor can be lifesaving (Whiskey and Taylor 2007).

Research Directions

Randomized controlled studies are needed that compare the efficacy and safety of antipsychotics with placebo and with other antipsychotics or with agents from different drug classes. These studies should also include individuals with conditions that are below the diagnostic threshold for bipolar I disorder or schizophrenia, such as bipolar disorder not otherwise specified (NOS), mood disorder NOS, and psychosis NOS, as antipsychotics are used off label for these patients with substantial symptoms and impairment. More studies are needed that assess efficacy and safety during longer developmental periods. Long-term studies are particularly needed in peripubertal patients in order to evaluate the potential impact of antipsychotics on pubertal development and maturation. Controlled trials are further needed that test the efficacy and safety of combination treatments, including both pharmacological and nonpharmacological augmentation strategies aimed at enhancing the efficacy and improving the tolerability and safety of antipsychotics. Ideally, studies would be conducted in antipsychotic-naive populations to remove potentially confounding order effects. Fasting assessments for important metabolic effects should always be included. Finally, research should include large practical trials that involve representative populations and settings that allow for a generalization of the findings.

Summary Points

- RCTs in youth have demonstrated efficacy of antipsychotics for schizophrenia, bipolar mania, aggressive behaviors associated with a variety of disorders, and Tourette's syndrome.

- While differences in antipsychotic efficacy (except for clozapine in refractory patients) are likely relatively small and difficult to predict, differences in adverse effects between antipsychotic agents are clinically relevant and easier to predict.

- Pharmacokinetic and pharmacodynamic profiles of antipsychotics can be used to predict the likelihood of adverse effects and drug-drug interactions that can manifest as overdose or rebound and withdrawal phenomena.

- Children and adolescents are likely to develop antipsychotic-induced sedation, acute extrapyramidal side effects (except for akathisia), withdrawal dyskinesia, hyperprolactinemia, age-inappropriate weight gain, and lipid abnormalities.

- Safety assessments need to use developmentally adjusted measures and thresholds.

- Treatment selection should be guided by individual patient factors (e.g., age, development, illness phase, target symptoms, and past response and side-effect pattern) and by medication factors, choosing early in the treatment algorithm medications with the lowest likelihood of causing relevant adverse effects.

- Education of patients and families about and proactive assessment of antipsychotic adverse effects in youth should be routine clinical practice.

- While adverse effects need to be balanced against efficacy gains, clinicians should be prepared to carefully change antipsychotic treatment or initiate interventions to reduce bothersome as well as physically problematic adverse effects to improve overall psychiatric and physical outcomes.

References

Aman MG, De Smedt G, Derivan A, et al: Double-blind, placebo-controlled study of risperidone for the treatment of disruptive behaviors in children with subaverage intelligence. Am J Psychiatry 159:1337–1346, 2002

Aman MG, Binder C, Turgay A: Risperidone effects in the presence/absence of psychostimulant medicine in children with ADHD, other disruptive behavior disorders, and subaverage IQ. J Child Adolesc Psychopharmacol 14:243–254, 2004

Aman MG, Arnold LE, McDougle CJ, et al: Acute and long-term safety and tolerability of risperidone in children with autism. J Child Adolesc Psychopharmacol 15:869–884, 2005

American Diabetes Association, American Psychiatric Association, American Association of Clinical Endocrinologists, et al: Consensus development conference on antipsychotic drugs and obesity and diabetes. J Clin Psychiatry 65:267–272, 2004

American Medical Association: Expert Committee Recommendations on the Assessment, Prevention, and Treatment of Child and Adolescent Overweight and Obesity: Recommendations for Treatment of Pediatric Obesity. Chicago, IL, American Medical Association, January 25, 2007. Available at: http://www.ama-assn.org/ama1/pub/upload/mm/433/ped_obesity_recs.pdf. Accessed March 18, 2008.

Ananth J, Parameswaran S, Gunatilake S: Side effects of atypical antipsychotic drugs. Curr Pharm Des 10:2219–2229, 2004

Anderson GM, Scahill L, McCracken JT, et al: Effects of short- and long-term risperidone treatment on prolactin levels in children with autism. Biol Psychiatry 61:545–550, 2007

Armenteros JL, Lewis JE, Davalos M: Risperidone augmentation for treatment-resistant aggression in attention-deficit/hyperactivity disorder: a placebo-controlled pilot study. J Am Acad Child Adolesc Psychiatry 46:558–565, 2007

Biederman J, Mick E, Hammerness P, et al: Open-label, 8-week trial of olanzapine and risperidone for the treatment of bipolar disorder in preschool-age children. Biol Psychiatry 58:589–594, 2005

Biederman J, Mick E, Spencer T, et al: A prospective open-label treatment trial of ziprasidone monotherapy in children and adolescents with bipolar disorder. Bipolar Disord 9:888–894, 2007

Blair J, Scahill L, State M, et al: Electrocardiographic changes in children and adolescents treated with ziprasidone: a prospective study. J Am Acad Child Adolesc Psychiatry 44:73–79, 2005

Buitelaar JK, van der Gaag RJ, Cohen-Kettenis P, et al: A randomized controlled trial of risperidone in the treatment of aggression in hospitalized adolescents with subaverage cognitive abilities. J Clin Psychiatry 62:239–248, 2001

Burris KD, Molski TF, Xu C, et al: Aripiprazole, a novel antipsychotic, is a high-affinity partial agonist at human dopamine D2 receptors. J Pharmacol Exp Ther 302:381–389, 2002

Calarge CA, Acion L, Kuperman S, et al: Weight gain and metabolic abnormalities during extended risperidone treatment in children and adolescents. J Child Adolesc Psychopharmacol 19:101–109, 2009

Campbell M, Small AM, Green WH, et al: Behavioral efficacy of haloperidol and lithium carbonate. A comparison in hospitalized aggressive children with conduct disorder. Arch Gen Psychiatry 41:650–656, 1984

Campbell M, Armenteros JL, Malone RP, et al: Neuroleptic-related dyskinesias in autistic children: a prospective, longitudinal study. J Am Acad Child Adolesc Psychiatry 36:835–843, 1997

Chang KD, Nyilas M, Aurang C, et al: Efficacy of aripiprazole in children (10–17 years old) with mania. Poster presented at the 54th annual meeting of the American Academy of Child and Adolescent Psychiatry, Boston, MA, October 2007

Chouinard G, Ross-Chouinard A, Annabel L, et al: The Extrapyramidal Symptom Rating Scale. Can J Neurol Sci 7:233, 1980

Connor DF, Fletcher KE, Wood JS: Neuroleptic-related dyskinesias in children and adolescents. J Clin Psychiatry 62:967–974, 2001

Correll CU: Real life switching strategies with second-generation antipsychotics. J Clin Psychiatry 67:160–161, 2006

Correll CU: Weight gain and metabolic effects of mood stabilizers and antipsychotics in pediatric bipolar disorder: a systematic review and pooled analysis of short-term trials. J Am Acad Child Adolesc Psychiatry 46:687–700, 2007

Correll CU: Antipsychotic use in children and adolescents: minimizing adverse effects to maximize outcomes. J Am Acad Child Adolesc Psychiatry 47:9–20, 2008a

Correll CU: Assessing and maximizing the safety and tolerability of antipsychotics used in the treatment of children and adolescents. J Clin Psychiatry 69(suppl):26–36, 2008b

Correll CU: Monitoring and management of antipsychotic-related metabolic and endocrine adverse effects in children and adolescents. Int Rev Psychiatry 20:195–201, 2008c

Correll CU, Carlson HE: Endocrine and metabolic adverse effects of psychotropic medications in children and adolescents. J Am Acad Child Adolesc Psychiatry 45:771–791, 2006

Correll CU, Kane JM: One-year tardive dyskinesia rates in children and adolescents treated with second-generation antipsychotics: a systematic review. J Child Adolesc Psychopharmacol 17:647–655, 2007

Correll CU, Leucht S, Kane JM: Lower risk for tardive dyskinesia associated with second-generation antipsychotics: a systematic review of 1-year studies. Am J Psychiatry 161:414–425, 2004

Correll CU, Penzner JB, Parikh UH, et al: Recognizing and monitoring adverse events of second-generation antipsychotics in children and adolescents. Child Adolesc Psychiatr Clin N Am 15:177–206, 2006

Correll CU, Nyilas M, Aurang C, et al: Long-term safety and tolerability of aripiprazole in children (10–17 y/o) with bipolar I disorder. Poster presented at the 54th annual meeting of the American Academy of Child and Adolescent Psychiatry, Boston, MA, October 2007

Correll CU, Schenk EM, DelBello MP: Antipsychotic and mood stabilizer efficacy and tolerability in adult and pediatric patients with bipolar I mania: a comparative analysis of acute, randomized, placebo-controlled trials. Bipolar Disord, in press

DelBello MP, Schwiers ML, Rosenberg HL, et al: A double-blind, randomized, placebo-controlled study of quetiapine as adjunctive treatment for adolescent mania. J Am Acad Child Adolesc Psychiatry 41:1216–1223, 2002

DelBello MP, Kowatch RA, Adler CM, et al: A double-blind randomized pilot study comparing quetiapine and divalproex for adolescent mania. J Am Acad Child Adolesc Psychiatry 45:305–313, 2006

DelBello MP, Findling RL, Earley WR, et al: Efficacy of quetiapine in children and adolescents with bipolar mania: a 3-week, double-blind, randomized, placebo-controlled trial. Poster presented at the 54th annual meeting of the American Academy of Child and Adolescent Psychiatry, Boston, MA, October 2007

DelBello MP, Findling RL, Wang PP, et al: Efficacy and safety of ziprasidone in pediatric bipolar disorder. Presented at the New Clinical Drug Evaluation Unit annual meeting, Phoenix, AZ, May 2008

Esposito D, Chouinard G, Hardy P, et al: Successful initiation of clozapine treatment despite morning pseudoneutropenia. Int J Neuropsychopharmacol 9:489–491, 2006

Expert Panel on Detection, Evaluation, and Treatment of High Blood Cholesterol in Adults: Executive summary of the Third Report of the National Cholesterol Education Program (NCEP) Expert Panel on Detection, Evaluation, and Treatment of High Blood Cholesterol in Adults (Adult Treatment Panel III). JAMA 285:2486–2497, 2001

Faulkner G, Cohn T, Remington G: Interventions to reduce weight gain in schizophrenia. Cochrane Database Syst Rev (1):CD005148, 2007

Fernandez JR, Redden DT, Pietrobelli A, et al: Waist circumference percentiles in nationally representative samples of African-American, European-American, and Mexican-American children and adolescents. J Pediatr 145:439–444, 2004

Findling RL, McNamara NK, Branicky LA, et al: A double-blind pilot study of risperidone in the treatment of conduct disorder. J Am Acad Child Adolesc Psychiatry 39:509–516, 2000

Findling RL, Steiner H, Weller EB: Use of antipsychotics in children and adolescents. J Clin Psychiatry 66(suppl):29–40, 2005

Findling RL, Robb AS, Nyilas M, et al: A multiple-center, randomized, double-blind, placebo-controlled study of oral aripiprazole for treatment of adolescents with schizophrenia. Am J Psychiatry 165:1432–1441, 2008

Fleischhacker C, Heiser P, Hennighausen K, et al: Clinical drug monitoring in child and adolescent psychiatry: side effects of atypical neuroleptics. J Child Adolesc Psychopharmacol 16:308–316, 2006

Fraguas D, Merchán-Naranjo J, Laita P, et al: Metabolic and hormonal side effects in children and adolescents treated with second-generation antipsychotics. J Clin Psychiatry 69:1166–1175, 2008

Gerbino-Rosen G, Roofeh D, Tompkins D, et al: Hematological adverse events in clozapine-treated children and adolescents. J Am Acad Child Adolesc Psychiatry 44:1024–1031, 2005

Glassman AH, Bigger JT Jr: Antipsychotic drugs: prolonged QTc interval, torsade de pointes, and sudden death. Am J Psychiatry 158:1774–1782, 2001

Gonzalez-Heydrich J, Raches D, Wilens TE, et al: Retrospective study of hepatic enzyme elevations in children treated with olanzapine, divalproex, and their combination. J Am Acad Child Adolesc Psychiatry 42:1227–1233, 2003

Greenhill LL, Solomon M, Pleak R, et al: Molindone hydrochloride treatment of hospitalized children with conduct disorder. J Clin Psychiatry 46(8 Pt 2):20–25, 1985

Guy W (ed): ECDEU Assessment Manual for Psychopharmacology (Publ ABM 76-338). Washington, DC, U.S. Department of Health, Education, and Welfare, 1976, pp 534–537

Haas M, Unis AS, Copenhaver M, et al: Efficacy and safety of risperidone in adolescents with schizophrenia. Poster presented at the annual meeting of the American Psychiatric Association, San Diego, CA, May 2007

Haase HJ: Zur Dosierung von Neuroleptika. Ein Leitfaden für Klinik und Praxis unter besonderer Berücksichtigung psychotisch Kranker. Erlangen, Germany, Perimed Fachbuch-Verlagsbuchhandlung, 1983

Hollander E, Wasserman S, Swanson EN, et al: A double-blind placebo-controlled pilot study of olanzapine in childhood/adolescent pervasive developmental disorder. J Child Adolesc Psychopharmacol 16:541–548, 2006

Hsieh MW, Everhart JE, Byrd-Holt DD, et al: Prevalence of neutropenia in the U.S. population: age, sex, smoking status, and ethnic differences. Ann Intern Med 146:486–492, 2007

Jensen PS, Buitelaar J, Pandina GJ, et al: Management of psychiatric disorders in children and adolescents with atypical antipsychotics: a systematic review of published clinical trials. Eur Child Adolesc Psychiatry 16:104–120, 2007

Kryzhanovskaya L, Schulz SC, McDougle C, et al: Olanzapine versus placebo in adolescents with schizophrenia: a 6-week, randomized, double-blind, placebo-controlled trial. J Am Acad Child Adolesc Psychiatry 48:60–70, 2009

Kumra S, Frazier JA, Jacobsen LK, et al: Childhood-onset schizophrenia: a double-blind clozapine-haloperidol comparison. Arch Gen Psychiatry 53:1090–1097, 1996

Kumra S, Herion D, Jacobsen LK, et al: Case study: risperidone-induced hepatotoxicity in pediatric patients. J Am Acad Child Adolesc Psychiatry 36:701–705, 1997

Kumra S, Kranzler H, Gerbino-Rosen G, et al: Clozapine and "high-dose" olanzapine in refractory early onset schizophrenia: a 12-week randomized and double-blind comparison. Biol Psychiatry 63:524–529, 2008a

Kumra S, Oberstar JV, Sikich L, et al: Efficacy and tolerability of second-generation antipsychotics in children and adolescents with schizophrenia. Schizophr Bull 34:60–71, 2008b

Laita P, Cifuentes A, Doll A, et al: Antipsychotic-related abnormal involuntary movements and metabolic and endocrine side effects in children and adolescents. J Child Adolesc Psychopharmacol 17:487–502, 2007

Lee JM, Okumura MJ, Davis MM, et al: Prevalence and determinants of insulin resistance among US adolescents: a population-based study. Diabetes Care 29:2427–2432, 2006

Luby J, Mrakotsky C, Stalets MM, et al: Risperidone in preschool children with autistic spectrum disorders: an investigation of safety and efficacy. J Child Adolesc Psychopharmacol 16:575–587, 2006

Malone RP, Cater J, Sheikh RM, et al: Olanzapine versus haloperidol in children with autistic disorder: an open pilot study. J Am Acad Child Adolesc Psychiatry 40:887–894, 2001

Malone RP, Maislin G, Choudhury MS, et al: Risperidone treatment in children and adolescents with autism: short- and long-term safety and effectiveness. J Am Acad Child Adolesc Psychiatry 41:140–147, 2002

Malone RP, Delaney MA, Hyman SB, et al: Ziprasidone in adolescents with autism: an open-label pilot study. J Child Adolesc Psychopharmacol 17:779–790, 2007

Martin A, L'Ecuyer S: Triglyceride, cholesterol and weight changes among risperidone-treated youths: a retrospective study. Eur Child Adolesc Psychiatry 11:129–133, 2002

McDougle CJ, Kem DL, Posey DJ: Case series: use of ziprasidone for maladaptive symptoms in youths with autism. J Am Acad Child Adolesc Psychiatry 41:921–927, 2002

Meyer JM: Drug-drug interactions with antipsychotics. CNS Spectr 12(suppl):6–9, 2007

Miral S, Gencer O, Inal-Emiroglu FN, et al: Risperidone versus haloperidol in children and adolescents with AD: a randomized, controlled, double-blind trial. Eur Child Adolesc Psychiatry 17:1–8, 2008

Nagaraj R, Singhi P, Malhi P: Risperidone in children with autism: randomized, placebo-controlled, double-blind study. J Child Neurol 21:450–455, 2006

National High Blood Pressure Education Program Working Group on High Blood Pressure in Children and Adolescents: The fourth report on the diagnosis, evaluation, and treatment of high blood pressure in children and adolescents. Pediatrics 114:555–576, 2004

Olfson M, Blanco C, Liu L, et al: National trends in the outpatient treatment of children and adolescents with antipsychotic drugs. Arch Gen Psychiatry 63:679–685, 2006

Pandina G, DelBello M, Kushner S, et al: Risperidone treatment of acute mania in bipolar youth. Poster presented at the 54th annual meeting of the American Academy of Child and Adolescent Psychiatry, Boston, MA, October 2007

Patel NC, Hariparsad M, Matias-Akthar M, et al: Body mass indexes and lipid profiles in hospitalized children and adolescents exposed to atypical antipsychotics. J Child Adolesc Psychopharmacol 17:303–311, 2007

Pool D, Bloom W, Mielke DH, et al: A controlled evaluation of loxitane in seventy-five adolescent schizophrenic patients. Curr Ther Res Clin Exp 19:99–104, 1976

Rajagopal S: Clozapine, agranulocytosis, and benign ethnic neutropenia. Postgrad Med J 81:545–546, 2005

Ratzoni G, Gothelf D, Brand-Gothelf A, et al: Weight gain associated with olanzapine and risperidone in adolescent patients: a comparative prospective study. J Am Acad Child Adolesc Psychiatry 41:337–343, 2002

Realmuto GM, Erickson WD, Yellin AM, et al: Clinical comparison of thiothixene and thioridazine in schizophrenic adolescents. Am J Psychiatry 141:440–442, 1984

Research Units on Pediatric Psychopharmacology Autism Network: Risperidone treatment of autistic disorder: longer-term benefits and blinded discontinuation after 6 months. Am J Psychiatry 162:1361–1369, 2005

Reyes M, Buitelaar J, Toren P, et al: A randomized, double-blind, placebo-controlled study of risperidone maintenance treatment in children and adolescents with disruptive behavior disorders. Am J Psychiatry 163:402–410, 2006

Safer DJ: A comparison of risperidone-induced weight gain across the age span. J Clin Psychopharmacol 24:429–436, 2004

Sallee FR, Kurlan R, Goetz CG, et al: Ziprasidone treatment of children and adolescents with Tourette's syndrome: a pilot study. J Am Acad Child Adolesc Psychiatry 39:292–299, 2000

Scahill L, Leckman JF, Schultz RT, et al: A placebo-controlled trial of risperidone in Tourette syndrome. Neurology 60:1130–1135, 2003

Shaw P, Sporn A, Gogtay N, et al: Childhood-onset schizophrenia: a double-blind, randomized clozapine-olanzapine comparison. Arch Gen Psychiatry 63:721–730, 2006

Shea S, Turgay A, Carroll A, et al: Risperidone in the treatment of disruptive behavioral symptoms in children with autistic and other pervasive developmental disorders. Pediatrics 114:e634–e641, 2004

Shim JC, Shin JG, Kelly DL, et al: Adjunctive treatment with a dopamine partial agonist, aripiprazole, for antipsychotic-induced hyperprolactinemia: a placebo-controlled trial. Am J Psychiatry 164:1404–1410, 2007

Sikich L, Hamer RM, Bashford RA, et al: A pilot study of risperidone, olanzapine, and haloperidol in psychotic youth: a double-blind, randomized, 8-week trial. Neuropsychopharmacology 29:133–145, 2004

Sikich L, Frazier JA, McClellan J, et al: Double-blind comparison of first- and second-generation antipsychotics in early onset schizophrenia and schizoaffective disorder: findings from the Treatment of Early Onset Schizophrenia Spectrum Disorders (TEOSS) study. Am J Psychiatry 165:1420–1431, 2008

Simpson GM, Angus JW: A rating scale for extrapyramidal side effects. Acta Psychiatr Scand Suppl 212:11–19, 1970

Snyder R, Turgay A, Aman M, et al: Effects of risperidone on conduct and disruptive behavior disorders in children with subaverage IQs. J Am Acad Child Adolesc Psychiatry 41:1026–1036, 2002

Spencer EK, Kafantaris V, Padron-Gayol MV, et al: Haloperidol in schizophrenic children: early findings from a study in progress. Psychopharmacol Bull 28:183–186, 1992

Sporn A, Gogtay N, Ortiz-Aguayo R, et al: Clozapine-induced neutropenia in children: management with lithium carbonate. J Child Adolesc Psychopharmacol 13:401–404, 2003

Tohen M, Kryzhanovskaya L, Carlson G, et al: Olanzapine versus placebo in the treatment of adolescents with bipolar mania. Am J Psychiatry 164:1547–1556, 2007

Van Bellinghen M, De Troch C: Risperidone in the treatment of behavioral disturbances in children and adolescents with borderline intellectual functioning: a double-blind, placebo-controlled pilot trial. J Child Adolesc Psychopharmacol 11:5–13, 2001

Wehmeier PM, Schuler-Springorum M, Heiser P, et al: Chart review for potential features of myocarditis, pericarditis, and cardiomyopathy in children and adolescents treated with clozapine. J Child Adolesc Psychopharmacol 14:267–271, 2004

Whiskey E, Taylor D: Restarting clozapine after neutropenia: evaluating the possibilities and practicalities. CNS Drugs 21:25–35, 2007

Woods SW, Martin A, Spector SG, et al: Effects of development on olanzapine-associated adverse events. J Am Acad Child Adolesc Psychiatry 41:1439–1446, 2002

Alpha-Adrenergics, Beta-Blockers, Benzodiazepines, Buspirone, and Desmopressin

Lawrence Scahill, M.S.N., Ph.D.
Yann Poncin, M.D.
Alexander Westphal, M.D.

With the exception of desmopressin, the medications reviewed in this chapter were developed and tested in adults and later adapted for use in pediatrics. They are a heterogeneous collection of drugs with specialized indications for children and adolescents. The evidence supporting the use of these drugs varies widely.

Alpha-Adrenergic Agonists

The alpha-adrenergic agents clonidine and guanfacine were developed for the treatment of hypertension.

Clonidine was introduced in pediatric psychopharmacology almost 30 years ago when Cohen and colleagues administered the drug to children with Tourette's syndrome (Cohen et al. 1979). Despite its rather widespread use for a range of conditions such as Tourette's syndrome, attention-deficit/hyperactivity disorder (ADHD), pervasive developmental disorders (PDD), and sleep disturbance, there are only two large-scale trials of clonidine in pediatric samples (Arnsten et al. 2007; Poncin and Scahill 2007). Guanfacine entered clinical practice in the early 1990s. Accumulated evidence to date suggests that it appears to be useful as a nonstimulant alternative for the treatment of ADHD

This work was supported by the following cooperative agreement grant from the National Institute of Mental Health: U10MH66764 (P.I., L. Scahill).

and the target symptoms of hyperactivity, impulsiveness, and distractibility in children with PDD.

Mechanism of Action

The historical view is that the alpha-agonist agents stimulate presynaptic receptors in the locus coeruleus, resulting in a turning down of the noradrenergic system. This regulatory effect on the noradrenergic system was presumed to result in decreased hyperactivity and impulsiveness. Clinical and preclinical studies have shown similarities and fundamental differences in the action of guanfacine. As is true for clonidine, early studies showed that guanfacine reduces norepinephrine release. However, a substantial body of preclinical work has also demonstrated that guanfacine has postsynaptic effects in prefrontal cortex (Arnsten et al. 2007). Because the prefrontal cortex is known to play an essential role in attention, planning, and impulse control, this preclinical evidence is potentially relevant to pharmacological treatment effects in children with ADHD.

Evidence

Clonidine

Several small trials with clonidine have been carried out in children with Tourette's syndrome, including placebo-controlled trials and head-to-head comparisons with another active drug. In a 12-week randomized trial of clonidine versus placebo in 47 subjects (ages 7–48 years old) with Tourette's syndrome, Leckman et al. (1991) showed that clonidine was more effective than placebo in controlling tics. When compared directly with the antipsychotic medication risperidone (n=9), clonidine (n=12) showed a similar reduction in overall tic severity and ADHD symptoms (Gaffney et al. 2002). The results of these studies suggest that at dosages ranging from 0.15 to 0.3 mg/day, clonidine exerts a moderate benefit on tics.

Two large-scale 16-week trials with clonidine have targeted ADHD (Palumbo et al. 2008; Tourette's Syndrome Study Group 2002). In both trials, clonidine was compared to placebo, methylphenidate only, and combined treatment (clonidine plus methylphenidate). Clonidine was introduced in the first 4 weeks for the clonidine-only group and the randomly assigned combined treatment group. Methylphenidate was not introduced until week 4 for the groups randomly assigned to methylphenidate only or to combined treatment. The Tourette's Syndrome Study Group trial in-

cluded 136 children with ADHD and tic disorder. Palumbo et al. (2008) included 122 children with ADHD but no tic disorder.

After subtracting out the placebo effect in the trial with children with ADHD and a tic disorder, the clonidine group showed a 21% improvement on a teacher rating compared to 16% for the methylphenidate group and 37% for the combined treatment group (calculated from graphic display of results). All three active treatments were superior to placebo. Although the magnitude of effect was larger on teacher ratings compared to parent ratings, the trend was similar for parent ratings (Tourette's Syndrome Study Group 2002). The placebo-adjusted improvement on teacher ratings in the Palumbo et al. (2008) study was 2% for clonidine only, 16% for methylphenidate only, and 32% for the combination of methylphenidate and clonidine (also calculated from graphic display of results). When compared to placebo, neither clonidine nor methylphenidate showed significant improvement. For the combined treatment group, there was a notable improvement in teacher ratings after methylphenidate was added at week 4. This improvement was stable from week 8 through week 16. The lower-than-expected benefit for methylphenidate alone in these two trials could be explained by the relatively conservative dosing strategy. The mean daily methylphenidate dosage in the Tourette's Syndrome Study Group trial was only 26 mg/day and 30 mg/day in the Palumbo et al. trial.

Although it was not a primary purpose of the Tourette's Syndrome Study Group trial, investigators evaluated the impact of study treatments on tics. There was no difference in measures of tic severity across the active treatment groups, which challenges the long-held view that stimulants invariably worsen tics in children with tic disorders. The dosage of clonidine was virtually identical across these two studies (0.24 mg/day in Palumbo et al., and 0.25 mg/day in the Tourette's Syndrome Study Group trial). The most common adverse effect of clonidine was sedation, especially early in treatment. When used in combination with methylphenidate, there was an attenuation of the sedative side effects of clonidine alone. Taken together, the results of these two trials indicate that the combination of clonidine and methylphenidate is generally well tolerated and for ADHD symptoms may be more effective than either drug treatment alone. Nonetheless, combined treatment with clonidine and methylphenidate would be indicated in children who do not show an adequate response to monotherapy.

Clonidine has also been examined for the treatment of hyperactivity in children with PDD. These trials were small and benefits modest. At doses similar to those described above, the efficacy of clonidine in children with PDD appears limited by the occurrence of adverse effects, particularly sedation (reviewed in Poncin and Scahill 2007).

Guanfacine

Evidence includes a handful of open pilot studies (Boon-Yasidhi et al. 2005; Chappell et al. 1995; Horrigan and Barnhill 1995; Hunt et al. 1995; Scahill et al. 2006a) and three placebo-controlled studies (Biederman et al. 2008; Cummings et al. 2002; Scahill et al. 2001). Most of these trials focused on the treatment of ADHD symptoms. The open-label trials, involving a total of approximately 100 patients, showed significant improvement in ADHD symptoms. The findings in the three placebo-controlled trials are inconsistent. In a study of 34 children with ADHD and tic disorders, guanfacine was superior to placebo for tics and on teacher ratings of ADHD symptoms (Scahill et al. 2001). However, Cummings et al. (2002) observed no difference between active drug and placebo in their study of 24 children with Tourette's syndrome. One important difference between these two trials is that Cummings et al. enrolled Tourette's syndrome subjects with and without ADHD. Thus, about half of the sample was low on ADHD symptom severity at baseline, making it difficult to assess improvement in ADHD measures in such a small study. These two trials used immediate-release guanfacine in dosages ranging from 1.5 to 3.5 mg/day given in three divided doses.

Biederman et al. (2008) conducted a 6-week multiple-dose, randomized industry-sponsored trial with a new once-daily formulation of guanfacine. Subjects (N=345) were randomly assigned to placebo or 2, 3, or 4 mg/day. The average age was 10.5 years, approximately three-fourths of the sample were boys, and 72% of the subjects had combined-type ADHD. All subjects assigned to active medication started at 1 mg with weekly increases of 1 mg until the randomized dosage level (2, 3, or 4 mg/day) was achieved for each subject. Of the 345 subjects enrolled, 38% (n=130) dropped out, with roughly equal attrition by treatment group. However, the reasons for dropout varied across groups. The rate of attrition due to adverse events was 23% for subjects in the 4 mg group compared to 1% for the placebo group, 10% for the 2 mg group, and 15% for the 3 mg group. This trend suggests a clear dose-dependent relationship. Across all active treatment groups, a similar percentage of subjects dropped out due to lack of efficacy.

The primary outcome measure was the Attention-Deficit/Hyperactivity Disorder Rating Scale IV scored by a clinician following an interview with the primary caretaker. Each dose of the extended-release guanfacine was superior to placebo, with a slight advantage for the 4 mg dosage. The 4 mg/day group had only 2 weeks at the full dosage, possibly obscuring the full benefit of this dosage as well as the full picture of adverse effects with the 4 mg dosage. Examination of efficacy by weight-adjusted dose suggested that 0.05 mg/kg/day is the threshold for clinically meaningful benefit and daily dosages in the range of 0.09–0.12 mg/kg appear to be optimal. Although there was improvement in both hyperactivity/impulsiveness and inattention, gains appeared greater in the hyperactive/impulsiveness dimension. Common adverse effects included sedation and fatigue.

The efficacy of combining methylphenidate and guanfacine has not been studied.

Clinical Management

The evidence suggests that treatment with clonidine or guanfacine may be justified for reducing hyperactivity, distractibility, and impulsiveness in children with ADHD, Tourette's syndrome, and possibly PDD. Some evidence supports the use of these drugs for the treatment of tics, though guanfacine has been less well studied than clonidine for this purpose. Pretreatment assessment includes the usual medical and psychiatric evaluations prior to the start of any medication, as well as rating scales for ADHD symptoms.

Adverse Events

Several areas of concern are specific to the alpha-2 agonists. Although blood pressure is rarely a clinically significant problem in healthy children treated with usual doses, blood pressure and pulse should be measured at baseline and during the dose adjustment phase. The placebo-controlled trial with guanfacine showed a slight drop in the average diastolic blood pressure and pulse at week 4 that resolved by week 8 (Scahill et al. 2001). In young children, it may be useful to enlist help from the school nurse to monitor blood pressure in the early weeks of treatment. Once the dose is established and it is clear that the child is tolerating the medication, only periodic monitoring of pulse and blood pressure is warranted. In a recent review, the Medical Advisory Board of the Tourette Syndrome Association noted the lack of consensus on the need for electrocardiograms (ECGs) before and after treatment with the alpha-2 agonists (Scahill et al. 2006b). In our center, we do not routinely obtain pretreatment ECGs before starting an alpha-2 agonist. A companion report from the Palumbo et al. (2008) trial supports the view that ECG monitoring is not required in clinical practice for healthy children (Daviss et al. 2008).

Another area that warrants attention is sleep. Sleep is a common complaint in children with ADHD, Tourette's syndrome, or PDD. Therefore, a sleep history and subsequent monitoring of sleep during treatment are appropriate. For children with a history of trouble falling asleep, the alpha-2 agonists can reduce sleep latency. Insomnia has been reported with guanfacine (Scahill et al. 2006a). A treatment-related adverse effect with clonidine or guanfacine is also midsleep awakening. This problem can often be managed by changing the hour of the bedtime dose—e.g., moving the dose closer to bedtime or giving it earlier in the evening. In other cases, it may be useful to lower or raise the bedtime dose.

Clonidine is roughly 10 times more potent than guanfacine. The usual dosage of clonidine falls in the range of 0.15–0.3 mg/day given in three or four divided doses. An appropriate starting dose of clonidine for a young child (ages 5–8 years) would be 0.025 mg at bedtime and 0.05 mg for school-age children and adolescents. The clonidine dose can be increased by the same increment every 3 or 4 days, first adding in the morning, then midday, then back to the bedtime dose. It is often necessary for one dose to be given in school.

Guanfacine dosages range from 1.0 mg to 3.0 mg/ day divided into two or three doses. The medication may be introduced with a 0.25 or 0.5 mg dose at bedtime, with dose increases following a pattern similar to that of clonidine. Given the longer half-life of guanfacine, three doses per day—with the middle dose given after school—is often effective. The optimal dosage with the new extended-release product appears to be 2–3 mg/day given in a single dose, though some children may benefit from an increase to 4 mg.

It may take several weeks to detect positive effects of clonidine or guanfacine. As suggested above, both drugs often require a 3- to 4-week dose adjustment phase. If adverse effects such as sedation occur during the early treatment phase, it may take even longer to achieve an effective dose. Parents should be reminded that positive effects may be delayed and that an adequate trial may take several weeks or longer. Parents should also be cautioned not to stop either drug abruptly to avoid possible rebound hypertension. This effect has been well documented with clonidine and is theoretically possible with guanfacine.

There is limited information to guide long-term treatment. Clinical experience with clonidine suggests that it is safe for long-term treatment. By extension, the same safety record could presumably be applied to guanfacine. To assess whether the perceived benefits of the medication are still present, a gradual decrease in the medication may be tried accompanied by regular symptom reports from parents and teachers. In children with tics or stereotypic behavior, assessment of these movements and repetitive behaviors is also warranted during the dose reduction.

Beta-Blockers

The beta-blockers were introduced for the treatment of hypertension and continue to be used for this reason, as well as for cardiac arrhythmias, migraine, and several other indications. Although used in practice for physical manifestations of anxiety, lithium-induced tremor, aggression, and akathisia, these psychiatric applications are not approved by the U.S. Food and Drug Administration (FDA). Currently, there are over 20 beta-blockers on the market, but propranolol, pindolol, and, to a lesser extent, nadolol are the most commonly used agents in psychiatry.

Mechanism of Action

These drugs are competitive antagonists of norepinephrine and epinephrine at beta-adrenergic receptors in a number of tissues, including brain. Beta-blockers differ in their affinity for beta-1 or beta-2 receptor subtypes. Both propranolol and pindolol are nonselective, meaning that they interact with both beta-1 and beta-2 receptors. The proposed mechanism is reduction of noradrenergic activity (Baumeister and Sevin 1990), resulting in turning down sympathetic discharge and overarousal, both centrally and peripherally (Ratey and Gordon 1993).

Propranolol is well absorbed after oral administration, but up to 70% of the oral dose is metabolized by the liver during first pass. Considerable individual variability in first-pass hepatic metabolism results in variability in dosing. Propranolol is highly protein bound and lipid soluble with a large volume of distribution and easily enters the central nervous system. Time to effect is 1–2 hours. The parent compound and major active metabolite, 4-hydroxypropranolol, have an elimination half-life of 3–7 hours (Hoffman 2001).

Pindolol has mild sympathomimetic effects and has also been of interest for a potential role in reducing the time to positive effect of antidepressants through its antagonist effect on serotonin type 1A (5-HT$_{1A}$) receptors (Blier 2001). Pindolol is well absorbed in the gastrointestinal system, with high bioavailability due to the absence of the variability imposed by first-pass hepatic metabolism. Pindolol also has relatively short duration of action with a half-life of 3–4 hours (Hoffman 2001).

Evidence

Anxiety

In adults, controlled trials have shown that the beta-blockers are effective for somatic symptoms of anxiety, such as tachycardia, tremors, palpitations, and diaphoresis (Pollack 1999). Based on this observation, propranolol has been used in the treatment of performance anxiety, though the evidence supporting this application is meager. Other anxiety disorders such as panic disorder, social phobia, and specific phobias have not shown a positive response to beta-blockers (Hidalgo et al. 2007). Although studies in adults with posttraumatic stress disorder (PTSD) provide some support for beta-blockers (Pitman et al. 2002), this strategy has not been attempted in children. There are no placebo-controlled studies of a beta-blocker in children for the treatment of anxiety.

Aggression

Aggression may occur in the context of multiple disorders, including intermittent explosive disorder, psychotic disorders, traumatic brain injury, autism, ADHD, and Tourette's syndrome. Beta-blockers have been used in adults and children with intellectual disabilities for the treatment of aggression or self-injurious behaviors. Pediatric trials include case studies and small controlled trials (see Schur et al. 2003 for a review). The agents in these reports include propranolol, nadolol, and pindolol. Although the evidence is limited, these reports suggest that the beta-blockers may be considered as an adjunct or as a primary treatment if other medications (e.g., an atypical antipsychotic) are unsuccessful.

Akathisia

Akathisia, described as an unpleasant sense of motor restlessness, is an adverse effect associated with traditional antipsychotics. It may also occur with the atypical antipsychotics and with serotonin reuptake inhibitors (Leo 1996; Sahoo and Ameen 2007). Untreated,

akathisia can lead to agitation and contribute to nonadherence with medication treatment. Several placebo-controlled studies in adults indicate that beta-blockers such as propranolol (80 mg/day in divided doses) can be helpful for the treatment of akathisia (Adler et al. 1991; Fischel et al. 2001). Case reports suggest that propranolol between 15 and 30 mg/day in three divided doses may be effective for children with drug-induced akathisia (Gogtay et al. 2002).

Adjunctive Treatment in Depression

The desensitization of the 5-HT$_{1A}$ autoreceptor by pindolol has been proposed to augment efficacy and to reduce the time to effect in antidepressant treatment of depression (Blier 2001). A meta-analysis of controlled studies failed to confirm augmentation effects but did support an accelerated time to response to an antidepressant (Ballesteros and Callado 2004). When used as an adjunct to accelerate response, pindolol at 2.5 mg three times a day is the typical dose. There are no reports on the use of pindolol in children for this purpose.

Clinical Management

Although the evidence for the use of beta-blockers in children is meager, these drugs may be useful for aggression and akathisia, and perhaps as an adjunct for the treatment of anxiety or depression in children who have failed behavioral or psychopharmacological approaches. General guidelines include obtaining baseline pulse and blood pressure and a history regarding cardiac disease, asthma, diabetes, or renal disease, as beta-blockers may be contraindicated in these conditions. A baseline ECG may be considered, depending on clinical history.

When behavioral approaches for the treatment of performance anxiety have been unsuccessful, propranolol may be considered. Clearly, a test dose should be given before an actual event to confirm tolerability. An initial dose of 10 mg could be given 30–60 minutes before the event. The dose can be increased to 40 mg if needed and tolerable. At this dose, effects on heart rate and blood pressure are not usually a problem. Nonetheless, monitoring blood pressure and pulse is warranted. The parents and the child should be informed that this strategy, although safe, is best regarded as an experimental intervention.

In the treatment of akathisia, propranolol between 20 and 80 mg/day in divided doses is generally successful. In the treatment of aggression, higher doses can be used, with a range extending to 320 mg daily for adolescents. The main limiting factor is significant changes in blood pressure and pulse rate. Children have lower normal systolic values and higher pulse rates than adults (blood pressure percentiles for children are available at the National Heart and Lung Institute Web site). Initial dosing is 10 mg/day for younger children and 10–40 mg/day for adolescents. Doses can be increased in 10–20 mg increments every 4 days until the maximum effect is obtained or side effects emerge. When discontinuing propranolol, the dose should be tapered by 10–20 mg every 4–5 days to prevent problems with rebound tachycardia. When used for aggression, the dose of pindolol would likely start with 5 mg twice a day and increase in 2.5–5 mg increments twice a day on a similar 4–5 day schedule to a 40 mg/day in two or three divided doses (Buitelaar et al. 1996). Studies in adults with depression used far lower doses of pindolol such as 2.5 mg three times a day (Blier 2001). Nadolol has also been used for aggression, with dosages ranging from 30 to 220 mg daily in divided doses. The initial dose is 10 mg bid followed by gradual increases.

Adverse Effects

Common side effects include dry mouth, dizziness, or tingling. The most common cardiovascular effects, such as bradycardia and orthostatic hypotension, appear to be dose related. Beta-blockers may also contribute to depressed mood, wheezing, sleep disturbance, nightmares, and rarely, hallucinations. Clinical monitoring includes blood pressure and pulse, mood, sleep, and change in mental status. Propranolol and pindolol are substrates and inhibitors of CYP2D6. Thus, caution is warranted when combining either drug with a potent 2D6 inhibitor such as fluoxetine or paroxetine (Ciraulo et al. 2006). For example, if propranolol is to be added in a patient already on fluoxetine, the dose should start low, with slow upward adjustment. If an antidepressant is to be added to ongoing treatment with a beta-blocker, sertraline might be considered due to its low level of 2D6 inhibition (Ciraulo et al. 2006).

Benzodiazepines

Although not well studied in children, benzodiazepines are used in pediatric populations for anxiety (as well as other nonpsychiatric indications). Lorazepam has FDA approval for anxiety or insomnia in children down to age 12 years. This approval reflects an earlier era when FDA policy did not require two positive randomized controlled trials in pediatrics for approval.

Of the benzodiazepines marketed in the United States, alprazolam, lorazepam, diazepam, oxazepam, and clonazepam are among the most commonly used for the treatment of anxiety.

Mechanism of Action

Benzodiazepines have a high affinity for specific sites on γ-aminobutyric acid type A ($GABA_A$) receptors. When a benzodiazepine binds to the $GABA_A$ receptor, it enhances the inhibitory activity of GABA. This enhancement of GABA is presumed to explain the sedative, antispasmodic, and anticonvulsant properties of benzodiazepines (Tallman et al. 2002).

Evidence

Although there is considerable research support for the use of benzodiazepines in adults with anxiety disorders, the evidence in children is limited and often negative (Rynn and Ryan 2008). Despite the positive findings in open trials with alprazolam and clonazepam, small controlled trials have failed to demonstrate efficacy for several benzodiazepines for anxiety (Graae et al. 1994; Simeon et al. 1992). One trial (Graae et al. 1994) was stopped early due to a high frequency of disinhibition and irritability. Other drawbacks include the possibility of dependence and loss of motor coordination.

Clinical Management

This class of medications should be considered for the treatment of pediatric anxiety disorders only when psychotherapeutic or other psychopharmacological approaches have failed or proven inadequate. They may also be used in a time-limited fashion while waiting for other pharmacological or psychotherapeutic treatments to take effect. Table 50–1 shows the usual starting dose for selected benzodiazepines. Diazepam is not listed as it is rarely used in children due to its extended half-life.

Benzodiazepines may be useful in emergency situations for severe agitation. The benzodiazepine of choice is lorazepam, which can be delivered by mouth or intramuscularly. It has the advantage of rapid onset, and it has no active metabolites. In prepubertal children, intramuscular injection of 0.5–2.0 mg may be sufficient. When treating agitation, close monitoring is warranted due to the potential for disinhibition and paradoxical worsening of the agitation.

TABLE 50–1. Pediatric oral dosing guidelines for benzodiazepines for anxiety

Drug	Available doses, mg	Starting dose, mg	Usual daily dose, mg (schedule)
Alprazolam	0.25, 0.5, 1.0, 2.0 ER: 1.0, 2.0, 3.0 Liquid 1 mg/mL	0.25–0.5	0.25–3.0 (in 3 or 4 divided doses or prn)
Lorazepam	0.5, 1.0, 2.0	0.25–0.5	0.5–6.0 (in 2 or 3 divided doses or prn)
Clonazepam	0.5, 1.0, 2.0	0.25–0.5	0.25–2 (in 2 or 3 divided doses or prn)

Note. ER=extended release; prn=as needed.

Understanding drug interactions with the benzodiazepines is complicated by the differences across the specific agents in the class. For example, diazepam, clonazepam, and alprazolam are vulnerable to CYP3A3/4 inhibition. Thus, ketoconazole, erythromycin, fluvoxamine, fluoxetine, and sertraline will slow down metabolism of these benzodiazepines. Because carbamazepine induces 3A3/4, drug levels of clonazepam, diazepam, and alprazolam will be decreased in the presence of carbamazepine. Lorazepam appears to be less prone to drug interactions.

Discontinuing Benzodiazepines

Because the use of benzodiazepines can lead to physiological dependence, discontinuation of treatment warrants careful consideration and monitoring. Moreover, in some cases it may be difficult to differentiate withdrawal effects from the reemergence of symptoms. There are no studies of discontinuation strategies in children. Studies in adults have included discontinuation alone, discontinuation with psychotherapy, and discontinuation with substitute pharmacotherapy (Voshaar et al. 2006). The findings of these studies indicate that subjects treated with a benzodiazepine daily for 8 weeks or more should have a gradual withdrawal. Taper may begin with 10% decrease per week with close monitoring of response. This may involve dividing tablets into quarters or even smaller increments to accomplish uneventful withdrawal. The longer the duration of treatment, the more painstaking the withdrawal should be.

Buspirone

Mechanism of Action

Buspirone selectively binds to the 5-HT$_{1A}$ receptor, where it acts as a partial agonist. It has weaker dopamine antagonist effects. It does not bind to benzodiazepine receptors and does not enhance GABA; therefore, buspirone is not an effective replacement for a benzodiazepine during withdrawal.

Evidence

Buspirone is approved by the FDA for the treatment of generalized anxiety disorder in adults. A recent meta-analysis concluded that buspirone is effective for the treatment of generalized anxiety, though less effective than benzodiazepines (Hidalgo et al. 2007). When selective serotonin reuptake inhibitors (SSRIs) were included as an active comparator, there was no difference between buspirone and the SSRIs (Chessick et al. 2006). Available evidence suggests that buspirone is superior to placebo, but this superiority has not been consistently demonstrated in all placebo-controlled trials (Hidalgo et al. 2007).

The evidence for the use of buspirone for the treatment of anxiety disorders in children comes from case reports and open-label trials (Rynn and Ryan 2008). There is also an open-label trial in 22 children with PDD targeting anxiety and irritability (Buitelaar et al. 1998). In that study, 9 of 22 subjects showed a positive response to buspirone on a global measure of change with dosages ranging from 15 to 45 mg/day in three divided doses. Given the limited evidence in pediatric samples and the modest effects in adult trials, buspirone deserves consideration for the treatment of mild anxiety. It may also be useful as an adjunctive treatment with SSRIs (Rynn and Ryan 2008).

Clinical Management

Buspirone is rapidly absorbed and extensively metabolized by CYP3A3/4. The half-life of 2–3 hours appears to be related to age, with younger children metabolizing buspirone more rapidly. However, buspirone and its metabolite 1-pyrimidinylpiperazine (1-PP) show significant variability in peak concentrations. Noting that buspirone is a substrate for CYP3A3/4, drugs that inhibit 3A3/4 (e.g., ketoconazole, erythromycin, some SSRIs) will increase the level of buspirone. The primary advantages of buspirone are that it does not cause dependence and there are no withdrawal effects upon discontinuation. When attempting to switch from a benzodiazepine to buspirone, the benzodiazepine must be tapered to avoid withdrawal effects.

Buspirone is generally well tolerated. Side effects are usually limited to nausea, headaches, dizziness, nervousness, and daytime somnolence. Agitation, excitation, insomnia, and trouble concentrating have been reported but appear to be uncommon. The dosage may begin with 5 mg/day, increasing in 5 mg increments every 3–5 days before moving to a twice-daily schedule. The usual dosage range in children is 15–30 mg/day in two or three divided doses. In cases showing a partial positive response and minimal adverse effects, the dosage can be increased to 45 mg/day. Benefit is unlikely to emerge much above this dosage, and dosages above 60 mg/day are not recommended.

Desmopressin

Desmopressin (DDAVP) was introduced for the treatment of nocturnal enuresis (see Chapter 28, "Elimination Disorders").

Mechanism of Action

DDAVP is an analogue of the naturally occurring hormone arginine vasopressin (AVP). AVP is a peptide secreted by the neurohypophysis that plays a primary role in the concentration of urine, and thus it contributes to water balance in the body. AVP decreases urine output by increasing uptake of water from the urine in the renal tubules. It also plays a role in regulation of blood pressure. One possible cause of nocturnal enuresis is inadequate secretion of AVP at night, resulting in urine production beyond bladder capacity. The antidiuretic effect of DDAVP is more potent than that of AVP, but it is far less potent as a vasopressor (Norgaard et al. 2007).

Evidence

Several placebo-controlled trials have shown a significant reduction in the number of "wet nights" (Lottmann et al. 2007). Using a benchmark of 50% improvement in dry nights, 60%–70% of children will show a positive response. Although relapse is not infrequent during treatment with DDAVP, evidence from at least one long-term trial suggests that continued treatment may result in return of sustained benefit (Lottmann et al. 2007). In a Cochrane review of 47 placebo-controlled trials involving 3,448 children, Glazener and Evans (2002) reported that DDAVP is effective, with a relatively rapid time to effect. However, the benefits may not endure and treatment effects wane when the medication is stopped. The authors concluded that behavioral interventions, such as the bell and pad alarm systems, may be more effective in the long-term. Therefore, DDAVP may be most appropriate as an adjunct to behavioral intervention and perhaps for short-term use, such as for camp or sleepovers.

DDAVP comes in three common formulations: intranasal spray, oral tablet, and sublingual melt tablet (MELT). These formulations appear to be equally effective. The new sublingual melt formulation (120 or 240 micrograms) was similar to 0.2 or 0.4 mg oral tablets when compared in a trial (Lottmann et al. 2007) with 221 children (mean age, 9.6 years). The study was a randomized, open-label crossover design with no placebo control. Although the difference was modest, the results suggested better compliance and greater preference for the sublingual tablets. Adverse effects were inconsequential and not different across treatment groups. The most common complaint was headache, which occurred in approximately 3% of cases.

Clinical Management

Prior to initiating therapy with DDAVP, there should be a careful review of sleeping habits, fluid intake, frequency of bedwetting, daytime urinary patterns, bowel habits, and interventions tried thus far. Evidence of a recent normal physical examination (especially a normal abdominal exam) and normal urinalysis should be confirmed or obtained (Reiner 2008; see Chapter 28, "Elimination Disorders"). Use of behavioral intervention with the bell and pad alarm system is often effective. It should be noted, however, that although the bell and pad system is often effective, it requires considerable commitment and effort to achieve success. In some cases, it may be appropriate to move to medication before going through an ill-fated trial with the bell and pad. All interventions for nocturnal enuresis should include the use of a diary to track the number of dry nights.

Bioavailability is highest with the intranasal formulation, followed by the sublingual and tablet preparations, respectively. In keeping with the differences in bioavailability, the dose equivalents are as follows: intranasal, 20–40 μg; sublingual tablet, 120–240 μg; and tablet form, 0.2–0.4 mg. The tablet is typically given twice a day. The advantage of the intranasal preparation is the rapid absorption. However, the intranasal preparation may be more vulnerable to dosing fluctuation. The choice of preparation may be based on family preference or cost.

Intranasal DDAVP is typically started at 20 μg (one spray in each nostril) via the intranasal route or 0.1 mg orally twice daily. This dose may be doubled after 1 week if treatment is not successful and the child is tolerating the medication. Following 3 months of successful treatment, the recommendation is to taper the medication (e.g., reduce by half for 2–4 weeks and then

discontinue) (Lottmann et al. 2007). The most common adverse effects of DDAVP include headaches, abdominal pain, nausea, dizziness, facial flushing, and epistaxis (for the intranasal spray). Education of parents and children about the importance of avoiding excessive water intake is warranted due to the remote potential of water intoxication with DDAVP. In most cases, water intoxication was associated with excessive water. Water intoxication is characterized by signs of hyponatremia such as abdominal pain and vomiting. If unchecked, hyponatremia can cause seizures.

In addition to DDAVP, there are several other pharmacological options for the treatment of enuresis. Thus, if DDAVP is not successful, these other treatments merit consideration (Reiner 2008).

Summary Points

- The alpha-2 agonists are commonly used in the treatment of ADHD symptoms across a range of conditions (ADHD, Tourette's syndrome, PDD). These drugs are generally well tolerated and may be especially useful in children who do show a positive response to stimulant medication. The use of clonidine in combination with methylphenidate appears justified in children who show a partial response to monotherapy. Combined treatment with a stimulant and guanfacine has not been studied.

- The use of beta-blockers is supported by clinical experience. This experience suggests that propranolol may be useful for the treatment of aggression when other treatments have not been successful. Propranolol or pindolol may also be useful for the treatment of drug-induced akathisia. Studies in adults suggest that pindolol may be useful as an adjunctive treatment for depression, but this has not been examined in pediatric populations.

- Benzodiazepines have only limited uses in children. When benzodiazepines are used in pediatric populations, treatment should be time limited.

- Buspirone also appears to have limited applications in children. Although it is well tolerated, evidence supporting efficacy in children is sparse.

- DDAVP is a safe and effective treatment for nocturnal enuresis. In some cases, the effectiveness wanes over time. In such cases, use of DDAVP may be reserved for short-term applications such as sleepovers and camp.

References

Adler LA, Angrist B, Weinreb H, et al: Studies on the time course and efficacy of beta-blockers in neuroleptic-induced akathisia and the akathisia of idiopathic Parkinson's disease. Psychopharmacol Bull 27:107–111, 1991

Arnsten AF, Scahill L, Findling RL: Alpha2-adrenergic receptor agonists for the treatment of attention-deficit/hyperactivity disorder: emerging concepts from new data. J Child Adolesc Psychopharmacol 17:393–406, 2007

Ballesteros J, Callado LF: Effectiveness of pindolol plus serotonin uptake inhibitors in depression: a meta-analysis of early and late outcomes from randomised controlled trials. J Affect Disord 79:137–147, 2004

Baumeister AA, Sevin JA: Pharmacologic control of aberrant behavior in the mentally retarded: toward a more rational approach. Neurosci Biobehav Rev 14:253–262, 1990

Biederman J, Melmed RD, Patel A, et al: A randomized, double-blind, placebo-controlled study of guanfacine extended release in children and adolescents with attention-deficit/hyperactivity disorder. Pediatrics 121:e73–e84, 2008

Blier P: Pharmacology of rapid-onset antidepressant treatment strategies. J Clin Psychiatry 62(suppl):12–17, 2001

Boon-Yasidhi V, Kim YS, Scahill L: An open-label, prospective study of guanfacine in children with ADHD and tic disorders. J Med Assoc Thai 88(suppl):S156–S162, 2005

Buitelaar JK, van der Gaag RJ, Swaab-Barneveld H, et al: Pindolol and methylphenidate in children with attention-deficit hyperactivity disorder: clinical efficacy and side-effects. J Child Psych Psychiatry 37:587–595, 1996

Buitelaar JK, van der Gaag RJ, van der Hoeven J: Buspirone in the management of anxiety and irritability in children with pervasive developmental disorders: results of an open-label study. J Clin Psychiatry 59:56–59, 1998

Chappell PB, Riddle MA, Scahill L, et al: Guanfacine treatment of comorbid attention-deficit hyperactivity disorder and Tourette's syndrome: preliminary clinical experience. J Am Acad Child and Adolesc Psychiatry 34:1140–1146, 1995

Chessick CA, Allen MH, Thase ME, et al: Azapirones for generalized anxiety disorder. Cochrane Database of Systematic Reviews 2006, Issue 3. Art. No.: CD006115. DOI: 10.1002/14651858.CD006115

Ciraulo DA, Shader RI, Greenblat DJ, et al: Drug Interactions in Psychiatry, 3rd Edition. Philadelphia, PA, Lippincott Williams & Wilkins, 2006

Cohen DJ, Young JG, Nathanson JA, et al: Clonidine in Tourette's syndrome. Lancet 2:551–553, 1979

Cummings DD, Singer HS, Krieger M, et al: Neuropsychiatric effects of guanfacine in children with mild Tourette syndrome: a pilot study. Clin Neuropharmacol 25:325–332, 2002

Daviss WB, Patel NC, Robb AS, et al: Clonidine for attention-deficit/hyperactivity disorder, II: ECG changes and adverse events analysis. J Am Acad Adolesc Psychiatry 47:189–198, 2008

Fischel T, Hermesh H, Aizenberg D, et al: Cyproheptadine versus propranolol for the treatment of acute neuroleptic-induced akathisia: a comparative double-blind study. J Clin Psychopharmacol 21:612–615, 2001

Gaffney GR, Perry PJ, Lund BC, et al: Risperidone versus clonidine in the treatment of children and adolescents with Tourette's syndrome. J Am Acad Child Adolesc Psychiatry 41:330–336, 2002

Glazener CM, Evans JH: Desmopressin for nocturnal enuresis in children. Cochrane Database of Systematic Reviews 2002, Issue 3. Art. No.: CD002112. DOI: 10.1002/14651858.CD002112

Gogtay N, Sporn A, Alfaro CL, et al: Clozapine-induced akathisia in children with schizophrenia. J Child Adolesc Psychopharmacol 12:347–349, 2002

Graae F, Milner J, Rizzotto L, et al: Clonazepam in childhood anxiety disorders. J Am Acad Child Adolesc Psychiatry 33:372–376, 1994

Hidalgo RB, Tupler LA, Davidson JR: An effect-size analysis of pharmacologic treatments for generalized anxiety disorder. J Psychopharmacol 21:864–872, 2007

Hoffman BB: Catecholamines, sympathomimetic drugs, and adrenergic receptor antagonists, in Goodman and Gilman's The Pharmacological Basis of Therapeutics, 10th Edition. Edited by Hardman JG, Limbird LE, Gilman AG. New York, McGraw-Hill, 2001, pp 215–268

Horrigan JP, Barnhill LJ: Guanfacine for treatment of attention-deficit hyperactivity disorder in boys. J Child Adolesc Psychopharmacol 5:215–223, 1995

Hunt RD, Arnsten AF, Asbell MD: An open trial of guanfacine in the treatment of attention-deficit hyperactivity disorder. J Am Acad Child Adolesc Psychiatry 34:50–54, 1995

Leckman JF, Hardin MT, Riddle MA, et al: Clonidine treatment of Gilles de la Tourette's syndrome. Arch Gen Psychiatry 48:324–328, 1991

Leo RJ: Movement disorders associated with the serotonin selective reuptake inhibitors. J Clin Psychiatry 57:449–454, 1996

Lottmann H, Froeling F, Alloussi S, et al: A randomised comparison of oral desmopressin lyophilisate (MELT) and tablet formulations in children and adolescents with primary nocturnal enuresis. Int J Clin Pract 61:1454–1460, 2007

Norgaard JP, Hashim H, Malmberg L, et al: Antidiuresis therapy: mechanism of action and clinical implications. Neurourol Urodyn 26:1008–1013, 2007

Palumbo DR, Sallee FR, Pelham WE, et al: Clonidine for attention-deficit/hyperactivity disorder, I: efficacy and tolerability outcomes. J Am Acad Adolesc Psychiatry 47:180–188, 2008

Pitman RK, Sanders KM, Zusman RM, et al: Pilot study of secondary prevention of posttraumatic stress disorder with propranolol. Biol Psychiatry 51:189–192, 2002

Pollack MH: Social anxiety disorder: designing a pharmacologic treatment strategy. J Clin Psychiatry 60(suppl):20–26, 1999

Poncin Y, Scahill L: Stimulants and nonstimulants in the treatment of hyperactivity in autism, in Clinical Manual for the Treatment of Autism. Edited by Hollander E, Anagostou E. Washington, DC, American Psychiatric Publishing, 2007, pp 131–147

Ratey JJ, Gordon A: The psychopharmacology of aggression: toward a new day. Psychopharmacol Bull 29:65–73, 1993

Reiner W: Pharmacotherapy in the management of voiding and storage disorders, including enuresis and encopresis. J Am Acad Adolesc Psychiatry 47:491–498, 2008

Rynn MA, Ryan J: Anxiety disorders, in Clinical Manual of Child and Adolescent Psychopharmacology. Edited by Findling RL. Washington, DC, American Psychiatric Publishing, 2008, pp 143–196

Sahoo S, Ameen S: Acute nocturnal akathisia induced by clozapine. J Clin Psychopharmacol 27:205, 2007

Scahill L, Chappell PB, Kim YS, et al: A placebo-controlled study of guanfacine in the treatment of children with tic disorders and attention deficit hyperactivity disorder. Am J Psychiatry 158:1067–1074, 2001

Scahill L, Aman MG, McDougle CJ, et al: A prospective open trial of guanfacine in children with pervasive developmental disorders. J Child Adolesc Psychopharmacol 16:589–598, 2006a

Scahill L, Erenberg G, Berlin CM, et al: Contemporary assessment and pharmacotherapy of Tourette syndrome. NeuroRx 3:192–206, 2006b

Schur SB, Sikich L, Findling RL, et al: Treatment recommendations for the use of antipsychotics for aggressive youth (TRAAY), part I: a review. J Am Acad Child Adolesc Psychiatry 42:132–144, 2003

Simeon JG, Ferguson HB, Knott V, et al: Clinical, cognitive, and neurophysiological effects of alprazolam in children and adolescents with overanxious and avoidant disorders. J Am Acad Child Adolesc Psychiatry 31:29–33, 1992

Tallman JF, Cassella J, Kehne J: Mechanism of action of anxiolytics, in Neuropsychopharmacology: The Fifth Generation of Progress. Edited by Davis KL, Charney D, Coyle JT, et al. Philadelphia, PA, Lippincott Williams & Wilkins, 2002, pp 993–1006

Tourette's Syndrome Study Group: Treatment of ADHD in children with tics: a randomized controlled trial. Neurology 58:527–536, 2002

Voshaar RC, Couvee JE, van Balkom AJ, et al: Strategies for discontinuing long-term benzodiazepine use: meta-analysis. Br J Psychiatry 189:213–220, 2006

Chapter 51

Medications Used for Sleep

Kyle P. Johnson, M.D.
Anna Ivanenko, M.D., Ph.D.

Prescription and nonprescription medications are being used for sleep problems by child psychiatrists and pediatricians at increasing rates, despite there being no U.S. Food and Drug Administration (FDA)–approved drugs for pediatric insomnia. We are beginning to see, only recently, published research on pharmacotherapy for pediatric sleep disorders. This chapter will summarize the use of medications for sleep disorders in children and adolescents. A recent survey of child and adolescent psychiatrists reveals that prescription or nonprescription medications are frequently used to manage insomnia in the following disorders: primary insomnia, depression, bipolar affective disorder, anxiety, posttraumatic stress disorder, delayed sleep phase syndrome, attention-deficit/hyperactivity disorder (ADHD), autism spectrum disorder, chronic pain, oppositional disorder, and mental retardation/developmental delay (Rosen et al. 2005). More than 75% of primary care pediatricians surveyed recommended nonprescription medications

for pediatric insomnia and greater than 50% had prescribed a medication specifically for sleep (Owens et al. 2003). Clinical situations in which medications were most commonly used were acute pain and travel, closely followed by children with special needs such as mental retardation, autism, and ADHD.

Medications for Insomnia

The regulation of sleep is related to neurotransmitters, including γ-aminobutyric acid (GABA), melatonin, histamine, and norepinephrine. Medications used to treat insomnia act at the receptors of these neurotransmitters. Benzodiazepines and benzodiazepine receptor agonists bind to the benzodiazepine receptor site, leading to modulation of the GABA receptor and its chloride ion channels. Antidepressants such as trazodone, mirtazapine, and amitriptyline exert this sedative effect through anticholinergic mechanisms. Antihistamines, available in a wide variety of compounds such as diphenhydramine, are sedating and often used to treat pediatric insomnia. Alpha-adrenergic agonists such as clonidine and guanfacine, although antihypertensives, are also prescribed for their sedative qualities.

Insomnia can be primary or can be a symptom of a number of medical and psychiatric conditions as well as other sleep disorders (secondary or comorbid insomnia). It is important to use sedating pharmacological agents only when behavioral interventions have been tried and found to be ineffective. Behavioral interventions for insomnia are discussed in Chapter 29, "Sleep Disorders."

The underlying diagnosis causing insomnia should influence the choice of medication. In many cases, treating the underlying condition will lead to improvement and resolution of insomnia. For example, use of a serotonin reuptake inhibitor in a child with major depressive disorder may be all that is necessary to treat the child's insomnia. However, the insomnia associated with a medical or psychiatric condition may be severe enough to warrant its own pharmacological treatment, at least in the short-term. Patients and their parents must understand that there are no FDA-approved drugs for pediatric insomnia; therefore, medicines prescribed for this purpose are being used off-label. A careful discussion of the risks, benefits, and alternatives is in order.

Below, we will discuss specific pharmacological agents that are often used to treat pediatric insomnia, whether or not the insomnia is associated with a medical or psychiatric condition.

Melatonin

In the United States, melatonin is a widely sold nutritional supplement, not a licensed drug. To date, there have been more placebo-controlled trials of melatonin in the treatment of pediatric insomnia than other licensed drugs (Smits et al. 2001, 2003; Weiss et al. 2006). Melatonin is now among the eight medications most commonly prescribed by British child psychiatrists (Clark 2004). Pediatricians in the United States frequently use melatonin as a first-line strategy in the treatment of insomnia (Owens et al. 2003). In a survey of members of the American Academy of Child and Adolescent Psychiatry, melatonin was a leading nonprescription medication prescribed for insomnia associated with ADHD and autism spectrum disorder (Rosen et al. 2005).

Melatonin is an indoleamine with sleep-promoting and chronobiotic properties. Chronobiotic properties refer to influencing the timing of sleep. In the United States, synthetic melatonin has been available since 1993 as an over-the-counter medication. Melatonin has been used to treat insomnia in a number of pediatric populations including typically developing children with initial insomnia, children with ADHD and comorbid insomnia, children with neurodevelopmental disabilities, and children with autism spectrum disorder (Garstang and Wallis 2006; Jan and Freeman 2004; Smits et al. 2003; Weiss et al. 2006). Additionally, melatonin has been used in the treatment of adolescents with delayed sleep phase syndrome, a circadian rhythm sleep disorder (Szeinberg et al. 2006). Optimal melatonin administration depends in part on what is being treated. Melatonin is relatively short acting, with a half-life of approximately 1 hour; therefore, it is much more effective in treating initial insomnia rather than sleep maintenance insomnia or terminal insomnia. For the treatment of initial insomnia, melatonin should be administered approximately 30 minutes before desired sleep-onset time. Melatonin is thought to be sedating in dosages of 1 mg and greater. Research studies have tended to use doses of 2.5–10 mg when treating initial insomnia. One potential strategy in treating initial insomnia with melatonin is to start with a dose of 1.5 mg and to increase in 1.5 mg increments every 4–5 days as indicated (Jan et al. 2007). Researchers have used doses as high as 10–15 mg in children with severe neurodevelopmental disabilities, without evidence of significant adverse events (Jan and Freeman 2004). If melatonin is to be used as a chronobiotic in an attempt to alter the circadian sleep-wake cycle, it can be given in smaller doses. In these cases, the timing of the administration is even more important. For example, in the treatment of delayed sleep phase syndrome, there is evidence that low-dose melatonin in the range of 0.3 mg is effective if given approximately 4–5 hours before the present habitual bedtime, which may not be the desired bedtime. This low dose of melatonin then can be progressively dosed earlier as the sleep phase is moved earlier (advanced). One particular use of low-dose melatonin is in children with total blindness. These children do not have access to the light-dark cycle; therefore, they tend to "free run," typically delaying their sleep-wake schedule over time. This leads to periods of time when they are extremely sleepy during the day and more awake and alert at night, causing significant impairment. Low-dose melatonin can be used to entrain their circadian rhythms, as demonstrated in adults (Lewy et al. 2005).

Sedative-Hypnotics

Benzodiazepines

Benzodiazepines act on the specific sites of GABA type A receptors (GABA$_A$) and produce hypnotic, myorelaxant, anxiolytic, and anticonvulsant effects. Benzodiazepines approved by the FDA for the treatment of insomnia in adults include temazepam, estazolam, quazepam, flurazepam, and triazolam. These medications vary mainly by elimination half-life, presence of active metabolite, and affinity for the benzodiazepine receptor subtype (Table 51–1).

Benzodiazepines are lipophilic, highly bound to plasma membranes, and eliminated by hepatic enzymes. Their effects on sleep architecture include suppression of slow wave sleep (stages 3 and 4), increase of sleep spindles and stage 2 sleep, mild suppression of rapid eye movement (REM) sleep, and reduction in frequency of nocturnal arousals.

Tolerance, next-day sedation, anterograde amnesia, cognitive and psychomotor impairments, and rebound insomnia are known side effects of benzodiazepines. There are virtually no pediatric clinical trials of benzodiazepines for insomnia and therefore no established data on their safety and effectiveness for this clinical indication. All benzodiazepines have abuse potential and should be used only with great caution, especially in the pediatric population.

Nonbenzodiazepine Benzodiazepine Receptor Agonists

The nonbenzodiazepine benzodiazepine receptor agonists include zolpidem and zaleplon. These medications bind preferentially to the omega-1 benzodiazepine receptor of the GABA$_A$ receptor complex. This preferential binding may explain the relative absence of anticonvulsant and myorelaxant effects as well as the preservation of stage 3 and 4 sleep (deep, slow wave sleep). These medications are FDA approved for the treatment of insomnia in adults only. Although the FDA-approved indication is for short-term insomnia, these medicines are often used long-term in adults with chronic, severe insomnia. Eszopiclone is a racemic isomer of zopiclone, a sedative-hypnotic used in Europe for many years. The precise mechanism of action is not known, but it is suspected to work at the benzodiazepine receptor of the GABA$_A$ receptor complex, much like zolpidem and zaleplon. These three medications differ primarily in their half-lives (Table 51–2).

Although there is little to no published research on the use of these medications in the treatment of insomnia in children or adolescents, there may be a role for their off-label use in certain cases of severe incapacitating insomnia.

New warnings have been issued regarding the sedative-hypnotic medications. In March 2007, the FDA requested that all manufacturers of sedative-hypnotic medications change their product labeling to include the risks of severe allergic reactions and complex sleep-related behaviors, including sleep driving and sleep eating.

Zolpidem.

Zolpidem (trade name Ambien) was the first benzodiazepine receptor agonist released in the United States. A noncontrolled-release formulation (referred to from here forward as zolpidem) was first released. The noncontrolled-release formulation is now available as a generic drug. Zolpidem has an onset of action of less than 30 minutes and a half-life of approximately 2.5 hours. The most common side effects experienced by adults in clinical trials included nausea, myalgia, dizziness, headache, and somnolence. There have been reports of parasomnias in adults taking zolpidem, including sleepwalking and sleep eating. It is very important that patients are instructed to take this medicine just as they are getting in bed with the intention to fall asleep.

More recently, a controlled-release formulation of zolpidem has been released (referred to from here forward as zolpidem CR). This controlled-release formulation was designed as a two-layer tablet, allowing biphasic absorption and a prolonged duration of effect.

TABLE 51–1. Pharmacological characteristics of benzodiazepines

Drug	Half-life, h	Onset of action, min	Active metabolites
Triazolam (Halcion)	1.5–5.5	10–20	No
Temazepam (Restoril)	8–22	45–60	No
Estazolam (ProSom)	10–24	15–30	No
Quazepam (Doral)	15–120	15–30	Yes
Flurazepam (Dalmane)	36–120	15–30	Yes

TABLE 51–2. Nonbenzodiazepine benzodiazepine receptor agonists

Name	Time of peak concentration (T_{max}), h	Half-life, h	Active metabolites
Zolpidem (Ambien)	1.6	2.5	None
Zolpidem CR (Ambien CR)	1.5	2.8	None
Zaleplon (Sonata)	1	1	None
Eszopiclone (Lunesta)	1	6	None

This design makes zolpidem CR effective for both initial and maintenance (middle of the night) insomnia. It comes in 6.25 mg and 12.5 mg tablet strengths. The most common side effects in adults taking zolpidem CR are headaches, somnolence, and dizziness.

Zaleplon.

Zaleplon (trade name Sonata) is FDA approved for the short-term treatment of insomnia in adults. It has a very short half-life of 1 hour, making it particularly effective for initial insomnia. It also has a unique role as an as-needed medicine for middle-of-the-night insomnia. Adult data suggest that it can be taken if the patient can stay in bed for at least 4 hours. Typical doses are 5 mg or 10 mg, but adults can take a dose up to 20 mg. It comes in capsule strengths of 5 mg and 10 mg. Common side effects include headache, dizziness, and somnolence.

Eszopiclone.

Eszopiclone (trade name Lunesta) is FDA approved for the treatment of insomnia in adults, without the disclaimer that it should be used only short-term. It comes in 1 mg, 2 mg, and 3 mg tablet strengths. Its half-life is 6 hours, which is significantly longer than that of zolpidem or zaleplon, potentially making eszopiclone an attractive medicine to treat insomnia in children. However, as with zolpidem and zaleplon, there are no significant pediatric studies.

While more data on the use of the nonbenzodiazepine benzodiazepine receptor agonists in children are gathered, a conservative approach is warranted. One should consider referring children who may be candidates for treatment with these medications to a sleep specialist.

Ramelteon

Ramelteon is a new class of hypnotic medication that is FDA approved for treatment of initial insomnia in adults, with no duration limitation. Ramelteon is a potent melatonin receptor agonist with higher affinity for melatonin MT_1 and MT_2 receptors than the MT_3 recep-

tor. The selective binding to these receptors, which are normally acted upon by endogenous melatonin, induces sleep and maintains the circadian rhythm underlying the normal sleep-wake cycle. Time to peak concentration is 0.75 hours. Ramelteon does have an active metabolite, M II. The half-life is approximately 1–2.6 hours for the parent compound and 2–5 hours for the active metabolite. It comes only in 8 mg tablet strength. A precaution listed in the labeling states that reproductive development may be affected in adolescents or children, given the possible effect of this medicine on the endocrine system. Ramelteon should not be prescribed to patients taking fluvoxamine since fluvoxamine is a major inhibitor of CYP1A2. Therefore, concurrent use of fluvoxamine and ramelteon will lead to significant increases in ramelteon plasma concentrations. Common side effects include nausea, dizziness, somnolence, fatigue, and depression.

Antihistamines

Antihistamines, although primarily indicated for treatment of allergies, motion sickness, and vertigo, are often prescribed to treat insomnia in children. Of the antihistamines, diphenhydramine hydrochloride, available over the counter, is most commonly recommended to induce sleep in children. Hydroxyzine hydrochloride is another antihistamine that has been prescribed for insomnia. Despite clinical trials demonstrating some efficacy with the use of these medicines, they are not ideal. Their half-lives are relatively long, leading to next-day sedation. Additionally, they appear to impair sleep quality, causing problems with next-day functioning. Side effects include loss of appetite, constipation, nausea, and even vomiting or diarrhea. Other anticholinergic side effects such as dry mouth are common, and there is a risk of confusion and paradoxical agitation especially in vulnerable children. It is our recommendation that these medications not be used to treat significant insomnia in children. The only potential role that we see for them is their use for one or two nights in cases of transient insomnia.

Chloral Hydrate

Chloral hydrate was one of the first synthetic agents used as a hypnotic. It has been prescribed to children with significant insomnia, although it is more commonly used as a preoperative anxiolytic/sedative. Chloral hydrate has a poor safety profile, in part due to its long half-life. It also is habit-forming and associated with tolerance. Therefore, it should not be used to treat insomnia in children. There are now other, much safer options available.

Other Medications With Sedating Properties

Antidepressants and Antipsychotics

There is no significant research evidence supporting the use of sedating antidepressants in the treatment of pediatric insomnia. Although a clinician could argue that using a sedating antidepressant (for example, mirtazapine) is appropriate when treating insomnia associated with clinical depression, it may not be the best choice. In our estimate, it may be more efficacious to treat the depression with a serotonin reuptake inhibitor such as fluoxetine while adding a sedating medication such as melatonin, a benzodiazepine, or a nonbenzodiazepine benzodiazepine receptor agonist in the short-term as the depression resolves.

There is no evidence supporting the use of antipsychotics in the treatment of pediatric insomnia, unless the insomnia is associated with a psychotic disorder. The potential risks far outweigh the benefits when considering use of an antipsychotic to treat primary insomnia or insomnia not associated with psychosis.

Alpha-Agonists

Alpha-agonists, particularly clonidine, are the most prescribed medications for insomnia in children, according to recent surveys of pediatricians and child and adolescent psychiatrists (Owens et al. 2003; Rosen et al. 2005), despite limited research data supporting their use and their problematic safety profiles (see Chapter 50, "Alpha-Adrenergics, Beta-Blockers, Benzodiazepines, Buspirone, and Desmopressin"). Several case series suggest the efficacy of clonidine in treating insomnia associated with neurodevelopmental disorders such as ADHD (Ingrassia and Turk 2005; Prince et al. 1996; Wilens et al. 1994). The mean dosage at bedtime in the case series of children with ADHD was approximately 0.15 mg (Prince et al. 1996). There

are no controlled studies using alpha-agonists to treat pediatric insomnia.

Medications for Excessive Daytime Sleepiness

Excessive daytime sleepiness (EDS) is a symptom associated with several pediatric sleep disorders. EDS is usually due to sleep deprivation, as is the case in sleep-disordered breathing, delayed sleep phase syndrome, severe insomnia, or insufficient sleep (simply not allowing enough time for sleep). In these cases, treating the underlying sleep disorder should lead to resolution of EDS. In other sleep disorders, such as narcolepsy and idiopathic hypersomnia, EDS is a primary symptom of the condition. In these cases, EDS causes significant distress and impairment, and pharmacotherapy is often indicated. Medicines often used by sleep specialists to treat EDS are discussed in this section. If EDS is due to behaviorally caused short sleep duration, then behavioral treatments are indicated.

Modafinil

Modafinil (brand name Provigil) is an alerting oral agent approved by the FDA for the treatment of adults with EDS associated with narcolepsy, shift work sleep disorder, and residual sleepiness despite the use of nasal continuous positive airway pressure (CPAP) in patients with obstructive sleep apnea. Modafinil has a Schedule IV designation by the U.S. Drug Enforcement Administration (DEA) and is not approved for any indication in the pediatric population. It is chemically and pharmacologically distinct from sympathomimetic amines and reportedly has fewer side effects (U.S. Modafinil in Narcolepsy Multicenter Study Group 2000). The exact mechanism of action remains unknown, but it appears to promote alertness by indirect activation of the frontal cortex via the hypothalamus and/or the tuberomammillary nucleus (Lin et al. 1996; Scammell et al. 2000).

In children, research has been limited to 1) a double-blind, placebo-controlled trial of modafinil in children with ADHD (Greenhill et al. 2006) and 2) a retrospective study in a small sample of children with narcolepsy and idiopathic hypersomnia (Ivanenko et al. 2003). The therapeutic dose reported in children and adolescents ranges from 100 to 600 mg/day. The most common side effects include headache, nausea, and anxiety. Modafinil does not seem to provoke any subsequent changes in sleep architecture. Psychotic symptoms associated with modafinil use have been reported in individuals with a history of psychiatric disorders. In 2007, a new warning was added to the labeling related to pediatric clinical trials data. In these clinical trials, a rash developed in 0.8% of patients treated with modafinil and 0% of patients treated with placebo. These dermatological reactions included Stevens-Johnson syndrome and multiorgan hypersensitivity.

Stimulants

Stimulants have a role in treating the EDS associated with narcolepsy and idiopathic hypersomnia. Amphetamine/dextroamphetamine is FDA approved for the treatment of narcolepsy in children as young as 6 years. Extended-release formulations are preferred since the daytime sleepiness in these conditions persists throughout the day. It is unlikely that stimulants used in this population would impair sleep at night.

Sodium Oxybate

Sodium oxybate (trade name Xyrem), also known as γ-hydroxybutyrate, is an FDA-approved drug for the treatment of narcolepsy in adults. It is available only through a centralized pharmacy as a Schedule III controlled substance. The drug is tightly controlled due to a history of diversion and abuse ("the date rape drug"). Sodium oxybate activates the $GABA_B$ receptors and suppresses dopaminergic neuronal activity, leading to an increase in slow-wave sleep and a decrease in awakenings at night. Improved sleep efficiency is the end result. Although not FDA approved for children, it has been reported to be effective in treating severe childhood narcolepsy-cataplexy (Murali and Kotagal 2006). Sodium oxybate should be used only in children and adolescents with documented narcolepsy with cataplexy or narcolepsy with significant EDS. It is our opinion that this medicine should be prescribed to children only by sleep specialists experienced in treating narcolepsy.

Medications for Restless Legs Syndrome

There are now two FDA-approved medications for the treatment of restless legs syndrome (RLS) in adults: ropinirole and pramipexole. This indication was not ex-

tended to children and adolescents, however. RLS does occur in children and adolescents and often requires treatment with medications, especially in moderate to severe cases. We recommend that children with suspected RLS be referred to a sleep medicine clinic for assessment with overnight polysomnography.

Dopaminergic Agonists

Ropinirole and pramipexole are dopamine agonists originally indicated for the treatment of Parkinson's disease. There is limited research in the area of pharmacological management of RLS in children. To date, it includes only case reports and case series. Levodopa (L-dopa) and pergolide, both dopaminergic agents, were found to be effective in a small cohort of children with RLS and/or periodic limb movements (Walters et al. 2000). It is important to note that pergolide was subsequently withdrawn from the U.S. market due to adverse reactions. More recent case reports have focused on the dopamine agonists eventually FDA approved for treatment of RLS in adults. Pramipexole was found to be effective in a number of children with RLS and/or periodic limb movements noted on polysomnogram (Martinez and Guilleminault 2004). There is one case report regarding the use of ropinirole to treat RLS in a child with ADHD (Konafal et al. 2005). It is important to note that there have been no placebo-controlled clinical trials in children or adolescents with RLS. It has been our experience that dopamine agonists are useful and often well tolerated in children with RLS.

Gabapentin

Gabapentin is an anticonvulsant that is often sedating and appears to increase slow wave sleep. Although not FDA approved for treatment of RLS, gabapentin has been found to be effective in adults (Garcia-Borreguero et al. 2002). Gabapentin may be particularly effective in treating RLS associated with neuropathies and pain. There are no clinical trials using gabapentin in children with RLS, but clinical experience demonstrates some utility in select cases.

Medications for Parasomnias

Parasomnias such as sleep walking and sleep terrors are relatively common in children. Treatment usually is comprised only of parent education and reassurance as well as institution of safety precautions. When these nocturnal behaviors occur frequently, disrupting the family, and especially if they put the child at risk for physical harm, pharmacotherapy may be indicated. The medication class of first choice is the benzodiazepines, which decrease slow wave (delta) sleep—the sleep stage from which parasomnias originate. Sleep specialists most commonly use low-dose clonazepam (0.125–0.5 mg) for this purpose, given approximately 1 hour before desired sleep-onset time.

Research Directions

The relative paucity of studies demonstrates the need for research in the area of pharmacological management of pediatric sleep disorders. Clinical trials of hypnotics in children and adolescents are clearly needed—this was the consensus opinion of a recent conference held on pharmacological management of pediatric sleep disorders. The consensus opinion called for initial concentration of pediatric insomnia studies to be on neuropsychiatric disorders, with the highest priority

set on pervasive developmental disorders (Mindell et al. 2006). It was the consensus opinion that research was needed in treating the insomnia often comorbid with ADHD, mood disorders, and anxiety disorders. There also was a call to study medical disorders with comorbid insomnia as well as primary sleep disorders.

Combined behavioral and pharmacological treatments should be studied against behavioral treatment alone and pharmacological treatment alone. Combined treatment may be the most efficacious. Additionally, appropriate doses of medications need to be determined for the pediatric population, likely based on weight, at least in younger children. Different formulations such as chewable tablets or liquid suspensions need to be developed, making medications easier to use especially in special needs populations.

Future research should use objective measures of sleep such as polysomnography and actigraphy (see Chapter 29, "Sleep Disorders"). Polysomnography is an important tool that allows accurate measurement of sleep architecture at baseline and clinical endpoints. Actigraphy is less expensive and invasive than polysomnography and can be used to determine sleep patterns that may change with treatment.

Summary Points

- There are no FDA-approved drugs for the treatment of pediatric insomnia.
- A number of placebo-controlled studies have demonstrated melatonin to be safe and effective in the short-term treatment of initial insomnia in children and adolescents.
- There is no role for the use of antipsychotics in treating insomnia unless the insomnia is related to a psychotic illness or a severe mood disorder.
- When choosing a medication to treat insomnia, the clinician must be guided by the underlying diagnosis.
- RLS does occur in children and may require pharmacotherapy. When RLS is suspected in a child, referral to a sleep clinic is indicated.

References

Clark A: Incidences of new prescribing by British child and adolescent psychiatrists: a prospective study over 12 months. J Psychopharmacol 18:115–120, 2004

Garcia-Borreguero D, Lorrosa O, de la Llave Y, et al: Treatment of restless legs syndrome with gabapentin: a double-blind, cross-over study. Neurology 59:1573–1579, 2002

Garstang J, Wallis M: Randomized controlled trial of melatonin for children with autistic spectrum disorders and sleep problems. Child Care Health Dev 32:585–589, 2006

Greenhill LL, Biederman J, Boellner SW, et al: A randomized, double-blind, placebo-controlled study of modafinil film-coated tablets in children and adolescents with attention-deficit/hyperactivity disorder. J Am Acad Child Adolesc Psychiatry 45:503–511, 2006

Ingrassia A, Turk J: The use of clonidine for severe and intractable sleep problems in children with neurodevelopmental disorders: a case series. Eur Child Adolesc Psychiatry 14:34–40, 2005

Ivanenko A, Tauman R, Gozal D: Modafinil in the treatment of excessive daytime sleepiness in children. Sleep Med 4:579–582, 2003

Jan JE, Freeman RD: Melatonin therapy for circadian rhythm sleep disorders in children with multiple disabilities: what have we learned in the last decade? Dev Med Child Neurol 46:776–782, 2004

Jan JE, Wasdell MB, Reiter RJ, et al: Melatonin therapy of pediatric sleep disorders: recent advances, why it works, who are the candidates and how to treat. Curr Pediatr Rev 3:214–224, 2007

Konafal E, Arnulf I, Lecendreux M, et al: Ropinirole in a child with attention-deficit hyperactivity disorder and restless legs syndrome. Pediatr Neurol 32:350–351, 2005

Lewy AJ, Emens JS, Lefler BJ, et al: Melatonin entrains free-running blind people according to a physiological dose-response curve. Chronobiol Int 22:1093–1106, 2005

Lin JS, Hou Y, Jouvet M: Potential brain neuronal targets for amphetamine-, methylphenidate-, and modafinil-induced wakefulness, evidenced by c-fos immunochemistry in the cat. Proc Natl Acad Sci USA 93:14128–14133, 1996

Martinez S, Guilleminault C: Periodic leg movements in prepubertal children with sleep disturbance. Dev Med Child Neurol 46:765–770, 2004

Mindell JA, Emslie G, Blumer J, et al: Pharmacologic management of insomnia in children and adolescents: consensus statement. Pediatrics 117:e1223–e1232, 2006

Murali H, Kotagal S: Off-label treatment of severe childhood narcolepsy-cataplexy with sodium oxybate. Sleep 29:1025–1029, 2006

Owens J, Rosen CL, Mindell JA: Medication use in the treatment of pediatric insomnia: results of a survey of community-based pediatricians. Pediatrics 111:e628–e635, 2003

Prince JB, Wilens TE, Biederman J, et al: Clonidine for sleep disturbances associated with attention-deficit hyperactivity disorder: a systematic chart review of 62 cases. J Am Acad Child Adolesc Psychiatry 35:599–605, 1996

Rosen CL, Owens JA, Mindell JA, et al: Use of pharmacotherapy for insomnia in children and adolescents: a national survey of child psychiatrists (abstract). Sleep 28(suppl): A79, 2005

Scammell TE, Estabrooke IV, McCarthy MT, et al: Hypothalamic arousal regions are activated during modafinil-induced wakefulness. J Neurosci 20:8620–8628, 2000

Smits MG, Nagtegaal EE, van der Heijden J, et al: Melatonin for chronic sleep onset insomnia in children: a randomized placebo-controlled trial. J Child Neurol 16:86–92, 2001

Smits MG, van Stel HF, van der Heijden K, et al: Melatonin improves health status and sleep in children with idiopathic chronic sleep-onset insomnia: a randomized placebo-controlled trial. J Am Acad Child Adolesc Psychiatry 42:1286–1293, 2003

Szeinberg A, Borodkin K, Dagan Y: Melatonin treatment in adolescents with delayed sleep phase syndrome. Clin Pediatr 45:809–818, 2006

U.S. Modafinil in Narcolepsy Multicenter Study Group: Randomized trial of modafinil as a treatment for the excessive daytime somnolence of narcolepsy. Neurology 54:1166–1175, 2000

Walters AS, Mandelbaum DE, Lewin DS, et al: Dopaminergic therapy in children with restless legs/periodic limb movements in sleep and ADHD. Pediatr Neurol 22:182–186, 2000

Weiss MD, Wasdell MB, Bomben MM, et al: Sleep hygiene and melatonin treatment for children and adolescents with ADHD and initial insomnia. J Am Acad Child Adolesc Psychiatry 45:512–519, 2006

Wilens TE, Biederman J, Spencer T: Clonidine for sleep disturbances associated with attention-deficit hyperactivity disorder. J Am Acad Child Adolesc Psychiatry 33:424–426, 1994

Electroconvulsive Therapy, Transcranial Magnetic Stimulation, and Deep Brain Stimulation

Daniel F. Connor, M.D.

This chapter discusses brain-based interventions in child and adolescent psychiatry. These include electroconvulsive therapy (ECT) for adolescents, repetitive transcranial magnetic stimulation, and deep brain stimulation. With the exception of ECT for adolescents, these brain-based interventions should currently be considered investigational procedures and not routinely prescribed for psychiatric disorders within the pediatric age range.

Electroconvulsive Therapy

ECT in adolescents is an uncommonly used treatment for severely disabling and treatment-resistant mood disorders in adolescents. Although ECT is a sometimes controversial and often misunderstood intervention, it can be very effective and even lifesaving in those who have severe depression, psychotic depression, or mania with risk of imminent harm to self or others (such as severe suicide risk or refusal to eat or drink) and when these conditions do not respond to inpatient hospitalization and psychiatric medication. It is also occasionally prescribed for catatonic states, schizophrenia, and rarely, for neuroleptic malignant syndrome (American Academy of Child and Adolescent Psychiatry 2004). ECT is generally considered a treatment of last resort.

ECT is the brief passage of electrical current through the brain via electrodes placed on the scalp that produces a grand mal seizure. It is as yet not entirely understood why the seizure is effective in relieving the symptoms of severe depression or mania in a majority of patients who undergo the procedure. Although ECT is well researched in adults with psychiatric disorders, published studies of ECT in adolescents are few and of uncontrolled methodology.

ECT was first administered to children and adolescents in the 1940s. Because of concerns about possible harmful effects, negative media portrayals, and the development of psychiatric medications, interest in the practice diminished. With the development of modern brief-pulse ECT machines and anesthesia techniques that diminish side effects, ECT is being again considered for adolescents with severe and treatment-refractory mood disorders. Guidelines for ECT in minors have now been published (American Academy of Child and Adolescent Psychiatry 2004; Weiner 2001).

Prevalence of Use

ECT is infrequently used to treat adolescents and is almost never used to treat prepubertal children. In 1980 a study from the National Institute of Mental Health revealed that only 500 of 33,384 patients who had been treated with ECT in the United States were between 11 and 20 years of age (Thompson and Blaine 1987). Another study identified all persons younger than age 19 years who received ECT in the Australian state of New South Wales between 1990 and 1999. Seventy-two patients ages 14–18 years underwent a total of 84 courses of ECT during this time period. This translates into a prevalence of 1.53/100,000 adolescents treated with ECT per year (Walter and Rey 2003).

Evidence of Effectiveness

There are no prospective randomized controlled trials of ECT in children or adolescents. Evidence of ECT effectiveness comes from clinical experience and retrospective case reports. These studies are outlined in Table 52–1.

Retrospective open case studies over the past 60 years suggest that ECT is an effective treatment for adolescents with treatment-resistant affective disorders and possibly for some adolescents with schizophrenia. Response rates range between 50% and 100%, with higher response rates generally reported for mood disorders as compared with psychotic disorders (American Academy of Child and Adolescent Psychiatry 2004). There appear to be no gender differences in response rates. With the exception of schizophrenia (i.e., higher ECT response rates are reported for adults),

these improvement rates in adolescents are very similar to ECT improvement rates in adults, suggesting (with limitations noted below) that teenagers may respond to ECT in a fashion similar to adults. Long-term ECT response rates in teenagers have yet to be systematically investigated. Little data are available on ECT effectiveness in prepubertal children.

There are significant limitations in the ECT effectiveness literature. No randomized controlled trials comparing ECT with sham (placebo) ECT in children or adolescents have been conducted. Given ethical concerns about ECT in the pediatric age range and concerns about the consequences of sham ECT given to youngsters with severe and disabling psychiatric disorders, it is doubtful that a placebo-controlled trial of ECT in children and adolescents can ever be completed.

Indications in Adolescents

Consensus psychiatric indications for ECT in adolescents are severe mood symptoms—depressive or manic—irrespective of their etiology. Mood symptoms occurring in the context of major depression, psychotic depression, schizoaffective disorder, schizophrenia, bipolar disorder, and organic brain disorder all may respond to ECT. In mood disorders (e.g., depression or mania), psychotic symptoms may respond as well. By extension from data on adults, some schizophrenic episodes in youth may respond to ECT, especially when mood symptoms are prominent. ECT may also be used to treat catatonia and neuroleptic malignant syndrome (American Academy of Child and Adolescent Psychiatry 2004). For patients to be eligible for ECT, their psychiatric symptoms must be severe, persistent, and significantly disabling.

Before the clinician recommends ECT, treatment refractoriness and the adequacy of previous psychological and pharmacological interventions must be documented. There is general agreement that patients considered for ECT must demonstrate a lack of response to several adequate psychopharmacology treatment trials. Treatment-resistant depression is defined as failure of at least two adequate antidepressant drug trials of at least 8–10 weeks' duration, each at a therapeutic dose and serum level (if available) without even mild improvement (American Academy of Child and Adolescent Psychiatry 2004; Ghaziuddin et al. 1996; Kutcher and Robertson 1995; Walter and Rey 1997). For bipolar disorder, failure of at least one antipsychotic–mood stabilizer/antidepressant combination treatment trial of at least 6 weeks' duration without even mild improvement is considered evidence for

TABLE 52–1. Electroconvulsive therapy (ECT) studies in children and adolescents

Study	Design	N	Age range, years	Diagnoses	Outcome[a]
Cohen et al. 1997	Retrospective	21	14–19	Depression, bipolar disorder, schizophrenia	100% depression, 75% mania, only partial response in schizophrenia
Ghaziuddin et al. 1996	Retrospective	11	13–18	Depression, bipolar depression, organic mood disorder	64% response rate
Kutcher and Robertson 1995	Retrospective	16	16–22	Bipolar depression, mania	Significantly better than those who refused ECT
Moise and Petrides 1996	Retrospective	13	16–18	Depression, bipolar disorder, mixed diagnoses	76% response rate
Paillere-Martinot et al. 1990	Retrospective	8	15–19	Schizophrenia, psychotic depression, mania, traumatic brain injury	88% overall response rate
Rey and Walter 1997	Review of 60 studies	396	7–18 (5 prepubertal)	Mixed diagnoses	63% depression 80% mania 42% schizophrenia
Schneekloth et al. 1993	Retrospective	20	13–18	Schizophrenia, schizoaffective disorder, psychotic depression, bipolar disorder	65% overall response rate
Stein et al. 2006	Review (4 new studies identified)	132	13–19 (2 prepubertal)	Depression, bipolar disorder, catatonia, schizophrenia spectrum	60%–80% depression 60% bipolar
Strober et al. 1998	Retrospective	10	13–17	Depression, bipolar depression	60% response rate
Walter and Rey 1997	Retrospective	42	14–17	Mixed diagnoses	100% mania 85% psychotic depression 51% all diagnoses
Total	All retrospective open studies	669	662 adolescent 7 prepubertal	Schizophrenia spectrum disorders, depression, bipolar disorder	Overall: 50%–100%

[a]Percent responding to ECT.

treatment refractoriness (American Academy of Child and Adolescent Psychiatry 2004; Kutcher and Robertson 1995; Walter et al. 1999).

In certain cases, the eligibility criteria concerning treatment refractoriness may be waived (Stein et al. 2006). For severely ill patients with life-threatening neuropsychiatric symptoms, waiting for a response to a psychopharmacological treatment trial may endanger the life of the adolescent. In other cases, a severely incapacitated patient might not be able to take medication. In another example, some adolescents are unable to achieve a therapeutic dose because they are not able to tolerate an adequate psychopharmacology trial. In these cases, earlier consideration of ECT may be necessary (American Academy of Child and Adolescent Psychiatry 2004). Given the safety and effectiveness of modern ECT and the morbidity, lifetime mortality rates, and seriousness of the psychiatric disorders for which ECT is considered in adolescents, the number of treatments prior to considering ECT should be limited.

Contraindications

There is insufficient information at present to draw firm conclusions about absolute contraindications for ECT in adolescents, but suggestions may be extrapolated from the adult literature. In adults, there are no absolute contraindications to ECT. ECT has been successfully given to adults with comorbid psychiatric disorders, mental retardation, central nervous system space-occupying lesions, seizures, a history of myocardial infarction, and active chest infection. ECT has been successfully given to pregnant women, especially if they have a history of previous ECT response. While these conditions remain relative contraindications, ECT may be safely administered after a prospective assessment of risk versus benefit from the procedure (American Academy of Child and Adolescent Psychia-

try 2004). Prepubertal children should not receive ECT because of a lack of scientific data in this age group.

Mechanism of Action

Most current work on the mechanism of action of ECT focuses on neurotransmitter and peptidergic systems. ECT causes a brief hypermetabolic state and a reversible disruption of the blood-brain barrier. As a result, an acute and transient increase in the plasma of a variety of neurotransmitters and neuropeptides occurs, and many of these molecules are associated with antidepressant effects (Prudic 2005; Sackheim et al. 1995). Some of the neurobiological effects of ECT are outlined in Table 52–2.

Clinical Assessment

The psychiatrist and clinical treatment team responsible for the patient should complete a full psychiatric assessment of the patient prior to considering ECT. The patient's family should be involved as needed. It should be determined whether the patient has the type of psychiatric disorder(s) known to be responsive to ECT treatment, whether the patient has not responded to an adequate trial of less invasive psychiatric treat-

TABLE 52–2. Neurobiological effects of electroconvulsive therapy (ECT)

Neurobiological system	Effect of ECT	Comment
Norepinephrine neurotransmission	↑	↓ Density of β-adrenergic receptors in cortex and hippocampus ↑ Noradrenergic function
Serotonergic neurotransmission	↑	↑ Electrophysiological and behavioral serotonergic responses mediated by the 5-HT$_2$ receptor
Dopamine neurotransmission	↑	↑ D$_1$ receptor density and ↑ second messenger potentiation No effects on D$_2$ receptor density
Acetylcholine neurotransmission	↓	↓ Muscarinic acetylcholine receptor density in cortex and hippocampus May be relevant for the cognitive side effects of ECT
γ-Aminobutyric acid neurotransmission	↑	May be relevant for raising the seizure threshold after serial ECT
Endogenous opioids: met-enkephalin	↑	Effects not clear
Endogenous opioids: β-endorphin	↑	Effects not clear
Brain-derived neurotrophic growth factor	↑	Possible relation to hippocampal neuroplasticity
Nerve growth factor	↑	Possible relation to hippocampal neuroplasticity
Neurotrophin	↓	Possible relation to hippocampal neuroplasticity

ments, and whether severity criteria are met. Collateral information from parents, caregivers, and other reliable informants should be obtained to supplement the clinical interview. Use of reliable and valid rating scales can document symptom severity. A standardized assessment of daily functioning (e.g., Vineland Adaptive Behavior Scales) should be completed to document impairment and illness severity criteria in the domains of self-care and interpersonal, family, peer, social, and academic/occupational functioning.

Because ECT should be considered only when previous adequate and appropriately prescribed treatments have proven ineffective, a thorough and complete review of past treatments is important. Documentation of previous pharmacotherapy for *each* medication prescribed should include 1) maximum dose prescribed, 2) duration of treatment, 3) patient adherence, 4) response of mood symptoms, and 5) tolerability, side effects, and treatment-emergent adverse effects. Combined medication strategies and augmentation therapies should be reviewed. If previous medication trials include agents known to have clinically meaningful serum levels, the adequacy of these levels should be examined. Likewise, the adequacy of previous treatments should be reviewed and include individual, family, and/or group psychotherapies and previous hospitalizations.

Because ECT may affect memory, an age-appropriate cognitive assessment is required before treatment, after treatment, and at 3–6 months posttreatment (American Academy of Child and Adolescent Psychiatry 2004). Cognitive testing should emphasize short-term memory and new knowledge acquisition.

Consultation with a second child and adolescent psychiatrist who is knowledgeable about and experienced in the use of ECT and not involved in the current treatment of the patient is recommended by ECT guidelines (American Academy of Child and Adolescent Psychiatry 2004; Walter et al. 1999, 2003). The second opinion should specifically review the adequacy of previous treatments prior to the consideration of ECT. ECT should not proceed unless the treating psychiatrist and consulting psychiatrist are in agreement.

Medical Evaluation

The objective of the pretreatment medical evaluation is to assess any medical condition that may increase the risk of anesthesia or ECT itself. The mortality rate associated with ECT in adults is approximately the same as that for anesthesia alone, or about 1 death per 10,000 patients treated (Walter et al. 2003). No deaths have been reported from ECT-related procedures in adolescents. Risks for adolescents appear to be similar to risks for adults. In adults, cardiovascular complications, arrhythmias, myocardial infarction, congestive heart failure, and cardiac arrest are the most common causes of peri-ECT mortality (Walter et al. 2003). Every patient considered for ECT should receive 1) a complete physical examination, 2) laboratory investigations appropriate for the findings from the medical history and physical examination, and 3) laboratory evaluation of physiological parameters that may influence the administration or tolerability of anesthesia (American Academy of Child and Adolescent Psychiatry 2004). Laboratory investigations may include complete blood count with differential, platelet count, electrolyte levels, liver and thyroid function tests, urinalysis, toxicology screen, and electrocardiogram. Female adolescents should have a serum or urine pregnancy test. Other laboratory and/or radiological tests should be obtained on a case-by-case basis. A review of current prescribed and nonprescribed drug use is mandatory. Most nonessential drugs are discontinued prior to ECT. ECT-drug interactions have been described (Kellner et al. 1991; Pritchett et al. 1994) and are given in Table 52–3.

ECT Procedures and Administration

ECT is administered to adolescents only as inpatients. Treatment tolerability, recovery from anesthesia, adverse events, and effectiveness are best monitored in the hospital. The team administering ECT consists of a psychiatrist, an anesthesiologist, and nursing staff experienced in ECT procedures and recovery from anesthesia. Patients generally fast for approximately 12 hours before the procedure.

ECT is administered by the placement of electrodes on the scalp while the patient is under generalized anesthesia and under the effect of a muscle relaxant (modified ECT). Traditionally, electrodes were placed on both temples, a procedure called *bilateral ECT*. Presently, many clinicians apply electrodes to the temporal and parietal regions of the nondominant hemisphere. *Unilateral ECT* results in less cognitive side effects such as memory problems and post-ECT confusion. However, unilateral ECT requires higher doses of electricity to achieve therapeutic effects than does bilateral ECT. The usual practice in depression is to begin ECT with unilateral electrode placement, and if response is inadequate, to change to bilateral lead placement. For severe and life-threatening illness in which a rapid

TABLE 52–3. Some drug interactions with electroconvulsive therapy (ECT)

Drug	Effect
Anticonvulsants	↓ Seizure length ↓ ECT effectiveness
Benzodiazepines	↓ Seizure length ↓ ECT effectiveness
Caffeine	↑ Seizure length
Lidocaine	↓ Seizure induction
Lithium	↑ Seizure length ↑ Potentiation of anesthetic and muscle relaxant medications ↑ Risk for organic brain syndrome and acute confusional states
Nicotine (high dose only)	↑ Seizure length
Selective serotonin reuptake inhibitors	↑ Seizure length
Theophylline	↑ Seizure length ↑ Risk of status epilepticus
Trazodone	↑ Seizure length
Venlafaxine	↑ Risk of cardiac asystole when combined with atropine and ECT

clinical response may be lifesaving, bilateral ECT may be used at the start. Mania may respond better to bilateral than unilateral ECT (American Academy of Child and Adolescent Psychiatry 2004). ECT is generally administered two to three times a week, and 6–12 treatments are usually given in a single course of treatment. However, the total number of ECT treatments should be determined by the patient's clinical response.

Since the goal of ECT is to produce a seizure of adequate duration using the lowest dose of electricity, modern ECT technique mandates the use of EEG monitoring to measure seizure quality and duration. The goal is to achieve a brief bilateral grand mal seizure lasting 30–90 seconds. Seizures lasting 180 seconds or more in adolescents are considered prolonged and should be terminated by use of intravenous diazepam or additional methohexital. ECT should be delivered with modern brief-pulse machines that are capable of delivering low-dose electrical current. Commonly used electrical variables to achieve an appropriate grand mal seizure include a wave frequency of 30–70 cycles per second, a pulse width of 0.5–2.0 milliseconds, and a total electrical charge of 32–576 millicoulombs (Walter et al. 2003).

Immediately after ECT, recovery takes place in a designated area monitored by a nurse skilled in the care of the unconscious patient. Vital signs, adverse events, and airway patency are monitored. Headaches are common during the recovery period and can be treated with acetaminophen. The patient should be observed over the next 24–48 hours for late-onset seizures (tardive seizures). If tardive seizures occur, neu-rological consultation is recommended. The patient should be monitored for any manic or hypomanic side effects that may occur during the recovery period.

Continuation Treatment

Continuation treatment—defined as treatment of 6 months or more beyond remission of the acute episode to prevent relapse—is a standard of care in all depression treatment. Risk factors that predict illness relapse include medication resistance, high symptom severity, psychotic features, and recurrent illness. After the course of ECT is completed, adolescents should be treated with an antidepressant and/or mood stabilizer to prevent relapse of the index mood disorder (American Academy of Child and Adolescent Psychiatry 2004). At present, there is no reported experience with maintenance ECT therapy for adolescents.

Adverse Effects in Adolescents

Modern ECT is generally well tolerated by patients, and side effects are usually mild and transient. The side effects of ECT in adolescents are the same as those described for adults and are presented in Table 52–4.

In the immediate post-ECT recovery period, headaches, nausea, vomiting, muscle aches and pains, confusion, and agitation may occur. The confusion and disorientation associated with awakening from the procedure generally clear within 1 hour. Occasionally, some patients may experience a manic switch after ECT.

TABLE 52–4. Adverse events of electroconvulsive therapy in adolescents[a]

Adverse event	Percentage
Headache	61%
Confusion	20%
Subjective memory problems	19%
Nausea/vomiting	15%
Muscle aches/pains	4%
Prolonged seizures (>180 seconds)	0.4%
Tardive seizures	0%
Fatalities	0%

[a]As reported in 826 patients <19 years.
Source. Walter and Rey 2003.

Adverse events that are of more concern include risks from generalized anesthesia, tardive seizures, prolonged seizures, and ECT effects on cognition. The anesthesia-related mortality rate is 1.1 per 10,000 inductions. Adolescents are not believed to be at more risk from anesthesia-related complications than adults. No fatalities have yet been reported in adolescents undergoing ECT procedures. Late seizures occurring up to 24 hours after the ECT session is completed are termed *tardive seizures.* Tardive seizures are uncommon but a potentially serious side effect of ECT, and consultation with neurology is advised. *Prolonged seizures* are defined as ECT-related seizures lasting longer than 180 seconds (3 minutes). Prolonged seizures are serious because they may be associated with inadequate oxygenation and increased risk for cerebral and cardiovascular hypoxia-related events such as infarcts (American Academy of Child and Adolescent Psychiatry 2004; Sackheim et al. 1995).

The possibility of ECT-related cognitive side effects is potentially of most concern. A pattern of memory loss for the time of the ECT series and extending back an average of 6 months accompanied by difficulties in learning new information has been described in adults (Blaine and Clark 1986). Few studies of cognitive side effects of ECT in the young have been completed. For all adolescents considered for ECT, it is mandatory that tests of cognition be completed prior to ECT, in the period immediately following a treatment course of ECT, and 3–6 months after treatment with ECT has stopped.

Legal Considerations

Psychiatrists who refer patients for ECT should be knowledgeable about their own institutional requirements and state laws pertaining to the delivery of ECT in minors. Some states have legislated age-related restrictions on the use of ECT. For example, in Texas and Colorado, ECT is not permitted in persons <16 years old. In Tennessee, ECT is not permitted in persons <14 years old. In California, ECT is not permitted in persons <12 years old. Most states require independent assessment of juveniles by one or more child and adolescent psychiatrists before ECT may be administered. An independent psychiatrist who is not involved in the treatment of the patient and is knowledgeable about the use of ECT in minors must conduct this assessment.

Informed Consent and Assent

Legal and ethical issues of informed consent to ECT from parent and patient are very important. Informed consent should be written. The rationale for ECT, alternative treatments to ECT, and the likely prognosis of the disease without treatment should be explained to the parents or guardians and the adolescent patient in easy-to-understand language, avoiding the use of technical jargon. The use of audiovisual aids may be helpful. Every effort should be made to obtain the informed consent of the adolescent. This may be difficult due to developmental immaturity and/or the presence of severe psychiatric symptoms. Informed consent is a process rather than a task to be completed at one moment in time. An adolescent initially unwilling or unable to consent to ECT may change his or her mind later as treatment proceeds or if side effects from medications become intolerable. When obtaining consent from the patient for ECT, it is helpful for the clinical treatment team to consider five ethical issues relevant to the treatment of minors: 1) the rights of the adolescent, including the right to refuse treatment; 2) the adolescent's relationship to the adults responsible for his or her well-being; 3) the teenager's developmental and cognitive capacity to understand the treatment; 4) the process of informed consent as it unfolds within the treatment alliance; and 5) the potential and risks for coercion of the minor either by adults in the teenager's environment or by the treatment process itself (Krener and Mancina 1994; Walter et al. 2003). Some states mandate a minimal waiting time between signing the consent document for ECT and commencing treatment. This waiting period is usually 72 hours, and during this period consent may be withdrawn. Additionally, parents and adolescents should clearly understand that consent for ECT may be withdrawn at any time.

Transcranial Magnetic Stimulation

Transcranial magnetic stimulation (TMS) is a noninvasive means of electrically stimulating the cerebral cortex. Introduced as a neurophysiological investigatory tool in the 1980s, TMS involves the induction of a brief, strong magnetic field caused by electrical current circulating within coils of the TMS device. When the TMS device is placed near the skull, a magnetic field penetrates the first few millimeters of cerebral cortex and activates neurons without causing a seizure or pain to the subject. The field volume is small, and the magnetic field strength decays exponentially with distance so that neuronal activation with TMS occurs in relatively specific cortical brain regions.

There are three types of TMS. *Single-pulse TMS* is best suited to diagnostic and research applications. *Paired-pulse TMS* is used to evaluate cortical excitability. *Repetitive TMS* (rTMS) has been used in therapeutic applications because it is capable of producing rapid bursts of pulses lasting approximately 60 seconds using an oscillatory magnetic field output (Curra et al. 2002; Quintana 2005). An advantage of the rTMS procedure in the clinical setting is that no anesthesia is needed. TMS has been used to investigate brain functioning and pathology in cortical motor areas and in corticospinal tract nerve conduction and as a diagnostic test.

Research in adults that suggested that TMS might be helpful in depression generated great enthusiasm for TMS as a possible treatment alternative to antidepressant drugs and ECT. Preliminary small studies of TMS generally reported positive results. Meta-analytic studies find that rTMS has a moderate effect size in adult depression (Herrmann and Ebmeier 2006). More investigation of the type of depressed patient who may benefit from rTMS is needed, and until more knowledge about this treatment accrues, rTMS should be considered an investigational procedure (Hirshberg et al. 2005).

To date, only two small case series (totaling nine subjects) have reported on the use of rTMS in adolescent depression (Loo et al. 2006; Walter et al. 2001). In the first case series, seven patients (ages 16–18 years) were treated with rTMS. Three patients had unipolar depression, three had schizophrenia, and one had bipolar disorder. Five of the seven patients improved. Tension headaches reported in one patient were the only adverse effects noted from the rTMS procedure (Walter et al. 2001). Another report included two new adolescent patients with depression. Both improved after a course of rTMS and reported no adverse effects of the procedure. Neuropsychological testing revealed no cognitive side effects after the course of rTMS was completed (Loo et al. 2006).

Deep Brain Stimulation

Deep brain stimulation (DBS) is a neurosurgical procedure in which stimulation electrodes are chronically implanted into specific areas of the brain, and an implanted, externally programmable pacemaker delivers high-frequency electrical pulses into explicit brain regions. The site of electrode placement differs depending on the disorder to be treated. DBS is most often used for intractable, treatment-resistant neurological disorders including dystonia, tremor, and movement disorders associated with Parkinson's disease. Its uses are being explored for depression, obsessive-compulsive disorder (OCD), and Tourette's disorder. DBS has been most extensively used in adult neurology for patients with movement disorders that are intractable to other less invasive treatments and that are very disabling (Wichmann and Delong 2006). DBS is currently approved for generalized dystonia in children 7 years and older. Its place in psychiatry is presently unclear. DBS should be considered an experimental procedure in children and adolescents with psychiatric disorders.

Research Directions

Although expert consensus and retrospective open study results suggest that adolescents respond to ECT in a fashion similar to adults, developmental considerations affecting ECT response rates have not yet been rigorously tested in well-designed studies. Future research should directly compare the response rates of adolescents receiving ECT with adults receiving ECT for the same diagnosis. The cognitive effects of ECT in adolescents require further investigation. The effectiveness and tolerability of rTMS for adolescent depression are in need of study.

Summary Points

- Open case studies over the past 60 years suggest that ECT is an effective short-term treatment for adolescents with affective disorders and possibly for some adolescents with schizophrenia. Response rates range between 50% and 100%, with higher response rates generally reported for mood disorders as compared with psychotic disorders. ECT may also be used to treat catatonia and neuroleptic malignant syndrome.

- With modern brief anesthetic techniques, there are no absolute contraindications to ECT. Recommendations for ECT should be based on an analysis of the patient's individual risks and possible benefits from the procedure.

- Psychiatric symptoms must be severe, disabling, and refractory to adequate previous medication trials to warrant consideration of ECT. An attempt to document patient compliance with previously prescribed medications is important before ECT is considered.

- Because ECT may affect memory function, all adolescents must undergo an age-appropriate cognitive assessment before treatment, after treatment, and at 3–6 months posttreatment. Cognitive testing should emphasize short-term memory functioning and new knowledge acquisition.

- Psychiatrists considering ECT for their adolescent patients should be familiar with the laws governing ECT use in the state where they practice and the need for a second independent psychiatric opinion before administering a course of ECT.

- TMS is a noninvasive means of electrically stimulating the cerebral cortex requiring no anesthesia, and it is currently under investigation as a possible therapeutic tool in depression.

- DBS is most often used for severe, intractable, and treatment-resistant neurological disorders, including dystonia, tremor, and movement disorders associated with Parkinson's disease.

References

American Academy of Child and Adolescent Psychiatry: Practice parameter for use of electroconvulsive therapy with adolescents. J Am Acad Child Adolesc Psychiatry 43:1521–1539, 2004

Blaine JD, Clark SM: Report of the NIMH-NIH Consensus Development Conference on electroconvulsive therapy: statement of the Consensus Development Panel. Psychopharmacol Bull 22:445–454, 1986

Cohen D, Paillere-Martinot ML, Basquin M: Use of electroconvulsive therapy in adolescents. Convuls Ther 13:25–31, 1997

Curra A, Modugno N, Inghilleri M, et al: Transcranial magnetic stimulation techniques in clinical investigation. Neurology 59:1851–1859, 2002

Ghaziuddin N, King CA, Naylor MW, et al: Electroconvulsive treatment in adolescents with pharmacotherapy-refractory depression. J Child Adolesc Psychopharmacol 6:259–271, 1996

Herrmann LL, Ebmeier KP: Factors modifying the efficacy of transcranial magnetic stimulation in the treatment of depression: a review. J Clin Psychiatry 67:1870–1876, 2006

Hirshberg LM, Chiu S, Frazier JA: Emerging brain-based interventions for children and adolescents: an overview and clinical perspective. Child Adolesc Psychiatr Clin N Am 14:1–19, 2005

Kellner C H, Nixon DW, Bernstein HJ: ECT—drug interactions: a review. Psychopharmacol Bull 27:595–609, 1991

Krener KP, Mancina RA: Informed consent or informed coercion? Decision-making in pediatric psychopharmacology. J Child Adolesc Psychopharmacol 4:183–200, 1994

Kutcher S, Robertson HA: Electroconvulsive therapy in treatment resistant bipolar youth. J Child Adolesc Psychopharmacol 5:167–175, 1995

Loo CT, McFarquhar T, Walter G: Transcranial magnetic stimulation in adolescent depression. Australas Psychiatry 14:81–85, 2006

Moise FN, Petrides G: Case study: electroconvulsive therapy in adolescents. J Am Acad Child Adolesc Psychiatry 35:312–318, 1996

Paillere-Martinot M-L, Zivi A, Basquin M: Utilisation de l'ECT chez l'adolescent. Encephale 16:399–404, 1990

Pritchett JT, Bernstein HJ, Kellner CH: Combined ECT and antidepressant drug therapy. Convuls Ther 9:256–261, 1994

Prudic J: Electroconvulsive therapy, in Kaplan and Sadock's Comprehensive Textbook of Psychiatry. Edited by Sadock BJ, Sadock VA. Philadelphia, PA, Lippincott Williams & Wilkins, 2005, pp 2968–2983

Quintana H: Transcranial magnetic stimulation in persons younger than the age of 18. J ECT 21:88–95, 2005

Rey JM, Walter G: Half a century of ECT use in young people. Am J Psychiatry 154:595–602, 1997

Sackheim HA, Devanand DP, Nobler MS: Electroconvulsive therapy, in Psychopharmacology: The Fourth Generation of Progress. Edited by Bloom FS, Kupfer DJ. New York, Raven, 1995, pp 1123–1141

Schneekloth TD, Rummans TA, Logan KM: Electroconvulsive therapy in adolescents. Convuls Ther 9:158–166, 1993

Stein DA, Weizman A, Bloch Y: Electroconvulsive therapy and transcranial magnetic stimulation: can they be considered valid modalities in the treatment of pediatric mood disorders? Child Adolesc Psychiatr Clin N Am 15:1035–1056, 2006

Strober M, Rao U, DeAntonio M, et al: Effects of electroconvulsive therapy in adolescents with severe endogenous depression resistant to pharmacotherapy. Biol Psychiatry 43:335–338, 1998

Thompson JW, Blaine JD: Use of ECT in the United States in 1975 and 1980. Am J Psychiatry 144:557–562, 1987

Walter G, Rey JM: An epidemiological study of the use of ECT in adolescents. J Am Acad Child Adolesc Psychiatry 36:809–815, 1997

Walter G, Rey JM: Has the practice and outcome of ECT in adolescents changed? Findings from a whole-population study. J ECT 19:84–87, 2003

Walter G, Rey JM, Mitchell PB: Practitioner review: electroconvulsive therapy in adolescents. J Child Psychol Psychiatry 40:325–334, 1999

Walter G, Tormos JM, Israel JA, et al: Transcranial magnetic stimulation in young persons: a review of known cases. J Child Adolesc Psychopharmacol 11:69–75, 2001

Walter G, Rey JM, Ghaziuddin N: Electroconvulsive therapy and transcranial magnetic stimulation, in Pediatric Psychopharmacology Principles and Practice. Edited by Martin A, Scahill L, Charney DS, et al. New York, Oxford University Press, 2003, pp 377–386

Weiner RD (ed): The Practice of Electroconvulsive Therapy: Recommendations for Treatment, Training, and Privileges, 2nd Edition. Washington, DC, American Psychiatric Publishing, 2001

Wichmann T, Delong MR: Deep brain stimulation for neurologic and neuropsychiatric disorders. Neuron 52:197–204, 2006

PART XI

PSYCHOSOCIAL TREATMENTS

Chapter 53

Individual Psychotherapy

Lenore Terr, M.D.

Individual psychotherapy is important for every child and adolescent psychiatrist to know and understand. Its associated techniques are also crucial to supervision, conferences, meetings with educators, community gatherings, and policy-setting agendas. One hundred years' worth of clinical case reports in the professional literature attest to the usefulness of child psychotherapy.

Several factors have delayed the conduct of the kind of research that might enable nonmanualized individual psychotherapy to reach the current criteria for being "evidence based." It is difficult to follow control subjects as long as some individual cases actually take in psychotherapy. It is even more difficult to locate the proper comparison groups and to offer the young people in them a good alternative to psychotherapy. "Blinding" is challenging, and "double blinding" is virtually impossible. Furthermore, interventional research on children is often difficult to have funded or institutionally approved. The proper parental and child consents (and/or assents) may be prob-

lematic to obtain (Group for the Advancement of Psychiatry 1989). All of this leads to just a few clinical case series and a handful of controlled research projects in a field that has existed for years.

Despite the difficulties in setting up a large contemporary research bibliography for psychotherapy, however, any well-trained mental health professional dealing with children should understand how to use psychotherapy and how to collaborate with a psychotherapist. This chapter will attempt to present and summarize psychotherapy, both as an idea and as a set of techniques.

Throughout the chapter, boldface words are defined by the author in Table 53–1, "Glossary of Terms."

Today's child and adolescent psychotherapy is eclectic, combining a number of Freudian principles (**psychodynamic psychotherapy**) with other ideas coming from the medical, educational, and non-Freudian psychological fields. Current individual psychotherapy consists of a half hour to 45 minutes spent between clinician and young patient, conversing and

TABLE 53–1. Glossary of terms

Term or phrase (in order of presentation)	Definition
Psychodynamic psychotherapy	Psychological treatment of a child, based on such Freudian principles as internal conflict, the unconscious, repetition compulsion, and transference
Uncovering psychotherapy	A type of treatment primarily utilizing exploration of defenses, conscience, secret wishes, and transference, in order to resolve internal unconscious conflict
Supportive psychotherapy	A type of treatment using the real relationship with the therapist, education, suggestions, and reinforcements to help a patient cope with the external world
Displacement	Defense mechanism in which the object of a conflict is moved over to someone else, an animal, even a thing or idea
Oedipal	The conscious or unconscious wish to marry the parent of the opposite sex and rid the self of the same-sexed parent
Id	The psychological space (and energies) occupied by primitive, raw sexual and aggressive drives, most of which are unconscious
Ego	The psychological space (and energies) occupied by ways of coping, ways of defending against the drives, thinking things through, dealing with loved ones and the world—both conscious and unconscious
Interpretation	The therapist's bringing together of ideas about the patient's defenses, wishes, conscience, and/or dealings with the world that makes unconscious mechanisms visible, and therefore, workable
Superego	The particular ways "conscience," ethics, ideals, morals, role models, operate in mentality—both conscious and unconscious
Clarification	The therapist's putting new words to something the patient already knows in a different way
Transference	The patient's particular defensive displacement toward the therapist, based on old attitudes and feelings about important others in the patient's life
Education	Teaching something to the patient
Suggestion	Guiding the patient to a conclusion the patient eventually makes, which can be unconscious on the patient's part—or entirely conscious
Modeling	Showing the patient—in the therapist's actions—how to act or be
Reinforcement	Responding to the patient's actions or story positively or negatively and thereby demonstrating how the therapist wants the patient to behave
Real therapist	Either being actual or telling the patient who the actual person treating him or her is
Diagnosis	The synthesis of history, observation, and tests, leading to the indication of a certain medical condition that is treated in a prescribed way
Formulation	The working psychological explanation for a patient's feelings, behavior, and thinking
Abreaction	The expression of emotion relating to a problem, particularly psychic trauma
Context	The perspective and understanding, particularly of a psychic trauma, in terms of history, geography, science, peer group, criminology, etc.
Correction	The imaginary or real solution to a traumatic event, even if it is an old one and/or virtually unsolvable
Denial in fantasy	Defense mechanism in which a painful reality is overlooked or forgotten by constructing a situation in one's imagination that negates or obscures the reality
Filial therapy	Treating a child through the parent (who takes the doctor's ideas home and tries them out on the young person)
Collaborative therapy	Treating a child while having another or others treat the parent(s) or sibling(s)

TABLE 53–1. Glossary of terms *(continued)*

Term or phrase (in order of presentation)	Definition
Countertransference	The doctor's unreasonable, personally based responses to a patient
Repetition compulsion	The need to refeel, retell, redream, or reenact (in conflicted or traumatized people)
Reenactment	Repetitive behavior (often related to past trauma) that replays a thought, a fear, or an original behavior from the event(s)
Ego ideal	Who and what a person wishes to become; or a person's better self

using play, art, word games, metaphor, and other forms of interaction. Sometimes a parent is present for the entire session. Frequently, a parent is seen for the first 5–15 minutes (or, less frequently, for the last few minutes). Most of the time, however, a parent is not in the room as the youngster is working with the practitioner.

Not only is contemporary psychotherapy used both for **uncovering** and for **supportive** purposes, but it is also used in more severe cases of pathology (character problems and psychic trauma, for instance) than it was first conceived to treat. For example, when Sigmund Freud, in 1909, indirectly treated his first modern-day child psychotherapy patient through the 5-year-old boy's father (who carefully implemented Freud's suggestions), the child, "Little Hans," was cured of his newly developed and mild problem, phobia of horses. Within a few sessions of working with the boy's major defense pattern (**displacement**) and his hidden fears and wishes (his fright of his father and his desire for an **Oedipal** victory), the phobia cleared. It took just a few good talks between the doctor and the parent, and then between the parent and the little boy. The problem was acute and it was mild. The psychotherapeutic answer was "Freudian," including an analysis of **id** (the boy's secret sexual and aggressive wishes) and **ego** (his "displacement" defense). The solution was ultimately simple (S. Freud 1909/1955). Today, however, when psychotherapy is being utilized with a child or adolescent, it may occur in much harsher settings than Freud's—and in much more confrontational situations (Terr 2008). Still, the technique works dramatically—as it did with Little Hans. And it may take no more time.

Anna Freud, Sigmund Freud's daughter, observed and commented on children's play, especially at her Hampstead, England, housing facility and school for children evacuated from the London blitz of World War II (A. Freud and Burlingham 1943). Before the war, Miss Freud expanded upon her father's ideas about the defenses, especially those developing in childhood

(A. Freud 1928). She thus helped child psychotherapy switch its emphasis from id to ego (A. Freud 1936/1946). She consistently preferred watching and listening to a child and carefully making remarks about the child's conflicts afterward. These spoken verbal interventions by the therapist are called **interpretations.**

In the next several years following the war, child psychotherapy adopted the concepts of ego, **superego,** and id. It followed adult psychiatry in separating the idea of uncovering (Freudian-minded psychotherapy) from support (ego building, conscience building, community-related helps, and education). But child psychiatry eventually came to incorporate both forms—uncovering and support—into its general approach to psychotherapy. To uncover with an adult, the therapist needed interpretation and **clarification.** The therapist also needed to maintain a neutral and relatively passive stance. This rather distant approach was intended to encourage **transference,** the displacement of old attitudes, especially about the patient's family or origin, to the therapist. To support a child, on the other hand, the therapist was taught to employ more **education, suggestion, modeling,** and positive or negative **reinforcement** (largely in the therapist's attitude toward the patient). The psychotherapist was also encouraged to be **real** with the patient in order to avoid potentially dangerous transference in seriously disordered children and to help very disturbed young people to learn how to act in society.

There is still discussion in our field as to what persona to adopt with what child. Over the years, we child psychotherapists have recognized that transference is not as pressing a phenomenon in the treatment of young children as it is in adults. This happens because children are still primarily involved in their families of origin and therefore do not consistently displace these feelings to their treating physician or counselor. We do not have to be as passive or neutral as Freud might have suggested. The corollary to this observation is the important idea that while knowing and understanding himself or herself well, the psychiatrist might remain "real" and inspire a good therapeutic relationship with the child (Harrison et al. 1970; Terr et al. 2005; Weiner and King 1977). No one rule, however, applies to all youngsters. In fact, not all child psychology is universal—various cultures offer different ways of raising children, and thus, of building young personalities. To keep these important cultural differences in mind, the treating psychotherapist must understand the child's racial, ethnic, and religious background and adjust his or her treatment of the young person to that understanding (Erikson 1950). Any child and adolescent psychotherapist, in fact, needs to be cautioned about the use of pure Freudian-derived psychotherapy. The clinician must be careful to include education, clarification, and other "supports" in any psychotherapy with children (Hartmann 1956). In other words, a contemporary child psychotherapist doesn't do either uncovering or supportive treatment with young people—he or she combines the two. The clinician doesn't automatically assume a single type of therapeutic persona with all children. The clinician is flexible.

D.W. Winnicott (1971b) taught us that the spirit of play must infuse psychotherapy. Not only must the therapist be playful, but the patient, if necessary, has to be shown how to play. Play reveals the inner world of the child, and it also releases considerable emotional energy (Levy 1939). Play also enables the therapist to interact entirely inside the pretend or the game (Kline 1932) and to insert new corrective ideas into the more hidden, playful life of the child.

Today's child psychotherapy takes in a broader age range of childhood than may have traditionally been considered. There are contemporary psychotherapeutic techniques geared to adolescents (Mishne 1986), as well as techniques specific to infants and toddlers (Fraiberg 1977). More kinds of disorders have fallen under the aegis of child psychotherapy, such as the (acute and chronic) posttraumatic conditions (see Terr 1991, 2003), problems of childhood personality (Kernberg et al. 2000; Thomas et al. 1968), physical and psychosomatic illness (Lewis and King 1994), congenital and hereditary differences and/or anomalies (Green and Solnit 1964), and disorders of attention and/or neurological integration (Silver 2003). Cognitive-behavioral techniques turn up frequently in the individual psychodynamic psychotherapies (Terr 2008). It would not be uncommon, for example, for a therapist exploring the inner reasons for an obsession to also work out a program to extinguish the accompanying compulsions in a child.

For an excellent reference on child psychotherapy through most of the twentieth century, see *The Process of Child Therapy* (Group for the Advancement of Psychiatry 1982). For a chart illustrating the major historical changes in the practice of child psychotherapy over the past 100 years, see Table 53–2. In summary, contemporary child and adolescent psychotherapy is increasingly eclectic, flexible, and able to treat (in many cases, with medications as well) all ages and conditions of childhood.

Which Child Needs Individual Psychotherapy?

In conducting a diagnostic evaluation of a child—and in initially interviewing parents and sometimes siblings—two important opinions are reached by the psychiatrist. One is the **diagnosis.** The second is the **formulation.** Each opinion is equally meaningful in deciding what to do with a mentally disordered or a developmentally disturbed young person (Jellinek and McDermott 2004; Shapiro 1989; Terr et al. 2006a). Because the formulation consists of a working psychological explanation of the patient's feelings, behaviors, and thinking, it expresses the "art" of the medical and mental health evaluation, as opposed to the "science," or the diagnosis. Both are essential to setting up a treatment program for a child. (See Chapter 6, "The Process of Assessment and Diagnosis," for a thorough discussion of diagnosis and formulation.)

For any proposed treatment, the child will need an understandable explanation, careful education about the condition, a coordinated treatment program to be carried out by the family, and meaningful follow-up over a long enough time to see if the program works. In other words, at least minimal individual supportive psychotherapy is necessary whenever the clinician treats a child. The child must know who the therapist is and how he or she will be working with the therapist.

Some cases clearly signal the need for individual nonmanualized psychotherapy. The use of maladaptive defenses defines a likely case for individual psychotherapy. Also, if a stress or series of stressors, or even worse, a traumatic event is affecting a child, this often requires psychotherapy. Trauma psychotherapy usually involves **abreaction:** helping the child define and express all the emotions inherent in what is taking or has taken place. It also involves understanding the event(s) in **context** and finding **corrections**—even fan-

TABLE 53–2. One hundred years of child psychotherapy

Early twentieth-century child psychotherapy	Early twenty-first-century child psychotherapy
Prekindergarten through late latency ages	All ages from birth into young adulthood
Children of the same culture as therapist	Children of all cultures
Talk emphasized	Talk plus all modes of play and art
Uncovering	Uncovering and supportive
Geared toward neurosis and problems of development	Potentially useful in any disorder or problem of development, as well as in prevention
Dealing with imagination	Dealing with imagination and reality
Therapist is entirely objective and distant	Therapist assumes various ways of being geared to the child and/or is real
Parents primary and must be engaged in therapy themselves	Parents important but are given advice, counseling, modeling—not necessarily therapy
Rules for administering therapy strict, largely Freudian	Rules for administering therapy loose and eclectic
Interpretation of internal id/ego conflicts and of transference	Interpretation of child's relationship to the real world, as well as id, ego, and/or transference
Insight is a goal	Insight is not necessarily a goal
Ethics—"first do no harm"	Ethics—"first do no harm"

tasized or historical ones—for such situations (Terr 2003; Terr, in press). For a summary of the types of cases for which psychotherapy is often warranted, see Table 53–3.

Here is an example of where psychotherapy is the preferred method of treatment: A child, who behaves well and is accomplished at school, appears angry much of the time at home. For several years, his mother and sisters have been the continuous objects of his rage. Neither "oppositional defiant disorder" nor "conduct disorder" encompass his strengths as well as his symptoms. Now the preadolescent boy is serving as president of his all-boys' sixth grade class. In school, he is easy to get along with and popular. His father is "too busy" to participate in the psychiatric evaluation. When asked about his activities with his dad, the boy lies: "He jogged with me lots of times last summer," he says. "In the winter, we played hockey." The boy's mother reports that there were no such games, play, or practice. In fact, the boy's father prefers the company of men his own age and hardly participates in family life. A divorce is being contemplated. At whom is the boy really angry—his mother who loves and protects him or his dad who usually doesn't give him "the time of day"? The boy is defending himself with **denial in fantasy** and displacement. He is developing attitudes about women that will not serve him well in the future. His phenomenological diagnosis does not suggest a type of treatment. His formulation, however,

leads directly to the consideration of individual psychotherapy. What moves the choice away from treatment with mood stabilizing drugs and a course of family therapy or anger management training? It is the psychological meaning to the preadolescent's behaviors. This meaning will direct the subsequent individual psychotherapy.

Another situation often calling for psychotherapy (again, considering the formulation but bearing in mind, too, the diagnosis) is slowdown, misdirection, or even an omission in social or emotional development. Babies who cannot feed properly, toddlers who cannot be toilet trained, smart youngsters who do not talk—all of this calls for close collaboration between parents, child, and doctor. In many such situations, the child will require some psychotherapy sessions by himself— or with a parent there to observe and/or participate (Fraiberg 1977; Gaensbauer in Terr et al. 2006c).

If a child's problems are related to a conflict around a developmental issue, such as attachment, autonomy, gender, self-esteem, getting older, sexuality, or identity, this kind of conflict usually requires treatment with psychotherapy. In addition, if a young person appears to be experimenting with a new line of behavior and in this way has come to a "fork in the road" (Schulman et al. 1977), he or she may require a brief course of individual therapy. Furthermore, if a child shows personality quirks that have hurt peer or family relationships or diminish the youngster's ability to concen-

TABLE 53–3. Cases for which individual psychotherapy may be warranted

Situations in the child	Situations affecting the family
Use of maladaptive defenses	Response to the child
Stressors	Stressors
Traumatic event	Response to child Traumatic event to the family Familial perpetration of trauma and/or neglect

Emotional or social development
   Slowdown
   Misdirection
   Omission
   Conflicts around a developmental issue
	Response to the child
	Parental naiveté or mistakes in rearing

Child psychiatric disorders
   Mood
   Attention
   Anxiety
	Response to the child
	Medication management
	Health management

Pediatric disorders
   Congenital defects and disorders
   Pre- or postsurgery
   The dying child
   Chronic illness (e.g., diabetes,
     neurological disorder, asthma)
	Parental guilt and/or grief
	Response to the child
	Health management

The child wants a therapist and/or therapy	Parents think therapy will help Parents will not allow medications for their child
Early personality problems	Response to the child Parent has personality disorder Parent has "superego lacunae" (Johnson 1949) Parental naiveté or mistakes Family perpetration of trauma and/or neglect

trate and work or to experience joy, that child may need psychotherapy. In other words, even when a child does not meet the criteria for a full disease or disorder, the clinician may consider psychotherapy as an option. Similar to the pediatrician's efforts, a good deal of the child mental health professional's work centers upon prevention.

Many common childhood psychiatric disorders—e.g., mood, attention, and anxiety disorders—often require first-line treatments with medication and/or cognitive-behavioral therapy. A number of children with these conditions, however, also need considerable attention, education, help with "Why me?" questions, observation for suicidality, and a deeper set of understandings of the interior conflicts and family difficulties that are associated with these conditions. Individual psychotherapy is often prescribed as an important addition to drugs and/or brief manualized treatments in these kinds of cases. Along the same line,

children with conditions along the autism spectrum need a great deal of educational and parental support. If the child is able to form a meaningful relationship with a psychotherapeutic clinician, long-term individualized treatment may greatly improve his or her prognosis.

The psychiatrist gathers clues from the child during the evaluation process that may lead to a decision in favor of psychotherapy. The child "gets" something the evaluator says, for instance, and responds with appropriate words and/or emotion. Or the child drops a huge "clue" for the psychiatrist that no one else has picked up before. Or the psychiatrist tries a simple interpretation and the child "sees" what is meant and offers feedback or an evident emotional response. Or the youngster actually asks the doctor to treat her. Or the physician notices that a bond with the child is forming. In these situations, the relationship serves as a cue for the psychiatrist to strongly consider individual therapy.

Parents, guardians, or institutions are often reluctant to medicate youngsters. Many adults fear unknown long-term effects and possible complications from giving drugs to children. In such situations, individual psychotherapy may be the child's only option. If it is appropriate for the child (in terms of both the diagnosis and formulation), psychotherapy may be tried (and may indeed be successful).

How Does a Child's Treatment Begin?

Once the decision to treat a child with psychotherapy is made, a time schedule is selected. Often this corresponds to the parents' or caregivers' ability to transport the child to the office, the youngster's schedule at home and school, and life circumstances. The clinician must consider these realities carefully, alongside what might be therapeutically optimal. Typically, once-weekly psychotherapy is about right for a school-age child. On the other hand, if the child or adolescent is entering treatment during a crisis period (serious illness of a parent, early in the wake of a trauma, suicidal thoughts), the clinician might consider two (or sometimes three) times a week to start and then cut back to once weekly within a month or two. Also, when emergencies arise during the course of psychotherapy, stepping up the frequency of sessions is often helpful.

Child patients should be given a developmentally tailored explanation so that they know what to expect. For example: "I'm a worry doctor." "I talk to children and play with them." "I help kids get along better at school." "I want to help you figure out how to make friends." "I've heard you're sad a lot, and I'd like to help you feel less depressed." For most children, it is important to let them know that this kind of doctor will not be undressing them, examining them, or giving them shots. The psychotherapist gears what is said at the beginning of therapy to what the child has expressed during the evaluation, as well as the child's stage of development. "I'm a talking doctor" is about all the clinician might say to a toddler. But with an adolescent, the clinician would have to offer a fuller explanation. When a psychiatrist will be prescribing medicine as well as psychotherapy, this must be discussed.

If the psychotherapist is also working with the child's parents, a sentence or two about confidentiality should be shared with the young patient. How much will the therapist say? Will the therapist listen to parents? Teachers? Who else? Why? If the therapist may

also have to go to court on a child patient's behalf, the doctor must fully explain that his or her notes will go to "a judge who decides things" or that the doctor may have to go to court and testify as well.

In beginning therapy with a child, the psychiatrist must make sure that the youngster has enough opportunity to ask questions and make statements about the treatment. Most young people do not have much to say at these early stages, however, and it's often a good idea to launch into play and/or talk about the child's life soon after the beginning of the first hour. A child patient must find out quickly in the early course of treatment that psychotherapy is often fun and funny, even though there will be painful moments as well.

Where Do Parents Fit Into Child and Adolescent Psychotherapy?

Parents need to understand—in an ongoing fashion—what the individual psychotherapy with their child is attempting to accomplish and where that accomplishment presently stands. They must know, therefore, the general outlines of the treatment as it is being carried out. The child patient should give a form of oral assent for the parents being told by the therapist why the child is being treated and what is currently happening in therapy. With an adolescent, it is often wise to tell the young patient what will be said to parents. Adolescents also benefit from an idea as to what their parents think about their general progress. This doctor-patient understanding about conveying general information back and forth should be established at the onset of psychotherapy and repeated as treatment proceeds. Child patients need to believe that the therapist will not give away the details of their secret lives and thoughts. Otherwise, it will be difficult to either establish or keep a trusting relationship.

It is best for both mothers and fathers to be engaged in facilitating their youngsters' psychotherapy. Even if one parent is busier than the other—or has moved out of the area—or has established a new, separate family—it is still important to enlist that parent's support, and from time to time, see that parent in the office. What does the more-or-less absent parent think of the child's progress? What has that parent observed over summers, on vacations, or when the child is with the new family? On the other hand, if there has been a total break between an absent parent and a child, there is no set rule about trying to reestablish the child-parent relationship. Often, trauma and/or neglect demand a continuation of such separations. Each case is considered individually. Any legal decisions to permanently terminate parental rights must be honored by the clinician until, at least, a time when the child has achieved legal adulthood and can decide how to proceed.

There are several ways to engage parents in the child's psychotherapy. In addition to occasionally giving a "temperature reading" on their youngster's progress, the clinician can ask parents about aspects of their child's life that the youngster currently does not understand, perceive, or choose to tell. The clinician can actually have parents in the same room reflecting on the realities of what their child is saying. This may be helpful for children with severe personality or social problems. Ordinarily, however, this approach will not work for more than a few sessions. If, on the other hand, the clinician routinely schedules the first several minutes of each of the child's sessions for one or more parents alone, then the child does not perceive this information sharing as tattling, refuting, or blaming.

Sometimes parents have a poor understanding or an almost total naiveté regarding how to be a parent. How does one play with a child? How does one talk? What does one say? In such instances, the clinician may include the parents in all of the child's sessions, from beginning to end, as a form of family therapy. Or the clinician may proceed as if the child were alone in individual therapy while the parent(s) watch, both for modeling from the psychiatrist and for new ideas about the child's thinking and experience directly from the young patient's mouth. These kinds of sessions often need active psychiatric "translation" of the child's behaviors for the parents, as well as a steady flow of comments and/or play between the psychiatrist and the child.

The "Little Hans" means of child treatment—by working only with a parent and then having the parent make the suggested therapeutic interventions and commentaries—has been elaborated by Erna Furman into what is known as **filial therapy.** This treatment can be especially useful in preschoolers or with crisis management situations, such as coping with a seriously ill adolescent or a health emergency in a latency-age child (Furman 1957).

Finally, **collaborative therapy** on behalf of children—based on the American "child guidance system" model, in which the child is assigned to one professional while the parents are assigned to another (Group for the Advancement of Psychiatry 1982)—has become less and less common with changes in the economics and practicalities of delivering services. Collaborative therapy can work, but it is expensive, and it also carries the potential to stir up conflict or competition among professionals, especially if there is a discrepancy in their status or their treatment philosophy (Group for the Advancement of Psychiatry 1982). The trick to this collaborative system is for all involved to communicate frequently. If the collaborators steadily keep the child in mind, complicated collaborative treatments may proceed smoothly. There must be a spoken or tacit understanding, however, about who will be leader.

Even the best individual psychotherapy with a child may fail if the parents or other treating professionals are not on board. Because the rest of this chapter will deal with what happens inside the clinician's office with the child patient alone, the author refers the reader to other chapters in this book that cover families and working with the various kinds of professional services that deal with children (Chapter 54, "Parent Counseling, Psychoeducation, and Parent Support Groups"; Chapter 56, "Family Therapy"; Chapter 61, "Systems of Care, Wraparound Services, and Home-Based Services"; Chapter 63, "School-Based Interventions"; and Chapter 64, "Collaborating With Primary Care").

The Therapist's Persona

Forming a therapeutic alliance with a child is essential to performing effective individual psychotherapy. This alliance, however, is not necessarily easy to obtain with the young and immature. At times, the relationship depends upon what kind of person—in the child's eyes—the therapist appears to be. All clinicians have options as to what traits in themselves they choose to emphasize with a specific child or adolescent patient in psychotherapy. Certainly, the clinician must be professional. This would include being calm, unhurried, willing to listen, nonjudgmental, relatively objective, focused on the patient, and committed to the basic principle behind the Hippocratic oath (actually enunciated by Florence Nightingale as, "First do no harm"). Beyond this professionalism, the child and adolescent psychiatrist must also consider how to "be" when with a certain specific child (Bugental 1964).

Sometimes a very calm, noncommenting, unemotional approach is exactly what is needed. A child going through a heated divorce, for instance, may respond well to this typically "psychoanalytic" persona in the clinician. It serves as a good foil to the overemotionality at home. A child with a life-threatening disease may also respond at his or her best to this impassive stance. Others around the child are showing their agony—perhaps crying, shrieking in frustration, being irritable. The unflappable physician in situations such as these becomes a stabilizing force in a childhood world falling apart.

Another choice for the physician-psychotherapist, however, is to emphasize the positive in his or her personality (Allen 1962). Never failing to notice something good about a child or the world outside the child becomes an important foil to years of neglect or negative criticism. This positive approach may work well for violent children, for children with histories of poor attachments, and for adolescents residing in institutions geared to delinquency. The psychiatric director of a California childhood residential care institution for latency-age children, for instance, set up a plan whereby his entire program could present a consistently positive persona to its young patients (Rosenfeld and Wasserman 1990). Numbers of children achieved success through experiencing this institutional approach.

Another approach is to become a "player"—with commentary of course—in the child's life. Play is usually similar—not opposite—to a child's previous life experience. Play and humor considerably lighten the load of the youngster's psychotherapy and make it more palatable (Terr 2003). Play also aids the therapeutic alliance (Terr et al. 2006c). The "player" is close to the actual persona of many child and adolescent clinicians. It works well in helping young patients express their deeper feelings and secret imaginings.

Although for adult patients, the classic psychodynamic psychotherapeutic persona is that of passive listener and occasional commentator, the child and adolescent psychotherapeutic persona is often more activist, serving as "tutor" or "coach." Most cognitive-behavioral therapists are seen by children as a kind of teacher as they educate and support, while sending their young patients off to do homework assignments until the next scheduled session. This, in most cases, does not destroy their doctor-patient relationship. Instead, it furthers the idea that the therapist is there to help the child. When a combination of individual work and behavioral modification is being attempted in nonmanualized individual therapy, the therapist frequently takes this same kind of tutorial approach. Habit disturbances, obsessional-compulsive symptoms, phobias, and some personality trait problems require that the psychotherapist employ a two-pronged technique: 1) uncovering (How did this particular problem arise? What basically is bothering the patient?) while 2) simultaneously coaching (How can the patient begin to extinguish his or her maladaptive habits, starting with the easiest?). Here, the therapist performs both as investigator and educator.

For example, a latency-age boy with encopresis, whose peer-given nickname was "Stink Bomb," was taken for short periods by his male psychiatrist into side-by-side stalls in a large public men's room at the hospital clinic where the doctor worked. They spoke out loud so anyone could hear. While training the youngster to push hard to defecate, the doctor simultaneously uncovered the boy's rage at his divorced father who lived in a distant city and the boy's paralyzing fear that to defecate meant to personally "explode." It took just a few months of this combination of uncovering and teaching to eradicate the symptom while strengthening the boy's adaptive abilities (see McDermott in Terr et al. 2005). Interestingly, at the end of his treatment, the patient voiced regret that his doctor would not be available to coach him at T-ball.

Taking a detective-like stance with a young patient is an interesting behavioral option for the child and adolescent psychotherapist. Not nosy or overly intrusive in these instances, the child psychiatrist allows the young patient to join in the work of investigation: "How can we find out what happened?" "Do you have any old friends from that neighborhood who knew you before?" The "mystery game" is a fascinating one for children making a difficult life transition, recovering from trauma, getting over a terrible illness, or trying to place into a foster care background. Understanding trauma puts the child's life stress into context. Understanding gives the trauma boundaries, and in fact, a possible solution. For instance, one child who could not sleep after watching the film *Nightmare on Elm Street* worked as a "detective" on the problem along with his doctor (see Dodson in Terr 2008). Doctor and patient first tried a number of behavioral techniques for the boy's intractable insomnia. None worked. But the doctor—willing to investigate further—decided, with the boy's permission, to write the film's conceiver and director, Wes Craven. Mr. Craven answered the letter. The boy, who had recently moved to a new home, new school, and new state, suddenly gained a new perspective on his problem. What had made Mr. Craven dream up the monster "Freddy Krueger" for the movies, in fact, had been entirely different and separate from what had been bothering the young patient. No longer did the boy have to fear Freddy Krueger. Freddy belonged to somebody else's imagination. This individual course of therapy was very brief, taking only a month or two. It is clear from these instances that individual, nonmanualized therapy does not have to be long-term, intensively insightful, or enormously expensive.

Although there are other possible personas for practicing clinicians, the "real doctor" is often the most useful, the most positive, and also the most potent role for a psychotherapist to take. For example, an adolescent spots the doctor's sports car out on the road. The doctor was speeding, the patient says. Was he? The truth is the best answer, whatever it is. "Are you pregnant?" a child asks of her therapist. This calls for truth. "I saw you coming out of a synagogue last Saturday. Are you Jewish?" An honest response is best. These realities about the therapist play into the treatment alliance and must be discussed with unvarnished truth and dignity. Their meaning to the child must be taken up as well.

Children may see their doctors on television. They can scan their physicians' Web sites and follow discussions about them in chat rooms on the Internet. Sometimes a child's peer at school is also visiting the same doctor, and an appointment is inadvertently scheduled back-to-back. Sometimes, the cultural chasm is so vast between doctor and young patient that the physician must admit to ignorance or ask questions that point to his or her naiveté. If the doctor's country of origin (even from generations ago) is at war with the patient's (across the ocean and also removed by time), it may still require an open talk and an indication that the psychiatrist is willing to accept further discussion.

Of course, **countertransference** (the therapist's feelings, often based on old unresolved conflicts that the patient's attitudes may bring to the surface) occasionally must be dealt with in order to save the therapeutic alliance with the child (Marshall 1979; Tsiantis et al. 1996). This, too, requires dealing with reality—often in small bits, but sometimes in one fell swoop (see Blos Jr. and Metcalf in Terr 2008). A thorough acquaintance with the concepts of transference and countertransference is important in doing psychotherapy with children (see Winnicott 1958). It is also important to be able to talk with a supervisor or with colleagues about these types of very personal responses to children.

Why is truthfulness and openness so important? Because the doctor-patient relationship in child psychotherapy is one of the main avenues to a child's improvement. Children change when they sense that their doctor cares enough about them to be real. They change when they believe that people can be honest with one another, no matter how painful that straight talk might be. They come to trust an adult who levels with them. They come to see that their intimate dialogues with others might safely be open and nonsecretive as well.

A good example from psychotherapy of a statement of a doctor's reality comes from a psychiatrist who was allergic to egg (see Deeney in Terr et al. 2005). The psychiatrist noticed himself becoming sick in his office, as a rebellious and sad adolescent patient with a Mohawk haircut repeatedly ran his fingers through his upright hair. Then, the boy spontaneously complained that the egg whites he had used to stiffen his "do" weren't effectively doing their job. Realizing that the boy's egg whites were leading him toward anaphylaxis, the psychiatrist told his patient that he needed to excuse himself to take some medicine. Upon returning, the psychiatrist explained what had happened, and the boy—for the first time in his treatment—expressed sincere empathy and offered to end the session early. From then on, the doctor-patient relationship turned around. The boy's psychotherapy became productive. As a matter of fact, the boy, now a young man, chose his life's work among the "helping" professions. The doctor's realistic and truthful explanation was given without hesitation or defensiveness. Briefly painful as it was for both doctor and patient, the "real" moment between them became an anchor for the boy's treatment and eventual cure.

The Doctor's Atmosphere

Individual child and adolescent psychotherapy requires a room in which to be alone with the young patient that is as appealing as possible. In certain instances, psychotherapy may also be conducted on walks with a young person (see Stewart or Zrull in Terr 2008), or it might occur in a child's hospital room (see Fine or Livingston in Terr 2008). In general, however, it usually takes place in an office furnished with enough shelves and drawers to house attractive and easy-to-use art supplies as well as a collection of toys. With these objects, a child patient will be able to express a multiplicity of feelings, problems, impulses, conflicts, and fantasies. This happens because children's play and art represent miniaturizations of life-sized situations.

A youngster's conflicts and concerns are often expressed in terms of animals (hence, animal puppets and small dinosaurs are important office equipment); vehicles (thus, a set of cars, fire and rescue equipment, pickup and tow trucks, police cars—and even a bus to the local prison—are helpful); a baby doll; older girl dolls, and if possible, a boy doll; a deck of cards; checkers; a doll house with miniature furniture and a small doll family; an army including men (and women) and their equipment; and some pop-culture items (e.g., a Little Mermaid, Star Wars figures, Hello Kitty, Power Rangers). Other kinds of objects, including some larger dolls and some movable ones—such as circus figures—and some simple games for two—such as cards or checkers—are also useful.

A toy (or choice of toys) may be purchased to suit a specific child's problem. All items should be kept clean, in good repair, and easily reachable by the child patient. If a child breaks something, the clinician should consider fixing it in front of the patient—this shows that situations (and people) can be made "right"—or at least put into working order. If a toy is irreparable, the therapist should try to buy another similar one in time for the child to see its replacement. If this is impossible, however, the therapist would be well-advised to tell the child that the toy will be replaced. Both doctor and patient must discuss the reality of what happened.

It is helpful for a well-equipped therapy office to be furnished with easily opening and closing toy cupboards and shelves so that adult patients, children's parents, and older adolescents can speak to their therapist without focusing on an office full of playthings. This does not mean that adults don't enjoy playing, too, or fiddling as they speak with something smoothly movable—such as small magnetic acrobats, tile puzzles, or tiny-ball-bearings-in-the-hole games. These things can be kept on open tables or a desktop. A nesting set of tables is a good furnishing for the psychotherapy office because children can pull these tables out and use them to arrange their play or artwork. Clay and finger paints, which have the capacity to ruin walls and carpeting, are best avoided. Attractive, washable baby rattles, blocks, and animals, on the other hand, are very useful, either for babies who accompany their parents to the office, or in observing and assessing the infants themselves.

In thinking about establishing a playful atmosphere, the therapist must also consider the needs and tastes of adolescents. For example: A doctor who had previously spent an unproductive, silent hour with a rebellious teenage girl, the daughter of an army sergeant deployed in Iraq, decided to suggest a game of pickup sticks at the beginning of the girl's second appointment. By the time the girl had won the game (which was new to her and therefore of considerable interest), she exposed her entire problem in a running mono-

logue that accompanied her play (see Massie, in Terr et al. 2006c). Suggesting play had broken the girl's initial negative transference. Without a handy game for teens in the office, this breakthrough might not have happened.

Children sometimes fantasize with toys in unique fashions far from the original intent of the toy (Waelder 1933). This often conveys meaning to the therapist. For instance, one angry boy used erasers to kick up chalk dust rather than to clean the clinician's chalkboard. The doctor turned to the boy, showing him how to bring the erasers together gently. They immediately created a mutually enjoyable, albeit dusty, game for two. In so doing, the psychotherapist was able to help the boy modify his violent behaviors in a larger world outside the office (see Teal in Terr 2008). The clinician can glean from this example that in individual psychotherapy, toys may be used to condense a child's problems into a nutshell, small enough to deal with.

Play does not only happen with toys and art. It happens with words. Words can be used playfully—as in word games like pig latin or William Steig's (1968) *CDB* language; codes or metaphors, especially ones that last for a while in treatment; rhymes; and little scenarios, set up and acted out by the child or adolescent patient. All of these plays on words charge the atmosphere with the spirit of fun and of bilateral discovery. For instance, a convicted juvenile rapist was treated during his 6-month sentence of "psychotherapy" by initially agreeing to call his crime—and his other serious problems with peers and authorities—"massive misunderstandings" (Terr et al. 2006c). Many years later, he contacted the psychiatrist for advice about helping his children through an impending divorce. "Don't worry," he said as if he had been in the office the day before, "[My divorce] was *not* a 'massive misunderstanding'!"

Not only does the psychotherapeutic office atmosphere reflect playfulness through the toys it contains and the words spoken there, but it also reflects a willingness to wait, if needed. The clinician may have to patiently "hold the fort" until a particular child responds—or to explain the next step in treatment and then accept a break in therapy while the patient thinks. Many a child psychotherapist has to patiently sit through a child's screaming tantrum, a refusal to talk, or even an avoidance of looking at the doctor. Sometimes monotonous games go on until a doctor fully appreciates the meaning of a young patient's behavior. Calmness and patience on the part of the psychotherapist are important characteristics to be developed in child and adolescent psychiatrists (see Sack in Terr

2008). They also become part of the doctor's atmosphere. Sooner or later, skilled therapists—and their patients—find their way out of such impasses (see Jetmalani in Terr 2008). The therapist thinks of something new, remembers something old, attends a conference, has a good talk with a colleague, or reads a book or a chapter. With effort and creativity, many of the "waiting games" played out in psychotherapy eventually benefit the patient.

The Doctor's Reading of the Child

Clinicians develop formulations about a youngster's problems during the evaluation phase. Later, clinicians may make shifts in the way they view the child's psychology (Group for the Advancement of Psychiatry 1982). Flexibility is required as any treatment moves along. As psychotherapy progresses, the therapist follows the child's leads, takes the child's tests, and enters the young person's fields of interest, seeking answers for the patient's dilemma. All of these methods of joining children on their personal journeys can work. Therapeutic collaboration works best when the clinician is finally able to "read" the child.

Children are likely to repeat a symptom in one form or another as long as that conflict or problem continues to exist. This **repetition compulsion,** one of Freud's most important observations of human behavior (S. Freud 1920/1955), gives the psychotherapist an opportunity to really "see" the child, even if other clues have previously been ignored or misunderstood. In other words, if the doctor misses what the child was conveying one time, he or she will have another chance to catch on. One of the beauties of doing play therapy in this context is that a child may repeat a certain theme endlessly in office play (Webb 2007). Not only does a child's play disclose these themes, but they are evident in drawings, poetry, songs, and other creative endeavors. They show up in dreams. And they show up in behaviors—both in the small, repeated habits children develop, as well as in their large-scale **reenactments.**

When a psychiatrist "gets" something about a child, the doctor has a number of choices. For instance, he or she may choose to continue to play it out with the child without leaving the arena of play. The doctor's therapeutic understanding may be interpreted directly to one of the characters in the child's play scenario, for instance. Or, as if the child were a screenwriter, the solution may be offered as an addition to the plot. Here, the treating doctor completely stays inside the play, the child's drawing, or the rhyming couplets. All help is offered to the fictional "characters" inside the child's creation.

On the other hand, the psychiatrist also has the option of moving outside the play and interpreting the child to himself. "You feel this way or that, but you can't express it because you're afraid of this or that," she might say, for instance. An interpretation is most often given, as in the above example. But a confrontation may be offered instead. "You actually *like* having a ghost in your life" (see Beitchman in Terr et al. 2006b) or "You'd rather have a *boy* therapist" (see Winters in Terr et al. 2006c).

Some children prefer being talked to inside of their play. Others prefer being directly approached as themselves. It may boil down to experiments of trial and error. But because of the repetition compulsion, the practitioner will get more than one chance to discover what works for a specific child. Sometimes, in fact, both techniques work for the very same individual.

"Getting" the child may come in a flash. Or it may come from careful listening and study. One doctor suddenly understood what his selectively mute boy-patient was trying to express to him when he accompanied his own children to the Disney film *The Little Mermaid* (see Jetmalani in Terr et al. 2006a). Another doctor watched her small Iranian patient, who was also selectively mute, search and search for the "right" doll to play with (see Rogers in Terr et al. 2005). Realizing that the little boy could not find the "right" doll, this psychiatrist fashioned a small nondescript doll from a rag—upon which the child quickly placed a head scarf. He named the doll "Grandma," eventually revealing his story of a wrenching removal from Iran, along with a total cutoff from his beloved grandmother. Once the boy was allowed to telephone his grandmother, he began speaking with everyone else. None of this would have happened without a doctor who could bridge their cultural gap. The practitioner did so with a piece of clean white cloth and some profound understanding.

Occasionally, a child patient leads the psychotherapist into a test that he or she must take (Terr 2008). Testing, like play, requires a sincere attempt on the psychiatrist's part to "get" the youngster. Like play, it also requires a technical decision—to stay inside or move outside the test. Adolescents are the most likely group to deliver such tests. Why? Because they *can.* And because psychotherapy so often feels to them like a deprivation. It takes away "their" time. It chips away at their developing selves—their defenses, deviant actions, and fears. In other words, doctors practicing psychotherapy are doing slow surgery, cutting out dysfunctional parts while their young patients are fully awake and unanesthetized. No wonder tests are administered by the patient in the hope that the doctor will fail.

Most of these child-given tests come early in the course of evaluation or therapy. But they may occur later as well. This is one of the main places where a clinician sees—and can interpret—transference. It also becomes an opportunity for the doctor to massively improve the relationship by playing along. As in the case of psychotherapeutic play, the clinician can sit apart, watch, and then comment on the test. Or the clinician can enter in and then correct the situation from inside the test itself. The important thing about a child-initiated test is to "get" the fact that an examination is taking place. Children may use a "bad" response as a quick way to achieve an exit from psychotherapy. They may decide to tell their parents, guardian, or school that their doctor is stupid. If the authorities in the child's life insist that the youngster wait it out, however, there is a high probability that the psychiatrist will be tested again. Because of the repetition compulsion, the doctor will receive a second chance.

Two case examples will be presented here: one, a severely neglected teenager, and the other, an ignored little boy.

Case Example

The adolescent girl—who had lived in succession with a drug-abusing mother; an unseeing, neglectful older sister; a middle sister who existed in chaos; and finally, a more stable paternal cousin—was undergoing psychotherapy with a male psychotherapist whom her grandmother had chosen for her (see Powers in Terr et al. 2006a). They had worked together briefly (on the girl's "conduct disorder") while she lived with her middle sister, but the chaos that drove her from her sister's home also disguised her silent dropout from psychotherapy. When she was forced to return 2 years later, and after about 3 months of grudging compliance, the girl suggested that she come to the doctor's office only twice a month (he had prescribed once a week). The psychotherapist considered this an unpassable "test." If he went along with the girl's request, he'd be seen by her as neglectful, like her mother and sisters (Silberschatz 2005). If he said "No," on the other hand, the girl would consider him one of the unthinking authorities who regularly stimulated rebellious feelings in her. The doctor refused to take the test. Musing aloud about both no-win options, he would not choose one side or the other. The patient argued, persuaded, cajoled, and finally left the office—for 2 weeks off, naturally. But when she came back, she announced that she had settled on a course of weekly

psychotherapy. Her attitude turned positive for the first time. She plunged into treatment. The test had been enunciated, interpreted, and passed by the doctor. As a result, the patient developed a meaningful relationship with him.

The second case illustrates a test given and taken without interpretation. It comes from a much younger child, a boy of 5 (see Stewart in Terr 2008).

Case Example

The kindergartener had a slightly older brother upon whom his parents doted. The patient himself was virtually ignored. At school the little boy hid under desks and curled into a fetal position. He feared bodily injury, saying that all his fluids might flow out of him. Two years of steady once-a-week psychotherapy led to some positive changes, but the boy still felt afraid of carnivorous animals and his school classmates. Then one day, he claimed he needed to interrupt his psychotherapeutic session to go to the bathroom. When his doctor came looking for him, he found the boy gripping his erect penis and smiling expectantly. The doctor instructed the child to return to the office at once. Over the next few months, this happened 4 or 5 more times. The doctor knew he was being tested, but the only response he could think of was to ask his patient to come back to the office. Then one day—on the same routine—the doctor found the boy standing atop a clinic bathroom sink, pants down, erect penis in hand, and a huge smile on his face. A new thought suddenly came to the psychiatrist. "That's a great one," the doctor said. The boy beamed at his psychiatrist, put his pants back on, climbed down from the sink, and never interrupted a session again. He improved afterward, so quickly in fact that his treatment was terminated in a few months' time. This is a situation in which the doctor—after thinking about this case for months—found a good solution in an instant. It was a "Eureka!" moment. The little boy's test was passed. Nor was any interpretation necessary. The child's masculinity had been confirmed for the very first time by, of all people, his psychiatrist.

Another way to show children that their doctors "get" them is to follow their interests. If a child in psychotherapy, for example, loves Harry Potter (main character in a series of books by J.K. Rowling), then it helps if the doctor reads some "Harry," too. If a child draws "Little Mermaids," it certainly aids the child to learn that the therapist has some ideas about young maidens-of-the-sea. Superheroes may be used to enhance children's treatments (Rubin 2007). It gives a child a new way of seeing himself, considering, for instance, what a character like Superman or Batman would do in the child's personal situation. Not only can pop culture and movie heroes be used in individual therapy, but depending upon the particular child, athletes, cancer survivors, and historical figures may be used as well. For example, one late-latency boy, whom the writer of this chapter treated for apathy, learning delays, and depression, became briefly interested in Julius Caesar (Terr 2008). How would Caesar have handled the politics of this young man's seventh-grade classroom? How would Caesar have planned to become friends with the boys he admired—or the girls? This patient gained 2 years' worth of academic reading skills during the 2 months he talked (and read) about Caesar. His grades went up dramatically. Despite years of receiving a number of diagnoses at a well-known clinic, taking a number of potent medications, and receiving tutoring in special classes, the idea of being like a great historical figure whom he liked and admired was what finally turned this particular adolescent around.

Individual child psychotherapy gears itself to the psychological needs of a specific youngster. Instead of aiming at a particular disorder, individualized therapy gives special attention to one particular child's ways of coping, internalized meanings, defensive choices, understandings of the world, and loves.

The Psychotherapeutic Response

In days past, psychotherapists felt the need to interpret a child's conflicts in terms of the youngster's secret wishes, defenses, past experiences, here-and-now behaviors, and/or transference. Whenever most of these elements could be brought together in a single comment, or group of comments, it was felt that the interpretation would be the most effective. The defenses were stressed as being more acceptable to children than the "naughty" desires. Therefore, if a psychotherapist could make an interpretation as an ego explanation (about coping and defense) rather than a comment about badness or mischief (the id), the child would handle it better (see Group for the Advancement of Psychiatry 1982).

Today, however, therapeutic statements to children cover a far wider gamut of issues than those noted above. Past realities in the child's life—the death of a peer's parent, an illness, a broken arm—loom larger today than they used to. Present realities—trouble at school, problems with classmates, joblessness at home, bullies in the neighborhood—are given far more room for exploration and discussion than they were in the past. What a child wishes for in the future and whom a child might wish to emulate as an **ego ideal** are also important (Terr 2003) as the clinician makes contemporary interpretations. How does the youngster envision what will happen next? Later in adulthood? How will he or she die? When? What about marriage, children, career? Discussing the future in terms of the youngster's present coping skills or behaviors often offers a new perspective to the child, and thus, a new way to combat old conflicts. These issues are taken into account right along with the classic issues—defenses and coping, secret unattainable desires, transference, and countertransference.

In current child psychotherapy, many of the doctor's responses to a youngster come as play rather than as speech. They come in the form of metaphor rather than as a direct hit. Some responses are conveyed as stories, supposedly about others but really about the young patient. All psychotherapeutic responses, however, carry one element in common: *They try to help the child make sense of his inner self or her external world.* And in so doing, they allow the child to reassess, consciously or unconsciously, how he or she wishes to be.

Psychotherapeutic commentary can be calculated—as in the instance of a young doctor watching a nonpsychotic hospitalized boy (with a psychotic identical twin brother) playing with "broken elevators" made up of blocks. After a consultation with his supervisor, the trainee came up with a carefully premeditated response—that elevator repairmen can fix certain elevators but have a much tougher time with others (see Zrull in Terr et al. 2005). This calculated response came about a week after the boy's play was first observed. It impressively relieved the young patient. Just as effective, however, is the doctor's quickly blurted-out or counterintuitive commentary. For example, a very angry boy seemed ready to destroy his psychiatrist's office. The psychiatrist knew that both the boy's teacher and his babysitter had quit their jobs that week. The doctor caught a similarity between how the boy responded to her and her symbolic stand-ins, the teacher and the babysitter. "Despite what may have happened with them," she unhesitatingly told her angry patient, "*I'm* not leaving!" The patient settled down and for the first time ever, he verbally expressed his ever-present sense of ambivalence about people, including his therapist. This was the key to the boy's psychology—and the crucial interpretation actually came from his own, not from the doctor's, mouth. But first, the psychiatrist said what immediately came to mind, putting the key into a door that the boy could now open by himself.

At times a verbal response to a child offers the youngster a solution to his own personal mystery. Dr. Louis Fine, for instance, wondered for years why so many children with congenital anomalies did poorly—especially in terms of depression—after rehabilitative surgeries aimed at giving them better functioning. The doctor solved the mystery by asking a number of youngsters about their postsurgical depressions. They were used to their congenital problems, they told him. Their problems had been with them forever. They liked their heavy shoes, with which they could kick their tormentors, or their wheelchairs and canes, with which they had always felt comfortable. Once Dr. Fine solved the mystery for one child (with his pointed commentary), he began solving the same mystery for others (with back and forth dialogue about these children's perceived dangers regarding their physical improvements). This consulting psychiatrist was thus able to solve similar dilemmas for many children by using very brief individual psychotherapies during their postsurgical hospitalizations (see Fine in Terr 2008).

With children it is sometimes appropriate to create a dramatic moment, a grand gesture that conveys to the child almost the entire meaning of the child's psychotherapeutic experience. Sometimes the doctor confronts the young child with exactly what he or she is doing or is wishing for (see Beitchman or Winters in Terr 2008). On the right occasion, on the other hand, it may be possible to say a poem, tell a story, or draw a picture that almost perfectly conveys to the young patient a sense of the doctor's understanding. Sometimes, using an already fixed method of working in psychotherapy, such as Winnicott's squiggle game (in which the doctor starts a doodle and the child finishes it [Winnicott 1971a]) or Gardner's mutual storytelling technique (in which the doctor and patient work out the beginnings of a story to which the doctor—or better yet, the patient—affixes a corrective ending [Gardner 1971]), creates just what was needed. Shapiro (1983), for instance, worked with a 5-year-old girl for only two sessions, using Winnicott's squiggle game. This psychotherapeutic approach completely relieved the young child's previously intractable insomnia. With children suffering from terrible experiences (Terr 2003), a story resembling the trauma can be started with the patient and the child is then asked to find a correction.

Letters to someone whom, the child feels, needs to receive this kind of communication is another dramatic way for a young psychotherapeutic patient to find comfort and self-awareness. Letters do not necessarily have to be sent in the mail. Letters to Santa, even

letters to God, for instance, have long been a childhood tradition. When this tradition is used on behalf of the individual youngster in psychotherapy, it may bring with it a sense of control and relief (Terr 2008).

Some gifted psychotherapists improvise just the "right" drama for the specific child. In fact, some of these little dramas are produced at the spur of the moment. One kindergarten-age girl, for instance, was brought to a Montreal emergency room because she had become afraid to eat. For a couple of days, she had refused all food, claiming she might inadvertently kill a living being, like a fly. "What is the worst thing that would happen," the doctor asked her, "if you *did* swallow a fly?" The youngster could not answer. So the psychiatrist did. "It would come out in your poo." (see Minde in Terr et al. 2006c). Entranced, the little girl's 2-year-old sister chanted, "Fly in the poo! Ha! Ha!" The doctor began to sing and dance, based on the toddler's chant. The entire family eventually joined in. The phobic kindergartener left the emergency room that night, cured.

If a child won't talk, the gifted psychotherapist might try a *soliloquy for two,* another dramatic gesture. In a soliloquy for two, the doctor tells a story about an imaginary child who, of course, is just like the patient herself (see Robson in Terr 2008). In a different context, if a child happens to give away something intimate about himself, the gifted psychiatrist might say something so dramatic it requires ongoing discussion. Consider, for instance, the phrase, "Your secret is safe with me" (actually from the 1942 film *Casablanca*). An institutionalized teenager, who was spotted feigning psychosis, heard this phrase coming from his psychiatrist, and the patient wished to discuss it. This adolescent was eventually able to leave the residential center where he was incarcerated because of the ongoing psychotherapeutic talks that followed from his doctor's provocative remark (see Livingston in Terr 2008). Many dramatic circumstances are so unique that they cannot be duplicated. Studying good books and research reports, watching others, and talking to peers can lead to calculated or instinctive solutions, where the impetus to create memorable moments for children can safely be followed.

Ending Treatment

If the clinician has the option of deciding when to end psychotherapy (and many times he or she does not), the doctor considers the original goals—have they been met?—and any secondary goals that arose during treatment—have they been met as well? After thinking these goals through, the clinician suggests an end date and may taper the frequency of sessions in order to assess how the young patient does without as much access to psychotherapy. Clinician and child talk about their relationship, what they each believe the treatment meant and accomplished, and what the child will do if a problem arises in the future.

Often the doctor makes sure that the child knows how to reach another good practitioner—or the same doctor—in the future, if one is needed. The doctor might also suggest yearly checkups for a while, if that option seems appropriate. Furthermore, the psychiatrist might make it clear that "booster shots" or briefer treatment periods may be necessary when the youngster enters a new phase of life. This is particularly common in cases of psychic trauma, where the old trauma is experienced differently as new developmental challenges arise (Terr 2003).

Frequently, psychotherapy ends prematurely by the doctor's standards. The young patient moves to a new city. The patient goes to a boarding school or college. The parents divorce. The family can no longer afford the therapy. Insurance plans change. Insurance carriers decide, "No more." Even improvement is sometimes cause for a premature termination, at least in the psychiatrist's opinion. The family sees the child's improvement as sufficient to stop the treatment—while the doctor still wishes to help strengthen and mature some of the child's underlying coping and defensive strategies.

In such cases, it is best to provide the young patient with two or three termination sessions—with some decreasing frequency of the sessions as well. If the doctor can successfully bargain with the family for a few hours to complete things, it is usually the most helpful way to end a child's therapeutic work.

Often when children take their summer breaks from school, parents decide that the time for ending treatment has come. If a child fails to reappear in the fall, it is worthwhile to make a phone inquiry and to ask for further in-person conversation with the family. But often, from the child's point of view, summer is a natural time to stop. School stops, as do certain sports and music lessons. In the case of therapy, however, missing the chance to say good-bye may lead to confusion later in life as to what those visits to the psychiatrist were all about. Unfortunately, even when termination with a child is handled with the greatest of skill, youngsters often still fail to understand why they went through a course of psychotherapy. Insight is, in fact, an almost-adult trait and a very difficult one for any young patient to develop.

Future Directions

Individualized, nonmanualized treatments for children must be rigorously studied in the future. Unfortunately, 100 years of stellar case reports are not enough. It will be necessary to set up good comparisons, with or without medications, to other therapies given for the same diagnoses. It will also be important to compare various age groups and various stages of childhood. Finding the funds and the approvals for such studies will be a problem, but it must be overcome. Otherwise a very useful way of working with children may eventually be discarded.

One interesting aspect of psychotherapy for study is the turning point. What accounts for almost instantaneous meetings of the mind between doctors and young patients? Daniel Stern (2004) has been studying this phenomenon, as have the author and her colleagues. Their interest in the instantaneous gesture and intuitive move in the well-trained and experienced clinician is one that may eventually lead in new and fruitful directions.

Most importantly, let us hope that innovative new studies allow us—with vigor and enthusiasm—to eventually supply an "evidence base" to this crucial field. The well-being of many children depends on it.

Summary Points

- Make a full diagnosis and formulation, suggesting psychotherapy where appropriate and potentially helpful.
- Find a way for the child's parents or guardians to participate.
- Pick a persona that will enhance the chances of success.
- Be willing to show your "realness" when called for.
- Outfit an office that is child friendly.

- Use a variety of techniques tailored to the particular child, such as conversation, play, art, and storytelling.
- Watch and listen, following the child's leads.
- Nurture the relationship with appropriate gestures and comments.
- Make therapeutic responses geared to the youngster's inner problems, problems with the real world, and/or problems in the relationship itself.
- Stay flexible.

References

Allen F: Positive Aspects of Child Psychiatry. New York, Basic Books, 1962

Bugental J: The person who is the psychotherapist. J Consult Psychol 11:272–277, 1964

Erikson E: Childhood and Society. New York, WW Norton, 1950

Fraiberg S: Insights from the Blind. New York, Basic Books, 1977

Freud A: Introduction to the Technique of Child Analysis. Washington, DC, Nervous and Mental Disease Publishing Company, 1928

Freud A: The Ego and the Mechanisms of Defense (1936). New York, International Universities Press, 1946

Freud A, Burlingham D: War and Children (Report 12). New York, Medical War Books, 1943

Freud S: Analysis of a phobia in a five-year old boy (1909), in The Standard Edition of the Complete Psychological Works of Sigmund Freud, Vol 10. Translated and edited by Strachey J. London, Hogarth, 1955, pp 3–147

Freud S: Beyond the Pleasure Principle (1920), in The Standard Edition of The Complete Psychological Works of Sigmund Freud, Vol 18. Translated and edited by Strachey J. London, Hogarth, 1955, pp 7–64

Furman E: Treatment of under-fives by way of parents. Psychoanal Study Child 12:250–262, 1957

Gardner R: Therapeutic Communications with Children: The Mutual Storytelling Technique. New York, Science House, 1971

Green M, Solnit A: Reactions to the threatened loss of a child: the vulnerable child syndrome. Pediatrics 34:58–66, 1964

Group for the Advancement of Psychiatry: The Process of Child Therapy. New York, Brunner/Mazel, 1982

Group for the Advancement of Psychiatry: How old is old enough? The ages of rights and responsibilities. Rep Group Adv Psychiatry 126:1–124, 1989

Harrison S, McDermott JF, Schrager J, et al: Social status and child psychiatric practice: the inference of the clinician's socioeconomic origin. Am J Psychiatry 127:652–658, 1970

Hartmann H: Notes on the reality principle. Psychoanal Study Child 11:31–53, 1956

Jellinek MS, McDermott JF: Formulation: Putting the diagnosis into a therapeutic context and treatment plan. J Am Acad Child Adolesc Psychiatry 43:913–916, 2004

Johnson A: Sanctions for superego lacunae of adolescents, in Searchlights on Delinquency. Edited by Eissler K. Oxford, England, International Universities Press, 1949, pp 225–254

Kernberg PF, Weiner AS, Bardenstein K: Personality Disorders in Children and Adolescents. New York, Basic Books, 2000

Kline M: The Psychoanalysis of Children. London, Hogarth, 1932

Levy D: Release therapy. Am J Orthopsychiatry 9:713–736, 1939

Lewis M, King R (eds): Consultation-liaison in pediatrics, in Child and Adolescent Psychiatric Clinics of North America. Philadelphia, PA, WB Saunders, 1994

Marshall R: Countertransference in the psychotherapy of children and adolescents. Contemp Psychoanal 15:599–629, 1979

Mishne JM: The treatment relationship: alliance, transference, countertransference, and the real relationship, in Clinical Work With Adolescents. Edited by Marks JM. New York, Free Press, 1986

Rosenfeld AR, Wasserman S: Healing the Heart: A Therapeutic Approach to Disturbed Children in Group Care. Washington, DC, Child Welfare League of America, 1990

Rubin LC (ed): Using Superheroes in Counseling and Play Therapy. New York, Springer, 2007

Schulman JL, de la Fuente ME, Suran BG: An indication for brief psychotherapy: the fork in the road phenomenon. Bull Menninger Clin 41:553–562, 1977

Shapiro T: The unconscious still occupies us. Psychoanal Study Child 38:547–567, 1983

Shapiro T: The psychodynamic formulations in child and adolescent psychiatry. J Am Acad Child Adolesc Psychiatry 28:675–680, 1989

Silberschatz G: The control mastery theory, in Transformative Relationships. Edited by Silberschatz G. New York, Routledge, 2005, pp 3–24

Silver L: Attention-deficit/Hyperactivity Disorder: A Clinical Guide to Diagnosis and Treatment for Health and Mental Health Professionals. Washington, DC, American Psychiatric Publishing, 2003

Steig W: CDB! New York, Aladdin, 1968

Stern D: The Present Moment in Psychotherapy and Everyday Life. New York, WW Norton, 2004

Terr L: Childhood trauma: an outline and overview. Am J Psychiatry 148:10–20, 1991

Terr L: Wild child: how three principles of healing organized 12 years of psychotherapy. J Am Acad Child Adolesc Psychiatry 42:1401–1409, 2003

Terr L: Magical Moments of Change: How Psychotherapy Turns Kids Around. New York, WW Norton, 2008

Terr L: Using contact to treat traumatized children. Psychoanal Study Child, in press

Terr L, McDermott JF, Benson RM, et al: Moments in psychotherapy. J Am Acad Child Adolesc Psychiatry 44:191–197, 2005

Terr L, Abright AR, Brody M, et al: When formulation outweighs diagnosis: 13 "moments" in psychotherapy. J Am Acad Child Adolesc Psychiatry 45:1252–1263, 2006a

Terr L, Beitchman J, Braslow K, et al: Children's turnarounds in psychotherapy: the doctor's gesture. Psychoanal Study Child 61:56–81, 2006b

Terr L, Deeney JM, Drell M, et al: Playful "moments" in psychotherapy. J Am Acad Child Adolesc Psychiatry 45:604–613, 2006c

Thomas A, Chess S, Birch HG: Temperament and Behavior Disorders in Children. New York, New York University Press, 1968

Tsiantis J, Sandler A-M, Anastasopoulos D, et al: Countertransference in Psychoanalytic Psychotherapy With Children and Adolescents. London, Karnac, 1996

Waelder R: The psychoanalytic theory of play. Psychoanal Q 2:208–224, 1933

Webb NB (ed): Play Therapy With Children in Crisis, 3rd Edition. New York, Guilford, 2007

Weiner MF, King JW: Self-disclosure by the therapist to the adolescent patient, in Adolescent Psychiatry, Vol 5. Edited by Feinstein S, Giovacchini P. New York, Jason Aronson, 1977, pp 449–459

Winnicott DW: Clinical varieties of transference, in Collected Papers: Through Pediatrics to Psychoanalysis. New York, Basic Books, 1958, pp 295–299

Winnicott DW: Playing and Reality. New York, Basic Books, 1971a

Winnicott DW: Therapeutic Consultations in Child Psychiatry. New York, Basic Books, 1971b

Chapter 54

Parent Counseling, Psychoeducation, and Parent Support Groups

Amy N. Mendenhall, Ph.D., M.S.W.
L. Eugene Arnold, M.D., M.Ed.
Mary A. Fristad, Ph.D., A.B.P.P.

Mental illness in children affects the entire family. Children are dependent on their parents to help recognize and meet their needs, so education and support for both the child and the caregivers about disorders and treatment are essential. Various parent and family interventions have been developed for families with a child with a serious emotional or behavioral disorder. Table 54–1 lists the distinguishing features of some of these programs.

This chapter describes three interventions that provide support and education to parents of children with serious emotional and behavioral disturbances: parent counseling, psychoeducation, and parent support groups. *Parent counseling* is a broad category of parent-focused work that combines a mixture of education and psychotherapy based on the needs of each parent. As a specific subset of parent counseling, *psychoeducation* is an explicit manualized intervention that focuses on education and skill building for both parents and children. *Parent support groups* are less formal than parent counseling and psychoeducation. They gather together parents experiencing similar situations to create a network of support. Despite these differences, the interventions have a common focus—to help parents of children with emotional and behavioral disorders in order to indirectly aid the children.

TABLE 54–1. Parent and family interventions

Intervention	Definition and distinguishing features	Relative importance of trained professional
Family assessment	Assesses child diagnosis, family needs, and necessary services and treatment	++++
Family therapy	Psychotherapeutic approach focusing on family interactions and relationships to promote change Classically based on a "systems" framework: may also include interventions from other theoretical models (e.g., behavioral)	++++
Multifamily psychoeducation groups[a]	Psychoeducation in context of multifamily group, providing knowledge, support, and skill building to families with a common problem	++++
Parent counseling[a]	Continuum of interventions to help parents understand their child and the mental illness; targets parent attitudes and behavior; includes advice, supportive therapy	++++
Parent management training	Teaches and coaches parents to change their child's problem behaviors, mainly using behavior modification strategies and techniques	+++
Parent support groups[a]	Creates a support network of parents experiencing similar situations; focus on self-help, identification, and guilt reduction	+
Psychoeducation[a]	Manualized approach focusing on education about the disorder; its treatment; accessing of services; and skill building in communication, problem solving, and symptom management	++++
Wraparound services	Creation of a network of community services and natural supports individualized to the needs of the child and family	++
Treatment of parent's own mental disorder	Parent is treated directly for a diagnosed mental disorder that impairs parenting	++++
Counseling in context of parent's treatment	Parent in treatment for own problem brings up difficulty with child during treatment	++++

[a]Interventions described in the current chapter.

Parent Counseling and Psychoeducation

What Is Parent Counseling?

Parent counseling or parent guidance has been used to more generally describe parent education and therapy separate from work with the child. It refers to an overall continuum of interventions aimed to help parents understand their children and their moods and behaviors. It sometimes targets parent attitudes and behaviors that may contribute to overall difficulties in the family.

Interventions range from basic education to psychotherapy and can include clarification, advice, persuasion, facilitation, and exploration of feelings (Arnold 1978). The decision of which intervention to use is made based on the nature of the problem, family personality and strengths, obstacles to effective parenting, and type of help the parents are willing to accept.

Regardless of the specific intervention, it should be accompanied by the sincere valuing of parents for their experience in caring for their children and their expertise in understanding their children and their needs (Arnold 1978). Recognizing parental expertise and beliefs can lead to better personalization of treatment, a stronger therapeutic relationship, and more positive

TABLE 54–2. Basic principles of parent counseling interventions

1. Education and therapy are provided to parents rather than directly to the child.

2. Parents are essential to treatment because they spend the most time with their child.

3. The experience and expertise parents have from caring for their children should be valued and utilized in treatment.

4. The appropriate choice of intervention depends on the problem, the circumstances, and the family.

5. The professional acts as a consultant to help parents identify problems and learn skills needed to manage their child's illness successfully on their own.

6. Help parents understand normal child development, their own child, and their child's needs and problems.

7. Help parents modify their own attitudes, behaviors, and parenting that may be unwittingly contributing to the problem.

8. Emphasize efficiency, effectiveness, and practicality to the exclusion of moral judgment or blame.

9. Assume that parent-child conflicts are two-way vicious cycles.

Source. Adapted from Arnold (1978).

outcomes. Table 54–2 lists basic principles of parent counseling, and Table 54–3 lists some tactics to use while working with parents in parent counseling. This chapter will focus on one specific type of parent counseling, psychoeducation, which refers to manualized educational programs for parents and children. Parent training, also an educational parent counseling approach, is covered in Chapter 55, "Behavioral Parent Training."

What Is Psychoeducation?

Psychoeducation integrates psychotherapeutic and educational methods with the intention of educating both the patient and the family to reach better outcomes for all (Lukens and McFarlane 2004). It teaches about diagnoses, course of illness, medications, other treatments, and symptom management. Psychoeducation is designed as an adjunctive treatment to medications or other treatment already in progress. It has been applied to many different areas within the health and mental health fields (Lofthouse and Fristad 2004). Growing literature on the effectiveness of psychoeducation has led to national and international recommendations to use psychoeducation for the treatment of schizophrenia and other mental illnesses (President's New Freedom Commission on Mental Health 2003).

History of Psychoeducation

Psychoeducation emerged from efforts to improve the prognosis of schizophrenia. Goldstein et al. (1978) pro-

TABLE 54–3. Tactics for working with parents in parent counseling

Help parents reframe the problem in a way that seems manageable and does not place responsibility solely on them.

Model appropriate parent-child behavior for parents to observe.

In cases where punishment has been excessively frequent or severe (which usually means it has been ineffective), guide parents in understanding the purpose of consequences and finding a humane consequence that works for their child.

Help parents understand the importance of counterbalancing punishment with rewards (both carrot and stick).

Provide parents with supplemental reading to reinforce topics discussed in sessions.

Refer parents to other services you cannot provide.

Encourage parents to seek therapy for themselves, not just for their child.

Encourage parents to be patient and to expect small increments of change rather than a quick cure.

Source. Adapted from Arnold (1978).

vided for recently discharged adults with schizophrenia and their families a program designed to help them understand the illness and its treatment and plan for future crises. The program was the first to combine medication and family intervention, and the combined program was found to be more effective than either separate intervention. Also during this time period, Carol Anderson and Gerald Hogarty (Anderson et al. 1980) developed the family psychoeducation approach combining psychoeducation and social skills training for families of individuals with schizophrenia. Miklowitz and Goldstein (1995) also successfully adapted the psychoeducation model to address bipolar disorder in adults. Success of these programs spurred a series of studies on the use of psychoeducation for schizophrenia, bipolar disorder, and other adult mental health disorders. Studies are now examining its use with children and adolescents, with some positive outcomes.

Theoretical Background of Parent Counseling and Psychoeducation

Parents are the primary caregivers and decision makers in their children's lives. Parents of a child with mental illness have the added responsibility of managing their child's symptoms and treatment. Educated parents are better positioned to help their child manage symptoms and to access services appropriate to their child's needs.

Psychoeducation combines several clinical approaches, including cognitive-behavioral, learning, narrative, systems, client-centered, stress and coping, and social support theories (Lukens and McFarlane 2004). Techniques such as role-playing encourage parents to practice applying new information and skills learned. Systems theory provides a framework to understand mental illness in relation to all relevant systems, including family, school or work, and social network. Group psychoeducation provides an atmosphere for social learning and support among group members. A biopsychosocial approach presents mental illness as a "no fault illness." Psychoeducation participants are specifically told they are not to blame for the illness; rather, they are taught how to separate themselves from the symptoms (Fristad et al. 1999).

Description of Parent Counseling and Psychoeducation

Parent counseling and psychoeducation can have very different structures, depending on the problem being addressed and the setting in which the interventions are being provided. The interventions can be delivered to individual families or in multifamily groups (Fristad 2006). Individual family psychoeducation consists of one family working one-on-one with the clinician to learn more about their child's diagnosis and treatment. Multifamily psychoeducation groups consist of multiple families in similar situations following a standardized format of education. A group of researchers at Ohio State University have developed and tested both individual family and multifamily psychoeducation interventions (Fristad 2006). Different strengths were found for each format, as listed in Table 54–4. McFarlane et al. (1995) found that multifamily group psychoeducation was even more effective in reducing relapse rates and increasing functioning in adults than individual or family psychoeducation; however, this has not been tested in families of children and adolescents.

Psychoeducation interventions usually consist of a set of sessions focused on providing information about mental illness and its treatment. These sessions are typically the same for every individual or group,

TABLE 54–4. Relative advantages of the two psychoeducation formats

Individual family psychoeducation	Multifamily psychoeducation groups
Easy for private practice clinician to implement	Cost-effective way to deliver services within a large clinic
Privacy	Opportunity to talk and share with both professionals and other families
Flexibility in scheduling	Development of support network
Flexibility to tailor topics to individualized needs	Identifying with and learning from other families' successes

with each session's topic area described in detail in a treatment manual. Information can be presented through lecture, discussions, video, and role-playing. Areas commonly covered are diagnosis, symptom management, communication, medication, other treatment, and skill building. Session length and duration may vary between different programs but are typically established prior to starting treatment. Typical session length is between 1 and 2 hours and treatment duration between 1 and 20 sessions. Some psychoeducation treatments have one or more built in "flex" sessions to be used as needed for specific parent and family concerns.

Psychoeducation is easily adapted to a variety of settings including hospitals, schools, mental health centers, jails or detention centers, and online Web sites. Format, length, duration, and treatment focus may vary based on the setting. The professionals leading the intervention may include psychiatrists or other physicians, psychologists, social workers, teachers, and nurses. Regardless of their profession, psychoeducation leaders serve as facilitators and teachers. They are responsible for developing the intervention to meet the needs, motivations, strengths, and weaknesses of the patients (Brown 1998).

Adaptation of psychoeducation for children and adolescents requires several changes in the content and format of the intervention. Fristad et al. (1996) suggest six adaptations to psychoeducational approaches based on children's developmental needs (Table 54–5).

Benefits of Parent Counseling and Psychoeducation

Education about specific disorders helps parents to understand their child's experiences and how to help them. Education about types of available treatments, classes of medications, side effects, and building a treatment team can promote treatment adherence and efficiency. Increased knowledge about the problem allows parents to react more appropriately.

Another benefit is a focus on the parents, their feelings, and their stress, which often have been neglected in pursuit of the child's treatment. The impact of mental illness on caregivers and families can be enormous, and psychoeducation tries to alleviate some of the difficulties of caring for a child with mental illness. Psychoeducation addresses these stresses not only by empowering parents with knowledge about their child's illness and treatment but also by promoting healthy communication, symptom management, parent health and mental health and by addressing parental needs. Parents are offered support, validation, and recognition of their own struggles (Fristad et al. 2003b).

TABLE 54–5. Age adjustments needed for psychoeducation with children and adolescents with mental illness, compared to programs with adults

Psychoeducational adjustments for children and adolescents	Reason for the adjustment
Clarification for the child and family about what the disorder is and what the child's traits are	With a much earlier age at onset than adults, children may not have had an opportunity to develop a healthy identity separate from symptoms.
Emphasis on social skills training	Children may not have had the opportunity to develop age-appropriate social skills due to early onset.
Assistance in adjusting environmental expectations	Education and intervention are often needed at school to help adjust the environment to one in which the child can succeed despite symptoms.
Emphasis on the importance of the home environment	Children are still dependent on their parents and so are particularly vulnerable to unhealthy home environments.
Greater intensity of treatment and longer follow-up	Earlier onset often leads to a more pernicious course and greater treatment resistance.
Developmentally appropriate group content	Children and adolescents differ in their developmental level, so separate content or groups are needed for the two ages.

Source. Adapted from Fristad et al. (1996).

Additionally, psychoeducation targets expressed emotion (EE), which may be a factor contributing to perpetuation of symptoms. EE refers to the type and quality of interactions and attitudes regarding a person who is mentally ill. The term emerged from a series of studies focused on relapse rates in adults with schizophrenia (Brown et al. 1972). A meta-analysis of 27 adult studies found that although EE is a general predictor of poor outcome, it can be modified (Butzlaff and Hooley 1998). High EE has also been found to be related to poor outcome in mood disorders in youth (Asarnow et al. 1993). Psychoeducation was developed to lower EE through parent support and education (Hooley 1998). It can help families adapt a strategy of problem-focused coping rather than emotion-focused coping, leading to better family communication and symptom management (Sloper 1999). Lowering negative EE through psychoeducation may lead to an improved environment for the child suffering from an emotional or behavioral disorder.

Research on Psychoeducation for Children's Mental Health

Family psychoeducation is an evidence-based practice in adult mental health. The application of psychoeducation has spread to children's mental health, and research on psychoeducation for various children's mental health disorders is ongoing. Table 54–6 lists examples of family psychoeducation as it has been applied to various mental disorders in children and adolescents. The table excludes psychoeducation interventions designed only for the child and not the parents or family.

As shown in Table 54–6, family or parent psychoeducation interventions have been designed for anxiety disorders, attention-deficit/hyperactivity disorder, depressive disorders, bipolar disorders, disruptive behavior disorders, and eating disorders. Programs have also been designed for general emotional and behavioral disturbances rather than for specific disorders. Across diagnoses, the active treatment components of these family psychoeducation interventions were all very similar and included medications, other forms of treatment, symptom management, parenting, and coping and communication skills. Some mood disorder interventions had pharmacotherapy and psychoeducation offered as a treatment package. Interventions followed structured formats most commonly led by a mental health professional and typically outlined in a treatment manual. Material was taught through a variety of

methods including lecture, video, role-playing, reading, and discussion. Most psychoeducation programs included both children and parents. Program length ranged from 1 session to 21 sessions. Most had 90-minute sessions. Study designs included case studies, open trials, and a few randomized controlled studies. Outcomes relate to level of knowledge and beliefs about mental illness, symptom severity, social functioning, and satisfaction with the intervention. Overall, the findings are supportive in several disorders for including psychoeducation as part of the treatment package for families of children with serious mental illness.

More research on psychoeducation interventions for children with psychiatric disorders is needed before their effectiveness is as well established as psychoeducation for families of adults with schizophrenia and bipolar disorder. However, ongoing research is testing various interventions with larger samples, more stringent research methods (randomized clinical trials), and a variety of disorders and populations. The following section provides a more detailed description of one of these psychoeducation interventions.

Example of a Psychoeducation Intervention: Multifamily Psychoeducational Psychotherapy for Children With Mood Disorders

Multifamily psychoeducational psychotherapy (MF-PEP) was developed by Fristad and colleagues as an adjunctive intervention for families of children ages 8–12 with mood disorders (Fristad et al. 2003a). The guiding principle of MF-PEP is that education, support, and skill building will lead to a better understanding of the illness, which in turn will lead to better treatment adherence, less conflict, and better outcomes for all. Eight 90-minute sessions are manualized with a nonblaming biopsychosocial model using systems and cognitive-behavioral techniques. Table 54–7 lists the weekly session topics for the parents and children.

Sessions start with children and parents together for a discussion of the day's content area, issues brought up in previous sessions, unanswered questions, and reports on the previous week's homework projects. Then the families separate into parent and youth groups for their separate lessons, and they rejoin for a wrap-up at the end of the session. Parents and children are assigned projects to complete between sessions to practice skills learned in the group.

The child group is led by two cotherapists, and the parent group by one therapist. Goals for the parent group are social support, information, and skill building (Goldberg-Arnold et al. 1999). Goals for the child group are meeting and interacting with other children who struggle with similar issues, increased awareness of symptoms and symptom management, increased affect regulation skills, and social skills building.

In a randomized controlled trial, 35 families with children diagnosed with a mood disorder (Fristad et al. 2002) were randomly assigned to MF-PEP or a 6-month waitlist control. Outcomes included improvement in parental report of family interactions, decreased negative interactions, increased support from parents, improvement in ability to obtain appropriate services, gain in social support, higher positive EE ratings, lower negative EE ratings, and increased knowledge. Immediately after treatment, families most commonly reported increased knowledge as the outcome of the treatment, while fewer parents reported change in behavior or attitude. Six months after treatment, although parents still reported a gain in knowledge, they most commonly reported a change in behavior and attitude. A larger ($N=165$) National Institute of Mental Health (NIMH)–funded randomized controlled trial found that youth who received MF-PEP had a significantly greater decrease in mood symptom severity at follow-up compared to waitlist control with improvement maintained through an 18-month follow-up period (Fristad et al., in press). Results suggest that MF-PEP helps parents become better consumers of the mental health system by increasing their knowledge about mood disorders and treatment, which then leads them to access higher quality services. Consequently, when children receive services appropriate for meeting their needs, the severity of their symptoms decreases (Mendenhall et al. 2009).

Starting a Multifamily Psychoeducation Group

Establishing a curriculum is the first step. Regardless of type of disorder, a curriculum for a new program should address several main content areas (Table 54–8). Addressing these areas provides families with a well-rounded education and skill development to help them successfully manage symptoms and access appropriate care. However, aspects of the programs should be specialized to the disorder being targeted. Table 54–9 lists some suggested adaptations to psychoeducation by disorder based on the studies previously summa-

rized. Integrated into the curriculum should be techniques for practicing and monitoring newly learned knowledge and skills. Techniques are often adapted from therapeutic approaches such as cognitive-behavioral therapy, narrative therapy, or learning theory. Table 54–10 describes some commonly used psychoeducational techniques.

When developing a group, logistical decisions—such as location, whether to include the youth, optimal group size, length of program, and duration of sessions—must also be made based on the setting and targeted disorder. Possible complications in implementing psychoeducation groups and how to address them should also be considered before starting the group. Table 54–11 lists some complications and options for possible solutions or responses.

For those seeking further guidance, many of the previously described psychoeducation programs have developed treatment manuals or other literature on their programs. Additionally, the Substance Abuse and Mental Health Services Administration (SAMHSA) developed an extensive tool kit for implementing family psychoeducation based on the adult literature and research; the tool kit is available at the Web site http://mentalhealth.samhsa.gov/cmhs/communitysupport/toolkits/family.

Though not based specifically on psychoeducation with families of children with mental illness, information from the site may be helpful in starting a group for this population.

Parent Support Groups
What Are Parent Support Groups?

Parent support groups bring together parents of children with similar symptoms or diagnoses in an environment designed to be safe for mutual sharing and learning. These groups are applicable in any setting or with any diagnosis and can be led by professionals or consumers. Such groups can alleviate parent burden by providing essential information, peer support, coping skills, and respite from the strain of life with a chronically ill child (Hellander et al. 2003). These goals match well with the three basic needs for which individuals join self-help groups: social support, practical information, and a sense of shared purpose or advocacy (Bennett et al. 1996; Koroloff and Friesen 1991; Madara 1997). A national survey of parents of children

TABLE 54–6. Studies of the use of psychoeducation in children's mental health

Study	Population	Design and sample	Active treatment protocol	Structure and duration	Outcomes
Anxiety disorders					
Copping et al. 2001	Children ages 3–17 who have experienced trauma and their caregivers	Open study $N=27$ (mean age=9.8; 48% female)	Psychoeducation and cognitive-behavioral therapy (CBT)	21 sessions of varying length, including 6 group psychoeducation sessions, 7 individualized CBT sessions, and 4 assessment sessions, followed by 4 treatment sessions	Reduction in conduct disorder ($P=.001$), problems in social relations ($P=.039$), and caregiver depression ($P=.006$) from pretest to posttest.
Attention-deficit/hyperactivity disorder (ADHD)					
Lopez et al. 2005	Children ages 6–17 with ADHD and their families	Open study $N=90$ (mean age=9.9; 29% female)	Psychoeducation through written materials and physicians and clinical assistants	Varied for each family	Parents utilized available education materials; they indicated satisfaction with intervention at the end of treatment.
Bipolar disorders					
Fristad 2006	Children ages 8–11 with major mood disorders and their families	RCT Waitlist control $N=35$ (54% depressive spectrum, 46% bipolar spectrum)	Adjunctive multifamily psychoeducational psychotherapy	6 sessions, 75 minutes in length, with separate parent and child groups	From pre- to posttreatment, immediate group (vs. waitlist group) had more knowledge ($P<.009$), more positive family interactions ($P<.05$), and increased perceived social support in children ($P<.003$).
Miklowitz et al. 2004	Adolescents with bipolar disorder ages 13–17 and family members	Open study $N=20$ (mean age=14.8; 45% female)	Family-focused psychoeducation and pharmacotherapy	21 sessions over 9 months with optional maintenance sessions	Improvements in depression symptoms (Cohen's $d=0.65$) and mania symptoms (Cohen's $d=0.79$) over 1 year.

TABLE 54–6. Studies of the use of psychoeducation in children's mental health (*continued*)

Study	Population	Design and sample	Active treatment protocol	Structure and duration	Outcomes
Bipolar disorders (*continued*)					
Pavuluri et al. 2004	Youth with early-onset bipolar spectrum disorder	Open study *N*=34 (mean age=11.3; 29% female)	Combination of psychoeducation, family-focused therapy, and CBT with pharmacotherapy	12 family sessions an hour in length	From pretest to posttest, children displayed reductions in symptom severity (*P*<.001) and increases in overall global functioning (*P*<.001). High levels of treatment adherence and satisfaction were also noted.
Depressive disorders					
Brent et al. 1993	Parents of adolescents with depressive disorder	Open study *N*=62	Psychoeducation	One 2-hour session	Improved knowledge from pretest to posttest (*P*<.001). Modification of dysfunctional beliefs about depression and its treatment.
Sanford et al. 2006	Adolescents ages 13–18 with major depressive disorder and their families	RCT Usual treatment control *N*=41 (mean age=15.9; 65% female)	Family psychoeducation and treatment as usual *vs.* treatment as usual	Twelve 90-minute family sessions in the home and 1 booster session at 3-month follow-up	Treatment group showed greater improvement in social functioning and adolescent-parent relationships from pretest to posttest than controls (*P*<.05, effect size >0.5). Parents reported greater treatment satisfaction than controls posttest (*P*<.01).
Disruptive behavior disorders					
Bradley et al. 2003	Parents of children ages 3–4 years who have trouble managing their child's behavior	RCT Waitlist control *N*=222 (mean age=3.8; 35% female)	Immediate multifamily psychoeducation based on the 1–2–3 Magic video *vs.* waitlist control	2-hour group meeting weekly for 3 weeks with booster session 4 weeks later	Improvement in parenting practices (*P*<.001) and child behavior from pretest to posttest compared to control group (*P*<.05).

TABLE 54–6. Studies of the use of psychoeducation in children's mental health *(continued)*

Study	Population	Design and sample	Active treatment protocol	Structure and duration	Outcomes
Disruptive behavior disorders *(continued)*					
Smith et al. 2006	93 parents and 102 adolescents with substance abuse and behavior disorder	Open study N=93 parents and 102 adolescents	Psychoeducation vs. control group	2-hour meeting weekly for 3 weeks with a booster session 4 weeks after	Substance abuse declined (P<.001); 85% did not relapse over the course of an entire year posttreatment.
Eating disorders					
Geist et al. 2000	Females ages 12–17 years with anorexia nervosa and their families	RCT Alternative treatment control N=25 (mean age=14.3; 100% female)	Family therapy vs. multifamily psychoeducation	8 total sessions every 2 weeks over 4 months	No significant differences between groups. Significant time effect found for both treatment groups for restoration of body weight (P<.001).
Holtkamp et al. 2005	Parents of adolescents in treatment for eating disorders	Open study N=153 (mean age=15.3)	Multifamily psychoeducation	Five 90-minute group sessions	Rated psychoeducation as helpful in coping with child's disorder and would recommend to others.
Psychosis					
Klaus et al. 2008	10-year-old boy with schizoaffective disorder and his parents	Case study	Adjunctive multifamily psychoeducational psychotherapy	8 sessions, 90 minutes in length	Improved mood symptoms, utilization of services, and social functioning.

TABLE 54–6. Studies of the use of psychoeducation in children's mental health *(continued)*

Study	Population	Design and sample	Active treatment protocol	Structure and duration	Outcomes
Serious emotional and behavioral disturbances in general					
Davidson and Fristad 2004	Families of children with mental illness	Open study $N=46$	Multifamily psychoeducation	8-week class led by other family members	Parents reported lower stress in relationships ($P=.02$), improved mental health ($P=.04$), more compliance with child's chores ($P=.04$), fewer child's self-harming acts ($P<.01$), and fewer public rages ($P=.01$) from pretest to posttest.
Ruffolo et al. 2005	Parents of children with serious emotional disturbance	RCT Usual treatment control $N=94$ (mean age=11.5; 25% female)	Multifamily psychoeducation and intensive case management vs. intensive case management	Open group format, 2-hour meetings twice a month	No statistically significant differences between groups in social support; behavior improved in both groups.
Pollio et al. 2005	Families of children receiving school social work services or related services	Open study $N=15$	Multifamily psychoeducation	Eight 90-minute sessions twice monthly or twelve 90-minute sessions weekly	High level of participation, satisfaction with the group experience.

Note. RCT=randomized controlled trial.

TABLE 54–7.   Weekly topic schedule for multifamily psychoeducational psychotherapy

Parents	Children
1. Welcome and overview of group and mood disorders	1. Welcome and overview of group and mood disorders
2. Medications	2. Medications
3. Systems of care	3. Symptom management techniques
4. Mood disorders and family life	4. Connection of thoughts, feelings, actions
5. Problem-solving skills	5. Problem-solving skills
6. Communication	6. Nonverbal communication
7. Symptom management techniques	7. Verbal communication
8. Review and graduate	8. Review and graduate

Source.   Adapted from Fristad et al. (2003b).

with emotional or behavioral disorders showed that 72% of respondents found emotional support to be the most helpful aspect of family support services (Friesen and Koroloff 1990). Approximately 70% of Americans suffering from mental disorders rely solely on self- and mutual-help options rather than specialized mental health care (Norcross 2000).

History of Parent Support Groups

During the 1970s and 1980s, the mental health recovery movement led to a boom in support groups and other consumer-led efforts to help individuals with mental illness and to promote change in the whole mental health system (Frese and Davis 1997). The recovery movement emerged as former patients and other advocates gathered together to protest issues such as involuntary hospitalization and the state of mental health treatment. The central philosophy was that individuals

TABLE 54–8.   Core psychoeducation content areas

Types of disorders and symptoms
Medication and side effects
Cognitive restructuring
Behavioral activation
Problem-solving skills
Relapse prevention
Daily routines
Communication skills
Social functioning
Treatment and services

with mental illness can and do recover. A key component in the recovery process is being around other people who offer hope, understanding, and support and who encourage self-determination and self-actualization (Carpenter 2002; Frese and Davis 1997). This emphasis on the importance of mutual help led to a growth in support groups and self-help programs. Now support groups exist for almost every problem or illness that has been identified in adults and children. Groups are held for individuals experiencing mental illness themselves and for family members and caregivers of adults or children with serious emotional or behavioral disorders.

Theoretical Background of Parent Support Groups

The theoretical assumption behind parent support groups is that parents need the opportunity to discuss their situation with other parents who have had similar experiences and therefore can understand what they are going through. These groups provide members with knowledge, support, and an outlet for their feelings. Two basic helping processes occur among support group members: giving help and support and receiving help and support (Roberts et al. 1999). Providing help to other group members allows participants to feel they have strengths to offer others, thus enhancing feelings of competence and usefulness. Help received can be in the form of knowledge and support, helping parents to be better prepared to manage their child's illness. Other key components include imparting information, group cohesiveness, universality of the problem, identification with others, altruism, catharsis, instillation of hope, interper-

TABLE 54–9. Potential psychoeducation adaptations by disorder

Disorder	Adaptation	Rationale for adaptations
Attention-deficit/ hyperactivity disorder	Share information with the school. Include tips to improve organizational skills, time management, and study skills.	Much impairment occurs at school. These skills are most often lacking.
Disruptive behavior disorders	Train parents in discipline strategies. Discuss and develop behavior contracts.	Parents often use inadequate methods to discipline these children. Discuss and implement limits on behavior to help youth understand what is acceptable.
Eating disorders	Include nutrition education and monitoring. Include weight monitoring.	Help youth and parents understand healthy eating patterns. Help monitor progress in weight normalization and potential relapses.
Mood disorders	Assess and treat parents for mood disorders. Use mood charts to monitor mood changes. Include pharmacotherapy as treatment component.	Parents of youth with mood disorders frequently have mood disorders as well, which makes parenting more challenging. Mood charts help to clarify the circumstances associated with mood changes. Pharmacotherapy is an important part of decreasing symptoms.
Posttraumatic stress disorder	Assess and treat parents for their own trauma response. Redefine (when appropriate) acting out behavior as a response to the trauma.	Parents have often experienced the same trauma. Correct attributions may assist the parents to empathically address difficult behavior.

sonal learning, self-understanding, adoption of an ideological framework, and advocacy (Citron et al. 1999). Of course, these components may not occur within every support group or for every member.

The impact of a support group is determined by the specific group environment and the process the group goes through together. The process may differ slightly depending on whether the group is time limited or open-ended. Time-limited groups occur for a set number of sessions and typically have the same members for the duration. Revolving open-ended groups are continuous, with members joining and leaving the group freely. In professionally led support groups, four phases of group process have been identified: exchanging information, developing intimacy, solidifying relationships, and terminating (Shulman 1992). Groups begin by superficially exchanging information; slowly they become more intimate as more personal information and experiences are shared. As members become more intimate, the relationships between members become stronger, so that sharing and advice become more profound. In revolving open-

ended groups, individual group members episodically terminate as new members join and the process repeats itself.

Description of Parent Support Groups

Support groups are typically affiliated or linked with social agencies, larger formal organizations, or consumer organizations—for example, community mental health agencies, a local National Alliance on Mental Illness (NAMI) chapter, a hospital, or a residential facility. The affiliation often provides the groups with financial and professional support, resources, recognition, and legitimacy, as well as referral of new members. Mental health professionals or agencies are the most common referral sources for family support groups (Heller et al. 1997).

Support groups for parents of children with emotional disorders can vary greatly in membership, format, and longevity (Koroloff and Friesen 1991).

TABLE 54–10. Examples of techniques used in psychoeducation

Psychoeducational techniques	Description of technique
Bibliotherapy	Using written materials, video, or Web sites to further educate families about mental illness.
Daily routine tracking	Tracking daily routines such as sleep-wake cycles, eating, and other daily activities to determine their effect on mood and behavior.
Mood chart	Tracking changes in mood, when they occur, and the circumstances that happen around the time of the changes.
Naming the enemy[a]	Helping the child and parents determine the difference between the child's symptoms and his or her own personality.
Thinking, feeling, doing[a]	Increasing insight of parents and child into the connections among their thoughts, feelings, and behavior.
Tool kit[a]	Develop a variety of pleasant or relaxing activities for the child to use in affect regulation.

[a]Techniques used in multifamily psychoeducational psychotherapy.

Groups can be professionally led and sponsored by a specific agency or can be completely consumer driven. Regardless of who leads the group, the support group facilitator has several roles to fulfill for the group to be successful. Table 54–12 outlines the role of a support group facilitator. Common issues the facilitator must handle during a support group include most of those listed in Table 54–11 for psychoeducation groups. One of the most difficult tasks is moderating parental sharing during discussion, especially to make sure other group members are not overwhelmed. In regard to such sharing, problems could arise in several ways: 1) members' reluctance to share enough to allow an appropriate response or to fit in as one of the group (playing observer role too long); 2) members sharing too much and scaring others or inducing guilt that they "do not have it so bad"; 3) members developing a "more unfortunate than thou" contest; and 4) members sharing successes to the extent that others feel inferior. Note that these are problems of quantity, not quality, and can be moderated or titrated by an assertive group leader. For example, in the first situation, the leader could comment that it seems difficult for that parent to talk about family problems and ask a more forthcoming group member to describe how hard it was to begin sharing. Additional group members could then be encouraged to comment on the topic of how hard it is to begin opening up.

Regardless of the type of support group, facilitators generally follow the same meeting format. The facilitator starts the meeting by introducing himself or herself and describing the purpose and expectations of the group. Group guidelines are then outlined and in-clude confidentiality, accepting other members, and being nonjudgmental. Then all present may introduce themselves for the benefit of new members. Next, the meeting core begins with either open discussion or individual extended turns. The meeting's discussion topic may be decided by the members, or there may be a predetermined topic for the session. The meeting is concluded with a summary of the discussion and a reminder of the next meeting date.

Internet support groups have recently emerged as another option for parents in need of support and information. They are often available on the Web sites of disorder-specific organizations (Table 54–13). A survey of caregivers of children with early-onset bipolar disorder reported that the main advantage of online support groups is convenience (Hellander et al. 2003). Groups are always available; parents can go online in their homes and receive immediate information and support. Additionally, some parents indicated that the anonymity of online interaction was more comfortable than face-to-face interaction.

Regardless of format, common problems with parent support groups are frequent dropouts and low membership, which can threaten the group's longevity. Common reasons for dropouts include not having enough time to attend, no longer finding the group helpful, having problems with transportation and parking, experiencing inadequate leadership, and lacking comfort with other members (Heller et al. 1997). Ironically, children in crisis can also prevent parents from attending support groups. These challenges must all be considered and addressed by group facilitators in order for a parent support group to thrive.

TABLE 54–11. Complications frequently faced by parent group and support group leaders

Complications	Possible responses, solutions, and alternatives
Arguing among members	Restate ground rules. Comment on strong feelings behind the opinions and point out potential learning experience for group if the reasons could be shared. Invite members to share why they have such strong feelings on the topic.
Crying	Empathize and encourage others to empathize. Offer tissues. Reflect their pain. Remind the group that one purpose of the group is to share such experiences.
Discussion of inappropriate topics	Change the topic. Remind group of its purpose and the ground rules. Ask if everyone feels comfortable with topic.
Discussion shifts away from scheduled topic	Restate topic. Ask group if they want to continue with diversionary topic or return to scheduled topic. Find connection between diversionary topic and scheduled topic.
Incomplete homework	Reassign. Complete as a group. Explore reasons not completed.
Late arrival	Ignore and continue discussion. Reintroduce everyone. Recap what has been discussed. Restate topic of discussion.
Nonparticipation	Invite the nonparticipant to comment on another member's comment. Suggest each parent share his or her story for 2 minutes.
Not enough time to cover topic	Ask if group wants to stay longer. Finish at following meeting. Adapt homework assignment if topic not finished.
Only one family attends group	Proceed the same, following the manual. Adapt to individual family psychoeducation for one session. Explore family's feelings about being the only family.
One parent dominates discussion	Set limits. Take turns for a set amount of time. Remind group of time. Thank parent for sharing and ask if others would also like to share.
Silence	Empathize with difficulty talking about the problems. Provide anecdote to start discussion. Use humor to break the ice. Suggest each parent share his or her story for 2 minutes.

Benefits of Parent Support Groups

Parent support groups can lead to positive outcomes in three ways. First, interaction with other parents of children with mental illness can be informative, relieving, and therapeutic. Through this interactive process, friendships and social connections form that can help improve parental mental health (Humphreys 1997).

Connecting with other parents helps parents realize they are not alone and allows them to share and compare experiences.

Second, the interaction of parents with differing levels of knowledge and experience with their child's mental illness provides a forum for knowledge and skill building. Parents can learn from each others' experiences with managing their children's symptoms, seeking services, and juggling responsibilities. One study found that parents who were involved in sup-

TABLE 54–12. Role and tasks of a support group facilitator

Manage logistics: Secure meeting location, set meeting date, arrange for food, remind members of dates.

Promote the group: Raise awareness in the community about the group; increase membership.

Moderate member sharing during the meeting: Ensure all members have an opportunity to share and no one monopolizes the discussion.

Listen: Be an attentive and empathic listener for all members.

Assess when members may need more help: Recognize members who need more help than the group can provide.

Create a safe environment: Ensure members do not feel threatened or uncomfortable sharing; stress confidentiality.

Refer members to resources: Have knowledge about local resources to refer members.

port groups reported more utilization of information and services than did parents not involved in support groups (Koroloff and Friesen 1991).

Third, parent support groups can help families develop effective advocacy skills and become more active in advocacy efforts (Humphreys 1997). Besides advocating for their own child, parents often become involved in advocating for better overall services at the community, state, or national level for all children with mental illness. As a result of these three benefits of support groups, parents are likely to be more comfortable in their roles as caregiver and case manager for their mentally ill child.

Research on Parent Support Groups for Children's Mental Health

Little research has been conducted on the effects of support group membership on parents of children with serious emotional or behavioral disturbances. Research on these parent support groups is difficult because of continually changing membership, inability to assign members in an experimental design, and difficulty accessing groups (King et al. 2000). Below are summaries of a few studies:

- One study explored the experience of implementing a parent support group in a children's inpatient hospitalization setting (Slowik et al. 2004). This open group met for 1 hour every 2 weeks for 9 months during the family visiting time. Each group meeting had three to seven members in attendance. Many discussion themes emerged in the groups, including the effects of the hospitalization on parents and siblings, relationships with and attitudes toward professionals, positive coping strategies, and the effects

and usefulness of the group. As a result of attending the group, parents felt less isolated and began to support each other and not rely exclusively on the experts. Parents also felt the doctors were more approachable at the group meetings. Doctors found it beneficial to interact with family members in a less formal setting and often learned more about the parents' experiences. Unit staff had to address several difficulties in setting up and running the group, including opposition from other staff, timing of the group, and engaging and maintaining a sufficient number of parents.

- In residential treatment, a parent support and education group was developed to provide parents with opportunities for support, learning new parenting skills, and improving their relationships with their children (Modlin 2003). Ten weekly meetings were held, with topics predetermined by staff to reflect the group members' needs. Parents indicated they had gained knowledge and support from participating. Success of the group led to its incorporation as a regular component of available services.

- Focusing on structure and organization rather than outcomes, a qualitative study conducted interviews and observed support groups to learn more about support groups for parents of children with special needs (King et al. 2000). Interviews were conducted with 20 parents, and six group meetings were observed. The researchers sought to understand the organizational characteristics and issues that affect the maintenance of self-help groups. The study found that challenges for groups include encouraging new leaders, attracting new members, obtaining funds or assistance to support their activities, and meeting the changing needs of members. Characteristics associated with group longevity included committed and effective leadership, community connections providing needed funds and

TABLE 54–13. Support groups and Internet resources

Organizations

American Self-Help Group Clearinghouse: Self-Help Group Sourcebook Online—
  http://mentalhelp.net/selfhelp

Anxiety Disorders Association of America (ADAA)—www.adaa.org

Autism Society of America (ASA)—www.autism-society.org

Child and Adolescent Bipolar Foundation (CABF)—www.bpkids.org

Children and Adults With Attention-Deficit/Hyperactivity Disorder (CHADD)—www.chadd.org

Depression and Bipolar Support Alliance (DBSA)—www.ndmda.org

Learning Disability Association of America (LDA)—www.ldaamerica.org

Mental Health America (MHA)—www.nmha.org

National Alliance on Mental Illness (NAMI)—www.nami.org

National Institute of Mental Health (NIMH)—www.nimh.nih.gov

Substance Abuse and Mental Health Services Administration (SAMHSA)—www.samhsa.gov

Publications

Kurtz LF: *Self-Help and Support Groups: A Handbook for Practitioners.* Thousand Oaks, CA, Sage, 1997

Nichols K, Jenkinson J: *Leading a Support Group: A Practical Guide.* New York, Open University Press, 2006

Schiff HS: *The Support Group Manual: A Session-by-Session Guide.* New York, Penguin, 1996

practical assistance, and group members' willingness to change the group to meet changing needs.

Research to date has been conducted in restrictive settings such as hospitals and residential placements, as groups in these settings are more readily accessible. Little research is available on support groups with a self-help format run by members, most likely due to the difficulty in accessing these groups. However, the studies described here do reveal that parents felt more knowledgeable and supported and less stressed following participation in parent support groups. Several studies examined support groups that incorporated education into their programs; therefore, it is difficult to separate out the unique benefit of the support, per se. As with the studies on psychoeducation, we see that the combination of support and education can be a powerful tool for parents of children with mental illness.

Research Directions

A summary of research on psychoeducation and parent support groups reveals that the literature on these interventions is promising but that several areas still emerge as directions for future research. The application of psychoeducation for families of children with mental illness has spread to various disorders, but there are still disorders for which its use has not been

fully explored, such as anxiety disorders. Also, many studies to date are exploratory. More randomized controlled trials must be conducted to determine treatment efficacy. The psychoeducation programs in Table 54–6 used a variety of formats, but little is known about how these various formats compare to each other. For example, research comparing individual family psychoeducation to multifamily psychoeducation for children's mental health would be an interesting and beneficial line of future research.

Research on parent support groups is less developed than that for psychoeducation. Researchers need to explore novel ways to access and study parent support groups in various settings and for various disorders. Once access is established, more studies are needed to determine the impact of professional and member-led parent support groups on parent and child outcomes. As use of the Internet continues to increase exponentially, research on the impact of Internet support groups will also be important.

Conclusion

Parent counseling, psychoeducation, and parent support groups all provide parents with support from professionals or from other parents in similar situations. These interventions aim to educate parents about their children's mental illness and how to manage and treat it. All these approaches view parents as essential to child outcomes and recognize parents as experts on their own family. Additionally, they encourage parents to take care of their own health to better help their child. Overall, these parent interventions focus on improving the mental health of children by focusing on the knowledge, beliefs, and behaviors of the parents. Together, these parent approaches paired with other treatment such as medication, psychotherapy, and school services can help to decrease the negative impact of symptoms and improve the quality of life for children and adolescents suffering from mental illness.

Summary Points

- Parent intervention is as important as child intervention because parents are responsible for recognizing and addressing their child's needs.

- Parent counseling and psychoeducation are adjunctive educational interventions aimed at providing parents with the knowledge and skills needed to be effective caregivers and case managers for their child with emotional or behavioral disorders.

- Parent support groups provide parents the opportunity to interact with and receive informational and emotional support from other parents in similar situations.

- Research on parent psychoeducation has been promising, with positive parent and child outcomes, but more randomized controlled studies are needed.

- Most research on parent support groups has occurred in restrictive placements such as hospitals and residential care. Studies have tentatively demonstrated that a combination of support and education can lead to positive outcomes for children in these settings. More research is needed on support groups in other settings.

- Parent interventions should be combined with other family or child-focused interventions—such as family therapy, individual therapy, medication, and school services—to systemically address the symptoms and impairment caused by the child's disorder.

References

Anderson CM, Hogarty GE, Reiss D: Family treatment of adult schizophrenic patients: a psychoeducational approach. Schizophr Bull 6:490–505, 1980

Arnold LE (ed): Helping Parents Help Their Children. New York, Brunner/Mazel, 1978

Asarnow JR, Goldstein MJ, Tompson M, et al: One-year outcomes of depressive disorders in child psychiatric inpatients: evaluation of the prognostic power of a brief measure of expressed emotion. J Child Psychol Psychiatry 34:129–137, 1993

Bennett T, DeLuca DA, Allen RW: Families of children with disabilities: positive adaptation across the life cycle. Soc Work Educ 18:31–44, 1996

Bradley SJ, Jadaa DA, Brody J, et al: Brief psychoeducational parenting program: an evaluation and 1-year follow-up. J Am Acad Child Adolesc Psychiatry 42:1171–1178, 2003

Brent DA, Poling K, McKain B, et al: A psychoeducational program for families of affectively ill children and adolescents. J Am Acad Child Adolesc Psychiatry 32:770–774, 1993

Brown GW, Birley JL, Wing JK: Influence of family life on the course of schizophrenic disorders: a replication. Br J Psychiatry 121:241–258, 1972

Brown NW: Psycho-Educational Groups. Philadelphia, PA, Accelerated Development, 1998

Butzlaff RL, Hooley JM: Expressed emotion and psychiatric relapse. Arch Gen Psychiatry 55:547–552, 1998

Carpenter M: "It's a small world": mental health policy under welfare capitalism since 1945. Sociol Health Illn 22:602–620, 2002

Citron M, Solomon P, Draine J: Self-help groups for families of persons with mental illness: perceived benefits of helpfulness. Community Ment Health J 35:15–30, 1999

Copping VE, Warling DL, Benner DG, et al: A child trauma treatment pilot study. J Child Fam Stud 10:467–475, 2001

Davidson KH, Fristad MA: The Hand-to-Family Education Program: a means of reducing parental stress and increasing support in families of children with brain disorders. Child and Adolescent Psychopharmacology News 9:7–9, 2004

Frese FJ, Davis WW: The consumer-survivor movement, recovery, and consumer professionals. Prof Psychol Res Pr 28:243–245, 1997

Friesen BJ, Koroloff NM: Family centered services: implications for mental health administration and research. J Ment Health Adm 17:13–25, 1990

Fristad MA: Psychoeducational treatment for school-aged children with bipolar disorder. Dev Psychopathol 18:1289–1306, 2006

Fristad MA, Gavazzi SM, Centolella DM, et al: Psychoeducation: a promising intervention strategy for families of children and adolescents with mood disorders. Contemporary Family Therapy: An International Journal 18:371–384, 1996

Fristad MA, Gavazzi SM, Soldano KW: Naming the enemy: Learning to differentiate mood disorder "symptoms" from the "self" that experiences them. J Fam Psychother 10:81–88, 1999

Fristad MA, Goldberg-Arnold JS, Gavazzi SM: Multifamily psychoeducation groups (MFPG) for families of children with bipolar disorder. Bipolar Disord 4:254–262, 2002

Fristad MA, Gavazzi SM, Mackinaw-Koons B: Family psychoeducation: an adjunctive intervention for children with bipolar disorder. Biol Psychiatry 53:1000–1008, 2003a

Fristad MA, Goldberg-Arnold JS, Gavazzi SM: Multifamily psychoeducation groups in the treatment of children with mood disorders. J Marital Fam Ther 29:491–504, 2003b

Fristad MA, Verducci JS, Walters K, et al: The impact of Multi-Family Psychoeducational Psychotherapy in treating children aged 8–12 with mood disorders. Arch Gen Psychiatry, in press

Geist R, Heinmaa M, Stephens D, et al: Comparison of family therapy and family group psychoeducation in adolescents with anorexia nervosa. Can J Psychiatry 45:173–178, 2000

Goldberg-Arnold JS, Fristad MA, Gavazzi SM: Family psychoeducation: giving caregivers what they want and need. Fam Relat 48:411–417, 1999

Goldstein MJ, Rodnick EH, Evans JR, et al: Drug and family therapy in the aftercare of acute schizophrenia. Arch Gen Psychiatry 35:1169–1177, 1978

Hellander M, Sisson DP, Fristad MA: Internet support for parents of children with early onset bipolar disorder, in Bipolar Disorder in Childhood and Early Adolescence. Edited by Geller B, DelBello M. New York, Guilford, 2003, pp 314–329

Heller T, Roccoforte JA, Hsieh KF, et al: Support groups for families of persons with mental illness: group benefits. Am J Orthopsychiatry 67:187–198, 1997

Holtkamp K, Herpertz-Dahlmann B, Vloet T, et al: Group psychoeducation for parents of adolescents with eating disorders: the Achen Program. Eat Disord 13:381–390, 2005

Hooley JM: Expressed emotion and psychiatric illness: from empirical data to clinical practice. Behav Ther 29:631–646, 1998

Humphreys K: Individual and social benefits of mutual aid self-help groups. Social Policy 27:12–19, 1997

King G, Stewart D, King S, et al: Organizational characteristics and issues affecting the longevity of self-help groups for parents of children with special needs. Qual Health Res 10:225–241, 2000

Klaus N, Fristad MA, Malkin C, et al: Psychosocial family treatment for a ten-year-old with schizoaffective disorder. Cogn Behav Pract 15:76–84, 2008

Koroloff NM, Friesen BJ: Support groups for parents of children with emotional disorders: a comparison of members and nonmembers. Community Ment Health J 27:265–279, 1991

Lofthouse N, Fristad MA: Psychosocial interventions for children with early onset bipolar spectrum disorder. Clin Child Fam Psychol Rev 7:71–88, 2004

Lopez MA, Toprac MG, Crismon ML, et al: A psychoeducational program for children with ADHD or depression and their families: results from the CMAP feasibility study. Community Ment Health J 41:51–66, 2005

Lukens EP, McFarlane WR: Psychoeducation as evidence-based practice: considerations for practice, research, and policy. Brief Treat Crisis Interv 4:205–225, 2004

Madara EJ: The mutual-aid self-help online revolution. Social Policy 27:20–26, 1997

McFarlane WR, Link B, Dushay R, et al: Psychoeducational multiple family groups: four-year relapse outcome in schizophrenia. Fam Process 34:127–144, 1995

Mendenhall AN, Fristad MA, Early TJ: Factors influencing service utilization and mood symptom severity in children with mood disorders: effects of multifamily psychoeducation groups (MFPGs). J Consult Clin Psychol 77:463–473, 2009

Miklowitz DJ, Goldstein MJ: The effectiveness of psychoeducation family therapy in the treatment of schizophrenic disorders. J Marital Fam Ther 21:361–376, 1995

Miklowitz DJ, George EL, Axelson DA, et al: Family focused treatment for adolescents with bipolar disorder. J Affect Disord 82(suppl):S113–S128, 2004

Modlin H: The development of a parent support group as a means of initiating family involvement in a residential program. Child and Youth Services 25:169–190, 2003

Norcross JC: Here comes the self-help revolution in mental health. Psychotherapy 37:370–377, 2000

Pavuluri MN, Graczyk PA, Henry DB, et al: Child- and family-focused cognitive-behavioral therapy for pediatric bipolar disorder: development and preliminary results. J Am Acad Child Adolesc Psychiatry 43:528–537, 2004

Pollio DE, McClendon JB, North CS, et al: The promise of school-based psychoeducation for parents of children with emotional disorders. Children and Schools 27:111–115, 2005

President's New Freedom Commission on Mental Health: Achieving the Promise: Transforming Mental Health Care in America. Rockville, MD, President's New Freedom Commission on Mental Health, 2003

Roberts LJ, Salem D, Rappaport J, et al: Giving and receiving help: Interpersonal transactions in mutual-help meetings and psychosocial adjustment of members. Am J Community Psychol 27:841–868, 1999

Ruffolo MC, Kuhn MT, Evans ME: Support, empowerment, and education: a study of multifamily group psychoeducation. J Emot Behav Disord 13:200–212, 2005

Sanford M, Boyle M, McCleary L, et al: A pilot study of adjunctive family psychoeducation in adolescent major depression: feasibility and treatment effect. J Am Acad Child Adolesc Psychiatry 45:386–395, 2006

Shulman L: The Skills of Helping: Individuals, Families, and Groups. Itasca, IL, FE Peacock, 1992

Sloper P: Models of service support for parents of disabled children: what do we know? Child Care Health Dev 25:85–99, 1999

Slowik M, Willson SW, Loh EC, et al: Service innovations: developing a parent/carer support group in an in-patient adolescent setting. Psychiatr Bull 28:177–179, 2004

Smith TE, Sells SP, Rodman J, et al: Reducing adolescent substance abuse and delinquency: pilot research of a family orientated psychoeducation curriculum. J Child Adolesc Subst Abuse 15:105–115, 2006

Chapter 55

Behavioral Parent Training

Linda J. Pfiffner, Ph.D.
Nina M. Kaiser, Ph.D.

Theoretical Underpinnings and Key Concepts

Behavior therapy has a long history of success in treating childhood problems. This approach is based on several core assumptions that highlight methodological rigor, empirical evaluation, a focus on observable behaviors as the most beneficial targets of intervention, and the importance of behavioral assessment in both design and ongoing evaluation of treatment plans. Behavior therapy approaches emphasize the importance of environmental and social contingencies in fostering and maintaining problem behavior—i.e., *contingency theory* (Patterson 1982). Contingency-based behavioral interventions involve one or more of four key concepts: Behavior is increased either by following it with something desirable (*positive reinforce-*

ment) or by removing something undesirable (*negative reinforcement*); behavior is decreased either by following it with something undesirable (*punishment*) or by removing something desirable (*extinction*). Current behavioral treatments also draw from social learning theory (Bandura 1977), which incorporates contingency theory into a more general model that also includes modeling and imitation and cognitive factors (e.g., cognitive appraisals and attributions).

Behavioral interventions usually begin with a *functional behavior analysis*, which involves specifying behaviors (positive behaviors to increase or negative behaviors to decrease) and then identifying each behavior's antecedents (variables setting the stage for or preceding the behavior) and consequences (variables maintaining the behavior). Based on this analysis, specific strategies for modifying antecedents and consequences are selected for a behavioral intervention plan with the goal of reducing problem behavior and promoting desired behavior. Maximally effective behavioral interventions consider the function of the problem behavior when attempting to reduce it. For example, if a child exhibits disruptive behavior in order to gain parental attention, a behavioral intervention might teach the child to gain attention through more appropriate behavior and reinforce this appropriate behavior when it occurs. Generally, the behavioral approach to intervention selects target behaviors for treatment that cause impairment in daily living (e.g., academic, social behavior) rather than targeting diagnostic symptoms per se, although it is important to note that these interventions often do have powerful direct and indirect effects on diagnostic symptoms. A behavioral approach can be very effective in modifying behavior and improving overall adjustment, whatever the underlying disorder.

Behavior therapy has been applied to a wide variety of childhood problems and within multiple different settings. Our main focus in this chapter will be on behavioral parent training (BPT), one of the most widely used forms of behavior therapy for disruptive behavior problems (also variously referred to as parent management training, parent training, or behavioral family therapy). In this approach, the therapist teaches parents skills to improve the quality of family relationships, promote positive child behaviors, and decrease child deviant behaviors. We include information about core components of parent training as well as adjunctive interventions used to address problems at school, with peers, and in the family system.

Rationale for Using Parent Training With Disruptive Behavior Disorders

Parent training programs largely are based on theory and data showing that families with a child displaying behavior problems tend to exhibit dysfunctional parent-child interaction patterns. One prominent pattern, described by Patterson (1982), is referred to as the "coercive process" and specifies that families with children having behavior problems learn to control one another through negative reinforcement. More specifically, children exhibit negative behaviors to the parent and the parent responds aversively to this behavior; this type of response from the parent in turn leads to an escalation of the child's negative behavior and so on until either the parent or the child gives in to the demands of the other, thereby reinforcing the other's negative behavior. One example of this type of pattern might be a child learning that unwanted parental demands (e.g., to do chores or homework) might be withdrawn if he or she provides a counterattack (e.g., arguing, refusing, exhibiting high levels of negative affect). Alternatively, a parent who discovers that the child complies when the parent engages in yelling or other extremely aversive behavior is more likely to employ this type of behavior in the future. Observational studies of family interaction (Dishion et al. 1991; Patterson et al. 1992) show that disrupted family management skills, most notably parent discipline and monitoring, appear to be key factors in antisocial behavior development. Subsequent studies consistently have found that problematic parenting practices (e.g., overly negative and controlling and lacking in warmth and positive involvement) are strongly related to disruptive behavior disorders (Johnston and Mash 2001). The importance of maladaptive parenting practices in perpetuating disruptive behavior problems is underscored by findings that the adverse effects of contextual factors on children such as stress, social disadvantage, divorce, and/or parent depression largely are mediated by these practices (Patterson et al. 1992).

Parent training for families of children with disruptive behavior disorders (DBDs) also is supported by accumulating data that children with these problems show dysfunctional responses to usual contingencies that disrupt these children's ability to regulate behavior according to typical consequences (for a review, see Luman et al. 2005). More specifically, children with DBDs appear to display a lack of sensitivity to partial reinforcement (Douglas and Parry 1983), elevated reward thresholds (Haenlein and Caul 1986), a marked aversion to delays in reinforcement (Sonuga-Barke 2005), and less avoidance or caution to cues of punishment or nonreward because of a weak inhibition system (Quay 1997). Children with conduct disorder have been shown to have a reward-dominant style, in that their behavior is motivated more by the possibility of gaining a reward than avoidance of punishment (O'Brien and Frick 1996). Together, these findings suggest that the families of children with DBDs are likely to benefit from parent training precisely because of this approach's focus on modification of external contingencies such as use of consistent, salient, and immediate rewards; well-delivered negative consequences; clear rules and directions; and predictable routines.

Parent training programs also can address attachment deficiencies between children and their parents. Lower levels of attachment are theorized to lead to emotional dysregulation and a lack of mutual responsiveness between parent and child (Harwood and Eyberg 2004; Herschell et al. 2002). Parent training addresses these emotional factors by fostering responsiveness, communication, and nurturance between parent and child. These processes in turn enable the child to develop secure attachments with others and improved emotional regulation.

Models of Parent Training

All models for delivering parent training involve a therapist working with parents to teach a variety of behavioral strategies; the parents then apply these strategies at home. Troubleshooting the use of each strategy occurs within the context of each individual family during each therapy session. Parent training may be offered in combination with behavioral school consultation and/or with child-focused interventions, such as skill-building groups or cognitive-behavioral interventions.

Parent training can be administered individually with parents, with families (parents and children together), or in groups of parents. The group format may be especially useful for parents who would benefit from receiving support from and/or sharing ideas with other parents. Reluctant parents often become more open to using a strategy after hearing firsthand about the success another parent has had with that particular strategy. However, not all parents benefit equally from a group experience. Groups seem to be most useful when members share very similar problems. Working with the individual family is indicated when more intensive and tailored interventions are needed; this may be the case when there are very severe child problems, for parents who have interpersonal styles that would be difficult for a group, or when a slower pace is desirable. In some cases, individual sessions interspersed with the group meetings are helpful.

Parent training is intended to be time limited. The number of sessions typically varies from 6 to 12 weeks, with some programs lasting as long as 20–25 weeks; duration generally depends on the severity of the problems and developmental level of the child (Forehand and McMahon 1981; Kazdin 1997; MTA Cooperative Group 1999; Webster-Stratton et al. 2004; Wells 2007). During sessions, the therapist presents specific strategies, discusses their rationale, has parents practice the skills (e.g., via role-plays), and instructs parents to implement the skills at home with their child

between sessions. If therapists opt to have parents practice skills in vivo with their child(ren), parents can be observed and coached by having the parents wear a "bug-in-the-ear" (wireless ear piece with radio transmission) while the therapist is behind a one-way mirror; alternatively, in-room coaching can be effective with young children. Programs in which parents observe videotaped examples of effective and ineffective parenting strategies with opportunity for discussion of the strategies also have substantial research support for efficacy (Webster-Stratton et al. 2004).

Baseline Assessments Prior to Starting Treatment

Initial assessments typically include the usual diagnostic work-up and gathering of information about functional impairment at home, at school, and with peers. This information ideally is obtained from the child's parents and teachers using a combination of empirically based and standardized rating scales, as well as more qualitative measures, including direct observation of the family interactions or school functioning (if possible). However, it is important to emphasize that behavioral forms of treatment are guided more by functional analysis of behavior and less by a diagnosis or symptoms per se. Therefore, parents typically are asked questions at the initiation of parent training about the frequency and specific types of behaviors of concern, as well as the antecedents (e.g., when they occur) and consequences (e.g., what happens after they occur) of each problem behavior. Parents often keep a chart of these behaviors during the first week or two prior to starting a behavior plan, and this chart then can serve as a baseline for comparison after specific strategies are implemented in order to determine if the program is having its intended effect. Assessment of target behaviors continues throughout behavioral treatment as an important guide to decision making about which strategies are most effective for each family.

Setting Treatment Goals

In behavioral approaches, setting goals for treatment is an individualized and collaborative process between parent and therapist. Usually, the parent's initial goal simply involves modifying the child's behavior. However, in parent training, treatment goals include the parents changing their own behavior. Although this goal does not always need to be explicitly stated, some discussion of this issue usually is helpful. It is important that the therapist communicates to the parents that they are not being blamed for their child's difficulties. Instead, parents are told that children's difficulties are multiply determined (including biological and environmental factors) and that children with behavioral challenges are more difficult to parent. The goal is to find the best "fit" between their child's personality and their parenting practices. We often tell parents of children having behavioral concerns that there is a need to become "superparents," providing a structured "superenvironment" that is more demanding than what average parents need to manage their children.

Initial treatment goals are set at levels that ensure that both the child and the parent experience some success at the outset (and consequently are motivated to continue). Thus, initial target behaviors and parenting strategies taught are relatively simple and easy to change (e.g., positive attention during nonconfrontational situations; compliance with nonprovocative commands). At treatment onset, parents typically are encouraged to target only one or two behaviors for change. A shaping process then is used so that as initial goals are reached, more difficult or complex behaviors and skills are added. Behaviors important to the child's family, social, and academic functioning generally are included as primary goals (e.g., following directions the first time asked, completing chores, completing homework, playing well with siblings), and both prosocial and antisocial behaviors are included. After parents have obtained some success with home-based targets, treatment goals may be expanded to incorporate problem behavior outside the home or with other adults.

Core Session Topics

Although a number of different approaches to parent training exist, all approaches generally involve some combination of the core topics we describe in Appendix 55–1 at the end of this chapter. Different approaches vary somewhat in the session time that is allocated to each topic, the order in which topics are presented, and/or supplemental topics that are also covered by the treatment package. In addition, we note that different clinicians may pick and choose specific topics to be

covered based on differences in the problems with which a given child and family present. For example, we have found that parents of children who are particularly impulsive or oppositional tend to need more instruction on effective discipline than do parents of children with mostly attentional problems. For each topic, we discuss and troubleshoot common parental concerns and questions.

Please note that we intend our descriptions of session topics to serve as an educational overview of each topic rather than step-by-step instructions. We reference a variety of excellent treatment manuals throughout this chapter that provide more explicit information on conducting BPT, and we encourage those interested in implementing this type of intervention to consult these manuals for further guidance.

Psychoeducation/ Background Information
Overview

The first session of BPT generally involves providing parents with background information and psychoeducation regarding childhood behavior problems, family interactions, and behavior therapy (see Appendix 55–1). In addition, parents are introduced to the Antecedent-Behavior-Consequence (A-B-C) model of behavior that sets the framework for all topics presented later.

Troubleshooting

As mentioned earlier, one question that often arises relates to why parents (as opposed to the child) participate in treatment, as the child is the identified patient. In response to these concerns, therapists typically acknowledge that the temperaments of children with externalizing problems make these children more difficult to parent; consequently, parent training is presented as a way for parents to obtain additional strategies for their parenting toolboxes that will help them more effectively manage their child's behavior.

Attending and Ignoring
Overview

The focus of this session is on improving the parent-child relationship, under the assumption that 1) this relationship has been negatively affected by negative parent-child interaction cycles and 2) children are more likely to comply with parental instructions in the context of a positive parent-child relationship. Parents thus are taught to spend "special time" with their child during which they actively attend to their child's behavior (see Appendix 55–1). After parents master this skill, they learn to generalize the attending skill and differentially attend to positive behaviors they would like to see increase and ignore negative behaviors that they aim to decrease.

Troubleshooting

During discussion of attending and ignoring, parents may raise the following concerns:

- *Why shouldn't I ask questions, praise my child, or be directive during special time?*

    Parents are encouraged to let the child direct the activity to the greatest extent possible in order for the child to feel that the activity is most pleasant and validating. Asking questions, praising, and redirecting the child all are subtle ways of controlling the situation and consequently are to be avoided during the attending/special time exercise.

- *How should I deal with misbehavior?*

    Parents are encouraged to ignore mild misbehavior during special time. Obviously, however, it is inappropriate to ignore behaviors that are unsafe, and parents should employ their usual system of consequences to cope with any such behaviors that occur.

- *How will I find time? What about my other kids?*

    Parents are encouraged to practice attending even if the special time lasts only for brief periods of time (5–10 minutes) or in the context of an activity that the child already is doing. Often, looking for opportunities to practice attending (rather than scheduling attending as a separate event) feels more manageable to parents. Parents with multiple children may find that all children are eager to have parents do attending with them; if this is the case, parents may choose to do special time with one child on one day and another child the next day.

- *I'm ignoring, but my child's behavior is getting worse!*

    It is important to warn parents that with ignoring, behaviors generally get worse before they get better; because the child often escalates in an attempt to obtain the parents' attention, the most unbearable behavior often occurs immediately before the child gives up. Once the child begins to behave appropriately, the parent is directed to resume attending.

Praise and Positive Reinforcement

Overview

As negative behavior generally is much more salient to parents than positive behavior, parents often unintentionally ignore positive behaviors when these behaviors do occur. Session content consequently focuses on reinforcing and rewarding positive behavior with praise and tangible reinforcers such as activities or token prizes (see Appendix 55–1).

Troubleshooting

The following issues or concerns may come up during a discussion of praise and positive reinforcement:

- *Giving rewards feels like bribing my child for things that he or she should be doing anyway.*

    Therapists may wish to point out that the child is not doing the task at the moment and that use of positive reinforcement can be helpful in getting the child to complete the task (and can consequently be faded out over time). It also may be useful to draw a parallel between this type of positive reinforcement and that experienced by parents in the workforce, few of whom likely would go to work if they were not paid.

- *My child is upping the ante and saying things like "I'll do it if you get me…"*

    Parents are encouraged to provide rewards only in the context of structured reward programs, as opposed to spontaneous rewards (particularly in situations in which the child is trying to manipulate the situation in order to obtain a reward). Giving in to this kind of request makes it more likely to happen in the future.

Token Economy or Point System

Overview

A crucial component of parent training programs for parents of school-age children involves working with parents to establish a home reward system in which the child earns tokens, points, or privileges for positive behavior; the child then can cash in earned tokens or points for activities or token reinforcers (see Appendix 55–1 and Figure 55–1).

 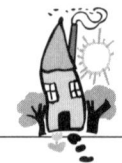 

NAME: Melissa S.

DATE:_____

TARGET BEHAVIORS	DAY				
	Monday	Tuesday	Wednesday	Thursday	Friday
Home Target Behavior <u>Getting ready in the morning:</u> (5 points each) 1. Out of bed by 7:00 2. Dressed by 7:15 3. Breakfast by 7:45 4. Brush teeth by 7:55 5. Get backpack and ready to leave for school by 8:05					
Daily Report Card Points					
TOTAL Points					
WEEKLY TOTAL	____ points				

Possible Daily Earnings = 40 points

Daily Rewards:	*Game with parent	10 points/15 minutes
	*8:30 bedtime	15 points
	*TV Time	20 points/30 minutes
Weekly Rewards:	*Dinner out	60 points
	*Trip to park	40 points/1 hour
	*Go to movie	80 points

FIGURE 55–1. Sample token economy for Melissa.

Vignette 1: Token Economy/Shaping and Fading/Integrating Home Challenge and Classroom Challenge

Melissa, a 7-year-old girl, was brought in to the clinic by her parents, Mr. and Mrs. Smith. The Smiths' primary concern was Melissa's need for excessive supervision when completing morning routine tasks, which made the entire family late to school and work on almost a daily basis; the Smiths indicated that they currently were giving Melissa four or more reminders for each task she needed to accomplish in the morning. In addition, Melissa's teacher reported that Melissa had difficulty completing her work independently in the classroom and that she required reminders to stay seated appropriately during class time. Mr. and Mrs. Smith set up a token economy system with five specific target behaviors for Melissa to accomplish during morning routine (see Figure 55–1). Melissa could earn 5 points for each behavior that she completed with two or fewer reminders from her parents, for a total of 25 points per day. In addition, Melissa's teacher agreed to implement a

daily behavior report card (Figure 55–2) in the classroom to help Melissa complete her work independently, remain seated during class time, turn in completed homework, and remember to bring the report card to the teacher each day (awarded with a bonus point). Melissa could earn an additional 15 points for successfully performing these behaviors.

Before beginning the program, the Smiths developed a reward menu with Melissa's assistance; as Melissa could earn up to 40 points each school day (for a total of 200 points per week), the Smiths assigned point values to each reward accordingly (see Figure 55–1). After posting the morning routine checklist and implementing the token economy, Mr. and Mrs. Smith reported an immediate improvement in Melissa's compliance with the morning routine. After 2 weeks, Melissa needed only one to two reminders for each morning routine behavior and consequently was regularly earning all 25 possible points every morning. At this point, Mr. and Mrs. Smith decided that because Melissa now was doing so well, they would change the criterion; now, Melissa would need to complete each task with one or

Name: Melissa S.   **Date:** _____

MY CHALLENGE

TARGET BEHAVIORS	TIME		
Completed classwork independently	0 1 2	0 1 2	0 1 2
Followed class rules	0 1 2	0 1 2	0 1 2
Turned in completed homework	0 1 2		
Gave challenge to teacher	1 bonus point		
DAILY TOTAL	=_____ **POINTS**		

Point Scale   0 = Needs Improvement
                    1 = Okay
                    2 = Super Job

Teacher signature: _____

FIGURE 55–2. Sample daily report card for Melissa.

fewer reminders in order to earn her points. After Melissa met this goal regularly, the Smiths then required Melissa to complete each morning routine behavior without any reminders in order to earn her points. The Smiths were able to phase out the token economy once Melissa was regularly completing the morning routine checklist independently, although they continued to praise her every morning for getting the checklist done on her own. Melissa's teacher continued to implement the daily behavior report card in the classroom throughout the remainder of the school year.

Troubleshooting

Parents often want to address a large number of behaviors and end up developing complicated programs that are difficult for the child to understand and for the parents to implement consistently (Table 55–1). It is best for parents to start with a simple system that focuses on increasing three or four positive behaviors and then revise the system as the child responds to the initial demands.

In addition, parents must set the criterion for earning the tokens or rewards low enough that the child is able to regularly obtain rewards; if the behaviors are too difficult relative to the child's current functioning, the child likely will become discouraged and the system will not work.

Giving Effective Instructions

Overview

Discussion of effective instructions shifts the focus from the consequences of behaviors to the antecedents of those behaviors. More specifically, parents discuss how to give instructions in a manner that maximizes the chance that the child will comply (see Appendix 55–1).

Troubleshooting

- *What do I do when my child does not comply?*

  Parents often want to jump ahead to a discussion of punishment, particularly in the context of this module, but it is important for them to master giving instructions in a maximally effective manner prior to implementing a punishment for noncompliance. To this end, parents are encouraged simply to practice giving effective instructions and to praise compliance without implementing any particular consequences for noncompliance.

Time-Out

Overview

Time-out, or time away from positive reinforcement (e.g., parental attention, another enjoyable activity) can be a powerful consequence for negative behavior. This session involves reviewing parents' past experiences with time-out, as well as discussion of mechanical and logistical issues of the time-out procedure (see Appendix 55–1 and Figure 55–3).

Vignette 2: Time-Out/Integrating Strategies
Kyle was a 10-year-old boy whose parents, Mr. and Mrs. Miller, reported concerns including aggressive behavior toward his younger sister and noncompliance with parental commands. The Millers decided to employ a time-out procedure to address both of these problem behaviors. They selected a time-out location (in the living room on the sofa, away from any distractions such as TV or toys) and decided that Kyle's time-outs would be 10 minutes long (1 minute for each year of his age). The Millers sat down with Kyle and explained that from now on, every time he displayed aggressive behavior toward his sister (e.g., hitting, kicking, pinching), he would earn an automatic time-out. In addition, Kyle now would be expected to follow parental instructions with only one reminder; if he did not follow the instructions after a warning was provided, he would earn a time-out. If Kyle chose not to serve this time-out, he would not be able to play video games or watch TV for the remainder of the day. Mr. and Mrs. Miller posted these rules on the refrigerator.

Later that day, Kyle was playing video games when Mr. Miller instructed him to pick up his shoes and put them away. Kyle ignored the instruction. After waiting 10 seconds for Kyle to comply, Mr. Miller stated, "I've asked you to pick up your shoes and put

TABLE 55–1. Troubleshooting token economies

Question	Solution
Is the target behavior defined very clearly?	Define target behavior in observable, positive terms.
Is the goal set too high?	Set goal at a level that allows the child to be successful immediately.
Is the child motivated by the reinforcer and not able to have it without earning it?	Make sure the child wants the reinforcer and can only get it when earned.
Does the child understand the program?	Have the child repeat all steps of the program, including goals and reinforcers.
Is the child overly anxious about the program or complaining that it is too hard?	Make sure goals are within the child's reach and ignore the child's complaining if it is intended to get the parents to stop the program.
Is the child interested in the reinforcer?	Make sure the child likes the reinforcer.
Is the reinforcer(s) given immediately and frequently?	Reinforcement needs to occur as often as necessary to ensure goals are met.
Are there other factors maintaining the problem behavior (e.g., getting peer attention, getting out of doing work, or getting someone else to do it for him or her)?	Address any competing factors directly.
Did the child do well for a while and then start to backslide?	Encourage parents to consider changing consequences to something more meaningful but to be consistent in keeping the program in place.
Are all caretakers supporting the program?	Communicate with caretakers in addition to the parents (e.g., grandparents, babysitters) so that everyone understands the program and can support it.

them away. If you do not pick up your shoes now, you will earn a 10-minute time-out." Kyle continued to ignore his father. Mr. Miller then informed Kyle that he had earned a 10-minute time-out and should proceed directly to the living room sofa to serve his time-out. When Kyle refused to do so, Mr. Miller calmly reminded Kyle that if he did not serve his time-out, he would be choosing to lose video games and TV for the remainder of the day. Although Kyle grumbled under his breath on his way to time-out, he served the time-out appropriately. At the end of the 10 minutes, Mr. Miller allowed Kyle to leave time-out and instructed him to pick up his shoes. Kyle complied, and then he was able to return to playing video games.

Troubleshooting

The following concerns often come up during a discussion of time-out:

- *I've tried time-out before and it did not work.*
  Discussion about the mechanics of time-out used in the past and how the time-out being recommended may differ from the procedure employed in the past likely will address these concerns. However, therapists should be prepared to troubleshoot

the time-out procedure with parents as they implement this strategy at home.

- *What if my child refuses to go to time-out?*
  Parents may handle time-out refusal in one of two ways. First, parents can modify the time-out procedure and use either an escalating or escalating-reducible time-out. In an escalating time-out, the child earns additional time in time-out for each refusal to go to time-out. In an escalating-reducible time-out, the duration of the child's time-out increases each time that he or she refuses to go to time-out, but the child has the chance to earn half off his or her time-out by proceeding to time-out and serving the time-out appropriately. An alternate way to handle time-out refusal involves implementing a backup consequence, such as removal of a favorite activity, should the child choose not to go to time-out.

Response-Cost Procedures

Overview

Parents also are taught punishment strategies that involve removing tokens, points, or privileges after the child demonstrates target negative behaviors; these strategies can be implemented either within the existing home reward system or separately (see Appendix 55–1).

Troubleshooting

Again, parents may get carried away with the number of behaviors that they want to address. Parents who employ response-cost procedures within the token economy must be cautioned to monitor the reward system in order to ensure that the child continues to earn rewards and remains motivated.

Parents also must be warned about punishment spirals that result in the child losing all of his or her tokens or points or losing activities or toys for unreasonably long periods of time. If a child continues to misbehave after the initial response-cost fine, the parent should implement a back-up consequence instead of continuing to fine the child tokens or points. Further, it may be helpful to discuss children's difficulty estimating time (as well as the fact that if parents take away toys or activities for extended periods of time, they are limiting their future response-cost options should the behavior recur).

Developing a Plan for Homework

Overview

Some programs include one or more sessions that specifically address homework time in the home environment (see Power et al. 2001). Key points of this session generally are related to the development of a plan to increase the structure of the time set aside for homework by making rules for this time explicit, thinking ahead about potential problems, and instituting consequences for specific homework target behaviors (see Appendix 55–1).

Troubleshooting

Homework assignments may not be clear, or needed materials may not get home. Using a homework assignment notebook containing daily assignments, materials, and due dates is advisable. Children and parents should be made aware of the teacher's procedure for assigning homework, and children should be reinforced for using the homework notebook. The teacher may also sign the notebook each day to ensure accuracy.

Parents also may be somewhat resistant to setting a specific and consistent time for homework in the context of other family activities. Although this is a valid concern, parents should be cautioned that children are

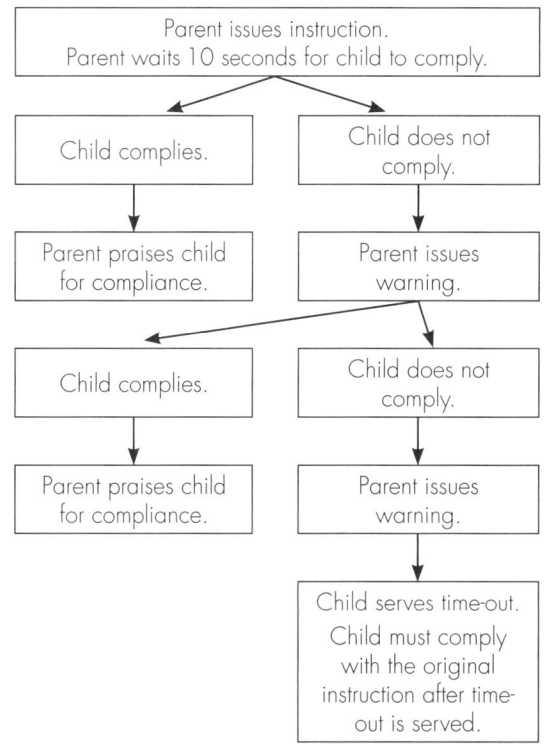

FIGURE 55–3.　Time-out flow chart.

likely to be most compliant with a homework hour that occurs at a routine time.

Home-School Report Cards

Overview

Many parent training intervention programs include a session teaching families to develop a daily behavior report card targeting between one and four problem behaviors that the teacher fills out and sends home with the child each day (Kelley 1990; see Appendix 55–1 and Figure 55–2). The child then can earn daily rewards at home based on his or her behavior at school. This type of program encourages better communication between parents and teachers and provides the child with incentives for positive behavior in the classroom. Degree of therapist involvement in developing these programs depends on the particular intervention model, as well as the type of service (i.e., group versus individual treatment) being provided. Some programs include regular school consultation meetings for the duration of treatment, and other programs may teach parents how to set up a classroom intervention with limited or no therapist contact with the school. The latter approach is more likely to be successful with reasonably skilled parents and with teachers who already are familiar with the approach.

Troubleshooting

Children may forget to bring home the daily behavior report card (DRC) or fail to bring it home on days with negative ratings. Usually this can be addressed successfully by treating the day as if the target goals were not achieved and therefore the daily home reward is not earned.

Parents and teachers may select too many behaviors on which to focus or set the bar for rewards too high. As with home-based interventions, home-school report cards must have a manageable number of behaviors (typically between two and four) and permit the child some success.

Managing Behavior in Public Places

Overview

Parents often report child misbehavior in public places outside the home setting in which the strategies that they have learned to use at home are not immediately available. Parents are encouraged to anticipate problem behavior by employing the A-B-C model before entering the public place in order to alter antecedents and minimize the chance that the child will engage in problem behavior (see Appendix 55–1).

Troubleshooting

Parents often raise concerns about feeling embarrassed about their child's misbehavior or about implementing punishment techniques in public; discussion of these concerns often may help parents to be more comfortable and less self-conscious about using available strategies. In the end, however, parents must realistically select strategies that they are willing and able to implement consistently.

When-Then

Overview

In addition to the formal rewards that parents have learned to use in their token economy systems, there are many activities that parents permit children to have for free that also can be used as rewards. During discussion of "Grandma's Rule" or Premack contingencies, parents learn to use more desirable activities as reinforcers for the completion of less desirable activities (see Appendix 55–1). For example, a parent might say, "If you do your homework, then you can watch TV."

Troubleshooting

Parents occasionally will attempt to use this strategy with desirable activities that they are not willing to withhold (e.g., family vacations or other outings); it is important to remind parents that they should employ this strategy only when the desired activity is one that they are willing and able to withhold if the child fails to complete the less desirable task.

Planning Ahead

During the final session, parents review the strategies that they have learned over the course of treatment and discuss ways to apply these strategies to future situations (see Appendix 55–1).

Supplemental Topics
Child Skills

BPT can be combined with child-focused skill-training treatments, such as social skills training, anger management, or organizational and study skills training, that permit direct skill instruction and practice for children (e.g., Abikoff and Gallagher 2007; Kazdin et al. 1992; Pfiffner and McBurnett 1997; Pfiffner et al. 2007). Parents also can be taught strategies, as part of BPT, for helping their child's skills develop in these domains (Table 55–2 contains details on addressing social and organizational problems). Session content generally includes two primary components. The first component involves working with the parents to address antecedents of skilled versus unskilled behavior on the part of the child and to structure the environment and provide the child with opportunities to be successful. Second, the parents also are taught to serve as skill coaches for their child by working with the child to focus on specific skills (for example, engaging in discussion with the child about what a specific skill may mean, cuing the child about when to use the skill, and rewarding the child for successfully demonstrating the skill).

Parent Stress Management

Parents usually are receptive to the idea that their own stress levels affect their child's behavior and that higher levels of parental stress are related to increased behavior problems on the part of the child (as well as

TABLE 55–2. Teaching parents about child skills

Social skills	Organizational skills
Discussing importance of providing children with opportunities to practice their social skills (e.g., one-on-one playdates and participation in activities)	Addressing antecedents of organized versus disorganized behavior
Structuring playdates in a manner that minimizes antecedents of problem behavior and makes playdates success experiences for the child:	Establishing an organizational structure at home that will encourage the child to be more organized:
• Selecting an easygoing or mild-mannered peer the child likes	• Modeling organizational skills
• Keeping the playdate brief	• Organizing the home environment (perhaps by implementing a system using boxes, labels, shelves, and visual cues such as colors and pictures)
• Planning an activity that both children will enjoy	Teaching parents to serve as skill coaches:
• Setting up a plan to reward positive behavior in advance of the playdate	• Demonstrating organizational skills for the child in a specific area (e.g., a backpack or desk) and then disorganizing the area and asking the child to reorganize it
Teaching parents to serve as skill coaches:	• Explaining the organizational process to the parent
• Discussing each skill and what it means with the child	• This strategy requires a time investment on the part of the parent that can be reduced over time, but any organization system established will continue to require monitoring and reinforcement on the part of the parent
• Cuing the child about when to use each skill	
• Rewarding the child for using each skill successfully	

Note. Please see the following references for additional information: Abikoff et al. 2007; Dawson and Guare 2004; Frankel and Myatt 2003; Pfiffner et al. 1997, 2007.

relational stress between the child and the parent). Likewise, parents usually agree that when they are able to manage their own stress levels, they also are better able to meet their child's needs. Parents may be engaged in discussion about their values and priorities and how these correspond to the manner in which they allocate their time. Further, parents also may be taught specific coping strategies to use when they are feeling pressured; these strategies may include relaxation, participating in pleasurable leisure activities, taking "time-out" when they can feel themselves getting upset or angry, engaging in good sleep hygiene and other healthy habits, and finding additional sources of support (for example, see Sanders et al. 2000; Webster-Stratton 1994).

Parent Cognitions and Emotion Management

Chronis et al. (2004) note that parental psychopathology and/or emotional dysregulation is one major moderator of treatment response for those participating in parent training. Clinicians recently have given more weight to the discussion of parents' own cognitions and

emotions, particularly as they pertain to the child. These interventions may include teaching parents cognitive restructuring techniques to help parents differentiate between unhelpful and helpful thoughts about the child or situation (for example, see Bloomquist 1996). Therapists generally make the point that some thoughts may cause the parents either to become angry with the child and escalate the situation (for example, age-inappropriate expectations or thoughts that the child is misbehaving intentionally) or to become discouraged and give up (for example, thoughts that attempts to exert control over the child are hopeless or that the parents themselves are bad parents), whereas other thoughts are more likely to help the parents remain calm and to deal with the child's behavior in a more rational manner. Parents are taught to identify the first type of thought as well as ways to respond to this kind of thinking that will be most effective in promoting calm and rational interactions with their child.

In addition, teaching parents mindfulness strategies also may help in addressing parent cognitions and emotions. More specifically, advocates of mindfulness in parent training argue that parents and children become enmeshed in automatic cycles and that being mindful of these interactions serves as a step toward

altering them. Dumas (2005) describes the following
key components of a mindfulness approach: 1) teaching parents to accept where the child and they themselves are in the moment without judging; 2) teaching
parents to distance themselves from situations that
could induce negative emotion; and 3) collaborating
with the parents to rationally develop and implement
a plan to meet goals relevant to both parents and child.

Monitoring Treatment Progress

In behavior therapy, treatment progress is monitored
each session by reviewing the "data," such as the
child's progress on behavior charts and DRCs (if used).
Written documents (e.g., charts or graphs of point to-
tals) can facilitate a more objective appraisal of gains
over time (although we note that gathering and constructing charts of such data can be time intensive for
the parents and/or therapist). Objective data can be
supplemented with more qualitative parent impressions regarding treatment progress (as well as teacher
impressions regarding school-based interventions). To
effectively monitor progress, parents should be asked
specific questions about how they are implementing
the programs (e.g., Which behaviors did you praise
this week? How often did you do special time? How
often did you catch yourself giving effective vs. ineffective instructions? Did you use the point system?
How calm were you when you gave the time-out?) and
about how their child is responding (e.g., How much
did your child seem to enjoy special time? How often
did your child complete his or her target behaviors?
What rewards did your child earn and how often?
How often did he or she earn a time-out? How well did
he or she take the time-out?). Brief behavior rating
scales also can be used to track progress, as can questionnaires regarding parents' understanding of social
learning principles and effective parenting practices.
Consumer satisfaction ratings also can be very helpful
for assessing parents' understanding of and perceptions about the usefulness of content covered during
each session. When such ratings are gathered each session, these data can alert the therapist to potential dissatisfaction that might lead to premature termination
or failure to follow through on programs at home. In
addition, observations of parent-child interactions can
be extremely useful in determining whether parents
are able to successfully implement the procedures and
also in evaluating the child's response.

Potential Adverse Effects or Complications

In general, this approach to treatment is associated
with a very low risk for any serious adverse effects,
making the risk-benefit ratio quite small. Instead, unwanted effects usually are mild and transient results of
parents using skills taught in an inappropriate manner
and can be addressed by making modifications to the
program. We discuss typical pitfalls in the above sections on troubleshooting session content (see "Core
Session Topics") and in Table 55–1. The most serious
complications may occur around the topic of punishment, as overly critical or potentially violent parents
may overuse these approaches to the exclusion of the
more positive ones. In these cases, an errorless learning
approach may be particularly helpful (Ducharme et al.
2000). *Errorless learning* is a success-based noncoercive
intervention that involves the gradual introduction of
more demanding requests so that child noncompliance
and associated consequences for noncompliance are
minimized throughout treatment. Likewise, children
presenting with aggressive behavior may become aggressive toward parents or other authority figures
when punishment is used. In these cases, reward-only
programs may be best, or there may be a need for additional intervention, such as collaborative family
problem-solving (Greene 2004) or medication.

A common complication in behavior therapy (as in
other forms of psychotherapy) is noncompliance or resistance to treatment, as indicated by failure to complete homework between sessions, poor attendance,
or other resistance to using recommended strategies.
In these cases, it is important to determine the contributing factors (e.g., he or she did not understand
homework, he or she was too busy, it was too difficult). Research shows that the relationship between
the therapist and parents greatly influences parental
compliance with behavioral treatment in the same
manner in which this type of relationship is important
to the success of other forms of psychotherapy. Thus,
even though a behavioral approach tends to be inherently directive, it is most effective in the context of a
collaborative parent-therapist relationship (see Webster-Stratton and Herbert 1993). Therapists' warmth,
humor, support, optimism, and knowledge are key
factors in establishing this type of relationship. A Socratic style of interaction in which the therapist asks
parents questions to facilitate their reaching desired
conclusions often improves parent-therapist collaboration and can increase parents' motivation to change.

It also is incumbent on the therapist to use the same reinforcement principles with parents that they are teaching parents to use with their children (e.g., praise their efforts!). Other procedures that also can improve compliance with treatment include making reminder phone calls, completing sessions only when homework is completed, scheduling sessions at convenient times, offering child care, and addressing transportation needs.

When to Expect Response

Children typically respond to initial strategies within the first few weeks of the time that parents put these strategies into practice (i.e., within the first several sessions of treatment). Some parents are surprised by how much change occurs with their use of contingent positive attention. More serious problems usually are not resolved until stronger reward-based and/or punishment programs are used. With a well-conceived behavior plan, initial improvement in specific target behaviors is expected within 1 week of starting the program. Continued improvement toward long-term treatment goals is achieved via a gradual shaping process of both child and parent behavior. For example, when the child successfully earns a reward for initial target behaviors (e.g., brushes teeth with only one reminder), the requirements for earning the reward are gradually increased (e.g., dresses and brushes teeth with one reminder) until the final goal is achieved (e.g., completes entire morning routine with one reminder; see Vignette 1). However, it is common for children (and parents) to backslide about halfway through the program. Troubleshooting usually can revamp a faltering program, and parents who had stopped using the program, thinking the child's gains were going to be durable without it, often see the importance of maintaining consistency.

When to Change to or Add a Different Treatment

In some cases, the ongoing weekly assessment of progress shows that desired effects are not being achieved. There are two critical areas to assess: 1) adherence to treatment (are the parents implementing the program consistently, or are the procedures only par-

tially implemented, explaining the poor response to treatment?) and 2) what exactly is the child's response, and how unsuccessful is the progress? In some cases, the treatment goals or behavioral criteria initially may have been too high and the child may display more success if the criteria are reduced to a more realistic level. Goals then can be increased more gradually via a shaping process. In other cases, unsuccessful programs may be helped by adding other strategies (e.g., adding response cost to a reward program) or adding a behavioral program in another setting for problems specific to that setting (e.g., school, peers). Parents may wish to consider adding medication if either severe behavior problems make it difficult to implement the program consistently or milder problems do not respond to tweaking of the behavioral program or cross-site implementation of the program. The combination of medication and behavioral treatments is considered the most potent intervention for many cases of attention-deficit/hyperactivity disorder (ADHD), improving symptoms and functioning across domains (MTA Cooperative Group 1999; Pelham 2002). Other forms of treatment also may be needed in order to address problems with the family system (marital therapy, cognitive-behavioral therapy for parental depression, treatment for parental ADHD); these adjunctive treatments can occur concurrently with BPT, or parent training can be terminated temporarily until gains in alternative treatments are achieved.

How Long to Continue Successful Treatment

Fading and termination of treatment usually are a collaborative decision between therapist and family. Many programs involve a set number of sessions, after which time a decision is made about whether additional treatment is needed. When most treatment goals are met, the frequency of individual sessions typically is reduced gradually in order to best maintain treatment gains (e.g., from once per week to once every other week and then once per month). Parents often become less motivated to come to sessions when their child is having success; termination thus often is initiated by the parents. After termination, booster sessions may be provided (and often are encouraged) during predictable transitional periods (start or change of schools) or at times of high stress. For more severe or chronic problems, a continued-care model may be necessary. For example, given that ADHD is considered a chronic disorder, it is likely that some sort of intervention may be needed throughout childhood, adolescence, and into adulthood. The precise nature and intensity of these interventions may vary somewhat depending upon environmental circumstances and developmental stage, but it seems reasonable to expect that maintenance of improvements following initial successful treatment will require continued intervention and troubleshooting from time to time.

Indications

BPT is strongly indicated for oppositional and conduct problems and ADHD based on numerous empirical studies and is recommended by the major professional organizations for psychiatry, pediatrics, and psychology (American Academy of Child and Adolescent Psychiatry 2007a, 2007b; American Academy of Pediatrics 2001; American Psychological Association Working Group on Psychoactive Medications for Children and Adolescents 2006). Both boys and girls spanning the full age range (toddler-adolescence) can benefit from this approach, although developmental considerations necessitate modifications across the ages (see the section "Developmental Issues" below). BPT also can be helpful for youth with comorbid internalizing problems such as anxiety or depression, although minor modifications may be made for children presenting primarily with these types of problems. Behavior therapy is indicated across all socioeconomic status (SES) levels and races and ethnicities. However, SES has been shown to moderate the efficacy of behavior therapy, with a generally less favorable response among families from lower SES levels (see the section "Factors Affecting Outcome" later in this chapter).

Contraindications

The demands of parent training can be substantial, as parents are required to learn specific procedures and complete homework each week to practice skills taught during group. As a result, the primary contraindications are parent psychopathology (ADHD, depression), marital discord, or some other type of family dysfunction that is sufficiently severe so that it prevents parents from participating or making the necessary time investment. Alternatives would be to

teach the skills in a more gradual manner, have the parents receive individual or couples counseling prior to parent training, or provide these interventions concurrently.

Developmental Issues

Parent training can be applied across developmental levels with various modifications. For the preschool level and early elementary school ages, parents and other caretakers assume dominant roles in socialization, and children typically are very responsive to parental and caretaker attention. Several behavioral programs have been developed for this age group. These interventions include the Incredible Years (Webster-Stratton et al. 2004), Parent Child Interaction Training (Eyberg et al. 1995), and Helping the Noncompliant Child (Forehand and McMahon 1981). Each of these programs follows a similar two-stage process. In the first, child-directed stage, parents are taught skills to foster a close, secure relationship with their child through use of traditional play therapy skills such as using attending and praising without questions, commands, and criticisms. In the second, parent-directed stage, parents are taught specific techniques for giving effective commands, labeled (or specific) praise, selective attention (ignoring), and time-out for more serious problems (e.g., hitting, tantrums).

At the elementary school level, there are greater expectations placed on children for independent functioning, and children develop the ability to delay gratification for longer periods of time, to work toward specific goals over time, and to understand the relationship between their behavior and contingencies. As exemplified by programs developed by Barkley (1987), Cunningham et al. (1995), Kazdin (2005), Patterson and Gullion (1968), and Webster-Stratton et al. (2004), interventions for this age group focus on daily and weekly reward programs or contracts as well as discipline techniques such as response cost (taking away privileges) and time-out. Treatment also often includes contact with schools and a focus on homework for the purpose of addressing academic problems.

Parent training without the direct involvement of the child may be less effective during adolescence due to teens' greater need for autonomy, increased risk-taking behaviors, reduced responsiveness to direct parent control, and greater influence of peer groups on values and behavior (relative to the influences of family or authority figures). For adolescents, contingency management and discipline (response cost and restitution through chores rather than time-out) continue to be part of the treatment, but there is a need for greater involvement of the adolescent in the problem-solving process. Treatment focuses on teaching teens and their parents effective skills for communication, negotiation, and family problem-solving (Dishion and Kavanagh 2003; Robin and Foster 1989). Formal behavioral contracts typically are used. Treatment for adolescents also focuses on improving parental monitoring and oversight of their teen's behavior. As with younger youth, treatment often includes consulting with the school to address academic and/or social problems in that setting.

Research Evidence for Efficacy and Effectiveness

Numerous outcome studies show strong and clinically meaningful effects of BPT for the disruptive behavior disorders during preschool and elementary school (Anastopoulos et al. 1993; Dishion and Patterson 1992; Kazdin 2005; Maughan et al. 2005; Nixon et al. 2003; Sonuga-Barke et al. 2001; Webster-Stratton et al. 2004). Gains occur in child compliance and reduction of problem behaviors, many of which place children in the nonclinical range of functioning relative to their same-age peers (Kazdin 1997). BPT also improves parenting skills, including use of effective commands, praise, attending, ignoring, and monitoring, and also decreases controlling and negative parenting. The extent of changes in parenting usually predicts the extent of improvement in child behavior (Dishion et al. 2003; Hinshaw et al. 2000). Gains made in parent training have been shown to be maintained several years post-treatment (Nock 2003). During adolescence, family-centered behavioral interventions (which include the teen in the treatment sessions) show positive effects (Dishion and Kavanagh 2003; Robin and Foster 1989).

BPT also has positive effects on parent functioning. Parents who participate in parent training often show reductions in parenting stress (Anastopoulos et al. 1993) and depression and greater confidence in their ability to manage their child's behavior (Herschell et al. 2002). Treatment effects can extend to untreated siblings (Herschell et al. 2002). Parent training also can be effective in alleviating marital distress that is caused by disagreements over childrearing since it can serve to unify the parents' approach (Beauchaine et al. 2005).

Parents typically report high levels of satisfaction with this form of intervention (Herschell et al. 2002).

The addition of components to address parents' problem solving, stress, depression, and marital discord shows increased effects of BPT on overall parent, child, and family functioning (Nock 2003).

Multicomponent Behavioral Interventions

The most potent treatment effects often are found when BPT is combined with school and/or child-focused interventions, as together these interventions can target the range of risk factors and settings contributing to child problems. In addition, such intervention combinations can synergize the effects of the individual components. The combination of parent training with school-based interventions such as those reviewed in Chapter 63 ("School-Based Interventions"; see also Pfiffner et al. 2006) and/or child-focused interventions, such as anger management training, problem solving, and social skills, as discussed earlier in the subsection "Child Skills" in the "Supplemental Topics" section), has been found to be effective in improving attention and externalizing problem behavior, parent-child interactions, and social skills in a number of studies across age groups (Kern et al. 2007; Nock 2003; Pelham 2002; Pfiffner et al. 1997, 2007; Webster-Stratton and Hammond 1997). Including a child component can reduce premature termination in BPT (Miller and Prinz 1990), suggesting that these adjunctive interventions exert a positive effect on parents' motivation for treatment. In addition, there is evidence that combining behavioral and medication treatments may permit a lower dose of medication when medication is needed (Hoza et al. 2007; Pelham 2002).

Factors Affecting Outcome

A number of studies have evaluated under which conditions and for whom behavioral interventions best work. Generally, the more difficult the living conditions and the more impaired the child functioning and parent functioning, the less favorable the outcome is. In particular, past research suggests that low SES predicts poorer outcome (Eamon and Venkataraman 2003). It is likely that the limited resources of families from lower levels of SES contribute to these families' greater likelihood of early termination from treatment. For example, transportation issues, need for daytime attendance (i.e., during working hours), lack of child care for siblings, and other such issues may present greater treatment barriers for these families relative to more affluent families. For families facing financial disadvantage, an individual approach to BPT that allows for more tailoring of treatment to individual family circumstances may be significantly more effective than group-based approaches (Harwood and Eyberg 2004; Lundahl et al. 2005). There is no evidence that low SES increases dropout differentially for behavior therapy versus other psychosocial treatments. There has been some question as to whether fathers need to attend parent training; outcome studies tend to show that having both parents attend may not affect post-treatment outcome but may improve maintenance of treatment gains (Miller and Prinz 1990). Generally we advise that all caretakers attend sessions but require only the primary caretaker to attend every week.

A number of other parent and family factors may affect outcomes. Single-parent families, high parent stress, and a lack of parent social support all predict less favorable outcomes (Harwood and Eyberg 2006; Nock 2003). As noted earlier, severe marital discord, parent psychopathology (e.g., depression, ADHD, antisocial behavior), and parental drug abuse or dependence all can reduce efficacy of parent training (Chronis et al. 2004). Parents' beliefs about their child and his or her capacity to change can also affect outcome. Parents who think that their child is behaving badly on purpose or that their child is destined to display negative behavior ("There is nothing I can do") often are less likely to feel motivated to implement new behavioral strategies. Further, perceived stigma about receiving mental health services may prevent parents from continuing to receive services or from accessing them at all.

A number of child factors also predict response to parent training. The severity and nature of symptoms and problems likely are the strongest predictor of whether or not (or to what degree) treatment produces desired change. For example, children with conduct disorder who are high on callous-unemotional traits show a poorer response to parent training in general than do children low on these traits, and these children show an especially poor response to time-out as compared to reward programs (Hawes and Dadds 2005). Children with very severe oppositional defiant disorder or explosive behavior also may respond less well to traditional parent training approaches and require a more collaborative family problem-solving model

(Greene 2004) relative to children presenting without these problems. For child-focused treatments, level of motivation and cognitive ability on the part of the child also are likely to be positively related to response.

Cultural and racial backgrounds affect treatment-seeking behavior, in that members of minority groups are less likely to seek or obtain services, and therefore much of the existing treatment outcome research is based largely on white samples (Forehand and Kotchick 1996). For families completing treatment, past research typically shows few differences in response to interventions after controlling for SES (Butler and Eyberg 2006), but this finding admittedly is based on small numbers of families. In light of differences in parenting across cultures, it seems important to take cultural factors into consideration. For example, in cultures involving extended family in child care and emphasizing communal parenting, it may be important for nonparent providers to take part in or observe the training. In order to address cultural conceptions regarding behavior and psychological functioning (and particularly the increased stigma that may be associated with psychological disorders or participation in mental health services), the language used to describe the treatment may require modification (e.g., "Understanding Your Child and Resolving Conflicts" or "Parent Coaching" instead of parent training; see Butler and Eyberg [2006]). Similarly, the types of reinforcers, activities, and privileges may need to be adapted depending on family and cultural values. Response to treatment also may benefit from a cultural match between therapist and family.

As noted earlier, there are a variety of process factors associated with implementation of parent training that also can affect outcome. As with any intervention, the therapist-client relationship influences outcome in behavior therapy (Webster-Stratton and Herbert 1993). Therapist warmth, knowledge of social learning principles and disruptive behavior disorders, likeability, and communication skills all are likely to contribute to more positive outcomes. Helpful therapist behaviors include active listening skills to guide and maintain parents' responses to open-ended questions, whereas overly supportive statements early in therapy may reinforce feelings of client helplessness, which might contribute to dropout (Harwood and Eyberg 2004). Compliance with treatment also can be enhanced using motivational strategies (Dishion et al. 2003; Nock and Kazdin 2005) and specific prompts (e.g., reminder phone calls between sessions that prompt parents to complete homework or to come to the next session).

Cost-Benefit Issues

Relative to long-term "traditional" individual therapy, behavior therapy is very cost-effective. The substantial gains of BPT reported above can result from as few as 8 to 12 parent training sessions. The cost-benefit of parent training may be especially favorable when it is administered in a group setting, which for many families is as effective as individual approaches (Chronis et al. 2004). Large community-based group parent training programs held in the child's neighborhood also provide a cost-effective and perhaps less stigmatizing approach than clinic-based services (Cunningham et al. 1995). Self-administered parent training (e.g., via workbooks, videos) does not appear to be sufficient for most families (Sanders et al. 2000; Webster-Stratton 1990).

Research Directions

As we have ample evidence for the efficacy of BPT, pressing clinical questions relate to how we can maximize effects and tailor current clinical approaches to best meet the needs of varied children, families, and circumstances. Novel interventions are being developed and evaluated to address factors that have been found to moderate outcomes; factors being considered include parent factors (e.g., concurrent depression or ADHD, the role of fathers in treatment), child factors (e.g., ADHD subtype, child age), SES, ethnicity, and family structure. In addition, we note that there also are important questions and controversies about best practices for sequencing BPT topics—and sequencing and combining various behavioral treatments (e.g., BPT, child skills training, school interventions) and behavioral and pharmacological treatments (see Pelham 2002, 2007). Finally, there is a great need for studies examining the exportability of evidence-based parent training from controlled research environments to real-world settings. Innovative methodologies for delivery of treatment (e.g., offering treatment in primary care and/or school settings; use of Web-based treatments; video-based media programs; interactive CD-ROMs) are needed to maximize accessibility. Policy research on the way in which parent training programs can best be provided and financed within systems of care (such as public and private health and mental health insurance, schools, community agencies) also is greatly needed (see Rosenblatt and Hilley 2007) so that the services are accessible to all families in need.

Summary Points

- BPT is a well-established and evidence-based treatment for all disruptive behavior disorders, can be adapted across developmental levels, and is useful for prevention of these conditions as well. The positive effects of BPT include reductions in children's deviant behavior and symptoms; improvement in child compliance, parenting skills, and the quality of parent-child interactions; and improvement in parents' stress, self-confidence, and well-being.

- BPT interventions employ functional behavior analysis—the Antecedent-Behavior-Consequence (A-B-C) model of behavior—in order to examine problem behaviors and identify potential antecedents and/or consequences maintaining those behaviors. BPT programs then include some combination of core topics that teach parents to alter either antecedents (attending, giving effective instructions, managing behavior in public places, planning ahead) or consequences (praise and positive reinforcement, time-out, token economy, when-then, response cost) to improve the behavior.

- Behavioral interventions designed to target school-based problems such as homework completion or school behavior can be taught during BPT sessions and therapist consultation with the child's teacher.

- Additional child problems, such as social or organizational skills deficits, can be addressed in additional parent sessions (often including the child) and in parallel skills-training group treatment for the child.

- Sessions also can be added to address concurrent parent stress management or maladaptive cognitions or emotions on the part of the parents; these sessions typically employ combinations of behavioral, cognitive-behavioral, and/or mindfulness techniques.

- Parent factors that often reduce positive outcomes include low SES, single-parent status, severe marital discord, and parent psychopathology (depression, ADHD, substance abuse). These issues may be addressed through adjunctive treatments or (in the case of limited financial resources) some alteration of the parent training protocol.

- Combinations of BPT with other cognitive-behavioral treatments and/or medication likely produce the most potent outcomes for children and families having the most impairment. In some cases of ADHD, behavioral treatments add benefit to medication and may minimize medication use and dose.

References

Abikoff H, Gallagher R: Assessment and remediation of organizational skills deficits in children with ADHD, in Attention Deficit Hyperactivity Disorder: Concepts, Controversies, New Directions. Edited by McBurnett K, Pfiffner L. New York, Informa Healthcare, 2007, pp 137–152

American Academy of Child and Adolescent Psychiatry: Practice parameters for the assessment and treatment of children, adolescents, and adults with attention deficit hyperactivity disorder. J Am Acad Child Adolesc Psychiatry 46:894–921, 2007a

American Academy of Child and Adolescent Psychiatry: Practice parameters for the assessment and treatment of children and adolescents with oppositional defiant disorder. J Am Acad Child Adolesc Psychiatry 46:126–141, 2007b

American Academy of Pediatrics: Clinical practice guideline: treatment of the school-aged child with attention-deficit/hyperactivity disorder. Pediatrics 108:1033–1044, 2001

American Psychological Association Working Group on Psychoactive Medications for Children and Adolescents: Psychopharmacological, Psychosocial, and Combined Interventions for Childhood Disorders: Evidence Base, Contextual Factors, and Future Directions. Report of the Working Group on Psychoactive Medications for Children and Adolescents. Washington, DC, American Psychological Association, 2006

Anastopoulos AD, Shelton TL, DuPaul GJ, et al: Parent training for attention-deficit hyperactivity disorder: its impact on parent functioning. J Abnorm Child Psychol 21:581–596, 1993

Anastopoulos AD, Rhoads LH, Farley SE: Counseling and training parents, in Attention Deficit Hyperactivity Disorder: A Handbook for Diagnosis and Treatment. Edited by Barkley RA. New York, Guilford, 2006, pp 453–479

Bandura A: Social Learning Theory. Englewood Cliffs, NJ, Prentice-Hall, 1977

Barkley RA: Defiant Children: A Clinician's Manual for Parent Training. New York, Guilford, 1987

Beauchaine T, Webster-Stratton C, Reid MJ: Mediators, moderators, and predictors of 1-year outcomes among children treated for early onset conduct problems: a latent growth curve analysis. J Consult Clin Psychol 73:371–388, 2005

Bloomquist ML: Skills Training for Children With Behavior Disorders: A Parent and Therapist Guidebook. New York, Guilford, 1996

Butler AM, Eyberg SM: Parent-child interaction therapy and ethnic minority children. Vulnerable Children and Youth Studies 1:246–255, 2006

Chronis A, Chacko A, Fabiano G, et al: Enhancements to the behavioral parent training paradigm for families of children with ADHD: review and future directions. Clin Child Fam Psychol Rev 7:1–27, 2004

Cunningham CE, Bremner R, Boyle M: Large group community-based parenting programs for families of preschoolers at risk for disruptive behaviour disorders: utilization, cost effectiveness, and outcome. J Child Psychol Psychiatry 36:1141–1159, 1995

Dawson P, Guare R: Executive Skills in Children and Adolescents. New York, Guilford, 2004

Dishion TJ, Kavanagh KK: Intervening in Adolescent Problem Behavior: A Family Centered Approach. New York, Guilford, 2003

Dishion TJ, Patterson GR: Age effects in parent training outcome. Behav Ther 23:719–729, 1992

Dishion TJ, Patterson GR, Kavanagh KK: An experimental test of the coercion model: linking theory, measurement, and intervention, in Preventing Antisocial Behavior. Edited by McCord J, Tremblay RE. New York, Guilford, 1991, pp 253–282

Dishion TJ, Nelson SE, Kavanagh KK: The family check-up with high risk young adolescents: preventing early onset substance use by parent monitoring. Behav Ther 34:553–571, 2003

Douglas V, Parry P: Effect of reward on delayed reaction time task performance of hyperactive children. J Abnorm Child Psychol 11:313–326, 1983

Ducharme JM, Atkinson L, Poulton L: Success-based, noncoercive treatment of oppositional behavior in children from violent homes. J Am Acad Child Adolesc Psychiatry 39:995–1004, 2000

Dumas JE: Mindfulness-based parent training: strategies to lessen the grip of automaticity in families with disruptive children. J Clin Child Adolesc Psychol 34:779–791, 2005

Eamon MK, Venkataraman M: Implementing parent management training in the context of poverty. Am J Fam Ther 31:281–293, 2003

Eyberg SM, Boggs SR, Algina J: Parent-child interaction therapy: a psychosocial model for the treatment of young children with conduct problem behavior and their families. Psychopharmacol Bull 31:83–91, 1995

Forehand R, Kotchick BA: Cultural diversity: a wake-up call for parent training. Behav Ther 27:187–206, 1996

Forehand R, McMahon R: Helping the Noncompliant Child: A Clinician's Guide to Parent Training. New York, Guilford, 1981

Frankel F, Myatt R: Children's Friendship Training. New York, Brunner-Routledge, 2003

Greene RW: Effectiveness of collaborative problem solving in affectively dysregulated children with oppositional defiant disorder: initial findings. J Consult Clin Psychol 72:1157–1164, 2004

Haenlein M, Caul W: Attention deficit disorder with hyperactivity: a specific hypothesis of reward dysfunction. J Am Acad Child Adolesc Psychiatry 26:356–362, 1986

Harwood MD, Eyberg SM: Therapist verbal behavior early in treatment: relation to successful completion of parent-child interaction therapy. J Clin Child Adolesc Psychol 33:601–612, 2004

Harwood MD, Eyberg SM: Child-directed interaction: prediction of change in impaired mother-child functioning. J Abnorm Child Psychol 34:335–347, 2006

Hawes DJ, Dadds MR: The treatment of conduct problems in children with callous-unemotional traits. J Consult Clin Psychol 73:737–741, 2005

Herschell AD, Calzada EJ, Eyberg SM, et al: Parent-child interaction therapy: new directions in research. Cogn Behav Pract 9:9–16, 2002

Hinshaw S, Owens EB, Wells KC, et al: Family processes and treatment outcome in the MTA: negative/ineffective parenting practices in relation to multimodal treatment. J Abnorm Child Psychol 28:555–568, 2000

Hoza B, Kaiser N, Hurt E: Multimodal treatments for childhood attention-deficit/hyperactivity disorder: interpreting outcomes in the context of study designs. Clin Child Fam Psychol Rev 10:318–334, 2007

Johnston C, Mash EJ: Families of children with attention-deficit/hyperactivity disorder: review and recommendations for future research. Clin Child Fam Psychol Rev 4:183–207, 2001

Kazdin A: Parent management training: evidence, outcomes, and issues. J Am Acad Child Adolesc Psychiatry 36:1349–1356, 1997

Kazdin A: Parent Management Training: Treatment for Oppositional, Aggressive, and Antisocial Behavior in Children and Adolescents. New York, Oxford University Press, 2005

Kazdin A, Siegel TC, Bass D: Cognitive problem-solving skills training and parent management training in the treatment of antisocial behavior in children. J Consult Clin Psychol 60:733–747, 1992

Kelley ML: School-Home Notes: Promoting Children's Classroom Success. New York, Guilford, 1990

Kern L, DuPaul GJ, Volpe RJ, et al: Multisetting assessment-based intervention for young children at risk for attention deficit hyperactivity disorder: initial effects on academic and behavioral functioning. School Psych Rev 36:237–255, 2007

Luman M, Oosterlaan J, Sergeant J: The impact of reinforcement contingencies on AD/HD: a review and theoretical appraisal. Clin Psychol Rev 25:183–213, 2005

Lundahl B, Risser HJ, Lovejoy MC: A meta-analysis of parent training: moderators and follow-up effects. Clin Psychol Rev 26:86–104, 2005

Maughan DR, Christianson E, Jenson WR, et al: Behavioral parent training as a treatment for children's externalizing behaviors and disruptive behavior disorders: a meta-analysis. School Psych Rev 34:267–286, 2005

Miller GE, Prinz RJ: Enhancement of social learning family intervention for childhood conduct disorder. Psychol Bull 108:291–307, 1990

MTA Cooperative Group: A 14-month randomized clinical trial of treatment strategies for ADHD. Arch Gen Psychiatry 56:1073–1086, 1999

Nixon RDV, Sweeney L, Erickson DB, et al: Parent-child interaction therapy: a comparison of standard and abbreviated treatments for oppositional defiant preschoolers. J Consult Clin Psychol 71:251–260, 2003

Nock MK: Progress review of the psychosocial treatment of child conduct problems. Clin Psychol Sci Pract 10:1–28, 2003

Nock MK, Kazdin A: Randomized controlled trial of a brief intervention for increasing participation in parent management training. J Consult Clin Psychol 73:872–879, 2005

O'Brien BS, Frick PJ: Reward dominance: associations with anxiety, conduct problems, and psychopathy in children. J Abnorm Child Psychol 24:223–240, 1996

Patterson GR: Coercive Family Process. Eugene, OR, Castalia Publishing, 1982

Patterson GR, Gullion ME: Living With Children: New Methods for Parents and Teachers. Champaign, IL, Research Press, 1968

Patterson GR, Reid JB, Dishion TJ: Antisocial Boys. Eugene, OR, Castalia Publishing, 1992

Pelham W: Psychosocial interventions for ADHD, in Attention Deficit Hyperactivity Disorder: State of the Science and Best Practices. Edited by Jensen P, Cooper J. Kingston, NJ, Civic Research Institute, 2002, pp 12-1–12-36

Pelham W: Against the grain: a proposal for a psychosocial first approach to treating ADHD: the Buffalo treatment algorithm, in Attention Deficit Hyperactivity Disorder: Concepts, Controversies, and New Directions. Edited by McBurnett K, Pfiffner L. New York, Informa Healthcare, 2007, pp 301–316

Pfiffner L, McBurnett K: Social skills training with parent generalization: treatment effects for children with attention deficit disorder. J Consult Clin Psychol 65:749–757, 1997

Pfiffner L, Barkley RA, DuPaul GJ: Treatment of ADHD in school settings, in Attention Deficit Hyperactivity Disorder: A Handbook for Diagnosis and Treatment. Edited by Barkley RA. New York, Guilford, 2006, pp 547–589

Pfiffner L, Mikami A, Huang-Pollock C, et al: A randomized controlled trial of integrated home-school behavioral treatment for ADHD, predominantly inattentive type. J Am Acad Child Adolesc Psychiatry 46:1041–1046, 2007

Power TJ, Karustis JL, Habboushe DF: Homework Success for Children With ADHD: A Family School Intervention Program. New York, Guilford, 2001

Quay H: Inhibition and attention deficit hyperactivity disorder. J Abnorm Child Psychol 25:7–13, 1997

Robin AL, Foster SL: Negotiating Parent Adolescent Conflict. New York, Guilford, 1989

Rosenblatt A, Hilley L: Attention deficit-hyperactivity disorder: organizing and financing services, in Attention Deficit Hyperactivity Disorder: Concepts, Controversies and New Directions. Edited by McBurnett K, Pfiffner L. New York, Informa Healthcare, 2007, pp 211–222

Sanders MR, Markie-Dadds C, Tully LA, et al: The Triple P-Positive Parenting Program: a comparison of enhanced, standard, and self-directed behavioral family intervention for parents of children with early onset conduct problems. J Consult Clin Psychol 68:624–640, 2000

Sonuga-Barke E: Causal models of attention-deficit/hyperactivity disorder: from common simple deficits to mul-tiple developmental pathways. Biol Psychiatry 57:1231–1238, 2005

Sonuga-Barke E, Daley D, Thompson M, et al: Parent-based therapies for preschool attention-deficit/hyperactivity disorder: a randomized, controlled trial with a community sample. J Am Acad Child Adolesc Psychiatry 40:402–408, 2001

Webster-Stratton C: Enhancing the effectiveness of self-administered videotape parent training for families of conduct problem children. J Abnorm Child Psychol 18:479–492, 1990

Webster-Stratton C: Advancing video-taped parent training: a comparison study. J Consult Clin Psychol 62:583–593, 1994

Webster-Stratton C, Hammond M: Treating children with early onset conduct problems: a comparison of child and parent training interventions. J Consult Clin Psychol 65:93–109, 1997

Webster-Stratton C, Herbert M: "What really happens in parent training?" Behav Modif 17:407–456, 1993

Webster-Stratton C, Reid MJ, Hammond M: Treating children with early onset conduct problems: intervention outcomes for parent, child, and teacher training. J Clin Child Adolesc Psychol 33:105–124, 2004

Wells K: Parent training in the treatment of ADHD, in Attention Deficit Hyperactivity Disorder: Concepts, Controversies and New Directions. Edited by McBurnett K, Pfiffner L. New York, Informa Healthcare, 2007, pp 191–197

APPENDIX 55–1. Core parent training topics

Topic	Key elements
Psychoeducation/ background information	What is behavior therapy/parent training? Why is this the treatment of choice for childhood behavior problems?
	If treatment is targeted toward parents of children with a specific disorder (e.g., attention-deficit/hyperactivity disorder, conduct disorder), provide information regarding core symptoms, diagnostic criteria, etiology, and empirically supported treatments.
	Parent-child coercive interaction cycles: negative behaviors on the part of both parent and child are reinforced and perpetuated.
	Antecedent-Behavior-Consequence (A-B-C) model: modifying behavior by altering either the *antecedents* (i.e., the way in which the situation is set up) or *consequences* (i.e., rewards or punishments) of any given behavior.
Attending and ignoring	Using attending skills during child-directed special time, with goal of improving parent-child relationship:
	• Child directs the activity.
	• Parent actively attends to child's behavior by narrating activity in a nondirective, noncoercive, and neutral manner (without interrupting or making suggestions).
	Expanding on attending during special time by differentially attending to positive and negative behaviors:
	• Attending to and praising positive behavior.
	• Ignoring mild negative behavior.
Praise/positive reinforcement	Delivering praise, rewards, or other positive reinforcement for positive behaviors that often are ignored, as they are less salient to parents than are negative behaviors.
	Effective vs. ineffective praise; examples of important aspects of effective praise include the following:
	• Specific: "I like the way you followed my instruction," rather than "Nice job."
	• Immediately follows positive target behavior each and every time it occurs.
	• Not contaminated by negative affect on the part of the parent.
	Need for consistency (and immediacy) in delivering praise or positive reinforcement.
	Developing a reward menu with child's assistance that provides multiple options, such as token prizes or activities that can be paired with verbal praise.
Token economy/ point system	Child earns tokens, points, or privileges for positive behavior at home that then can be cashed in for rewards such as small toys, stickers, or valued activities.
	• Generate lists of daily and weekly rewards.
	• Select clearly observable and specific target behaviors that include both difficult and relatively easy tasks in order to ensure that the child earns rewards and remains motivated.
	• Assign points or token values to each behavior (behaviors can all earn the same number of points or can be weighted by importance or difficulty level).
	• Set point or token costs for each reward based on the total number of points or tokens that the child can earn in any given day and week.
	Use reward menu from list of daily and weekly rewards.

APPENDIX 55–1. Core parent training topics *(continued)*

Topic	Key elements
Giving effective instructions	Effective vs. ineffective instructions; effective instructions involve the following: • Getting the child's attention. • Keeping the command brief, specific, and framed as what the child should do (vs. what he or she should *not* do). • Phrasing commands as statements rather than questions or "let's" statements. • Using a neutral voice. • Giving the child time (up to 10 seconds) to respond. • Giving praise if the child complies or implementing a consequence if the child does not comply. Need for attention to phrasing and consistency.

Time-out	Time-out from positive reinforcement or enjoyable activity as a consequence for two or three specific target negative behaviors (such as noncompliance with commands or rule violations such as physical aggression or destruction of property).
	Discussion and troubleshooting of parents' past experience with time-out.
	Mechanics of three-step procedure (see Figure 55–3), including the following:
	• Give an instruction.
	• Wait 5–10 seconds for the child to comply (counting aloud can improve compliance).
	• If the child does not comply, issue a warning (e.g., "I've asked you to pick up your shoes. If you do not pick up your shoes now, you will earn a 5-minute time-out").
	• If the child does not comply, inform the child that he or she has earned a time-out and should proceed directly to the prespecified time-out location.
	• Child must serve minimum time in time-out and is only permitted to leave time-out if he or she has served the last moment or two of the time-out appropriately; avoid reinforcing negative behavior by approaching or engaging with the child in time-out when he or she is displaying disruptive behavior.
	• For noncompliance, child must complete original instruction following release from time-out; if child resists, time-out cycle should be repeated until child follows through on instruction in order to ensure that he or she does not use time-out to avoid following parental directions.
	• For rule violations, no warning is necessary prior to assigning time-out (as long as parent has discussed this with child in advance).
	Specific logistical issues:
	  • Location for time-out: safe, easily monitored, no potential for positive reinforcement.
	  • Duration of time-out may vary according to child's age (e.g., 1 minute for each year) or type of time-out procedure parents have chosen.
	  • Behaviors that earn time-out.

APPENDIX 55–1. Core parent training topics *(continued)*

Topic	Key elements
Response-cost procedures	Removal of tokens, points, or privileges when child displays target negative behaviors. Can be done in several ways: • Within token economy system. • Can provide prespecified number of tokens/points at the beginning of day or week and then assess a fine each time the behavior occurs (i.e., subtract fined tokens from the initial amount). • Can directly fine child tokens or points he or she has already earned. • Can add a separate line to the token economy for rule infractions and then total points earned minus points lost at the end of the week. • Separate from token economy system: Parents can take away privileges, activities, or toys. Parents should continue to frame the token economy system in a positive manner to the child even after adding a response-cost component and also ensure that the child continues to earn rewards even if tokens are being subtracted for negative behavior.
Developing a plan for homework	Increasing structure for homework time by making rules explicit and planning ahead for potential problems: • Ensuring necessary materials are available. • Using an assignment system so that parents are aware of work needing to be completed. • Prespecifying a location for homework that is free of distractions. • Setting a consistent time for homework (or designating a "homework hour," during which time child must engage in quiet activities even if schoolwork is completed). Discussing with parents what their role or level of involvement in homework should be. Extending the token economy to the homework time, with tokens earned and lost for specific homework-related behaviors.
Home-school report cards	Teaching parents to work collaboratively with teachers in developing and implementing a daily behavior report card that targets between one and four specific school-based problem behaviors. Parents provide the child with rewards at home for positive behavior at school. Teacher involvement can vary in time commitment or intensity; teachers may track the precise number of times a problem behavior occurs or provide a Likert rating of how well the child is doing on each target over the course of the school day.
Managing behavior in public places	Employing the A-B-C model before entering the public place in order to minimize possible problem behavior. Anticipating potential problems and restructuring antecedents accordingly. Setting expectations for behavior and conveying these to the child in advance. Having preplanned consequences in place and communicating these to the child in advance. Rewarding positive behavior. Assigning consequences (e.g., modified time-out) for negative behavior.
When-Then/If-Then/ "Grandma's Rule" (Premack contingencies)	Using more desirable activities as reinforcers for completion of less desirable activities: "When/if you do what I want you to do, *then* you do what you want to do"; for example, parents using this strategy might tell their child, "When you finish your homework, then you can watch TV."

APPENDIX 55–1. Core parent training topics *(continued)*

Topic	Key elements
Planning ahead/ anticipating future behavior problems	Reviewing strategies learned to date. Applying the A-B-C model to new problems. Troubleshooting existing interventions: making sure rewards are motivating for the child, interventions are manageable in size for both child and parents, and reward and punishment (e.g., time-out, response cost) procedures are being implemented consistently.

Note. Please see the following references for additional information: Anastopoulos et al. 2006; Barkley 1987; Bloomquist 1996; Forehand and McMahon 1981; Kazdin 2005; Pelham 2002; Pfiffner et al. 2007; Wells 2007.

Chapter 56

Family Therapy

Richard Wendel, D.Min.
Karen R. Gouze, Ph.D.

What is the place of family therapy in child and adolescent psychiatric practice? The practice parameters of the American Academy of Child and Adolescent Psychiatry (AACAP) repeatedly emphasize the critical role families play in the treatment of child and adolescent psychiatric disorders. The Practice Parameter on Family Assessment (American Academy of Child and Adolescent Psychiatry 2007) states: "A family assessment is always indicated in the psychiatric evaluation of a child or adolescent" (p. 922); "The family assessment must recognize and describe family strengths as well as identify family problems" (p. 922). The 10 "principles" of the family assessment parameter call for a high level of skill in family assessment and treatment in child and adolescent psychiatry. AACAP regards the family assessment and treatment as indispensable for child and adolescent mental health practice.

This chapter will present a short history of family therapy and introduce key concepts in the field. A re-

view of family therapy models will provide the background for the presentation of integrative module-based family therapy, a treatment approach that is especially applicable for practice in child and adolescent psychiatric settings (Gouze and Wendel 2008; Wendel et al. 2005).

Historically, individual and family therapy arose from two distinct traditions. Individual therapies, by definition, focus on an individual patient. Some of these therapies restrict contact with family members (i.e., psychoanalysis), while others allow for some involvement. Early family therapies focused on social processes and argued that individual problems resulted from familial factors. As individual and family therapies matured and were influenced by empirical studies, each grew to include the other. Contemporary family therapy addresses problems in both individuals and relationships. The either/or of individual versus family pathology has given way to seeing multiple or bidirectional influences. For example, an angry child may struggle with regulating his or her own affect and/or he or she may dysregulate due to an overbearing or inconsistent parent. Family therapies take seriously transactional patterns that may either complicate or be used to aid treatment. Thus, family therapies work with individuals and dyads as well as with families. In this sense, family therapy recognizes several patients: the child or adolescent, other relevant family members (e.g., the parents), and the family (disordered family processes). Current family therapies and family-based treatments developed within an evidence-based and pathology-focused (i.e., *Diagnostic and Statistical Manual of Mental Disorders* [DSM]) milieu. These interventions are designed to work with the family in order to lessen the child's presenting problem. The goal is the eradication or stabilization of psychiatric pathology and the enhancement of healthy development in the patient.

History

Around the time of World War I, the child guidance movement, with its hope for early intervention, was a major contributor in the development of treatments involving children and families. After World War II, the field of social psychology rapidly developed. Studies focused on small group dynamics and the impact of social role and interactional forces that influence human behavior. Gestalt psychology drew upon a wide variety of theories and interventions that addressed human experience and the social world. In the post–World War II era, family therapy developed in response to the perceived failure of individually based and psychoanalytic approaches to effectively treat a variety of psychiatric problems. The focus shifted to social influences and interactions as well as to forms and patterns of communication.

Virginia Satir, Theodore Lidz, John Bowlby, Nathan Ackerman, and the Mental Research Institute headed by Gregory Bateson were key contributors of this early tradition and played major parts in the formation of family therapy theory. Early forms of marriage counseling contributed significantly by establishing a focus on the interaction of dyads. The decades after World War II were periods of creative enthusiasm, exuberance, and pioneering efforts in the behavioral sciences. Development of family therapy practice was driven by theory rather than empirical research. Primarily, it was the charisma of the founders and the

force of their personalities that popularized early models and approaches to treatment. Rarely were systematic outcomes of interventions subjected to empirical testing. Nevertheless, these pioneers drove home the point that including the family in the assessment and treatment of individual psychopathology made theoretical and practical sense. Clearly, they pointed out, the onset and maintenance of individual psychopathology do not occur in a vacuum; rather, human beings are fundamentally social creatures whose development is intricately tied to the bidirectional forces between individuals and their environments. Subsequent generations of family-oriented clinicians strove to identify the "active ingredients" contributing to change in different approaches and methods. Many early models of family therapy are no longer practiced. The basic sciences of family studies, family psychology, and developmental child psychology, along with the now established research traditions in family and couples therapy, provide a firm foundation for current treatments. Furthermore, since the 1970s, longitudinal research in couples therapy has led to increasing knowledge about the factors contributing to troubled versus well-functioning relationships. To a significant degree, this knowledge about "couples" translates into family "dyads." For instance, we know a great deal about how healthy couples upregulate positive affects and downregulate negative affects, and we have many intervention techniques to help troubled dyads improve their emotion regulation (Fruzzetti and Iverson 2006; Valiente and Eisenberg 2006). This work can be extrapolated to helping parents and children regulate affects. Currently, the research traditions in and related to family therapy readily link to evidence-based medicine and empirically supported treatments. What the clinician now needs is a road map to help him or her navigate the terrain.

Traditional Models

This section describes briefly some of the classic or traditional models of family therapy. It is beneficial to recognize their names and the key concepts associated with them. Structural family therapy, represented by Salvador Minuchin of the Philadelphia Child Guidance Clinic, emphasizes aspects of family structure. Family boundaries that are too rigid, disengaged, diffuse, or enmeshed are areas of intervention (Cuffe et al. 2005). Triangles, coalitions, and over- and underinvolvement are also concerns. Often, we see one parent overtly or covertly aligned with a child against the other parent, thus weakening overall parental effectiveness. A triangle exists when the emotionality between two persons spills over to a third. For example, a father has longstanding anger toward his wife because she is forgetful. In response, the father is overly harsh toward his son for his forgetfulness. A coalition is a recognized voting bloc within family. For instance, a coalition exists when a father always supports his son's interests. A triangle may be unconscious or covert, while a coalition is overt. Identifying triangles and changing negative parenting are important in order to increase parental effectiveness and improve parent-child interactions. This approach emphasizes strong parental participation and the need for clear parental leadership and communication across boundaries. Problems are thought to arise when family boundaries or structures are outside of an expected range.

Strategic family therapy, a historically important model that is now rarely used, views problem formation in terms of failed solutions and interventions in terms of paradoxical injunctions. For example, parents become concerned that their child's school performance is declining and so increase their surveillance of the child's homework and studies. The child becomes anxious and resents what he or she sees as parental pressure and continues to fail. A strategic intervention would encourage the parents to do more of the same (paradoxical injunction) until they become frustrated and open to different solutions.

Historically, Bowen family systems therapy is noteworthy for its equal regard for both the individual and familial dimensions contributing to human problems. This model assesses and intervenes through seven interlocking concepts: differentiation of the self, emotional triangles, nuclear family emotional process, multigenerational transmission, family projections, sibling positions, and emotional cutoffs. The centerpiece of this approach is a self that is sufficiently secure to be both less reactive to others and able to form viable relationships with other family members. This is achieved by helping family members to calmly make *I-statements* and not react beyond a normal range in response to others. This concept is known as *differentiation of self*. The *nuclear family emotional process* entails both emotional triangles and the overall process of reactivity (heightened anxiety) to others. Insufficient differentiation of self leads to excessive emotional reactivity. The *multigenerational transmission process* refers to how anxious relating is passed from one generation to another. The *family projection process* describes intergenerational patterns that assign roles to family members. For instance, the oldest female may be expected to become the family switchboard (the one who communicates and coordinates social contact). *Emotional cutoffs* are often seen as an indicator of anxiety, that is, when the conflict or reactivity is so great that family members cease to relate.

Experiential family therapies, represented by Carl Whitaker and Virginia Satir, demonstrate that a keen awareness of the here-and-now experience of family members is beneficial to treatment. This attunement to the emotional reactions of family members guides assessment and intervention. These models brought to the field an appropriate emphasis on in-session interaction. An example would be asking a conflicted parent-child dyad to talk about a problem in session. This allows the clinician to see firsthand the strengths and weaknesses of the relationship.

Key Terms and Organizing Metaphors

Family therapy has developed its own descriptive vocabulary that aids the clinician in maintaining the dual focus on the identified patient and the relevant social forces. The *identified patient* is the person (the child or adolescent) originally presenting for treatment. Family therapy uses this term to remind clinicians that other family members and the family as a whole, in some sense, are "patients" requiring assessment and intervention. For instance, there are strong associations between the emergence of conduct problems in young people and parents who are inconsistent or use overly harsh punishment (Buehler and Gerard 2002). It is quite difficult to address the primary problems of the identified patient without addressing the family parental dysfunction.

The interlocking nature of family interactions is, perhaps, best captured in the term *circular causality*. *Linear causality* seeks to identify, in a sequential fashion, when and how a certain problem began. For instance, the child's behavior problems increased when a parent moved out of the household. However, many human difficulties arise within a social or interactional context, and a specific moment of change when the problem emerged cannot be identified. For instance, trying to find a first cause to a family argument often fails because each participant can cite a previous grievance (in some cases, going back years). Employing circular causality frees the clinician from evaluating who (or what) started the problem. Family therapists often refer to a *nag-withdrawal pattern*. A parent may say, "Yes, I nag you (try to get you to talk) because you are so withdrawn." Whereas, the young person may say, "I tune you out because you nag me all the time." Seeing the circular causality prevents the useless search for a first cause or perpetrator and allows for interventions that address how both individuals may be a little right and a little wrong—but can change the cycle if they choose.

Related to circular causality, family therapists are alert to *interactive, bidirectional,* or *transactional processes.* For example, the escalation of *negative affective reciprocity* (perceiving negative emotion from someone and amplifying one's response) has been found to be frequently associated with lower levels of attachment and relational stability (Gottman 1994). Helping dyads understand this interactive process and teaching them to resist increasing their retaliatory responses helps them create and sustain a stable and satisfying bond. Because families are made up of interlocking dyads, helping dyads construct stable and beneficial relationships is an important focus for clinical intervention.

Emotion (or *affect*) *regulation* deals with how well-functioning individuals downregulate negative emotion and upregulate positive emotions (related to mastery and achievement, which build emotional security and self-esteem). Family therapists also focus on how dyads regulate affect. For instance, a mother may model the downward spiral of negative emotion (e.g., anxiety) and not know what to do when her child does the same. In this example, helping the mother to both downregulate her negative mood and learn how to respond to her child when the same is present is important. Also, we frequently see parental differences with one parent more able or less able to respond to the child's affective expression. Working on two levels provides a powerful advantage for clinicians.

The notion of clinical *constraints* was developed by Breunlin et al. (1992). It asks the questions, "Why can't people solve their own problems? What is constraining a person or a family from overcoming the difficulty?" By thinking in terms of constraints, the clinician is guided to potential sources of problems and can readily develop a workable intervention focus.

From the beginning, family therapy has thought in terms of several parallel and sometimes intertwined *developmental trajectories.* Besides the developmental needs of the identified patient, family therapists consider the developmental processes of couple and family formation and how parent-child interactions are affected by them and how interactional styles must change with maturation. For instance, one child may become symptomatic when the youngest sibling enters school and the mother returns to work. Helping the family and the identified patient to adapt to the change is an important clinical consideration.

Since the 1990s, family therapists have focused on the kinds of stories or *narratives* families tell. These stories identify family cultures and often reflect the kinds of images, roles, and cognitive constructions family members have of one another. For example, if parents see a child as troublesome, this child may often be blamed for things he or she did not do. This process may also discourage him or her from trying to differentiate from the ascribed role. Helping the family shift the narrative to more constructive images (Freeman et al. 1997; White and Epston 1990) is important. Within the last decade, we have seen some crossover between cognitive-behavioral therapy (CBT) and narrative (family) therapies (Dattilio 2005) in theory formation and intervention. This is a fruitful area of exploration and practice.

The Social Environment for Children and Adolescents

D. W. Winnicott, an early major figure in child psychiatry, emphasized the significance of the social environment for the child in terms of two interlocking processes. The first is the developmental process from *absolute dependence through relative dependence to independence* (Winnicott 1960/1965, 1963/1965). The second process is the profoundly beneficial influence of an *emotionally facilitating environment.* Winnicott posited that the adequacy of this social environment is essential for normal human development and psychological growth. Perhaps more than anything else, it is the dependence of infants, children, and adolescents and the sensitivity and reactivity of young people to their environment that distinguish working with children and adolescents from the treatment of adults. Winnicott's theory is now firmly established in the literature. There are a variety of regulatory processes, biologically based and environmentally shaped, that influence emotional outcomes from health and vitality to the manifestation of behavioral disorders. A critical component of Winnicott's theory is the *holding environment*: that is, the provision of a safe and need-fulfilling social context within which the infant and young child can develop. The creation of this holding environment requires an early and primary parental preoccupation in order to facilitate the growth of children, which gradually recedes as the child matures. This is one reason why the family is so important to child and adolescent mental health practice. Adults may be able to be treated without reference to their family (although many rightly question this), but the dependency of children requires the assessment and involvement of the family.

Approaching the Complexity of Youth in Families

Assessment and treatment of the family involve more layers than the assessment of each member of a family. It also requires an analysis of the effects of one or more members of the family on the identified patient. Historically, practitioners of family therapy and family-based therapies added a level of assessment and intervention generally referred to as *systems* (Berman and Heru 2005). More recently, scholars use the terms bidirectional influence, transactional processes, or interactive processes to describe how the patient and his or her social world actively affect each other. This influence is more powerful than many think. In practical terms, "sick kids can make families dysfunctional" and "dysfunctional families can make kids sick." Also, and often overlooked, strengths in the family and in individuals can be brought to bear to improve treatments (American Academy of Child and Adolescent Psychiatry 2007). For example, if a clinician is seeing a patient within a frustrated but strongly attached family, the love and care they have for one another can be called upon to enhance treatment. Simply saying, in this instance, "I understand how upsetting this problem is for all of you and how tired and frustrated you are, but I also see that you really care for one another. I am sure we can work together to improve things," can have a powerful facilitative effect on treatment.

For some clinicians, sensitivity to transactional influences comes naturally. For others it may take a great deal of effort, even a paradigm shift. Therapists with these skills think in terms of patterns, sequences, and shared responsibility for problems and solutions and readily invite family members to sessions. Effective family therapy requires a working alliance not just with the identified patient but also with other pertinent family members. In the beginning of treatment, clinicians cannot be sure who is negatively affecting the patient and who might be called upon to enhance the outcome.

General Principles

Successful family-based treatments share specific characteristics. In therapies for individuals, when the patient enters the consultation room, it is reasonable for the clinician to ask, in a variety of ways "What is the problem?", whereas working with dyads and families requires different tactics. Families, by definition, involve multiple people, often with different experiences and perspectives on the "problem." So clinicians who ask, "What is the problem?" are likely to hear the most verbal and most frustrated person, probably a parent, launch into a *problem-saturated description* (White and Epston 1990), such as portrayed in the clinical vignette later in this chapter, in the section "Implementing IMBFT." The neediness and frustrations of family members are often overwhelming, and beginning therapists find themselves unable to redirect the speaker, quickly losing control of the session. At the same time, the child who is the identified patient is likely to become flooded with negative emotion and either fight back or shut down. Either way, therapists with an individual therapy orientation find themselves in an alienating situation. Family therapists actively use a technique known as *joining* to do three things. First, they avoid the "What's wrong?" question. Second, family therapists begin with relationship-building small talk with each person in the room. Third, they postpone (interrupting if necessary) the serious talk until everyone in attendance has had a chance to enter the process (in as low stress an atmosphere as possible). Following this joining with the family, the therapist solicits each person's view of the problem in turn. Only after everyone's story has been heard is it wise to move on to the next stage.

Family therapists listen to the description of the problem from each family member and note points of agreement and disagreement. Discrepancies are expected, and family therapists begin to construct in their own mind a view of the problem that is clinically workable and most likely to be shared by all. This may be done in one session or several. When family therapists together with the family and identified patient have generated a shared explanation of the problem (*shaping a workable presenting problem*), then and only then can they begin to think in terms of solutions and interventions. It should be noted that family therapists routinely delay formal assessment until they have built a working alliance with each pertinent family member. This may be difficult in many clinical settings and may work better if diagnostic assessment and treatment are separated. This relational style models good relationship formation and has been found to be one of the most powerful "common factors" (Bachelor and Horvath 1999; Blatt et al. 1996; Sprenkle and Blow 2004) in good psychotherapeutic practice. This working relationship with all family members also enhances assessment cooperation. As assessment comes to a close, family therapists move to *create a shared tenable treatment plan*. This requires, in most cases, agreement among all family members present; otherwise, a misalliance may be created leading to treatment dropout or nonadherence.

Indications

In the last decade and a half, family therapy and family-based treatments have moved from theoretical models to more empirically supported or evidence-based practice. Treatment effectiveness summaries highlight that family therapy and family-based approaches are effective in the treatment of externalizing disorders, particularly for alcohol and substance abuse and conduct disorder, as well as the secondary features of attention-deficit/hyperactivity disorder (ADHD) (Diamond and Josephson 2005; Pinsof and Wynne 1995, 2000; Rowe at al. 2006; Sprenkle 2002). There is also suggestive evidence that depression, anxiety problems, and eating disorders can be addressed effectively with family treatments. Since Diamond and Josephson's review, Wood et al. (2006) have done a study of family-based CBT for anxiety disorders that shows superior outcomes compared to individual CBT alone for the identified patient. See other chapters in this text for more details on treatment of specific disorders.

In evaluating the effectiveness of family treatments, the clinician must keep two important points in mind. First, it is sometimes said that family therapies are less established than treatments for individuals. However, the lag in evidence-based studies is due more to the complexity of the subject matter, with many added trajectories of influence in family research, than to weaker intervention potential. Also, many studies that "compare" family treatment to individual therapies use a generic or nonspecific family

treatment as a comparison group rather than an empirically supported family treatment. Such studies are minimally informative, since family therapy and family treatments have been moving in a more focal, integrative, and evidence-based direction.

More Recent Models

The more recent models take into account the lessons of the earlier generations of family therapy as well as current thinking and empirical data in the fields of family therapy research and child and adolescent psychiatry and psychology. *Functional family therapy* is most often associated with James Alexander (Alexander and Parsons 1982). Functional family therapists observe how symptoms and behaviors function and then seek to remedy the manifesting problems. This model has been shown to reduce behavior problems in children and adolescents. The 1990s saw *solution-focused family therapy* grow in popularity. This model deemphasizes problems and instead focuses on solutions. When families want to talk about problems, solution-focused clinicians explore exceptions to the problem (i.e., identify times or circumstances in which the problem does not exist). *Narrative family therapy* (Freeman et al. 1997) focuses on the stories families tell and how these narratives both define roles of family members and constrain the family from seeking alternative narratives (leading to more adaptive behaviors). *Emotionally focused therapy* (EFT) has received empirical support for the treatment of couples and depression in adults (Bradley and Johnson 2005; Dessaulles et al. 2003; Greenberg and Johnson 1988; Johnson and Greenberg 1985) and is growing in influence. EFT draws from the experiential family therapy tradition and focuses on how both individual members and dyads in families regulate affects. One of the central interventions in EFT is helping individuals and dyads transform the expression of *hard emotions* (defensive or secondary affects such as anger, suspicion, resentment, retaliation) into *soft emotions* (primary or vulnerable feelings such as hurt, shame, fear) in order to downregulate negative affects and improve empathy, attachment, and cooperative problem-solving.

Psychoeducational Therapies

Some family-based treatments are not designed to change or treat conditions so much as to help a family manage them. Medical family therapy (McDaniel et al.

1992, 2004; Rolland and Walsh 2005) strives to help patients and their families cope with a variety of medical conditions. John Rolland (1994) has done extensive work with families with significant medical conditions. Parent management training (Kazdin 2005) has gained both use and empirical support. This approach focuses on the identified patient's behavior but also actively includes the family, addressing strengths and weaknesses that may affect outcomes. (See Chapter 54, "Parent Counseling, Psychoeducation, and Parent Support Groups," and Chapter 55, "Behavioral Parent Training," respectively, for parent psychoeducational and behavioral therapies.) Barkley (2006) and colleagues have designed treatment protocols to address the secondary deficits of ADHD. Webster-Stratton and colleagues (Webster-Stratton 2005; Webster-Stratton and Reid 2003) have developed successful parent-based programs designed to manage conduct problems in young children.

Current Models

Newer models of family therapy have been developed that fit the kind of clinical challenges we face today. To provide context, we highlight three current models and their zeitgeist.

In 1997, Jay Lebow wrote an influential article that signified a dramatic change in family therapy practice, which he described as an "integrative evolution in couple and family therapy." He called attention to empirically supported treatments, evidence-based practice, and best practice standards that have led clinicians to "do what works" rather than be loyal to and practice within a preferred theoretical model. In fact, many of these treatments require a multimodal integrative approach. Lebow's article emphasized a shift that had already begun to take place. Henggeler and colleagues, in the 1980s and 1990s, developed multisystemic therapy, an integrative approach that involves individual, family, school, and community interventions (Henggeler et al. 1986, 1992). In 1992, Breunlin and colleagues published their approach to family therapy, which incorporates the learned wisdom of the traditional models into six assessment and intervention domains called *metaframeworks*. In 1995, Pinsof developed a problem-centered integrative model designed to synthesize family, individual, and biological therapies. Integrative module-based family therapy (Gouze and Wendel 2008; Wendel et al. 2005) is within this trajectory and aims to create an evidence-based practice that addresses the biopsychosocial world of the patient. All of these integrative models strive to *view disorders within empirically identified biological, familial, dyadic, and individual processes*. In this sense, today's integrative practice hopes to capture both the art of earlier therapies and the science of contemporary evidence-based treatment.

Integrative Module-Based Family Therapy

The integrative module-based family therapy (IMBFT) approach (Gouze and Wendel 2008; Wendel et al. 2005) combines previous integrative family therapy models (e.g., Breunlin et al. 1992), empirically supported and best practice approaches to family treatment, and theoretical and empirical literature from the fields of developmental psychology and psychopathology, family studies, and psychiatry to provide a road map for assessment and treatment of families.

IMBFT identifies 10 critical modules for assessment and treatment that can be used by clinicians in planning and executing treatment decisions. A module is a critical domain for assessment and intervention. After assessment directs the clinician to an initial module for intervention, the clinician seeks out an empirically supported or best practice treatment for the identified problem. The 10 modules are as follows:

1. **Psychiatric/biological module** (intervention in this module would include psychopharmacology)—This module entails assessing the psychiatric status of the identified patient (i.e., the child or adolescent) initially presented for assessment and treatment using standard criteria from the *Diagnostic and Statistical Manual of Mental Disorders*, 4th Edition, Text Revision (DSM-IV-TR; American Psychiatric Association 2000). The assumption is that successful family intervention requires a complete understanding of the child or adolescent's more biologically based difficulties. For example, family intervention with a child with moderate to severe ADHD might necessitate pharmacological intervention for ADHD before significant progress can be made through family therapy. Similarly, identifying the biological bases of disorders in participating family members, particularly parents, may be a prerequisite for improvement through family therapy. A depressed or substance abusing parent, for example, may require adjunctive individual treat-

ment before progress can be made with the identified patient through family intervention.

2. **Attachment/relationship module**—This module is derived from a large body of literature (Egeland and Erikson 1993; Lieberman et al. 1991) that demonstrates the relationship between secure parent-child attachments and healthy child development. This attachment relationship provides a secure base (Bowlby 1988) from which children can explore the environment and functions as a template for future relationships (Cassidy 1999; Lyons-Ruth et al. 1998). As children and adolescents grow, their relationships with their parents serve as a fundamental source of self-esteem. When family relationships are fractured, it is difficult to move past the negative aspects of these relationships unless this module is addressed first.

3. **Family structure module**—Since the work of Minuchin and colleagues (Minuchin 1974; Minuchin and Fishman 1981), family structure has been seen as an important contributor to the formation and maintenance of individual pathology within families. A family with an oppositional defiant child, for example, is often a family with a poorly developed parenting dyad. Assessment of and intervention in this module requires attention to roles, hierarchies, family alliances, and boundaries.

4. **Family communication module**—From the inception of family therapy, every model, in its own way, has dealt with the type, method, and content of communication in families. Healthy families communicate clearly, express and respond to emotional content, are attuned to nonverbal messages, and are able to problem-solve without avoidance or escalating into conflict. The questions within the assessment template help the clinician to identify strengths and problems of communication in families.

5. **Developmental module**—Since Freud, the concept of stages of development and barriers to development as an organizing theme have been central to understanding the emergence of psychopathology. Traditional family therapy models that address family of origin issues (e.g., Bowen) also adhere closely to the notion that impediments to healthy individuation are developmental in nature. Assessment and intervention within this module necessitate an understanding of normal family processes (see Chapter 40, "Family Transitions: Challenges and Resilience," and Walsh

2003) and child development. An example of the need for treatment within this module might be the emergence of symptoms as a child begins to negotiate the demands of adolescence.

6. **Affect regulation module**—As elaborated earlier in the description of emotionally focused therapy, affect regulation is a critical aspect of psychiatric health. Poor affect regulation is, almost by definition, indicative of poor psychological functioning. Note, for example, the number of diagnoses that have irritability as a core symptom. The ability to regulate affect has been shown to be critical to the mental health of individual members of the family (Kovacs et al. 2006; Valiente and Eisenberg 2006). Not only do individual family members who themselves affectively dysregulate contribute to high levels of negative emotionality, but the reverse is also true. Families that have the ability to regulate affect contribute to greater stability in psychiatrically impaired members (Anderson and Reiss 1982; Anderson et al. 1986). Children and adolescents learn to regulate their own affects within the context of their families, making this a critical area of intervention for children and adolescents who present with affective disturbances.

7. **Behavior regulation module**—Assessment and intervention within this module are often central for children and adolescents with externalizing disorders. It draws upon the vast array of empirically supported treatments in the parenting literature (Eyeberg and Boggs 1998; Kazdin 2005; Webster-Stratton 1990), multisystemic therapy (Henggeler et al. 1992), and the work of Gerald Patterson and associates (Patterson 1982; Snyder et al. 2007) that demonstrate that treatment of externalizing disorders often requires behavioral intervention at the family level (Cummings and Davies 1994). Parental monitoring of behavior programs, providing structure for accomplishing tasks (e.g., homework), and setting of household rules are examples of interventions that fall under this module.

8. **Cognitive/narrative module**—This module draws upon literature in two areas: the narrative family therapy tradition described earlier and cognitive-behavioral therapies as cornerstones of treatment. This module is addressed first if family stories or myths continue to support maladaptive behavior in an individual child or adolescent—e.g., "He's the lazy one in the family." Or it might be the first module engaged in interven-

tion if cognitive restructuring is required to shift a family's focus from a problem-oriented view of a child to the things he or she does right. *Reframing*—a time-honored technique in family therapy, in which a more positive perspective is placed on what is otherwise seen as a maladaptive behavior—falls in this category. An example might be when a parent complains that an anxious child is driving her crazy with her clingy behavior and the therapist reframes this as the child's need to be close to her mother.

9. **Mastery module**—Mastery is a core concept in developmental psychology and psychopathology. Winnicott, Freud, and Erickson all identify mastery as central to the growing child's development of self-esteem and a core self. The mastery module is critical to address in families in which individual members' failures of mastery—e.g., inability to hold a job, poor school performance, inability to make friends—are contributing to or serving to maintain mental health problems.

10. **Community module**—This broad module encompasses the need for family therapists to be sensitive to the role that culture, socioeconomic level, immigration status, religion, race, and gender play in creating conditions that produce or maintain psychopathology. Even when this module is not the prime focus of intervention, it is critical that it be considered as a frame for working within all the other modules.

Implementing IMBFT

A step-by-step assessment instrument and sample assessment questions for each module can be found in Tables 56–1 and 56–2. Assessment of the family across all 10 dimensions provides the clinician with a focus for beginning intervention. After assessing all 10 modules, using the assessment template, the clinician chooses a focus for beginning intervention based on two criteria. The first concern is to focus on the most acute problem area. Second, the therapist must assess whether leaving a particular problem area unresolved will interfere with progress in another module and thereby block therapeutic progress. For example, if familial relationships are badly fractured and there is poor behavior regulation, it is likely that some repair of the attachments will have to precede the behavioral intervention or the behavioral intervention will fail. This is why most parenting programs begin with instructing parents to play with their children before

teaching discipline techniques such as time-out (e.g., Eyeberg and Boggs 1998; Webster-Stratton 2005). Once a module is selected as the focus for beginning intervention, the clinician is encouraged to search the literature (e.g., Medline and PsycINFO) to determine the best practice or empirically supported treatments that are applicable (see also Chapter 30, "Evidence-Based Practices"). Table 56–3 provides a sample of empirically based and best practice interventions to guide treatment for each of the modules. Following the choice of module and subsequent intervention, it is critical that the clinician assess progress using standard outcome techniques such as ratings of symptoms, standard checklists, or regular reviews with the family concerning progress toward shared therapeutic goals. When treating children and adolescents, depending upon the presenting problems, it is often important for the clinician to get measures from outside the family—e.g., teachers. IMBFT was designed to be flexible, and therefore, responsive to changing clinical presentations or new barriers that interfere with treatment. As the clinician proceeds, ongoing evaluation of outcomes and barriers guides the clinician toward new modules or dimensions of intervention. As the therapist moves to address new symptoms or overcome barriers, he or she can easily reassess with the assessment template and choose new modules as points of intervention. This systematic approach provides a heuristic frame for treatment that is readily accessible even to less experienced family therapists.

Clinical Vignette

You welcome a plainly dressed mother with a serious and distressed look on her face and a young teenage male wearing clothes that look slept in with his underwear showing atop his low-slung pants. He doesn't make eye contact, avoids a handshake, drops into your consultation chair, and begins to stare out the window. His mother turns to you and says, "See, he has no respect for others. You gotta straighten him out." That is only the beginning, as the mother launches into a 10-minute monologue about how her son won't talk "normally" to his parents. He yells and "starts a fight if you say anything to him." He isn't doing well in school. He has been caught with cheap whiskey in his room, and "last week he was arrested for driving without a license." She enacts a dramatic pause and exclaims, "And he's only 14." As you realize that the teenager is actually in the room, you notice that his mood is sullen and he has been shaking his head in disgust. When you try to ask him what he makes of what his mother has just said, he replies, "Yeah whatever…" as his mother begins to yell at him. The teen interrupts her and shouts, "I was just going to see Brandy." Even though it is unpleasant, you decide to let the two of them argue, just

TABLE 56–1. Integrative module-based family therapy: step-by-step assessment

1. Patient identification

    a. Age and gender

    b. Cultural and/or social variables

    c. Family composition (members of household, pertinent extended family)

2. Diagnostic assessment and indicators

    a. DSM-IV-TR symptoms in the identified patient

    b. Diagnostically unanswered questions

    c. Current or tentative diagnosis

    d. Medications (if any)

Until the patient is psychiatrically stable, supportive and psychoeducational interventions are indicated.

3. Diagnostic assessment of psychosocial indicators

    a. *Attachment/relationship*: How strained or conflicted are the relationships within the family? It is difficult to form a viable treatment plan until at least there is an understanding that improving relationships and managing conflict are priorities. Rate from stable (7) to unstable (1). List strengths and weaknesses in the family.

          Strengths   Weaknesses

    b. *Family structure*: Are there indications that structural issues (excessive discipline, inconsistent discipline, poor parental leadership, etc.) are exacerbating the presenting problem? Rate from stable (7) to unstable (1). List strengths and weaknesses in the family.

          Strengths   Weaknesses

    c. *Family communication*: Do family members speak directly to one another? Are the messages clear? Do family members feel heard? Do family members hear and respond to one another's feelings? Do family members interrupt one another? Do family members use feeling words, and is the emotion vocabulary sufficiently broad? Is parenting done through imperatives with no explanation? Do family members speak with I-statements? Can family members discuss emotionally charged issues without avoidance or conflict? Can family members perceive and respond to nonverbal cues? Rate from stable (7) to unstable (1). List strengths and weaknesses in the family.

          Strengths   Weaknesses

    d. *Developmental issues*: How pertinent are individual and/or family developmental issues to the presenting problem? Rate from stable (7) to unstable (1). List strengths and weaknesses in the family.

          Strengths   Weaknesses

    e. *Affect regulation*: Are individuals able to regulate affects? Are there relationships within the family that are prone to dysregulation? Rate from stable (7) to unstable (1). List strengths and weaknesses in the family.

          Strengths   Weaknesses

TABLE 56–1. Integrative module-based family therapy: step-by-step assessment *(continued)*

    f. *Behavior regulation*: Are there individuals in the family who are prone to behavioral dysregulation? Are there specific relationships where this is more common? Who in the family is best able to regulate the behavior of the ones who lose control? Rate from stable (7) to unstable (1). List strengths and weaknesses in the family.

              Strengths   Weaknesses

    g. *Cognitive/narrative concerns* (family narratives): Is there evidence of cognitive distortions, exaggerated thoughts, or opinions about one another based more on emotion than facts? Rate from stable (7) to unstable (1). List strengths and weaknesses in the family.

              Strengths   Weaknesses

    h. *Mastery*: Is the family successful in helping members achieve mastery, self-efficacy, and self-esteem? Is this related to the presenting problem? Rate from stable (7) to unstable (1). List strengths and weaknesses in the family.

              Strengths   Weaknesses

    i. *Community* (race, gender, worldview, religion, culture, sexual orientation, etc.): Are there relevant community issues that make achieving therapeutic goals difficult? Rate from stable (7) to unstable (1). List strengths and weaknesses in the family's community context.

              Strengths   Weaknesses

Formulation

In light of the psychiatric diagnosis and the assessment of relevant psychosocial dimensions, describe how the presenting problem has become difficult for this particular patient and his or her family to manage. Or, how is the Axis I diagnosis embedded within the familial context? What strengths within the family may be used to further clinical goals? What weaknesses complicate treatment?

Treatment plan

Domains of high concern generally require initial attention. Evidence-based medicine, empirically supported treatment, and best practice standards aid treatment planning. If treatment is not progressing, consider ways to strengthen the alliance with critical family members in order to aid treatment adherence. Please describe the (proposed or to-date) treatment plan.

Please assess how well the patient and the family agree with the treatment plan.

Source. Adapted from Gouze and Wendel 2008.

so you can hear something from the teen and watch how they relate. After about 5 minutes you learn that the teen isn't the only one shouting at home. Apparently mom and dad fight regularly because dad goes out and no one knows where he is. The teen's older brother left for college earlier in the year and hasn't come home for a visit.

How and where does one begin? First of all, it is generally best to not allow the problem-saturated description to take over the therapeutic process. The clinician will have to interrupt the mother and state that

the problems will be fully addressed later, but at this point it is more important for him or her to get to know both the mother and her son. This would begin the three-step joining process described earlier in the section "General Principles." As the therapist builds a relationship and rapport with both the mother and the teen, several questions emerge: Do we assess for substance abuse? Depression? ADHD? Conduct disorder? Do we have individual sessions with the teen or conjoint clinical hours with the teen and mom? What about dad? Clearly, there is no simple one-, two-, or

TABLE 56–2. Sample assessment questions for integrative module-based family therapy modules

Psychiatric and related medical conditions module
- Standard psychiatric diagnostic questions guided by DSM-IV-TR, such as "Does your child have difficulty completing tasks?" "Does he or she get easily distracted?" "Does he or she seem sad most days?" "Does he or she have difficulty being left with a babysitter?"
- Describe your child's medical history—any hospitalizations, medical conditions, current or past medications?

Attachment/relationship module
- Who in the family has the closest relationship with your child?
- What is your relationship with your parents? Are you close?
- Whom do you go to for support with your parenting?
- Who is the best listener in the family?

Family structure module
- Who is most likely to enforce the rules in your family?
- How are chores assigned to the children? Who assigns them? Who makes sure they are done?
- Do parents usually agree about how things should be done? If they disagree, how do they decide?
- If you are planning a family outing, how do you decide where to go?

Family communication module
- Do family members feel heard?
- Can family members tell what others are feeling?
- How do parents present and explain their directives?

Developmental module
- Your child is starting school in the fall. How do you feel about this transition?
- What was school like for you? (Ask other children in the family, How do you guys feel about school? Do you do well?)
- What are your hopes and dreams for your child?
- How will having all your children in school all day change your life? What will you do with your free time during the day?

Affect regulation module
- Who has the worst temper in your family? Anyone else with a bad temper? What does that person do when he or she is angry?
- How do people in your family calm down after a fight? How long does it take to restore positive relationships? How is that accomplished?
- Do you think of your family as a pretty calm family or a very emotional one? Tell me more about that.

Behavior regulation module
- What are the rules about acceptable and unacceptable behavior in your family?
- What kinds of rewards and consequences do you use?
- Do the adults in your family follow rules and model good behavior, or do the adults push the limits (e.g., ignore parking regulations or lie about children's ages to get them into the movies less expensively)?

Cognitive/narrative module
- Do you have favorite family stories or traditions that would help me understand your family?
- Do you think of different members of the family in particular ways? If they were characters in a novel, how would you describe each of them?
- How do different family members react to your child when he or she is nervous? Do you all seem to follow the same script when this happens?

Mastery module
- Are you pleased with your performance in school? Who else in your family has opinions about how you do in school?
- What other things are you good at? Do you do sports or music or art?
- Do you feel effective as a parent? What kinds of things make you feel more or less effective?

TABLE 56–2. Sample assessment questions for integrative module-based family therapy modules *(continued)*

Community module
- What were gender roles like in your own family of origin? How have you worked these out in your current family?
- Are you involved with a religious or community group of any type?
- What has it been like for you to immigrate to this country? How do you feel that this affects your relationship with your children?

Source. Adapted from Gouze and Wendel 2008.

three-step algorithm. By applying the 10 modules of IMBFT (see Tables 56–1 and 56–2), the clinician begins to form a road map for intervention. Step 1 (see Table 56–1) involves soliciting descriptive information of the identified patient and his family. It is important to see the "problem" within the larger familial context. Asking questions like "Please describe a typical day from rising until bedtime for the family" or "Are there times when the 'problem' isn't a problem?" can be quite informative. The clinician should be attuned to family transitions known to be times of increased vulnerability. Be sure to ask more than one person and note differences and similarities in accounts. This type of discussion helps the clinician do two things. First, it provides important information without stimulating a problem-saturated description and helps the family therapist to begin to form a view of overall family life and functioning. Secondly, it allows the clinician to indirectly consider DSM indications.

As the atmosphere calms down, the therapist can seek more specific information related to Axis-I pathology (Step 2). In the above vignette, conduct disorder, ADHD, depression with agitation, and drug abuse need to be considered and viewed within overall family function. Table 56–2 provides sample questions the clinician can ask to determine the primacy of the other nine modules: attachments, family structure, communication, development, affect regulation, behavior regulation, cognitive/narrative concerns, mastery, and community. Ranking from low concern (1) to high concern (7) helps focus all of the information. In reviewing these scales, the therapist notes that modulating affect and behavior regulation are areas of concern. Also, the strained attachments suggest that cooperation and treatment adherence is unlikely until the familial relationships improve. Why are mom and dad fighting (see Buehler and Gerard 2002)? Are they modeling hostile and impulsive interactional styles? Where does the dad go? Who is he with? Is the teen doing what dad does? Do mom and dad exhibit positive and consistent parental structure focusing more on re-

wards than punishments? Why are the family attachments strained? Did this happen recently or is it longstanding? Who in the family is best able to help regulate the teen's affects and what are the differences between the one who is best and worst at regulating the teen's emotional response? Why hasn't the older brother come home from college? Questions such as these help the clinician construct a formulation in which the problem is seen within overall family functioning.

Before the family therapist moves toward a treatment plan, session configuration needs to be considered. In this case, family or dyadic sessions are more appropriate but the marital and familial climates are significant complicating factors. The clinician must guard against allowing the parents to prematurely focus on the teen's problems, which would be likely to stimulate an outburst confirming the parents' views and agenda but alienating the identified patient. The clinician could meet separately with each and corroborate accounts. Perhaps a better plan would be to invite other family members so accounts can be verified or dismissed. The clinician would have to exert more session management so as not to let the emotional level escalate. As the clinician formulates the case and considers treatment foci and options, the next step is entering into a discussion with the family and seeking agreement. In this example, emotionally focused therapy may be applied in order to downregulate negative affective interaction and promote more empathic familial communication (Efron 2004). After there is some improvement in the family's affective and behavioral regulation and their relationships with one another, the therapist might shift to a focus on delays in developmental success and achievement of mastery for the teen. It is hard to focus and apply oneself within an emotionally labile and hostile atmosphere. As a clinician identifies the priority modules (Table 56–1) and intervenes accordingly, he or she is able to engage in a cycle of reassessment that will lead to a new focus until treatment is complete.

TABLE 56–3. Examples of best practice and empirically supported treatments per module

Psychiatric and related medical conditions module
- Medical family therapy for treatment of somatizing patients (McDaniel et al. 1992, 1995)
- Eating disorders (Le Grange et al. 2005, 2007)
- Other chapters in this text
- Practice parameters of the American Academy of Child and Adolescent Psychiatry
- Practice guidelines of the American Psychiatric Association

Attachment/relationship module
- Attachment interventions (Egeland and Erikson 1993; Lieberman et al. 1991).
- Relationship-based therapies (Diamond 2005; Diamond and Stern 2003; Donaldson et al. 2005; Efron 2004; Lieberman et al. 2006)

Family structure module
- Family structure interventions (Minuchin 1974; Minuchin and Fishman 1981)

Family communication module
- Communication and problem solving (Gottman 1999)
- Working with intense affect (Johnson 1996)

Developmental module
- Family therapies that focus on the family of origin (e.g., Bowen family systems)
- Attention to "developmental oscillations" (Breunlin et al. 1992)

Affect regulation module
- Reducing intensity of expressed emotion in families (Anderson et al. 1986; Bradley and Johnson 2005; Denton et al. 2002; Diamond and Stern 2003; Efron 2004; Fristad et al. 2003; Fruzzetti and Iverson 2006; Johnson and Greenman 2006; Kovacs et al. 2006; Valiente and Eisenberg 2006)

Behavior regulation module
- Parent training and related behavioral interventions with parents and children (Eyeberg and Boggs 1998; Forehand and McMahon 1981; Kazdin 2005; Webster-Stratton 1990)
- Family intervention to improve limit setting and reduce coercive cycles of discipline (Patterson 1982)
- Multisystemic family therapy (Henggeler et al. 1986, 1992, 1993; Schoenwald and Henggeler 2005)
- Functional family therapy (Alexander and Parsons 1982; Sexton and Alexander 2005)
- Collaborative problem-solving (Greene and Ablon 2006)

Cognitive/narrative module
- Use of narrative structure to rewrite the family story (Freedman and Combs 1996; White and Epston 1990)
- Use of externalization to understand a problem-saturated story (Freeman et al. 1997)
- Extension of cognitive-behavioral techniques from individual to family (Reinecke and Clark 2004; Reinecke et al. 1996; Wood et al. 2006)

Mastery module
- Academic skill encouragement (Martinez and Forgatch 2002)
- Skills training for externalizing children (Bloomquist 2006)
- Psychoeducational approaches (Anderson et al. 1986)

Community module (social context, gender, culture, sexual orientation, etc.)
- Sensitivity to culture (Bean et al. 2001, 2002; Keiley et al. 2002; Kim et al. 2004; Silk et al. 2004)
- Sensitivity to race (Mandara and Murray 2002)
- Sensitivity to gender (Haddock et al. 2000; Laird 2000)
- Sensitivity to sexual orientation (Bepko and Johnson 2000; Bernstein 2000; Kurdek 2004; Sanders and Kroll 2000; Solomon et al. 2004)
- Sensitivity to religion (Josephson and Peteet 2004)

Source. Adapted from Gouze and Wendel 2008.

Summary Points

Clinicians are encouraged to

- Build a relationship with all family members and encourage each one to tell his or her story.
- Assess through 10 modules (psychiatric/biological, attachment/relationship, family structure, family communication, developmental, affect regulation, behavior regulation, cognitive/narrative, mastery, community).
- Choose a focus.
- Form a feasible shared treatment plan.
- Learn (know) what works based on empirically supported treatments or best practice standards.
- Craft interventions.
- Assess progress toward goals, and make treatment shifts when necessary.

References

Alexander JF, Parsons BV: Functional Family Therapy: Principles and Procedures. Carmel, CA, Brooks and Cole, 1982

American Academy of Child and Adolescent Psychiatry: Practice parameter for the assessment of the family. J Am Acad Child Adolesc Psychiatry 46:922–937, 2007

American Psychiatric Association: Diagnostic and Statistical Manual of Mental Disorders, 4th Edition, Text Revision. Washington, DC, American Psychiatric Association, 2000

Anderson CM, Reiss DJ: Approaches to psychoeducational family therapy. International Journal of Family Psychiatry 3:501–517, 1982

Anderson CM, Reiss DJ, Hogarty GE: Schizophrenia and the Family: A Practitioner's Guide to Psychoeducation and Management. New York, Guilford, 1986

Bachelor A, Horvath A: The therapeutic relationship, in The Heart and Soul of Change: What Works in Therapy. Edited by Miller SD. Washington, DC, American Psychological Association, 1999, pp 133–178

Barkley RA: Attention-Deficit Hyperactivity Disorder: A Handbook for Diagnosis and Treatment, 3rd Edition. New York, Guilford, 2006

Bean RA, Perry BJ, Bedell TM: Developing culturally competent marriage and family therapists: guidelines for working with Hispanics. J Marital Fam Ther 27:43–54, 2001

Bean RA, Perry BJ, Bedell TM: Developing culturally competent marriage and family therapists: treatment guidelines for non-African-American therapists working with African-American families. J Marital Fam Ther 28:153–164, 2002

Bepko C, Johnson T: Gay and lesbian couples in therapy: perspectives for the contemporary therapist. J Marital Fam Ther 26:409–419, 2000

Berman E, Heru AN: Family systems training in psychiatric residencies. Fam Process 44:321–335, 2005

Bernstein AC: Straight therapists working with lesbians and gays in family therapy. J Marital Fam Ther 26:443–454, 2000

Blatt SJ, Sanislow CA, Zuroff DC, et al: Characteristics of effective therapists: further analysis of data from the National Institute of Mental Health treatment of depression collaborative research program. J Consult Clin Psychol 64:1276–1284, 1996

Bloomquist ML: Skills Training for Children With Behavior Problems: A Parent and Practitioner Guidebook, Revised Edition. New York, Guilford, 2006

Bowlby J: A Secure Base: Parent-Child Attachment and Healthy Human Development. New York, Basic Books, 1988

Bradley B, Johnson SM: EFT: an integrative contemporary approach, in Handbook of Couples Therapy. Edited by Harway M. Hoboken, NJ, Wiley, 2005, pp 179–193

Breunlin DC, Schwartz RC, MacKune-Karrer B: Metaframeworks: Transcending the Models of Family Therapy. San Francisco, CA, Jossey-Bass, 1992

Buehler C, Gerard JM: Marital conflict, ineffective parenting, and children's and adolescents' maladjustment. J Marriage Fam 64:78–92, 2002

Cassidy J: The nature of the child's ties, in Handbook of Attachment: Theory, Research, and Clinical Applications. Edited by Cassidy J, Shaver PR. New York, Guilford, 1999, pp 3–20

Cuffe SP, McKeown RE, Addy CL, et al: Family and psychosocial risk factors in a longitudinal epidemiological study of adolescents. J Am Acad Child Adolesc Psychiatry 44:121–129, 2005

Cummings EM, Davies P: Children and Marital Conflict: The Impact of Family Dispute and Resolution. New York, Guilford, 1994

Dattilio FM: The restructuring of family schemas: a cognitive-behavior perspective. J Marital Fam Ther 31:15–30, 2005

Denton WH, Walsh SR, Daniel SS: Evidence-based practice in family therapy: adolescent depression as an example. J Marital Fam Ther 28:39–45, 2002

Dessaulles A, Johnson SM, Denton WH: Emotion-focused therapy for couples in the treatment of depression: a pilot study. Am J Fam Ther 31:345–353, 2003

Diamond G: Attachment-based family therapy for depressed and anxious adolescents, in Handbook of Clinical Family Therapy. Edited by Lebow JL. New York, Wiley, 2005, pp 17–41

Diamond G, Josephson A: Family based treatment research: a 10-year update. J Am Acad Child Adolesc Psychiatry 44:872–887, 2005

Diamond G, Stern RS: Attachment-based family therapy for depressed adolescents: repairing attachment failures, in Attachment Processes in Couple and Family Therapy. Edited by Johnson SM, Whiffen VE. New York, Guilford, 2003, pp 191–212

Donaldson D, Spirito A, Esposito-Smythers C: Treatment for adolescents following a suicide attempt: results of a pilot trial. J Am Acad Child Adolesc Psychiatry 44:113–120, 2005

Efron D: The use of emotionally focused family therapy in a children's mental health center. Journal of Systemic Therapies 23:78–90, 2004

Egeland B, Erikson M: Attachment theory and findings: implications for prevention and intervention, in Prevention in Mental Health: Now, Tomorrow, and Ever? Edited by Kramer S, Parns H. Northvale, NJ, Jason Aronson, 1993, pp 21–50

Eyeberg SM, Boggs SR: Parent-child interaction therapy: a psychosocial intervention for the treatment of young conduct-disordered children, in Handbook of Parent Training: Parents as Co-Therapists for Children's Behavior Problems. Edited by Briesmeister JM, Schaeffer CE. New York, Wiley, 1998, pp 61–97

Forehand RL, McMahon RJ: Helping the Noncompliant Child: A Clinician's Guide to Parent Training. New York, Guilford, 1981

Freedman J, Combs G: Narrative Therapy: The Social Construction of Preferred Realities. New York, WW Norton, 1996

Freeman J, Epston D, Lobovits D: Playful Approaches to Serious Problems: Narrative Therapy With Children and Their Families. New York, WW Norton, 1997

Fristad MA, Goldberg-Arnold JS, Gavazzi SM: Multifamily psychoeducation groups in the treatment of children with mood disorders. J Marital Fam Ther 29:491–504, 2003

Fruzzetti AE, Iverson KM: Intervening with couples and families to treat emotion dysregulation and psychopathology, in Emotion Regulation in Couples and Families: Pathways to Dysfunction and Health. Edited by Snyder DK, Simpson JA, Hughes JN. Washington, DC, American Psychological Association, 2006, pp 249–267

Gottman JM: What Predicts Divorce?: The Relationship Between Marital Processes and Marital Outcomes. Hillsdale, NJ, Lawrence Erlbaum Associates, 1994

Gottman JM: The Marriage Clinic: A Scientifically Based Marital Therapy. New York, WW Norton, 1999

Gouze KR, Wendel R: Integrative module-based family therapy: application and training. J Marital Fam Ther 34:269–286, 2008

Greenberg LS, Johnson SM: Emotionally Focused Therapy for Couples. New York, Guilford, 1988

Greene RW, Ablon JS: Treating Explosive Kids: The Collaborative Problem-Solving Approach. New York, Guilford, 2006

Haddock SA, Zimmerman TS, MacPhee D: The power guide: attending to gender in family therapy. J Marital Fam Ther 26:153–170, 2000

Henggeler SW, Rodick JD, Borduin CM, et al: Multisystemic treatment of juvenile offenders: effects on adolescent behavior and family interaction. Dev Psychol 22:132–141, 1986

Henggeler SW, Melton GB, Smith LA: Family preservation using multisystemic therapy: an effective alternative to incarcerating juvenile offenders. J Consult Clin Psychol 60:953–961, 1992

Henggeler SW, Melton GB, Smith LA, et al: Family preservation using multisystemic treatment: long-term follow-up to a clinical trial with serious juvenile offenders. J Child Fam Stud 2:283–293, 1993

Johnson SM: The Practice of Emotionally Focused Marital Therapy: Creating Connection. New York, Brunner/Mazel, 1996

Johnson SM, Greenberg LS: Emotionally focused couples therapy: an outcome study. J Marital Fam Ther 11:313–317, 1985

Johnson SM, Greenman PS: The path to a secure bond: emotionally focused couple therapy. J Clin Psychol 62:597–609, 2006

Josephson AM, Peteet JR (eds): Handbook of Spirituality and Worldview in Clinical Practice. Washington, DC, American Psychiatric Publishing, 2004

Kazdin AE: Parent Management Training: Treatment for Oppositional, Aggressive, and Antisocial Behavior in Children and Adolescents. New York, Oxford University Press, 2005

Keiley MK, Dolbin M, Hill J, et al: The cultural genogram: experiences from within an MFT training program. J Marital Fam Ther 28:165–178, 2002

Kim EY-K, Bean RA, Harper JM: Do general treatment guidelines for Asian American families have applications to specific ethnic groups? The case of culturally competent therapy with Korean Americans. J Marital Fam Ther 30:359–372, 2004

Kovacs M, Sherrill J, George CJMS, et al: Contextual emotion-regulation therapy for childhood depression: description and pilot testing of a new intervention. J Am Acad Child Adolesc Psychiatry 45:892–903, 2006

Kurdek LA: Are gay and lesbian cohabiting couples really different from heterosexual married couples? J Marriage Fam 66:880–900, 2004

Laird J: Gender in lesbian relationships: cultural, feminist, and constructionist reflections. J Marital Fam Ther 26:455–467, 2000

Le Grange D, Binford R, Loeb KL: Manualized family based treatment for anorexia nervosa: a case series. J Am Acad Child Adolesc Psychiatry 44:41–46, 2005

Le Grange D, Crosby RD, Rathouz PJ, et al.: A randomized controlled comparison of family-based treatment and supportive psychotherapy for adolescent bulimia nervosa. Arch Gen Psychiatry 64:149–1056, 2007

Lebow J: The integrative revolution in couple and family therapy. Family Process 36:1–17, 1997

Lieberman AF, Weston DR, Pawl JH: Preventive intervention and outcome with anxiously attached dyads. Child Dev 62:199–209, 1991

Lieberman AF, Ghosh IC, Van Horn P: Child-parent psychotherapy: 6-month follow-up of a randomized controlled trial. J Am Acad Child Adolesc Psychiatry 45:913–918, 2006

Lyons-Ruth K, Bruschweiler-Stern N, Harrison AM, et al: Implicit relational knowing: its role in development and psychoanalytic treatment. Infant Ment Health J 19:282–289, 1998

Mandara J, Murray CB: Development of an empirical typology of African American family functioning. J Fam Psychol 16:318–337, 2002

Martinez CR, Forgatch MS: Adjusting to change: linking family structure transitions with parenting and boys' adjustment. J Fam Psychol 16:107–117, 2002

McDaniel SH, Hepworth J, Doherty WJ: Medical Family Therapy: A Biopsychosocial Approach to Families With Health Problems. New York, Basic Books, 1992

McDaniel SH, Hepworth J, Doherty W: Medical family therapy with somatizing patients: the co-creation of therapeutic stories, in Integrating Family Therapy: Handbook of Family Psychology and Systems Theory. Edited by Mikesell RH, Lusterman D-D, McDaniel SH. Washington, DC, American Psychological Press, 1995, pp. 377–388

McDaniel SH, Campbell TL, Hepworth J, et al: Family Oriented Primary Care: A Manual for Medical Providers, 2nd Edition. New York, Springer-Verlag, 2004

Minuchin S: Families and Family Therapy. Cambridge, MA, Harvard University Press, 1974

Minuchin S, Fishman CH: Family Therapy Techniques. Cambridge, MA, Harvard University Press, 1981

Patterson GR: Coercive Family Process. Eugene, OR, Castalia Publishing, 1982

Pinsof WM: Integrative Problem-Centered Therapy: A Synthesis of Family, Individual, and Biological Approaches. New York, Basic Books, 1995

Pinsof WM, Wynne LC: The effectiveness of marital and family therapy: an empirical overview, conclusions, and recommendations. J Marital Fam Ther 21:585–613, 1995

Pinsof WM, Wynne LC: Toward progress research: closing the gap between family therapy practice and research. J Marital Fam Ther 26:1–8, 2000

Reinecke MA, Clark DA: Cognitive Therapy Across the Lifespan: Evidence and Practice. New York, Cambridge University Press, 2004

Reinecke MA, Dattilio FM, Freeman A (eds): Cognitive Therapy With Children and Adolescents. New York, Guilford, 1996

Rolland JS: Families, Illness and Disabilities: An Integrative Treatment Model. New York, Basic Books, 1994

Rolland JS, Walsh F: Systemic training for healthcare professionals: the Chicago Center for Family Health approach. Fam Process 44:283–301, 2005

Rowe CL, Gómez LC, Liddle HA: Family therapy research: empirical foundations and practical implications, in Family Therapy: Concepts and Methods, 7th Edition. Edited by Nichols MP, Schwartz RC. New York, Allyn and Bacon, 2006, pp 399–440

Sanders GL, Kroll IT: Generating stories of resilience: helping gay and lesbian youth and their families. J Marital Fam Ther 26:433–442, 2000

Schoenwald SK, Henggeler SW: Multisystemic therapy for adolescents with serious externalizing problems, in Handbook of Clinical Family Therapy. Edited by Lebow JL. New York, Wiley, 2005, pp 103–127

Sexton TL, Alexander JF: Functional family therapy for externalizing disorders in adolescents, in Handbook of Clinical Family Therapy. Edited by Lebow JL. New York, Wiley, 2005, pp 164–191

Silk JS, Sessa FM, Morris AS, et al: Neighborhood cohesion as a buffer against hostile maternal parenting. J Fam Psychol 18:135–146, 2004

Snyder J, Schrepferman L, Brooker M, et al.: The roles of anger, conflict with parents and peers, and social reinforcement in the early development of physical aggression, in Anger, Aggression, and Interventions for Interpersonal Violence. Edited by Cavell TA, Malcolm KT. Mahwah, NJ, Lawrence Erlbaum, 2007, pp. 187–214

Solomon SE, Rothblum ES, Balsam KF: Pioneers in partnership: lesbian and gay male couples in civil unions compared with those not in civil unions and married heterosexual siblings. J Fam Psychol 18:275–286, 2004

Sprenkle DH (ed): Effectiveness Research in Marriage and Family Therapy. Alexandria, VA, American Association for Marriage and Family Therapy, 2002

Sprenkle DH, Blow AJ: Common factors and our sacred models. J Marital Fam Ther 30:113–129, 2004

Valiente C, Eisenberg N: Parenting and children's adjustment: the role of children's emotional regulation, in Emotion Regulation in Couples and Families: Pathways to Dysfunction and Health. Edited by Snyder DK, Simpson JA, Hughes JN. Washington, DC, American Psychological Association, 2006, pp 101–121

Walsh F (ed): Normal Family Processes: Growing Diversity and Complexity. New York, Guilford, 2003

Webster-Stratton C: Long-term follow-up of families with young conduct problem children: from preschool to grade school. J Clin Child Psychol 19:144–149, 1990

Webster-Stratton C: The incredible years: a training series for the prevention and treatment of conduct problems in young children, in Psychosocial Treatments for Child and Adolescent Disorders: Empirically Based Strategies for Clinical Practice. Edited by Hibbs ED, Jensen PS. Washington, DC, American Psychological Association, 2005, pp 507–555

Webster-Stratton C, Reid JM: The incredible years parents, teachers and children training series: a multifaceted treatment approach for young children with conduct problems, in Evidence-Based Psychotherapies for Children and Adolescents. Edited by Kazdin AE, Weisz JR. New York, Guilford, 2003, pp 224–240

Wendel R, Gouze KR, Lake M: Integrative module-based family therapy: a model for training and treatment in a multidisciplinary mental health setting. J Marital Fam Ther 31:357–370, 2005

White M, Epston D: Narrative Means to Therapeutic Ends. New York, WW Norton, 1990

Winnicott DW: The theory of the parent-infant relationship (1960), in The Maturational Processes and the Facilitating Environment: Studies in the Theory of Emotional Development. New York, International Universities Press, 1965, pp 37–55

Winnicott DW: From dependence towards independence in the development of the individual (1963), in The Maturational Processes and the Facilitating Environment: Studies in the Theory of Emotional Development. New York, International Universities Press, 1965, pp 83–92

Wood JJ, Piacentini JC, Southam-Gerow M, et al: Family cognitive behavioral therapy for child anxiety disorders. J Am Acad Child Adolesc Psychiatry 45:314–321, 2006

Chapter 57

Interpersonal Psychotherapy for Depressed Adolescents

Meredith L. Gunlicks-Stoessel, Ph.D.
Laura Mufson, Ph.D.

Interpersonal psychotherapy for depressed adolescents (IPT-A; Mufson et al. 2004a) is a time-limited, manualized psychotherapeutic intervention adapted from interpersonal psychotherapy for adults (IPT; Weissman et al. 2000). IPT is based on the principle that regardless of the underlying cause, depression occurs within an interpersonal context. The goal of treatment, therefore, is to decrease depressive symptoms by focusing on current interpersonal difficulties and helping the individual improve his or her relationships and communication patterns.

The theoretical basis for IPT comes from the work of Adolf Meyer, Harry Stack Sullivan, and other interpersonal theorists who have stated that interpersonal interactions form the basis of personality and functioning and that psychopathology develops out of and is perpetuated by problems in these interactions (Meyer 1957; Sullivan 1953). Consistent with these principles, IPT focuses on helping patients become aware of their current communication patterns and the types of responses these patterns elicit from others. They can then observe that by altering their communication patterns, the nature of their relationships is changed, and this, in turn, can lead to improvements in mood. Attachment theory is also relevant for IPT. Bowlby (1978) proposed that people have a tendency and need to develop strong bonds to significant others. When these bonds are disrupted in some way, the individual experiences emotional distress, including symptoms of depression. IPT addresses the role of attachment in depression by targeting interpersonal conflicts, transitions, and grief in relationships that may affect the patient's attachment experiences and contribute to the development of depression.

IPT was originally designed as an intervention for nonpsychotic depressed adults treated as outpatients, and there is strong support for its use (Weissman et al. 2000). IPT-A is designed to treat adolescents, ages 12–18 years, with nonpsychotic, unipolar depression. Depressed adolescents with comorbid anxiety disorders, attention-deficit/hyperactivity disorder, and oppositional defiant disorder have been successfully treated with IPT-A, though IPT-A is most effective when depression is the primary diagnosis and the comorbid diagnoses are limited. IPT-A is not recommended for adolescents who are mentally retarded, actively suicidal or homicidal, psychotic, bipolar, or are actively abusing substances.

Course of Treatment

IPT-A is designed to be delivered once a week for 12 weeks, although the treatment schedule can be more flexible, if necessary. If a crisis occurs or supplementary sessions are needed for other reasons, the treatment duration can be extended or sessions can be temporarily scheduled for more than once a week. However, it is crucial to keep the treatment time-limited, even when negotiating additional sessions, by restating the treatment contract with those modifications.

IPT-A is an individual treatment that recommends, but does not require, parental participation. Parental session attendance can range from none to several sessions, although nonattendance is strongly discouraged. Parental absence from sessions is sometimes necessary, however, depending on the family's circumstances. It is recommended that parents attend at least one session in the beginning of treatment in order to be educated about depression and the IPT-A treatment, and at least one session at the end of treatment in order to learn about the adolescent's warning signs of depression and strategies for managing potential recurrence. Parental participation can also be helpful in the middle phase of treatment, as parental participation provides adolescents with opportunities to practice learned skills with their parents.

IPT-A is divided into three treatment phases: initial, middle, and termination. Each session begins with the therapist assessing the adolescent's depressive symptoms and asking the adolescent to rate his or her mood using a 1–10 scale. Any changes in depressive symptoms that occurred since the last session are noted and linked to interpersonal events that happened during the week. The symptom review and mood ratings are useful ways for both the therapist and adolescent to monitor treatment progress. Following the review of symptoms, the therapist and adolescent focus on tasks that are specific to the adolescent's current phase of treatment.

Initial Phase (Sessions 1–4)

Confirm the Depression Diagnosis and Suitability of IPT-A

Prior to entering IPT-A, the adolescent should have already completed a full psychiatric evaluation to assess current symptoms and diagnoses, as well as psychiatric, family, developmental, medical, social, and academic history (Mufson et al. 2004a). However, it is important to confirm the depression diagnosis in the first session, using a clinical interview.

Provide Psychoeducation About Depression

The therapist should provide the adolescent and his or her family with information about depression, including its associated symptoms and behaviors. For example, many families do not realize that irritability is a symptom of depression. They also may not realize that a decline in academic performance may be a function of reduced concentration, anhedonia, fatigue, and other symptoms of depression, rather than an indication that the adolescent is being oppositional or lazy. It is also useful to place depression in the context of a medical illness that can be treated. This can decrease the stigma often associated with depression, take the blame off of the adolescent for causing the depression, and provide an optimistic prognosis that the depression will improve with treatment.

Psychoeducation also includes assigning the adolescent the *limited sick role*. This involves explaining that like someone with a medical illness, adolescents who have symptoms of depression may not be able to do as many things or do things as well as they did before the depression developed. The goal of the limited sick role is for the adolescent to try to do as many of his or her usual activities as possible, with the awareness and acceptance that he or she might not do these things as often or as well as before the depression developed. It is important for the family to understand the limited sick role so that they can be more supportive of the adolescent's efforts in these activities and less critical of the outcomes.

Explain the Theory and Goals of IPT-A

The therapist should explain the theory and structure of IPT-A to the adolescent and family so that they know what to expect. This includes educating the family about the premise that depression occurs within an interpersonal context. Specifically, regardless of what initially caused the depression, depression affects people's relationships, and relationships affect people's moods. Thus, the treatment will focus on improving the adolescent's relationships by teaching communication and interpersonal problem-solving skills that can lead to a reduction in the adolescent's depressive symptoms.

Conduct the Interpersonal Inventory

The interpersonal inventory is used to identify the interpersonal issues that are most closely related to the adolescent's depression. First, the adolescent identifies the significant relationships in his or her life by completing a *closeness circle.* A closeness circle is a series of four concentric circles that resembles a bull's-eye. The adolescent writes his or her name in the innermost circle and places the names of the people in his or her life in the other circles according to the closeness of their relationship. People to whom the adolescent feels closest, even if the relationship is not always positive, are put in the circle closest to the adolescent, with other people placed in the middle or outer circle. Once the closeness circle has been completed, the therapist and adolescent discuss each relationship in more depth, placing particular emphasis on the relationships that the adolescent feels are most related to his or her mood in either positive or negative ways. For each relationship, the therapist should ask about the frequency and content of their interactions, terms and expectations for the relationship, positive and negative aspects of the relationship, ways in which the relationship is associated with the adolescent's depression, and changes the adolescent would like to make in the relationship (Mufson et al. 2004a).

Identify the Interpersonal Problem Area(s)

Based on the interpersonal inventory, the therapist helps the adolescent link the status and quality of his or her relationships to his or her depressive symptoms. The therapist identifies common themes or problems in the adolescent's relationships, and together with the adolescent, identifies one of four interpersonal problem areas that will be the focus of treatment: grief due to death, interpersonal role disputes, interpersonal role transitions, or interpersonal deficits. Generally, only one interpersonal problem area is identified, but it is also possible to identify a secondary problem area.

Grief due to death.

Grief is selected as the problem area when an adolescent experiences the death of a loved one and the loss is associated with normal bereavement or prolonged grief, significant depressive symptoms, and impairment in functioning. The goal of IPT-A for adolescents with this problem area is to facilitate the delayed normal mourning process and to develop or improve other relationships that can provide the support, nurturance, companionship, or guidance that has been lost (Mufson et al. 2004a).

Interpersonal role disputes.

An interpersonal role dispute involves the adolescent and at least one significant other having different expectations about the terms and/or guidelines for behavior within their relationship (Weissman et al. 2000). Interpersonal role dispute is selected as the problem area if the adolescent's depressive episode coincides with a relationship conflict. The goal of treatment is to help the adolescent develop skills to attempt to resolve the dispute. If resolution is not possible, the goal is to help the adolescent develop strategies for coping with the relationship (Mufson et al. 2004a).

Interpersonal role transitions.

A role transition occurs when a life change requires an alteration of behavior from an old role to a new role (Weissman et al. 2000). Role transitions may be biologically determined (transitioning from childhood to puberty) or a result of social and cultural practices (transitioning from middle school to high school). In addition to these more normative transitions, adolescents may also experience unexpected changes that require them to take on new social roles, such as a change in family structure due to parents' separation or divorce. An adolescent may develop symptoms of depression in response to a role transition if the role is unexpected or undesired, the adolescent is not psychologically or emotionally prepared for the new role, or the adolescent misses the old role. Depression may also exacerbate the adolescent's ability to successfully negotiate a transition. For adolescents experiencing a role transition, the goal of IPT-A is to help them mourn the loss of the old role and develop the skills they need to manage the new role more successfully (Mufson et al. 2004a).

Interpersonal deficits.

Interpersonal deficits refer to underdeveloped social and communication skills that impair the adolescent's ability to have positive relationships (Weissman et al. 2000). Deficits may include difficulty initiating or maintaining relationships, verbally expressing one's feelings or needs, or eliciting information from others to establish communication. The goal of treatment is to develop the interpersonal skills needed to have more satisfying relationships and reduce social isolation (Mufson et al. 2004a). Due to the time-limited nature of IPT-A, it is best suited for adolescents whose interpersonal deficits are less pervasive or are a consequence of their depression or a specific stressor.

Make the Treatment Contract

Once the problem areas have been identified, the adolescent and therapist make a verbal treatment contract regarding the adolescent's and therapist's roles in treatment, the interpersonal problem area(s) that will be the focus of treatment, and the practical details of the treatment. This includes explaining to the adolescent that for the treatment to be most helpful, the adolescent will need to bring in information about relationships and interpersonal interactions each week for the therapist and adolescent to discuss and problem-solve. The therapist also informs the adolescent that his or her parent(s) may be invited to attend a treatment session to work on the identified problem area(s).

Middle Phase (Sessions 5–9)

During the middle phase of treatment, the therapist and adolescent begin to work directly on the identified interpersonal problem area(s). This is accomplished by identifying effective strategies for managing the problem and practicing and implementing the strategies. Some of the therapeutic techniques used during this phase of treatment are specific to the identified problem area(s), and others are used across problem areas. It is best to start with an interpersonal issue that is relatively simple and has a high likelihood of success. This generates hope that the strategies learned can help facilitate change in relationships and improved mood.

General Techniques

Encouragement of affect and linkage with interpersonal events.

These techniques are used to help the adolescent become aware of, acknowledge, and accept negative emotions about events and relationships and understand how emotions affect relationships (Weissman et al. 2000). It is our experience that adolescents tend to present in one of two ways. Some adolescents experience their emotions intensely and can readily express them but do not seem to be aware of how the emotions are related to the events in their lives. Other adolescents can easily describe events in their lives but do so without any mention of emotion. For both types, it is important to help them link interpersonal events with their mood. If the adolescent describes a change in mood without an awareness of the cause, the therapist and adolescent may review the week in great detail to unearth an event or relationship that may have led to the change in mood. If the adolescent describes a difficult interaction with a significant other without awareness of the feelings associated with it, the therapist may ask the adolescent how the event made the adolescent feel and how it affected his or her depressive symptoms. This educates the adolescent about the link between interpersonal events and mood and helps the adolescent become more comfortable and skilled in identifying, understanding, and communicating his or her feelings.

Communication analysis.

Communication analysis is used to explore the adolescent's patterns of interacting with others in order to identify ways in which his or her communication is problematic and skills the adolescent needs to master to have more satisfying relationships. Communication analysis involves asking the adolescent to describe a recent interpersonal event in great detail. The therapist may ask the adolescent questions, such as the following (Mufson et al. 2004a): "How did the discussion start?" "When and where did it take place?" "What exactly did you say?" "What did the other person say back?" "Then what happened?" "How did that make you feel?" "How do you think it made the other person feel?" "Is that the outcome you wanted?" Through this process, the therapist helps the adolescent recognize the impact of his or her words on others, the feelings that arose during the interactions, and the feelings he or she conveys verbally and nonverbally.

Once the therapist and adolescent have an understanding of the interaction, they discuss how doing things differently at various points might have led to a different outcome and different emotional experience. Some common communication techniques to be taught and modeled include 1) selecting an optimal time to initiate a conversation, 2) communicating feelings and opinions directly ("I statements"), 3) attempting to see the problem from the other person's perspective, 4) being specific when talking about a problem and focusing on the present problem at hand (avoid "you always" or "you never"), and 5) generating some solutions prior to the conversation and being willing to compromise (Mufson et al. 2004a).

Decision analysis.

Decision analysis is similar to problem-solving techniques that are used in other models of therapy but is focused more specifically on addressing interpersonal problems. It involves selecting an interpersonal situation that is causing the adolescent problems, determining the goal, generating a list of alternative strategies (some of these may come out of the communication analysis), evaluating the pros and cons of each potential solution or strategy, and selecting a strategy to try first in session and then, if it looks promising, outside of the session (Mufson et al. 2004a). Once the adolescent has tried the strategy, the therapist and adolescent should evaluate the outcome and determine if there is a need to select an alternative strategy.

Role-playing.

Role-playing is a way for adolescents to practice the communication and interpersonal problem-solving skills that they have learned in order to feel more comfortable using them in real life. To be most helpful, the therapist and adolescent should not simply talk about what it would be like to have the conversation using the new strategies; they should actually act it out. It can be useful to give the adolescent the opportunity to play both roles, in turn, so the adolescent can better understand the other person's perspective. This also helps the therapist understand the adolescent's experience of the other person. It is also useful to try the role-play more than once, with different outcomes to the interactions, both positive and negative, so that the adolescent can become more skilled in handling different kinds of situations that might develop. Once the adolescent is able to role-play the interaction effectively, the therapist should encourage the adolescent to try having the conversation with the other person prior to the next therapy session. The therapist and adolescent can then use communication analysis in the next therapy session to process how the conversation went and determine if further action is needed.

Problem Area–Specific Techniques

Grief due to death.

The treatment goal for adolescents with the identified problem area of grief is to facilitate the delayed normal grieving process. This involves detailed discussions of the adolescent's relationship with the deceased, including both positive and negative aspects of the relationship and conflicts in the relationship. The therapist should also gently encourage expression of affect about the relationship and its loss, and help the adolescent to connect current depressive symptoms and behaviors to feelings surrounding the death. As the treatment progresses, the therapist helps the adolescent develop skills for communicating thoughts and feelings about the loss with other people in the adolescent's life. The idea is to help the adolescent develop new relationships or further develop existing relationships to fill in the support that was lost with the death of the loved one.

Interpersonal role disputes.

An adolescent may present with interpersonal role disputes that may be in one of three stages: renegotiation, impasse, or dissolution (Weissman et al. 2000). An adolescent and significant other are in the *renegotiation stage* if they are still communicating with one another and are attempting to resolve the conflict. They are in the *impasse stage* if they are no longer attempting to negotiate the conflict and social distancing (or "the silent treatment") has occurred. In the *dissolution stage,* the adolescent and significant other have already decided that the dispute cannot be resolved, and they have chosen to end the relationship. For adolescents whose disputes are in the renegotiation or impasse stages, the goal of treatment is to help the adolescent define and resolve the dispute. This involves working with the adolescent and the other person, if possible, to describe the dispute, identify existing patterns of communication, teach new communication skills, and generate solutions to the dispute (Mufson et al. 2004a). If complete resolution of the problem does not appear to be possible, the therapist works with the adolescent to develop strategies for coping with a relationship that cannot be changed. This may include developing other relationships that the adolescent can use as a means of support. It is often helpful to point out that although a relationship may not be changeable, simply decreasing the frequency or intensity of conflict can lead to improved mood. If the dispute is in the dissolution stage, treatment focuses on mourning the loss of the relationship. This involves discussing the dispute and lost relationship, developing an understanding of what occurred, and helping the adolescent establish new relationships.

Interpersonal role transitions.

For adolescents experiencing an interpersonal role transition, treatment involves identifying and defining the transition, helping the adolescent give up the old role and accept the new one, and helping the adolescent develop a sense of competence in the new role (Mufson et al. 2004a). The therapist should provide the adolescent and parents, when possible, with information about the effect that transitions can have on functioning. The therapist then explores with the adolescent the meaning of the transition, feelings and expectations about the old and new roles, and gains and losses associated with the transition. The therapist also helps the adolescent learn and practice new communication and interpersonal problem-solving skills that can be used to manage the new role and develop relationships that can provide ongoing support during the transition.

Interpersonal deficits.

For adolescents with interpersonal deficits, treatment begins with helping the adolescent identify and label repetitive interpersonal problems and connect these problems with his or her depressive symptoms (Mufson et al. 2004a). If the adolescent does not have many current relationships, the therapist can review past relationships to look for patterns of difficulty as well as strengths upon which to build. The therapist can also use his or her own relationship with the adolescent to explore the adolescent's interpersonal deficits. The therapist then helps the adolescent learn and practice new skills for developing and maintaining relationships, such as how to initiate and sustain a conversation, ask a peer to join in an activity, or share feelings with someone. The therapist works with the adolescent to identify existing relationships that he or she would like to build upon and/or new relationships that the adolescent would like to develop. It is important with these adolescents to focus on strengths as much as on deficits. The therapist should draw attention to skills the adolescent has used in other relationships or in the therapy session to help the adolescent build a sense of confidence and competence and to reinforce positive communication patterns.

Termination Phase (Sessions 10–12)

The termination phase of IPT-A is similar to the termination phases of other therapy models. This phase involves reviewing the course of the adolescent's depressive symptoms and how these symptoms have changed. The therapist and adolescent should also review the changes that occurred in the adolescent's communication style and relationship functioning,

link these changes to the improvement in the adolescent's mood, and highlight the skills and strategies the adolescent found particularly useful. It is also helpful to discuss anticipated future difficult situations and review strategies that the adolescent can use to negotiate those situations. As part of termination, it is also important to discuss the adolescent's feelings about ending treatment and the relationship with the therapist. Finally, the therapist and adolescent should discuss the possibility of recurrence of depression, the warning symptoms of depression that are particular to that adolescent, and strategies for managing a recurrence (Mufson et al. 2004a). It is recommended that parents attend a session during the termination phase in order to review the adolescent's progress, plans for managing future interpersonal difficulties, warning signs for recurrence of depression, and strategies for managing the depression, should it recur.

The following case example illustrates the IPT-A techniques and course of treatment.

Case Example

Tianna is a 14-year-old African American girl who had recently begun ninth grade in a new high school. She was referred for treatment by her school counselor for possible depression after three incidents in which other students reported finding Tianna crying in the bathroom. Tianna lives with her mother, older sister, and younger brother. Her depressive symptoms reportedly began approximately 6 months prior to the evaluation and included irritability, reduced interest in spending time with peers, insomnia, fatigue, and decreased appetite. Her mother also described her as more quiet and isolative around the house. Tianna had consistently been a strong student, and this had not changed with the onset of her depressive symptoms. On the basis of the clinical evaluation, she was diagnosed with major depressive disorder.

Initial Phase

During the first session, the therapist met with Tianna and her mother to hear their perspectives on Tianna's depressive symptoms and to confirm the depression diagnosis. The therapist provided them with information about depression, including describing depression as a medical illness that can be treated. The therapist assigned the limited sick role, which for Tianna meant trying to continue socializing with peers and communicating with her family, despite her reduced interest in doing so—but also not being too critical of herself at times when she does not feel able to socialize. The session ended with the therapist explaining the theory and structure of IPT-A and addressing Tianna's and her mother's questions.

The next three sessions were spent completing the interpersonal inventory. In the closeness circle,

Tianna identified her mother, sister, brother, two aunts who lived close by, and one friend from middle school as the important people in her life. With respect to her mother and siblings, Tianna described their relationships as distant. Tianna noticed that her mother and siblings were more talkative than she was. She felt that she spent a lot of time listening to them talk about the events of the day and their problems, but they did not reciprocate. Whenever she tried to talk, one of her family members would interrupt her or talk over her. Consequently, Tianna kept her problems to herself. She felt overlooked by her family, and this left her feeling depressed. She spent increasing amounts of time in her room to avoid her family.

Tianna also talked about her two aunts who lived close by. She reported seeing them a few times a week and stated that she had fun with them, but she had never used them as a means of support in coping with problems at home or elsewhere. In terms of peers, Tianna continued to see and talk regularly with one friend from middle school who did not go to her high school. Tianna stated that most of the kids at her new school seemed nice, but she had not developed friendships with any of them.

After the interpersonal inventory, Tianna and the therapist developed an interpersonal formulation of Tianna's depression. Tianna's primary interpersonal problem area appeared to be interpersonal deficits. She was having difficulty expressing her feelings, problems, and needs with her immediate and extended family; she had only one existing friendship; and she was having difficulty developing new social connections at her high school. The therapist and Tianna discussed how Tianna's difficulty talking about her feelings and problems with her family left her feeling depressed. Her depression caused her to withdraw even more, and her withdrawal then prevented her from getting support from family and friends. The therapist and Tianna made a treatment contract to work on communication skills that would help Tianna better express her feelings and needs so that she could have more satisfying relationships.

Middle Phase

During the middle phase of treatment, the therapist and Tianna worked to develop a better understanding of Tianna's difficulty expressing herself and soliciting support from others. This involved conducting communication analysis on several interactions Tianna had with her mother and siblings to examine how and what Tianna communicated to her family and how these interactions made her feel. Through these analyses, the therapist and Tianna became aware that Tianna tended to wait for one of her family members to ask her how she was doing rather than initiating a conversation when she needed support. In addition, if Tianna's mother or siblings interrupted her when she was talking, Tianna tended to just let the other person talk. These interactions left

Tianna feeling depressed and angry. The therapist and Tianna discussed how Tianna could initiate a conversation with her mother or siblings when she needed some support, at a time when her mother or siblings seemed like they might be particularly receptive to listening to her (e.g., letting mom relax a bit after she gets home from work before trying to talk to her). Tianna practiced initiating a conversation and expressing her feelings using a role-play, and she was asked to try the conversation at home. Tianna attempted the conversation and reported back to the therapist that when she tried to talk to her mother, her sister came in and interrupted the conversation. Tianna and the therapist discussed and practiced having Tianna explain to her sister that when she interrupts it makes Tianna feel ignored and unimportant. Tianna also had the idea of telling her sister that she would like to hear what her sister has to say and proposing that her sister have a turn to talk when Tianna is finished.

The therapist also worked with Tianna to help her enhance her relationships with her aunts and develop friendships at her new high school. This included having Tianna talk to her aunts about her depression and the difficulties she had been having communicating with her mother and siblings. The therapist and Tianna also conducted communication analysis regarding interactions Tianna had with her friend. Through the course of these analyses, the therapist was able to highlight the communication skills Tianna used in this relationship that could be applied toward developing relationships at her new school. Tianna identified two girls with whom she would like to initiate friendships, and Tianna and the therapist role-played having conversations with them. As changes in Tianna's relationships began to occur, Tianna's depressive symptoms began to improve. The therapist pointed out the link between the improvements in Tianna's relationships and her improved mood.

Termination Phase

During the termination phase, the therapist and Tianna reviewed the course of Tianna's depressive symptoms, noting that Tianna felt better when she was able to talk more to her family members and friends about her problems and needs. They discussed the interpersonal strategies that Tianna found most helpful, including directly expressing her feelings and needs and selecting an appropriate time to initiate a conversation. During this discussion, Tianna and the therapist also discussed the strategies that Tianna could continue to use after treatment had ended. Tianna also discussed her feelings about ending treatment. Tianna's mother joined Tianna and the therapist for the last session. Together they reviewed Tianna's progress in treatment, discussed Tianna's warning signs for recurrence of depression, and discussed how to seek help should the depression recur.

Group Psychotherapy

IPT-A has been adapted to be delivered in a group format (Mufson et al. 2004c). Group IPT-A consists of a combination of individual and group therapy sessions delivered over the course of 14 weeks. Two to three individual pregroup sessions are conducted with each adolescent and his or her parent(s) to collect information about the adolescent's depressive symptoms and significant relationships and to identify the interpersonal problem area(s). There are 12 group sessions. Adolescents participate in group exercises in which they coach each other to use better communication and problem-solving skills. In addition, they report to each other on their experiences trying the new techniques outside of the group, which provides opportunities for adolescents to learn from each other's successes and mistakes. Parents are also invited to participate in a single family session midtreatment and posttreatment. The midtreatment session provides the adolescent with an opportunity to practice newly learned communication skills with his or her parents. The post-treatment session is used to review with parents the adolescent's progress and to discuss strategies for managing potential recurrence of depression.

Empirical Support

The efficacy and effectiveness of IPT-A for reducing adolescents' depressive symptoms have been examined in three randomized controlled clinical trials (Mufson et al. 1999; Mufson et al. 2004b; Rossello and Bernal 1999). Depressed adolescents treated with IPT-A demonstrated fewer depressive symptoms, better social functioning, and better global functioning at the completion of treatment than adolescents in control conditions. Based on the empirical support for treatment efficacy, IPT-A meets the American Psychological Association Division 12 criteria for a "well-established" psychotherapy for depression in youth.

A modified version of group IPT-A, entitled Interpersonal Psychotherapy—Adolescent Skills Training (IPT-AST) has also been developed as a prevention intervention for adolescents with elevated symptoms of depression (Young et al. 2006). In a clinical trial, adolescents who received IPT-AST had significantly fewer depressive symptoms and depressive diagnoses and had better overall functioning posttreatment than adolescents who received school counseling (Young et al. 2006).

Research Directions

Applications and adaptations of IPT-A that are being developed and empirically tested include use with depressed adolescents who are engaging in nonsuicidal self-injury, depressed pregnant teenagers, prepubertal youth with symptoms of depression and anxiety, bipolar adolescents, and offspring of bipolar parents. An adaptation of IPT-A that includes greater and more structured parent involvement is being evaluated for use with depressed adolescents with higher levels of family relationship problems. A combined treatment of IPT-A and medication is also being tested in an open clinical trial for adolescents with treatment-resistant depression.

Summary Points

- IPT-A is based on the observation that depression occurs within an interpersonal context. The goal of treatment is to decrease depressive symptoms by helping the adolescent improve his or her relationships and communication patterns.

- As part of the psychoeducation about depression, the therapist should assign the adolescent the limited sick role. This involves encouraging the adolescent to try to do as many of his or her usual activities as possible, with the understanding that he or she might not do these things as often or as well as before the depression developed.

- To identify the interpersonal issues that are most closely related to the adolescent's depression, the therapist conducts an interpersonal inventory. The adolescent identifies the significant relationships in his or her life by completing a closeness circle, and the therapist probes each relationship in depth.

- Based on the interpersonal inventory, the therapist identifies one of four interpersonal problem areas that will be the focus of treatment: grief due to death, interpersonal role disputes, interpersonal role transitions, or interpersonal deficits.

- During the middle phase of treatment, adolescents learn to use exploration of affect, communication analysis, decision analysis, and role-plays to acquire and practice skills for managing their interpersonal problems.

- Adolescents are encouraged to try the interpersonal skills they have learned outside of the therapy setting. This "work at home" is not predetermined by the therapist but rather grows out of each therapy session's specific focus and content.

- During the termination phase of treatment, the therapist should highlight interpersonal skills gained, promote generalization of specific strategies, and help the adolescent identify warning signs of depression that might indicate that he or she should seek treatment again.

References

Bowlby J: Attachment theory and its therapeutic implications. Adolesc Psychiatry 6:5–33, 1978

Meyer A: Psychobiology: A Science of Man. Springfield, IL, Charles C Thomas, 1957

Mufson L, Weissman MM, Moreau D, et al: Efficacy of interpersonal psychotherapy for depressed adolescents. Arch Gen Psychiatry 56:573–579, 1999

Mufson L, Dorta KP, Moreau D, et al: Interpersonal Psychotherapy for Depressed Adolescents, 2nd Edition. New York, Guilford, 2004a

Mufson L, Dorta KP, Wickramaratne P, et al: A randomized effectiveness trial of interpersonal psychotherapy for depressed adolescents. Arch Gen Psychiatry 61:577–584, 2004b

Mufson L, Gallagher T, Dorta KP, et al: A group adaptation of interpersonal psychotherapy for depressed adolescents. Am J Psychother 58:220–237, 2004c

Rossello J, Bernal G: The efficacy of cognitive-behavioral and interpersonal treatments for depression in Puerto Rican adolescents. J Consult Clin Psychol 67:734–745, 1999

Sullivan HS: The Interpersonal Theory of Psychiatry. New York, WW Norton, 1953

Weissman MM, Markowitz JC, Klerman GL: Comprehensive Guide to Interpersonal Psychotherapy. New York, Basic Books, 2000

Young JF, Mufson L, Davies M: Efficacy of Interpersonal Psychotherapy-Adolescent Skills Training: an indicated preventive intervention for depression. J Child Psychol Psychiatry 47:1254–1262, 2006

Cognitive-Behavioral Treatment for Anxiety Disorders

Deborah C. Beidel, Ph.D., A.B.P.P.
Teresa Marino Carper, M.S.

Historically, psychiatric descriptions of childhood anxiety disorders date back to case reports in the early part of the twentieth century (e.g., Little Hans, Little Albert, Little Peter; see Beidel and Turner 2005). These descriptions, although differing in theoretical orientation, share a common theme—anxiety in children is not simply a "developmental phase." Rather, anxiety symptoms can be serious, distressful, and functionally impairing. Yet, despite their importance, the notion that children would outgrow their fears limited scientific investigation. Until the early 1990s, there were few randomized controlled trials (RCTs) addressing the pharmacological or psychological treatment of anxiety disorders in children. Since that time, there has been an explosion of interest in treatment, primarily from pharmacological and cognitive-behavioral perspectives. In this chapter, we review cognitive-behavioral treatment (CBT) for anxiety disorders.

Empirical Support

To date, most RCTs demonstrate that CBT is superior to waitlist and no-treatment control conditions (Table 58–1), and CBT is considered an efficacious treatment for child anxiety disorders. Today, controlled trials exist for all of the anxiety disorders, and data consistently support the efficacy of CBT.

Theoretical Underpinnings and Key Concepts

Anxiety is best conceptualized as multidimensional. The tripartite model (Lang et al. 1983) consists of three

TABLE 58–1. Randomized controlled trials examining the efficacy of cognitive-behavioral therapy (CBT)

Author	Participants	Active treatment	Control treatment	Results
Barrett et al. 1996	79 children with SAD, OAD, or SP	CBT; CBT plus family management	Waitlist	CBT plus family management>CBT alone>waitlist
Barrett 1998	60 children with SAD, OAD, or SP	Group CBT; group CBT plus family management	Waitlist	Group CBT=group CBT plus family management>waitlist
Beidel et al. 2000	67 children with SP	Group CBT (SET-C)	Nonspecific active condition (Testbusters)	Group CBT>nonspecific active condition
Beidel et al. 2007	139 children/adolescents with primary diagnosis of SP	Group CBT (SET-C) or fluoxetine	Placebo	Group CBT>fluoxetine>placebo
Bernstein et al. 2000	47 adolescents with school refusal plus anxiety or depression	CBT plus imipramine	CBT plus placebo	CBT plus imipramine>CBT plus placebo
Dadds et al. 1997	128 children with DSM-IV anxiety diagnosis	Group CBT (Coping Koala)	Monitoring group	Group CBT=monitoring group posttreatment; group CBT>monitoring group at 6-month follow-up
Flannery-Schroeder and Kendall 2000	37 children with GAD, SAD, or SP	CBT; group CBT (Coping Cat)	Waitlist	CBT=group CBT>waitlist
Hayward et al. 2000	35 female adolescents	Group CBT	Waitlist	Group CBT>waitlist
Kendall 1994	47 children with OAD, SAD, or avoidant disorder	CBT (Coping Cat)	Waitlist	CBT>waitlist
Kendall et al. 1997	94 children with OAD, SAD, or avoidant disorder	CBT (Coping Cat)	Waitlist	CBT>waitlist
Shortt et al. 2001	71 children with SAD, GAD, or SP	Family-based group CBT (FRIENDS)	Waitlist	Family-based group CBT>waitlist
Silverman et al. 1999b	56 children/adolescents with OAD, GAD, or SP	Group CBT	Waitlist	Group CBT>waitlist
Spence et al. 2000	50 children/adolescents with SP	CBT; CBT with parental involvement	Waitlist	CBT with parental involvement>CBT>waitlist

Note.   GAD=generalized anxiety disorder; OAD=overanxious disorder; SAD=separation anxiety disorder; SET-C=Social Effectiveness Therapy for Children; SP=social phobia.

symptom classes: physiological arousal, subjective (cognitive) distress, and behavioral avoidance. Depending upon theoretical orientation, intervention may begin by addressing any one of these elements. However, successful outcome depends on making changes across all three dimensions.

There is now virtually uniform agreement that the key ingredient in CBT is the behavioral intervention commonly known as *exposure,* a procedure whereby the individual is placed in contact with the object or situation that elicits fear or distress. Graduated exposure is based on a classical conditioning paradigm whereby situations that elicit a low level of fear are introduced first, followed over time by situations that elicit more intense fear. As the number of times that the child confronts the situations increases, even former "high fear" items no longer elicit distress. An example of a successful hierarchy for a child with selective mutism is presented in Table 58–2. In many instances, graduated exposure is combined with cognitive strategies such as *cognitive restructuring* (see the penultimate paragraph of this section) in an attempt to elicit and change negative thoughts that may be part of the fear complex.

An alternative to graduated exposure is intensive exposure. Underlying this approach is Mowrer's two-factor theory (Mowrer 1947). Mowrer hypothesized that fears may be acquired by classical conditioning but are maintained by operant conditioning, where escape or avoidance behaviors eliminate physical and psychological distress. For example, Jackie has a fear of dogs. When playing outside, Jackie sees a dog and becomes anxious. If Jackie runs away, the anxiety dissipates. In turn, the feeling of relief increases the likelihood that in the future, Jackie will run away the next time she sees a dog. Using this theory, elimination of fearful behavior is based on an *extinction* model,

whereby a person is exposed to a feared object or event, but escape or avoidance is prohibited. The individual remains in contact with the feared stimulus until physiological arousal and subjective distress extinguish (dissipate), a process known as *within-session habituation.* When using intensive exposure, the therapist does not begin with objects or situations that elicit low levels of fear. Rather, the child or adolescent is exposed initially to the most fear-producing stimuli and contact is maintained until elicited fear dissipates. Over repeated treatment sessions, physiological and psychological distress are further reduced and ultimately eliminated *(between-session habituation),* and the situation loses its ability to elicit fearful responses.

Exposure strategies have been misunderstood and mistakenly associated with *implosion therapy,* which uses horrific, frightening, and psychodynamic cues in order to maximize anxiety arousal, which in turn was presumed to enhance rapid extinction. Empirical studies demonstrate that such cues are often ineffective, and in many instances, may be countertherapeutic. Extremely high anxiety in itself is not the primary goal of exposure. However, significant increase in arousal ratings of subjective distress or physiological measures should occur when the feared object or situation is introduced and when increased arousal in the presence of the stimulus is significantly related to outcome (e.g., Lang et al. 1983). The choice to use a graduated or intensive approach often depends on the particular characteristics of the child or adolescent and the disorder (see the next section, "Developmental and Gender Considerations," in this chapter).

In the case of children with social phobia, an additional important consideration is their documented lack of social skill (Beidel and Turner 2005). When present, this deficit must be addressed during the course of treatment. In these instances, interventions that com-

TABLE 58–2. Hierarchy for a child with selective mutism

1. Whisper aloud to Mom and Dad so a friend can hear.
2. Talk aloud to Mom and Dad so a friend can hear.
3. Whisper aloud to a friend.
4. Talk aloud to a friend.
5. Talk aloud to two friends.
6. With Mom present, say one word aloud to an unfamiliar adult.
7. With Mom present, say one sentence aloud to an unfamiliar adult.
8. Say "hello" to next-door neighbor when parents are not present.
9. Say "hello" to teacher at school.
10. Say "hello" to a classmate.

bine *social skills training* with exposure are effective. Social Effectiveness Training for Children (Beidel et al. 2000, 2007), for example, combines social skills training, peer generalization, and graduated exposure to treat children and adolescents with social phobia.

Another behavioral intervention is *relaxation training,* a procedure where children learn to decrease their physiological and subjective arousal by engaging in either muscle tension-relaxation sequences or through cognitive meditation. Relaxation training is sometimes used as part of a multifaceted component for children with generalized anxiety disorder (e.g., Kendall 1994) but is rarely used as the sole intervention.

In contrast to a behavioral approach, cognitive conceptualizations of anxiety begin with the premise that emotional disorders result from maladaptive thought patterns. The goal of treatment is to restructure faulty cognitions. Cognitive restructuring is based on the theory that negative thoughts can affect the emotional and behavioral response to the anxiety-provoking situations. Cognitive restructuring, which often is used in conjunction with exposure, teaches children to recognize negative self-thoughts and then to replace those thoughts with less anxiety-provoking self-statements.

Parents play an important role in successful treatment of children with anxiety disorders. First, they may inadvertently behave in a manner that maintains the disorder. Through verbal instruction or modeling, parents may communicate that the world is a fearful place (Barrett et al. 1996; Turner et al. 2003). Additionally, parents often reinforce anxious behaviors (Silverman and Kurtines 1996) by attending to children's anxious statements in an attempt to reassure them or by providing physical affection when a child expresses fear. Therefore, an important element of most treatment programs is contingency management, whereby parents are trained to reinforce (reward) "brave" behavior and ignore anxious or fearful behaviors.

Developmental and Gender Considerations

CBT requires consideration of the child's developmental stage. Although chronological age is a useful starting point, clinicians also need to consider social aptitude, cognitive ability, emotional maturity, and idiosyncratic needs.

Young children may not have the mental faculties necessary to engage in cognitive restructuring (Alfano et al. 2002). Fortunately, the elimination of this compo-

nent from some CBT programs, resulting in a program utilizing primarily exposure procedures, does not reduce its efficacy (Spence et al. 2000). When cognitive restructuring is included in the treatment program, its implementation will vary as a function of developmental level. With younger children, tasks such as filling in cartoon thought-bubbles or completing sentence prompts are often used to identify thoughts. Using child-friendly terms instead of psychological jargon is also recommended (e.g., "thinking traps" instead of "cognitive distortions," and "clues" as opposed to "evidence"). Older children and adolescents typically have more sophisticated metacognitive capabilities and therefore can use cognitive restructuring techniques similar to those used with adults. However, working with more mature children presents a unique set of challenges. As cognitive skills develop, worries become more intricate and complex.

As noted earlier, exposure to feared stimuli is essential for successful outcome, and the exposure paradigm must be developmentally appropriate. Due to cognitive immaturity, younger children often have difficulty understanding the rationale behind intensive exposure, which is therefore typically reserved for adolescents. With younger children, graduated exposure procedures are recommended and are efficacious. Younger patients may also require more parental involvement with exposure tasks to be completed outside of the session (i.e., homework), whereas adolescents may be more autonomous with scheduling and completing homework assignments. Similarly, the use and type of reinforcers require consideration of developmental stage and individual preferences (e.g., stickers, toys, and other tangible items for preadolescents vs. extra time allowed on the phone or allowing a friend to visit for adolescents).

Gender may also influence treatment. Boys have a greater tendency to underreport symptoms (Ollendick et al. 1985), perhaps as a result of gender role expectations. Boys may also deny fear, minimizing fear intensity and its impact on functioning.

Indications and Contraindications

Although CBT is generally efficacious for the treatment of anxiety disorders (see the earlier section "Empirical Support"), there are instances where certain elements may be contraindicated. Cognitive restructuring requires the ability "to think about thinking," sometimes known as metacognition. This ability may not be present in young children (Alfano et al. 2002); therefore, this CBT element is not appropriate for very young children. Similarly, older children who appear to lack metacognitive abilities may require skills training prior to cognitive restructuring. Children with pervasive developmental disorders are not optimal candidates for CBT, as they may have difficulty comprehending and actively participating in treatment.

Certain comorbid conditions suggest caution in the use of CBT. Severe depressive symptoms, including lack of motivation and inability to concentrate, can directly interfere with treatment. In these cases, the depression must be addressed first. Symptoms of conduct disorder are also likely to impede the fundamental processes involved in CBT, thus reducing the effectiveness of treatment.

Finally, successful CBT requires parents who are willing and able to participate in the process. When parents are not invested in the treatment or interfere with treatment by "rescuing" their child from anxiety-provoking situations, parent training with psychoeducation is a necessary first step.

Positive Outcomes That May Be Expected

Efficacious CBT decreases physical and cognitive symptoms and improves behavioral functioning. Improvement in primary symptoms often leads to improvement in comorbid conditions and improved academic and family functioning. In the case of anxiety-based school refusal, the child returns to the school environment. For social phobia, expected outcomes include increased socialization.

Factors Affecting Outcome

Several factors likely impact CBT's efficacy. Chronological age may be a factor, but findings regarding the nature of this effect have been inconsistent. An early meta-analysis of the efficacy of CBT on different childhood disorders revealed that age, as an indicator of cognitive development, had a positive impact on treatment outcome; that is, older children were generally more responsive to CBT (Durlak et al. 1991). However, in a more recent investigation (Southam-Gerow et al. 2001),

age predicted *less* favorable treatment outcome for children with anxiety disorders. This disparity may have to do more with the nature of the specific treatment program than the composition of the treated sample. CBT programs developed for preadolescents may need substantial modification for use with adolescents.

Baseline psychopathology also may affect treatment outcome. Comorbid symptoms of depression and trait anxiety in particular, or higher levels of childhood internalizing disorders in general, were negatively associated with treatment efficacy (Berman et al. 2000; Southam-Gerow et al. 2001). Similarly, among children with obsessive-compulsive disorder treated with CBT family interventions, higher baseline severity significantly predicted poorer long-term results (Barrett et al. 2005).

Few data are available that specifically examine the number of treatment sessions necessary for optimal treatment response. Outcome data from controlled trials indicate that many children demonstrate significant improvement after 12–16 weeks of treatment. In a recent trial comparing behavioral and pharmacological treatment for youth with social phobia (Beidel et al. 2007), fluoxetine appeared to achieve its maximum effectiveness by week 8, whereas behavior therapy (in the form of social skills training and graduated exposure) continued to exert an effect through week 12, suggesting 3 months may allow for consolidation of treatment gains.

In addition to duration, frequency of the treatment sessions also affects treatment response. Specifically, massed treatment sessions (frequent and temporally close applications of the intervention, perhaps occurring two to three times per week) achieve superior outcome in a shorter period of time than once weekly sessions. Finally, in order for treatment to be efficacious, patients need to attend to exposure stimuli. Distraction during the exposure session reduces treatment efficacy (e.g., Grayson et al. 1982).

Parental psychopathology also may impact successful treatment of the child. Symptoms of depression, fear, hostility, psychoticism, paranoia, and obsessive-compulsive tendencies have all been negatively associated with treatment outcome (Berman et al. 2000; Southam-Gerow et al. 2001). Additionally, higher levels of overall family dysfunction predict poorer prognosis (Barrett et al. 2005). In contrast, sociodemographic variables do not seem to significantly affect treatment outcome. Efficacy appears consistent across ethnicity, gender, and socioeconomic status (Berman et al. 2000; Ferrell et al. 2004; Pina et al. 2003; Southam-Gerow et al. 2001).

Economic Cost-Benefit Issues

When taking into account both direct and indirect expenses, the total cost of anxiety disorders (of all ages) in 1990 was approximately $42.3 billion dollars (Greenberg et al. 1999). The current cost would likely be significantly higher. This burden could be mitigated considerably by early detection, accurate diagnosis, and effective intervention.

Given the chronicity of anxiety disorders, data from adult studies suggest that early effective intervention may offset later costs to society and to the individual. In comparison to combined or eclectic interventions, CBT tends to be less expensive and require a shorter treatment period. Among children, group CBT appears to be less expensive than and as equally effective as individual CBT (Manassis et al. 2002), indicating that it may be a quality cost-effective alternative.

Baseline Assessments

Various empirical assessment strategies, including diagnostic interviews, behavioral assessments, self-report, and informant-based questionnaires, are used to determine baseline functioning. The Anxiety Disorders Interview Schedule for Children (Silverman and Albano 1996) was developed specifically to assess anxiety disorders. Administered to parents and children, it provides a composite score for each symptom and assesses the presence of other childhood disorders in order to facilitate differential diagnosis (see also Chapter 7, "Diagnostic Interviews").

Behavioral assessment includes direct observation, behavioral avoidance tests, and self-monitoring. With direct observation, the clinician assesses a child's behavior in varied naturalistic settings. Behavioral avoidance tests incorporate direct observation in structured situations where the child approaches a feared stimulus, and subsequent behaviors are recorded. Self-monitoring requires children to record thoughts, emotional distress, and antecedents and consequences to anxious episodes.

Standardized self-report instruments are an integral part of a comprehensive assessment. Well-validated instruments include the Multidimensional Anxiety Scale for Children (MASC; March et al. 1997), the Screen for Child Anxiety Related Emotional Disorders (SCARED; Birmaher et al. 1999), and the Fear Survey

Schedule for Children—Revised (FSSC-R; Ollendick 1983). Additionally, several well-validated measures exist for social phobia, such as the Social Phobia and Anxiety Inventory for Children (SPAI-C; Beidel et al. 1995), the Social Anxiety Scale for Children—Revised (SASC-R; La Greca and Stone 1993), and the Social Anxiety Scale for Adolescents (SAS-A; La Greca and Lopez 1998). (See also Chapter 8, "Rating Scales.")

Setting Treatment Goals and Monitoring Progress

CBT is considered successful if there are clearly observable changes in physical and subjective distress and behavioral avoidance. Enhancing social skills is an important goal for children with social phobia. Additional treatment goals may include improved sleep and appetite as well as improved ability to concentrate and a reengagement in pleasant activities.

A distinguishing feature of CBT is assessment not only before and after treatment, but also throughout therapy. Self-monitoring allows the child and/or parent to record daily the occurrence or frequency of problematic behavior. These forms, reviewed at each treatment visit, provide immediate feedback regarding treatment efficacy or the lack of behavioral change, which signals a need to modify the intervention.

Adverse Effects and Complications

Parental assumptions or negative biases that reinforce caution and behavioral avoidance and that discourage risk-taking behaviors are called the *protection trap* (Silverman and Kurtines 1996). These actions are counterproductive to CBT's goals and method of intervention, which encourage the child (in a controlled fashion) to approach feared situations or objects. In many instances, one of the therapist's first objectives is to correct misperceptions and educate the parent about the crucial role of exposure for effective intervention. Similarly, parents may fail to understand that anticipatory anxiety is often more severe than the distress experienced when actually contacting the feared stimulus or that anxiety during exposure sessions is actually less than what the child (and parent) imagined would occur, particularly in the case of gradual exposure. Without this understanding, parents often work at cross-purposes with the therapist, reinforcing the child for anxious and avoidant behaviors rather than for positive approach behaviors.

Another complication occurs when exposure sessions are too short to allow habituation to occur. Depending upon the type of exposure selected (graduated or intensive) and the age of the patient (child or adolescent), sessions may last from 30 to 90 minutes. If exposure is discontinued prior to habituation, sensitization to the feared stimulus and an increase in fear may occur, thereby leading to a worsening of the child's condition.

The effect of CBT in children may be attenuated when depression is present (Hayward et al. 2000). Depressive symptoms such as excessive fatigue and poor concentration may prevent active engagement in activities such as exposure and cognitive restructuring. The use of antidepressant medication may alleviate neurovegetative symptoms, following which CBT may be implemented effectively.

Research Directions

Despite its established efficacy, few controlled comparisons have compared CBT to conditions other than waitlist comparison groups. Among those that have (Beidel et al. 2000, 2007; Last et al. 1998; Silverman et al. 1999a, 1999b), results have been mixed. Further studies examining outcome of CBT in comparison to active placebo or other active interventions are needed. Furthermore, even though group outcome data have established CBT's efficacy, a subset of children do not have an optimal outcome and a few fail to achieve even minimal benefit. Although extending the length of treatment is one possibility, other ways of enhancing outcome need to be considered. In addition, there has been insufficient attention to moderator and mediator variables that might impact CBT's efficacy.

Finally, what data exist (Barrett et al. 2001; Beidel et al. 2006; Kendall et al. 2004) indicate that the effects of CBT are long-lasting. However, the studies are few and the sample sizes are small. Much more work is necessary to examine the long-term outcome of these interventions on effectiveness variables including adult milestones such as occupational adjustment and the establishment of long-term, stable interpersonal relationships.

Summary Points

- CBT is a term for a group of interventions that share a commitment to empiricism and focus on behavior change.

- Exposure is the key ingredient for all forms of CBT.

- CBT is efficacious for various childhood anxiety disorders.

- Whereas developmental factors play a role in the manner in which CBT is implemented, the intervention is equally efficacious across age, gender, race and ethnicity, and socioeconomic status.

- The presence of comorbid depression may attenuate the efficacy of CBT, and consideration should be given to treating the depression prior to initiating treatment for the anxiety disorder.

References

Alfano C, Beidel DC, Turner SM: Cognition in childhood anxiety: conceptual, methodological, and developmental issues. Clin Psychol Rev 22:1209–1238, 2002

Barrett PM: Evaluation of cognitive-behavioral group treatments for childhood anxiety disorders. J Clin Child Psychol 27:459–468, 1998

Barrett PM, Rapee RM, Dadds MR, et al: Family enhancement of cognitive style in anxious and aggressive children. J Abnorm Child Psychol 24:187–203, 1996

Barrett PM, Duffy AL, Dadds MR, et al: Cognitive-behavioral treatment of anxiety disorders in children: long-term (6-year) follow-up. J Consult Clin Psychol 69:135–141, 2001

Barrett PM, Farrell C, Dadds MR, et al: Cognitive-behavioral family treatment of childhood obsessive-compulsive disorder: long-term follow-up and predictors of outcome. J Am Acad Child Adolesc Psychiatry 44:1005–1014, 2005

Beidel DC, Turner SM: Childhood Anxiety Disorders: A Guide to Research and Treatment. New York, Routledge/Taylor and Francis Group, 2005

Beidel DC, Turner SM, Morris TL: A new inventory to assess childhood social anxiety and phobia: the Social Phobia and Anxiety Inventory for Children. Psychol Assess 7:73–79, 1995

Beidel DC, Turner SM, Morris TL: Behavioral treatment of childhood social phobia. J Consult Clin Psychol 68:1072–1080, 2000

Beidel DC, Turner SM, Young BJ: Social effectiveness therapy for children: five years later. Behav Ther 37:416–425, 2006

Beidel DC, Turner SM, Sallee FR, et al: SET-C vs fluoxetine in the treatment of childhood social phobia. J Am Acad Child Adolesc Psychiatry 46:1622–1632, 2007

Berman SL, Weems CF, Silverman WK, et al: Predictors of outcome in exposure-based cognitive and behavioral treatments for phobic and anxiety disorders in children. Behav Ther 31:713–731, 2000

Bernstein GA, Borchardt C, Perwien AR: Imipramine plus cognitive-behavioral therapy in the treatment of school refusal. J Am Acad Child Adolesc Psychiatry 39:276–283, 2000

Birmaher B, Brent DA, Chiappetta L, et al: Psychometric properties of the Screen for Child Anxiety Related Emotional Disorders (SCARED): a replication study. J Am Acad Child Adolesc Psychiatry 38:1230–1236, 1999

Dadds MR, Spence SH, Holland DE, et al: Prevention and early intervention for anxiety disorders: a controlled trial. J Consult Clin Psychol 65:627–635, 1997

Durlak J, Fuhrman T, Lampman C: Effectiveness of cognitive-behavior therapy for maladapting children: a meta-analysis. Psychol Bull 110:204–214, 1991

Ferrell C, Beidel DC, Turner SM: Assessment and treatment of socially phobic children: a cross cultural comparison. J Clin Child Psychol 33:260–268, 2004

Flannery-Schroeder EC, Kendall PC: Group and individual cognitive-behavioral treatments for youth with anxiety disorders: a randomized clinical trial. Cognit Ther Res 24:251–278, 2000

Grayson JB, Foa EB, Steketee G: Habituation during exposure treatment: distraction vs attention-focusing. Behav Res Ther 20:323–328, 1982

Greenberg PE, Sisitsky T, Kessler RC, et al: The economic burden of anxiety disorders in the 1990s. J Clin Psychiatry 60:427–435, 1999

Hayward C, Varady S, Albano AM, et al: Cognitive-behavioral group therapy for social phobia in female adolescents: results of a pilot study. J Am Acad Child Adolesc Psychiatry 39:721–726, 2000

Kendall PC: Treating anxiety disorders in children: results of a randomized clinical trial. J Clin Child Psychol 62:100–110, 1994

Kendall PC, Flannery-Schroeder E, Panichelli-Mindel SM: Therapy with youths with anxiety disorders: a second randomized clinical trial. J Consult Clin Psychol 65:366–380, 1997

Kendall PC, Safford S, Flannery-Schroeder E, et al: Child anxiety treatment: outcomes in adolescence and impact on substance use and depression at 7.4 year follow-up. J Am Acad Child Adolesc Psychiatry 72:276–287, 2004

La Greca AM, Lopez N: Social anxiety among adolescents: linkages with peer relations and friendships. J Abnorm Child Psychol 26:83–94, 1998

La Greca AM, Stone WL: Social Anxiety Scale for Children–Revised: factor structure and concurrent validity. J Clin Child Psychol 22:17–27, 1993

Lang PJ, Levin DN, Miller GA: Fear behavior, fear imagery, and the psychophysiology of emotion: the problem of affective response integration. J Abnorm Psychol 92:276–306, 1983

Last CG, Hansen C, Franco N: Cognitive-behavioral treatment of school phobia. J Am Acad Child Adolesc Psychiatry 37:404–411, 1998

Manassis K, Mendlowitz SL, Scapillato D, et al: Group and individual cognitive behavioral therapy for child anxiety disorders: a randomized trial. J Am Acad Child Adolesc Psychiatry 41:1423–1430, 2002

March JS, Parker JDA, Sullivan K, et al: The Multidimensional Anxiety Scale for Children (MASC): factor structure, reliability, and validity. J Am Acad Child Adolesc Psychiatry 36:554–565, 1997

Mowrer OH: On the dual nature of learning: a reinterpretation of "conditioning" and "problem solving." Harv Educ Rev 17:102–148, 1947

Ollendick TH: Reliability and validity of the Revised Fear Survey Schedule for Children (FSSC-R). Behav Res Ther 21:685–692, 1983

Ollendick TH, Matson JL, Helsel WJ: Fears in children and adolescents: normative data. Behav Res Ther 23:465–467, 1985

Pina AA, Silverman WK, Fuentes RM, et al: Exposure-based cognitive-behavioral treatment for phobic and anxiety disorders: treatment effects and maintenance for Hispanic/Latino relative to European-American youths. J Am Acad Child Adolesc Psychiatry 42:1179–1187, 2003

Shortt AL, Barrett PM, Fox TL: Evaluating the FRIENDS program: a cognitive-behavioral group treatment for anxious children and their parents. J Clin Child Psychol 30:525–535, 2001

Silverman WK, Albano AM: The Anxiety Disorders Interview Schedule for Children (ADIS-C/P). San Antonio, TX, Psychological Corporation, 1996

Silverman WK, Kurtines WM: Anxiety and Phobic Disorders: A Pragmatic Approach. New York, Plenum, 1996

Silverman WK, Kurtines WM, Ginsburg GS, et al: Contingency management, self-control, and education support in the treatment of childhood phobic disorders: a randomized clinical trial. J Consult Clin Psychol 67:675–687, 1999a

Silverman WK, Kurtines WM, Ginsburg GS, et al: Treating anxiety disorders in children with group cognitive-behavioral therapy: a randomized clinical trial. J Consult Clin Psychol 67:995–1003, 1999b

Southam-Gerow MA, Kendall PC, Weersing VR: Examining outcome variability: correlates of treatment response in a child and adolescent anxiety clinic. J Clin Child Psychol 30:422–436, 2001

Spence SH, Donovan C, Brechman-Toussain M: The treatment of childhood social phobia: the effectiveness of a social skills training-based, cognitive-behavioral intervention, with and without parental involvement. J Child Psychol Psychiatry 41:713–726, 2000

Turner SM, Beidel DC, Roberson-Nay R, et al: Parenting behaviors in parents with anxiety disorders. Behav Res Ther 41:541–554, 2003

Chapter 59

Cognitive-Behavioral Therapy for Depression

Mark A. Reinecke, Ph.D.
Rachel H. Jacobs, Ph.D.

Cognitive-behavioral therapy (CBT) has been found to be efficacious in treating depressed children and adolescents. CBT is based upon Beck's (1963, 1983) models of depression and psychotherapy and is designed to address maladaptive cognitions and patterns of behavior that contribute to low mood. Early meta-analyses reported high mean effect sizes for CBT with depressed youth (Lewinsohn and Clarke 1999; Michael and Crowley 2002; Reinecke et al. 1998). More recent meta-analyses found smaller mean effect sizes but still presented positive evidence for the efficacy of CBT (Klein et al. 2007; Weisz et al. 2006). Klein et al. (2007) found several moderators of treatment outcome effect sizes. Studies that yielded significantly smaller effect sizes employed intent-to-treat statistical analyses, compared CBT to active treatments rather than controls, and delivered the intervention in clinical rather than research settings. Overall, recent randomized controlled trials have subjected cognitive-behavioral interventions to more rigorous testing. Taken together, current evidence suggests that CBT can be effective for the treatment of major depression among youth, that improvements in mood are associated with improved psychosocial functioning, and that CBT can be effective in reducing suicidal ideation among depressed adolescents.

Cognitive Vulnerability

A range of cognitive, biological, social, and environmental factors have been implicated as risk factors for depression (Chapter 18, "Depression and Dysthymia").

Social and contextual factors, family environment, temperament, and genetic and neurohormonal factors all contribute to how an individual responds to stressful life events. The practice of CBT with depressed youth is based on the assumption that by targeting factors implicated in the etiology and maintenance of depression, symptoms can be alleviated.

Cognitive diathesis-stress models (e.g., Abramson et al. 1989; Beck 1967) posit that depression is precipitated by a cognitive vulnerability that in interaction with a negative life event, leads to the onset of a depressive episode. It is hypothesized that cognitive vulnerabilities are latent and, like software on a computer that has not been booted up, do not operate without being activated by stress. These cognitive vulnerabilities are organized as *schemas:* stable cognitive structures that include representations of the self and others and that guide the processing of information (Beck 1963, 1983).

Depressed children and adolescents demonstrate many of the same biases and distortions characteristic of depressed adults. They demonstrate negative thoughts about themselves, the world, and their future, attending selectively to negative events. For example, they may view themselves as unlovable, undesirable, or flawed. Moreover, they may view others as unreliable, unsupportive, and uncaring. Depressed youth anticipate rejection and tend to ruminate about their problems. Deficits in rational problem-solving and problem-solving motivation also are manifest. Specifically, they anticipate that their attempts to solve life's problems will be unsuccessful, choosing to either avoid addressing problems directly or approach them impulsively. Perfectionistic standards can impede both treatment and overall sense of self-esteem. A negative attributional style includes viewing losses or failures as stemming from personal characteristics that are broad, stable, and unchanging. These proposed cognitive vulnerabilities are all targets of CBT intervention.

General Characteristics of CBT

CBT is **formulation based** and prescriptive. Specific intervention strategies are selected based on an understanding of the cognitive, social, and environmental variables contributing to a particular child's distress. Thus, the techniques used in CBT are individually tai-

lored and strategically directed toward rectifying maladaptive beliefs and attitudes, as well as alleviating social skill deficits. An essential characteristic of CBT is its **time-limited** nature. Treatment is not typically open-ended or long-term. In contrast, it attempts to bring about meaningful symptomatic improvement within 12–16 sessions. In community practice, however, comorbidities and the particular strengths and weaknesses of the patient and family may require longer interventions. Active and focused treatment is organized in accord with an **agenda**. **Homework** assignments allow for practicing cognitive and behavioral skills during the week. The therapeutic relationship is characterized by **collaboration**. That is, the cognitive-behavioral therapist, the patient, and the youth's caregivers work together to address cognitive deficits, distortions, and deficiencies, as well as help the child to learn social skills and adaptive coping strategies for affect regulation. The therapist works with the child to understand the child's experience, the meanings he or she ascribes to events, and the ways he or she attempts to cope with daily challenges. Negative thoughts are seen as hypotheses to be explored, rather than facts to be accepted. Working together, therapist and child test the utility and validity of these beliefs. In many cases it is also important to understand parental beliefs, expectations, and attributions, as they directly influence the child's developing sense of self and others. Table 59–1 summarizes common CBT targets, whereas Table 59–2 summarizes specific CBT interventions. We refer the interested reader to Friedberg and McClure (2002), Reinecke et al. (2003; Reinecke and Curry 2008), and Stallard (2002) for more detailed descriptions of CBT with children and adolescents.

Psychoeducation is the first component of a successful CBT intervention. Children and adolescents are typically brought to treatment by their parents and may be confused, anxious, and even angry. CBT therapists educate parents and children about the nature of depression, its causes, and the rationale for specific interventions. A model of how CBT will apply to the specific problems the child is experiencing is presented. The child or adolescent is reassured that human emotions, such as depression, are normal and expected. The clinician explains how biological and developmental vulnerabilities, life events, cognitive processes, and moods interact in contributing to distress. This provides a structure for understanding the child's difficulties. **Mood monitoring** is introduced to increase the child's awareness and understanding of emotions. Mood diaries are one tool that can be used later in treatment as the child is taught to recognize

TABLE 59–1. Common targets of cognitive-behavioral intervention with youth

Cognitive	Automatic thoughts (self, world, future) and images
	Perceptions
	Cognitive distortions
	Memories
	Schemata, assumptions
	Goals, wishes, plans, standards (example: perfectionism)
	Problem solving (rational skills and motivation)
	Attributions
Social and behavioral	Social skills
	Communication skills
	Conflict resolution/ negotiation
	Maladaptive coping
	Attachment difficulties (insecure, disorganized, fearful)
	Supports (peers, family, adults)
Environmental	Stressors (major and minor)
	Cues and reinforcers

TABLE 59–2. Specific interventions commonly used in cognitive-behavioral therapy (CBT)

1. Introducing CBT model and treatment rationale
2. Goal setting
3. Mood monitoring
4. Activity scheduling (Pleasant/Social/ Mastery)
5. Rational problem-solving and problem-solving motivation
6. Rationally disputing automatic thoughts, replacing with adaptive self-statements
7. Cognitive distortions
8. Affect regulation
9. Social skills
10. Assertiveness
11. Communication and compromise
12. Attachment security
13. Parent training
14. Booster sessions and relapse prevention

cues that trigger certain emotions. With younger children, emotion cards, games, and books allow for the identification of feelings. Perhaps the most important part of CBT psychoeducation is communicating a sense of hope to the family, offering them a vision of a more positive future and an introduction to the tools that are likely to bring this about.

The therapist and child work together toward specific **goals**. The CBT therapist guides the parent(s) and child to develop a list of meaningful, specific, and concrete goals on which they can agree.

Activity scheduling allows the depressed child or adolescent to engage in activities that give a sense of pleasure or accomplishment. Social activities, in particular, are encouraged. The therapist begins by brainstorming a list of activities the child may enjoy. Activities on this list should be safe, active, inexpensive, readily available, legal, and genuinely enjoyable. Once a list of approximately 10 activities has been generated, the patient is asked to increase the amount of pleasant activities in which he or she participates each day and to note his or her mood. The adolescent is taught to use self-reward for trying to use a new strategy. The child's

parents are taught to use tangible rewards such as stickers or activities enjoyed together (for example, a trip to the museum with mom). The use of contingent reinforcement helps the child or adolescent recognize his or her efforts and learn the importance of rewarding and praising oneself for a good effort. Punishment or removal of rewards is deemphasized.

Social skills are another focus of treatment, as depressed youth are often withdrawn and behave in ways that alienate peers and family. Using modeling and role-play, the therapist and patient practice concrete skills such as starting a conversation, asking questions, smiling, and maintaining eye contact.

Problem solving is a critical component of CBT with depressed youth, as they often demonstrate poor problem-solving skills and low motivation to address their problems. First, it is acknowledged that everyone has problems. The therapist can begin by presenting common problems experienced by other children and adolescents (curfew disputes, grades, difficulties with friends), and the patient is encouraged to identify a specific problem and to generate a range of possible solutions. After generating a list of potential solutions, the therapist and the patient discuss the pros and cons of each and select the best course of action. A formal model of problem solving is introduced using the acronym RIBEYE: Relax, Identify the problem, Brainstorm possible solutions, Evaluate their strengths and weaknesses, say Yes to one (or two), and Encourage yourself for success. As Frauenknecht and Black (2004) note, the CBT therapist's goal is to teach problem-solving skills that can be used in a range of settings. This is done by providing the child with graduated experiences in therapy (again using modeling and role-play) and integrating this with in vivo practice. Generalization of skills is most likely to occur when explicit attempts are made to bring it about. Young children may enjoy playing games that involve problem solving or acting out problem scenarios with puppets.

Affect regulation and distress tolerance strategies help the child or adolescent modulate negative moods. Depressed youth can be taught specific strategies for coping with emotionally arousing situations. Using a blank emotions thermometer, the therapist asks the adolescent to describe his or her feelings when he or she is "about to lose it…your feelings are going out of control." The patient is then asked to identify thoughts, physiological sensations, and behavioral cues that occur just before his or her moods escalate to this level. This typically takes the form of feelings of agitation, tension, and thoughts such as "I can't take this!" As anchors are placed on the thermometer, the patient comes to identify cues of mood escalation, noting that action will be needed to prevent an outburst. The therapist and the teen then work collaboratively to develop a list of cognitive, behavioral, and social strategies that can be introduced before mood escalation. Example strategies include relaxation exercises, leaving the situation, adaptive self-statements (e.g., "It's no big deal," "there's nothing here I can't handle"), seeking social support, and distraction. By anticipating situations that may lead to an emotional outburst, the adolescent can prepare for them and avoid the negative consequences that typically accompany such outbursts.

With younger children, the therapist helps the child identify how a particular emotion manifests in his or her body (we have found coloring exercises to be helpful). They are also led to recognize their "bugs" or what leads them to feel a particular negative emotion such as sadness or anger. The child is taught to "Stop—and think!" before simply reacting emotionally to the situation.

Changing automatic thoughts or cognitive distortions is accomplished by teaching youth to identify and change such patterns. First, the child or adolescent must become aware of these thoughts. Based upon **Socratic questioning**, guided discovery is a process by which a therapist, by patiently asking a series of gentle questions, guides the patient to recognize errors in logic and to see how maintaining a particular belief may be maladaptive. By avoiding direct confrontation,

the therapist maintains the collaborative rapport and demonstrates how the patient can come to a new, more adaptive way of thinking about his or her predicament. The therapist is simultaneously modeling a rational way of thinking and a systematic method of approaching life's problems. Simply pointing out a child's maladaptive thoughts and cognitive distortions (e.g., "*Nobody* likes me," "I'm too stupid to do *anything*") and suggesting more positive alternative thoughts is not likely to be effective. Rather, the child or teen must recognize that the negative beliefs are, in fact, untrue and then develop skills for evaluating the validity of thoughts that can be used in a range of situations. To promote the generalization of these skills to new settings, homework is assigned in which the CBT therapist encourages children and adolescents to apply cognitive techniques learned in the therapy session to problems they encounter at home and at school. As they become adept at identifying maladaptive thoughts during sessions, teens are asked to complete a three-column mood log at home as a homework task. A useful strategy with children is showing them pictures of a somewhat ambiguous situation, with cartoon thought-bubbles above the character's heads. The therapist gently guides the child in disputing negative beliefs and in using positive thought-bubbles.

Adaptive counterthoughts allow the patient to "talk back" to negative cognitions. Using automatic thoughts the adolescent has identified, the CBT therapist then teaches the adolescent specific strategies for rectifying maladaptive thoughts. Upsetting thoughts are seen as questions or hypotheses to be tested, and evidence is sought to ascertain their validity and utility. Specifically, patients are taught to ask: 1) What is the evidence that supports the thought? 2) Is there any contradictory evidence? Is there any evidence I have overlooked or anything that might lead me to think the thought may not be true? 3) Is there another way of looking at the situation? 4) If the negative thought is true, is it really so big a deal? 5) What's the solution? What can be done to handle this?

Relaxation training gives the child or adolescent a means of coping adaptively when confronted with stressful situations. Relaxation techniques are taught including controlled breathing, guided imagery (e.g., relaxing on a warm beach), muscle relaxation, and adaptive self-statements (e.g., "It's OK. I can handle this."). With children, relaxation techniques may be more creative. For example, one child with whom we worked did not enjoy breathing exercises; however, he found it relaxing to blow bubbles on his back porch. For him, this was a relaxing activity he enjoyed that regulated his breathing, without seeming like "a corny breathing thing."

Taking stock involves helping the child or adolescent consolidate skills learned over the course of treatment. The therapist, parent, and child review the gains that have been made and determine which strategies have been the most helpful. Identifying associations between the use of these strategies and positive changes is emphasized. Ways of coping with future problems are discussed. Periodic booster sessions may be scheduled.

Specific CBT Protocols for Adolescent Populations

The Adolescent Coping With Depression Course (CWD-A; Clarke et al. 1990) is a group treatment designed for adolescents with depression. The course is designed to have a classroom rather than clinical feel. Each participant is given a student workbook (available at: http://www.kpchr.org/public/acwd.html). A leader's manual (also available at this Web site) guides the therapists through lectures, discussions, role-plays, and homework. Major topics include social skills, relaxation, changing unpleasant cognitions, resolving conflicts, and planning for the future. The CWD-A can be adapted for use in individual therapy, although the authors stress that much can be gained from a group of adolescents learning together and from one another. A parallel course has been developed for the parents of depressed adolescents (Lewinsohn et al. 1991). Parents become familiar with what their teens are learning and join their sessions, allowing families to practice their communication skills. The first study evaluating the efficacy of the CWD-A course (Lewinsohn et al. 1990) compared three conditions: the treatment of adolescents alone, the treatment of adolescents with a parallel parent group, and a waitlist control. Adolescents who received the CWD-A course demonstrated significant reductions in depression relative to those in the control condition. These gains were maintained over a 2-year follow-up period. The parent training component did not appear to facilitate clinical improvement. The CWD-A has been refined over the past 15 years, and it can be quite effective for treating mild to moderate depression among some teens.

The Treatment for Adolescents With Depression Study (TADS) Team was a multisite, randomized con-

trolled trial that examined the effectiveness of individual CBT in comparison to fluoxetine, placebo, and the combination of fluoxetine and CBT (Treatment for Adolescents With Depression Study Team 2003, 2004). The CBT protocol included eight skills considered essential (introduction to treatment rationale, mood monitoring, goal setting, pleasant activities, problem solving, automatic thoughts and cognitive distortions, realistic counterthoughts, and taking stock) with an additional five optional skills (social interaction, assertion, communication and compromise, relaxation, and affect regulation). Treatment occurred on an individual level with optional family sessions. After 12 weeks, TADS CBT did not lead to more improvement in depression than the other TADS treatments (Treatment for Adolescents With Depression Study Team 2004). Youth who received active treatments maintained their gains over the 36 weeks. At the end of 36 weeks of treatment, CBT, fluoxetine, and their combination yielded similar levels of clinical improvement (Treatment for Adolescents With Depression Study Team 2007). Youth receiving CBT demonstrated a somewhat greater and more rapid reduction in suicidal ideation than did youth receiving fluoxetine. These findings suggest that when suicidal ideation is present, careful monitoring of suicidality and a referral for CBT may be appropriate (Emslie et al. 2006). Overall, the combination of CBT and fluoxetine resulted in more rapid alleviation of depressive symptoms than fluoxetine or CBT alone (Treatment for Adolescents With Depression Study Team 2004). The combination of CBT and fluoxetine was also effective in improving global functioning, global health, and quality of life (Vitiello et al. 2006). The TADS CBT treatment manuals (Curry et al. 2005) can be found at https://trialweb.dcri.duke.edu/tads/manuals.html.

Specific CBT Protocols for Childhood Depression

The ACTION treatment and workbook (Stark et al. 2004) outlines a gender-specific, developmentally sensitive program for depressed girls. The treatment program is based on a self-control model in which youth use coping, problem solving, and/or cognitive restructuring strategies to address their depression. Strengths of the ACTION program include its engaging activities as well as use of ACTION kits that help the child remember the central therapeutic concepts. Earlier iterations of ACTION (Stark and Kendall 1996) outline a protocol for both girls and boys. Research with earlier versions of the treatment protocol suggests that it may be efficacious for alleviating depression among prepubertal youth (Stark 1990; Stark et al. 1987).

The Primary and Secondary Control Enhancement Training (PASCET; Weisz 1990; Weisz et al. 1993; a detailed description is available in Kazdin and Weisz 2003) is based on a two-process model of control, wherein primary control involves enhancing reward and reducing punishment by adjusting objective conditions, while secondary control involves adjusting oneself to more adaptively deal with situations that are more difficult to change. Core CBT techniques are delivered through group meetings with additional individual meetings to fit the lessons of treatment to the individual child's situation. The PASCET program was compared to a no-treatment control (Weisz et al. 1997). After treatment, the CBT group showed greater reductions than the control group in depressive symptoms.

Factors Affecting Outcomes

Predictors of poor response to CBT include greater severity of depression, higher levels of cognitive distortion (Brent et al. 1998; Clarke et al. 1992), and greater hopelessness (Brent et al. 1998; Curry et al. 2006). In TADS, younger adolescents who were less chronically depressed and demonstrated higher functioning were more likely to benefit from 12 weeks of CBT treatment. Lower levels of suicidal ideation and higher expectancies for treatment were also predictive of 12-week positive outcomes. There is mixed evidence regarding the effect of comorbidity on depression outcomes, with some studies finding a lack of evidence of effect (e.g., Weersing and Weisz 2002) and some finding that comorbidity predicts poor treatment response (e.g., Clarke et al. 1995; Curry et al. 2006). Family income may also moderate the effect of CBT in adolescents (Curry et al. 2006). There is much work remaining to be done exploring "what treatment, for whom?"

Research has not yet supported the use of CBT with very young children (e.g., ages 3–5 years) or among youth with a severe learning disability or developmental delay. The effectiveness of CBT in treating youth with psychotic features has also not been established. Preliminary findings indicate that a combined treatment approach of CBT and fluoxetine can be effective

in alleviating suicidal ideation and in reducing the risk of suicidal gestures among depressed adolescents (Treatment for Adolescents With Depression Study Team 2004). Indeed, CBT appears to be effective in addressing the slight increase in suicidal ideation observed among youth receiving fluoxetine (Treatment for Adolescents With Depression Study Team 2004).

Common Mistakes

Clinicians often make mistakes when learning to implement CBT. Although CBT protocols tend to be straightforward, attention must be given to individual, familial, and developmental factors. Maladaptive beliefs, attitudes, and behaviors are learned and function in a social context. Although CBT emphasizes rectifying intrapsychic cognitive processes that maintain the child's depression, care should be taken to address ways in which parents, teachers, and peers may inadvertently be modeling or reinforcing these maladaptive patterns. Attention should be given to environmental factors, such as parental participation in treatment, parental mood, parenting practices (including cultural practices), parental attitudes and beliefs, and parental motivation for treatment. Consideration of cultural factors and ethnic minority status will enhance treatment. In treating depressed children, it is helpful to discuss low motivation as part of the disorder. Activity scheduling is helpful in alleviating some mood symptoms, which then may increase motivation. Last, the family as well as clinician must be patient with the change process.

Findings from the TADS project indicate that 12 weeks of treatment may be insufficient for many adolescents. If treatment is continued for 36 weeks, however, approximately 80% of youth will demonstrate significant improvement.

Nonspecific factors, including therapeutic warmth, responsiveness, and empathy, go a long way in forging an effective treatment alliance. Consistency in completing homework assignments is a strong predictor of outcome. The completion of homework encourages both the child and the family to generalize interventions "out of the office" and apply them in day-to-day life. It is vital to continue practicing each cognitive and behavioral skill until it is learned well, rather than exposing the child to a plethora of techniques all at once. The old adage "less is more" applies here. Progress must be assessed systematically. Objective assessment can help the clinician step back and reformulate the case if current interventions are not leading to clinical improvement. Attention to these common pitfalls will aid the clinician in implementing CBT effectively with youth.

Research Directions

Studies to date, although promising, have primarily been conducted in university and medical center settings. The effectiveness of CBT within community settings has received little study. At the same time, relatively little is known about which specific components of CBT programs bring about positive change or the mechanisms of clinical improvement. In other words, we do not know which strategies are necessary and/or sufficient for clinical improvement and what processes mediate clinical improvement. We do not know whether different strategies or techniques are helpful for different individuals. CBT also needs more testing head to head with other active treatments. Questions of generalizability and cultural sensitivity are important, as few trials have evaluated CBT among large samples of ethnic minority children and adolescents (for exceptions see McClure et al. 2005; Rossello and Bernal 1999).

Summary Points

- CBT seeks to ameliorate cognitive and behavioral vulnerability factors associated with low mood.
- CBT is characterized by collaboration between the clinician and the patient.
- When a clinician is conducting CBT with youth, attention must be given to developmental and environmental factors.
- Suicidal ideation must be assessed regularly.
- CBT techniques must be implemented with the individual patient in mind.
- For moderately depressed youth, 12–18 sessions of CBT (either individual or group) can be effective for reducing levels of depression.
- Individual CBT appears to be effective for the treatment of moderate to severe depression and in reducing suicidal ideation.
- A combination of CBT and fluoxetine appears to offer the best opportunity for rapid improvement for more severely depressed youth.

References

Abramson L, Metalsky G, Alloy L: Hopelessness depression: a theory based subtype of depression. Psychol Rev 96:358–372, 1989

Beck AT: Thinking and depression, 1: idiosyncratic content and cognitive distortions. Arch Gen Psychiatry 9:324–333, 1963

Beck AT: Depression: Causes and Treatment. Philadelphia, University of Pennsylvania Press, 1967

Beck AT: Cognitive therapy of depression: new perspectives, in Treatment of Depression: Old Controversies and New Approaches. Edited by Clayton P, Barrett J. New York, Raven Press, 1983, pp 265–284

Brent D, Kolko D, Birmaher B, et al: Predictors of treatment efficacy in a clinical trial of three psychosocial treatments for adolescent depression. J Am Acad Child Adolesc Psychiatry 37:906–914, 1998

Clarke G, Lewinsohn P, Hops H: Leader's Manual for Adolescent Groups: Adolescent Coping With Depression Course, 1990. Available at: http://www.kpchr.org/public/acwd/CWDA_manual.pdf. Accessed June 16, 2009.

Clarke G, Hops H, Lewinsohn PM, et al: Cognitive-behavioral group treatment of adolescent depression: prediction of outcome. Behav Ther 23:341–354, 1992

Clarke G, Hawkins W, Murphy M, et al: Targeted prevention of unipolar depressive disorder in an at-risk sample of high school adolescents: a randomized trial of a group cognitive interview. J Am Acad Child Adolesc Psychiatry 34:312–321, 1995

Curry J, Wells KC, Brent DA, et al: Treatment for Adolescents With Depression Study (TADS) Cognitive Behavior Therapy Manual. Durham, NC, Duke University, 2005. Available at: https://trialweb.dcri.duke.edu/tads/manuals.html. Accessed June 16, 2009.

Curry J, Rohde P, Simons A, et al: Predictors and moderators of acute outcome in the Treatment for Adolescents With Depression Study (TADS). J Am Acad Child Adolesc Psychiatry 45:1427–1439, 2006

Emslie G, Kratochvil C, Vitiello B, et al: Treatment for Adolescents With Depression Study (TADS): safety results. J Am Acad Child Adolesc Psychiatry 45:1440–1455, 2006

Frauenknecht M, Black D: Problem-solving training for children and adolescents, in Social Problem Solving: Theory, Research, and Training. Edited by Chang E, D'Zurilla T, Sanna L. Washington, DC, American Psychological Association, 2004, pp 153–170

Friedberg RD, McClure JM: Clinical Practice of Cognitive Therapy With Children and Adolescents: The Nuts and Bolts. New York, Guilford, 2002

Kazdin AE, Weisz JR: Evidence-Based Psychotherapies for Children and Adolescents. New York, Guilford, 2003

Klein JB, Jacobs RH, Reinecke MA: A meta-analysis of CBT in adolescents with depression. J Am Acad Child Adolesc Psychiatry 46:1403–1413, 2007

Lewinsohn P, Clarke G: Psychosocial treatments for adolescent depression. Clin Psychol Rev 19:329–342, 1999

Lewinsohn P, Clarke G, Hops H, et al: Cognitive-behavioral treatment for depressed adolescents. Behav Ther 21:385–401, 1990

Lewinsohn PM, Rohde P, Hops H, et al: Leader's Manual for Parent Groups: Adolescent Coping With Depression Course, 1991. Available at: http://www.kpchr.org/public/acwd/CWDA_parent_manual.pdf. Accessed June 16, 2009.

McClure EB, Connell AM, Zucker M, et al: The adolescent depression empowerment project (ADEPT): a culturally sensitive family treatment for depressed African American girls, in Psychosocial Treatments for Child and Adolescent Disorders: Empirically Based Strategies for Clinical Practice, 2nd Edition. Edited by Hibbs ED, Jensen PS. Washington, DC, American Psychological Association, 2005, pp 149–164

Michael KD, Crowley SL: How effective are treatments for child and adolescent depression? A meta-analytic review. Clin Psychol Rev 22:247–269, 2002

Reinecke MA, Curry JF: Adolescents, in Adapting Cognitive Therapy for Depression: Managing Complexity and Comorbidity. Edited by Whisman M. New York, Guilford, 2008, pp 394–416

Reinecke MA, Ryan N, DuBois D: Cognitive-behavioral therapy of depression and depressive symptoms during adolescence: a review and meta-analysis. J Am Acad Child Adolesc Psychiatry 37:26–34, 1998

Reinecke MA, Dattilio FM, Freeman A (eds): Cognitive Therapy With Children and Adolescents: A Casebook for Clinical Practice, 2nd Edition. New York, Guilford, 2003

Rossello J, Bernal G: The efficacy of cognitive-behavioral and interpersonal treatments for depression in Puerto Rican adolescents. J Consult Clin Psychol 67:734–745, 1999

Stallard P: Think Good, Feel Good: A Cognitive Behaviour Therapy Workbook for Children and Young People. New York, Wiley, 2002

Stark KD: Childhood Depression: School-Based Intervention. New York, Guilford, 1990

Stark KD, Kendall PC: Treating Depressed Children: Therapist Manual for ACTION. Ardmore, PA, Workbook Publishing, 1996

Stark KD, Reynolds WM, Kaslow NJ: A comparison of the relative efficacy of self-control therapy and a behavioral problem-solving therapy for depression in children. J Abnorm Child Psychol 15:91–113, 1987

Stark KD, Schnoebelen S, Simpson J, et al: Treating Depressed Children: Therapist Manual for ACTION. Ardmore, PA, Workbook Publishing, 2004

Treatment for Adolescents With Depression Study Team: Treatment for Adolescents With Depression Study (TADS): rationale, design, and methods. J Am Acad Child Adolesc Psychiatry 42:531–542, 2003

Treatment for Adolescents With Depression Study Team: Fluoxetine, cognitive-behavioral therapy, and their combination for adolescents with depression: Treatment for Adolescents With Depression Study (TADS) randomized controlled trial. JAMA 292:807–820, 2004

Treatment for Adolescents With Depression Study Team: The Treatment for Adolescents With Depression Study (TADS): Long-term effectiveness and safety outcomes. Arch Gen Psychiatry 64:1132–1143, 2007

Vitiello B, Rohde P, Silva S, et al: Functioning and quality of life in the Treatment for Adolescents With Depression Study (TADS). J Am Acad Child Adolesc Psychiatry 45:1419–1426, 2006

Weersing VR, Weisz JR: Mechanisms of action in youth psychotherapy. J Child Psychol Psychiatry 43:3–29, 2002

Weisz JR: Development of control-related beliefs, goals, and styles in childhood and adolescence: a clinical perspective, in Self-Directedness and Efficacy: Causes and Effects Throughout the Life Course. Edited by Schaie KW, Rodin J, Schooler C. New York, Erlbaum, 1990, pp 103–145

Weisz JR, Sweeney L, Proffitt V, et al: Control-related beliefs and self-reported depressive symptoms in late childhood. J Abnorm Psychol 102:411–418, 1993

Weisz JR, Thurber CA, Sweeney L, et al: Brief treatment of mild-to-moderate child depression using primary and secondary control enhancement training. J Consult Clin Psychol 65:703–707, 1997

Weisz JR, McCarty CA, Valeri SM: Effects of psychotherapy for children and adolescents: a meta-analysis. Psychol Bull 132:132–149, 2006

Chapter 60

Motivational Interviewing

Paul Nagy, M.S., L.P.C., L.C.A.S., C.C.S.

Dealing with resistant and risk-taking youth can be a special challenge for the child and adolescent mental health specialist. It may be particularly difficult to motivate change when the young patient is engaged in behaviors, such as substance abuse, sexual risk-taking, or driving fast cars, that are positively reinforced by social, developmental, or biological conditions. Motivational interviewing (MI) is an effective approach for raising problem awareness and facilitating change exploration with individuals who may be resistant, stuck, or not yet "ready" to make behavioral changes. MI uses a client centered, collaborative approach that follows a particular set of principles and uses a certain set of skills and techniques (Miller and Rollnick 1991). While MI has been primarily studied with adults, it is now being used with children and adolescents seen in a variety of settings including pediatric practice, schools, juvenile justice settings, and emergency rooms (Feldstein and Ginsburg 2006).

This chapter provides a brief description of MI, a summary of the research supporting the use of MI

with children and adolescents, and practical guidelines and strategies for implementing MI. It addresses developmental issues, as well as implications for future research and recommendations for further study.

MI Described

MI is "a client-centered, directive method for enhancing intrinsic motivation for change by exploring and resolving ambivalence" (Miller and Rollnick 2002, p. 25). The interpersonal model presented by Carl Rogers (1957) and further supported by Truax and Carkaff (1967) and Gordon (1970) provides the theoretical basis of MI. When the client experiences a safe and comfortable therapeutic environment, he will more likely engage with the therapist in an open examination of his life to determine how to resolve his problems. This is accomplished by showing the client respect and by applying a certain set of principles and skills (Miller and Rollnick 1991). MI posits that resistance to behavior change may be due to a lack of awareness or concern about a problem or to a conflict of opposing desires expressed as ambivalence. Ambivalence is viewed as normal rather than pathological, and a primary goal of MI is to identify, explore, and resolve ambivalence (Miller and Rollnick 1991). An assumption of MI is that people need to want to change and will more likely initiate and sustain change when they determine for themselves that change will improve their lives.

MI uses a cluster of counseling skills referred to as OARS—Open-ended questions, Affirmations, Reflective listening, and Summaries. MI assumes that client awareness and concern will be facilitated by using these skills while examining an individual's particular values, interests, and concerns in a collaborative, nonjudgmental manner (Miller and Rollnick 2002).

According to the principles of MI, both motivation and resistance are influenced by the therapist's style. Motivation is seen as key to change; it is useful to view it as a dynamic state, rather than a personality trait, because it can be modified and influenced by therapist style (Miller and Rollnick 1991). That resistance is also influenced by therapist style explains why confrontational approaches are ineffective. The MI therapist communication style is based on a spirit that emphasizes collaboration, evocations, and respect for patient autonomy (Miller and Rollnick 2002). The MI therapist is directive, exercising skills and techniques that confront patient choices in relation to his or her own personal goals.

Stages of Change Model

The stages of change model (Prochaska and DiClemente 1982) suggests that change is based on a client's level of awareness and concern about a particular problem, as well as the degree of commitment for change. These stages include *precontemplation* (is not aware of the need for change or is resistant to change), *contemplation* (has some ambivalence and is willing to consider change but not yet willing to make a commitment), *preparation* (is planning change and willing to plan goal-oriented steps), *action* (is actively taking steps to change), and *maintenance* (has achieved change goals and works to maintain changes). MI suggests that applying different approaches in order to meet people where they are in the change process

leads to better therapeutic outcomes (Miller and Rollnick 1991).

A primary goal of MI is to elicit self-motivational statements by building on "change talk," which is categorized by recognition of a problem, statements of concern, intention to change, and optimism about change (Miller and Rollnick 2002). Another goal of MI is targeting interventions to a client's expressed level of readiness. Interventions and techniques that can be used with adolescents at a precontemplation level of readiness are shown in Table 60–1. The following case example illustrates an adolescent who vacillates between stages of readiness.

Case Example
A marijuana-using patient in his third MI session communicated that he had decided that the time had come to quit using marijuana. His expressed motivation for quitting included several factors. The most heavily weighted factor was an emotional one: his younger brother had expressed concern and regret that the patient was no longer attending his soccer games because he was choosing to get high with friends after school. The patient also indicated that he wanted to get serious about planning for college and was now concerned that his drug use was interfering with his completion of college applications.

The following week, the patient presented as if the discussion we had had the prior week had never occurred as he stated that he had no intention of stopping his marijuana use. He said that his brother was really not all that bothered about his missing the soccer games. Also, he no longer wanted to apply to colleges as most of his friends were planning to take a year off and he would now do the same. As a result, we again focused on exploring the pros and cons of his behavior rather than planning for change.

MI Principles
Express Empathy

Empathy is the ability to view the world through the eyes of another by seeing, feeling, and understanding things as if living the same life experience. Expression of empathy works to reduce defensiveness by reassuring patients that they are understood and not "crazy" for having their particular set of thoughts and feelings. Effective communications of empathy enable patients to risk more honesty and open exploration of their problems (Miller and Rollnick 1991).

TABLE 60–1. Stage of change interventions

Precontemplation	Interventions	Techniques
Doesn't see the need for change or is unwilling to consider change	Build rapport Promote awareness of risk Educate about risk behavior Explore pros and cons Review behaviors in situational context Emphasize personal choice Promote self-efficacy Encourage future awareness Plan for the future	Icebreakers Assessment instruments and personal feedback reports Client education Pros and cons Functional analysis FRAMES (Miller and Sanchez 1994) Imagine benefits of change or identify indicators for future awareness Goal setting and establishing a plan

Develop Discrepancy

Motivation for change occurs when clients recognize a faulty connection between their behavior and their self-image, desires, or goals. In MI, the therapist's task is to gently but directly guide the patient toward evaluating whether or not behavior choices are consistent with personal values and aspirations. MI encourages individuals to examine whether or not they are living with full integrity, and if not, to consider making the changes that would enable a more congruent sense of self.

Roll With Resistance

Resistance is common when working with adolescent patients. Rolling with resistance is best accomplished by using a collaborative and friendly style and by not arguing with or provoking the patient. MI techniques that may help in overcoming patient resistance include simple reflections, amplified reflections, double-sided reflections, shifting focus, agreement with a twist, reframing, and siding with the negative (Miller and Rollnick 2002). Van Bilsen (1991) refers to the "Columbo" technique for dealing with resistance. Based on the TV series character, the therapist acts incompetent in a way that leads the patient toward wanting to be helpful to the therapist.

Support Self-Efficacy

The client must come to believe in his own capacity for change. The MI therapist helps the patient identify his assets and strengths by guiding him to call up past victories that might inform his ability to handle new challenges. Troubled adolescents may be so used to critical judgments and negative attention that they have lost hope or perspective. When the adolescent's positive attributes and achievements are noticed, it enhances confidence and capability for determining and pursuing a chosen destiny.

Research Support for MI

The literature describing the use of MI with adolescents is limited but growing. Studies to date have suggested efficacy while also informing the potential benefit of incorporating MI into other standard treatments. MI has primarily been evaluated in studies of brief intervention models for alcohol- and drug-using youth based on MI principles and techniques (Feldstein and Ginsburg 2006). These models are very brief (one to five sessions), and while abstinence is an expressed outcome, reduction in harmful alcohol use and drug using patterns is the primary target. The approach in each of these brief intervention programs is raising patient awareness of the problem while eliciting motivation, by providing personal feedback about the ways in which the behavior might be interfering with expressed personal goals. Further goal setting is then conducted to modify the behavior in an effort to reduce harm while also informing and encouraging future behavior that might enhance progress toward personal goals.

Some sample findings include those from the Cannabis Youth Treatment (CYT) study. This study compared a variety of standardized treatments and found that a five-session motivational therapy combined with cognitive-behavioral therapy had results comparable to those of other, longer-term interventions for the treatment of cannabis abuse (Dennis et al. 2004). This particular intervention is being further evaluated at multiple sites in modified formats through a number of other federal grant projects underway to evaluate and improve on motivationally based interventions targeted to adolescents (www.samhsa.gov). Aubrey (1998) used a one-session motivational interviewing technique incorporated into a feedback and assessment session for adolescents preparing for drug treatment. At 6-month follow-up, the adolescents receiving this one pretreatment session attended more sessions and reported greater reduction in substance use compared to those inducted in the usual way. A comparison of a 1-hour motivational session to an education-as-usual session was studied by McCambridge and Strang (2004) to evaluate efficacy for reducing substance consumption and enhancing perceived risk. In this study, the experimental group demonstrated greater reduction in their use of tobacco, alcohol, and cannabis compared to a control group. Studies have also been conducted by Colby et al. (1998), Monti et al. (1999), Barnett et al. (2001), and Spirito et al. (2004) to evaluate the effectiveness of MI in changing alcohol use behavior in adolescents and young adults treated in emergency settings. While postdischarge behaviors between both conditions were similar, those receiving the MI intervention demonstrated a greater decrease in drinking and driving episodes, alcohol-related injuries, and alcohol-related problems.

In studies of MI with tobacco users, Colby et al. (1998) and Brown et al. (2003) found small effects in helping adolescent users quit. Masterman and Kelly (2003) found that in a sample of 56 randomly assigned high school students, MI showed significant short-term reduction in smoking frequency and quantity compared to a standard educational approach.

MI has also begun to be tested in pediatric settings with older youth. Berg-Smith et al. (1999) used MI with a large sample of 13–17 year olds with high levels of lipoprotein cholesterol. The MI group displayed higher rates of dietary adherence. Channon et al. (2003) showed that glycemic control was improved in a pilot study of 22 diabetic patients ages 14–18 years.

Based on the evidence at hand, it appears that MI approaches do make a difference. However, as these outcomes suggest, there is a need for more studies that might inform possibilities for achieving fuller and longer-term outcomes. At the very least, MI seems to demonstrate its efficacy as an engagement and support strategy. Adolescents in practice settings report high acceptance, and it should certainly be considered in combination with other therapies.

Rationale: Developmental Issues Favoring MI

MI seems to be a particularly good match with adolescents due to normal developmental pulls toward identity formation, independence, acceptance, and connection (Berg-Smith et al. 1999; Channon et al. 2003), as well as the fact that MI is typically brief, focused, and personalized. There are additional advantages in working with children and adolescents:

- **Lack of readiness for change is the norm**—Adolescents are often reluctant to engage with the therapist primarily because someone in authority thinks meeting with the therapist is a good idea. It is even more likely that the adolescent will be defensive if the identified problem behavior is instrumentally serving the adolescent.

- **Avoids labels and promotes acceptance**—Adolescents may rebel when labeled with a diagnosis. Brief interventions that use MI techniques offer feedback about behavior without judgment, labels, or expectations. Patients are presented with facts in plain speaking terms and without the use of jargon or labels.

- **Validates versus discounts the payoffs**—Adolescents have a need to feel heard, understood, and accepted. MI communicates an understanding of the ways in which target behaviors have served the patient's needs and desires.

- **Collaborative versus authoritative**—MI's collaborative and friendly style enhances adolescent comfort and cooperation.

- **Positive reinforcement**—MI promotes a strategy of "catching the adolescent doing something right." Particular attention is given to assessing, acknowledging, and building on patient strengths and progress.

- **Emphasizes autonomy and self-determination**—MI's emphasis on accepting responsibility for personal choices fits well with the adolescent's developmental need for asserting independence.

- **Positive relational connection**—The MI therapist's warm and genuine style fits with an adolescent's emotional need for meaningful, trusting, and valued connection. Adolescent brains are particularly sensitive to the kind of reinforcing limbic activity that can be generated by a positive human connection with the therapist.

- **Works to reduce defensiveness**—MI provides an effective way of "getting in the door" with the more resistant, angry, and negative patients (Project MATCH Research Group 1997).

Practice Challenges to Using MI

The clinician using MI in practice may experience a number of challenges:

- **The adolescent's brain may not cooperate with the adolescent's intention**—Due to the gradual maturation of the prefrontal cortex, there are limitations to the adolescent's capacity for reasoning, decision making, and impulse control (Galvan 2005; Giedd 2004). Adolescents have an enhanced drive toward reward seeking and risk taking (Galvan 2005). The immature prefrontal system cannot be expected to reliably mediate emotional drive and reward-seeking behaviors. Adolescents are naturally at risk for alcohol and drug use, risky sexual activity, and other forms of risk-taking behaviors. High emotional needs for peer acceptance, stimulation, or excitement may lead to increased vulnerability for risk taking, pending full brain maturation. Sole reliance on cognitive-behavioral strategies that instruct on ways to "think through behavior" may not work unless coupled with a strategy for enhancing motivation and resisting temptation by helping the adolescent emotionally connect with the target behavior change.

- **Adolescent insight may be an oxymoron**—The capacity for awareness and insight is more limited in young patients who are not adequately equipped with the cognitive and reasoning abilities for effective decision making. Highly valued behavior is harder to change. Even when risk can be acknowledged, adolescents may view themselves as invincible and therefore immune from harm. For example, a young heroin user was encouraged by the therapist to learn from a friend's fatal overdose and was advised on a plan to avert a similar fate. He responded by saying that he was "smarter" than his friend and therefore invulnerable to any such risk.

- **Discrepancies may not exist**—Attempts to help an adolescent examine discrepancies with risk-taking behavior will backfire if an adolescent concludes that no such discrepancies exist. For example, if an adolescent's substance use is reinforced by an important peer group, or if the assessed positives strongly outweigh the negatives, guiding the adolescent toward change-oriented goals becomes a particular challenge. Ideally, personal feedback and factual information promote discrepancy, but in the absence of any external motivators, adolescents are less likely to consider change.

- **Enablers**—In some instances, certain key individuals in an adolescent's life may interfere with the change process. For some young substance abusers, parents or other individuals in authority approve of or willfully enable substance use. A parent may provide a young substance abuser with alcohol, or a law enforcement officer, judicial officer, or school-based authority may be unwilling to implement consequences.

- **Peer and cultural influence factors**—Peer approval is a powerful motivator for adolescents. When risk-taking behaviors are reinforced by peers, and there is an absence of an alternative peer system in place to support change, persuasion in favor of change will be difficult. Cultural factors may promote risky or unhealthy behaviors. For example, individuals who have succeeded financially by breaking the rules or living a high-risk lifestyle may be viewed by society as role models.

- **Stimulus control**—Attempts at making healthy behavior choices can be greatly compromised in the face of opportunities to engage in risk-taking activities. If the adolescent's environment is inadequately structured to support the change, the adolescent's chances for success will be fewer.

- **Professional responsibility versus patient autonomy**—Clinicians working with children and adolescents walk a tightrope in working to maintain the therapeutic alliance without compromising patient safety. An authority role has to be assumed to some extent and can confuse the patient treated by an MI-oriented therapist. Another important consideration is whether or not harm reduction should even be a goal when working with young patients. Developmental and risk-related complications can occur from even a moderate amount of alcohol use, so is it really okay to help underage drinkers learn to drink moderately? It is also difficult to argue in favor of having just a little bit of unprotected sex or just a few fast driving episodes. A related concern is that the patient may interpret the therapist's willingness to work on a harm reduction plan as the therapist's approval of the behavior.

- **Adolescent problems are complex and usually require more intensive treatment**—MI has been shown to work most effectively as a short-term intervention. It seems to best fit those adolescents who are in the early versus more established stages of risk-taking behavior or those who do not also have a severe psychiatric illness. Adolescents in clinical settings typically present with a myriad of issues and treatment needs. MI cannot serve as a substitute for other services that may be required.

- **It usually takes a village to effectively help an adolescent**—MI is an individually focused model. The treatment of certain adolescent disorders may require a professional team approach and can often involve a number of system agents as well.

- **Different approaches are used by other team members**—The theoretical orientation and roles of team members may vary. In some cases, using an MI approach may cause resentment toward colleagues whose role it is to prescribe treatment and mandate adherence. When an MI therapist collaborates with a team of other providers or with natural change agents such as parents, school counselors, or probation officers, the patient may become less trusting of the therapist.

Guidelines for MI With Adolescents

- **Safety first**—While MI is based on the belief that the patient is responsible for personal choice (Miller and Rollnick 1991), the clinician is obligated to ensure that he follows the privacy and confidentiality laws of the state that governs his practice. The health and safety of the patient trumps treatment fidelity. Parents and patients alike should know the boundaries and limits of professional responsibility and confidentiality. It is particularly important to educate parents as to their ongoing responsibilities respective to their child's risky behavior so that they do not assume the therapist is solely responsible for determining and acting on risk. Risky behaviors must be carefully assessed respective to the child's demonstrated capacities. Even when an adolescent is communicating his intention to refrain from risky behavior, the clinician should still be questioning whether a direct intervention is necessary. When confidentiality needs to be broken, it is best practice for the therapist to in-

form the patient about the assessed need and collaboratively plan for disclosure.

- **Always express care, concern, and collaboration**—It may be helpful if the therapist informs the patient about his allegiance to the MI model with a written contract defining the parameters of this collaborative effort. Untrusting patients may particularly need reassurance that you plan to "play it straight" with them. Describing ways in which you plan to demonstrate how you're on their side can help. Also, addressing how it may be possible that there may be differences between you and the client. Young patients may interpret agreement as the only way of showing you care about them. When offering unwelcome feedback to patients, it should be delivered in a manner consistent with the spirit of MI as seen in the following example.

Case Example

Counselor: "Susan, while I see that you think I am making too much of the situation, one reason I share my concerns with you about having unprotected sex is that I want to ensure that I have done all I can to provide you an opportunity to make informed decisions about your behavior choices. I want to honor my commitment to caring for you in the fullest way possible, even if we disagree about whether you may be creating a difficult situation for yourself."

- **Pay attention to process as much as content**—While patients may verbalize cooperation and behave compliantly, engagement is something that should be continually assessed and not taken for granted. Rapport building and therapeutic joining are essential.

- **Focus on building a positive relationship**—In some cases, relational leverage may be the only means of gaining the trust and credibility to help young patients honestly examine their lives.

Case Example

A 16-year-old male referred for MI was unwilling to take medication recommended by his psychiatrist for his ADHD. After two MI sessions focused on the expressed reasons for the adolescent's concerns about taking the medicine, the adolescent presented at the third session indicating he would now be willing to discuss a plan for taking his medication. He said that this was because the therapist had showed himself to be a stand-up guy by not telling him what he should do. He further shared that he now trusted enough that if the therapist advised him to take the medicine, he would be willing to believe it might help (even though he still didn't want to do it). In this instance, it wasn't words of persuasion that led to his willingness to take a risk but that the therapist was seen as a partner in helping him evaluate this decision.

- **Control what can be controlled**—While the therapist cannot control therapy outcome, behavior of the therapist can be controlled. In MI, process is as important as content.

- **Inform and honor choices**—The therapist is advised to acknowledge up front the power the adolescent has for determining his choices. Emphasizing patient responsibility is a key technique of MI and is demonstrated in the FRAMES technique (Miller and Sanchez 1994). This technique empowers the adolescent by providing feedback and offering choices while reminding the patient that he is responsible for deciding which option is best.

  Case Example

  Counselor: "George, I believe I've done all I can to inform you about the potential risks associated with your continued use of marijuana. From what we have discussed, it seems pretty clear that you will not likely get your driving privileges reinstated by your parents as you would like if you continue smoking. However, this really is your choice to make, and I'll be happy to continue helping you to evaluate whether your choice is ultimately getting you what you want."

- **Stay out of the way of the adolescent hearing his own voice**—In MI, the therapist creates an open and welcoming space for patients to know themselves better. Sharing a diagnostic interpretation or giving unsolicited advice will usually interfere with the MI goal of helping patients arrive on their own accord at the best way for getting what they want.

  Case Example

  Counselor: "While I might have some suggestions about how to best achieve your goal of completing the requirements for your high school diploma, you seem to know yourself pretty well, so I am wondering what you might think about how to get this done."

- **Boosting ambivalence is an outcome**—In working with young substance users, the ultimate goal is abstinence. However, given that these behaviors have alternative reinforcing payoffs, the therapist is advised to focus on enhancing ambivalence by working on strategies for discovering discrepancy. As illustrated in the case example of an adolescent who could not imagine wanting a life without marijuana, using pros and cons appropriate to exploring his behavior was effective when he indicated that a possible benefit to giving up marijuana was that he could pass a drug test for a job he wanted.

- **Stay hopeful**—Working with unwilling adolescents can be exhausting. Given the expected setbacks, the therapist needs to continually maintain perspective to deal effectively with countertransference and to trust in the process. Having regular supervision or collaborating with colleagues can help prevent burnout.

Strategies for MI With Children and Adolescents

- **Be prepared and be a good host**—Adolescents often arrive to an initial appointment angry and defensive (Nuckols et al. 1994). The therapist can be a good host by having a waiting room and office setting conducive to teenagers and young adults.

- **Conduct the initial interview with care**—The adolescent cannot be expected to understand the purpose of therapy or the responsibilities each of you brings to the relationship. A formal role induction may enhance the patient's orientation. This induction might include a review of specific reasons you are aware of as to why the adolescent is there. It is recommended that a detailed discussion of the legal and professional limits of confidentiality as well as an overview of the possible range and scope of services be offered in this initial interview. Specific detail as to what you will do with any information shared by the adolescent, and the conditions under which any such information might be shared with others, is important to the induction process (Powers and Mantano 1996). Describing the MI approach may also serve to increase patient buy-in.

- **Ease your way in the door**—After establishing rapport and inquiring about the adolescent's priorities, discussion of other topics becomes easier. When conducting an assessment, it can be strategic to begin by inquiring about less threatening topics first. For example, it may be helpful to ask questions about personal hobbies or favorite subjects at school before asking questions about alcohol or drug use.

- **Talk about the change process**—Discussing change as a dynamic and shifting process provides a frame for discussions about goal setting and measuring progress. Identifying readiness indicators with the patient can inform the treatment planning process, and interventions can be staged accordingly.

- **Consider the adolescent's worldview and validate, validate, validate**—Ensuring that the adolescent feels heard and understood is essential to successful engagement. Discounting the adolescent's experience, on the other hand, could present real problems. For example, it is certain to affect the therapist's credibility if he responds to an adolescent about the reported experience of how much fun it is to get high with his friends by telling him he just "thinks" he's having fun because he's having an "artificial" experience. The MI therapist must effectively communicate an understanding and acceptance of the patient's expressed reality.

- **When providing personal feedback, stick to facts and inform decisions fully and honestly**—In MI, personal feedback about behavior should be specific and shared objectively and factually. Ideally, permission will be requested of the young client before offering any specific advice related to the feedback. When advice is shared, it should be expressed with authority but without judgment.

- **Carefully look for and acknowledge successes**—MI is grounded in the idea that motivation can be influenced by recognizing the patient's strengths and achievements. The use of affirmations is an important skill to master in doing MI with children and adolescents.

Case Example

Counselor: "Joe, you certainly have shown a willingness to explore the issue of your drinking by acknowledging your parents' concerns. It seems that you really are committed to not having your alcohol use affect your relationship with your parents or complicate your life in other ways."

- **Be a good role model**—I once received feedback from a patient that by arriving late to the appointment and appearing stressed and distracted, I was no longer inspiring him to consider the benefits of furthering his education, as he didn't see any advantage to becoming a professional like me. The power of positive example can be one of the most influential tools we have at our disposal. In trying to motivate patients toward a healthy lifestyle, taking care of our own can be a good place to start.

- **Work fervently to help make change worthwhile**—One of the principal challenges in promoting behavior change with others is that the change may not seem to be worth it. The MI therapist helps patients envision the benefits of change while also helping them benefit from the fruits of their labor.

Case Example

Counselor: "Debbie, as you continue to do your part to work on your goal of getting your driving privileges back, I certainly will do all I can to help your parents see you in a more trusting light if you continue on the path of remaining alcohol and drug free."

- **Ask for and respond to feedback**—Orienting the patient to the MI approach and asking for feedback about the helpfulness of the therapy could prove useful. Taping and reviewing sessions with experienced MI supervisors might help better ensure MI skill mastery.

- **Be creative**—Creating discrepancy with adolescents sometimes calls for creative thinking. As an example, a 15-year-old was invited to bring in his prized guitar to a session so that he could play some songs he had written. A "discrepancy moment" came up when he was unable to recall a song he had recently written while under the influence of marijuana. Discrepancy may prove to be more of an experience than a thought.

- **Avoid the traps**—Client resistance is usually a cue that the therapist's approach may be a problem. There are a number of potential traps that a therapist can fall into that can evoke client resistance. These include asking too many questions, giving advice without permission, focusing prematurely on topics the adolescent would prefer to avoid, and using labels to describe problem behaviors (Miller and Rollnick 1991). Any of these traps will interfere with efforts to establish a meaningful relationship with the young patient. The beginning MI therapist would be well advised to tape sessions and use a self-assessment tool to remain conscious of these traps and improve MI skills.

Research Directions

While there is growing evidence to support the efficacy of MI, particularly as used in brief intervention models developed for high-risk populations, there is an opportunity to improve MI applications to achieve positive longer-term outcomes. There is a need for further study to determine the effectiveness of MI for treatment populations such as younger children with behavioral and disruptive disorders; children and adolescents with acute or chronic health illnesses, including obesity; depressed, anxious, and more severely mentally ill youth; patients with anorexia or bulimia; and youth with conduct disorder, including those adjudicated to the juvenile justice system. Models for integrating MI with other standard treatments such as those developed for the Cannabis Youth Treatment study (Dennis et al. 2004) might improve outcomes for co-occurring as well as stand-alone conditions. Another need is the development of brief intervention approaches for enabling parents of risk-taking teens.

Summary Points

- MI uses a client-centered, collaborative approach based on a therapist style that is warm and friendly. The therapist uses a range of counseling skills such as open-ended questions, affirmations, reflective listening, and summaries.

- MI is guided by principles of empathy, developing discrepancy, rolling with resistance, and supporting self-efficacy, and it is typically structured as a short-term intervention designed to provide personal feedback and explore consistency of behavior choices with personal goals and values.

- MI focuses on enhancing motivation for behavior change by guiding goal setting and eliciting change talk consistent with these goals.

- Motivating change in adolescents is a unique challenge given developmental and practical issues.

- MI provides a set of principles, skills, and techniques that enhance possibilities for facilitating behavior change by reducing resistance and resolving ambivalence.

- MI has been shown to improve client engagement and self-efficacy.

- MI is a particularly good fit with children and adolescents because of its emphasis on collaboration, acceptance, and personal autonomy.

References

Aubrey L: Motivational interviewing with adolescents presenting for outpatient substance abuse treatment. (Doctoral dissertation, University of New Mexico). Dissertation Abstracts International 59:1357, 1998

Barnett NP, Monti PM, Wood MD: Motivational interviewing for alcohol-involved adolescents in the emergency room, in Innovations in Adolescent Substance Abuse Interventions. Edited by Wagner EF, Waldron, HB. Amsterdam, The Netherlands, Pergamon, 2001, pp 143–168

Berg-Smith SM, Stevens VJ, Brown KM, et al: A brief motivational intervention to improve dietary adherence in adolescents. Health Educ Res 14:399–410, 1999

Brown RA, Ramsey SE, Strong DR, et al: Effects of motivational interviewing on smoking cessation in adolescents with psychiatric disorders. Tob Control 12(suppl):3–10, 2003

Channon S, Smith VJ, Gregory JW: A pilot study of motivational interviewing in adolescents with diabetes. Arch Dis Child 88:680–683, 2003

Colby SM, Monti PM, Barnett NP, et al: Brief motivational interviewing in a hospital setting for adolescent smoking: a preliminary study. J Consult Clin Psychol 66:574–578, 1998

Dennis M, Godley SH, Diamond G, et al: The Cannabis Youth Treatment (CYT) Study: main findings from two randomized trials. J Subst Abuse Treat 27:197–213, 2004

Feldstein SW, Ginsburg JID: Motivational interviewing with dually diagnosed adolescents in juvenile justice settings. Brief Treat Crisis Interv 6:218–233, 2006

Galvan A: Earlier development of the accumbens relative to orbitofrontal cortex might underlie risk-taking behavior in adolescents. J Neurosci 26:6885–6892, 2005

Giedd JN: Structural magnetic resonance imaging of the adolescent brain. Ann NY Acad Sci 1021:77–85, 2004

Gordon T: Parent Effectiveness Training. New York, Wyden, 1970

Masterman PW, Kelly AB: Reaching adolescents who drink harmfully: fitting intervention to developmental reality. J Subst Abuse Treat 24:347–355, 2003

McCambridge J, Strang J: The efficacy of single-session motivational interviewing in reducing drug consumption and perceptions of drug-related risk and harm among young people: results from a multisite cluster randomized trial. Addiction 99:39–52, 2004

Miller WR, Rollnick S: Motivational Interviewing: Preparing People to Change Addictive Behavior. New York, Guilford, 1991

Miller WR, Rollnick S: Motivational Interviewing: Preparing People for Change, 2nd Edition. New York, Guilford, 2002

Miller WR, Sanchez VC: Motivating young adults for treatment and lifestyle change, in Alcohol Use and Misuse by Young Adults. Edited by Howard G, Nathan PE. Notre Dame, IN, University of Notre Dame Press, 1994, pp 55–81

Monti PM, Colby SM, Barnett NP, et al: Brief intervention for harm reduction with alcohol-positive adolescents treated in a hospital emergency department. J Consult Clin Psychol 67:989–994, 1999

Nuckols CC, Porcher AG, Toft D: Helping Chronically Addicted Adolescents: Problems, Perspectives and Strategies for Recovery. Bradenton, FL, Human Services Institute, 1994

Powers R, Mantano R: Substance use and abuse, in Treating Adolescents. Edited by Yalom I. San Francisco, CA, Jossey-Bass, 1996, pp 77–152

Prochaska JO, DiClemente, CC: Transtheoretical Therapy: Toward a more integrative model of change. Psychotherapy: Theory, Research, and Practice 19:276–288, 1982

Project MATCH Research Group: Matching alcoholism treatments to client heterogeneity: Project MATCH posttreatment drinking outcomes. J Stud Alcohol 58:7–29, 1997

Rogers CR: The necessary and sufficient conditions of therapeutic personality change. J Consult Psychol 21:95–103, 1957

Spirito A, Monti PM, Barnett NP, et al: A randomized clinical trial of a brief motivational intervention for alcohol-positive adolescents treated in an emergency department. J Pediatr 145:396–402, 2004

Truax CB, Carkaff RR: Toward Effective Counseling and Psychotherapy. Chicago, IL, Aldine, 1967

Van Bilsen PJGH: Motivational interviewing: perspectives from the Netherlands, with particular emphasis on heroin-dependent clients, in Motivational Interviewing: Preparing People to Change Addictive Behavior. Edited by Miller WR, Rollnick S. New York, Guilford, 1991, pp 214–224

Chapter 61

Systems of Care, Wraparound Services, and Home-Based Services

Yann Poncin, M.D.
Joseph Woolston, M.D.

Systems of care (SOCs) and wraparound services represent philosophies of care rather than programs with clearly specified elements of treatment. An SOC recognizes the importance of family, school, and the community at large in a child's overall health. The informal and formal supports and services available in a given community and their linkage comprise the SOC, and coordinating access to services within the larger community is an integral part of an SOC. Wraparound services are one approach to working with families using an SOC philosophy. Wraparound "wraps" services in the community around a child and family, according to the individualized needs of the family. Wraparound

has a specifically defined clinical and theoretical orientation and is concerned with the process of how a child and family are engaged to create a service plan that accesses or creates the relevant services available in the community. Core features of wraparound and SOCs include engagement with the family from a strength-based and culturally competent perspective and respecting the family's own perception of their needs and goals, along with helping them to obtain services to meet those goals (Walker and Bruns 2006). The wraparound process became the favored approach to implementing the SOC philosophy when SOC programs first emerged; therefore, the two terms are closely linked.

Historical Roots: Emergence of SOCs and Wraparound Services

An early progenitor of SOCs is the child guidance movement, which emerged at the turn of the nineteenth century and led a shift from a punishment model to a corrective model ("guiding" children) that emphasized advocacy in multiple life domains (Jones 1999). Congress passed the Mental Retardation Facilities and Community Mental Health Center (CMHC) Construction Act in 1963 in order to create a national network of community mental health centers. Because the act did not specifically address children, only half of the centers had children's services. The indirect costs of child services, such as consultation with schools, were poorly reimbursed, if at all. Once the planned transition of the responsibility for managing CMHCs moved to the states, few states had a child mental health system or expertise (Lourie 2003).

Unclaimed Children (Knitzer 1982), which described the inadequacies of the national response to children with serious emotional disturbances and their families, served as a rallying point for advocates. This concern, coupled with philosophical and financial concerns about the overutilization of institutionalized care, ultimately facilitated congressional funding of the Child and Adolescent Service System Program (CASSP) in 1984 and later the Comprehensive Community Mental Health Services for Children and Their Families Program. These new programs, along with state and foundation funding, led to the development of community-based services for youth with significant emotional disturbances.

At the time CASSP was funded, children who had the most significant difficulties were also those least likely to get the range of services they might need. Mental health, education, child welfare, and juvenile justice each had elements of mental health services, or had children with mental health needs within their purview, but were largely disconnected from one an-

other (Lourie 2003). CMHCs had the ability to manage children with mild to moderate problems, but services were inadequate for more disturbed children with multiple needs. For families to access child welfare's financial resources for services, they often had to forego their parental rights. A goal of CASSP was to enable children with special needs to access services without resorting to the juvenile justice or child protective service systems (Lourie 2003). Improved communication and collaboration among agencies was another goal. The guiding principle of the CASSP was the SOC, a multiagency approach to the delivery of services. The three core values of an SOC are the child and family's needs, community-based services with decision making remaining at the community level, and care that is culturally competent and responsive to the family's cultural, racial, and ethnic characteristics (Stroul 2003). CASSP included expectations of interagency efforts to meet children's needs, using state-level discussions among existing disconnected agencies. Another goal of CASSP was to develop and strengthen mental health resources for children, given that half of states had no budget dedicated to children's mental health. With the focus on empowering families in forging individualized care plans, wraparound services and intensive home-based services also became common features of an SOC approach (Burns et al. 2000). Tables 61–1 and 61–2 highlight the key features of an SOC.

SOCs and community-based services developed as the result of the interaction of social, legal, cultural, therapeutic, political, and economic changes. In providing wraparound care, a team is organized around a child and family, and interventions are determined collaboratively to access and link a range of community services and agencies. Advocacy for both children and families is essential. The term *wraparound* was reportedly first used by Lenore Behar in North Carolina in the early 1980s (VanDenBerg 1999), following a lawsuit that resulted in the state's requirement to provide less restrictive services in the community (Behar 2003). The Individuals with Disabilities Education Act (IDEA), for example, which was passed in 1975, reinforced ideas of inclusion and "least restriction" (see Chapter 63, "School-Based

TABLE 61–1. System of care: core values

Core values	Core values in action
Child and family centered	The family determines the mix of services.
Community based	Management and decision making are at the community level.
Culturally competent	Agencies and individuals are responsive to cultural and ethnic differences.

Source. Adapted from Stroul 2003.

TABLE 61–2. System of care: guiding principles

Children with emotional disturbances should receive services that address their emotional, social, educational, and physical needs.

Services should be individualized for the child and family.

Services should be developmentally appropriate and least restrictive.

Caregivers should be fully integrated into the planning and treatment process.

Services should be integrated and linked to one another.

Case management should be provided to coordinate care as needed.

Early identification and intervention should be promoted to ameliorate outcomes.

A smooth transition to adult services should be ensured.

The rights of children with emotional disturbances should be protected and efforts at advocacy promoted.

All children with emotional disturbances should receive services regardless of race, sex, physical disability, religion, or other characteristics.

Source. Adapted from Stroul 2003.

Interventions"). The Supreme Court's Olmstead decision (*Olmstead v. L.C.* 1999) found that the institutionalization of individuals with disabilities could be a form of discrimination that is prohibited by the Americans with Disabilities Act (ADA). Another factor increasing interest in community-based care is cost. Although it has proved difficult to compare long-term outcomes or collateral or consequential costs, monies required for institutionally based care (hospital or residential treatment) are much greater than those required for community-based care (Brown and Hill 1996).

Wraparound Services

Wraparound services are helpful when children and families have significant emotional and behavioral difficulties and have experienced treatment failures. Children and their families who are served by wraparound may be involved in foster care, child protective services, juvenile justice, residential treatment facilities, and special education, among other agencies. Approximately 200,000 children in the United States are served by wraparound services (Faw 1999).

A consensus group of experts in 1998 came to define the key elements of wraparound services (Table 61–3). As can be seen in Table 61–3, many aspects of wraparound involve developing a particular perspective and attitude, rather than specifying well-defined components of care. Three key characteristics of wraparound are 1) strength-based orientation, 2) the value placed on cultural competence, and 3) integration of the family as an active participant in building a treatment plan. Traditional mental health treatment uses a deficit model,

where a problem is identified and ameliorating the problem becomes the focus of treatment. A strength-based approach, one that uncovers positive coping mechanisms and resiliency factors, can be especially helpful in engaging with and helping families who come to receive wraparound or SOC services, as these families have significant needs and are often accustomed to working with multiple (poorly coordinated) agencies and services from the perspective of failure.

Wraparound Services in Practice

Examples of well-known early wraparound services and those programs serving specific populations are listed in Table 61–4. The characteristics of wraparound programming and SOCs depend on local ecologies and other factors. Some of the key elements for the process used by wraparound services are described in Table 61–5. Examples of informal and formal community supports are in Table 61–6. Implementing a wraparound approach presents challenges. Development of cultural competence requires team or individualized training and ongoing supervision. Enhancement of coordination among agencies and services requires systems change at the policy and leadership levels that must filter down to (or up from) the individual workers in the agencies and systems to be linked.

Wraparound Services and Research Considerations

Although outcome research has been limited, a number of studies have examined qualitative and quantitative outcomes and have shown positive results. Lack

TABLE 61–3. Key elements to a wraparound process

The youth and family must be full and active partners at every level and in every activity of the wraparound process. They must have a voice.

The wraparound approach must be a team-driven process involving the family, child, natural supports, agencies, and community services working together to develop, implement, and evaluate the individualized plan.

Wraparound services must be located in the community, with all efforts toward serving the identified youth in community, residential, and school settings.

The process must be culturally competent, building on the unique values, preferences, and strengths of children and families and their communities.

Services and supports must be individualized and built on strengths, and must meet the needs of children and families across life domains to promote success, safety, and permanence in home, school, and community.

Wraparound plans must include a balance of formal services and informal community and family supports.

There must be an unconditional commitment to serve children and their families.

Plans of care should be developed and implemented based on an interagency, community-based collaborative process.

Wraparound child and family teams must have flexible approaches and adequate and flexible funding.

Outcomes must be determined and measured for the system, for the program, and for the individual child and family.

Source. Adapted from Burns and Goldman 1999.

of clarity in how adherent these studies were to the core elements of wraparound services and what exact approaches were used makes conclusive interpretations difficult. From a research perspective, there are several challenges. Wraparound services are highly individualized, applied to a variety of populations, and generally reserved for families who present with a complex range of function and psychosocial distress. Moreover, those elements that make up the so-called core elements of wraparound services remain somewhat unsettled. The key elements of wraparound services as determined by experts set the foundation on which measures of model fidelity were developed. Epstein et al. (1998) developed the Wraparound Observation Form (WOF) and Bruns et al. (2004) developed the Wraparound Fidelity Index (WFI).

Evidence Base in SOCs and Wraparound Services

Randomized controlled studies by Clark et al. (1996, 1998) and Evans et al. (1996, 1998) have found benefits to wraparound services. Other less methodologically rigorous studies also support the wraparound approach (Eber et al. 1996; Hyde et al. 1996; Pullmann et al. 2006; Yoe et al. 1996).

Evidence for wraparound services also points in a negative direction (Bickman et al. 2003; Carney and

Buttell 2003; Toffalo 2000). The Fort Bragg Study (Bickman et al. 2003) found that subjects receiving wraparound services did not differ in a number of domains compared with those receiving treatment as usual. The treatment as usual in this sample, however, was more intensive than that available in many communities. Even with adequate methodological rigor, studies involving wraparound can be difficult to generalize to other populations and localities.

Home-Based Services

Home-based services are often an integral part of a system of care. Because of the resources, staffing, funding, and intensity of treatment required, home-based services are typically reserved for families who have children at risk of being placed out of home, whether in a hospital, residential, correctional facility, foster care, or other location. The Adoption Assistance and Child Welfare Act of 1980 was passed with the intent to strengthen permanency planning for children. States were required to make reasonable efforts to prevent removal of youth from their family, to return them to their family, or to make permanency planning occur within a reasonable amount of time if attempts to remain with the family are unsuccessful. In 1993, Congress passed legislation establishing Title IV, Part

TABLE 61–4. Examples of wraparound services and systems of care (SOCs)

Program	Location	Features
Alaska Youth Initiative (AYI)	Alaska	Early wraparound system. Alaska was a CASSP-designated state and had received funds from NIMH to implement SOCs for children. Based on Kaleidoscope programs in Chicago. Kaleidoscope had the principle of unconditional care and individualized services in the community. AYI initially served out-of-state returnees from residential treatment centers.
Washington Youth Initiative	Washington	Replication of AYI. For out-of-state children and in-state children in long-term residential treatment centers.
Project Wraparound	Vermont	Replication of AYI. For children at risk of out-of-home placement.
Project Milwaukee	Milwaukee	Example of Medicaid managed care behavioral carve-out. For children under court order in juvenile justice or child protective services.
La Grange, IL, school district	Illinois	Example of school-based wraparound program with goal of having child in less restrictive school settings by improving collaboration between schools and families.
Program UPLIFT (Uniting Partners to Link and Invest in Families Today)	Santa Clara County, California	Example of wraparound provided through private agency. Serves children in lieu of residential placement.
Fostering Individualized Assistance Program	Florida	Designed to improve permanency outcomes of children placed in foster care.

Note. CASSP=Child and Adolescent Service System Program; NIMH=National Institute of Mental Health.
Source. Adapted from Goldman and Faw 1999; VanDenBerg 1999.

B-2, of the Social Security Act, creating funding for family preservation and family support programs.

The first program with which the term *family preservation* became associated was the Homebuilders program in Tacoma, Washington, developed in 1974 to prevent foster care placement. Homebuilders worked with the entire family using a treatment approach based on crisis intervention theory (Kinney and Dittmar 1995). Nowadays, intensive home-based family preservation refers to a wide array of treatment services and interventions with significantly different treatment models and implementation strategies. They differ from traditional treatment approaches in a number of ways. Services are provided in the home and community, at a time of day that more flexibly meets the family's schedule. Treatment is often time-limited, usually lasting 1–6 months, although longer periods are common. Caseloads for therapists are small (two to eight families). Therapists have frequent in-home or in-community contact with families, and care providers or their proxies are available to families on a 24-hour basis to respond to crises and treatment needs.

Home-Based Services and Mental Health

Home-based services generally serve children who are involved with child welfare, juvenile justice, and/or mental health. The specific home-based service provided and its focus will depend on the primary problem and the population served. The examples of home-based services below are those that have been used to help children with mental health needs that are well known and systematically evaluated and/or widely disseminated.

Massachusetts Mental Health Services Program for Youth

Although the Mental Health Services Program for Youth (MHSPY) is limited to Massachusetts (Grimes and Mullin 2006), it is an example of services delivered with an SOC and wraparound philosophy and in

TABLE 61–5. Implementation of a wraparound approach

What	Who	Role

Community team (informal and formal stakeholders)	Leaders of
	    Agencies, public and private
	    Schools
	    Parent groups
	    Advocacy groups
	    Business
	    Higher education
	    Clergy
		Provide services or support to the family according to the care plan.

Identification and referral	"Subcommittee" of a community team	To determine which families will receive services, often decided by consensus vote. Test scores have been used.
Referral sources	Will vary by wraparound system May include a large referral pool or only those children who are in state custody or at risk of out-of-home placement	Work collaboratively with wraparound teams and help identify children suited for the wraparound process.
Resource coordinator (or case manager or individualized service coordinator)	An agency brokers the services and is responsible for hiring resource coordinators who have bachelor's level or higher education The agency oversees the wraparound process and manages flexible funds	Identify key individuals in child and family's life. Perform strength-based assessment. Conduct child and family team meetings. Help family team create individualized service plan. Evaluate helpfulness of current services. Develop crisis plan. Arrange services not currently being used or available. Manage flexible funds. Provide direct services. Evaluate progress. Arrange for transition.
The family	Parent and child	Parent and child must be actively engaged and listened to, and once a plan is co-constructed with them, the parent and child agree to the plan and commit to it.
Strengths discovery	Resource coordinator with family	Informal or formal assessment of strengths to determine which services will be tailored.
Child and family team	Child, family, extended family, friends, professionals, neighbors (usually consisting of 4–10 members)	No more than half the team should be professionals to encourage family ownership of the process.
Team meetings	Child and family team	Review strengths and develop individualized service plan.

TABLE 61–5. Implementation of a wraparound approach *(continued)*

What	Who	Role
Review of major life domains	Child and family team Child may or may not be present, depending on developmental and emotional considerations	Examination of the following areas: Living arrangements Family—structure, needs, function Social Emotional and psychological Educational Legal Financial Spiritual Medical Cultural Safety
Creating a service plan	Resource coordinator with child and family team	Life domains are prioritized according to the most need. These are often voted on, and the family has ultimate say in deciding what these are. Brainstorming of ideas to meet the needs. Ideal plan focuses on informal supports as these are longer lasting than formal supports, which will end. Detailed crisis plan with action steps for each team member is established.
Review of plan	Community team	Review plan for consistency with individual and community values and consider safety issues. Review budget to determine how needs can be met. If team disagrees with plan, the plan is not stopped, but it is sent back for revision to the child and family team.
Implementation of plan	Coordinator and child and family team	Coordinator implements the plan and meets with the child and family team every few weeks initially and then at least every quarter thereafter. Major changes are undertaken only with the input of the child and family team.
Outcomes	Resource coordinator and others	Normally, quantitative measures of behavioral change, reduction in drug use, school attendance, and out-of-home placement are used along with qualitative feedback from families.

Source.   Adapted from VanDenBerg and Grealish 1996.

TABLE 61–6. Potential sources of community support

Home life: Family, friends, family friends, grandparents, extended family, foster care agency, independent living center, group home, respite care

School: Teacher, special education teacher, paraprofessional aide, guidance counselor, school social worker, school psychologist, principal, peer groups, parent-teacher organization and other parent groups, sports activities, school programs and groups, student mentors, student tutors, alternative education, therapeutic day schools, general equivalency diploma programs

After-school programs: Community centers, recreation centers, sports leagues, any organized leisure activities

Mental health and allied services: Social worker, psychologist, psychiatrist, nurse, art therapist, recreation therapist, therapeutic mentor, social skills training, individual therapy, group therapy, family therapy, in-home services, intensive outpatient services, partial hospital, speech and language therapist, occupational therapist

Legal: Probation officer, attorney, guardian ad-litem, case manager

Employment: Vocational and job training agencies, job internships, employment

Spiritual: Church, mosque, pastors, ministers, imams, meditation, members of the congregation

Complementary: Complementary alternative medicine and other approaches

Economic: Flexible funding support

which clinical data are tracked. The MHSPY is a collaboration among various agencies, including child welfare, medical assistance, mental health, education, and juvenile justice. Eligible children are Medicaid enrolled, have a serious emotional disturbance, have significantly impaired function, are at risk of out-of-home placement, and are eligible for services from one of the participating state agencies. A parent or guardian consents to services. When a family is deemed eligible for services, a family coordinator, who is a nonprofessional, is assigned to make a home visit with the purpose of addressing any family concerns about the process. Once the family chooses to proceed, the referral is brought to a community-based team, which is made up of various agency and relevant school district representatives, to prioritize referrals. Any child who meets eligibility criteria can be enrolled, and no child is discharged except for completion of services. Funds from multiple agencies are blended together to purchase individualized services—from the least to most restrictive—according to the child and family's need. After enrollment, a care manager is assigned. The care manager is a mental health clinician with training in family therapy and team communication. The care manager is not the child or family's primary therapist. The care manager is responsible for direct clinical intervention, which includes home-based work to identify the family's needs, coordination of care among formal and informal supports, and case administration, such as payment authorization or creation of new services. The care manager views the family from a

strength-based perspective and assesses the family's major life domains (see Table 61–5 and VanDenBerg and Grealish 1996). The care manager helps to identify individuals who will become part of the care planning team, which meets monthly to help create and implement an individualized service plan. Members of the team may include informal and formal supports, such as friends, relatives, teachers, state agency representatives, pediatricians, and other clinicians. Care managers receive supervision weekly through individual, group, and peer support along with 24-hour backup supervision. The clinical associate director and medical director of the MHSPY facilitate supervision. The MHSPY collects clinical data on enrolled children at baseline and every 6 months. Data collected over 4 years suggest that enrollees have improved clinical functioning and a reduction in risk to themselves and others (Grimes and Mullin 2006).

Multisystemic Therapy

Multisystemic therapy (MST) is a home-based, family-focused program, meant to treat youth who have serious behavioral problems. It was developed and refined serving the juvenile justice population and has been available for more than two decades. An adapted model has been applied to populations with primarily mental health needs (Multisystemic Therapy Services 2007).

MST uses an ecological model as a guiding principle that places a child in the inner circle of expanding concentric circles that include child, family, peers, school, neighborhood, community, and culture. MST teams consist of two to four therapists. A therapist works with two to four families at a time. A supervisor conducts weekly clinical team supervision and individual supervision for cases in crisis. The duration of treatment ranges from 3 to 5 months. Discharge criteria are outcome based and must show that there has been an improvement in the problem behavior. MST has a rigorous quality assurance program, and for agencies to provide MST services, they must adhere to this program (Multisystemic Therapy Services 2007).

MST has a robust evidence base from randomized clinical trials for use with juvenile offenders and substance-abusing youth at risk for out-of-home placement. The evidence for populations with psychiatric problems as a primary concern is less established. In one large controlled trial, MST was associated with a reduced number of days of inpatient psychiatric hospitalization, improvement in externalizing symptoms, improved family relationships, and increased school attendance (Schoenwald et al. 2000). However, longer-term follow-up revealed few differences over time compared with the control group (Henggeler et al. 2003). Another controlled study, comparing MST to existing continuum of care services (the latter ranging from outpatient to home-based to out-of-home placement), showed a short-term decrease in out-of-home placements and externalizing symptoms (Rowland et al. 2005).

Intensive In-Home Child and Adolescent Psychiatric Service

The Intensive In-Home Child and Adolescent Psychiatric Service (IICAPS; Woolston et al. 2007), developed at Yale in 1997, is a home-based intervention for children and adolescents with serious emotional and behavioral problems. Most of the youth served are at risk of requiring institutional care or have exhausted traditional outpatient services. The in-home, or family, component of IICAPS represents the view that the family is essential to and has the power to make and sustain change in a child's life. Families agree to participate voluntarily in treatment, be partners in the work, and colead treatment planning. Families are more likely to feel comfortable and empowered if services are provided in their own home. This also circumvents obstacles for families who have difficulty attending clinic-based care. In the home, the IICAPS team can see firsthand the multiple social and interac-

tion factors—both strengths and vulnerabilities—that influence the vicious cycle of significant emotional disturbance for the child and family. Teams can provide direct psychiatric evaluation and treatment, parenting skills training, family management skills training, problem-solving skills training, 24/7 mobile crisis emergency services, and intensive case management.

IICAPS teams consist of a senior clinician with a master's level degree, usually in social work, and a mental health counselor with a bachelor's degree. All individual clinicians receive 15 hours of initial training. A more senior mental health clinician supervises the teams weekly. A child and adolescent psychiatrist serves as the medical director and coleads interdisciplinary treatment rounds. Clinicians each treat 6–8 families for 4–6 months or longer, depending on need. The team is available 24/7 for mobile crisis interventions. Programmatically, IICAPS has a nested structure: 6–8 cases to a team, 4 teams to a rounds group, 1–4 rounds groups to a program, 15 programs to a network. IICAPS has expanded from Yale to 14 sites in Connecticut. The model is manualized, and adherence to the model at the team level is ascertained by clinician fidelity to the IICAPS tools and structures of treatment. At the program level, each site must demonstrate the use of specified tools for engagement, assessment, treatment, and quality assurance. IICAPS uses a Web-based system to collect data, with the goal of determining the effectiveness of IICAPS in both improving function and reducing out-of-home placement. IICAPS has yet to be evaluated empirically. A controlled trial is currently under way that randomly assigns children and families referred to IICAPS to one of two arms: treatment in the community as usual, supplemented with the assistance of a case manager to broker services, or IICAPS services.

As detailed in the case vignette below, IICAPS is an in-home service and reflects a system of care philosophy. IICAPS provides direct treatment and not coordination of care per se. Additional therapeutic and community supports are determined according to the child's and family's needs and are enlisted in the service of treatment.

Case Vignette: Stages of IICAPS Treatment

Julia is a 12-year-old girl referred to IICAPS after her second psychiatric hospital admission. She lives with her maternal grandmother, her grandmother's fiancé, a 21-year-old half sister, and a 2-year-old niece. Child protective services had placed Julia in her grandmother's care at age 4 for reasons of neglect. Julia entered outpatient treatment at age 6 after an aggressive outburst at school resulted in Julia being sent to the emergency room. Over the years, Julia has had general outpatient services, parent management training, intensive outpatient services, partial hospital treatment, medication management, and inpatient psychiatric hospitalization. She has carried a number of diagnoses, including bipolar disorder, intermittent explosive disorder, attention-deficit/hyperactivity disorder, mood disorder not otherwise specified, posttraumatic stress disorder, psychotic disorder not otherwise specified, and borderline intellectual functioning. Although she has been suspended from school a number of times, she has not been identified for special education. Her institutional care to date has helped with acute behaviors and maintaining safety, but it has not addressed the domains in Julia's social ecology that promote the symptoms that lead to her hospitalization. In some areas, hospitalization has even worsened Julia's function by exacerbating symptoms of trauma and abandonment.

After a referral from the hospital to IICAPS was accepted, the senior clinician (master's degree in social work) and the mental health counselor (bachelor of arts) set up an appointment within the week and reviewed the tools and processes they would use to engage the family and co-construct a treatment plan for the *assessment and engagement phase* of treatment. The tools and objectives of this phase include developing the immediate action plan; defining and rating the initial main problem; creating a genogram; cataloging strengths and vulnerabilities in four domains; and creating the eco-domain map.

At the first meeting, the family and team developed an *immediate action plan*, which included safety planning—that is, identifying what behaviors were considered an emergency for Julia and how the family would access help in a crisis. At the first visit, the team also learned that the electricity had been turned off and that the grandmother's fiancé, the main breadwinner, had relapsed into substance use and was working only sporadically. The team and family decided that the mental health counselor would meet with Julia individually while the senior clinician would meet with Julia's grandmother and the fiancé. All would meet together for family work, which would include the sister. The team and family arranged a schedule for three home visits per week. The team first helped the family get the electricity turned on (for reasons of medical necessity) and establish a payment plan with the company. The grandmother, however, remained guarded with the team and often confused their role with the role of child protective services, with which the family was involved. On several occasions, at the appointed visit times, no one answered the door. Three weeks into treatment, Julia was rehospitalized after an aggressive outburst toward her 21-year-old half sister, whom she threatened to kill. The team attended team rounds on the inpatient unit, met with Julia, and continued to meet with her grandmother at home. After Julia's discharge, the team renewed their home visits as scheduled. After continuous and ongoing efforts at engagement with the family, the grandmother

warmed up to the team, appreciating their demonstration of commitment and support.

With Julia home, the family and team began to co-construct the treatment plan. *Co-construction* is a key philosophical element of IICAPS. The family takes the lead in establishing main problems and goals, and the IICAPS team, through their increasing familiarity with the family's psychosocial function, contributes as well. The team helped the family discuss and discover their *strengths and vulnerabilities in each of four domains*—child, family, school, and physical environment—and to review the impact of these on the main problem. The IICAPS model defines the *main problem* as the behavior that leads to a higher level of care, such as hospitalization. The strengths and vulnerabilities in each domain were mapped out on paper as an *eco-domain map*. This is a graphical representation of the multiple connections between the main problem and the strengths and vulnerabilities in each domain. The team and family then cocreated goals and action steps in each of the four domains to address the main problem. Goals and action steps were limited to one or two per domain and were phrased in the family's own words. Often families list too many goals and action steps, which dilutes efforts to address the very serious behaviors related to the main problem.

Julia's main problem was that "she gets angry and hits people." One child domain goal was that "Julia will not hit others," with one of the action steps being "Julia will go to her room when she is becoming upset." In the family domain, one goal was that "family members will respect each other and not yell." The action step included, "Grandmother will spend nice, alone time with Julia." For the school domain, the goal was "Julia will attend school." The action steps included, "Team and family will meet with school to get more information about Julia's function and abilities at school." In the physical environment domain, which highlights therapeutic and natural supports in the community, the family identified their minister as helpful and concerned. He, along with other church members, was enlisted as support. The team and grandmother also thought that Julia would benefit from a therapeutic mentor, someone who could provide individual support to Julia while taking her out into the community. The grandmother also mentioned needing help with day-to-day household chores; the team agreed to help the grandmother look into free daycare services for the 2-year-old through another community organization. The team and family also decided that a meeting bringing together all the services involved in the family's life—child protective services, outpatient treatment team, and school, among others—would be helpful. The team wrote the treatment plan, and all members—the family, Julia, clinical team, team supervisor, and medical director—reviewed and signed the plan.

During treatment, the team met weekly with their supervisor and presented Julia's case in multidisciplinary team rounds every 4 weeks. In rounds, the team, supervisors, and the child psychiatrist contributed to the biopsychosocial formulation and the team's conceptualization of the case.

The next phase after assessment and engagement, which may take weeks or months, is the *work and action phase,* in which the main problem and goals are established, as described above, and a treatment plan is signed. These are regularly reevaluated and rated by the family and team. The focus remains on developing problem-solving skills, parent management skills, and family management skills as they relate to the main problem. The purpose is to help the child stay out of institutional care, to function better in all aspects of the social ecology, and to improve the developmental trajectory.

The last phase of treatment is the *ending and wrap-up phase,* in which the course of treatment and goals are re-reviewed and therapeutic and community supports are consolidated prior to discharge.

Functional Family Therapy

Functional family therapy (FFT) uses principles of systems theory and behavior modification to improve the interactions, communication, and problem solving within a family. FFT has existed for close to 40 years and targets youth between 11 and 18 years of age. It focuses on youth with disruptive behaviors, conduct disorder, and substance use, who may have a number of additional psychiatric diagnoses. It is often used in juvenile justice populations and as an alternative to out-of-home placement or incarceration (Alexander et al. 2002; Sexton and Alexander 2000). FFT is provided in 8–12 sessions over 3 months, including up to 30 direct service hours. FFT therapists have a master's degree in a human services field. FFT also examines the multiple systems involved in a child and family's life. FFT first discovers the family's strengths and then helps empower the family to be self-sufficient as they interact with or access multiple systems in the community (Alexander et al. 2002; Sexton and Alexander 2000).

Brief Strategic Family Therapy

Brief strategic family therapy (BSFT) is a 12- to 15-session problem-focused intervention delivered over 3 months. Its target population is school-age children and adolescents who have behavioral problems. Generally, it has been delivered in the office but has also been used as an in-home service. BSFT focuses on the family system and the patterns of interaction that influence each member. The therapist's goal is to help identify which family interactions lead to the child's

problem behaviors. BSFT is manualized and has been empirically validated for the treatment of substance abuse and conduct problems and has also been modified to serve the cultural needs of Hispanic youth (Szapocznik et al. 2002).

Multidimensional Treatment Foster Care

Multidimensional treatment foster care (MTFC) is a program designed for youth who require out-of-home care. Children are placed in a foster family setting for 6–9 months. The MTFC team consists of a program supervisor, a family therapist, an individual therapist, a child skills trainer, and a daily telephone contact person. The foster parents undergo training and become part of the team. They attend a weekly meeting and provide a daily phone report, Monday through Friday. Foster parents have access to staff 24/7. The MTFC team meets weekly to review the child's progress, including the daily reports, and to adjust the treatment plan as indicated. The birth parents receive parent training and family therapy in preparation for their child's return home. The skills they learn resemble the approach to the child in the foster home. The goal of treatment is to have the child return home. MTFC has been shown to reduce out-of-home placements and juvenile delinquency (Chamberlain et al. 2007a, 2007b).

Nurse-Family Partnership

The nurse-family service is delivered in the home as both treatment for the parent and prevention for the child. In this program, nurses visit low-income, first-time mothers weekly or biweekly from the prenatal period until the child reaches the age of 2 years. Nurses focus on the mother's health and the environment, and they educate mothers about developmental expectations and caregiving issues. Family members are engaged and access to services in the community is facilitated as needed. Senior nurses supervise the home visitors, each of whom carries a caseload of approximately 25. A 15-year follow-up study demonstrated a reduction in maternal behavior problems, maternal arrests, running away by children, arrests of children, and alcohol use by children. A reduction of child abuse and neglect also occurred, but the reduction was limited if high rates of domestic violence were present (Olds 2007).

Summary Points

- The SOC philosophy recognizes the importance of family, school, and the community at large in a child's overall health and functioning.

- An important goal of SOCs is for the various agencies and treatment providers involved in a child's life to be linked to one another.

- Wraparound is a community-based service that implements an SOC philosophy. Wraparound services help provide and obtain services in the community by working with and advocating for a child and family.

- The wraparound process includes a focus on the child's and family's strengths, cultural competence, and co-construction with the family of a treatment plan. A case manager is assigned to and works with the family to help negotiate community services.

- Wraparound services have been used with youth in foster care, juvenile justice, schools, and mental health settings. Wraparound services are often used to work with families who have children at risk for out-of-home placement.

- Home-based services are delivered in the community to the family and usually include 24/7 team availability, small caseload, and intense short-term treatment of 6 weeks' to 9 months' duration.

- Multisystemic therapy is a well-known home-based service that has robust evidence of efficacy for youth who are in juvenile justice or who use substances, and to a lesser degree, youth who have mental illness.

- Mental health services programs for youth, intensive in-home child and adolescent psychiatry service, brief strategic family therapy, functional family therapy, multidimensional treatment foster care, and nurse-family partnerships are programs that are, or have elements of, home-based services and that are promising for the treatment or prevention of mental illness.

References

Adoption Assistance and Child Welfare Act of 1980 (Pub. L. No. 96-272)

Alexander J, Barton C, Gordon D, et al: Book Three: Functional Family Therapy. Boulder, Center for the Study and Prevention of Violence, Institute of Behavioral Science, University of Colorado, 2002

Behar LB: Using litigation to improve child mental health services: promises and pitfalls. Adm Policy Ment Health 30:199–218, 2003

Bickman L, Smith CM, Lambert EW, et al: Evaluation of a congressionally mandated wraparound demonstration. J Child Fam Stud 12:135–156, 2003

Brown RA, Hill BA: Opportunity for change: exploring an alternative to residential treatment. Child Welfare Journal 75:35–57, 1996

Bruns EJ, Burchard JD, Suter JC, et al: Assessing fidelity to a community-based treatment for youth: the Wraparound Fidelity Index. J Emot Behav Disord 12:79–89, 2004

Burns BK, Goldman SK: Executive summary, in Promising Practices in Wraparound for Children With Severe Emotional Disorders and Their Families (Systems of Care: Promising Practices in Children's Mental Health series, Vol IV). Edited by Burns BK, Goldman SK. Washington, DC, Center for Effective Collaboration and Practice, American Institutes for Research, 1999, pp 11–18

Burns BJ, Schoenwald SK, Burchard JD, et al: Comprehensive community-based interventions for youth with severe emotional disorders: multisystemic therapy and the wraparound process. J Child Fam Stud 9:283–314, 2000

Carney MM, Buttell F: Reducing juvenile recidivism: evaluating the wraparound services model. Res Soc Work Pract 13:551–568, 2003

Chamberlain P, Leve LD, DeGarmo DS: Multidimensional treatment foster care for girls in the juvenile justice system: 2-year follow-up of a randomized clinical trial. J Consult Clin Psychol 75:187–193, 2007a

Chamberlain P, Reid J, Fisher PA, et al: Multidimensional Treatment Foster Care, 2007b. Available at: http://www.mtfc.com. Accessed September 25, 2007.

Clark HB, Lee B, Prange ME, et al: Children lost within the foster care system: can wraparound service strategies improve placement outcomes? J Child Fam Stud 5:39–54, 1996

Clark HB, Prange ME, Lee B, et al: An individualized wraparound process for children in foster care with emotional/behavioral disturbances: follow-up findings and implications from a controlled study, in Outcomes for Children and Youth With Emotional and Behavioral Disorders and Their Families: Programs and Evaluation Best Practices. Edited by Epstein MH, Kutash K, Duchnowski A. Austin, TX, Pro-Ed, 1998, pp 513–542

Eber L, Osuch R, Redditt CA: School-based applications of the wraparound process: early results on service provision and student outcomes. J Child Fam Stud 5:83–99, 1996

Epstein MH, Jayanthi M, McKelvey J, et al: Reliability of the Wraparound Observation Form: an instrument to measure the wraparound process. J Child Fam Stud 7:161–170, 1998

Evans ME, Armstrong MI, Kuppinger AD: Family centered intensive case management: a step toward understanding individualized care. J Child Fam Stud 5:55–65, 1996

Evans ME, Armstrong MI, Kuppinger AD, et al: Preliminary outcomes of an experimental study comparing treatment foster care and family centered intensive case management, in Outcomes for Children and Youth With Emotional and Behavioral Disorders and Their Families: Programs and Evaluation Best Practices. Edited by Epstein MH, Kutash K, Duchnowski A. Austin, TX, Pro-Ed, 1998, pp 543–580

Faw L: The state wraparound survey, in Promising Practices in Wraparound for Children With Severe Emotional Disorders and Their Families (Systems of Care: Promising Practices in Children's Mental Health series, Vol IV). Edited by Burns BK, Goldman SK. Washington, DC, Center for Effective Collaboration and Practice, American Institutes for Research, 1999, pp 79–83

Goldman SK, Faw L: Three wraparound models as promising approaches, in Promising Practices in Wraparound for Children With Severe Emotional Disorders and Their Families (Systems of Care: Promising Practices in Children's Mental Health series, Vol IV). Edited by Burns BK, Goldman SK. Washington, DC, Center for Effective Collaboration and Practice, American Institutes for Research, 1999, pp 35–78

Grimes KE, Mullin B: MHSPY: a children's health initiative for maintaining at-risk youth in the community. J Behav Health Serv Res 33:196–212, 2006

Henggeler SW, Rowland MD, Halliday-Boykins C, et al: One-year follow-up of multisystemic therapy as an alternative to the hospitalization of youths in psychiatric crisis. J Am Acad Child Adolesc Psychiatry 42:543–551, 2003

Hyde KL, Burchard JD, Woodworth K: Wrapping services in an urban setting. J Child Fam Stud 5:67–82, 1996

Individuals With Disabilities Education Act (Pub. L. No. 94-142), 1975

Jones K: Taming the Troublesome Child: American Families, Child Guidance, and the Limits of Psychiatric Authority. Cambridge, MA, Harvard University Press, 1999

Kinney J, Dittmar K: Homebuilders: helping families help themselves, in Home-Based Services for Troubled Children. Edited by Schwartz IM, AuClaire P. Lincoln, University of Nebraska Press, 1995, pp 29–54

Knitzer J: Unclaimed Children: The Failure of Public Responsibility to Children and Adolescents in Need of Mental Health Services. Washington, DC, The Children's Defense Fund, 1982

Lourie IS: A history of community child mental health, in The Handbook of Child and Adolescent Systems of Care: The New Community Psychiatry. Edited by Pumariega AJ, Winters NC. San Francisco, CA, Jossey-Bass, 2003, pp 1–16

Multisystemic Therapy Services: Complete Overview: Research on Effectiveness. Mt. Pleasant, SC, Multisystemic Therapy Services, 2007. Available at: http://www.mstservices.com/complete_overview.php. Accessed September 23, 2007.

Olds DL: Preventing crime with prenatal and infancy support of parents: the Nurse-Family Partnership. Victims and Offenders 2:205–225, 2007

Olmstead v L. C. 527 U.S. 581, affirmed in part, vacated in part, and remanded (1999)

Pullmann MD, Kerbs J, Koroloff N, et al: Juvenile offenders with mental health needs: reducing recidivism using wraparound. Crime Delinq 52:375–397, 2006

Rowland MD, Halliday-Boykins CA, Henggeler SW, et al: A randomized trial of multisystemic therapy with Hawaii's felix class youths. J Emot Behav Disord 13:13–23, 2005

Schoenwald SK, Ward DM, Henggeler SW, et al: Multisystemic therapy versus hospitalization for crisis stabilization of youth: placement outcomes 4 months post referral. Ment Health Serv Res 2:3–12, 2000

Sexton TL, Alexander JF: Functional Family Therapy. Washington, DC, U.S. Department of Justice, Office of Juvenile Justice and Delinquency Prevention, 2000. Available at: http://www.ncjrs.gov/pdffiles1/ojjdp/184743.pdf. Accessed October 1, 2007.

Stroul BA: Systems of care: a framework for children's mental health care, in The Handbook of Child and Adolescent Systems of Care: The New Community Psychiatry. Edited by Pumariega AJ, Winters NC. San Francisco, CA, Jossey-Bass, 2003, pp 17–34

Szapocznik J, Robbins MS, Mitrani VB, et al: Brief strategic family therapy, in Comprehensive Handbook of Psychotherapy: Integrative/Eclectic, Vol 4. Edited by Kaslow FW. Hoboken, NJ, Wiley, 2002, pp 83–109

Toffalo DAD: An investigation of treatment integrity and outcomes in wraparound services. J Child Fam Stud 9:351–361, 2000

VanDenBerg JE: History of the wraparound process, in Promising Practices in Wraparound for Children With Severe Emotional Disorders and Their Families (Systems of Care: Promising Practices in Children's Mental Health series, Vol IV). Edited by Burns BK, Goldman SK. Washington, DC, Center for Effective Collaboration and Practice, American Institutes for Research, 1999, pp 19–26

VanDenBerg JE, Grealish EM: Individualized services and supports through the wraparound process: philosophy and procedures. J Child Fam Stud 5:7–21, 1996

Walker JS, Bruns EJ: The wraparound process: Individualized, community-based care for children and adolescents with intensive needs, in Community Mental Health: Challenges for the 21st Century. Edited by Rosenberg J, Rosenberg S. New York, Routledge, 2006, pp 47–57

Woolston JL, Adnopoz J, Berkowitz SJ: IICAPS: A Home-Based Psychiatric Treatment for Children and Adolescents. New Haven, CT, Yale University Press, 2007

Yoe JT, Santarcangelo S, Atkins M, et al: Wraparound care in Vermont: program development, implementation, and evaluation of a statewide system of individualized services. J Child Fam Stud 5:23–37, 1996

Chapter 62

Milieu Treatment

Inpatient, Partial Hospitalization, and Residential Programs

Theodore A. Petti, M.D., M.P.H.

Inpatient hospital units (IU), partial hospital (PH) or day treatment (DT) programs, and residential treatment centers (RTCs) (sometimes grouped as "restrictive" or "intensive" services) play a critical role for children and adolescents (youth) with severe and/or persistent mental illness requiring extensive or intensive health and psychiatric services. Federal reports sometimes combine residential and inpatient statistics, while PH/DT is now pooled with outpatient treatments. A common set of values and expectations allows these programs to be considered together. A therapeutic milieu is central to each. This chapter describes common features across these milieu treatments (MTs) and considers each modality by defining the intervention and describing its structure, clinical role, and related issues.

Historical Context

Therapeutic milieus began as orphanages and boarding schools for youngsters with mental handicaps and psychiatric illness and evolved into child care institutions and group foster homes to assist emotionally disturbed and socially deviant children. The past 15 years were marked by proliferation of unregulated facilities and generated critical media attention concerning lack of community contact and serious abuses (Teich and Ireys 2007). Behavior problems were the predominant focus of IUs that began in the early 1920s. Ascendancy of a managed mental health care model and other forces led to their decreased use in the 1990s. Closing of mostly for-profit programs and publicly funded state and county units has resulted (Parmelee and Nierman 2006). Managed care has not lessened problems of access to and appropriate use of IU care across geographical areas but has resulted in decreased use and shortened lengths of stay (LOS) (Case et al. 2007; Cuellar et al. 2001). PH/DT programs began after 1963 as a movement against the perceived antitherapeutic effects of institutional care and for cost-effective treatments and for a greater family and community role. Blader and Foley (2007) provide a more detailed historical perspective of MTs.

Common Issues

The current political, fiscal, and clinical environments require a sufficiently flexible organizational structure to allow accommodation and adaptation to rapid regulatory and funding changes while being stable enough to provide predictability for all involved staff.

Parent or Sponsoring Body, Structure, and Administrative Issues

Programs offering MTs have various types of governing bodies and range from simple to multiple hierarchical layers. Administration links to the governing body serve to define how a program functions. The administrative structure must deal with regulatory and certifying body authorities and demands by funders of care (Whitted 2004). With managed care's impact, funders appear to exert a disproportionate influence (Cuellar et al. 2001). Expectations of accountability should facilitate use of evidence-based practice (EBP).

Full census for many programs determines solvency and viability; fluctuations represent threats to consistent staffing levels and sustaining morale. Professional staff members devote time to justify initial admission, continued stay, and level of treatment, thus raising expenses and lowering staff availability for direct clinical work. Requirements to evaluate outcome by regulatory and certifying bodies are particularly difficult for most milieu programs due in part to the heterogeneous nature of populations served, diversity of programs, and the difficulties in developing operational definitions and measurement of delivered services. Epstein (2004) systematically reviewed studies measuring treatment effects. Basic methods suggested for studying MT service outcomes are change analysis, decision analysis,

and outcome prediction (Lyons et al. 2001). Most studies have employed change analysis (i.e., the differences between measures before and after service delivery) with standardized measures properties.

Outcome reviews are available for each type of program, but few generalizations can be made beyond concluding that some youth can benefit from such intensive treatments. But return to a dysfunctional or abusive family with high expressed emotion or failure to comply with agreed on aftercare recommendations can easily eradicate any benefits from even highly effective MT. In addition, long-term positive benefit is unlikely when aftercare services are limited, unavailable, or inaccessible, or not culturally sensitive to family needs. Conclusive evidence demonstrating MT's effectiveness is lacking (Tse 2006; Whittaker 2004) and may explain MT absence from most practice guidelines. Summarizing multiple outcome studies, Epstein (2004) concluded that most RTC- and IU-treated children and adolescents improve, but studies are limited by admitting the most disturbed youth, with practical and ethical questions making studies difficult to design and implement.

Factors essential for providing effective MT care are listed in Table 62–1. Community resources have expanded significantly, but services to adequately address MT and other needs of youth continue (Lieberman 2004). With increasing emphasis on crisis stabilization, reliance on medication, and shorter LOS, concern about recycling youth among the types of acute IUs, outpatient care, RTC, intermediate care, and readmission to acute settings has been voiced. One study (Case et al. 2007) demonstrated increased IU readmission with slight decreases in LOS and inevitable subsequent disruption of care.

Clinical Issues

Quality assurance and continuing quality improvement efforts represent links between administrative and clinical issues. Need to maintain well-trained and motivated staff, meet fiscal goals, and nurture constructive relationships with referral sources are common objectives. Surprisingly, admission criteria (illness severity, consideration of dangerousness and safety, and need for separation from the family) of MT program types appear to poorly differentiate between residential, IU, and PH/DT. Criteria for MT care have been widely described and are compared in Table 62–2.

Formal education occurs in most programs. Exceptions are PH/DT programs provided after school or on weekends focusing on social skills and relationships.

TABLE 62–1. Essential milieu factors for patient assessment, safety monitoring and assurance, and transition to community

Patient assessment

Estimation of ability to form therapeutic alliance

Determination of critical factors prior to admission

    Child and family functioning

    Consistency of discipline within family

    Family perceived stress

    Contact with delinquent peers for those with disruptive disorders

    Extent of drug and/or alcohol use or abuse

Consideration of multiple domains in the life of mentally ill child and family

Safety monitoring and assurance

Protection of vulnerable populations of youth (e.g., autism spectrum, developmentally delayed, prior abuse or neglect)

Monitoring extent of

    Contact with delinquent peers

    Potential harm to self or others

    Adherence of patient and family to program rules and recommendations

    Appropriate assessment of biopsychosocial risk factors (i.e., predisposing, precipitating, perpetuating, and preventive factors)

Transition to community

Interdisciplinary functioning, coordination, and communication

Availability of aftercare by other services in the continuum of care

    Transitional psychosocial services for step-down processes within the mental health system

    Physicians and related professionals for medication management

Education components vary from structured, certified school programs offering academic credit to certified teachers working with school books and assignments that families bring for the few hours a day the child spends in the school setting. Many children and adolescents admitted for MT are certified as requiring special education (Carman et al. 2004). Legal requirements for an individualized education plan must be heeded when the youngster is expected to be in a program for an extended duration and requires special services. Youth in MT may have language delays, other developmental disabilities, and psychiatric disorders that impair learning and academic achievement. These issues represent significant, difficult-to-address assessment and treatment challenges during acute psychiatric admissions, but they are more likely to be addressed during intermediate to long-term IU and RTC stays. Funding sources for such services vary. Programs depend increasingly upon local public school systems to fund and/or provide school personnel to meet educational requirements. Flexibility and collaboration are necessary (Carman et al. 2004; Kiser

et al. 2006). Coordinating the school with other milieu components remains a challenge. Educating the child and family about the illness and its treatment is a basic component of care. Social skills training, including anger management, is present in virtually all programs, though labels and emphasis may differ.

Nonpsychiatric health care concerns may differ between programs, with some devoted to psychosomatic illness or eating disorders. Pediatrician or nurse practitioner involvement ranges from regular to as-needed consultations. Nursing staff to varying extents play a critical role in health and mental health care for juveniles receiving MT. The participation of physical, occupational, art, and music therapists varies depending upon the facility and populations served.

Managing highly aggressive, violent, destructive youth is an expectation for all MT staff and relates directly to concerns about staff morale, regulations, and fiscal and regulatory issues. Aggressive youth influence everyone's perception of providing, working, or residing in a safe environment. The American Academy of Child and Adolescent Psychiatry (2002) practice param-

TABLE 62–2. Comparative criteria for milieu treatment programs

Criteria	Acute inpatient	Partial hospital	Day treatment	Residential treatment center
Danger to self and/or others				
High risk	2	2	1	0
Low risk	0	2	2	2
Moderate to severe psychopathology	2	2	2	1
Need for constant observation	2	0	0	0
Need for 24-hour care	2	0	0	1
Unstable home environment	2	1	1	2
Unstable home environment, but manageable most of the time and not dangerous to self and/or others	0	2	2	1
Dangerous when nonadherent to treatment	2	2	1	2
Comprehensive evaluation required	1	1	1	1

Note.   2=generally applicable; 1=sometimes applicable; 0=not applicable.

eter addresses this issue. An extensive seclusion and restraint literature regarding how to address violent and agitated behavior provides multiple perspectives of seclusion and restraint from therapeutic to dangerous (Day 2007; Masters 2007; Mohr 2007). Regulatory agencies and advocacy groups are extensively involved in this critical area secondary to highly publicized adverse effects associated with mechanical and other forms of restraint (Nunno et al. 2007). Stricter federal policy is the result (Centers for Medicare and Medicaid Services 2006). Multiple approaches have reduced the incidence of aggression and agitation that often precede seclusion and restraint, lowered the incidence of seclusion, and eliminated mechanical restraint in some settings (Greene et al. 2006; Nunno et al. 2007; Petti et al. 2003a, 2005). Colton (2007) demonstrated through five case studies how leadership served to reduce seclusion and restraint in MT program types through organizational and cultural change.

Perceptions vary about interventions widely accepted and employed across MT programs, such as seclusion and restraint, time-out, level systems, and as-needed (prn) medications (Mohr et al. 2009). Contrary to earlier studies advocating time-out, hospitalized children prefer medication to time-outs or seclusion (Petti et al. 2003b). The terms *chemical restraint* and *prn sedation* to describe psychotropic use targeted for reduction in MT settings (Dean et al. 2006) deserve further thoughtful consideration before they are accepted as valid. Limiting orders of seclusion and both mechanical and personal (holding) restraint through regulations and accrediting guidelines and by returning the

initiation of restrictive interventions to mental health professionals may have had the greatest impact on reducing seclusion and restraint rates (Petti et al. 2005).

Various types of aggression, especially in the presence of mental retardation and developmental delay, are highly correlated with oppositional defiant or noncompliant behavior, a frequent reason for MT admission and germane to the functioning of the milieu. Though aggression was significantly associated with use of seclusion and restraint, noncompliant behavior was significantly associated with number of psychiatric medications at discharge and hospital LOS in one study (Sukhodolsky et al. 2005). A challenge is to adapt the extensive EBPs for treating disruptive and defiant behavior and to modify the milieu especially for youth with mental retardation and developmental disabilities in order to reduce aggression and improve outcome. Aggression and violence will continue to demand considerable attention until more effective interventions are found to lessen or eliminate agitation in impulsive youngsters with severe mental illness. Psychotropic medications scheduled within a framework of 14 recommendations are suggested as the means to decrease agitation and aggression in MT settings (Pappadopulos et al. 2003). However, scarce empirical data for this approach exists (Schur et al. 2003).

Sexual perpetrators are a subset of aggressive youngsters referred with increasing frequency for intensive, restrictive care. Of equal concern are referrals of youngsters who, having been sexually or physically abused, represent potential victims to peers, or rarely, by deviant staff. The literature in the care of sexual predators and victims in residential care and group settings has been reviewed and recommendations have been made (American Academy of Child and Adolescent Psychiatry 1999).

Elopement risk has lessened as a safety factor since programs have increased their security. Dynamics related to elopement from treatment programs are similar to those found in youth who exhibit self-injurious behavior (e.g., self-cutting, head banging, and ingesting foreign objects) (Petti et al. 2005). Effective communication among staff and between staff and patients is the best way to prevent elopement and other risky behaviors. Suicidal youth represent a critical additional safety risk factor for MTs (American Academy of Child and Adolescent Psychiatry 2001; Ash and Nurcombe 2007). Safety factors for consideration when admitting or discharging youngsters representing potential danger to self and others are described in Table 62–3. The Suicide Risk Scale (SRS), a 15-item self-report true-false scale, approximates suicide risk. The scale was used in one study with juvenile detention and adolescent inpatients, and results indicated that measures of depression severity remain significant predictors of suicidality (Sanislow et al. 2003).

Dialectical behavior therapy (DBT) is increasingly being employed in MT programs. DBT has been especially useful for parasuicidal and suicidal youth by targeting impulsive aggression, noncompliance, and engagement in therapy. Demonstrated to be feasible in outpatient and acute and intermediate hospital settings (Katz et al. 2002, 2004; Petti et al. 2005), DBT should be of value in MT care. It can be conducted in 2 weeks with follow-up in community settings. A DBT focus is expected to work best on a unit with staff trained in its principles and capable of assisting the youth in using and developing the ability to generalize the skills to other settings (Katz et al. 2002, 2004).

Recurrence of seclusion and restraint, sexualized behavior, and issues concerning safety are all threats to a program's integrity as related to licensure and certification. MT programs for mentally ill or developmentally delayed children and teens are under the observation of multiple entities. These range from the Center for Medicare and Medicaid Services to The Joint Commission (formerly known as the Joint Commission on the Accreditation of Healthcare Organizations or JCAHO), various state agencies, and related oversight bodies (Teich and Ireys 2007). Safety and outcome evaluation issues are raised by these regulatory and certifying bodies with demands for a structure and process to assure safety and demonstrate efficacy of the MT program. National accrediting bodies

TABLE 62–3. Risk factors for suicidal behavior warranting admission and conditions for safe discharge

Admission risk factors

Clearly abnormal mental state of a suicide attempter or someone with suicidal ideation

Stated persistent wish to die

Adequate supervision and support not possible outside therapeutic milieu

Unresolved biopsychosocial risk factors unlikely to change sufficiently to allow safe return home

Discharge safety factors

Crisis issue resolved to acceptable extent

Suicidal potential deemed minimal

Sanitized home environment

  No firearms

  Medication secured

Family-related issues addressed

  Parental psychiatric illness

  Dysfunctional family patterns

Aftercare in place

  Appropriate education of family and patient

  Realistic transition plan agreed on by all concerned

    Psychosocial interventions

    Medication monitoring

for non-mental-health-related programs providing MTs are also developing (Friedman et al. 2006).

Required master treatment plans are expected to reflect the multidisciplinary and interdisciplinary nature of staff and programming and vary depending upon program type and populations served. Critical elements include targeted psychiatric symptoms, medical issues, education and psychoeducation, and discharge or disposition. Accrediting, certifying, and other bodies have differing expectations and criteria for an acceptable plan; often programs struggle to develop plans that balance such competing interests.

The Milieu

Therapeutic milieus are generally characterized by their predominant environment, social organization, or culture, with a multidisciplinary professional and paraprofessional team devoted to diagnosis and treatment of children with major mental illness. The milieu and its operation are based upon program philosophy, leadership, history, culture, staff, and average LOS. The physical environment may determine the manner in which the milieu functions, as safety and aesthetic issues can impact morale and outcomes. Recognized as mediators for change by their ability to contain the child in a structured environment, MTs allow to varying degree the opportunity to comprehensively assess complex child and family-related issues (Tse 2006).

The Child or Adolescent Requiring Milieu Treatment

Youngsters admitted to MT programs differ from other children with emotional illness by the degree of stress they place on the home, school, and community. They have not benefited from, or had access to, individualized community services (Friedman et al. 2006). Over 20% of IU patients are diagnosed with comorbid medical conditions (Case et al. 2007), and most have complex comorbid psychiatric disorders and family dynamics. The out-of-home facilities where they are admitted range from small group homes for disruptive youth to comprehensive RTCs and highly sophisticated university acute hospital units.

The Family

The opportunity for contact between hospitalized youngsters or those in residential care with their family or others is inconsistent across programs. In the absence of research, The Joint Commission, Child Welfare League, and other interested bodies have clearly defined expectations about residents' rights to have visits and/or contact with parents or family members. Restrictions need to be reasonable, detailed in the treatment plan, explained to the child and family, and reviewed monthly. Parents are expected to be integral to treatment planning and ongoing care for all MT programs, though this is not universal and infrequently includes parent management training or other EBPs (Tse 2006).

Role in a System of Care

The MTs play a critical role in the array of services necessary to provide effective care. The provision of service with long-term involvement by some MT programs can differentiate successful from unsuccessful response to treatment (Whittaker 2004). Recommen-

TABLE 62–4. Recommendations for assuring effective milieu treatment

Optimize safety for patient, peers, and staff

Family and patient collaboration in treatment plan development

Ongoing family involvement
   Transportation
   Funding

Treatment plan addresses factors identified in case formulation

Financial support for duration of required treatment

Discharge when lesser level of care will suffice and is appropriate

dations for the most efficacious MT are detailed in Table 62–4 (Leichtman et al. 2001; Lyons and Schaefer 2000; Whittaker 2004).

Family involvement, vitally needed in treatment plan development and implementation, is a problem for those without adequate transportation and child care for other children, poor and rural families, and those living a distance from the facility. MT programs depend on other aftercare services to provide appropriate transition services to the general community. Even in a program with significant resources allotted to discharge planning, for example, one-third of adolescents consecutively discharged from a comprehensive RTC were homeless within 5 years, over one-sixth in the first year (Embry et al. 2000).

Residential Treatment Centers

RTCs provide 24-hour mental health and related care for youth who are often indistinguishable from those served in hospitals or PH/DT programs. The federal government defines RTCs as "psychiatric organizations (exclusive of psychiatric hospitals) that provide residential services primarily to persons under age 18 who have been diagnosed as exhibiting moderate or severe emotional illness or psychiatric disorders" (Stroup et al. 1988, p. 2). Teich and Ireys (2007) found little consistency of definition from state to state noting that several differing state agencies share responsibility for handling complaints, licensing, and oversight. They categorized 71 facility types from the 3,628 facilities described by informants from 38 reporting states. Burgeoning private, largely unlicensed, or unaccredited residential programs are considered problematic for youth with mental health special needs; there is a dearth of accurate numbers of such programs and of youth being served—and benefited or harmed—at these facilities (Friedman et al. 2006).

Presenting problems include family issues, 72%; aggression, 66%; school coping, 57%; depression, anxious mood, and delinquent behavior, 55% each (Pottick et al. 2004). The 8% of total mental health services for RTC-treated children account for almost 25% of expended national child mental health dollars (Teich and Ireys 2007). This does not count cost of the private, largely unregulated programs described as programs, camps or schools for behavior disordered youth (Friedman et al. 2006).

The increased number of mentally ill children using, and facilities providing, residential care is considered secondary to decreased LOS in acute IUs and fewer long-term state and other psychiatric hospital beds (Manderscheid et al. 2004). From 16 randomly selected New York State RTCs, Dale et al. (2007) report a significant increase in children formally served by the juvenile justice and mental health systems. To meet the changing needs, some RTCs have managed to become integral components within systems of care and to partner with managed care organizations (MCOs) to develop innovative strategies linking all the positive features of a system of care with family involvement and sophisticated technology. They have changed and modified their programs to provide increasingly shorter LOS and greater flexibility in keeping parents actively involved (Petti 2006).

Residential Care

Some RTCs provide more comprehensive services than hospital units, and others resemble group homes or halfway houses. These 24-hour facilities are not considered hospitals because nursing and medical care is not available around the clock. Some operate for only 5 days a week or have prolonged closures during which services are not provided. Some operate with 2 or 3 shifts of staff, while others have live-in houseparents or counselors.

RTCs may be differentiated from psychiatric IUs by their group living and individual treatment focus. RTC youth view themselves as being a "resident" of the facility as contrasted to a hospitalized sick person. Less regression has been expected in residential compared to hospital treatment, where total care and

meeting of dependency needs are paramount. RTCs expect "healthy" as contrasted to the "sick" behavior allowed and expected during a hospital stay by parents, the court, advocates, community workers, and staff. These differences may diminish with the shortened LOS allowed for inpatient programs but may hold for intermediate and longer-term IUs. RTCs offer services for the resident to become self-sufficient. A "honeymoon period" (Blader and Foley 2007) is not generally expected. Located in communities, traditional RTCs are better able to facilitate the transition back to the residents' home communities and local schools since they frequently are integrated with community public schools and their residents often spend time in the community schools.

Per diem RTC costs, except for the most specialized units, are significantly less than comparable IU costs but more than most community programs. Typical annual costs to families for private residential facilities range from $30,000 to $80,000 with some families required to make nonrefundable payments in advance (Friedman et al. 2006). Because some of these non–mental health residential programs have been accused of maltreatment and even death of their charges, the Alliance for the Safe, Therapeutic and Appropriate use of Residential Treatment (A START; http://astart.fmhi.usf.edu) was established (Friedman et al. 2006). This group has developed "Warnings for Parents Considering a Residential Placement for Their Child or Adolescent" that lists 11 recommendations concerning residential programs (Alliance for the Safe, Therapeutic and Appropriate use of Residential Treatment 2006).

Lyons et al. (1998) comment upon the multiple non-mental-health-related reasons for RTC placement and report that more than one-third of residents in randomly selected Illinois RTCs had risk profiles suggesting that those youth might be better served in community placements since they represented no danger to themselves or others and had limited overall dysfunction and psychopathology. Older teens were the most likely to inappropriately remain. However, many others disagree. Leichtman and Leichtman (1996) cogently argue that some youngsters need long-term placement for a variety of reasons, including the need and opportunity for stability in their lives. This needy subpopulation of youth may be defined by absence of a supportive discharge environment and the child or adolescent's inability to benefit from intensive treatment (Leichtman et al. 2001). After the Illinois child welfare system changes (Parmelee and Nierman 2006), youth remaining in residential care were those who had not responded to the range of community-based services and had no viable placement alternatives due to their higher levels of required mental health interventions (Lyons and McCulloch 2006).

Contrary to arguments that mental health services are disproportionately provided to white mentally ill juveniles compared to those of minority races (who are purported to be relegated to juvenile justice facilities), data indicate that admission rates for African Americans to mental health RTCs exceeded those for whites, overall and for both males and females (Milazzo-Sayre et al. 2000). African American female admission rates were higher than for Hispanic females. In 1997, RTC residents in the organized mental health sector were 65% white, 20% black, and 12% Hispanic (Pottick et al. 2004), similar to findings of those children in child welfare.

RTCs have often been classified by their functional orientation (e.g., therapeutic communities, token economies, chemical dependency programs, psychoeducational, and community-based residential group care). Some are behaviorally oriented, others are psychodynamic/psychoanalytic, and many are cognitive-behaviorally based. A limited number serve youth with eating disorders or co-occurring mental illness or chemical dependency, while others serve dually diagnosed mental illness and mental retardation or related developmental issues. Some are built around the facility's education program with schools on site, some have their residents attend school in the community, and others have both. Many offer both outpatient and PH/DT programs (Milazzo-Sayre et al. 2000; Stroup et al. 1988). Practical aspects of working or consulting in residential programs have been detailed (Cohen 2006; Fujita and Arnold 2006).

Outcome and Quality Assessment

Outcome studies of RTCs suggest relative effectiveness while in care. Factors associated with outcomes identified in several studies (Kutash and Rivera 1995) include absence of psychosis, organic etiology for the psychiatric disorder, below-average level of intelligence, antisocial and bizarre behavior, dysfunctional family, insufficient duration of residence to allow for consolidation of gains, and adequate aftercare services. Defining an adequate residential care LOS is difficult and may relate to our overall difficulty in evaluating the cost and benefits of RTC care. Residential care data on the extent to which children are helped or harmed and the number actually served are considered glaringly absent (Friedman et al. 2006).

Controlled and randomized studies have been problematic to implement. Curry (2004) suggested employing research designs that compare between-treatment, within-program, and across-program designs. Noting that residential treatment is not an isolated event in the life and treatment of a youth, he provides results of comparative outcome studies and emphasizes the need to control for the postdischarge environment. Curry (2004) suggests that EBP methods can be and have been adapted for RTCs, with special adaptations made for those with substance abuse, abuse, or neglect histories and facility factors.

Comparison and other studies evaluating different RTC types and treatments have been reported (Curry 2004; Epstein 2004), including an intensive short-term residential program (Leichtman et al. 2001) developed at the Menninger Clinic that employed standardized measures to demonstrate outcome effectiveness. Lyons and Schaefer (2000) found that the most dangerous youth were the most severely ill and benefited most from residential care. Lyons and McCulloch (2006) recently described a model for using outcomes research as an effective means to monitor residential treatment by identifying RTC site strengths, weaknesses, treatment progress trajectories, and trends. Use of the Child Functional Assessment Rating Scale (CFARS), the main tool for a Residential Treatment Outcomes System (RTOS) evaluation, allows system-wide assessment with generated data that administrators and providers can report via a Web-based system efficiently and quickly. It allows comparison within and between providers and monitoring of individual patient progress or deterioration compared to a reference group.

Subramaniam et al. (2007), in a prospective study of adolescents following stays in a substance abuse–treating RTC, reported that a Beck Depression Inventory (BDI) baseline score of ≥11 predicted significantly poorer substance use outcome as measured by the mean percentage of days of non-nicotine substance use after discharge in 90-day blocks for 1 year. A drug career ≥2 years predicted later opioid use. The authors' conclusions suggested the need to treat the comorbid depression for improved outcomes.

Inpatient Hospitalization

Psychiatric IU care has been defined as the most restrictive and expensive MT. Usually reserved for the most severely ill who require round-the-clock medical and nursing supervision, IUs may exist within psychiatric, pediatric, general, or freestanding child and adolescent psychiatric hospitals and be obligated to serve within a system of care, be selective in caring for special populations, or be available to all within a certain age range or residential area. In 1997, 286,176 youth under age 18 were admitted for organized mental health IU care. Over two-thirds were ages 13–17, and 30% were ages 6–12 years (Pottick et al. 2004). Age ratios in IU community hospital discharges between 1900 and 2000 ($N=29,590$) were similar to the 1997 figures, as were primary payer source 43% to 37% public insurer; 48% to 55% private insurance; and 9% other for both. More white (78%–67%) and fewer black (14%–16%) and Hispanic (4%–14%) youth were seen in community hospitals (Case et al. 2007; Pottick et al. 2004).

The number of discharges and population-based discharge rates with a mental health diagnosis from community hospitals between 1990 and 2000 for children 17 years and younger has remained relatively stable. Mean charges per stay and total LOS decreased by half, and a 63% decrease in median LOS from 12.2 to 4.5 days was found (Case et al. 2007). Other, nonclinical variables may best predict LOS for youth, contributing between 22% and 30% to the variance. Leon et al. (2006) reported the most consistent, largest LOS predictor was the hospital itself. Clinical predictors accounted for only 7% of variance, with suicide risk predicting decreased LOS; increased LOS was predicted by danger to others and consistency of symptoms across multiple contexts. Snowden et al. (2007) reported that although factors influencing IU admission decisions in a large foster care population were due to illness level related to safety and were clinically appropriate, multiple context issues (e.g., family problems) also play a significant role.

Inpatient Care

Acute IU care, the most common form of hospital-based care, now comprises several functions as listed in Table 62–5. Intermediate- and long-term IUs are becoming uncommon. Comprehensive assessment using resources of larger pediatric, psychiatric, or general hospitals is ideal. Intermediate-term facilities offer patients and families opportunities for more extensive assessment and consolidation of gains needed for successful transition to less restrictive settings.

Conduct disturbance, broadly defined, most frequently precipitates preadolescent admission (Blader 2006). Table 62–6 lists frequency of presenting problems to acute IUs. Coded severity of psychiatric illness has increased over the past decades. Contemporary is-

TABLE 62–5. Acute inpatient psychiatric unit functions

Assessment
Minimize potential for harm
   Separation from family and community
   Monitoring behavior
Case formulation and diagnosis
Treatment plan development and brief implementation
Stabilization of symptoms and crisis
Disposition planning
Transition to less restrictive setting

sues including potential undertreatment of minority youth, "diagnostic upcoding" (i.e., coding more serious psychiatric disorders or self-harm to justify admission or greater reimbursement), discrepancies in admissions between publicly and privately insured youth, the highly significant increase in disposition to home, and significant decreases in both referral to another facility (12% to 7%) and discharges against medical advice (5% to 2%) have been considered (Case et al. 2007).

Providing therapy beyond resolving the precipitating crisis in acute IUs is challenging. Emphasis on therapeutic intervention is expected from longer-term facilities, although most youth so hospitalized are seldom candidates for traditional therapies. Altering negative cognitions and training in social skills through cognitive, behavioral, and psychodynamic approaches within the milieu are standard in most treatment plans. DBT was equally effective in highly significantly reducing suicidal ideation, depressive symptoms, and parasuicidal behavior at 1-year follow-up when administered to suicidal adolescents in 10 daily sessions on one acute hospital unit compared to treatment as usual (psychodynamically oriented crisis assessment and

TABLE 62–6. Frequency of presenting problems to acute specialty mental health inpatient programs

Depressed or anxious mood (including self-harm)	65%
Suicidality	55%
Aggression	49%
Family problems	47%
Alcohol or drug use	26%
Delinquent behavior	25%

Source. Pottick et al. 2004.

treatment) on a matched unit. For both groups, mean LOS was 18 days, prn medications were employed, and symptom improvement was evident at discharge. The DBT group had significantly fewer behavioral incidents during hospitalization (Katz et al. 2004). Thus, positive therapeutic interactions employing traditional and innovative means can occur with lasting benefit, given sufficient time.

Efforts devoted to family work depend on family availability, motivation for positive change, and complex family factors (Blader 2006). Aftercare is often difficult to implement. The concern for "institutionalizing" the patients in intermediate or longer-term care is real, particularly when patients feel more comfortable in the protective and nurturing environment than in the community environment. Aggression and violence are common foci of attention. Current quandaries for acute IU psychiatrists involve prescribing psychotropics and readmissions, as shown in the case example below.

Case Example

Thirteen-year-old Jennie's hospitalization following a suicide attempt was prolonged. On the basis of a case formulation of her mild to moderate depression, her treatment team concluded that intensive family work and social skills training were needed to prevent recurrence of her hopelessness; antidepressant medication demanded by the MCO to secure continued stay beyond 3 days for crisis stabilization was deemed unwarranted. Sertraline was prescribed in part to secure additional approved days. Hospital discharge was delayed because a physician to monitor medication within reasonable distance from her home could not be located.

The aftercare problem—given the shortage of child and adolescent psychiatrists, the reluctance of primary care physicians to prescribe psychotropic medications in light of U.S. Food and Drug Administration (FDA) warnings, and the pressure by MCOs to prescribe medication and discharge once danger or other reason for hospital justification are lessened—makes EBP difficult to implement and the likelihood for readmission higher than previously experienced. Attention to parental attitudes toward aftercare treatment and specific aspects of psychopathology may improve aftercare adherence to discharge recommendations (Burns et al. 2008).

Outcome and Quality Assessment

Readmissions to acute IUs are a potential measure of outcome. Defining outcomes and factors specific to IU care has been difficult. Blader (2004) followed for 1 year after IU discharge 109 school-age children. Predictors for readmission, 81% occurring within 90 days, included more severe conduct problems, disengaged parent-child relations, and harsh parental discipline. He concluded readmissions might best be prevented by attention to the immediate postdischarge period with efforts directed to family factors and severe conduct symptoms. The findings are consistent with those reported by Kolko (1992) for symptom abatement in formerly hospitalized elementary school– and middle school–age children at 2, 4, and 6 months after discharge. He suggested attending to factors improved in the higher functioning youngsters: internalizing and externalizing symptom decreases, parental disciplinary effectiveness, adaptive involvement in recreation and leisure activities, positive peer interaction, and improved satisfaction with relationships. Interventions most likely to improve functioning were as follows: parent management training; exposure to group activities fostering prosocial behavior; cognitive-behavioral skills training; aftercare planning; and clarifying parent versus child variables, diagnoses, and other factors that contribute to outcome. Masters (2005) provided an example of using components of cognitive-behavioral therapy, an evidence-based treatment that can be implemented within 5 hospital days.

Studies of multisystemic therapy (MST; see Chapter 61, "Systems of Care, Wraparound Services, and Home-Based Services") suggest that intermediate- or long-term IU care can be dramatically decreased. But for adolescents in psychiatric crisis (average age of 13 years, 64% African American, 65% male), acute hospitalization was subsequently required in 44% of MST-assigned cases (Henggeler et al. 1999), thus supporting the role of IUs in a total system of care. A similarly designed study of youth presenting for psychiatric hospitalization for dangerous behavior toward self or others found both standard IU care and MST effective, with MST superior to IU care in reducing suicide attempts but no different in related symptoms (Huey et al. 2004).

Partial Hospitalization and Day Treatment

Multiple variations of PH or DT have been described. PH and DT are defined as less than 24-hour hospital-level daily care targeted to diagnose and treat psychiatric disorders for which preventing relapse or hospitalization and improvement in the condition could be expected (Daily and Reddick 1993). The American Association for Partial Hospitalization has defined partial hospitalization as clinical services offering active ambulatory treatment within a stable therapeutic milieu that is time limited, therapeutically intensive, coordinated, and structured. Broadly defined, partial hospitalization refers to less than 24-hour care provided in a hospital setting; while DT is care provided as school-based for at least 5 hours a day and involves integrated education, counseling, and family services. Data for PH/DT no longer are differentiated from "less than 24-hour care programs" (Milazzo-Sayre et al. 2000).

PH/DT programs have been underutilized for children and teens with severe psychiatric disorders, often due to their absence under insurance coverage, residence in rural areas, or poor access to programs not located in schools. Additional problems include the absence of criteria for admission and clear definitions of outcome and reluctance to maintain seriously ill youngsters in the community. Many parents express reluctance to engage in regular family therapy. With the emergence of MCOs, PH and DT programs were expected to grow and become more prominent components of the child and adolescent mental health service system, but this has rarely occurred.

Partial Hospital and Day Treatment Care

PH and DT programs offer the intensive MT of an IU or RTC setting while maintaining the youngster in home and community. DT programs are the most common, including evening and after-school programs. They may be freestanding, part of a hospital clinic or IU, school, or RTC. Most are highly structured, attend to their patients' educational needs, and provide multimodal treatments. They attempt to avoid the regression frequently found when psychiatrically ill children and adolescents enter other MTs. Patients are expected to have sufficient self-control to avert dangerous behavior, thus not requiring the structure needed to as-

sure safety of severely ill youth. However, quick access to the IU or RTC as indicated is facilitated when the PH/DT unit is integrated with or a component of a more restrictive program. Care exceeding multiple outpatient visits per week is provided in partial hospitalization on a variable but short-term crisis focus as an IU alternative; partial hospitalization often serves as a step-down from an IU or RTC setting. Therapeutic school DTs often are of longer duration and funded by school systems for out-of-district placements.

PH/DT programs are meant for patients who can be managed safely in an intensive setting without need for 24-hour care. Specialized MTs for substance abuse and chemical dependency, eating disorders, victims of abuse, and those with medical disorders and comorbid psychiatric difficulties are available employing the PH model of care. Tse (2006) suggests that DT programs may be the only place where disruptive children and their families find acceptance. Conduct and attention-deficit/hyperactivity disorders are common diagnoses found in referred children (Grizenko 1997). Parents or caretakers must be able to regularly participate in family counseling, training, and therapy and to adequately provide support and control over their children during evenings and weekends. Reliable transportation must be available. PH restrictive practice (i.e., seclusion and restraint) depends upon the hospital configuration; DT restrictive practice is generally limited to those methods acceptable and available in most school or home environments holds. Personal ("therapeutic") holding of young children and quiet rooms are used in some DT programs; chemical and manual restraints are not. Medication use on an as-needed basis is available in some settings, particularly PHs.

Understanding the interplay among family, environment, and the child is central to PH/DT successful program operation. Programs strive to provide the MT structure of IUs and RTCs while maintaining active, community, and family functional links. The academic domain is secondary to the social-emotional domain in many PH/DT programs even when set in educational settings; the school experience serves as a core for therapeutic interactions. Physician involvement depends upon PH/DT type and psychiatric functions. Those settings serving as alternatives to or step-downs from IU care require more medical input and greater psychiatrist involvement; other settings mainly employ the psychiatrist as a consultant to provide diagnostic assessment and medication monitoring. Practical aspects of work in and consulting to PH and DT programs are detailed by Kiser et al. (2006).

Outcome and Quality Assessment

Studies of PH/DT programs suffer from similar problems faced by the other MTs. Studies measuring successful reintegration into regular school settings report effectiveness in 65%–70% of DT cases successfully discharged (Kutash and Rivera 1995). A comparison of PH programs to each other and to other forms of MT results in fair evidence for efficacy and effectiveness. Outcome studies suggest the following: a portion of children can benefit from this service or be reintegrated into school settings; individual and family functioning improves; gains are not generalized to the school setting; and families play critical roles posttreatment as measured by standardized scales (Grizenko 1997; Kutash and Rivera 1995).

Though DT programs for preschoolers (sometimes called "therapeutic nurseries") have been used extensively since the 1950s, Tse (2006) commented on the paucity of related literature. Her review of research reports on psychosocial intervention outcome data with preschool children (published between 1974 and 2004) identified one published controlled study reporting no long-term benefits and five studies reporting quantitative outcomes. She offered a list of prevention and efficacy studies that should improve DT for disruptive preschoolers that apply as well to all youngsters.

Research Directions

Clinical questions and controversies expected to be addressed in the next 5 years for MTs must include the issues of greatest need:

1. Overcoming barriers to translating EBP into MT settings and incorporating related systematic evaluation
2. Improving aftercare services so that gains made in MT settings will be maintained
3. Determining modifiable factors related to failed return to home or other placements
4. Decreasing readmission rates
5. Expanding and evaluating use of standardized measures for MTs
6. Moving toward more manualized, time-limited treatments for families and patients
7. Regulating non–mental health residential facilities
8. Reducing impulsive aggression and violence
9. Eliminating deaths from seclusion and restraint in mental health MTs

Summary Points

- Milieu treatments are critical components of a mental health system of care.
- The evidence base for MT effectiveness needs immediate attention.
- Mental health MTs are heavily regulated, monitored, and affected by managed care.
- Aftercare following discharge must be enhanced.
- Standardized instruments can be effectively used for assessment, monitoring, and outcome.
- Alternatives to seclusion and restraint must be developed and evaluated.

References

Alliance for the Safe, Therapeutic and Appropriate use of Residential Treatment: A START Factsheet. Available at: http://astart.fmhi.usf.edu/AStartDocs/factsheet.pdf. Accessed June 16, 2009.

American Academy of Child and Adolescent Psychiatry: Practice parameters for the assessment and treatment of children and adolescents who are sexually abusive of others. J Am Acad Child Adolesc Psychiatry 38(suppl): 55S–76S, 1999

American Academy of Child and Adolescent Psychiatry: Practice parameters for the assessment and treatment of children and adolescents with suicidal behavior. J Am Acad Child Adolesc Psychiatry 40(suppl):24S–51S, 2001

American Academy of Child and Adolescent Psychiatry: Practice parameter for the prevention and management of aggressive behavior in child and adolescent psychiatric institutions, with special reference to seclusion and restraint. J Am Acad Child Adolesc Psychiatry 41(suppl): 4S–25S, 2002

Ash P, Nurcombe B: Malpractice and professional liability, in Lewis's Child and Adolescent Psychiatry: A Comprehensive Textbook, 4th Edition. Edited by Andres M, Volkmar FR. Philadelphia, PA, Lippincott Williams & Wilkins, 2007, pp 1018–1032

Blader JC: Symptom, family, and service predictors of children's psychiatric rehospitalization within one year of discharge. J Am Acad Child Adolesc Psychiatry 43:440–451, 2004

Blader JC: Which family factors predict children's externalizing behaviors following discharge from psychiatric inpatient treatment? Arch Gen Psychiatry 47:1133–1142, 2006

Blader JC, Foley CA: Milieu-based treatment: Inpatient and partial hospitalization, residential treatment, in Lewis's Child and Adolescent Psychiatry: A Comprehensive Textbook, 4th edition. Edited by Andres M, Volkmar FR. Philadelphia, PA, Lippincott Williams & Wilkins, 2007, pp 865–878

Burns CD, Cortekk MA, Wagner BM: Treatment compliance in adolescents after attempted suicide: a 2-year follow-up study. J Am Acad Child Adolesc Psychiatry 47:948–957, 2008

Carman GO, Dorta N, Kon D, et al: Special education in residential treatment. Child Adolesc Psychiatr Clin N Am 13:381–394, 2004

Case BG, Olfson M, Marcus SC, et al: Trends in the inpatient mental health treatment of children and adolescents in US community hospitals. Arch Gen Psychiatry 64:89–96, 2007

Centers for Medicare and Medicaid Services: Medicare and Medicaid programs; hospital conditions of participation: patients' rights; final rule. Fed Regist 42 CFR Part 482, Dec 8, 2006, pp 71377–71428

Cohen P: Chemical dependency program, in Community Child and Adolescent Psychiatry: A Manual of Clinical Practice and Consultation. Edited by Petti TA, Salguero C. Washington, DC, American Psychiatric Publishing, 2006, pp 205–218

Colton D: Leadership's and program's role in organizational and cultural change to reduce seclusions and restraints, in For Our Own Safety: Examining the Safety of High-Risk Interventions for Children and Young People. Edited by Nunno MA, Day DM, Bullard LB. Washington, DC, Child Welfare League of America, 2007, pp 143–166

Cuellar AE, Libby AM, Snowden LR: How capitated mental health care affects utilization by youth in the juvenile justice and child welfare systems. Ment Health Serv Res 3:61–72, 2001

Curry JF: Future directions in residential treatment outcome research. Child Adolesc Psychiatr Clin N Am 13:429–440, 2004

Daily S, Reddick C: Adolescent day treatment: an alternative for the future. Adolesc Psychiatry 19:523–540, 1993

Dale N, Baker AJL, Anastasio E, et al: Characteristics of children in residential treatment in New York State. Child Welfare 86:5–27, 2007

Day DD: A review of the literature on the therapeutic effectiveness of physical restraints with children and youth. in For Our Own Safety: Examining the Safety of High-

Risk Interventions for Children and Young People. Edited by Nunno MA, Day DM, Bullard LB. Washington, DC, Child Welfare League of America, 2007, pp 27–44

Dean AJ, McDermott BM, Marshall: PRN sedation-patterns of prescribing and administration in a child and adolescent mental health inpatient service. Eur Child Adolesc Psychiatry 15:277–281, 2006

Embry LE, Evens C, Stoep AV, et al: Risk factors for homelessness in adolescents released from psychiatric residential treatment. J Am Acad Child Adolesc Psychiatry 39:1293–1299, 2000

Epstein RA Jr: Inpatient and residential treatment effects for children and adolescents: a review and critique. Child Adolesc Psychiatr Clin N Am 13:411–428, 2004

Friedman RM, Pinto A, Behar L et al: Unlicensed residential programs: the next challenge in protecting youth. Am J Orthopsychiatry 76:295–303, 2006

Fujita M, Arnold V: Community residential programs, in Community Child and Adolescent Psychiatry: A Manual of Clinical Practice and Consultation. Edited by Petti TA, Salguero C. Washington, DC, American Psychiatric Publishing, 2006, pp 219–230

Greene RW, Ablon JS, Martin A: Use of collaborative problem solving to reduce seclusion and restraint in child and adolescent inpatient units. Psychiatr Serv 57:610–612, 2006

Grizenko N: Outcome of multimodal day treatment for children with severe behavior problems: a five-year follow-up. J Am Acad Child Adolesc Psychiatry 36:989–997, 1997

Henggeler SW, Rowlan MD, Randall J, et al: Home-based multisystemic therapy as an alternative to the hospitalization of youths in psychiatric crisis: clinical outcomes. J Am Acad Child Adolesc Psychiatry 38:1331–1339, 1999

Huey SJ Jr, Henggeler SW, Rowlan MD, et al: Multisystemic therapy effects on attempted suicide by youths presenting psychiatric emergencies. J Am Acad Child Adolesc Psychiatry 43:183–190, 2004

Katz LY, Gunasekara S, Miller AI: Dialectical behavior therapy for inpatient and outpatient parasuicidal adolescents. Adolesc Psychiatry 26:161–178, 2002

Katz LY, Cox BJ, Gunasekara S, et al: Feasibility of dialectical behavior therapy for suicidal adolescent inpatients. J Am Acad Child Adolesc Psychiatry 43:276–282, 2004

Kiser L, Heston JD, Paavola M: Day treatment center/partial hospital setting, in Community Child and Adolescent Psychiatry: A Manual of Clinical Practice and Consultation. Edited by Petti TA, Salguero C. Washington, DC, American Psychiatric Publishing, 2006, pp 189–203

Kolko DJ: Short-term follow-up of child psychiatric hospitalization: clinical description, predictors, and correlates. J Am Acad Child Adolesc Psychiatry 31:719–727, 1992

Kutash K, Rivera VR: Effectiveness of children's mental health services: a review of the literature. Education Treatment Children 18:443–477, 1995

Leichtman ML, Leichtman ML: Short-term residential treatment and its limits. Treatment Today Spring:12–14, 1996

Leichtman ML, Leichtman ML, Barber CC, et al: Effectiveness of intensive short-term residential treatment with severely disturbed adolescents. Am J Orthopsychiatry 71:227–235, 2001

Leon SC, Snowden J, Bryant FB, et al: The hospital as predictor of children's and adolescents' length of stay. J Am Acad Child Adolesc Psychiatry 45:322–328, 2006

Lieberman RE: Future directions in residential treatment. Child Adolesc Psychiatr Clin N Am 13:279–294, 2004

Lyons JS, McCulloch JR: Monitoring and managing outcomes in residential treatment: practice-based evidence in search of evidence-based practice. J Am Acad Child Adolesc Psychiatry 45:247–251, 2006

Lyons JS, Schaefer K: Mental health and dangerousness: characteristics and outcomes of children and adolescents in residential care. J Child Fam Stud 9:67–73, 2000

Lyons JS, Libman-Mintzer LN, Kisiel CL, et al: Understanding the mental health needs of children and adolescents in residential treatment. Prof Psychol Res Pr 29:582–587, 1998

Lyons JS, Terry P, Martinovich Z, et al: Outcome trajectories for adolescents in residential treatment: a statewide evaluation. J Child Fam Stud 10:333–345, 2001

Manderscheid R, Atay JE, Male A, et al: Highlights of organized mental health services in 2000 and major national and state trends, in Mental Health in the United States, 2002. DHHS Publ No SMA-3938. Edited by Manderscheid RW, Henderson MJ. Rockville, MD. Center for Mental Health Services, Substance Abuse and Mental Health Services Administration, 2004, pp 243–279

Masters KJ: A CBT approach to inpatient psychiatric hospitalization. J Am Acad Child Adolesc Psychiatry 44:708–711, 2005

Masters KJ: Modernizing seclusion and restraint, in For Our Own Safety: Examining the Safety of High-Risk Interventions for Children and Young People. Edited by Nunno MA, Day DM, Bullard LB. Washington, DC, Child Welfare League of America, 2007, pp 45–66

Milazzo-Sayre LJ, Henderson MJ, Manderscheid RW, et al: Persons treated in specialty mental health programs, United States, 1997, in Mental Health, United States, 2000. Edited by Manderscheid RW, Henderson MJ. Rockville, MD, Center for Mental Health Services, 2000, pp 172–217

Mohr WK: Physical restraints: are they ever safe and how safe is safe enough? in For Our Own Safety: Examining the Safety of High-Risk Interventions for Children and Young People. Edited by Nunno MA, Day DM, Bullard LB. Washington, DC, Child Welfare League of America, 2007, pp 69–86

Mohr WK, Martin A, Olson JN, et al: Beyond point and level systems: moving toward child-centered programming. Am J Orthopsychiatry 79:8–18, 2009

Nunno MA, Day DM, Bullard LB (eds): For Our Own Safety: Examining the Safety of High-Risk Interventions for Children and Young People. Washington, DC, Child Welfare League of America, 2007

Pappadopulos E, MacIntyre JC, Crismon L, et al: Treatment recommendations for the use of antipsychotics for aggressive youth (TRAAY), part II. J Am Acad Child Psychiatry 42:145–161, 2003

Parmelee DX, Nierman P: Transitions from institutional to community systems of care, in Community Child and Adolescent Psychiatry: A Manual of Clinical Practice and Consultation. Edited by Petti TA, Salguero C. Washington, DC, American Psychiatric Publishing, 2006, pp 249–257

Petti TA: Future directions, in Community Child and Adolescent Psychiatry: A Manual of Clinical Practice and Consultation. Edited by Petti TA, Salguero C. Washington, DC, American Psychiatric Publishing, 2006, pp 269–275

Petti TA, Somers J, Sims LA: Chronicle of seclusion and restraint in an intermediate-term care facility. Adolesc Psychiatry 27:83–116, 2003a

Petti TA, Stigler K, Gardner-Haycox J, et al: Perceptions of PRN psychotropic medications by hospitalized child and adolescent recipients. J Am Acad Child Adolesc Psychiatry 42:434–441, 2003b

Petti TA, Blitsch M, Blix S, et al: Deliberate foreign body ingestion in hospitalized youth: a case series and overview. Adolesc Psychiatry 29:249–287, 2005

Pottick K, Warner L, Isaacs M, et al: Children and adolescents admitted to specialty mental health care in the United States, 1986 and 1997, in Mental Health in the United States, 2002. DHHS Publ No SMA-3938. Edited by Manderscheid RW, Henderson MJ. Rockville, MD, Center for Mental Health Services, Substance Abuse and Mental Health Services Administration, 2004, pp 314–326

Sanislow CA, Grilo CM, Fehon DC, et al: Correlates of suicide risk in juvenile detainees and adolescent inpatients. J Am Acad Child Adolesc Psychiatry 42:234–240, 2003

Schur SB, Sikich L, MacIntyre JC, et al: Treatment recommendations for the use of antipsychotics for aggressive youth (TRAAY), part I: a review. J Am Acad Child Psychiatry 42:132–144, 2003

Snowden JA, Leon SC, Bryant FB, et al: Evaluating psychiatric hospital admission decisions for children in foster care: an optimal classification tree analysis. J Child Adolesc Psychol 36:8–18, 2007

Stroup A, Witkin M, Atay J, et al: Residential Treatment Centers for Emotionally Disturbed Children 1983 (Mental Health Statistical Note No 188). Rockville, MD, National Institute of Mental Health, 1988

Subramaniam GA, Stitzer MA, Clemmey P: Baseline depressive symptoms predict poor substance use outcome following adolescent residential treatment. J Am Acad Child Adolesc Psychiatry 46:1062–1069, 2007

Sukhodolsky DG, Cardona L, Martin A: Characterizing aggressive and noncompliant behaviors in a children's psychiatric inpatient setting. Child Psychiatry Hum Dev 36:177–193, 2005

Teich JL, Ireys HT: A national survey of state licensing, regulating, and monitoring of residential facilities for children with mental illness. Psychiatr Serv 58:991–998, 2007

Tse J: Research on day treatment programs for preschoolers with disruptive behavior disorders. Psychiatr Serv 57:477–486, 2006

Whittaker JK: The reinvention of residential treatment: an agenda for research and practice. Child Adolesc Psychiatr Clin N Am 13:267–278, 2004

Whitted BR: Legal issues in residential treatment. Child Adolesc Psychiatr Clin N Am 13:295–307, 2004

PART XII

CONSULTATION

Chapter 63

School-Based Interventions

Heather J. Walter, M.D., M.P.H.

The substantial gap between children's mental health service needs and available resources has been well documented in the United States. Although over 10% of all children and adolescents have a psychiatric disorder associated with significant functional impairment—and an estimated 25%–50% of youth engage in risky behaviors such as unprotected sexual activity, substance use, and violent conflict resolution—only 20% of children and adolescents in need of mental health services receive them (President's New Freedom Commission on Mental Health 2003).

Lack of access to services poses a major barrier to meeting the mental health needs of young people. Providing mental health services in schools increasingly is considered a logical way to surmount this barrier, as schools require attendance, are highly accessible to children and their families, comprise a milieu that can be structured to achieve therapeutic outcomes, and employ professionals capable of providing a spectrum of services in a setting that may be less stigmatizing than clinics or hospitals. Strong support for the expan-

sion of school mental health services has been expressed in policy statements from the federal government (e.g., President's New Freedom Commission on Mental Health 2003; U.S. Department of Health and Human Services 1999; U.S. Public Health Service 2000) and from professional health care organizations (e.g., American Academy of Child and Adolescent Psychiatry 2005; American Academy of Pediatrics 2004; Tolan et al. 2001). These statements converge in their recommendation that schools provide a broad range of preventive, early intervention, and clinical mental health services for enrolled students.

History

For more than a century, clinicians have collaborated with school personnel to improve the mental health of students. Since the 1950s, a number of psychiatrists have made seminal contributions to the interface between psychiatry and education, notably Caplan (1970), Berlin (1975), Comer (1992), and Berkovitz (1998, 2001). During this time, mental health consultation and service to schools underwent five major periods of expansion that were stimulated by broad sociocultural movements. First, the community mental health movement after World War II advanced the idea that schools were appropriate community-based sites for the delivery of mental health services. Second, the civil rights movement in the 1960s led to educational rights legislation prohibiting discrimination against and providing services to students with mental disabilities. Third, the dramatic change in social mores in the 1960s through the 1980s led to students' increased involvement in risky behaviors and pressure on schools to intervene with preventive interventions. Fourth, the growth of the school-based health clinic movement in the 1990s led to recognition of the high prevalence of mental health problems among students attending the clinics (Lear et al. 1991; Walter et al. 1995) and the corresponding need for increased mental health services. Most recent is the move toward greater academic accountability in the school setting (as exemplified by the "No Child Left Behind" legislation), which is leading to a call for parallel accountability in the social-emotional domain of education.

Models of School Consultation and Clinical Care

Consultation

Case Consultation

In the consultation model, clinicians advise school personnel about appropriate educational and/or therapeutic approaches to and/or services for students with developmental, cognitive, emotional, behavioral, or social problems. The consultation may be direct or indirect. In direct consultation, the clinician assesses the student and suggests to school personnel appropriate interventions that are typically provided by professionals other than the consultant. In indirect consultation, the clinician does not assess the student but rather assesses an issue (e.g., behavioral, social) articulated by school personnel and makes general recommendations to school personnel about resolving the problem. Because in this model the clinician typi-

cally is paid by the school to provide consultative services to school personnel, role, boundary, and confidentiality issues must be clarified at the outset to protect all involved parties and conform to federal, state, and local regulations.

Systems Consultation

In this model, clinicians are paid by the school to advise school personnel about the creation of a milieu that is conducive to learning. Individual students' needs typically are not addressed in this type of consultation; rather, the focus of consultation may include creating a positive school environment, valuing diversity in the school, improving attendance, building school connectedness among students and parents, fostering teacher and staff morale, developing and coordinating mental health programs, and planning for crisis situations. The principles of organizational psychology often are brought to bear in this type of consultation.

Clinical Care

School-Based Health Centers

In the past decade, there has been exponential growth in school-based health centers, rising to around 1,500 centers located in nearly every state. About 60% of these centers are said to include mental health services (National Assembly on School-Based Health Care 2000). Centers typically are staffed by a multidisciplinary team of providers and are funded by a variety of mechanisms (e.g., grants, contracts, state and local allocations, fee-for-service). Centers with mental health practitioners can provide a broad range of mental health services including assessment; individual, group, and family psychotherapy; pharmacotherapy; and prevention and health promotion activities. Mental health services delivered in school settings offer a number of advantages, including enhanced access (Diala et al. 2002; Weist et al. 1999), reduced stigma (Nabors and Reynolds 2000), increased generalization and maintenance of treatment effects (Weare 2000), enhanced clinical productivity (Flaherty and Weist 1999), and more ecologically grounded roles for mental health clinicians (Atkins et al. 2001).

Studies of the school-based health center model have suggested that students using the centers need and are receiving services that they otherwise might not have received (e.g., Walter et al. 1996; Weist et al. 1999) and that they respond favorably to therapeutic interventions (e.g., Evans 1999; Nabors and Reynolds

2000; Weist et al. 1996). Clinic users also have been shown to have better attendance, fewer discipline referrals, and higher test scores than nonusers, suggesting the potential academic side effects of this model (Jennings et al. 2000).

School-Linked Health Centers

In this model, schools are linked with hospitals or community clinics that are contracted to provide medical and mental health services to students at convenient locations off-site from the school. In some settings, this model better suits the community's needs and preferences and can be more cost-effective and therefore sustainable due to fee-for-service billing capability (Jennings et al. 2000).

Expanded School Mental Health Programs

Over the past several decades, schools have attempted to respond to the need for broader mental health services by gradually expanding the array of programs available on-site. According to a School Health Policies and Programs Study (Brener et al. 2001), 94% of schools nationwide provide crisis intervention; 93% provide referrals for physical, sexual, or emotional abuse; 87% provide activities targeted at violence prevention; 84% provide counseling or case management for students with mental or emotional problems; 77% provide suicide prevention activities; 76% provide alcohol and drug use prevention activities; and 67% provide activities targeted at tobacco use prevention. Yet despite what appears to be an encouraging array of programs, funding constraints, competing academic priorities, limited evidence of program effectiveness, and lack of program coordination combine to perpetuate a pervasive marginalization and fragmentation of mental health and social services in the school setting (Taylor and Adelman 2000). Proponents of expanded school mental health (Weist and Albus 2004) espouse the belief that all students should have access to a broad range of preventive, early intervention, and clinical treatment services. To achieve this goal, schools must partner with community organizations to coordinate and integrate the variety of existing programs and funding streams into a coherent whole. Although schools with expanded mental health programs have been suggested to have favorable therapeutic and academic outcomes, this model remains underresearched and underutilized at present.

School Characteristics
Climate

The milieu of a school is a key factor influencing the desirability and effectiveness of mental health interventions. The milieu derives from several interrelated components (Brookover et al. 1979), including the sociodemographic composition of the student body and school personnel (social inputs); the size, structure, and processes of the school (social structure); and attitudinal characteristics, such as the norms, expectations, and feelings about the school shared by students and staff (social climate). The school climate literature supports several key components of a positive climate, including a supportive, welcoming atmosphere; respectful peer and adult relationships; a variety of learning experiences; high expectations for achievement and self-regulation; fair and effective discipline; participation in extracurricular activities; and parent/community involvement (Libbey 2004). Research suggests that the social climate of a school has a substantial impact on students' academic achievement that can surpass expectations based on social inputs or structure (Brookover et al. 1979). For example, schools with high expectations for student achievement and schoolwide recognition for academic success can be more effective than schools without this climate, especially in large schools with predominantly disadvantaged student populations. The social climate may affect mental health as well (Rutter et al. 1979); for example, high-conflict schools have been shown to produce an increase in the severity of externalizing symptoms in their students (Hoglund and Leadbeater 2004; Kasen et al. 1990).

Connectedness

Perceptions of a positive school climate have been strongly associated with a sense of connectedness to the school—that is, the sense of bonding and commitment a student feels as a result of perceived caring from teachers and peers (Comer 1980; Thompson et al. 2006). School connectedness has been shown to predict a variety of positive health outcomes, including higher levels of emotional well-being, less substance abuse, less aggression and victimization, better health, decreased levels of suicidal ideation, decreased depressive symptoms, and decreased deviant behavior and teen pregnancy (Blum et al. 2002; Bond et al. 2007; Bonny et al. 2000; Catalano et al. 2004; Eccles et al.

1997; Jacobson and Rowe 1999; McNeely and Falci 2004; Resnick et al. 1997; Wilson 2004). Connectedness also has been shown to exert protective effects in the context of a negative school climate; that is, highly connected students in either positive or negative school climates engage in fewer risky behaviors (Wilson 2004). The theoretical basis for these associations lies in attachment, control, and social development theories. Attachment theory suggests that positive interactions between a child and caregivers build the foundation for bonding. Control theory (Hirschi 1969) postulates that bonding and resultant commitment to caring adults create informal controls that reduce problem behaviors. Social development theory (Catalano and Hawkins 1996) suggests that children are socialized through perceived opportunities for and development of skills for appropriate interactions, practice in appropriate interactions, and perceived rewards for appropriate interactions. Once bonding and commitment to school are established through socialization, these factors inhibit behavior inconsistent with the norms and values of the school.

Personnel

Understanding the roles of school personnel is necessary to develop collaborative relationships and make effective use of the limited resources available in schools. Teachers have the most extensive involvement with students, providing instruction approximately 6 hours per day to approximately 25 students at the elementary level and six to eight times that many at higher grade levels. Special education teachers have received training for and are credentialed to provide alternative instruction to smaller groups of students with a variety of disabilities (e.g., learning, language, developmental, cognitive, physical). Aides often do not have advanced education or training but assist classroom teachers or individual students.

Student support staff typically are employed on a part-time basis and have narrowly defined responsibilities within the school. School psychologists primarily assess students for eligibility for special education services and develop individual education plans for eligible students as indicated. They also may have limited capacity to consult with teachers around classroom management techniques and to provide individual and/or group therapy to students. School social workers participate in special education assessments and program planning and have limited capacity to provide therapies to students and their families. They may address social problems in social skills groups.

The primary role of guidance counselors is to assist students in college or vocational planning, although they sometimes provide therapy to students.

School nurses address acute health needs of students and maintain health records. Speech therapists address communication difficulties individually with the student or in groups and may address social problems as well. Occupational therapists focus on skills of daily living and strategies for dealing with sensory integration difficulties.

School principals manage all services within their building, and superintendents manage and coordinate activities in all schools within a school district. Administrators report to a school board, which is elected in public schools and appointed in private, parochial, or charter schools. School boards generally are charged with fiscal responsibility for the schools in their purview, and as such, they can exert considerable influence over the allocation of funds and resources for external consultants and programs.

In public schools, the special education administration is responsible for implementing the state's interpretation of the federal educational rights legislation, as delineated in the state's administrative or school code. Special education administrators and school administrators may have competing agendas because special education administrators often are responsible for determining the special education needs of students, whereas school administrators may be concerned about finding adequate resources to meet those needs.

Educational Rights of Students With Mental Disabilities

The foundation for all legislation pertaining to the educational rights of children with disabilities, including mental disabilities, rests in the Fourteenth Amendment to the U.S. Constitution, which prohibits discrimination through its equal protection clause. Despite this federal protection, through the first half of the twentieth century, many states either completely excluded children with disabilities from public school systems and placed them in institutions or relegated them to segregated classes in schools where they received little attention. The U.S. Supreme Court decision in *Brown v. Board of Education* (1954) rectified this inequity, asserting that education is a "right that must be made available to all on equal terms." Throughout the next four decades, the U.S. Congress took steps to end discrimination in schools against children with disabilities, guided by the principle that all such children must receive a free and appropriate public education in the least restrictive environment.

Americans With Disabilities Act and Section 504 of the Rehabilitation Act

The Americans With Disabilities Act (ADA) prohibits the denial of educational services to students with disabilities and prohibits discrimination against all such students once enrolled. If parents suspect their child has a disability, they can request an evaluation to see what accommodations might be helpful. Accommodations are environmental changes designed to overcome impediments to learning posed by the disability. Accommodations can be formalized in a written 504 Plan. This type of plan derives from Section 504 of the Rehabilitation Act of 1973, which mandates inclusion without discrimination for any person who has a "physical or mental impairment that substantially limits a major life activity." Typical accommodations relevant to common psychiatric disorders are presented in Table 63–1. A behavioral intervention plan (BIP) also can be written into a 504 Plan for students with disruptive behavior. A BIP derives from the findings of a functional behavioral assessment, which identifies the disruptive behaviors with their precipitants, functions, and settings. The BIP specifies 1) behavioral goals based on functional alternatives to disruptive behaviors and 2) behavioral interventions designed to help the student achieve the behavioral goals. Table 63–2 contains a sample functional behavioral assessment and BIP.

Individuals With Disabilities Education Act

The Education for All Handicapped Children Act (EAHCA; 1975) mandated the provision of special education and related services to meet the unique needs of children with physical or mental disabilities. Although Section 504 had established the principle of educational inclusion on civil rights grounds, for the first time the EAHCA provided federal funds to support the efforts of states to develop individualized special education programs. A number of amendments have been made to the EAHCA since its passage. Whereas EAHCA had applied only to children between 6 and 21 years old, initial amendments extended the protections to children younger than age 6 years. Subsequent amendments expanded the list of protected disabilities, specifically defined special education and related services, and increased early intervention services for young children. The most recent amendments provide for increased related services, delineate specific guidelines for school-based discipline of children with disabilities, and expand parental rights in the special education process. There can be considerable local variation in the interpretation of the federal educational rights legislation.

According to the provisions of the Individuals With Disabilities Education Act (IDEA), a child is eligible for special education services if he or she meets criteria for one or more categories of disability (Table 63–3) and if the disability substantially interferes with his or her educational progress. States have a responsibility to actively "find" children with suspected disabilities, who can be identified by their parents, by teachers or other professionals, or through school-based global screening (e.g., vision/hearing tests, group achievement tests). A number of psychiatric disorders correspond to IDEA disability designations (see Table 63–3).

A child with a suspected disability should undergo a special education evaluation to determine his or her eligibility for special education services. A special education evaluation is a comprehensive individual analysis of all suspected areas of disability conducted by a multidisciplinary team of school-based professionals (Table 63–4). The request for a special education evaluation should be made in writing and may specify the reasons for the request (e.g., child is performing below grade level academically or is having attention, behavioral, social, emotional, developmental, or communication problems). Although requests from parents or professionals outside the school do not guarantee an evaluation, the "child find" requirement makes it difficult for a school to refuse such a request. If the school does refuse, then parents have the right to appeal the decision (Table 63–5).

If the school conducts a special education evaluation, then it must be completed within a specified time period (the federal guideline is 60 working days). When the evaluation has been completed, the school-based team will schedule an eligibility meeting to present the findings to the parents. If there is disagreement about the findings from the evaluation, then the parents may obtain an independent evaluation to present as evidence during any of the various appeal

TABLE 63–1. Typical classroom accommodations for students with mental health problems

Mental health problem	Examples of accommodations
Inattention/hyperactivity/ impulsivity	Provide preferential seating
	Minimize distractions
	Establish work/play/work routine
	Establish time-to-completion goals
	Use visual/graphic organizers
	Provide verbal and visual cues to stay on task
	Assign a study/monitoring partner
	Use small-group instruction
	Simplify and repeat directions; give concrete examples
	Have student repeat directions and ask clarifying questions
	Vary routine tasks to increase novelty
	Organize student's workspace
	Allow for active modes of responding
	Plan for transitions by posting schedules
	Provide duplicate materials
	Affix materials to student's desk
	Remind student of materials needed for homework
	Remind student to turn in homework
	Reinforce double-checking
	Specify personal space
	Establish a waiting routine
Anger/oppositionality	Create behavioral intervention plan
	Model appropriate expressions of anger
	Allow self-time-outs for de-escalation
	Provide "redo" opportunities for misbehavior
	Establish clear rules and routines
	Provide immediate contingent rewards and consequences
Separation anxiety	Create desensitization schedule
	Provide desirable activity for student upon entering school
	Provide times during day to convey brief messages to family member
	Have parent send notes to school to be read as a reward for staying at school
Social anxiety	Allow student to observe others before performing task
	Provide practice in smaller or more relaxed setting
Generalized anxiety	Provide progressive mastery experiences
	Help student examine other perspectives
	Provide student with competing responses to negative thoughts
Communication problems	Obtain student's full attention before giving verbal instruction
	Speak in short, simple, and positively phrased sentences
	Pause between sentences

TABLE 63–1. Typical classroom accommodations for students with mental health problems *(continued)*

Mental health problem	Examples of accommodations
Communication problems *(continued)*	Allow sufficient time for the student to formulate a response while maintaining eye contact, and restate response
	Provide cloze phrases (e.g., "You have a fork, but for ice cream, you need a _____.")
	Offer choices verbally and visually (e.g., "Would you like the pen or pencil?")
	Respond promptly to requests that are stated verbally
	Model verbal requests for incomplete communication attempts
	Explicitly model and encourage use of pragmatic language skills (e.g., greetings, turn- and leave-taking)
	Positively reinforce appropriate use of eye contact during verbal exchanges
	Maintain consistent expectations for communication behaviors, and reinforce frequently with verbal praise
Pervasive developmental disorder	Provide autism consultant to teacher
	Provide classroom aide for student
Social interaction problems	Pair student with a buddy to model social skills
	Teach social skills incrementally
	Provide explicit guidance about making and keeping friends
Sensory processing problems	Minimize adverse sensory inputs

options that are available for conflict resolution (see Table 63–5).

If the findings from the special education evaluation indicate that the child has a disability and would benefit from special education, the school-based team will develop a written individualized education program (IEP) for the child in collaboration with his or her parents (Table 63–6). In addition to special education (i.e., instructional) services, the IEP may specify relevant modifications and accommodations and/or related services, as well as the setting in which they will be provided (Table 63–7). Specific accommodations (e.g., environmental changes designed to overcome impediments to learning posed by the disability) and/or related services (e.g., noninstructional services required to assist a child with a disability to benefit from special education) may be recommended for inclusion in the IEP. Modifications (e.g., curricular changes that can reduce learning expectations) should only be recommended with caution, as they may have the unintended consequence of reducing the child's opportunity to learn critical instructional content. According to the provisions of IDEA, the educational setting must be both appropriate to the child's needs and least restrictive of his or her interactions with peers without

disabilities. If the parents disagree with the educational program proposed in the IEP, then they can appeal as outlined previously. The child remains in the current placement until the disagreement is resolved.

The IEP is reviewed and revised annually; however, if the parents believe that the child is not progressing adequately, they may request an IEP review at any time to consider changes in services. Every 3 years, a comprehensive reevaluation is conducted by the school-based team to determine whether the child continues to meet eligibility criteria for special education services and what services should be provided.

Children with an IEP are afforded special disciplinary considerations. For example, children with an attention or tic disorder may not be able to sit still or quietly. Children whose disruptive behavior is a manifestation of their disability should have a BIP (see Table 63–2) written into their IEP, with the goal of preventing suspensions or expulsions. If the number of consecutive days of suspension exceeds 10 in a given school year or if more than 10 nonconsecutive days of suspension constitute a pattern, then a manifestation determination review (MDR) must be conducted by the school to determine whether the behavior resulting in the suspensions was related to the child's dis-

TABLE 63–2. Functional behavioral assessment and behavioral intervention plan for disruptive behavior

Functional behavioral assessment

Define behavior (physical aggression)

Describe behavior (e.g., Brian pushes, hits, trips other students, usually smaller students, especially when no adults are watching)

Describe antecedents (unstructured time in hallways, when unsupervised, when around students who provoke him)

Describe consequences (teacher and peer attention, verbal reprimand, after-school detention, in-school suspension)

Hypothesize function of behavior (power seeking, expression of anger, retribution)

Related information (low grades, few friends, disrupted family life)

Behavioral intervention plan

Specify goal (e.g., Brian will decrease aggressive incidents toward peers)

Specify interventions

   Remediate skills deficits (model, practice, and reinforce the following: anger recognition and management skills, problem-solving skills, communication skills, friendship skills, personal space skills)

   Remediate performance deficits (teach importance of personal safety, provide rewards [praise, tokens, privileges] for control of aggression)

   Manipulate antecedents (pair with adult in hallways, monitor and intervene with provocations)

   Provide other supports (skill-building services from school social worker, speech pathologist; daily home-school report card)

Specify persons responsible (teachers, social worker, speech pathologist)

Evaluate outcome (criterion: no fighting in next 6 weeks)

ability. If the behavior was related to the child's disability, then the child may not be excluded for more than 10 days and the IEP and BIP must be revised to address the behavior problem. If the behavior was not related to the child's disability, the child may be excluded for more than 10 days, provided that he or she receives a free and appropriate public education during the removal period. The IEP must be revised to document this change in services. If the parents disagree with the decision of the MDR, then they may appeal the decision. Children suspected of having disabilities who become subject to discipline before they have been evaluated for special education services are entitled to the same protections as children already found eligible.

A student with a disability may be expelled and transferred to a temporary alternative placement under several conditions: 1) if the student carries a weapon to school or a school function; possesses, uses, or sells illegal drugs or controlled substances at school or a school function; or has inflicted serious bodily injury on another person while at school or a school function; 2) if the hearing officer determines that maintaining the current placement is substantially likely to result in injury to the child or others; and 3) if the student commits vi-

olations of school policies other than the above if students without disabilities are subject to the same disciplinary measures.

Interventions in the School Setting

Preventive Interventions

Universal Prevention Programs

Universal prevention programs are targeted at the general population of students and can be general or specific in content (as delineated below). A listing of effective school-based universal prevention programs can be found in *Safe and Sound: An Educational Leader's Guide to Evidence-Based Social and Emotional Learning (SEL) Programs* (Collaborative for Academic, Social, and Emotional Learning 2003); in *Teen Risk-Taking: Promising Programs and Approaches* (Eisen et al. 2000); and at the Web site for the National Registry of Evidence-Based Programs and Practices, http://www.nrepp.samhsa.gov.

TABLE 63–3. Individuals With Disabilities Education Act (IDEA) disability designations and examples of corresponding psychiatric disorders

IDEA	Diagnostic and Statistical Manual of Mental Disorders (DSM)
Autism	Pervasive developmental disorders
Deaf-blindness	N/A
Deafness	N/A
Emotional disturbance[a]	Mood, anxiety, behavior, somatization, psychotic, eating, and elimination disorders
Hearing impairment	N/A
Mental retardation	Mental retardation
Multiple disabilities	N/A
Orthopedic impairment	N/A
Other health impairment[b]	Attention-deficit/hyperactivity disorder, sensory processing difficulties
Specific learning disability	Disorders of reading, mathematics, written expression
Speech-language impairment	Communication disorders
Traumatic brain injury	N/A
Visual impairment	N/A

[a]One or more of the following characteristics that are exhibited to a marked degree over an extended period of time that adversely affect a child's educational performance: 1) an inability to learn that cannot be explained by intellectual, sensory, or health factors; 2) an inability to build or maintain satisfactory interpersonal relationships with peers and teachers; 3) inappropriate types of behavior or emotions under normal circumstances; 4) a pervasive mood of unhappiness or depression; or 5) a tendency to develop physical symptoms or fears associated with personal or school problems. The term does not apply to children who are socially maladjusted, unless it is determined that they have an emotional disturbance.
[b]An acute or chronic health problem that results in limited alertness with respect to the educational environment and adversely affects a child's educational experience.

TABLE 63–4. Typical components of a special education evaluation

Usual components

Cognitive abilities

Communication abilities

Academic performance

Social/emotional status

Medical history/current health status

Vision/hearing screenings

Motor abilities

Additional components as indicated

Intelligence testing

Speech/language testing

Achievement testing

Neuropsychological testing

Physical examination

Occupational therapy evaluation

Physical therapy evaluation

Psychiatric assessment

General Prevention Programs.

Social-emotional skills. Key social-emotional skills include self-awareness, self-regulation, interpersonal skills, and decision making (Elias et al. 2006). A large body of evidence links social-emotional competencies to improved school-related attitudes (e.g., motivation, connectedness to school), behaviors (e.g., attendance, disciplinary actions), and performance (e.g., grades, test scores, graduation rates), as well as to reduction in risky behaviors and improved mental health (Zins et al. 2004).

Catalano et al. (2002) examined a database of 161 social-emotional skills curricula and ultimately designated 22 school-based programs as effective. Favorable results included improvements in interpersonal skills, quality of peer and adult relationships, and academic achievement, as well as reductions in problem behaviors such as school misbehavior and truancy, alcohol and drug use, high-risk sexual behavior, and violence and aggression.

School connectedness. Two exemplary examples of school connectedness curricula are the Seattle Social Development Project (SSDP) and the Gatehouse

TABLE 63–5. Typical appeal options for Individuals With Disabilities Education Act (IDEA) conflict resolution

Discuss the issue informally with the school staff, principal, superintendent, and/or director of special education.

File a written complaint with the state board of education. A full investigation must follow. If the parent disagrees with the findings of the investigation, then he or she can request a review by the U.S. Department of Education.

Request impartial mediation with a trained mediator appointed at no cost by the state board of education.

Request a due process hearing with a hearing officer appointed by the state board of education. The parent has the right to legal counsel.

Appeal to a court of law. The court may award attorneys' fees should the parent prevail in the decision.

Project. The SSDP (Catalano et al. 2004; Hawkins et al. 2008) targeted elementary school students and focused on teacher training, child skill development, and parent training. By twelfth grade, students in the intervention condition reported more school commitment, school attachment, and school achievement; fewer disciplinary actions; and lower levels of high alcohol use, violence, and risky sexual behavior. By age 27, adults who had participated in the intervention as students reported better educational and economic attainment, mental health, and sexual health. The Gatehouse Project (Bond et al. 2004) targeted high school students and focused on developing cognitive and interpersonal skills and creating an environment that enhanced connectedness. By tenth grade, students with good school and social connectedness were less likely to experience mental health problems, less likely to be involved in risky behaviors, and more likely to have good educational outcomes (Bond et al. 2007).

Mental health. Durlak and Wells (1997) used a meta-analysis to examine 177 primary prevention programs designed to prevent behavioral and social problems in young people, primarily in school settings. The findings indicated favorable effects on internalizing and externalizing behaviors greater in magnitude than many other established treatment approaches in medicine and the social sciences. Interventions using behavioral approaches produced larger effects than those using nonbehavioral approaches. Greenberg et al. (2001) reviewed more than 130 prevention programs for school-age children and concluded that multiyear programs are more likely to produce enduring benefits; programs that focus on the individual, family, and school are more effective than those that focus solely on the child; the school climate should be a central focus of intervention; and success is enhanced by combining emphases on changing students', teachers' and families' behavior, home-school relationships, and neighborhood support.

Specific Prevention Programs.

Suicide. According to a Cochrane Library review of school-based suicide prevention curricula targeted at general populations of students (Guo and Harstall 2002), there is insufficient evidence to either support or refute these programs. A subsequent review (Gould et al. 2003) went beyond curricula to examine the effects of other approaches to suicide prevention and intervention. The authors concluded that screening for suicidality is fraught with problems related to low specificity of the screening instrument, poor acceptability among school administrators, and paucity of referral sites; gatekeeper training is effective in improving skills among school personnel and is highly acceptable to administrators but has not been shown to prevent suicide; peer helpers have not been shown to be either efficacious or safe; and postvention is promising but underinvestigated.

Since the publication of that review, one study (Aseltine and DeMartino 2004) has shown some promise. The Signs of Suicide prevention program combines a curriculum to raise awareness of suicide with a brief screening for depression and other risk factors associated with suicide. The curriculum promotes the concept that suicide is directly related to mental illness, typically depression, and is not a normal reaction to stress. Students are taught to recognize the signs of suicide and depression in themselves and others, and they are taught the specific action steps necessary for responding to those signs. Evaluation of this program in a randomized, controlled, posttest-only design among high school students demonstrated significantly lower rates of suicide attempts and greater knowledge and more adaptive attitudes about depression and suicide among students in the intervention group.

Aggressive/disruptive behavior. A number of school-based programs targeting the prevention of aggressive and disruptive behaviors have been implemented and evaluated (e.g., Bauer et al. 2007; Botvin et

TABLE 63–6. Typical components and related services of an individualized education program

Usual components	Comments
Present level of educational performance	Can include social/emotional/behavioral performance
Educational goals and objectives with measurable benchmarks	Can include social/emotional/behavioral goals and with measurable benchmarks
Educational modifications and accommodations	See Table 63–1
Special education	Should be of sufficient intensity to meet educational goals
Placement and participation specifications	Placement should be least restrictive setting; mental health problems may preclude participation in standardized testing
Transition services planning	Posteducational planning process should consider student's mental health needs
Transfer of rights planning	Student must be apprised of rights when reaching age of majority

Related services as indicated	Comments
Adapted physical education	—
Assistive technology	Can include keyboarding devices for communication or motor impaired students
Audiology	—
Behavioral intervention plan	See Table 63–2
Counseling services	For transition or transfer of rights planning
Extended school-year services	To prevent academic regression in cognitively impaired students
Home-based support	—
Medical services	—
Occupational therapy	Can include training in penmanship, activities of daily living; may also include special cushions, devices, or techniques to address sensory sensitivities
Orientation/mobility services	—
Parent counseling/training	To enhance parent-teacher collaboration
Physical therapy	Can include development of gross and fine motor skills
Psychological services	For specialized testing
Recreation	To enhance social skills
School health services	For medication administration, vital sign or other checks, nutrition services
School social work services	For individual, group, or family therapy
Speech/language services	For testing and therapy (pragmatics as well as articulation)
Transportation services	For students incapable of using school bus or public transportation

al. 2006; Cooke et al. 2007; Dolan et al. 1989; Durant et al. 2001; Flannery et al. 2003; Fraser et al. 2005; Grossman et al. 1997; Ialongo et al. 2001; Twemlow et al. 2001; van Lier et al. 2004). These programs typically targeted elementary school students, and the curricula converge in their focus on problem-solving, communi-cation, and conflict resolution skills; appropriate expression of anger; and empathy. Although outcomes from these programs have been mixed, some studies have demonstrated favorable outcomes in aggressive behaviors and discipline referrals. According to Dusenbury et al. (1997), the most effective conflict resolu-

TABLE 63–7. Typical educational placement options (least to most restrictive)

Regular classroom

Regular classroom with consultative services to teacher

Regular classroom with modifications/ accommodations/supports

Regular classroom with pull-out resource services

Special education classroom with some pull-out regular education

Special education classroom

Special (therapeutic) school

Home/hospital services

tion programs teach students how to manage anger, control aggressive responses, understand how conflict is generated, and avoid or diffuse potentially violent confrontations.

Substance use.   According to a recent Cochrane Library review (Faggiano et al. 2005) of school-based substance use prevention curricula, skill-based programs appear to be effective in deterring early-stage drug use. In contrast, another Cochrane Library review (Thomas and Perera 2006) of school-based cigarette smoking prevention curricula concluded that there is little strong evidence that such programs are effective in the long-term in preventing smoking initiation. Tobler et al. (2000) classified 207 drug prevention programs as either noninteractive (knowledge/ affective/decision making/values) or interactive (social influences/life skills) and found that noninteractive approaches have minimal impact in comparison to interactive approaches. Greater benefits were achieved by interactive approaches that included training in refusal skills, goal setting, assertiveness, communication, and coping, as well as community, media, and family components. According to Dusenbury and Falco (1995), the most effective substance abuse prevention programs provide information about the risks associated with substance use, teach students how to refuse offers to experiment with substances, and correct misperceptions about the prevalence and acceptability of substance use.

Early/unprotected sexual activity.   A number of school-based programs targeting the prevention of early and/or unprotected sexual activity have been implemented and evaluated (e.g., Aarons et al. 2000; Aten et al. 2002; Lieberman et al. 2000; Siegel et al. 2001). Abstinence-oriented programs target the delay

of sexual debut by teaching students how to avoid situations in which they are vulnerable to having unintended intercourse and how to refuse offers to engage in intercourse if they do not feel ready. Safe sex-oriented programs target correct, consistent condom use by teaching students how to refuse intercourse if barrier protection is unavailable and how to use barrier protection correctly. Although the findings from program evaluations have been mixed, some studies have demonstrated favorable effects on the target outcomes, with abstinence-oriented programs having the greatest effect on sexually uninitiated students.

Depression.   A number of school-based programs targeting the prevention of depression have been implemented and evaluated (Clarke et al. 1993; Gillham et al. 2007; Merry et al. 2004; Pattison and Lynd-Stevenson 2001; Shochet et al. 2001; Spence at al. 2003, 2005). These curricula generally provide psychoeducation about the link among beliefs, feelings, and behaviors and about pessimistic cognitive styles, as well as training in cognitive restructuring, coping, problem-solving, communication, and relaxation skills. In a recent meta-analysis (Horowitz and Garber 2006) of the findings from 12 such programs, the effect size was found to be 0.12 and 0.02 at postintervention and follow-up, respectively, casting doubt on the effectiveness of these programs. This opinion was echoed in a recent qualitative review (Spence and Shortt 2007). Nonetheless, if these low-cost programs can prevent even a few cases of depression, they may ultimately prove to be cost-effective according to Horowitz and Garber (2006).

Multiple risk factors.   An innovative school-based program targeting multiple risky behaviors is the social development curriculum (Flay et al. 2004). This curriculum focuses on teaching students social competence skills necessary to manage situations in which high-risk behaviors occur. In a randomized trial of this curriculum among inner-city minority elementary school students and their teachers and parents, the curriculum was found to significantly reduce the rate of increase in violent behavior, provoking behavior, school delinquency, drug use, and recent sexual intercourse and condom use—however, all these effects were found only among boys. A more recent study (Beets et al. 2009) of a program (the Positive Action program) targeted at multiple risky behaviors found that the program, focused on social and character development in elementary school students, significantly reduced involvement in drug use, violence, and sexual activity among intervention students compared to controls.

Selective Prevention Programs

Selective prevention programs targeted students who are at high risk for developing emotional, behavioral, or social problems. School personnel must be able to identify vulnerable students, who can then be screened for underlying psychopathology and provided with appropriate services (Mattison 2000). Specially trained teachers, social workers, guidance counselors, and nurses can play key roles in this gatekeeping process. High-risk students fall into several categories: students who are performing poorly in school because of excessive absenteeism, frequent referrals for disciplinary actions, or academic failure; students who are engaging in multiple risky behaviors; and students who are exposed to psychosocial adversity. Undetected psychiatric disorders often underlie the overt presentation in high-risk students (reviewed in Mattison 2000). Thus, students who are habitually absent often have anxiety, mood, or conduct disorders. Students who are repeatedly referred for disciplinary actions often have high rates of externalizing psychopathology and learning or language disorders. Students who are failing academically often have diminished cognitive and/or attention abilities, learning or language disorders, or behavioral problems. Students who are involved in risky behaviors or are exposed to adverse psychosocial circumstances often have undetected mood, anxiety, and disruptive behavior or adjustment disorders.

Screening

Consulting psychiatrists can advise school personnel regarding the use of appropriate rating scales to screen for symptomatic students (Weist et al. 2007). Rating scales can be administered universally, for example, to entire populations of older students to screen for depression (e.g., Clarke et al. 1995; Shaffer et al. 2004), suicidality (e.g., Shaffer et al. 2004), anxiety (e.g., Chemtob et al. 2002; March et al. 1998; Masia-Warner et al. 2005), or involvement in risky behaviors (Vaughan et al. 1996) or to teachers of entire populations of younger students to screen for attention or disruptive behavior problems (e.g., Casat et al. 1999). Universal administrations of rating scales generate a substantial service burden, however, because resources must be expended to follow up with students who screen "positively." Alternatively, rating scales can be used selectively with high-risk students who have been identified by school personnel. This approach generates a smaller service burden, but students whose problems are covert may be missed. In any case, several protocols should be in place before the implementation of a screening program: to train gatekeepers to understand and appropriately use the rating scales; to obtain parental consent and to notify parents of screening results; to protect the confidentiality of students' responses; to initiate appropriate school-based services if indicated; and to provide appropriate, timely, and convenient linkages to external service providers for students in need of additional assessment.

Indicated Prevention Programs

Indicated prevention programs targeted students who exhibit symptoms of emotional, behavioral, or social problems but do not meet the full diagnostic criteria for a specific disorder. Most of the programs of this type have targeted students with symptoms of aggression, depression, anxiety, or trauma and were designed for delivery in group settings by trained school personnel in collaboration with clinicians. Only a small number of such programs have been rigorously evaluated.

The largest body of evidence pertains to school-based violence prevention programs for aggressive students (Conduct Problems Prevention Group 2004; Eddy et al. 2003; Lochman and Wells 2004; Tremblay et al. 1995). A Cochrane Library review (Mytton et al. 2006) of randomized controlled trials of these programs suggested that they appear to produce meaningful reductions in aggressive and violent behaviors, especially when delivered to mixed-gender groups. According to the Conduct Problems Prevention Group (2004), the most effective programs have multiple components that address parent, youth, and environmental processes that contribute to aggressive behavior. Their Fast Track program is an example of a multicomponent program, as it targets poor parenting practices, deficient social problem-solving and emotional coping skills, poor peer relations, weak academic skills, disruptive classroom environments, and poor home-school relations. Despite the comprehensiveness of this approach, by the end of elementary school, the program had a significant influence on conduct problems in the home and community, but no effect on conduct problems at school (Conduct Problems Prevention Group 2004).

The evidence of the effectiveness of programs targeting mood, anxiety, or trauma symptoms is more limited. Only a few effective programs targeting symptoms of depression have been reported. In a recent meta-analysis of the findings from eight such programs, Horowitz and Garber (2006) found the effect size to be 0.18 and 0.25 at postintervention and follow-up, respectively, suggesting the promise of these programs in improving subsyndromal depression. Two programs found to be effective are the Coping With Stress course for high school students (Clarke et al. 1995) and the Depression Prevention Program for elementary school students (Gillham et al. 1995). Both programs focused on helping students develop cognitive skills to identify and challenge negative or irrational thoughts related to depressed mood. At follow-up, the Coping With Stress course was found to significantly reduce the occurrence of major depression and dysthymia, and the Depression Prevention Program was found to significantly reduce depressive symptoms among students receiving the program compared to those in control groups.

An effective program targeting elementary school students with symptoms of anxiety, as well as students meeting the full diagnostic criteria for anxiety disorders, is the Coping Koala Program (Dadds et al. 1997, 1999). The program focuses on relaxation exercises, cognitive restructuring, exposure, and contingent rewards. At both 6-month and 2-year follow-up, reductions were observed in the proportion of intervention subjects meeting diagnostic criteria for anxiety disorders as compared with control subjects.

The effects of indicated programs targeting elementary school students exposed to trauma were examined by Chemtob et al. (2002), Kataoka et al. (2003), and Stein et al. (2003). The programs focused on educating students about common reactions to trauma, restoring a sense of safety, grieving losses, managing anxiety, adaptively expressing anger, challenging negative thoughts, and achieving closure. After treatment, students in these studies reported significant reductions in trauma-related symptom severity.

An innovative indicated prevention program targeted elementary school students with concurrent internalizing and externalizing symptoms was evaluated by Weiss et al. (2003). The yearlong program comprised individual, small group, and classroom sessions with students, plus sessions with parents and teachers. The student sessions focused on developing social, communication, affect recognition/expression, self-monitoring, relaxation, and cognitive reattribution skills. The parent and teacher sessions focused on using appropriate praise and punishment, improving adult-child communication, strengthening the adult-child relationship, and supporting the students in skills development. At follow-up, intervention subjects exhibited greater improvement in both internalizing and externalizing symptoms than did control subjects.

Clinical Interventions

Clinical interventions target students who are found on clinical assessment to meet diagnostic criteria for specific psychiatric disorders. The literature regarding effective programs is limited, focusing primarily on the treatment of attention-deficit/hyperactivity disorder (ADHD).

The effects of school-based, nonpharmacological interventions for the treatment of ADHD were examined by DuPaul and Eckert (1997) in a meta-analysis of 63 outcome studies. They concluded that contingency management and tutoring were more effective than cognitive-behavioral strategies in reducing ADHD behaviors and enhancing academic performance.

In addition to the results from the Coping Koala Program noted above, findings from two pilot studies (Ginsburg and Drake 2002; March et al. 1998) and one randomized controlled trial (Masia-Warner et al. 2005) also suggest the effectiveness of school-based programs for the treatment of anxiety disorders. The pilot programs were designed for delivery in group settings by trained school personnel in collaboration with clinicians. Both of the programs focused on relaxation exercises, cognitive restructuring, and gradual exposure, and both were associated at follow-up with reductions in the proportions of subjects meeting diagnostic criteria for their primary anxiety disorder. The randomized trial targeted high school students with impairing social anxiety disorder. Twelve clinician-delivered group sessions focused on psychoeducation, realistic thinking, social skills, exposure, and relapse prevention. These sessions were supplemented by individual meetings to identify individual treatment goals, parent and teacher psychoeducation meetings, peer assistance to support learned skills, and social events to practice learned skills. At 9-month follow-up, students in the intervention group demonstrated significantly greater reductions than controls in social anxiety and avoidance, as well as significantly improved overall functioning. In addition, 67% of treated subjects, compared to 6% of controls, no longer met criteria for social phobia following treatment.

A study (Mufson et al. 2004) suggested the potential of school-based programs for the treatment of depression. In this study, high school students with major depressive disorder, dysthymia, depressive disorder not otherwise specified, or adjustment disorder with depressed mood received 12 sessions of interpersonal therapy delivered by trained school-based health center clinicians. The therapy focused on developing strategies for dealing with problems in grief, role dispute, role transition, and interpersonal deficit domains. Compared to treatment as usual, students receiving this treatment showed greater symptom reduction and improvement in overall functioning.

Crisis Interventions

A crisis at school occurs when the integrity of the school environment is threatened by an event to such a degree that the school's internal resources are deemed insufficient or exhausted (Arroyo 2001). Events that may precipitate a crisis include the suicide of a student or school staff member, a natural disaster, or violence that directly affects the school community.

The primary goals when creating a plan to effectively manage a crisis are to help the school resume a normal routine as quickly as possible and address the needs of students and staff beyond the immediate crisis period. Successful plans involve collaborations with organizations beyond the school, such as departments of health and mental health, law enforcement agencies, and other organizations skilled in crisis response. Crisis response plans should be highly organized and centralized in the school or district administrative office. The roles, responsibilities, and required training of both school staff and other collaborators should be specified in the plan, and the plan should contain a framework for the coordination of and communication with all of the collaborative entities. It also should contain guidelines for interacting with the media.

Immediately after a crisis, interventions should focus on providing 1) social and emotional support to students and school personnel and 2) information about normal responses to traumatic events to school personnel, parents, and other caretaking adults. Teachers can be provided with guidelines about developmentally appropriate ways to discuss the events with students and how to model appropriate coping strategies. After the immediate crisis period, school personnel should be taught to recognize the signs and symptoms of trauma-related disorders in students, and arrangements should be made for the appropriate treatment or referral of students or staff.

Research Directions

Important questions for research in school-based intervention are as follows:

- **Theoretical models**—Which theoretical models most powerfully and parsimoniously predict students' connectedness to school, social-emotional competence, and avoidance of risky behaviors? What are the interrelationships among these constructs themselves, as well as among these constructs, mental health, and academic success?
- **Services**—Which models are most feasible, desirable, and effective in increasing students' access to mental health services in the school setting? What factors predict effective utilization of school-based mental health services? What are the most important barriers to the effective utilization of school-based mental health services?
- **Outcomes**—Which preventive, early identification, and clinical interventions are most feasible, desirable, and effective in the school setting? Which program components contribute most powerfully to favorable outcomes? What factors mediate and moderate intervention effectiveness? Do effective preventive, early identification, and clinical interventions enhance academic success? Are school-based preventive, early identification, and clinical interventions cost-effective? How can feasible, desirable, and effective interventions be widely disseminated? What are the barriers to the widespread adoption of preventive, early identification, and clinical interventions in the school setting?

Useful Web Sites

The following are some useful Web sites on school-based interventions:

www.schoolpsychiatry.org
www.aboutourkids.org
http://idea.ed.gov
http://csmh.umaryland.edu
http://smhp.psych.ucla.edu

Summary Points

- The educational rights of children with mental disabilities are protected by federal law.

- Students with psychiatric disorders may be eligible for classroom accommodations, curricular modifications, special education, and related services to overcome impediments to learning imposed by their mental disabilities.

- There are effective school-based interventions for the promotion of social-emotional competency, school connectedness, and mental health.

- There are effective school-based interventions for the prevention of aggressive and/ or disruptive behavior, substance use, early or unprotected sexual activity, and multiple risky behaviors.

- There are effective school-based interventions for the treatment of subsyndromal and syndromal disruptive behavior, mood, anxiety, and posttraumatic stress disorders.

- Students with problems at school often have undetected, untreated psychiatric disorders.

- Students can be effectively screened with standardized rating scales for the presence of psychiatric disorders.

References

Aarons SJ, Jenkins RR, Raine TR, et al: Postponing sexual intercourse among urban junior high school students: a randomized controlled evaluation. J Adolesc Health 27:236–247, 2000

American Academy of Child and Adolescent Psychiatry: Practice parameter for psychiatric consultation to schools. J Am Acad Child Adolesc Psychiatry 44:1068–1084, 2005

American Academy of Pediatrics: Policy statement, school-based mental health services. Pediatrics 113:1839–1845, 2004

Arroyo W: School crisis consultation. Child Adolesc Psychiatry Clin N Am 10:55–66, 2001

Aseltine RH, DeMartino R: An outcome evaluation of the SOS suicide prevention program. Am J Public Health 94:446–451, 2004

Aten MJ, Siegel DM, Enaharo M, et al: Keeping middle school students abstinent: outcomes of a primary prevention intervention. J Adolesc Health 31:70–78, 2002

Atkins M, Adil J, Jackson M, et al: An ecological model for school-based mental health services, in 13th Annual Conference Proceedings: A System of Care for Children's Mental Health: Expanding the Research Base. Tampa, FL, University of South Florida, 2001, pp 119–122

Bauer NS, Lozano P, Rivara FP: The effectiveness of the Olweus bullying prevention program in public middle schools: a controlled trial. J Adolesc Health 40:266–274, 2007

Beets MW, Flay BR, Vuchinich S, et al: Use of a social and character development program to prevent substance use, violent behaviors, and sexual activity among elementary-school students in Hawaii. Am J Public Health 99: 1438–1445, 2009

Berkovitz IH: School consultation, in Handbook of Child and Adolescent Psychiatry, Vol 7. Edited by Noshpitz JD, Adams PL, Bleiberg E. New York, Wiley, 1998

Berkovitz IH (ed): School Consultation/Intervention: Child and Adolescent Psychiatric Clinics of North America. Philadelphia, PA, WB Saunders, 2001

Berlin IN: Psychiatry and the school, in Comprehensive Textbook of Psychiatry II. Edited by Freedman AM, Kaplan HI, Sadow BJ. Baltimore, MD, Williams & Wilkins, 1975, pp 2253–2255

Blum RW, McNeely CA, Rinehart PM: Improving the Odds: The Untapped Power of Schools to Improve the Health of Teens. Technical Report. Minneapolis, Center for Adolescent Health and Development, University of Minnesota, 2002

Bond L, Patton G, Glover S, et al: The gatehouse project: can a multilevel school intervention affect emotional well-being and health risk behaviors? J Epidemiol Community Health 58:997–1003, 2004

Bond L, Butler H, Thomas L, et al: Social and school connectedness in early secondary school as predictors of late teenage substance use, mental health, and academic outcomes. J Adolesc Health 40:357e9–357e18, 2007

Bonny AE, Britto MT, Klosterman BK, et al: School disconnectedness: identifying adolescents at risk. Pediatrics 106:1017–1021, 2000

Botvin GJ, Griffin KW, Nichols TD: Preventing youth violence and delinquency through a universal school-based prevention approach. Prev Sci 7:403–408, 2006

Brener ND, Martindale J, Weist MD: Mental health and social services: results from the school health policies and programs study 2000. J Sch Health 71:305–312, 2001

Brookover WB, Beady C, Flood P, et al: School Social Systems and Student Achievement: Schools Can Make a Difference. New York, Praeger, 1979

Brown v Board of Education of Topeka, 347 U.S. 483 (1954)

Caplan G: The Theory and Practice of Mental Health Consultation. New York, Basic Books, 1970

Casat CD, Norton HJ, Boyle-Whitesel M: Identification of elementary school children at risk for disruptive behavioral disturbance: validation of a combined screening method. J Am Acad Child Adolesc Psychiatry 38:1246–1253, 1999

Catalano RF, Hawkins JD: The social development model: a theory of antisocial behavior, in Delinquency and Crime: Current Theories. Edited by Hawkins JD. New York, Cambridge University Press, 1996, pp 149–197

Catalano RF, Berglund ML, Ryan JAM, et al: Positive youth development in the United States: research findings on evaluations of positive youth development programs. Prevention and Treatment 5, Article 15, 2002

Catalano RF, Haggerty KP, Oesterle S, et al: The importance of bonding to school for healthy development: findings from the social development research group. J Sch Health 74:252–261, 2004

Chemtob CM, Nakashima JP, Hamada RS: Psychosocial intervention for postdisaster trauma symptoms in elementary school children, a controlled community field study. Arch Pediatr Adolesc Med 156:211–216, 2002

Clarke GN, Hawkins W, Murphy M, et al: School-based primary prevention of depressive symptomatology in adolescents: findings from two studies. J Adolesc Res 8:183–204, 1993

Clarke GN, Hawkins W, Murphy M, et al: Targeted prevention of unipolar depressive disorder in an at-risk sample of high school adolescents: a randomized trial of a group cognitive intervention. J Am Acad Child Adolesc Psychiatry 34:312–321, 1995

Collaborative for Academic, Social, and Emotional Learning: Safe and Sound: An Educational Leader's Guide to Evidence-Based Social and Emotional Learning (SEL) Programs. Chicago, IL, 2003. Available at: http://www.casel.org/downloads/Safe%20and%20Sound/1A_Safe_&_Sound.pdf. Accessed June 18, 2009.

Comer JP: School Power: Implications of an Intervention Project. New York, Free Press, 1980

Comer JP: School consultation, in Psychiatry, Vol 2. Edited by Michels R, Cooper AM, Guze SB. Philadelphia, PA, Lippincott, 1992, pp 1–10

Conduct Problems Prevention Group: The effects of the fast track program on serious problem outcomes at the end of elementary school. J Clin Child Adolesc Psychol 33:650–661, 2004

Cooke MB, Ford J, Levine J, et al: The effects of city-wide implementation of "second step" on elementary school students' prosocial and aggressive behaviors. J Prim Prev 28:93–115, 2007

Dadds MR, Spence SH, Holland DE, et al: Prevention and early intervention for anxiety disorders: a controlled trial. J Consult Clin Psychol 65:627–635, 1997

Dadds MR, Spence SH, Holland DE, et al: Early intervention and prevention of anxiety disorders in children: results at 2-year follow-up. J Consult Clin Psychol 67:145–150, 1999

Diala CC, Mentaner C, Walrath C, et al: Racial/ethnic differences in attitudes toward seeking professional mental health services. Am J Public Health 91:805–807, 2002

Dolan LJ, Jaylan T, Werthamer L, et al: The Good Behavior Game Manual. Baltimore, MD, The Johns Hopkins Prevention Research Center, 1989

DuPaul GJ, Eckert TL: The effects of school-based interventions for attention-deficit/hyperactivity disorder: a meta-analysis. Sch Psychol Rev 26:5–27, 1997

Durant RH, Barkin S, Krowchuk DP: Evaluation of a peaceful conflict resolution and violence prevention curriculum for sixth-grade students. J Adolesc Health 28:386–393, 2001

Durlak JA, Wells AM: Primary prevention mental health programs for children and adolescents: a meta-analytic review. Am J Community Psychol 25:115–152, 1997

Dusenbury L, Falco M: Eleven components of effective drug abuse prevention curricula. J Sch Health 65:420–425, 1995

Dusenbury L, Falco M, Lake A, et al: Nine critical elements of promising violence prevention programs. J Sch Health 67:409–414, 1997

Eccles JS, Early D, Frasier K: The relation of connection, regulation, and support for autonomy to adolescents' functioning. J Adolesc Res 12:263–286, 1997

Eddy JM, Reid JB, Stoolmiller M, et al: Outcomes during middle school for an elementary school-based preventive intervention for conduct problems: follow-up results from a randomized trial. Behav Ther 34:535–552, 2003

Education for All Handicapped Children Act of 1975 (Pub. L. No. 94-142)

Eisen M, Pallitto C, Bradner C, et al: Teen Risk-Taking: Promising Programs and Approaches. Washington, DC, Urban Institute, 2000

Elias MJ, Arnold H: The Educator's Guide to Emotional Intelligence and Academic Achievement: Social-Emotional Learning in the Classroom. Thousand Oaks, CA, Corwin Press, 2006

Evans SW: Mental health services in schools: utilization, effectiveness and consent. Clin Psychol Rev 19:165–178, 1999

Faggiano F, Vigna-Taglianti FD, Versino E, et al: School-based prevention for illicit drugs' use. Cochrane Database Syst Rev 2:CD003020, 2005

Flaherty LT, Weist MD: School-based mental health services: the Baltimore models. Psychol Sch 36:379–389, 1999

Flannery DJ, Vazsonyi AT, Liau AK, et al: Initial behavior outcomes for the peacebuilders universal school-based violence prevention program. Dev Psychol 39:292–308, 2003

Flay BR, Graumlich S, Segawa E, et al: Effects of 2 prevention programs on high-risk behaviors among African American youth: a randomized trial. Arch Pediatr Adolesc Med 158:377–384, 2004

Fraser MW, Galinsky MJ, Smokowski PR, et al: Social information-processing skills training to promote social competence and prevent aggressive behavior. J Consult Clin Psychol 73:1045–1055, 2005

Gillham J, Reivich K, Jaycox L, et al: Prevention of depressive symptoms in school children: two-year follow-up. Psychol Sci 6:343–351, 1995

Gillham J, Reivich KJ, Freres DR, et al: School-based prevention of depressive symptoms: a randomized controlled study of the effectiveness and specificity of the Penn resiliency program. J Consult Clin Psychol 75:9–19, 2007

Ginsburg GS, Drake LK: School-based treatment for anxious African-American adolescents: a controlled pilot study. J Am Acad Child Adolesc Psychiatry 41:768–775, 2002

Gould MS, Greenberg T, Velting DM, et al: Youth suicide risk and preventive interventions: a review of the past 10 years. J Am Acad Child Adolesc Psychiatry 42:386–405, 2003

Greenberg MT, Domitrovich CE, Bumbarger B: The prevention of mental disorders in school-aged children: current state of the field. Prevention and Treatment 4, Article 1, 2001

Grossman DC, Neckerman HJ, Koepsell TD, et al: Effectiveness of a violence prevention curriculum among children in elementary school: a randomized controlled trial. JAMA 277:1605–1611, 1997

Guo B, Harstall C: Efficacy of suicide prevention programs for children and youth. Edmonton, Alberta, Canada: Alberta Heritage Foundation for Medical Research, 2002

Hawkins JD, Kosterman R, Catalano RF, et al: Effects of social development intervention in childhood 15 years later. Arch Pediatr Adolesc Med 162: 1133–1141, 2008

Hirschi T: Causes of Delinquency. Berkeley, University of California Press, 1969

Hoglund WL, Leadbeater BJ: The effects of family, school, and classroom ecologies on changes in children's social competence and emotional and behavioral problems in first grade. Dev Psychol 40:533–544, 2004

Horowitz JL, Garber J: The prevention of depressive symptoms in children and adolescents: a meta-analytic review. J Consult Clin Psychol 74:401–415, 2006

Ialongo N, Poduska J, Werthamer L, et al: The distal impact of two first-grade preventive interventions on conduct problems and disorder in early adolescence. J Emot Behav Disord 9:146–160, 2001

Jacobson KC, Rowe DC: Genetic and environmental influences on the relationships between family connectedness, school connectedness, and adolescent depressed mood: sex differences. Dev Psychol 35:926–939, 1999

Jennings J, Pearson G, Harris M: Implementing and maintaining school-based mental health services in a large, urban school district. J Sch Health 70:201–205, 2000

Kasen S, Johnson J, Cohen P: The impact of school emotional climate on student psychopathology. J Abnorm Child Psychol 18:165–177, 1990

Kataoka SH, Stein BD, Jaycox LH, et al: A school-based mental health program for traumatized Latino immigrant children. J Am Acad Child Adolesc Psychiatry 42:311–318, 2003

Lear JG, Gleicher HB, St. Germaine A, et al: Reorganizing health care for adolescents: the experience of the school-based adolescent health care program. J Adolesc Health 12:450–458, 1991

Libbey HP: Measuring student relationship to school: attachment, bonding, connectedness, and engagement. J Sch Health 74:274–283, 2004

Lieberman LD, Gray H, Wier M, et al: Long-term outcomes of an abstinence-based, small-group pregnancy prevention program in New York City schools. Fam Plann Perspect 32:237–245, 2000

Lochman JE, Wells KC: The coping power program for preadolescent aggressive boys and their parents: outcome effects at the one-year follow-up. J Consult Clin Psychol 72:571–578, 2004

March JS, Amaya-Jackson L, Murray MC, et al: Cognitive-behavioral psychotherapy for children and adolescents with posttraumatic stress disorder after a single-incident stressor. J Am Acad Child Adolesc Psychiatry 37:585–593, 1998

Masia-Warner C, Klein RG, Dent HC, et al: School-based intervention for adolescents with social anxiety disorder: results of a controlled study. J Abnorm Child Psychol 33:707–722, 2005

Mattison RE: School consultation: a review of research on issues unique to the school environment. J Am Acad Child Adolesc Psychiatry 39:402–413, 2000

McNeely C, Falci C: School connectedness and transitions into and out of health-risk behavior among adolescents: a comparison of social belonging and teacher support. J Sch Health 74:284–292, 2004

Merry S, McDowell H, Wild CJ, et al: A randomized placebo-controlled trial of a school-based depression prevention program. J Am Acad Child Adolesc Psychiatry 43:538–547, 2004

Mufson L, Dorta KP, Wickramaratne P, et al: A randomized effectiveness trial of interpersonal psychotherapy for depressed adolescents. Arch Gen Psychiatry 61:577–584, 2004

Mytton J, DiGuiseppi C, Gough D, et al: School-based secondary prevention programmes for preventing violence. Cochrane Database Syst Rev 3:CD004606, 2006

Nabors LA, Reynolds MW: Program evaluation activities: outcomes related to treatment for adolescents receiving school-based mental health services. Children's Services: Social Policy, Research, and Practice 3:175–189, 2000

National Assembly on School-Based Health Care: Creating Access to Care for Children and Youth: SBHC Census 1998–1999. Washington, DC, National Assembly on School-Based Health Care, 2000

Pattison C, Lynd-Stevenson RM: The prevention of depressive symptoms in children: immediate and long-term outcomes of a school-based program. Behav Change 18:92–102, 2001

President's New Freedom Commission on Mental Health: Achieving the Promise: Transforming Mental Health Care in America. Final Report. (DHHS Publ No SMA-03-3832.) Rockville, MD, U.S. Department of Health and Human Services, 2003

Rehabilitation Act of 1973. Pub. L. No. 93-112, 93rd Congress, H. R. 8070, September 26, 1973

Resnick MD, Bearman PS, Blum RW, et al: Protecting adolescents from harm: findings from the National Longitudinal Study of Adolescent Health. JAMA 278:823–832, 1997

Rutter M, Maughan B, Mortimore P, et al: Fifteen Thousand Hours: Secondary Schools and Their Effects on Children. Cambridge, MA, Harvard University Press, 1979

Shaffer D, Scott M, Wilcox H, et al: The Columbia suicide screen: validity and reliability of a screen for youth suicide and depression. J Am Acad Child Adolesc Psychiatry 43:71–79, 2004

Shochet IM, Dadds MR, Holland D, et al: The efficacy of a universal school-based program to prevent adolescent depression. J Clin Child Psychol 30:303–315, 2001

Siegel DM, Aten MJ, Enaharo M: Long-term effects of a middle school- and high school-based human immunodeficiency virus sexual risk prevention intervention. Arch Pediatr Adolesc Med 155:1117–1126, 2001

Spence SH, Shortt AL: Research review: can we justify the widespread dissemination of universal, school-based interventions for the prevention of depression among children and adolescents? J Child Psychol Psychiatry 48:526–542, 2007

Spence SH, Sheffield JK, Donovan CL: Preventing adolescent depression: an evaluation of the problem solving for life program. J Consult Clin Psychol 71:3–13, 2003

Spence SH, Sheffield JK, Donovan CL: Long-term outcome of a school-based, universal approach to prevention of depression in adolescents. J Consult Clin Psychol 73:160–167, 2005

Stein BD, Jaycox LH, Kataoka SH, et al: A mental health intervention for schoolchildren exposed to violence: a randomized controlled trial. JAMA 290:603–611, 2003

Taylor L, Adelman HS: Toward ending the marginalization and fragmentation of mental health in schools. J Sch Health 70:210–215, 2000

Thomas R, Perera R: School-based programmes for preventing smoking. Cochrane Database Syst Rev 3:CD001293, 2006

Thompson DR, Iachan R, Overpeck M, et al: School connectedness in the health behavior in school-aged children study: the role of student, school, and school neighborhood characteristics. J Sch Health 76:379–386, 2006

Tobler NS, Toona MR, Ochshorn P, et al: School-based adolescent drug prevention programs: 1998 meta-analysis. J Prim Prev 20:275–337, 2000

Tolan PH, Anton BS, Culbertson JL, et al: Developing Psychology's National Agenda for Children's Mental Health. Report of the APA Working Group on Children's Mental Health to the Board of Directors. Washington, DC, American Psychological Association, 2001

Tremblay RE, Pagani-Kurtz L, Masse LC, et al: A bi-modal preventive intervention for disruptive kindergarten boys: its impact through mid-adolescence. J Consult Clin Psychol 63:560–568, 1995

Twemlow SW, Fonagy P, Sacco FC, et al: Creating a peaceful school learning environment: a controlled study of an elementary school intervention to reduce violence. Am J Psychiatry 158:808–810, 2001

U.S. Department of Health and Human Services: Mental Health: A Report of the Surgeon General. Executive Summary. Rockville, MD, U.S. Department of Health and Human Services, Substance Abuse and Mental Health Services Administration, Center for Mental Health Services, National Institute of Health, National Institute of Mental Health, 1999

U.S. Public Health Service: Report of the Surgeon General's Conference on Children's Mental Health: A National Action Agenda. Rockville, MD, U.S. Department of Health and Human Services, Substance Abuse and Mental Health Services Administration, Center for Mental Health Services, National Institute of Health, National Institute of Mental Health, 2000

van Lier PAC, Muthen BO, van der Sar RM, et al: Preventing disruptive behavior in elementary schoolchildren: impact of a universal classroom-based intervention. J Consult Clin Psychol 72:467–478, 2004

Vaughan RD, McCarthy JF, Walter HJ, et al: The development, reliability, and validity of a risk factor screening survey for urban minority junior high school students. J Adolesc Health 19:171–178, 1996

Walter HJ, Vaughan RD, Armstrong B, et al: School-based health care for urban minority junior high school students. Arch Pediatr Adolesc Med 149:1221–1225, 1995

Walter HJ, Vaughan RD, Armstrong B, et al: Characteristics of users and non-users of health clinics in inner-city junior high schools. J Adolesc Health 18:344–348, 1996

Weare K: Promoting Mental, Emotional and Social Health: A Whole School Approach. London, Routledge, 2000

Weiss B, Harris V, Catron T, et al: Efficacy of the RECAP intervention program for children with concurrent internalizing and externalizing problems. J Consult Clin Psychol 71:364–374, 2003

Weist MD, Albus KE: Expanded school mental health: exploring program details and developing the research base. Behav Mod 28:463–471, 2004

Weist MD, Paskewitz DA, Warner BS, et al: Treatment outcome of school-based mental health services for urban teenagers. Community Ment Health J 32:149–157, 1996

Weist MD, Myers CP, Hastings E, et al: Psychosocial functioning of youth receiving mental health services in the schools versus community mental health centers. Community Ment Health J 35:69–81, 1999

Weist MD, Rubin M, Moore E, et al: Mental health screening in schools. J Sch Health 77:53–58, 2007

Wilson D: The interface of school climate and school connectedness and relationships with aggression and victimization. J Sch Health 74:293–299, 2004

Zins JE, Bloodworth MR, Weissberg RP, et al: The scientific base linking social and emotional learning to school success, in Building Academic Success on Social and Emotional Learning: What Does the Research Say? Edited by Zins JE, Weissberg RP, Wang MC, et al. New York, Teachers College Press, 2004, pp 3–22

Chapter 64

Collaborating With Primary Care

L. Read Sulik, M.D.
Jon Dennis, M.D., M.P.H.

Child and adolescent psychiatrists are in great demand in every community throughout the United States as the number of children and adolescents requiring access to care for mental health needs continues to increase, while the number of child and adolescent psychiatrists practicing in the United States has grown little in the last two decades. A recent report identifies great disparity across the United States of child psychiatrists available, with rural and poor populations clearly having the greatest shortage and therefore the worst access to care (Thomas and Holzer 2006). The shortage of child mental health professionals is a likely contributing factor to the Surgeon General's estimate that only 20% of the children with a mental illness obtain any care at all (U.S. Public Health Service 2000).

Due to very long waits to see a child and adolescent psychiatrist (or in some locales, barriers due to managed care), families are turning to primary care physicians (PCPs) for at least initial care for common mental

health problems—yet most pediatricians report that they do not feel prepared to address the psychosocial problems and mental health needs of their patients, citing inadequate training and experience as well as the lack of referral resources as the greatest barriers for providing mental health care in their clinics (Horwitz et al. 2007; Trude and Stoddard 2003). In recognition of these needs for further assistance, there has been an increased effort, particularly in the past several years, to provide tools for PCPs to improve their ability to identify, assess, diagnose, and treat mental illness and other psychosocial problems (Jellinek and Froehle 2002; Wolraich and Drotar 1996).

As pediatricians and family physicians become more involved in providing mental health services, protocols and algorithms for assessment and treatment will need to be further developed and implemented just as in other areas of medicine, such as asthma and diabetes management. Earlier identification and earlier intervention with implementation of evidence-based protocols for care should lead to improved clinical outcomes and reduced use of expensive inpatient hospitalization, emergency room visits, and out-of-home placements. Bringing mental health services into the primary care clinic in a more integrated manner improves access to care (Blount 1997; Connor et al. 2006; Jayabarathan 2004). PCPs can provide "primary" mental health care services, such as anticipatory guidance, mental health screening, earlier identification, and earlier intervention (Jellinek 1997).

We are in the midst of a global paradigm shift that is leading to the expanded role of the pediatrician and family physician in the delivery of mental health care to children (Gadit 2007; Rockman et al. 2004; Samy et al. 2007; Sved Williams et al. 2006; World Health Organization 2001). Treating mental health problems adequately in primary care settings requires knowledge, experience, and comfort in 1) recognition of signs and symptoms, 2) assessment, 3) appropriate use of psychotropic medications and indications, and 4) referral for psychotherapy and other treatment interventions. Without the assistance of child and adolescent psychiatrists in guiding appropriate responses of PCPs to new information on risks associated with medications (Rappaport et al. 2005), a widespread reduction in prescribing appropriately to those patients in need of treatment can lead to a resurgence of negative outcomes.

Expectations for the role of primary care in the mental health care of children include the following:

1. As part of the care of the well child and routine health maintenance, the PCP will provide anticipatory guidance to promote mental health and draw attention to early warning signs of mental health problems.
2. The PCP will screen for and identify signs, symptoms, and risks of mental health problems.
3. Mental health evidence-based assessment and diagnosis will be provided in the primary care setting by PCPs skilled in mental health diagnosis or in collaboration with collocated mental health care professionals.
4. Children and adolescents in need of mental health care will be able to receive evidence-based mental health treatment in the primary care clinic.
5. As part of evidence-based mental health treatment protocols, the PCP will be involved in follow-up care and monitoring for treatment effectiveness (symptom change and improvement in functioning).
6. The PCP will be able to monitor for patient safety (assessing for suicide risk) and for the safety of treatments prescribed (monitoring for adverse events associated with medications or other interventions).
7. The PCP will be part of a multidisciplinary team providing an integrated approach to the mental health care of the child.
8. The primary care clinic is the overall medical home as well as the mental health home for children and adolescents, where services involving various mental health and medical specialists can be coordinated.
9. The degree of collaboration between PCPs and child and adolescent psychiatrists and other mental health specialists exists on a continuum according to the level of acuity of the patient. This may range from the PCP primarily managing the mental health care of the child to the other end of the spectrum in more severely ill patients, where the mental health care is primarily managed by the mental health specialists.

How prepared are we for these emerging expectations? A 2004 survey of a random sampling of Fellows of the American Academy of Pediatrics would suggest that the PCP is not prepared. Many respondents indicated it was the pediatrician's responsibility to identify common mental health problems, such as attention-deficit/hyperactivity disorder (ADHD), anxiety, and depression, but far fewer reported that they actually do this in their practice (Horwitz et al. 2007). For instance, only 25% of respondents reported that they believe pediatricians should be managing depression in children and adolescents, and far fewer indicated that they actually do. Barriers to identifying, treating, and managing mental health problems in the primary care clinic included lack of training in identifying and in treating these problems and lack of confidence in their own skills in using counseling and medications. Finally, the lack of availability of referral services and the long waiting periods for referrals were also reported to significantly affect respondents' comfort levels.

With the increased expectations, PCPs must not only seek additional training and education to improve their own skill sets but must also regularly seek consultation from and work collaboratively with child and adolescent psychiatrists, psychologists, and other mental health professionals.

The roles of the child and adolescent psychiatrist must expand to include mentor, educator, consultant, and collaborator with PCPs. In order to be successful, the child and adolescent psychiatrist must concentrate on establishing relationships with colleagues in primary care, assisting PCPs in triaging and referring patients of higher levels of acuity, and helping PCPs to know which patients they should be able to manage and when and how to consult with a child and adolescent psychiatrist or other mental health professional. The child and adolescent psychiatrist must become much more aware of the culture and needs of the primary health care setting and have realistic expectations of what can and cannot be appropriately identified and treated in an outpatient clinic.

Understanding the Primary Care Clinic Setting

Case Example

Jack is a 13-year-old who was seen along with his mother in the pediatric clinic by Dr. Rosen due to concerns about school. He is scheduled for a 15-minute appointment, and Dr. Rosen is already almost 60 minutes behind schedule. As Dr. Rosen is reading the chart outside the door, his nurse walks by and states, "That mom has called three times today, so make sure you see the note I left you on the chart before you go in there."

On the top of the chart is a Post-It note that says, "The mom wants to see you without the patient first and wants a drug screen done today." Dr. Rosen notices in the chart that Jack has been seen in the clinic six times during the last year by several different partners for a variety of vague complaints.

Dr. Rosen puts his head in the door and asks the mom to step out into the hall. She tells him that Jack is completing the seventh grade but may be at risk of failing; he missed over 30 days of school this year. She now can't seem to get him to go to school at all, he doesn't do his homework, and "he has stopped caring about anything at all." She worries that he is using drugs and says, "I just don't want him to go down the same path as his brother" (who used drugs and dropped out of school).

Dr. Rosen walks into the exam room with Jack's mother. Jack does not look up or make eye contact, despite attempts to ask Jack about school. He then proceeds to say, "I don't know," to most of the things that Dr. Rosen asks during the visit.

Dr. Rosen's nurse rings the phone in the exam room to let him know he is now 70 minutes behind and two patients are still waiting in rooms. Dr. Rosen excuses the mom from the room and asks to talk to Jack briefly. Jack says that he is living at home with his mom, his older unemployed brother, his younger sister (who fights with him all the time), and his stepfather. He says, "I can't stand him," and states that he and his stepfather fight "constantly." Jack states that he can't concentrate at school and that he received A's and B's through elementary school but is now

"failing almost everything." Dr. Rosen asks if Jack is feeling depressed, and Jack says, "No. I'm not depressed," adamantly and angrily. Dr. Rosen asks Jack, "Do you ever have any suicidal thoughts?" and Jack replies, "Doesn't everybody?"

Dr. Rosen steps out of the office and states to his nurse, "Let's get a urine drug screen on him and get him in to see child psychiatry." Jack and his mother are instructed to wait in the room while the nurse tries to secure an appointment. After calls to the four child psychiatrists in the community and six other child psychiatry offices within a 2-hour radius, she learns that no one can see Jack. She finds most are not taking new patients and only one would even schedule an intake appointment, but it was 6 months away.

As this case exemplifies, the PCP is often caught "off guard" by the presentation of mental health concerns. Referring a patient for assessment and care is not often an immediate option. The role of the PCP involves prevention, screening, education, assessment, treatment, monitoring, and referral. Now many PCPs must initiate assessment and treatment but should be doing this in consultation and collaboration with mental health professionals. Collaborative models are not usually taught in training programs. Child and adolescent psychiatrists involved in collaboration with primary care clinics may be in the role of consulting not only on cases but also on clinic policies and procedures as well, such as on protocols for phone triage for clinic nurses or for ADHD assessments.

In the case above, mental health screening at routine and acute visits might have helped identify problems much earlier. Also, clinic protocols in place for nurses and for physicians would assist in knowing how to schedule patients when a mental health concern is identified and also what tools to have available for the physician to help with a clinic-based mental health assessment. PCPs may need assistance in knowing how to screen, what screening tools to use, how to interpret self-report and parental-report questionnaires, and how to assimilate the information into an appropriate diagnostic formulation. Most PCPs have not received training on the Axis V diagnostic formulation (American Psychiatric Association 2000) and would benefit from help in thinking about the formulation of a case. PCPs do not typically feel comfortable or have the skills to interview patients or even parents in regard to mental health concerns and therefore may need mentoring, teaching, and even modeling of interview skills. In addition, the entire clinic staff may need education and training on interacting and working with families of children with mental illness.

If a child and adolescent psychiatrist were not available to immediately evaluate this patient, could the pediatrician be guided by a consultant in the approach to assessment and initiation of treatment? If so, how would the consultant be paid? If the pediatrician knew he could contact his consulting child and adolescent psychiatrist, perhaps at a predetermined time when the consultant would be available, then the case could be discussed over the telephone and an approach to evaluation could be determined. Once the diagnosis is made clear, further consultation might allow the pediatrician to initiate care so that the patient does not decompensate further while awaiting a referral appointment. Finally, with consultation availability, the pediatrician may be able to monitor the patient more effectively, knowing when to bring the patient back for follow-up visits and what to do at those follow-up visits.

Approaches to Education and Improving Skills of the Primary Care Physician

How can the child and adolescent psychiatrist assist the PCP in improving skills needed to provide mental health care to children? Improving knowledge and skills in order to create a change in physician behavior and clinical practice requires more than attending continuing medical education lectures or reading a journal article or textbook chapter. It is critical to develop training, consultation, and mentoring models with child psychiatrists and other mental health professionals.

Collaborative Care

Optimal mental health care requires collaboration between the PCP and mental health specialists such as the child and adolescent psychiatrist, child psychologist, other psychotherapists such as licensed clinical social workers, case managers, schoolteachers, and school-based mental health professionals. At the time of a mental health assessment in a primary care clinic, the physician must determine the acuity of the patient so that the appropriate level of care required can be determined. If a PCP is able to determine that he or she can manage the patient initially, then adequate follow-up and monitoring will provide the opportunity for reassessment of the need for a higher level of care. Collaborative mental health care can be considered along a spectrum of the following five levels:

1. **Primarily primary care**—The pediatrician or family physician identifies and treats the child with a mental illness with a mild level of acuity. In this situation, the primary care clinic is the primary site for the mental health care of the patient. The PCP educates the child and family, manages the overall care, prescribes any treatments, and monitors the treatments prescribed. An example would be a child with ADHD who is responsive to usual medications and who is without comorbid features.

2. **Primarily primary care with consultation**—The primary care provider consults with a child psychiatrist or a psychologist regarding approaches to assessment, diagnosis, and treatment. The psychiatrist may be consulted to inquire about medications: which ones to consider, when to consider them, appropriate dosing and titration, recommended length of treatment, and how to appropriately monitor. Consultation can occur at the assessment, at the initiation of treatment, or any time during the course of treatment, such as in a child with ADHD who is unresponsive to stimulants, atomoxetine, clonidine, or guanfacine or in a child with exacerbation of a previously controlled depression.

3. **Shared care**—The PCP identifies, assesses, and then refers for an emergency consultation with a child and adolescent psychiatrist but then shares in the ongoing care of the patient. Communication is critical when a patient is shared. Additional mental health specialists such as psychologists and other therapists may be consulted and share in the care of the patient. Sharing care implies that the required ongoing monitoring of the symptoms of the mental illness and the response to medications and therapy is a responsibility of *all* the providers involved and that there is ongoing communication about the patient among the providers. Examples here might be a child with depression comanaged for cognitive-behavioral therapy, a child requiring psychiatry evaluation due to inadequate response to selective serotonin reuptake inhibitor (SSRI) therapy, or a child with increased suicidal risk.

4. **Shared care and higher levels of care**—The patient may require a higher level of care, such as more frequent follow-up visits, closer monitoring, and even hospitalization, partial hospitalization, or day treatment. Additional community support services may be required, such as a mental health case manager. In this situation, the responsibility for management is shifting to the mental health specialists, but the primary care provider is still actively involved as a treatment team member and is

sharing in the overall care, as in a patient with depression following hospital discharge.

5. **Primarily mental health care**—The patient is referred to mental health specialty care for ongoing treatment and management. The child and adolescent psychiatrist would be the primary medical provider managing the child's mental illness due to the level of severity, the level of complexity of the individual and family problems, higher levels of concern regarding safety, and/or the coexistence of other complicating conditions. The responsibility for ongoing care and management is with the child and adolescent psychiatrist and other mental health specialty team members, but the PCP is included in communication and is informed of changes in level of care, such as hospitalization, changes in medications, or other treatment plan changes. Examples would be children with bipolar affective disorder, schizophrenia, or severe ADHD unresponsive to usual medications.

A Collaborative Model

The CentraCare Integrative Behavioral HealthCare Initiative at CentraCare Health System in St. Cloud, Minnesota, is a comprehensive integrative care program for behavioral health services in primary care clinics (Sulik 2006; Sulik et al. 2007). Several features of our current program provide examples of stages of collaborative care. As depicted in Figure 64–1, in our system, we have Diagnostic Assessment for Referral and Triage (DART) therapists—who are master's level–psychologists, therapists, or social workers—in the primary care clinics to provide a comprehensive diagnostic assessment in order to triage the patient to an appropriate level of care. Patients are referred to the DART therapist based on positive mental health screens or by direct physician referral due to physician or parent concern.

For patients with mild and even low-moderate levels of acuity, if the DART therapist determines that the patient may require medical intervention, he or she will consult with the pediatrician about scheduling a return appointment or referring the child back for an appointment to assess for medication. The pediatrician has available protected consultation time that can be scheduled with an on-call child and adolescent psychiatrist if there are specific questions or if the pediatrician needs a consultation about the patient's diagnosis, medications, monitoring, or additional treatment interventions that

may be required. The DART therapist may have already referred the patient to an individual therapist and provided information to the patient and family. If the DART therapist has assessed the level of acuity to be high, he or she may refer the patient to a therapist for individual therapy and refer the patient to a child and adolescent psychiatrist. When an emergent appointment with the child and adolescent psychiatrist is not available, he or she may refer the patient back to the PCP for initial care and facilitate communication between the PCP and the child and adolescent psychiatrist. The DART therapist assesses the level of acuity and triages the patient to an appropriate level of care, thereby improving the availability of child and adolescent psychiatrists for the patients at higher levels of need. The DART therapist is a resource to the PCP not only to assist in the initial assessment but also to provide some case management services to facilitate connection with community and clinic resources as required.

During the first year after implementation of the CentraCare Integrative Behavioral Healthcare Initiative in the pediatric clinic, 324 patients were referred to the DART therapist for evaluation (Sulik et al. 2007). Only 37 (11%) of these patients required referral to the child and adolescent psychiatrist for an emergency evaluation and treatment, and 40 patients (12%) were referred back to the PCP to initiate treatment. A total of 127 (36%) were referred to a therapist but at the time of evaluation were not requiring treatment with medications. This model of mental health screening for common mental health problems at well visits and the availability of a clinic-based mental health professional conducting mental health assessments and triaging to appropriate levels of care has led to earlier identification and improved access to care while decreasing the number of unnecessary referrals to the child and adolescent psychiatrist.

If Jack (in the case example described earlier) presented to our CentraCare pediatric clinic, the patient and parent could have been screened before the appointment via an electronic questionnaire covering depressive symptoms, school performance, and drug use. Significant findings on screening questionnaires or in interview would prompt a referral for the DART therapist. After the patient and parent were seen by the DART therapist, the PCP would complete the evaluation for depressive symptoms and assess the level of safety risk. If the patient was found to be depressed and in need of medication, the PCP would initiate treatment with an SSRI. The DART therapist would evaluate the patient for seriousness of symptoms and comorbidities and would make an appointment with a

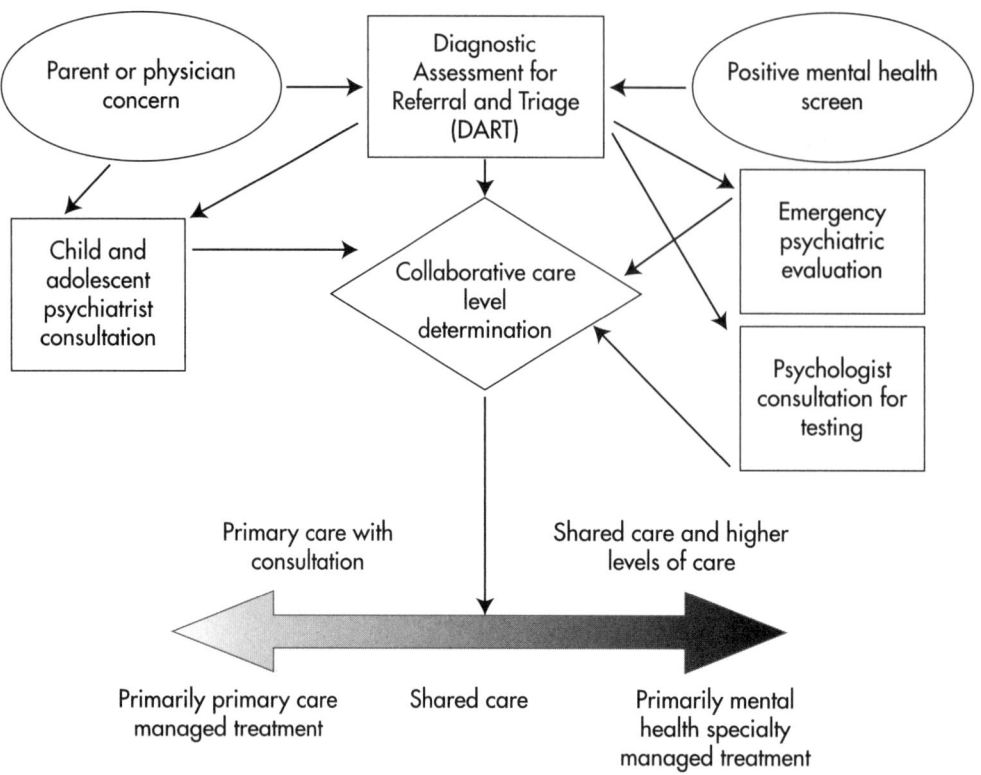

FIGURE 64–1.   CentraCare Integrative Behavioral HealthCare Initiative.

psychologist or psychiatrist as deemed necessary, and if indicated, the DART therapist would ensure referral to drug rehabilitation treatment as well. The primary pediatrician would follow the patient weekly for the first 4–6 weeks as medication was started. If a medication trial was unsuccessful, the pediatrician would be able to consult one of the child psychiatrists by phone at a predetermined time allotted for this. Psychotherapy would be initiated by one of the psychologists in the collocated child and adolescent behavioral health clinic, who would communicate via a common electronic record with the pediatrician and child and adolescent psychiatrist. Visits to the pediatrician for medication evaluation would become less frequent as counseling progresses and the patient stabilizes.

Core Principles of Collaborative Care in the Primary Care Setting

The resources available to assist the PCP vary across communities. Providing the mental health care in the primary care clinic requires that the pediatrician or family physician do the following:

1. Establish local or regional connections with mental health professionals who may be needed to participate as team members in the patient's care. Some access to child and adolescent psychiatrists and licensed psychologists or licensed clinical social workers is necessary. Additional professionals may include county social services mental health case managers, school psychologists, a neuropsychologist if indicated, special education teachers and educational case managers, school nurses, chemical dependency counselors, and possibly inpatient treatment staff. Most primary care clinics do not employ their own mental health professionals, and therefore clinics must have a consultative and collaborative relationship with professionals who are practicing independently or who are employed by another agency.

2. Establish clear and regular communication, preferably via a common electronic chart, so that information is available to the emergency room, psychologist, and PCP on a timely basis.

3. Establish a mental health professional in the clinic to provide triage assessments, crisis counseling, case management services, and patient and family education. This has several important benefits, including removing some of the burden from the practicing physician, ensuring that referrals are

properly made, and having flexible time to deal with crises that inevitably require more time than a physician can free up.

4. Establish screening protocols, mechanisms, and treatment and evaluation pathways so that all providers are on the same track, providing similar standards of care.

5. Have continuing education, in either lecture or case discussion format, as a continuing point of connection between psychiatry, psychology, and the primary physician.

Components of Collaborative Care in the Primary Care Setting

Screening

It is critical that the screening and triage occur parallel to the physician's usual visit. It is unlikely that physicians would be able to take extra time in an already packed schedule to ask questions for a detailed mental health screen. This screening can be done in several ways, preferably via electronic forms, so that the results of a standard mental health screen are available at the time of a routine well child exam or the nursing personnel can initiate screening on a patient with chronic vague complaints or psychosocial presenting issues according to a protocol. Ideally, positive results on a screen could result in the nursing personnel initiating a referral to mental health triage, based on protocol. Some suggestions for screening instruments for the 0–4 years age group include the Ages and Stages Questionnaire (ASQ; Squires et al. 1998), Ages and Stages Questionnaire Socio-Emotional (ASQ-SE; Beligere et al. 2005), or the Pediatric Screening Checklists (PSC; Jellinek et al. 1999). Screening tools for the 5–12 years age group include the PSC, the Strength and Difficulty Questionnaire (SDQ; Glazebrook et al. 2003), or the Vanderbilt Behavioral Evaluation Tool (Williams et al. 2004). Adolescent screening tools include the PSC, the Patient Health Questionnaire—Adolescent Version (PHQ-A; Johnson et al. 2002), or the Vanderbilt Behavioral Evaluation Tool.

Consultation

A good relationship with good communication is essential. The informal "curbside consult" requires famil-

iarity and trust between the physicians. PCPs can begin the process of creating relationships with child and adolescent psychiatrists and psychologists by inviting local or regional individuals to a meeting to discuss the process. Clinical case or round table discussions have been held monthly between a child and adolescent psychiatrist and a group of pediatricians with CME credit provided. Although this may be limited to 1 hour every month or even less, the relationship may be established for the continuation of "informal" consults to continue to support the pediatrician. A novel approach to making consultation available has been implemented in Massachusetts, where the state legislature has funded the availability of six regional consultation teams made up of child and adolescent psychiatrists, clinical social workers, and case managers who provide various levels of consultation and resource coordination to PCPs in their region (Sarvet 2006). In this program, the Massachusetts Child Psychiatry Access Program (MCPAP) and PCPs can seek consultation regarding mental health care of a child or adolescent or request that a patient be seen for a psychiatric evaluation and returned to the PCP with recommendations for care.

Documentation

When a consultation occurs in the MCPAP or in the CentraCare program, the PCP documents in the patient's chart the results of a consultation with a child and adolescent psychiatrist or psychologist. The notation includes the professional consulted, the reason for the consultation, a reference to the case being summarized, and the resulting discussion of the diagnosis and recommendations for treatment. In our clinics at CentraCare, the note is copied to the consulting child and adolescent psychiatrist via the electronic medical record. Much discussion has ensued among child and adolescent psychiatrists in Minnesota on whether or not they, too, should document the consultation. Since they do not necessarily have a patient chart in which to record the documentation, the consensus seems to be to abide by the wording in the legislative action to request the PCP to document the consultation. However, each physician and clinic may choose to do this differently, perhaps by suggesting a shared form that the consulting psychiatrist completes and then sends to the PCP to place in the chart.

Communication

Consent for release of information should be obtained during the initial mental health evaluation so that all providers can communicate with one another regarding ongoing care. The PCP who is prescribing psychotropic medications and is sharing the care of the patient with a therapist must have ongoing communication with the therapist to insure optimal coordination of care. Physicians need to communicate to the therapist that ongoing communication is desired and is expected but also commit to communicating regularly with the therapist. Physicians may consider using a communication document that summarizes important information to be shared. When the PCP is sharing care with a child and adolescent psychiatrist, communication on medication changes is critically important.

Triage

In order for the collaborative spectrum of care to be effective, the patient must be assessed for acuity so that the appropriate level of collaborative care can be provided. An acuity assessment allows the physician to determine what additional resources are going to be necessary in the ongoing care of the patient. Acuity is determined based on the severity of symptoms, the degree of impairment in functioning, and a determination of safety. Acuity is assessed not only during an initial evaluation but also throughout the course of treatment because the level of acuity may change, and the patient may move to a different level of care as a result.

Follow-Up

In our setting, the pediatrician often has called the child and adolescent psychiatrist for a follow-up consultation after initiating treatment or to simply provide an update to determine if there are any other treatment modalities needed. During these consultations, the psychiatrist guides the pediatrician on how often to see a patient for follow-up, what to assess, and what information to provide at the follow-up visits. The PCP must communicate clearly with other team members regarding follow-up plans. It should be agreed upon who will see the patient and how often the patient will be seen.

Financial Viability

In our clinic, the initial screening involves utilization of an electronic device, with push buttons, which involved some initial grants for start-up costs. However, the reimbursement of the screening makes this financially viable. This is currently charged by the PCP under code 96110. The financing for the DART involves reimbursable mental health visits charged by the DART therapist, under the supervision of the child and adolescent psychiatrist. Under our current cost structure, the DART therapist must see at least 12 cases per week in order to break even; currently, after 1½ years, our pediatric department DART therapist is seeing 17 cases per week, and we are looking to add a second DART therapist. This is in a department of 19 pediatricians, with 14 equivalent full-time positions. Consultation from the child and adolescent psychiatrist currently involves scheduled phone consultation. Under current reimbursement guidelines from at least three of our third-party payers, this time is reimbursable.

Summary Points

- PCPs are increasingly expected to conduct mental health screening and provide mental health assessments and mental health treatment in the primary care clinic.

- Child and adolescent psychiatrists are increasingly involved in teaching, mentoring, and providing consultation to PCPs in order to improve access to mental health care for children and adolescents.

- Collaborative care of children's mental health includes mental health screening, mental health diagnostic assessments, and determination of where on a collaborative care continuum the child falls.

- The level of collaborative care is determined by the patient's acuity and can range from primary management of the patient by the PCP to a sharing of care between the PCP and the child and adolescent psychiatrist and other mental health specialists; finally, some patients' mental health care is primarily managed by the mental health specialists involved.

- PCPs and primary care clinic staff need to improve their understanding of mental health issues in children and adolescents and improve skills needed to identify and treat mental health disorders in the primary care clinic.

- Child and adolescent psychiatrists need to improve their understanding of the primary care setting and recognize how to provide support to PCPs and their staff in order to better treat mental illness in children and adolescents in the primary care clinic setting.

- Improved collaboration between PCPs and child and adolescent psychiatrists can improve access to mental health care for children and hopefully reduce 1) the dependency on use of more intensive levels of mental health services and 2) overall cost in providing improved care due to earlier identification and earlier intervention.

References

American Psychiatric Association: Diagnostic and Statistical Manual of Mental Disorders, 4th Edition, Text Revision. Washington, DC, American Psychiatric Association, 2000

Beligere N, Bandepalli C, Helin R, et al: Parents report of social and emotional status of the premature infants. Ages and Stages Questionnaire (ASQ) on Social and Emotional (S/E) Assessment ASQ: SE. J Dev Behav Pediatr 26(6):472, 2005

Blount A: Beyond philosophy: primary care and behavioral health integration. Behav Healthc Tomorrow 6:41–45, 1997

Connor DF, McLaughlin TJ, Jeffers-Terry M, et al: Targeted child psychiatric services: a new model of pediatric primary clinician—child psychiatry collaborative care. Clin Pediatr (Phila) 45:423–434, 2006

Gadit AA: Shared care model for mental health: is it a viable option for Pakistan? J Coll Physicians Surg Pak 17:185–186, 2007

Glazebrook C, Hollis C, Heussler H, et al: Detecting emotional and behavioural problems in paediatric clinics. Child Care Health Dev 29:141–149, 2003

Horwitz SM, Kelleher KJ, Stein RE, et al: Barriers to the identification and management of psychosocial issues in children and maternal depression. Pediatrics 119:e208–e218, 2007

Jayabarathan A: Shared mental health care: bringing family physicians and psychiatrists together. Can Fam Physician 50:341–346, 2004

Jellinek MS: DSM-PC: bridging pediatric primary care and mental health services. J Dev Behav Pediatr 18:173–174, 1997

Jellinek MS, Froehle MC (eds): Bright Futures in Practice: Mental Health. Arlington, VA, National Center for Education in Maternal and Child Health, 2002

Jellinek MS, Murphy JM, Little E, et al: Use of the Pediatric Symptom Checklist to screen for psychosocial problems in pediatric primary care: a national feasibility study. Arch Pediatr Adolesc Med 153:254–260, 1999

Johnson JG, Harris ES, Spitzer RL, et al: The patient health questionnaire for adolescents: validation of an instrument for the assessment of mental disorders among adolescent primary care patients. J Adolesc Health 30:196–204, 2002

Rappaport N, Prince JB, Bostic JQ, et al: Lost in the black box: juvenile depression, suicide, and the FDA's black box. J Pediatr 147:719–720, 2005

Rockman P, Salach L, Gotlib D, et al: Shared mental health care: model for supporting and mentoring family physicians. Can Fam Physician 50:397–402, 2004

Samy DC, Hall P, Rounsevell J, et al: "Shared Care–Shared Dream": model of shared care in rural Australia between mental health services and general practitioners. Aust J Rural Health 15:35–40, 2007

Sarvet B: The Massachusetts Child Psychiatry Access Project (MCPAP). Paper presented at American Academy of Child and Adolescent Psychiatry Meeting, San Diego, CA, October 2006

Squires JK, Potter L, Bricker DD, et al: Parent-completed developmental questionnaire: effectiveness with low and middle income parents. Early Child Res Q 13:345–354, 1998

Sulik LR: A tale of two sides: integrating mental health and primary care—The CentraCare Integrative Behavioral HealthCare Initiative. Paper presented at American Academy of Child and Adolescent Psychiatry Meeting, San Diego, CA, October 2006

Sulik LR, Tilstra D, Moritz D, et al: The CentraCare Integrated Behavioral HealthCare Initiative. Poster presentation at the American Academy of Pediatrics Meeting, Orlando, FL, June 2007

Sved Williams A, Dodding J, Wilson I, et al: Consultation-liaison to general practitioners coming of age: the South Australian psychiatrists' experience. Australas Psychiatry 14:206–211, 2006

Thomas CR, Holzer CE 3rd: The continuing shortage of child and adolescent psychiatrists. J Am Acad Child Adolesc Psychiatry 45:1023–1031, 2006

Trude S, Stoddard JJ: Referral gridlock: primary care physicians and mental health services. J Gen Intern Med 18:442–449, 2003

U.S. Public Health Service: Report of the Surgeon General's Conference on Children's Mental Health: A National Action Agenda. Washington, DC, Department of Health and Human Services, 2000

Williams J, Klinepeter K, Palmes G, et al: Diagnosis and treatment of behavioral health disorders in pediatric practice. Am Acad Pediatrics, 2004

Wolraich ML, Drotar D (eds): The Classification of Child and Adolescent Mental Health Diagnoses in Primary Care: Diagnostic and Statistical Manual for Primary Care (DSM-PC), Child and Adolescent Version. Elk Grove Village, IL, American Academy of Pediatrics, 1996

World Health Organization: The World Health Report 2001. Mental Health: New Understanding, New Hope. Geneva, Switzerland, World Health Organization, 2001

Chapter 65

Juvenile Justice

Louis Kraus, M.D.
Kayla Pope, M.D., J.D.

Historical Overview of the Juvenile Justice System

Treatment of the juvenile justice population has evolved over time. The current system reflects the constant tension between the need to limit the destructive behavior of delinquent youth and the recognition that their behaviors are influenced by many factors that are beyond their control and place them at risk—the concept of police power versus *parens patriae*. Prior to the nineteenth century, children were seen as property of their parents and were accorded few protections from parental abuse and neglect. With respect to criminal matters, children above the age of 7 years old were treated as adults and were presumed to be responsible for their actions. These attitudes began to change in the late nineteenth century in response to industrialization,

with its effects on the family and community structure and the increase in social problems including delinquent behavior. From this social context a rehabilitative ideal emerged under the influence of social reformers who believed that children who engaged in delinquent behavior were the victims of poverty, poor social training, and economic instability. By adopting a rehabilitative model, these reformers believed that delinquent children could be made into productive members of society. It was out of this movement that the first juvenile court came into existence in Chicago, Illinois, in 1899.

Over the last 100 years, the juvenile courts have undergone considerable change. The courts have moved away from a model of parens patriae to a more adversarial system as a result of a series of cases that recognized juvenile rights during the adjudicatory process. The first of these cases was *Kent v. United States* (1966), which established that juveniles have certain rights during a juvenile court proceeding, including the right to have a lawyer present during interrogation and to be present during the waiver proceeding. This was followed by *In re Gault* (1967), where a 15-year-old juvenile was brought before the court on a petition stating that he was a delinquent minor in need of care. On appeal, the U.S. Supreme Court held that all juveniles were entitled to certain due process rights including notice of charges being brought against them, right to counsel, right to confront witnesses, and privilege against self-incrimination.

Legal and Ethical Issues in Working With Juvenile Offenders

During each stage of the process, from arrest to adjudication, there are unique issues raised in working with juvenile offenders. Increasingly, there is awareness of how developmental issues play a role in the ability of a juvenile to effectively engage with the justice system, and research on developmental differences has helped to shape policies and procedures when working with this population.

Arrest and Interrogation

During the arrest and interrogation process, maturational issues can undermine a youth's ability to effectively protect his or her rights. In most systems, police employ the same interrogation practices used with adults in their interactions with juveniles. These tactics are designed to lower the defenses of the juvenile and to encourage him or her to cooperate with the investigator and to waive Miranda rights. For Miranda waivers to be valid, they must be done knowingly, intelligently, and voluntarily. Research that has examined juvenile's ability to understand the Miranda warning has found that juveniles under the age of 15 years old having significantly less understanding and appreciation of the significance of the Miranda warning. These youth have difficulty understanding the adversarial nature of the interrogation process and abstract concepts such as rights (Grisso 1981; Redlich et al. 2003). As a result, they are more apt to waive their rights, especially if they are innocent (Kassin and Norwick 2004; Redlich and Drizin 2007).

Younger children have less legal knowledge and understanding of the legal system (Carter et al. 1996) and are more suggestible than older children and adults (Bruck and Melnyk 2004). Younger children are more likely to confess to police and to provide false confessions (Goldstein et al. 2003). These findings were supported by a study that used hypothetical interrogations to evaluate juveniles' responses to interrogation practices. Younger children were more likely to falsely confess when presented with false evidence by the interrogator, and half of the youth were willing to sign a confession without asking any questions of the investigator (Redlich and Goodman 2003). For youth with mental illnesses and substance abuse issues, the risk of waiving their rights and making false confessions is even greater.

Competency and Criminal Responsibility

In order for a juvenile to stand trial, he or she must be able to understand the nature of the proceedings and to assist in his or her own defense. With juveniles, competence can be challenged on many grounds, including immaturity. Approximately one-third of 11- to 13-year-olds and one-fifth of 14- to 15-year-olds failed to meet the standard for competence needed to participate in an adult criminal proceeding (Grisso et al. 2003). In reality, juvenile courts apply a more relaxed standard in assessing a youth's ability to participate in a criminal proceeding.

In assessing competency, there are several factors to consider (Geraghty et al. 2007):

1. Ability to understand the nature of the charges and the potential consequences.
2. Ability to understand the nature and process of the proceeding. This requirement focuses on whether the child understands that the purpose of the proceeding is to determine guilt and what the sentence might be if he or she were determined to be guilty. This requirement also entails that the youth be able to understand the mechanics of the process and the roles of the different participants in the proceeding.
3. Ability to cooperate with counsel. For youth to meet this requirement, they must be able to communicate effectively with their attorney and have the ability to understand and evaluate the advice given to by the attorney.

In evaluating a youth's competence, the clinician should consider age, intelligence, capacity for abstract thinking, emotional maturity, psychiatric status, and any physical disability that interferes with communication. Depression or psychosis can interfere with a youth's reality testing as well as ability to recall information accurately. However, neither mental illness nor mental retardation will automatically result in a finding of incompetence (Geraghty et al. 2007). Evaluations of competency are usually conducted by a psychiatrist or a psychologist. Instruments have been developed to assist in the evaluation.

Waiver to Adult Court

Youth who commit criminal offenses may be transferred to adult courts for adjudication. In making the determination of whether a youth should be transferred, the court considers future dangerousness and amenability to treatment. Several factors have been associated with the likelihood to commit future acts, including a history of violence, male gender, being age 13–18 years old, and the age at which the first violent act occurred, with the younger the age making it more likely that the child will engage in additional violent acts. Youth engaging in a variety of criminal acts are at greater risk for recidivism. Environmental predictors include exposure to violence, carrying a weapon, and gang participation.

In assessing the likelihood that treatment will rehabilitate the youth, the evaluator should consider whether the youth has any diagnosable mental health or substance abuse disorders, the history of the youth's treatment for these disorders, and the youth's compliance with treatment. The evaluator should also consider the timeline for effective treatment in relation to the time available to deliver treatment, given the offense and the age of the offender. Jurisdictions are divided on whether the court should consider whether resources are available in the community (Grisso 1998).

Judicial waiver is available in most states and allows the judge discretion in deciding whether to transfer a juvenile to adult court. In most states, it is necessary for there to be probable cause that the juvenile committed the offense prior to transfer, and in all states a hearing must take place to establish the basis for the transfer. Many states now have statutes that mandate transfer of a juvenile for specific offenses or if a crime is committed after a certain age. Critics of these automatic waivers argue that it places first-time offenders within the adult courts and removes any consideration of rehabilitation for many offenders who would benefit from treatment (Kruh and Brodsky 1997). Automatic waiver to adult court also precludes the possibility of any psychiatric assessment and carries with it an assumption of guilt.

Juvenile Death Penalty

Executing juveniles was legally permissible in the United States until the Supreme Court ruling in *Roper v. Simmons* in March 2005. The Court applied a *standards of decency test* and looked at state and federal trends in sentencing and executing minors, noting that many states had made it unconstitutional to execute minors and that federal law excluded defendants under the age of 18 from execution. The majority decision also quoted the Supreme Court decisions not allowing the execution of mentally retarded individuals. Of great interest was the Court's reliance on science and their use of research on brain development to guide them in evaluating juveniles' ability to make informed and measured decisions (Giedd et al. 1999). Based on this research, the Court concluded that the developmental differences between adults and adolescents were significant enough to make juvenile offenders ineligible for death.

The Juvenile Justice Population

Based on data from the Office of Juvenile Justice and Delinquency Prevention, there were 2.2 million juveniles arrested in the United States in 2003. Of those arrested, 71% were male, 32% were under the age of 15, and 96 million were placed in the custody of the juvenile justice system. The arrest rate of females continues to increase, and females are committing crimes at younger ages. It is estimated that the likelihood that a female will spend time in prison at some point in her life is six times higher if she was born in 2001 than if she was born in 1974.

Minorities continue to be overrepresented in the juvenile justice population. Minorities account for 34% of the juvenile population, yet they represent 62% of juveniles who are incarcerated. Custody rates are highest for African American youth, who represent 17% of the juvenile population but 55% of arrests for violence. Further, black youth are twice as likely to be held in secure detention and are more likely to be petitioned to adult court for offenses involving persons and drug-related offenses (Poe-Yamagata and Jones 2000). Racial disparity is also seen in sentencing and placement of offenders, with minority youth being more likely to be sentenced to adult court (Males and Macallair 2000) and more likely to be sent to an adult prison (Snyder and Sickmund 2000). Race is often the key factor in determining outcomes in the adjudicative process (Pope et al. 2002).

In evaluating the causes for disproportionate minority treatment within the juvenile justice system, factors include racial stereotyping and cultural insensitivity, demeanor and attitude of minority youth, lack of culturally appropriate services to help minorities, and misuse of discretionary authority. A variety of socioeconomic factors are also thought to play a role and include poverty, exposure to violence, poor schools, and family disintegration (Hsia et al. 2004).

Special Needs of the Juvenile Justice Population
Mental Health and Substance Abuse

A study by the Northwestern Juvenile Project (Teplin et al. 2002) surveyed juvenile detainees within the Cook County Juvenile Detention Center. A total of 1,829 subjects, ages 10–18 years, were evaluated using the Diagnostic Interview Schedule for Children (DISC). Females and minorities were oversampled to assure sufficient numbers. Nearly two-thirds of males and three-quarters of females met diagnostic criteria for one or more psychiatric disorders—higher than the rates for youth in the general population, which are estimated to be between 6% and 38%. When conduct disorder was excluded because of the overlap with delinquent behavior, prevalence rates decreased only slightly. The most common disorders among both males and females were substance abuse (51% for males and 47% for females) and disruptive behaviors (oppositional defiant disorder and conduct disorder, 41% of males and 46% of females). Of all respondents, 93% reported at least one trauma, with 11% of participants meeting criteria for posttraumatic stress disorder (PTSD) within the last year. Females were significantly more likely to be diagnosed with a mood or anxiety disorder. In females, 22% met criteria for major depressive disorder (13% of males) and 31% met criteria for an anxiety disorder, with separation anxiety being the most common. Overall, females were more likely than males to have two or more disorders. There were also racial differences in prevalence rates of disorders, with non-Hispanic white males having the highest rates of disorders (82%) and African Americans the lowest rates (65%). When this was broken

down, African Americans and Hispanic males had higher rates than non-Hispanic whites of both affective disorders and anxiety disorders, whereas non-Hispanic whites had higher rates of substance abuse, attention-deficit/hyperactivity disorder (ADHD), and disruptive behaviors. Among females, there was less variation in prevalence rates between ethnic groups. Females across all races had significantly higher rates of single and comorbid disorders, including depression, anxiety disorders, and substance abuse.

The prevalence of disorders was also evaluated by the age of juveniles. In general, the prevalence for all disorders increased among males and females as they grew older. With respect to onset of comorbid mental health and substance abuse disorders, 25% of the males and the females reported that their mental health disorders preceded the onset of substance abuse disorders by over a year, and two-thirds of the females and one-half of the males reported onset within the same year. Only 10% of the females and 20% of the males reported substance abuse preceding mental health issues.

Suicide Risk

From 1950 to 2002, the suicide rate for young people (ages 15–24) tripled from 2.7 per 100,000 to 9.9 per 100,000 (Arias et al. 2003; Kochanek et al. 2002). Among this group, children and adolescents who are incarcerated are at the highest risk for serious suicide attempts (Gray et al. 2002). Several risk factors have been identified that place incarcerated youth at increased risk for suicide attempts: depression, history of impulsivity and drug abuse (Sanislow et al. 2003), history of abuse (Morris et al. 1995), and not living with a biological parent before incarceration (Rohde et al. 1997).

To better understand the phenomenon of youth suicide while youth are in detention, a retrospective case study was undertaken to identify individual and institutional risk factors associated with successful suicide attempts (Hayes 2004). The study evaluated 79 cases of suicide and found that 42% occurred in secure facilities, 37% in short-term detention centers, 15% in residential treatment, and 6% in reception/diagnostic centers. The vast majority of the victims had been confined for nonviolent offenses (70%), and all of the suicides occurred within the first 4 months of incarceration, with 40% occurring within the first 72 hours. The Hayes study and others have demonstrated the importance of early screening of youth to identify those at risk of suicide attempts, with facilities that screen within the first 24 hours having the lowest suicide rates (Gallagher and Dorbin 2005). Research also supports the need for staff to be alert to the signs of suicidality, as 16% of the suicides occur while the youth are under close observation for suicide precautions.

Mental Health Screening and Assessment

Early evaluation of confined youth is important to ensuring their safety while they are being detained. They are at highest risk for suicide during this early period. Other benefits associated with evaluating youth during their confinement (Vincent et al. 2007) include identifying mental disorders that threaten the health and welfare of detained juveniles and the staff. Untreated mental disorders can result in increased levels of unpredictable behavior due to aggression or psychosis. Another reason for early evaluation is to prevent future acts of delinquency. Treatment of underlying disorders that interfere with emotional and behavioral control will help juveniles in developing better coping skills and making better decisions. Finally, evaluation of youth and documentation of mental disorders help inform the need for resource allocation.

Screening tools are generally used for initial evaluations. In selecting a screening tool, the time required to administer the test as well as the skill level needed by the person giving the test should be considered. The Massachusetts Youth Screening Instrument—Version 2 (Grisso and Barnum 2006) is a 52-item self-report scale that evaluates mental and emotional problems and identifies areas of crisis in need of immediate attention. The instrument is appropriate for youth ages 12–17 years old. It can be self-administered or can be read by nonclinical staff and takes 10–15 minutes to complete. The Global Appraisal of Individual Needs—Short Screener (GAIN-SS; Dennis et al. 2002) is a 20-item screening instrument designed to identify adolescents in need of additional assessment. It is a self-report instrument that can be completed in under 5 minutes. The GAIN-SS was developed for general use but has been validated in the juvenile justice setting and is used by systems across the country. It has four subscales: internal disorder, behavioral disorders, substance abuse, and crime/violence. Screening tests should be completed in conjunction with a comprehensive clinical evaluation.

For youth in need of further evaluation, several assessment tools are commonly used. The Present State Voice Version of the DISC is frequently used in the juvenile justice setting. It screens for more than 30 DSM-IV (American Psychiatric Association 1994) diagnoses and provides information on current levels of impairment. It does not require any special training to administer, can be completed in 60 minutes, and is computer scored. The one drawback with this instrument is that it requires a minimal reading ability, which can be problematic given the high prevalence of learning disabilities in this population. The Practical Adolescent Dual Diagnosis Interview (PADDI; Estroff and Hoffman 2001) can be used to diagnose mental health and substance abuse disorders and provides information on level of severity. The PADDI must be administered by an adult but does not require any special training. Scoring and interpretation must be done by a trained professional. The test takes 20–40 minutes to complete.

Neuropsychological Testing

Two areas of cognitive deficits are frequently found in juvenile offenders: executive functioning and verbal ability (Kraus 2007). Deficits in executive functioning can be due to maturation but can also be caused by injury to this region during the prenatal period or after birth. Executive functioning is involved in decision making and regulating behavior. Youth with deficits will exhibit problems with impulsivity, regulating emotional responses, and difficulty in organizing and executing activities and in sustaining attention. They may also display increased levels of aggression, poor insight into their behavior, and rage reactions (Teichner and Golden 2000).

Deficits in verbal ability have been associated with delinquency even in the absence of deficits in executive functioning (Dery et al. 1999). Juveniles who are delinquent are more likely to have lower verbal IQs than nonverbal IQs. Verbal deficits may interfere with the development of self-control strategies (Vermeiren et al. 2000). Verbal skills are necessary for seeking help, resolving conflict, and managing emotions and behaviors. Verbal deficits can also interfere with the development of a child's understanding of what is acceptable behavior. Finally, verbal deficits can undermine a child's ability to be successful in school.

In a study looking at the differences between recidivists and nonrecidivists, 44% of the variance was attributable to a diagnosis of conduct disorder, low verbal IQ, and the absence of depressive symptoms. Further, low verbal IQ was also associated with higher recidivism rates among younger offenders (Vermeiren et al. 2000).

Psychopharmacological Treatment of Aggression and Conduct Disorder

The treatment of aggression in this population can present challenges. Often acute aggression will be present at the time of entry into a facility, before an evaluation of the youth has been conducted. In addressing aggression, it is recommended that behavioral interventions be attempted to redirect the youth and de-escalation techniques be implemented. When these interventions fail, pharmacological interventions should be considered (see Chapter 37, "Aggression and Violence"). In treating chronic aggression, it is necessary to characterize it as proactive or reactive. Perpetrators of proactive aggression do not respond to pharmacological interventions, and behavioral techniques should be used that help to socialize the child and assist him or her in comprehending social rules and norms. Reactive aggression is characterized by defensive or impulsive acts and responds well to psychopharmacological interventions, especially mood stabilizers. It is important to identify underlying mental health diagnoses (ADHD, mood disorders, anxiety disorders, and so forth) and focus treatment on these disorders. The physician should not use psychotropic medication as "chemical restraint."

Medical Needs

There are unique considerations for the medical needs of youth in juvenile justice (Morris 2007). Several medical conditions predispose children to violent and aggressive behavior, and testing or further investigation may be warranted. During the prenatal period, exposure to lead (Needleman et al. 1990), alcohol (Fast et al. 1999), or other illicit substances (Lester et al. 1998) has been associated with increased levels of aggression and impulsive behavior in children. During the postnatal period, juvenile delinquents are more likely than members of the general population to have a history of head trauma (Otnow-Lewis 1998). Similarly, a history of physical abuse has also been associated with delinquency, which may extend beyond the effects of the assault to more subtle neurobiological findings that impair social and emotional adjustment (Otnow-Lewis 1998). Finally, temporal-limbic epilepsy has also been associated with violent and aggressive behavior.

Youth who engage in delinquent behavior also engage in other high-risk behaviors, including illicit drug use (Morris 2007), and are at increased risk for diseases, including HIV and Hepatitis B and C. Delinquent youth also are more likely to engage in high-risk sexual behavior with multiple partners (Morris 1995) and are at increased risk for sexually transmissible diseases. Youth should be evaluated for these diseases and treated appropriately during confinement. Youth should also be counseled during their confinement on the risks associated with their drug use and risky sexual behavior.

Educational Needs

In 1989, school districts across the United States began adopting a zero-tolerance policy, which mandated expulsion from school for drugs, fighting, and gang-related activities (Skiba and Noam 2002). By 1993, most schools had adopted such policies, and many had broadened them to include smoking and classroom disruption. In 1994, zero tolerance became mandated by the federal government with the adoption of the Gun-Free Schools Act, which required a 1-year expulsion for any child bringing a firearm onto school property. Critics of these policies have observed that time missed from school weakens the youth's connection to the school and increases the likelihood of dropouts. Schools have also overreacted at times, resulting in students being unreasonably expelled. For many students, especially students with disabilities, suspension is a strong predictor of academic failure and dropout (Closson and Rogers 2007).

There is also a high prevalence of learning disabilities among juvenile delinquents, estimated to be between 20% and 70% (Closson and Rogers 2007; Quinn et al. 2005). In one study of youth who had been incarcerated in the Chicago area, it was found that nearly all of the students who became incarcerated had a history of severe academic difficulties and reported attending school an average of 58% of the time. These youth were also found to have failed at least a quarter of their classes and on average were reading at a sixth-grade level (Balfanz et al. 2003). Given all of these factors, it is not surprising that few youth who are incarcerated will complete high school. One study that looked at this issue estimated high school completion to be as low as 12% among these youth (Balfanz et al. 2003).

Problems in educating the juvenile justice population include obtaining appropriate diagnostic information; inadequate assessment in the school system and the juvenile justice system (Kraus 2007); difficulties in continuing education during confinement with students who present with a variety of learning disabilities; varying lengths of stay; and poor communication between juvenile justice and school systems, making it difficult to pick up instruction where the youth left off and ensuring that the youth will be at the same place as his class following return to the program (Closson and Rogers 2007). Recommendations to improve the quality of instruction for youth during confinement include transferring educational records when youth are incarcerated, developing a continuum of services that can be offered within the facility to meet the needs of the individual students, and paying greater attention to transition planning prior to returning the youth to the community (Closson and Rogers 2007).

Treatment Options for Justice-Involved Youth

Innovative Courts

While the trend in the juvenile justice system has been away from rehabilitation and toward punishment, there are efforts underway that focus on understanding the causes of delinquency and developing innovative ways to address these problems. Innovative courts are designed to address some of the core reasons for juvenile delinquency. Juveniles identified at the time of arrest as having specific problems are diverted to programs that have corresponding expertise. Youth courts, also known as peer courts or peer juries, often are used with first-time offenders. Although the courts vary, most are staffed with previous offenders and community volunteers. Peers serve as judge, jury, and counsel. Offenders who are convicted are given community service. These programs have proven to be effective in reducing recidivism among first-time offenders and have been favorably received by communities (Butts et al. 2002).

The first youth mental health court was created in Santa Clara, California, in 2001 in response to the community's awareness that 50%–70% of the juveniles involved in criminal behavior had significant mental health problems. There was recognition that mentally ill youth were unlikely to comply with treatment in the absence of sanctions and would likely continue to engage in criminal behavior in the absence of treatment. The courts have oversight of mental health treatment as well as accountability for delinquent behavior. Youth who enter the program are evaluated and then are given a treatment plan. Youth remain on probation, and failure to comply with the treatment plan constitutes a violation of probation. The effectiveness of mental health courts in addressing recidivism is not

known. The Bazelon Center has expressed concern that this system may encourage the arrests of youth based on their need for services (Kessler 2007).

Drug courts attempt to divert juveniles who have significant substance abuse issues that drive their delinquent behavior. Given that over 60% of offenders are imprisoned for drug-related crimes and over 70% of incarcerated individuals have substance abuse issues (Drug Court Clearinghouse and Technical Assistance Project 1999), making substance abuse treatment a focus of court services seems to be warranted. Outcomes from drug courts have been promising. On average, 70% of drug-dependent offenders remained in or graduated from treatment programs (Drug Court Clearinghouse and Technical Assistance Project 1999). Recidivism rates for juveniles who were diverted to drug courts were significantly decreased, averaging one arrest, as compared to juveniles sent to traditional courts, who averaged 2.3 arrests. Six months after court entry, only 11% of drug court participants had been rearrested as compared to 46% of traditional court juvenile offenders (Belenko 2001). Furthermore, 80% of youth in drug courts either returned to or remained in school.

Community-Based Programs

Community-based treatment programs provide services to youth and their families in their homes and communities and serve as an alternative to incarceration, recognizing the importance of families in providing long-term support and helping juveniles remain integrated into their communities. These programs include multisystemic therapy (MST), functional family therapy (FFT), and multidimensional treatment foster care (MTFC) (for further discussion of these programs, see Chapter 61, "Systems of Care, Wraparound Services, and Home-Based Services").

Research Directions

The majority of youth who enter juvenile correctional facilities are in need of a variety of services, most of which exceed what the facility is able to offer. It is important to have ongoing research and to be able to use the information gleaned from this research to identify youth at risk, justify ongoing treatment needs, and assist in structuring the most appropriate treatment interventions. There is an ongoing need for advocacy on both the state and national levels. There continues to be a relative paucity of funding for these youth, who are the most at-risk population that we have.

Summary Points

- Based on statistics from the Office of Juvenile Justice and Delinquency Prevention, 2.2 million juveniles were arrested in 2003. Of those arrested, 71% were males and 32% were under the age of 15.

- Youth within the juvenile justice system have a higher prevalence of mental illness, learning disabilities, and cognitive delays as compared with age-appropriate peers.

- Juveniles within the court system have the same constitutional rights as their adult counterparts.

- Based on a U.S. Supreme Court decision in March 2005 (*Roper v. Simmons*), juveniles can no longer be executed for capital offenses. This decision involves juveniles who were 16 and 17 years of age.

- Arrested females under the age of 16 are the most rapidly increasing group of delinquents.

- There is a significant minority overrepresentation within the juvenile justice population. Minorities account for 34% of the U.S. juvenile population but represent 62% of juveniles incarcerated nationally.

- Children and adolescents who are incarcerated are at the highest risk for serious suicide attempts. Risk factors include depression and situational distress.

- Innovative court models include drug courts and mental health courts.

- Treatment options need to focus beyond simply incarceration, with a greater focus on community-based options. Three community-based treatment options that have been implemented with some success include multisystemic therapy, functional family therapy, and multidimensional treatment foster care.

References

American Psychiatric Association: Diagnostic and Statistical Manual of Mental Disorders, 4th Edition. Washington, DC, American Psychiatric Association, 1994

Arias E, Anderson R, Kung H, et al: Deaths: Final Data for 2001. National Vital Statistics Report. Hyattsville, MD, National Center for Health Statistics, 2003

Balfanz R, Spiridakis K, Curran-Nield R, et al: High poverty, secondary schools, and the juvenile justice system: how neither helps the other and how that could change. New Dir Youth Dev 99:71–89, 2003

Belenko S: Research on Drug Courts: A Critical Review. New York, The National Center on Addiction and Substance Abuse at Columbia University, 2001

Bruck M, Melnyk L: Individual differences in children's suggestibility: a review and synthesis. Appl Cogn Psychol 18:947–996, 2004

Butts J, Buck J, Coggeshall M: The Impact of Teen Courts on Young Offenders. Washington, DC, The Urban Institute, 2002

Carter CA, Bottoms BL, Levine M: Linguistic and socioemotional influences on accuracy of children's reports. Law Hum Behav 20:335–358, 1996

Closson M, Rogers KM: Educational needs of youth in the juvenile justice system, in The Mental Health Needs of Young Offenders: Forging Paths Toward Reintegration and Rehabilitation. Edited by Kessler L, Kraus L. Cambridge, UK, Cambridge University Press, 2007, pp 230–241

Dennis M, Titus J, White M, et al: Global Appraisal of Individual Needs: Administration Guide for the GAIN and Related Measures. Bloomington, IL, Chestnut Health Systems, 2002

Dery M, Toupin J, Pauze R, et al: Neuropsychological characteristics of adolescents with conduct disorder: association with attention-deficit-hyperactivity and aggression. J Abnorm Child Psychol 27:225–236, 1999

Drug Court Clearinghouse and Technical Assistance Project: Looking at a Decade of Drug Courts. Washington, DC, Report of Office of Justice Programs, Drug Court Technical Assistance Project at the American University, 1999

Estroff TW, Hoffman NG: PADDI: Practical Adolescent Dual Diagnosis Interview. Smithfield, RI, Evince Clinical Assessments, 2001

Fast DK, Conry J, Loock CA: Identifying fetal alcohol syndrome among youths in the criminal justice system. J Dev Behav Pediatr 20:370–372, 1999

Gallagher CA, Dorbin A: The association between suicide screening practices and attempts requiring emergency care in juvenile justice facilities. J Am Acad Child Adolesc Psychiatry 44:485–493, 2005

Geraghty TF, Kraus L, Fink P: Assessing children's competence to stand trial and to waive Miranda rights: new directions for legal and medical decision making in juvenile courts, in The Mental Health Needs of Young Offenders: Forging Paths Toward Reintegration and Rehabilitation. Edited by Kessler L, Kraus L. Cambridge, UK, Cambridge University Press, 2007, pp 79–122

Giedd JN, Blumenthal J, Jeffries NO, et al: Brain development during childhood and adolescence: a longitudinal MRI study. Nat Neurosci 2:861–863, 1999

Goldstein N, Condie L, Kalbeitzer R, et al: Juvenile offenders Miranda rights comprehension and self-reported likelihood of offering false confessions. Assessment 10:359–369, 2003

Gray D, Achilles J, Keller T, et al: Utah Youth Suicide Study, phase I: government agency contact before death. J Am Acad Child Adolesc Psychiatry 41:427–434, 2002

Grisso T: Juvenile's Waiver of Rights: Legal and Psychological Competence. New York, Plenum, 1981

Grisso T: Forensic Evaluations of Juveniles. Sarasota, FL, Professional Resource Press, 1998

Grisso T, Barnum R: Massachusetts Youth Screening Instrument: User's Manual and Technical Report. Sarasota, FL, Professional Resources Press, 2006

Grisso T, Steinberg L, Cauffman E: Juveniles' competence to stand trial: a comparison of adolescents' and adults' capacities as defendants. Law Hum Behav 27:333–363, 2003

Hayes L: Juvenile Suicide in Confinement: A National Survey. Alexandria, VA, National Center on Institutions and Alternatives, 2004

Hsia HM, Bridges GS, McHale R: Disproportionate Minority Confinement, Update 2002. Washington, DC, U.S. Department of Justice Programs, Office of Justice Programs, Office of Juvenile Justice and Delinquency Prevention, 2004

In re Gault, 387 U.S. 1 (1967)

Kassin SM, Norwick RJ: Why people waive their Miranda rights: the power of innocence. Law Soc Rev 28:211–221, 2004

Kent v United States, 383 U.S. 541 (1966)

Kessler CL: Innovative problem-solving court models for justice-involved youth, in The Mental Health Needs of Young Offenders: Forging Paths Toward Reintegration and Rehabilitation. Edited by Kessler L, Kraus L. Cambridge, UK, Cambridge University Press, 2007, pp 386–401

Kochanek KD, Murphy SL, Anderson RN, et al: Deaths: Final Data for 2002. National Vital Statistics Report. Hyattsville, MD, National Center for Health Statistics, 2002

Kraus R: Psychological testing in juvenile justice settings, in The Mental Health Needs of Young Offenders: Forging Paths Toward Reintegration and Rehabilitation. Edited by Kessler L, Kraus L. Cambridge, UK, Cambridge University Press, 2007, pp 289–308

Kruh IP, Brodsky SL: Clinical evaluations for transfer of juveniles to criminal court: current practices and future research. Behav Sci Law 15:151–165, 1997

Lester BM, LaGasse LL, Seifer R: Cocaine exposure and children: the meaning of subtle effects. Science 282:633–644, 1998

Males M, Macallair D: The Color of Justice: An Analysis of Juvenile Adult Court Transfers in California. Washington, DC, Building Blocks for Youth, 2000

Morris R: Health risk behavior survey from thirty-nine juvenile correctional facilities in the United States. J Adolesc Health 17:334–344, 1995

Morris R: Medical issues regarding incarcerated youth, in The Mental Health Needs of Young Offenders: Forging Paths Toward Reintegration and Rehabilitation. Edited by Kessler L, Kraus L. Cambridge, UK, Cambridge University Press, 2007, pp 256–270

Morris R, Harrison E, Knox G, et al: Health risk behavioral survey from 39 juvenile correctional facilities in the United States. J Adolesc Health 17:334–344, 1995

Needleman HL, Schell A, Bellinger, et al: The long-term effects of exposure to low doses of lead in childhood: an 11-year follow-up report. N Engl J Med 322:83–88, 1990

Otnow-Lewis D: Guilt by Reason of Insanity: A Psychiatrist Probes the Minds of Killers. New York, Fawcett Columbine, 1998

Poe-Yamagata E, Jones M: And Justice for Some: Differential Treatment of Minority Youth in the Justice System. Washington, DC, Youth Law Center, 2000

Pope CE, Lovell R, Hsai HM: Disproportionate Minority Confinement: A Review of the Research Literature from 1989 through 2001 (Bulletin). Washington, DC, U.S. Department of Justice, Office of Justice Programs, Office of Juvenile Justice and Delinquency Prevention, 2002

Quinn MM, Rutherford RB, Leone PE, et al: Youth with disabilities in juvenile corrections: a national survey. Except Child 71:339–345, 2005

Redlich A, Drizin S: Police interrogation of youth, in The Mental Health Needs of Young Offenders: Forging Paths Toward Reintegration and Rehabilitation. Edited by Kessler L, Kraus L. Cambridge, UK, Cambridge University Press, 2007, pp 61–78

Redlich AD, Goodman GS: Taking responsibility for an act not committed: the influence of age and suggestibility. Law Hum Behav 27:141–156, 2003

Redlich AD, Silverman M, Steiner H: Factors affecting preadjudicative and adjudicative competence in juveniles and young adults. Behav Sci Law 21:1–17, 2003

Rohde P, Seeley J, Mace D: Correlates of suicidal behavior in a juvenile detention population. Suicide Life Threat Behav 27:164–175, 1997

Roper v Simmons, 543 U.S. 551 (2005)

Sanislow C, Grilo C, Fehon D, et al: Correlates of suicide risk in juvenile detainees and adolescent in-patients. J Am Acad Child Adolesc Psychiatry 42:234–240, 2003

Skiba RJ, Noam GG: Zero tolerance, zero evidence: an analysis of school disciplinary practices. New Dir Youth Dev 92:17–43, 2002

Snyder HN, Sickmund M: Minorities in the Juvenile Justice System, 1999. Washington, DC, U.S. Department of Justice, Office of Justice Programs, Office of Juvenile Justice and Delinquency Prevention, 2000

Teichner G, Golden CJ: The relationship of neuropsychological impairment to conduct disorder in adolescence: a conceptual review. Aggress Violent Behav 5:509–528, 2000

Teplin LA, Abram KM, McClelland GM, et al: Psychiatric disorders in youth in juvenile detention. Arch Gen Psychiatry 59:1133–1143, 2002

Vermeiren R, De Clippele A, Schwab-Stone M, et al: Neuropsychological characteristics of three subgroups of Flemish delinquent adolescents. Neuropsychology 16:49–55, 2000

Vincent GM, Grisso T, Terry A: Mental health screening and assessment in juvenile justice, in The Mental Health Needs of Young Offenders: Forging Paths Toward Reintegration and Rehabilitation. Edited by Kessler L, Kraus L. Cambridge, UK, Cambridge University Press, 2007, pp 271–288

Index

Language disorders (*continued*)
auditory processing disorder, 198
clinical evaluation of, 200
in DSM, 64, 198
in HIV disease, 497
listening comprehension problems, 198
oral expression problems, 198
pragmatic disorders, 198
Laurence-Moon/Bardet-Biedl syndrome, 385
Law of equal segregation, **566**
Law of independent assortment, **566,** 575
Laxative abuse, 115, 117, 388, 399
LDs. *See* Learning disabilities or disorders
LDX (lisdexamfetamine dimesylate), 254
Lead poisoning, 155, 231, 992
Lead serum level, **673**
Learning disabilities or disorders (LDs), 32, 191–201
aggression and, 557
clinical evaluation of, 200
comorbidity with, 192
anxiety disorders, 300, 314
attention-deficit/hyperactivity disorder, 207, **208,** 683
child abuse, 485
depression, 191
definitions of, 139–140, 191–193
DSM, 63, 64, 139, 191–192, **193**
federal government, 139, 192, 193, **193**
delinquency and, 992
diagnosis of, 139–140
differential diagnosis of
anxiety disorders, **311**
intellectual disability, 153
educational programs for children with, 192
etiology of, 193
functional significance of, 192
identification of, 139–141, 192, 193–194
aptitude-achievement discrepancy model for, 139, 192, 193
classroom-based evaluation, 193–194
communication disorders, 141, 197–198
disorder or written expression, 141, 197
goal of, 194

mathematics disorder, 140–141, 196–197
psychological testing, 139–141, 193
reading disorder, 140, 194–196
Response to Intervention model for, 194
nonverbal, 199
not otherwise specified, 139, 198–200
problems associated with, 192
stress due to, 191
summary points related to, 201
of youth in milieu treatments, 941
Learning, neuropsychological assessment of, 145
Least restrictive environment, 926
Legal issues, 637–646. *See also* Ethical issues
best interests of the child standard, 638, 639, 644, 645
child psychiatrist as expert witness, 643, 645, 813
civil commitment, 641
civil litigation, 642, 645
confidentiality, privilege, and duty, 640–641, 813
conflicts of interest and dual agency, 639, 645
evolving concepts of status of children, 637–639
forensic evaluation of children, 34, 483, 491, 643–644
informed consent and competence, 641
legal standard of proof, 642–643
overview of legal system, 642–643
professional liability, 641–642
related to child abuse and neglect, 491, 644
child as witness, 644–645
mandated reporting, 50, 480, 483, 488, 491, 644
related to child custody and divorce, 33–34, 48, 600, 643–644
related to substance abuse, 587
responding to a subpoena, 642
school-related, 645–646
summary points related to, 646
termination of parental rights, 643, 644, 814
use of electroconvulsive therapy in minors, 801
in working with juvenile offenders, 988–989

arrest, interrogation, and confessions, 988
competency and criminal responsibility, 988–989
juvenile death penalty, 989
waiver to adult court, 989
Legislation, federal
Adoption Assistance and Child Welfare Act of 1980, 928
Americans With Disabilities Act, 645, 927, 961
Best Pharmaceuticals for Children Act, 676
Child Abuse Prevention, Adoption, and Family Services Act of 1988, 479
Child Abuse Prevention and Treatment Act of 1974, 644
Education for All Handicapped Children Act, 638, 646, 961
Emergency Medical Treatment and Active Labor Act, 584
Gun-Free Schools Act, 992
Health Insurance Portability and Accountability Act (HIPAA), 658
Individuals With Disabilities Education Act (IDEA), 193, 268, 646, 926, 961, 963, **965**
Mental Retardation Facilities and Community Mental Health Center Construction Act of 1963, 926
No Child Left Behind Act, 958
Rehabilitation Act of 1973, Section 504, 331, 645, 961
Social Security Act, 929
Uniform Marriage and Divorce Act, 644
U.S. Food and Drug Administration Modernization Act of 1997 (FDAMA), 676, 701
Leiter International Performance Scale—Revised (Leiter-R), 142, **154**
Length of stay (LOS) in inpatient hospital units, 940, 947
Lennox-Gastaut syndrome, 732
Lesbians. *See* Homosexuality
Lesch-Nyhan syndrome, **114**
Lethargy, drug-induced
stimulants, 684
valproate, 730
Leukopenia, drug-induced
clozapine, 765
lamotrigine, 734
mirtazapine, 717

indications for, 132

localization of findings on, 123–124

summary points related to, 132

Neurological "soft signs," in attention-deficit/hyperactivity disorder, 212

Neurontin. *See* Gabapentin

Neuropsychological testing, 135–138, 144–147

of aggressive youth, 559

of executive function, 146

indications for, 135, 144–145

of juvenile offenders, 991

of language, 145

of learning and memory, 145

of motor output, 146

in obsessive-compulsive disorder, 351

obtaining consent for, 136

persons qualified to perform, 136

purposes of, 144

reporting results of, 138

of sensory input, 145

of spatial and manipulatory ability, 145

standards for, 136–138

summary points related to, 146–147

tests for, 135–136

batteries of, 136, 146

psychometric properties of, 136–138

scores on, 136–137

using current tests, 136

training for, 144

Neuroticism, suicide and, 533

Neurotransmitters. *See also specific neurotransmitters*

in conduct disorder, 231

drug pharmacodynamics and, 675

in eating disorders, 402–403

electroconvulsive therapy effects on, **798**

magnetic resonance spectroscopy of, 130

in obsessive-compulsive disorder, 352, 360

in sleep regulation, 787

in tic disorders, 422

Neurotrophin, electroconvulsive therapy effects on, **798**

Neutropenia

antipsychotic-induced, **758, 761**

management of, 770

monitoring risk of, 765

benign ethnic (cyclic), 765

Nevirapine, **499**

New York Teacher Rating Scale, **560**

Niacin, for dyslipidemia, 770

NICE (National Institute for Clinical Excellence) practice guidelines, 469

for eating disorders, 407, 409

NICHCY (National Dissemination Center for Children with Disabilities), **166**

Nicotine replacement therapy (NRT), 252, 253

Nicotinic agents, for attention-deficit/hyperactivity disorder, 694–695

Night terrors, 35, 63, 456

Nightmares, 35, 456, 459

beta-blocker–induced, 694, 780

NIH (National Institutes of Health), 676

NIMH. *See* National Institute of Mental Health

NIMH Diagnostic Interview Schedule for Children, Version IV (DISC-IV), 54, **84**

NIMH—Global Obsessive Compulsive Scale, 357

NLD (nonverbal learning disability), 199

NMS (neuroleptic malignant syndrome), 755

No Child Left Behind Act, 958

No-suicide contracts, 536, 586

Nocturia. *See also* Enuresis

bupropion-induced, 693

Nomological network, 81

Nonadherence. *See* Treatment adherence

Nonbenzodiazepine benzodiazepine receptor agonists, for insomnia, 787, 789–790, **790**, 791

Nondisjunction, chromosomal, 569

Nonnucleoside reverse transcriptase inhibitors, **499**, 500

Nonsteroidal anti-inflammatory drugs, interaction with lithium, 501, 728

Nonverbal learning disability (NLD), 199

Noonan syndrome, **114**

Noradrenergic and specific serotonergic antidepressant (NaSSA), **713**, 716. *See also* Mirtazapine

Norepinephrine, 675

in conduct disorder, 231

electroconvulsive therapy effects on, **798**

in sleep regulation, 787

Norepinephrine-dopamine reuptake inhibitor (NDRI), **713**, 714. *See also* Bupropion

Norepinephrine receptor occupancy of drugs

bupropion, 714

duloxetine, 716

mirtazapine, 716

paroxetine, 710

tricyclic antidepressants, 718

venlafaxine, 717

Norepinephrine transporter occupancy, of tricyclic antidepressants, 718

Norfluoxetine, 709

Norpramin. *See* Desipramine

Northwestern Juvenile Project, 990

Nortriptyline, 718

for attention-deficit/hyperactivity disorder, 690–691

dosing of, 691, **692**

pharmacokinetics and pharmacodynamics of, **719**

Nose, assessment of, 113

NRT (nicotine replacement therapy), 252, 253

NSDUH (National Survey on Drug Use and Health), 242, 243

Nucleoside and nucleotide reverse transcriptase inhibitors, **499**

Nucleotides, 565, **566**, 567

Numbing, in abused children, 485

Nurse-family partnership, 935

Nurses

role in milieu treatments, 941

in schools, 960

Nutrition. *See* Diet

Nutritional deficiencies, 117, **118**

eating disorders and, 399, 404

Nutritionist, 406

OAD. *See* Overanxious disorder

Obesity/overweight, 35, 383–394

body mass index and, 383, **766**, 768

clinical description of, 383

course of, 388

cultural factors and, 383, 393

epidemiology of, 383–384

ethical concerns and, 393

etiology of, 385–386

environmental factors, 385–386

medical and genetic factors, 385

evaluation of, 388–389

medical evaluation, 388

psychiatric evaluation, 388–389, **390–391**

readiness to change, 389

TG-CBT (traumatic grief–cognitive behavioral therapy), 512–513
Theory of mind, autism and, 174, 182
Therapeutic drug monitoring, 117
Therapeutic milieu, 943–944. *See also* Milieu treatment programs
Therapeutic relationship, 674, 814–816
  for behavioral parent training, 856–857, 860
  collaborative, for cognitive-behavioral therapy, 908
  for motivational interviewing, 916, 918, 919, 920
  with parents, 5, 6, 28, 674
  for pharmacotherapy, 674
  for psychotherapy, 814–816
  for telepsychiatry, 656
Therapists. *See* Child and adolescent psychiatrists
Thimerosal in vaccines, 180
Thinking, feeling, doing technique, **838**
Thioridazine
  adverse effects of
    hypotension, 613
    QTc interval prolongation, 119, 672, 760
    cardiovascular risk assessment before initiation of, 119
  for early-onset schizophrenia, 375, **750**
  for tic disorders, **756**
Thiothixene, for early-onset schizophrenia, 375, **750**
Thorax, assessment of, 113
Thought disorder
  mania with, 372
  pragmatic deficits and, 198
  in schizophrenia, 369
3di (Developmental, Dimensional and Diagnostic Interview), 177
Throat, assessment of, 113
Thrombocytopenia, valproate-induced, 730
Thymine, 567–568, 571–573
Thyroid disorders. *See also* Hypothyroidism
  lithium use in, 727
Thyroid screening tests, 119, 310
Thyroid-stimulating hormone (TSH), 119, 310, **673**
  hyperprolactinemia and, 764
  lithium effects on, 727–728
Thyroxine (T₄), 119, 310
Tic disorders, 417–429
  in adults, 418–419
  advocacy group for, 428

age at onset of, 65, 418
assessment of, 422–423
comorbidity with, 418, 420
  attention-deficit/hyperactivity disorder, 418, 420
  autism spectrum disorders, 418
  obsessive-compulsive disorder, 351, **352**, 418, 420
complex tics, 418
diagnostic criteria for, 419
  chronic motor or vocal tic disorder, **419**
  Tourette's disorder, **419**
  transient tic disorder, **420**
differential diagnosis of, 419, **421**
in DSM, 63, 64, 65, 66, 419
epidemiology of, 420
genetics of, 420–422
neuroanatomy and neurophysiology of, 422
neuropsychological assessment of, 146
PANDAS and, 353, **353**, 419
premonitory urges in, 418
rating scales for, 423
research directions related to, 428
simple tics, 418
during sleep, 418
summary points related to, 428–429
suppression of tics, 417–418
symptoms of, 417–418
treatment of, 423–428
  behavioral interventions, 424
  observation, 423
  pharmacotherapy, 424–428
    alpha-2-adrenergic agonists, 425, **427,** 775, 776
    antipsychotics, 425, **426, 749,** 753, **756–757**
    in child with attention-deficit/hyperactivity disorder, 214, 425, 428, 684–685
    in child with obsessive-compulsive disorder, 425
    dopamine antagonists, 425, **426**
twin studies of, 420
types of, 417
use of stimulants in child with, 214, 425, 428, 684–685
Tic Rating Scale, 423
Time-outs, 851–852, **853,** 866
Timeline
  of critical events in family, 597, 603

of moods, 267
Title IX of the Education Amendments of 1972, 646
TMS. *See* Transcranial magnetic stimulation
Tobacco use. *See* Smoking/tobacco use
Toddler(s)
  clinically salient behaviors of, 8, **9**
  diagnosing autism in, 176
  with difficult temperament, 4
  examining for child abuse, 482
  fears of, 299
  observing parents' interactions with, 6, 8
  separation anxiety in, 325
  sleep of, 449
  social communication skills of, 174
Toddler assessment, 3–13
  biopsychosocial formulation based on, 6
  comprehensive, 6
  developmental history, 7, **7**
  diagnostic issues regarding disorders of early childhood, 5
  family history, 7, **7**
  formal procedures for, 8–12
    caregiver-report checklists, 10–12, **11**
    diagnostic interviews, 10
    parent-child relationship assessments, 8–10
    parent symptoms, 12
  goals of, 5–6
  history of presenting problem, 6, **7**
  key elements of, **7**
  medical history, 7, **7,** 112
  observations, 6, 8, **9**
  parent interview for, 6
  psychological testing, 143, 155, **155**
  relational approach to, 4–5
  research directions related to, 12
  self-regulatory skills, 6
  settings for, 5
  social history, **7,** 8
  summary points related to, 12–13
Tofranil. *See* Imipramine
Toilet training history, 438
Token economy or point system, 849–851, **850, 852,** 865
Tool kit technique, **838**
Topamax. *See* Topiramate
Topiramate, 725, 735–736
  adverse effects of, 735–736
  baseline assessments before initiation of, 735
  for bipolar disorder, 290, **291,** 735